28

Infections

Edited by David Isaacs, Kim Mulholland

MORTALITY AND MORBIDITY IN INFECTIOUS DISEASE

THE GLOBAL PERSPECTIVE

Worldwide, infections are responsible for the majority of deaths and loss of good health in children. In 2005, infectious diseases were estimated to have caused about 6.7 million of a total of 10.1 million deaths among the estimated global child population of under-5-year-olds of 616.2 million.[1,2] These deaths occurred disproportionately in resource limited countries, where it is also estimated that five groups of infections caused the death of more than 7 million children: acute respiratory infections (ARIs); diarrheal diseases; congenital infections including human immunodeficiency virus (HIV) and hepatitis B; malaria; and vaccine-preventable diseases including measles.[1,2] Although there has been improvement worldwide in the all cause under-5 child mortality rate from 1990 to 2005 (from 95 to 76 per thousand) there is little reason to believe the proportion of deaths attributable to infection has changed much over this time, except that the numbers of children dying as a result of HIV have considerably increased.[2,3] This and other factors means that there has been far less improvement in under-5 mortality in sub-Saharan Africa where the decline between 1990 and 2005 has been only from 188 to 169 per thousand. Indeed there are countries most heavily affected by HIV such as Botswana and South Africa where HIV has reversed previous trends with the estimated under-5 mortality rising from 58 to 120 per thousand and 60 to 68 per thousand respectively.[2] The relationship between infection, malnutrition and socially determined factors such as wars and orphanhood is subtle but important, as poor nutrition, poverty and social dislocation greatly multiply the impact of infections. To a considerable extent this explains why infections are so much more important as a cause of death and disability in resource limited compared to resource rich countries.[4] The rising incidence of HIV infection in resource limited countries has added another multiplier and these relations are shown schematically in Figure 28.1, contrasting sub-Saharan Africa with South Asia in the early years of the new millenium.[2,3]

Malnutrition underlies a substantial proportion of the deaths from diarrheal diseases, respiratory infections, measles and malaria, while HIV is of particular importance in sub-Saharan Africa and some parts of Asia.[2,3] In contrast, in Western Europe and other resource rich countries, malnutrition plays little role as a cofactor for the effects of infection, except in children with serious constitutional diseases such as malignancies or congenital immunodeficiencies. However, a growing population of immunocompromised children (very low birth weight babies, children with congenital immunodeficiencies or HIV infection and children on powerful immunocompromising therapies) represents an increasingly important source of deaths due to infections, often with organisms that are usually innocuous for immunocompetent children. It has been estimated that infections are responsible for around 17% (37 000) of 214 000 deaths under 5 years old that take place among 78 million children annually in resource rich countries.[1,2] Proportionately, the burden of infections is far higher in primary care. In England and Wales, infectious diseases are responsible for 40% of all new episodes of illness presenting to general practitioners with annual rates of around 730 episodes per 1000 population. Rates are even higher for infants (children before their first birthday).[5] Mortality statistics and data on acute consultations need to be supplemented by estimates of the burden of disability (morbidity) and to allow for the varying implications of the disability or death of an individual at different ages. This can be done by use of a measure such as disability adjusted life years (DALYs).[1,6] Combining estimates of chronic disability and mortality statistics, this measure calculates the likely numbers of healthy years of life lost because of specific diseases and conditions and, by 'weighting', an allowance is made for the different significance of ill-health and mortality among infants, elderly persons and adults providing for dependants. Estimates of the burden of disease experienced (Table 28.1 and Figure 28.1)[1] further emphasize the importance of infectious disease in resource limited

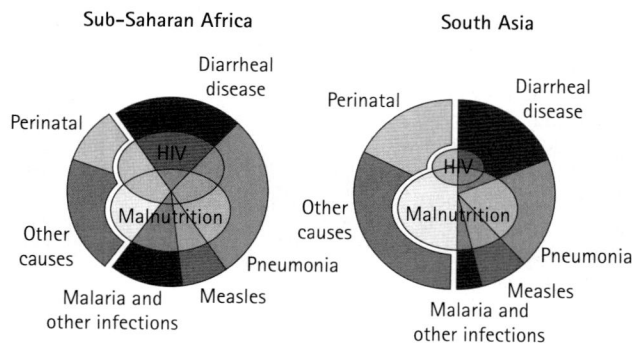

Sub-Saharan Africa

South Asia

Fig. 28.1 Principal causes of death in children under age 5, sub-Saharan Africa and South Asia, circa 2000.

Table 28.1 Estimated distribution of burden of disease (combined mortality and chronic morbidity) in children in resource limited countries – 1990. (Source World Bank 1993[1])

	Total DALYs lost (million)			
	Age under 5 years		Age 5–14 years	
Perinatal conditions	13.5		Nil	
Communicable disease	63.3		33.9	
Congenital STDs (HIV and syphilis)		(2.0%)		(4.0%)
Diarrheal diseases		(32%)		(15%)
Tuberculosis		(1.0%)		(11%)
Other vaccine-preventable disease		(20%)		(18%)
Malaria		(8%)		(9%)
Intestinal helminths		Nil		(27%)
Respiratory infections		(35%)		(16%)
Noncommunicable disorder	20.8		16.9	
Injuries	6.2		9.7	
Total	103.8		60.5	

countries and the particular contribution to mortality in children under age 5 played by respiratory disease, diarrheal disease, the five vaccine-preventable diseases (diphtheria, measles, pertussis, polio and tetanus), and in older children by tuberculosis and intestinal helminths.[1]

HIV AND AIDS

Since the 1990s there has been an inexorable rise in the global importance of HIV. In 2006, the United Nations AIDS program and WHO estimated that 39.5 million persons worldwide were infected with HIV, of whom 2.3 million were children under the age of 15, and 530 000 children became infected with HIV.[2,3] The majority of childhood infections occur through mother-to-child transmission, with a smaller number from unscreened blood transfusions in resource limited settings. The distribution of deaths varies dramatically by global region, with the highest numbers and rates in sub-Saharan Africa where the rates have reversed previous improving trends in child mortality rates (Figs. 28.2 and 28.3). HIV rarely kills children directly, but by lowering the child's immunocompetence it leaves the infected child increasingly vulnerable to other infections. In addition, HIV infection affects children by making them lose their parents to HIV prematurely and it is estimated that 15.2 million children (under age 18) were living having lost one or more parents to HIV.[3] Since the appreciation that the risk of mother-to-child transmission of HIV infection can be reduced to under 2%, screening for HIV infection has resulted in a fall in early AIDS cases in France, Italy, Spain and the UK, the countries most affected in Western Europe (Fig. 28.4).[7] The fall in early pediatric AIDS has taken place despite rising levels of HIV infection in mothers in the UK, notably in London, but also in the rest of the UK (Fig. 28.5).[8]

THE UK

Infections remain an important cause of death in UK children. Conventional death registration data indicate that in 2005 infections (including infections of the central nervous and respiratory systems) were the main cause of death in 127 children in England and Wales (Table 28.2). The figure rises to 199 if sudden infant death syndrome is included. This represents a considerable change over time. In 1995 there were 193 deaths where infections were the main cause, with the figure including SIDS being 537.

Recent trends in a number of important infections in the UK are shown in Figures 28.4–28.14. Trends in vertically acquired HIV

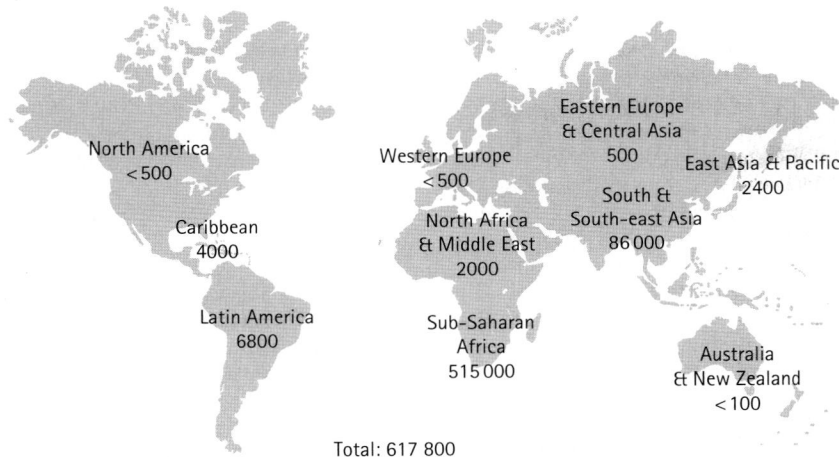

Fig. 28.2 New HIV infections in children globally and by region in 2001.
Source: Joint United Nations Programme on HIV–AIDS (UNAIDS).

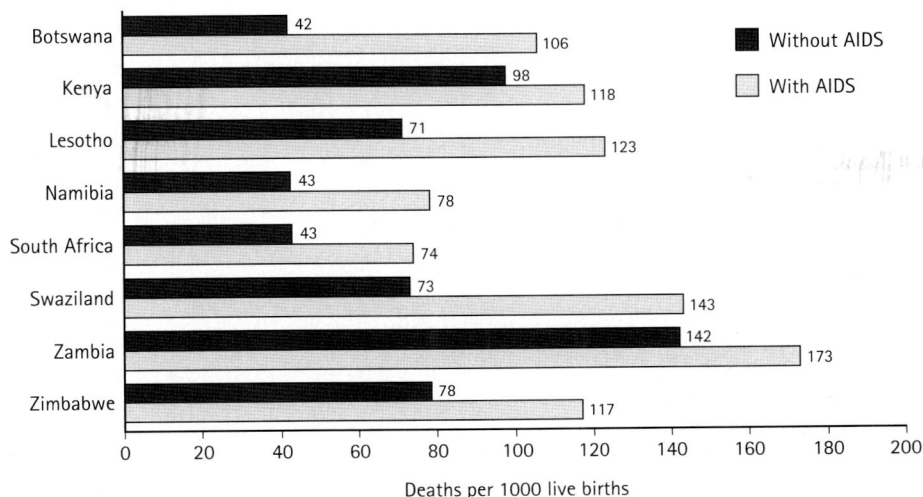

Sources: UNICEF (2005); United Nations Population Division, World Population Prospects: The 2004 Revision, database

Fig. 28.3 Estimated impact of HIV and AIDS on under-5 mortality rates 2002–2005.
Source: Joint United Nations Programme on HIV–AIDS (UNAIDS).

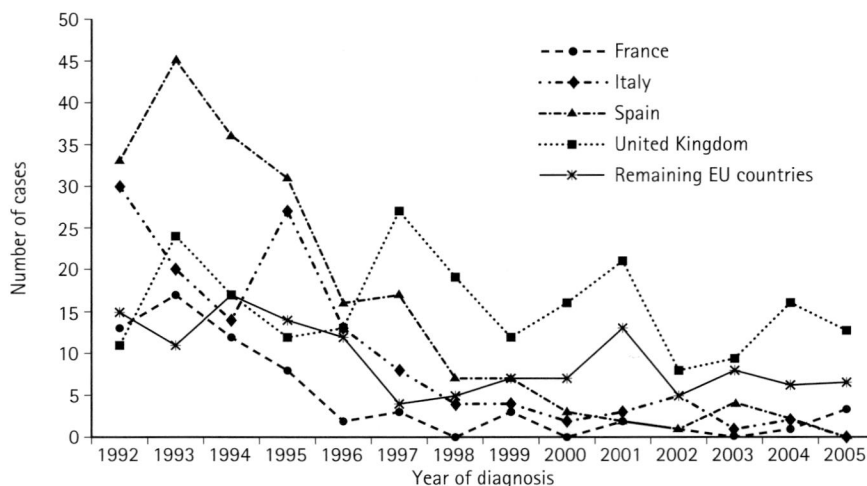

Fig. 28.4 Mother-to-child HIV transmission in European countries. AIDS cases in children aged less than 1 year at diagnosis. 2002–2005.
Source: EuroHIV European Centre for the Epidemiological Monitoring of AIDS.

infection (Figs 28.4 and 28.5) have already been mentioned.[7,8] The introduction of immunization against *Haemophilus influenzae* type b (Hib) in 1992 led to a dramatic decline in invasive infections attributed to this organism (Fig. 28.6). However, a booster dose of Hib was added when it became clear that primary immunization alone was insufficient and numbers began to rise again after 2000 (Fig. 28.6).[9] There has been heightened awareness of meningococcal infections as the most important single cause of septicemic and meningitic infections in immuno-competent children. The introduction of a conjugate vaccine against type C meningococcal infections has resulted in a fall in cases attributed to this infection in the earliest targeted groups, the under-1-year-olds and teenagers (Fig. 28.7).[10] Immunization was highly effective in reducing the incidence of measles in the 1970s (Fig. 28.8). However, measles vaccination coverage is incomplete. Sero-epidemiological investigations in England in the early 1990s indicated a growing number of suscep-tible (antibody negative) older children and hence an increasing risk of a substantial measles epidemic in school age children, with its inevitable morbidity and mortality, and more recently there have been significant

outbreaks.[11,12] To pre-empt further larger epidemics a UK-wide initia-tive immunized 8 million schoolchildren (90% of those eligible) in 1994. Transmission of indigenous measles was almost entirely inter-rupted and confirmed notifications fell dramatically. Hence the risk of an epidemic was averted, at least temporarily.[12] Subsequent declines in measles, mumps and rubella (MMR) vaccination following unwarranted parental concern over the safety of vaccine left more children under-protected (Fig. 28.9) and substantial outbreaks of measles followed in the late 1990s and early 2000s.[13,14] Trends in whooping cough (pertus-sis) in the late 1980s and early 1990s, following the collapse of profes-sional and public confidence in pertussis vaccine, had provided earlier evidence of what can happen if myths about immunization are allowed to prevail over science (Fig. 28.10).[15,16] The rate of diphtheria and polio-myelitis declined dramatically in the UK following the introduction of immunization in the 1940s and 1950s rather as it did for *Haemophilus* in the 1990s. In contrast, control of another illness for which there is a vaccine, tuberculosis,[17] has been less successful with an overall rise in notifications in the 1990s, which particularly reflects trends in London

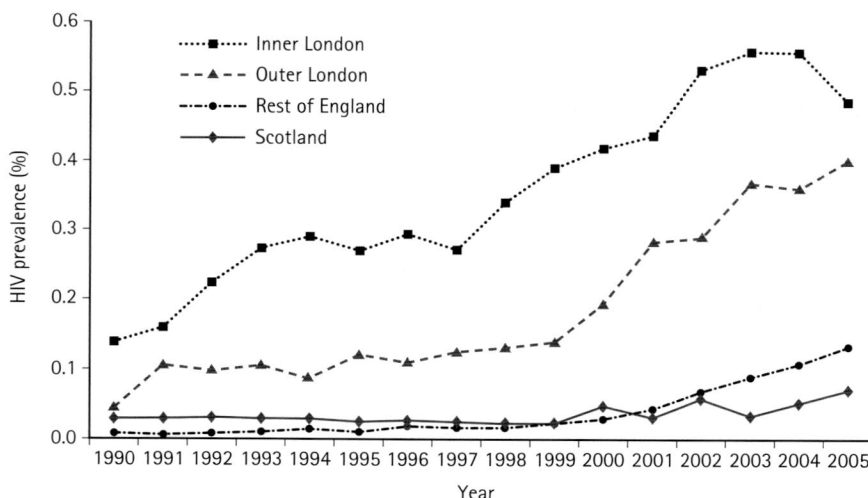

Fig. 28.5 Trends in prevalence of HIV infection in pregnant women in the UK by area of residence 1990–2005.
Source: UK Unlinked Anonymous HIV Monitoring Programme – Health Protection Agency, University College London Institute of Child Health, Health Protection, Scotland.

Table 28.2   Deaths due to infections in children aged 14 years and under; England and Wales 1990–2005. (Source of original data: Office of National Statistics)

ICD-9 code	ICD-10 code		1990	1991	1992	1993	1994	1995	1996	1997
001–009	A00–A09	Intestinal infectious disease	18	20	12	23	22	28	17	35
036	A39	Meningococcal infection	108	110	87	102	85	107	112	100
038	A40–A41	Septicemia	24	21	26	28	33	50	44	39
030–041*	A30–A49*	Other bacterial infection*	13	10	10	12	9	9	11	8
042–044	B20–B24	HIV	0	0	0	6	8	4	11	5
052	B01	Chickenpox	3	5	3	6	3	2	7	2
055	B05	Measles	1	0	1	0	0	0	0	0
042–079*	A80–B34	Other viral diseases*	31	24	16	24	27	26	22	23
001–139	A00–B99	All infectious and parasitic disease	212	199	170	227	203	250	240	230
320–322	G00–G03	Meningitis	52	59	53	49	19	28	32	36
323	G04–G05	Encephalitis	9	8	3	4	10	7	2	8
466–469	J20–J22	Acute bronchitis and bronchiolitis	59	65	31	44	38	27	34	34
480–486	J10–J18	Pneumonia	135	127	83	137	124	104	115	129
487	J10–J11	Influenza	4	3	0	2	2	4	2	2
798–799	R95–R99	SIDS	1090	927	466	431	421	371	394	384
All cause mortality		All cause	4491	4264	3495	3386	3167	3023	2973	2970
Population	Population denominator		9 529 400	9 659 000	9 777 400	9 866 500	9 913 900	9 921 300	9 921 800	9 956 900

ICD-9 code	ICD-10 code		1998	1999	2000	2001	2002	2003	2004	2005
001–009	A00–A09	Intestinal infectious disease	44	45	40	4	3	3	7	10
036	A39	Meningococcal infection	86	84	69	85	49	59	33	46
038	A40–A41	Septicemia	38	48	46	20	19	23	27	16
030–041*	A30–A49*	Other bacterial infection*	16	18	8	42	40	27	44	31
042–044	B20–B24	HIV	5	1	1	8	2	4	3	1
052	B01	Chickenpox	6	3	2	2	1	2	7	2
055	B05	Measles	0	1	0	0	1	0	0	0
042–079*	A80–B34	Other viral diseases*	23	15	20	16	18	31	20	17
001–139	A00–B99	All infectious and parasitic disease	232	238	201	187	144	155	150	135
320–322	G00–G03	Meningitis	43	35	35	32	29	40	29	29
323	G04–G05	Encephalitis	7	5	1	2	7	5	11	6
466–469	J20–J22	Acute bronchitis and bronchiolitis	34	32	22	33	19	16	24	14
480–486	J10–J18	Pneumonia	125	122	87	63	69	73	53	73
487	J10–J11	Influenza	6	8	3	5	5	16	1	15
798–799	R95–R99	SIDS	310	300	271	95	81	101	104	95
All cause mortality		All cause	2826	2767	2495	2523	2377	2407	2248	2242
Population	Population denominator		9 970 100	9 972 500	9 905 500	9 970 100	9 972 500	9 685 352	9 637 426	9 589 141

*Contains other totals not shown above.

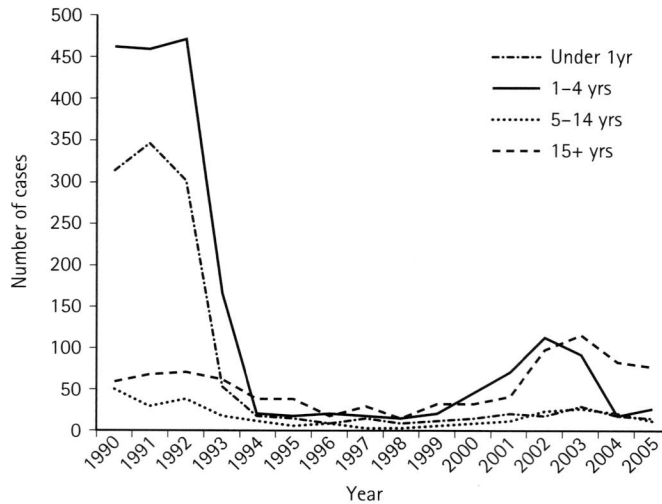

Fig. 28.6 Invasive Hib infections by age group, 1990–2005. Supplied by the Health Protection Agency Centre for Infections and relying on laboratory reporting, reporting by clinicians, genitourinary medicine (GUM) clinic returns (KC60) (gonorrhea), tuberculosis notifications, COVER Vaccination coverage statistics, reports through the Royal College of General Practitioners Research Unit (influenza).

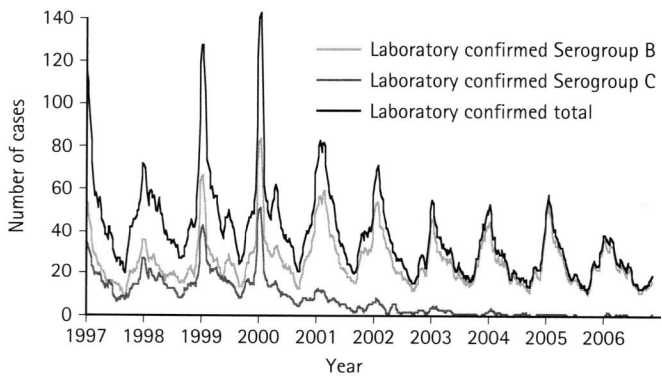

Fig. 28.7 Laboratory confirmed cases of meningococcal disease. England & Wales Five Weekly Moving Averages: 1997–2006. Supplied by the Health Protection Agency Centre for Infections and relying on laboratory reporting, reporting by clinicians, genitourinary medicine (GUM) clinic returns (KC60) (gonorrhea), tuberculosis notifications, COVER Vaccination coverage statistics, reports through the Royal College of General Practitioners Research Unit (influenza).

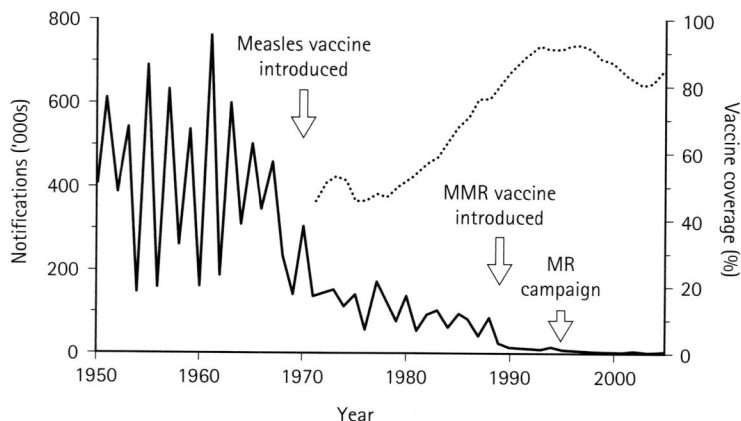

Fig. 28.8 Annual measles notification and vaccine coverage in England and Wales 1950–2005. Supplied by the Health Protection Agency Centre for Infections and relying on laboratory reporting, reporting by clinicians, genitourinary medicine (GUM) clinic returns (KC60) (gonorrhea), tuberculosis notifications, COVER Vaccination coverage statistics, reports through the Royal College of General Practitioners Research Unit (influenza).

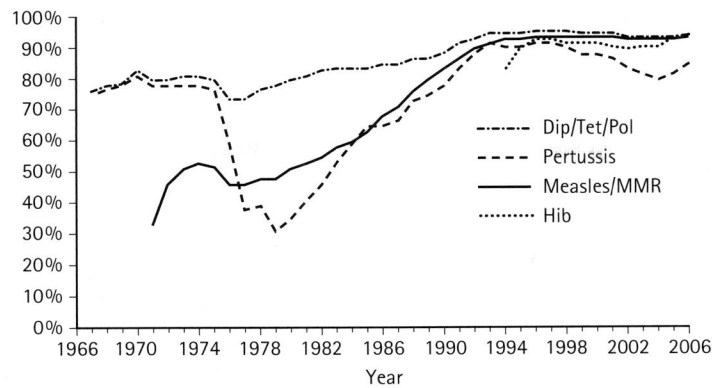

Fig. 28.9 Two year vaccine coverage in England and Wales 1966–2005/6. Supplied by the Health Protection Agency Centre for Infections and relying on laboratory reporting, reporting by clinicians, genitourinary medicine (GUM) clinic returns (KC60) (gonorrhea), tuberculosis notifications, COVER Vaccination coverage statistics, reports through the Royal College of General Practitioners Research Unit (influenza).

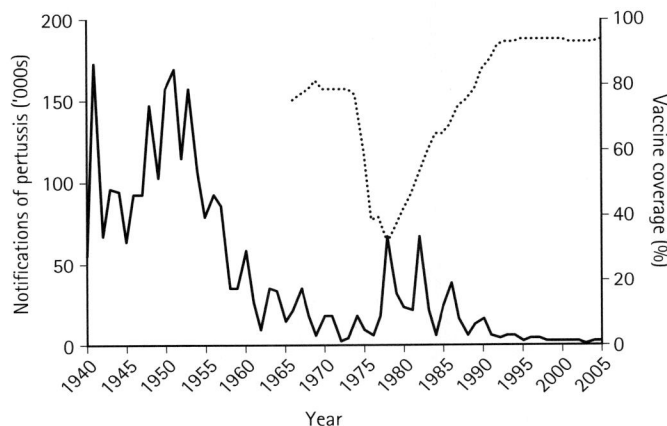

Fig. 28.10 Whooping cough cases and vaccine coverage in England and Wales 1940–2005. Supplied by the Health Protection Agency Centre for Infections and relying on laboratory reporting, reporting by clinicians, genitourinary medicine (GUM) clinic returns (KC60) (gonorrhea), tuberculosis notifications, COVER Vaccination coverage statistics, reports through the Royal College of General Practitioners Research Unit (influenza).

and imported cases (Fig. 28.11). Influenza epidemics occur every winter though they vary in their severity and the proportion of infections that occur among children (Fig. 28.12). Food poisoning has become the commonest notifiable infection in children. Sharply increasing trends in notified numbers of cases of food poisoning in the 1980s and 1990s were mirrored by trends in national laboratory reporting of salmonellosis. Since 1997, however, salmonella reports have declined while reports of *Campylobacter* spp. have risen (Fig. 28.13). Though numbers are far less than for campylobacter or salmonella, the emergence of *Escherichia coli* O157 since the 1980s is of concern because of the severe disease and specific renal pathology that often follows this infection. Not all countries see this subtype of verocytotoxigenic *E. coli* (VTEC): in Australia for example the predominant subtype is *E. coli* O111.[18]

Sexually transmitted diseases are now appreciated to be a substantial problem among adolescents in the UK. Rates of gonorrhea rose by over 50% between 1995 and 2000 (Fig. 28.14) with the highest percentage rise among adolescents.[19] The highest incidences of gonorrhea and chlamydia seen among genitourinary medicine clinic attenders are in females aged 16–19 years.[8,19] After intensive campaigns the rates of gonorrhea are now declining.[8] Chlamydia is the more important, because of its widespread distribution and serious sequelae of pelvic inflammatory disease, infertility and ectopic pregnancies. It is clear that the chlamydia infections seen in genitourinary medicine clinics are only

a fraction of those prevalent in the teenage population and campaigns in the UK are now aiming to control this infection through opportunistic screening in primary care.[20]

General practitioner (GP) reporting provides the least-selected surveillance data in the UK on the nature and burden of infectious disease in children in the community, particularly on conditions such as chickenpox or influenza that are unlikely to be investigated microbiologically or to lead to hospital admission. These data show that respiratory tract infections (mainly upper tract infections) account for over 80% of new GP consultations for infectious diseases in children.[5]

EMERGING AND RE-EMERGING INFECTIONS

In the 1960s and 1970s it was often stated that improving social conditions and medical treatments were leading to a relentless decline in the importance of infectious diseases. Emerging and re-emerging infections such as HIV and tuberculosis (Figs. 28.1 and 28.11), high profile nosocomial outbreaks of legionnaires' disease and food poisoning in the UK, and most recently the appearance of severe acute respiratory syndrome (SARS) and highly pathogenic avian influenza (H5N1) have changed medical opinion. In addition, the deliberate release of organisms such as anthrax in the USA has brought a new threat to health from infections.[21] It is now realized that infections remain important threats to the health

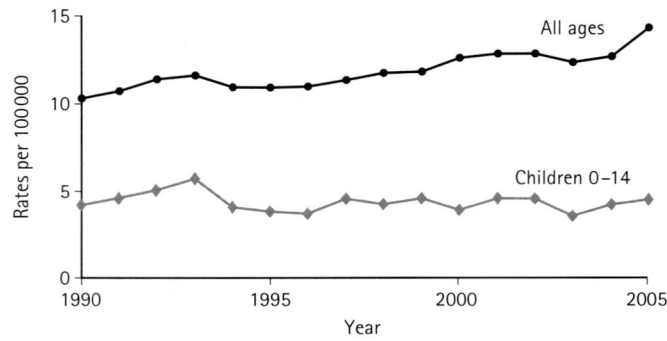

Fig. 28.11 Tuberculosis notification rates per 100 000 population in England and Wales 1993–2005. Supplied by the Health Protection Agency Centre for Infections and relying on laboratory reporting, reporting by clinicians, genitourinary medicine (GUM) clinic returns (KC60) (gonorrhea), tuberculosis notifications, COVER Vaccination coverage statistics, reports through the Royal College of General Practitioners Research Unit (influenza).

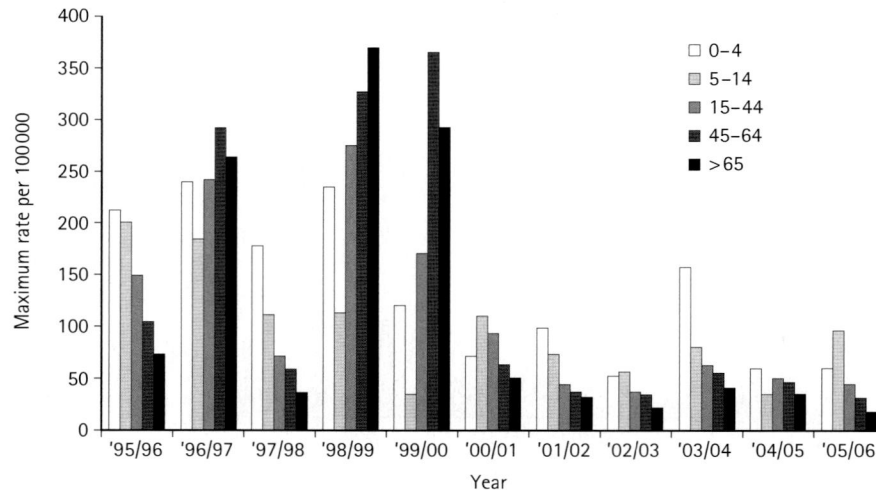

Fig. 28.12 Rates of influenza reports 1990–2006 by age group (RCGP). Supplied by the Health Protection Agency Centre for Infections and relying on laboratory reporting, reporting by clinicians, genitourinary medicine (GUM) clinic returns (KC60) (gonorrhea), tuberculosis notifications, COVER Vaccination coverage statistics, reports through the Royal College of General Practitioners Research Unit (influenza).

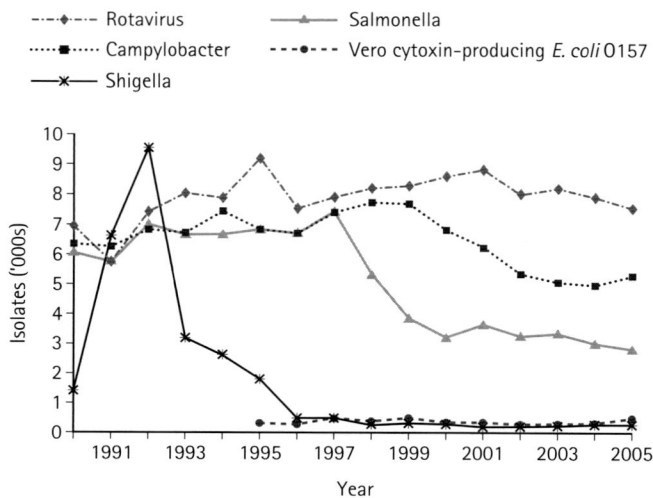

Fig. 28.13 Laboratory reporting of selected gastrointestinal pathogens in England and Wales 1977–2005. Supplied by the Health Protection Agency Centre for Infections and relying on laboratory reporting, reporting by clinicians, genitourinary medicine (GUM) clinic returns (KC60) (gonorrhea), tuberculosis notifications, COVER Vaccination coverage statistics, reports through the Royal College of General Practitioners Research Unit (influenza).

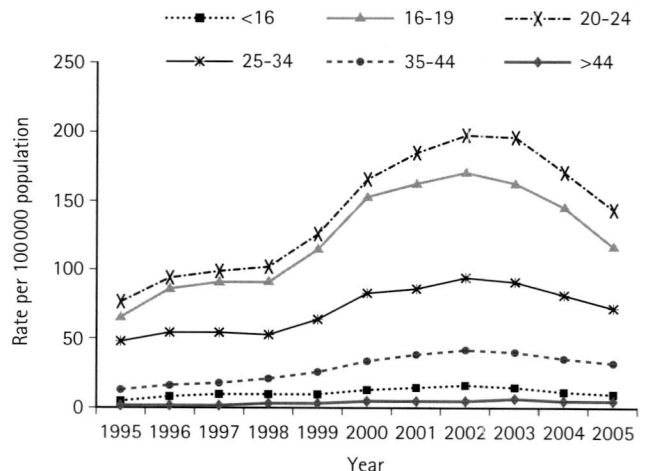

Fig. 28.14 Rates of uncomplicated gonorrhea seen in genitourinary medicine clinics by age group in the UK 1995–2005.

of children and adults in every country. Following a lead from the United States Centers for Disease Control and Prevention (CDC), in 1995 the World Health Organization established a Division of Emerging Viral and Bacterial Disease Surveillance and Control (www.who.int/emc/index.html). Some countries and regional bodies (for example the European Union and WHO's Western Pacific Region) have been establishing or strengthening infrastructures to detect and respond to emerging or re-emerging infections and in 2005 the International Health Regulations were radically revised so that they would detect any new threat. The new regulations require all governments to strengthen surveillance and to report any potential previous public health emergency of international concern (the previous regulations only required countries to report cases of cholera, plague and yellow fever).[22] Some emerging infections are new or involve newly recognized pathogens (Table 28.3),[23] examples being human herpesvirus types 6 and 7, variant Creutzfeldt–Jakob disease, and *Clostridium difficile* O27.[24] Other infections derive from animal infections that have only latterly come to affect humans, such as HIV, Lassa fever, avian influenza virus type A/H5N1 and SARS. Yet a third group is established infections whose incidence, pathogenicity or antimicrobial resistance has recently increased, for example dengue fever, methicillin resistant *Staphylococcus aureus* infection (MRSA) and tuberculosis (both drug susceptible and multiply resistant *Mycobacterium tuberculosis*).

Table 28.3 New and emerging infections – new and newly recognized agents identified since 1973. (Source: European Centre for Disease Prevention and Control)

Year of report	Agent	Disease
1973	Rotavirus	Major cause of infantile diarrhea worldwide
1975	Parvovirus B19	Fifth disease; aplastic crisis in hemolytic anemia
1976	*Cryptosporidium parvum*	Acute enterocolitis
1977	Ebola virus	Ebola hemorrhagic fever
1977	*Legionella pneumophila*	Legionnaires' disease
1977	Hantaan virus	Hemorrhagic fever with renal syndrome (HFRS)
1977	*Campylobacter* sp.	Enteric pathogens distributed globally
1980	Human T cell lymphotropic virus-I (HTLV I)	T cell lymphoma leukemia
1981	*Staphylococcus* toxin	Toxic shock syndrome associated with tampon use
1982	*Escherichia coli* O157:H7	Hemorrhagic colitis; hemolytic uremic syndrome
1982	HTLV II	Hairy cell leukemia
1982	*Borrelia burgdorferi*	Lyme disease
1983	HIV	HIV disease including AIDS
1983	*Helicobacter pylori*	Peptic ulcers
1988	Human herpesvirus-6 (HHV-6)	Roseola infantum and encephalitis
1989	*Ehrlichia chaffeensis*	Human ehrlichiosis
1989	Hepatitis C	Parenterally transmitted non-A, non-B hepatitis
1990	Human herpesvirus-7 (HHV-7)	Roseola infantum and encephalitis
1991	Guanarito virus	Venezuelan hemorrhagic fever
1992	*Vibrio cholerae* O139	New strain associated with epidemic cholera
1992	*Bartonella* (=*Rochalimaea*) *henselae*	Cat-scratch disease; bacillary angiomatosis
1993	Sin nombre hantavirus	Hantavirus pulmonary syndrome
1994	Sabiá virus	Brazilian hemorrhagic fever
1994	Hendra virus infection	Severe respiratory illness, neurologic syndrome
1995	Human herpesvirus-8 (HHV-8)	Kaposi sarcoma
1997	Bovine spongiform encephalopathy (BSE) agent (a prion)	New variant Creutzfeldt–Jakob disease
1997	Influenza A, H5N1	Severe respiratory illness
1999	Nipah virus, West Nile virus in USA	West Nile fever, meningitis, encephalitis, acute flaccid paralysis
2001	Human metapneumovirus (hMPV)	From asymptomatic infection to severe bronchiolitis
2003	SARS coronavirus (SARS CoV)	Severe acute respiratory syndrome (SARS)
2003 (USA)	Monkeypox virus (previously seen in Africa from 1970s)	Similar to smallpox, but usually milder
2004	Simian foamy retroviruses	No evidence of pathology
2005	Human retroviruses, HTLV3 and HTLV4	Immunodeficiency?
Islands in the Indian Ocean 2006	Chikungunya virus (previously first described in Tanzania in 1956)	Joint pains which may or may not be accompanied by muscle pain, high fever, conjunctivitis, and a rash.
Past decade	Emergence of: multidrug resistant organisms (MDROs), including methicillin resistant *Staphylococcus aureus* (MRSA), vancomycin resistant enterococci (VRE) and certain Gram negative bacilli (GNB) including those producing extended spectrum beta-lactamases (ESBLs)	Sepsis, pneumonia, surgical infection, ventilator-associated pneumonia (VAP), etc.
	Clostridium difficile type O27	
	Extended spectrum drug resistant *M. tuberculosis* (XDR-Tb)	
	Drug resistant *Streptococcus pneumoniae* (DRSP)	Meningitis, pneumonia, sepsis

Of particular importance to children are HIV, diphtheria, pertussis, *E. coli* O157 causing hemolytic uremic syndrome (HUS) and avian influenza (A/H5N1), and sexually transmitted infections in adolescents.

The reasons for emergence and re-emergence are almost as varied as the organisms themselves (Table 28.4).[25] Failure of public health programs can be an important cause. Diphtheria reappeared in the 1990s as an epidemic in Russia because of a collapse in vaccine production and the emergence of mistaken reasons among the public and professionals for refusing immunization. A similar phenomenon affecting pertussis occurred in the UK in the 1970s and 1980s from the mistaken impression that the vaccine was more dangerous than the disease (see Fig. 28.10).[15,26] Both *E. coli* O157 and various salmonellas have been spread efficiently through industrialized production and distribution of foods.[27] An outbreak of HUS due to contaminated commercial hamburgers occurred in the USA in 1993[28] and in 1995 an outbreak of gastrointestinal disease in children due to *S. agoma* in north London was traced to defective production in a factory in Israel. Changes in behavior can result in disease emergence. International trends towards earlier menarche and sexual debut are causing younger females to be exposed to STDs with a consequent rise in pelvic inflammatory disease, ectopic pregnancy and secondary infertility.[20,29]

EFFECTIVE INTERVENTIONS

In 1990, at a World Summit for Children, government leaders including that of the UK committed their administrations to 27 goals to improve the health and lives of children. There have been some major achievements towards these goals and subsequent aspirational targets such as the Millenium Goals.[2] More than 60 countries have reached their national goals of reducing mortality rates of children < 5 years by a third or more. Polio has been eradicated in more than 175 countries and deaths from diarrheal illnesses have been more than halved.[2]

Interventions designed to prevent or treat infections may be assessed by measuring their resulting health gain as healthy years of life and comparing their costs relative to other interventions. Thus it is possible to come up with 'best buys' for countries, and this has been undertaken for resource limited countries by the World Bank using the 'DALY' measure.[1,6] Interventions targeted against acute respiratory infections, diarrheal disease, malaria and the six vaccine-preventable diseases represent four of the six top interventions for health gain in children under age 5, and five out of six of those targeted at children aged 5–14 years[30] (Tables 28.5 and 28.6). While new technologies and developments are necessary, greater health gains can come from the application of established interventions of proven effectiveness such as the early detection and treatment of acute respiratory infections, and the use of oral rehydration therapy (ORT) for gastrointestinal infections.[30] Immunization represents a success story. By 1990, the Expanded Program of Immunization (EPI) reached a goal of immunizing 80% of children in most countries with an estimated benefit of 3 million lives saved in 1995. A particular priority has been polio immunization. The EPI, supported by Rotary International, had, by 1995, eliminated wild polio from 145 countries, including all of the Americas.[30] However, the 80% target remains unachieved in sub-Saharan Africa where overall immunization rates are static and there have been outbreaks extending out of West Africa into

Table 28.4 Factors in infectious disease emergence and re-emergence relevant to child and adolescent health (Adapted from Morse 1995[25])

Factor	Example of specific factors	Examples of disease (more than one factor may be driving the emergence of an infection)
Ecological changes including: those due to economic development and land use, distribution of animal populations and climate changes	Agriculture: dams, changes in water ecosystems; deforestation/reforestation; flood/drought; famine; changes in animal distribution; climate changes	Schistosomiasis (dams); Rift Valley fever (dams, irrigation); Argentine hemorrhagic fever (agriculture); West Nile virus (bird movement), highly pathogenic avian influenza Hantaan–Korean hemorrhagic fever (agriculture); hantavirus pulmonary syndrome, southwestern US, 1993 (weather anomalies)
Human demographics, behavior	Societal changes and events: population growth and migration (movement from rural areas to cities); practices of keeping animals and contact with wild animals, war or civil conflict; urban decay; sexual behavior; intravenous drug use; preference for 'fast foods'; use of high-density facilities	Introduction of HIV; spread of dengue; spread of HIV and other sexually transmitted diseases, appearance of zoonoses [highly pathogenic avian influenza (H5N1), SARS (corona virus)], meningococcal disease, cholera increases in food poisoning (*Salmonella enteritidis*)
International travel and commerce	Worldwide movement of goods and people; air travel	'Airport' malaria; dissemination of mosquito vectors; rat-borne hantavirusues; antibiotic-resistant gonorrhea; introduction of cholera into South America; dissemination of O139 *V. cholerae*
Technology and industry	Globalization of food supplies; changes in food processing and packaging; organ or tissue transplantation; drugs causing immunosuppression; widespread use of antibiotics	Hemolytic uremic syndrome (*E. coli* contamination of hamburger meat), *S. agoma* in kosher snacks; transfusion-associated hepatitis (hepatitis B, C), opportunistic infections in immunosuppressed patients, Creutzfeldt–Jakob disease from contaminated batches of human growth hormone (medical technology)
Microbial adaptation and change	Microbial evolution, response to selection in environment	Antibiotic-resistant bacteria (multiply resistant *M. tuberculosis*), 'antigenic drift' in influenza virus; zidovudine-resistant HIV
Breakdown in public health measures	Curtailment or reduction in prevention programs; inadequate sanitation and vector control measures, immunization myths	Whooping cough in the UK, resurgence of tuberculosis in the US; cholera in refugee camps in Africa; resurgence of diphtheria in the countries of the former Soviet Union

Table 28.5   Main cause of disease burden in children in demographically developing countries in 1990 and the cost-effectiveness of the interventions available for their control. (Adapted from Morse[25])

Disease and injuries	Number of DALYs lost* millions (% total)	Main intervention	Cost-effectiveness ($ per DALY)
Respiratory infections	98 (14.8)[†]	Integrated management of the sick child	30–100
Perinatal morbidity and mortality	96 (14.6)	a. Prenatal and delivery care b. Family planning	30–100 20–150
Diarrheal disease	92 (14.0)	Integrated management of the sick child	30–100
Childhood cluster (diseases preventable through immunization)	65 (10.0)	Expanded Program on Immunization (EPI) EPI-plus[†]	12–30
Congenital malformation	35 (5.4)	Surgical operations	High (unknown)
Malaria	31 (4.7)	Integrated management of the sick child	30–100
Intestinal helminths	17 (2.5)	School health program	20–34
Protein-energy malnutrition	12 (1.8)	Integrated management of the sick child	30–100
Vitamin A deficiency	12 (1.8)	EPI-plus[†]	12–30
Iodine deficiency	9 (1.4)	Iodine supplementation	19–37
Subtotal	467 (71.0)	–	–
Total DALYs lost	660 (100)	–	–

*DALYs lost (for specific diseases and the total) are taken from the 1993 World Development Report (World Bank 1993[1]).
[†]EPI-plus includes the six vaccines of the Expanded Program on Immunization (EPI), plus the vaccine against hepatitis B and vitamin A supplementation.

Table 28.6   The global balance sheet – child health 1990–2000. (Source WHO 2001[22])

Goal	Gains	Unfinished business
Infant and under-5 mortality (U5MR): reduction by one third in infant mortality and U5MR	More than 60 countries achieved the goal of U5MR At the global level, U5MR declined by 14%	U5MR rates increased in 14 countries (nine of them in sub-Saharan Africa) and were unchanged in 11 others Serious disparities remain in U5MR within countries: by income level, urban vs. rural, and among minority groups
Polio: *global eradication* by 2000	More than 175 countries are polio free	Polio is still endemic in 20 countries
Routine immunization: *maintenance of a high level of immunization coverage*	Sustained routine immunization coverage at 75% [three doses of combined diphtheria/pertussis/ tetanus vaccine (DPT3)]	Less than 50% of children under 1 yr of age in sub-Saharan Africa are immunized against DPT3
Measles: *reduction by 95% in measles deaths and 90% in measles cases by 1995 as a major step in global eradication in the longer run*	Worldwide reported measles incidence has declined by nearly two thirds between 1990 and 1999	In more than 15 countries, measles vaccination coverage is less than 50%
Neonatal tetanus: *elimination* by 1995	104 of 161 resource limited countries have achieved the goal Deaths caused by neonatal tetanus declined by 50% between 1990 and 2000	27 countries (18 in Africa) account for 90% of all remaining neonatal tetanus
Deaths due to diarrhea: *reduce them by 50%*	This goal was achieved globally, according to World Health Organization (WHO) estimates	Diarrhea remains one of the major causes of death among children
Acute respiratory infections (ARIs): *reduction of ARI deaths by one third in children under 5*	ARI case management has improved at health center level The effectiveness of *Haemophilus influenzae* type b and pneumococcus vaccines is established	ARI remains one of the greatest causes of death among children Vertical, single-focus ARI programs seem to have had little global impact

other parts of Africa. Because of economic or social reasons there are at least some war-torn countries where polio elimination looks difficult or impossible. The infection is also proving hard to eradicate in India.[31,32] This makes the goal of global polio elimination, and its prize of release of resources currently committed to polio immunization, look difficult.[2]

SURVEILLANCE TO INFORM PUBLIC HEALTH ACTION

Given adequate resources and will, many infectious diseases can be prevented or contained, but eradication of all infection-related morbidity

and mortality is unachievable as many microorganisms have extensive animal and environmental reservoirs. Interventions can prevent infections or ameliorate the effects of disease. Knowledge as to which interventions are effective must be combined with timely surveillance data on the epidemiology of infection and susceptibility so as to allow rational decisions to be made on resource allocation for public health action. Equally, surveillance provides the basis for health protection, for example in detecting and directing action on deliberate release of biological agents.[21]

Data for surveillance of the commoner infectious diseases in the UK are derived from mortality statistics, disease notifications and laboratory reporting although in recent years enhanced surveillance to answer specific public health questions has become far more important (Table 28.7).[7-14,19,24,33] An infection may be made statutorily notifiable in the UK, either because there is a need for rapid information for effective local control or for the purpose of monitoring national immunization programs. Often taken for granted, these systems are among the best in the world. Routine reporting is supplemented by special or enhanced surveillance systems for rare and/or more important infections such as HIV and congenital rubella syndrome. An example of this is active reporting by clinicians through the British Paediatric Surveillance Unit (BPSU) of the Royal College of Paediatrics and Child Health (RCPCH), whereby researchers combine reports from RCPCH members with data from other systems to give optimal coverage.[33] Other innovative mechanisms are using primary care mechanisms through general practice or NHS Direct. Surveillance of infectious disease mortality and morbidity in England and Wales is undertaken by the Office for National Statistics (ONS) and by the Centre for Infections and Local and Regional Services of the Health Protection Agency (HPA) and the Public Health Service-Wales. In Scotland this function is performed by Health Protection Scotland though public health policy is coordinated by national departments of health and enacted by local specialists in public health medicine. In Wales it is performed by the Communicable Diseases Surveillance Centre (CDSC) of the Public Health Service Wales and in Northern Ireland by CDSC (Northern Ireland). The HPA and ONS collaborate closely to obtain, analyze and interpret data from several sources which often overlap, but which are also complementary allowing validation of reports (Table 28.7). From these national reporting centers data and information are routinely reported to the European Centre for Disease Prevention and Control and the World Health Organization. The legal basis of these reporting mechanisms is established under the European Union Legislation and the new (2005) International Health Regulations.[22,34]

ACKNOWLEDGMENTS

In the preparation of this section the assistance is gratefully acknowledged of a large number of colleagues in the European Centre for Disease Prevention and Control; the United Nations Special Program on AIDS; the European HIV Centre (EUROHIV) at INVS, Paris; the Office for National Statistics; the Registrar General's Office, Scotland; the Department of Health and Social Security, Northern Ireland; the Centre for Infections of the Health Protection Agency; the Royal College of General Practitioners Research Unit; Health Protection Scotland; the Communicable Disease Surveillance Centre of the Public Health Service, Wales; and the Communicable Disease Surveillance Centre (Northern Ireland).

Table 28.7 Infectious disease morbidity and mortality: principal sources of data in the UK

Data source	Collected by	Type of information
Mortality data	OPCS, GRS, DHSS	Death entries from medical practitioners
Statutory notifications	OPCS, LGAs, SHHD, DH	Currently (1995) list of 39 IDs; selected because need for rapid local information for control, or to monitor national immunization program; clinical diagnoses
Laboratory reports	Cfl and HPA from routine and specialist laboratories	Wide range of microbiologically confirmed infections
General practitioners	Computerized reporting by GPs including the RCGP from weekly returns from 40 practices	Wide range of infectious diseases presenting in general practice; clinical diagnoses
NHS Direct	Daily outputs from NHS Direct systems	Wide range of infectious diseases presenting as syndromes through the NHS Direct centers
Computerized hospital discharge data	ONS and SHHD from individual hospitals and health boards	All diagnoses categorized by ICD code; combination of clinical and microbiological
Enhanced surveillance systems	From many sources to Cfl, HPS, CDSC-PHS (Wales), CDSC NI	A wide variety of conditions answering specific questions: e.g. levels of MRSA in hospitals, rates of completion of treatment courses by those with tuberculosis, performance of antenatal screening for HIV
Consultant pediatricians	British Paediatric Surveillance Unit	Changing 'menu' of rare infections and infection-related disorders; specified case definitions
Consultant clinicians (genitourinary medicine)	HPA Centre for Infections	HIV and AIDS cases including detailed demographic data
Public health specialists	HPA Centre for Infections	Significant outbreaks and incidents

CDSC-PHS (Wales), Communicable Disease Surveillance Centre of the Public Health Service, Wales; CDSC NI, Communicable Disease Surveillance Centre (Northern Ireland); Cfl, Health Protection Agency Centre for Infections; DH, Department of Health; DHSS, Department of Health and Social Security, Northern Ireland; GRS, General Registrar's Office for Scotland; HA, health authority; HB, health board; HPS, Health Protection Scotland; ID, infectious disease; LGA, local government authority; ONS, Office for National Statistics; OPCS, Office of Population Censuses and Surveys; PHLS, Public Health Laboratory Service; RCGP, Royal College of General Practitioners; SHHD Scottish Home and Health Department.

CLINICAL PROBLEMS

THE CHILD WITH FEVER

The most useful temperature measurement is the core or central temperature which has a normal range in young adults of 36.4–36.9 °C, and fluctuation around these values of up to 0.4 °C. Infants have a rectal temperature above 37 °C which falls by about 0.8 °C during sleep and rises before waking.[35] There is a circadian rhythm in childhood with the highest temperature at 6 P.M. The peripheral temperature is normally 0.5 °C lower than that recorded centrally.[36] What is regarded as fever varies. Studies of infants define fever as a central temperature of greater than 38 °C. Antipyretic agents have the same effect on fever of either bacterial or viral origin and the response should not be used as a distinguishing feature. There are a number of different devices available for temperature measurement. Electronic probes are widely used in hospital for oral (central), axillary (peripheral) or rectal (central) sites. Tympanic membrane thermometers are moderately accurate providing they are inserted correctly but are not recommended in young infants. Other methods using strips or chemical dots are of variable accuracy. Mercury thermometers, sometimes regarded as the 'gold standard', are not recommended because of the risks from broken glass and the toxic effects of the metal.

Although a central temperature reading is of value in the sick child, and measurement of the temperature difference between core and periphery is of particular value in the shocked patient, for most purposes a peripheral reading is adequate.

The commonest cause of fever in childhood is viral infection, usually resolving within a week of onset. Persistence of fever demands thorough investigation; the term pyrexia or fever of unknown origin (PUO, FUO) is normally applied when fever has been present for 14 days.

FEVER IN THE NEWBORN

Fever during the neonatal period may be the presenting sign of bacterial infection. If investigation is delayed until other signs occur, such as lethargy, anorexia or apnea, infection may be far advanced before treatment is started. It is generally accepted that any febrile newborn should have cultures of blood, cerebrospinal fluid (CSF) and urine taken, and then should be started on empirical antibiotics.[37] Other investigations such as a peripheral white blood count (WBC), serum C-reactive protein (CRP) and serum procalcitonin (PCT) may indicate the likelihood of bacterial infection.[38] If an infant is tachypneic then a chest X-ray (CXR) should be performed.

Infections presenting within 48 h of birth are likely to have resulted from maternal transmission with bacteria such as group B streptococcus (GBS, *Streptococcus agalactiae*), *S. pneumoniae* and *Escherichia coli*. Later infections in the neonatal period are more likely to be nosocomial, and are more common in the preterm infant undergoing intensive care. Typical organisms are *Staphylococcus aureus* and *S. epidermidis*. However, maternally acquired infections with organisms such as GBS, and those acquired in the community, are also seen later in the neonatal period.

Viral infections, either congenital or acquired, may also be associated with fever. Babies who acquire herpes simplex virus (HSV) infection from their mothers at birth may present after 2–7 days with fever and nonspecific signs of sepsis, and HSV should be considered in the differential diagnosis. Clinical features may include skin, eye or mouth lesions, pneumonitis, hepatitis, encephalitis and disseminated intravascular coagulopathy (DIC). Other viruses that commonly present with fever in the neonatal period include enteroviruses, influenza and respiratory syncytial virus.

FEVER DURING INFANCY AND CHILDHOOD

The commonest cause of fever in this group is viral infection, which tends to be short lived. The challenge for the pediatrician is to determine whether the fever is the result of a viral or bacterial infection. In a series of 292 infants < 2 months old admitted to hospital with a history of fever, 19 (6.5%) were described as having serious bacterial infection (SBI), although 5 of the 19 were afebrile at the time of admission.[39] In a prospective study of children 3–36 months of age, pathogenic bacteria were isolated in blood culture from 60/519 (12%) with a fever greater than 39.5 °C (method of temperature measurement not described). The risk of bacterial infection was found to be higher among infants with an elevated white blood count.[40] In the young infant the signs of SBI are relatively nonspecific and it is generally accepted that children < 3 months old require hospital admission. The strategy described by Baraff et al is widely accepted.[41]

The infant is assessed as toxic or nontoxic based on level of activity, responsiveness, feeding and peripheral perfusion. Toxic infants need to be evaluated urgently for bacteremia or meningitis and started on antibiotics. Nontoxic infants should have blood cultures and lumbar puncture and can be classified as low risk if they have normal CSF and urinalysis, and a WBC between 5 and 15 000/mm³. The well looking infant in the high risk group should also be started on antibiotics. A CXR should be performed in the presence of abnormal respiratory signs.

Guidance on many aspects of fever in the infant and child is published by the National Institute for Clinical Excellence.[42]

The typical signs of viral upper respiratory infection include coryza, inflamed tympanic membranes, tonsillitis and fever. Bacterial tonsillitis and otitis media are difficult to differentiate from viral causes.

A good history and thorough examination are essential if a speedy diagnosis is to be achieved. Direct questions should be asked about the following:

1. previous immunizations;
2. family members with fever;
3. travel abroad;
4. consumption of unpasteurized milk (to exclude listeriosis, brucellosis), or raw eggs (*Salmonella* spp.);
5. history of congenital heart disease;
6. symptoms of this illness (abdominal pain, urinary frequency and dysuria);
7. signs noticed, e.g. rash, joint swelling.

Examination should take note of rash, lymphadenopathy, hepato- and splenomegaly, chest signs, heart murmurs, abdominal masses and tenderness. The bones and joints should be assessed for swelling and tenderness.

When fever has been persistent – over a week for instance – and no cause has been found, serious consideration should be given to hospital admission to confirm pyrexia and to initiate investigations. The physical signs and investigations required to exclude conditions producing FUO or PUO are given in Table 28.8.

However, certain basic investigations should be performed, of which urine and blood culture are arguably the most important.

FEVER AND NEUTROPENIA

The neutropenic child with fever is in a similar clinical situation to the neonate with fever, in that there is no time to wait for culture results. Antibiotics should be started after blood cultures have been taken. The antibiotics chosen must cover infections due to staphylococci and Gram negative enteric bacilli. Neutropenic children are also at risk of fungal infection, and empirical antifungal therapy is indicated if fever persists despite antibiotics and negative cultures.

THE CHILD WITH A RASH

In some cases a rash will be diagnostic, and in others the diagnosis will only be reached in conjunction with the history and appropriate investigations. Failure to recognize certain rashes could cost the life of a child, as in meningococcal infection or varicella in an immunocompromised child.

If an infectious cause is suspected, certain information should be obtained by history: prior infectious disease and/or rashes; recent contact with infectious disease; prior immunization; foreign travel; prodromal illness; fever.

In the general examination, note should be taken of the child's general state, the temperature, appearance of conjunctivae, ears and throat. Careful auscultation of the chest should be performed; all groups of lymph glands as well as liver and spleen should be examined.

Once this has been done, interest should return to the rash, which should be described carefully (e.g. hemorrhagic, macular, papular):

1. macules – flat and impalpable;
2. papules – circumscribed, elevated lesions;
3. vesicles – circumscribed, elevated, filled with clear fluid, and normally less than 0.5 cm in diameter;
4. pustules – elevated lesions containing a purulent exudate;
5. petechiae and other hemorrhagic spots – cannot be blanched by compression and may be flat or raised; the term purpura usually refers to the larger lesions with a diameter greater than 0.5 cm.

The distribution may be an important clue to certain infections, and it may be relevant whether or not the rash is itchy.

INFECTIOUS RASHES IN THE NEWBORN

Rashes are common in the neonatal period. Neonatal urticaria, or erythema toxicum, is characterized by a mixture of erythematous macules and white or yellow papules that usually develop over the first few

Table 28.8 Causes of pyrexia of unknown origin

Disease	Signs	Investigations
Bacterial		
Brucellosis	Lymphadenopathy, splenomegaly	Antibody titers
Bacterial endocarditis	Murmur, splinter hemorrhages	Blood culture × 3, *Brucella, Coxiela* titers
Leptospirosis	Hematuria, jaundice, conjunctivitis	Blood culture, serology
Osteomyelitis	Bone swelling, tenderness, redness, immobility	Blood culture, bone aspirate culture, bone radioisotope scan
Pelvic abscess	Abdominal tenderness, tender mass rectally	Leukocytosis on full blood count
Pyelonephritis	Loin tenderness	Urine microscopy and culture
Tuberculosis	Pneumonia, meningitis	Tuberculin test, culture gastric washings ± cerebrospinal fluid, chest X-ray
Typhoid fever	Abdominal tenderness, rose spots, splenomegaly	Blood culture
Septic arthritis	Swelling, tenderness, immobility at single joint	Joint aspirate culture
Psittacosis	Chest crackles, tachypnea	Chest X-ray, serology
Listeriosis	Arthritis, meningism	Blood culture, cerebrospinal fluid culture
Virus		
Cytomegalic inclusion disease	Lymphadenopathy, hepatosplenomegaly	Urine culture, etc., blood and urine PCR
Human immunodeficiency virus	Lymphadenopathy, failure to thrive, chronic infection, e.g. candida	T4/T8 lymphocyte ratio, HIV antibody, HIV PCR
Infectious mononucleosis	Tonsillitis, hepatosplenomegaly	Paul–Bunnell/Monospot, Epstein–Earr viral antibody
Hepatitis	Icterus, hepatomegaly	Hepatitis A, hepatitis B serology, hepatitis B and C PCR
Parasite		
Malaria	Splenomegaly, hepatomegaly, encephalopathy	Thick or thin blood film
Toxoplasmosis	Cervical, supraclavicular lymphadenopathy	Smear from biopsy specimen, serology
Miscellaneous		
Crohn's disease	Abdominal tenderness and mass	GI endoscopy or barium study of GI tract. Exclude *Yersinia* and *Campylobacter* infection
Diabetes insipidus	Polyuria, polydipsia	Dilute urine following water deprivation
Juvenile rheumatoid arthritis		
1. Systemic	Fever, characteristic maculopapular rash, lethargy, arthritis, pericardial effusion	No diagnostic test
2. Monoarticular/polyarticular	Fever not a consistent sign	
Kawasaki disease	Cervical lymphadenopathy, bilateral conjunctival injection, red, fissured lips and tongue, maculopapular rash, swelling and desquamation of hands and feet	No diagnostic test
Malignancy	Includes anemia, lymphadenopathy, splenomegaly, abdominal mass, bone pain	Full blood count, blood film, lymph node biopsy, bone marrow trephine, vanillylmandelic acid
Leukemia		
Lymphoma		
Neuroblastoma		
Factitious fever (Munchausen by proxy)	Pyrexia only recorded by parent	None

days and may persist until the end of the second week. Staphylococcal infection of the newborn may be difficult to distinguish from neonatal urticaria. Although erythematous lesions are seen with staphylococcal infection, pustules and vesicles predominate. When there is uncertainty as to the diagnosis, a Gram stain of vesicle fluid should be performed. Plentiful polymorphs as well as Gram positive cocci should be seen in the presence of staphylococcal infection; eosinophils predominate in neonatal urticaria.

Vesicles are also seen in neonatal varicella and herpes simplex virus (HSV) infection. In the former, a history of maternal varicella will be elicited. In the latter, however, a history of past or current genital herpes is obtained in only a quarter of cases. The vesicles of HSV tend to be larger and less opaque than those of staphylococcal infection. Urgent treatment of neonatal HSV is essential. Rapid diagnosis can be achieved by rapid viral identification tests such as immunofluorescence on vesicle fluid or by electron microscopy if available. PCR of vesicle fluid, if available in a timely way, can also be diagnostic.

Other rashes associated with infection may be petechial or purpuric as a result of thrombocytopenia, as seen in congenital cytomegalovirus (CMV) or congenital rubella infections. In such cases the rash is usually just one of several clinical features of congenital infection.

INFECTIOUS RASHES IN INFANCY AND CHILDHOOD

These will be described under descriptive headings.

Vesicular rashes
Varicella

Lesions normally appear without a prodromal illness and progress rapidly (within a few hours) from papules to vesicles surrounded by an erythematous base. Crops of vesicles appear over 3 days, predominantly on the trunk and proximal limbs. Vesicles may also develop on mucous membranes.

Herpes zoster

Lesions similar to those seen in varicella infection may develop over specific dermatomes or cranial nerves. Although the immunosuppressed are at increased risk from zoster, this condition is also seen in normal children.

Herpes simplex virus (HSV)

HSV infection in childhood may be primary, usually associated with gingivostomatitis, may be secondary (reactivation) as with cold sores and other recurrent herpetic lesions, or may occur as eczema herpeticum, a spreading vesicular rash in association with eczema (caused by HSV but sometimes confusingly called Kaposi's varicelliform eruption). Pyrexia is followed by the appearance of crops of vesicles on the eczematous skin, which may occur over several days. Rapid diagnosis, e.g. with immunofluorescence, and treatment with antivirals is essential because untreated severe infection may be fatal.

Hand, foot and mouth
This is caused by enteroviruses, the commonest being Coxsackie virus type 16, and occurs in epidemics. It is associated with a papular–vesicular eruption of the mouth, hands, feet and sometimes buttocks.

Impetigo
This condition usually presents as a red macule and then becomes vesicular. The small vesicles burst to leave a honey-colored crust. Both streptococcal and staphylococcal impetigo occur most commonly around the mouth.

Molluscum contagiosum
This is caused by a pox virus. Flesh-colored papules with a central dimple are firm initially, but become softer and more waxy with time. Lesions are 2–5 mm in size and may occur anywhere. Molluscum is more severe in HIV infection.

Maculopapular rashes
Measles
Measles rash is blotchy, red or pink in color, raised in places, and starts behind the ears and on the face, spreading downwards. The lesions tend to become confluent on the upper part of the body and remain more discrete lower down. The rash fades, usually after 2–3 days. The skin becomes brown and although desquamation occurs this is not usually seen on the hands and feet, as it is in scarlet fever.

Rubella
Rubella results in a pink rash which progresses caudally. The lesions are normally discrete and the rash develops more quickly and disappears earlier than in measles. Desquamation is not a characteristic.

Scarlet fever
The eruption is dark red and punctiform. The rash tends to be most prominent on the neck and in the major skinfolds. A distinctive feature is circumoral pallor as a result of the rash sparing the area around the mouth. Desquamation of the hands and feet is common after 1–2 weeks. True scarlet fever is associated with inflammation of the tongue (white and red strawberry tongue). Scarlatina refers to the rash, which may occur alone in milder streptococcal infection and is often short lived.

Kawasaki disease
Although several features are required for the diagnosis of this condition, which is of unknown etiology, the rash may be confused with that of scarlet fever. Discrete red maculopapules are seen on the feet, around the knees and in the axillary and inguinal skin creases. Desquamation of the hands and feet is a common feature (Fig. 28.15).

Erythema infectiosum or fifth disease
Infection caused by parvovirus B19 is associated with a rash which develops in two stages. The cheeks appear red and flushed, giving rise to a 'slapped cheek' appearance. A maculopapular rash develops 1–2 weeks later, predominantly over the arms and legs which, as it fades, appears lace-like.

Roseola infantum
The main cause is human herpes virus 6 (HHV-6). Roseola infantum is characterized by a widespread morbilliform (measles-like) rash, seen in its most florid form on the trunk. The lesions tend to be discrete. As the rash appears the fever, which is normally present over the previous

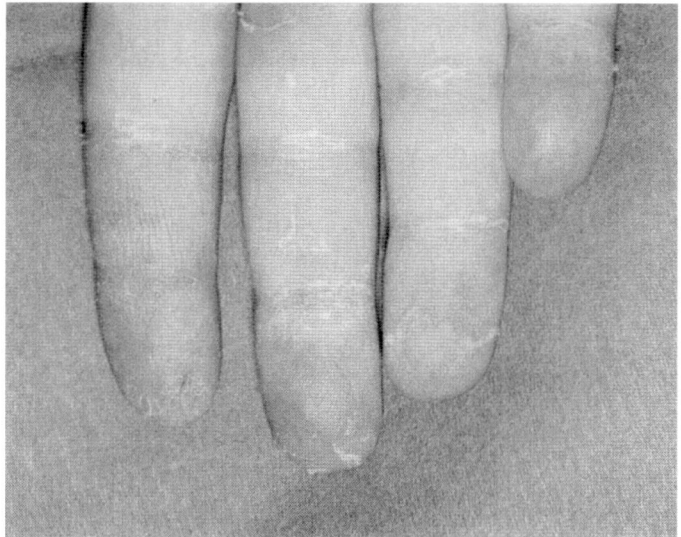

Fig. 28.15   Kawasaki disease: finger desquamation starting at the tips.

4 days, resolves and the child looks well (in contrast to measles, in which the child is febrile and unwell when the rash appears).

Viral infections
Many viral infections, particularly those associated with the enteroviruses, may cause maculopapular rashes.

Petechial and purpuric rashes
Meningococcal infection
The first sign of meningococcal septicemia may be a petechial or purpuric rash anywhere on the body and often localized (Fig. 28.16). On occasions these lesions may be preceded by or accompany a maculopapular rash which may blanch (Fig. 28.17). The petechiae will not blanch, and although it is conventional to make a microbiological diagnosis on blood culture and PCR, bacteria can often be seen on Gram stain and cultured on scrapings of the skin lesions.

Meningococcal petechiae can be confused with those seen on the face around the eyes following events that result in a transient rise in venous pressure such as vomiting. Rarely petechial rashes are associated with septicemia caused by other bacteria, such as *S. pneumoniae*, *S. aureus* and *Haemophilus influenzae* type b.

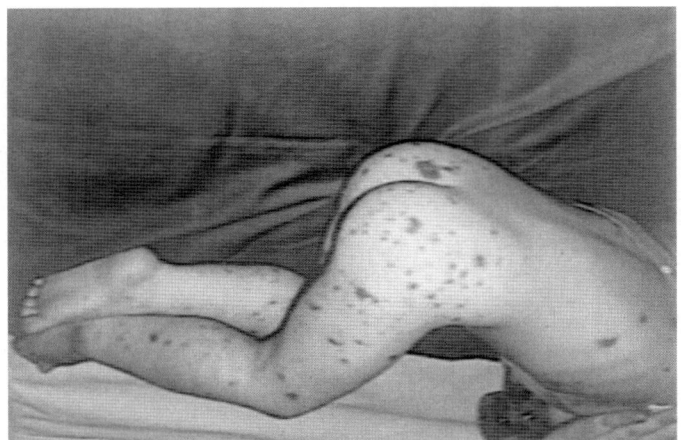

Fig. 28.16   Purpuric rash of meningococcemia.
(Courtesy of Department of Medical Illustration, University of Aberdeen.)

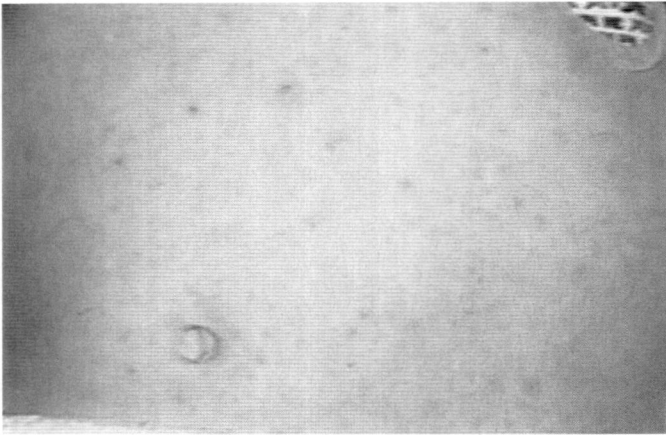

Fig. 28.17   Maculopapular/morbilliform rash of early meningococcemia. (Courtesy of Department of Medical Illustration, University of Aberdeen.)

Henoch–Schönlein purpura

This condition often follows an upper respiratory tract infection but no single infective agent has been implicated. Hemorrhagic macules and papules develop on the buttocks and extensor surfaces of the limbs, particularly the knees and ankles. The lesions come in crops and fade over a few days leaving a brown pigmentation.

Idiopathic thrombocytopenic purpura (ITP)

A purpuric rash sometimes associated with frank bleeding is seen in this condition. Even post-infective cases are often referred to as ITP, and rubella infection is considered to be the commonest infectious cause.

Leukemia

Children with leukemia may present with a hemorrhagic rash as a result of thrombocytopenia but in addition, the pallor of severe anemia will usually be obvious.

FEVER AND INCREASED RESPIRATORY RATE

The combination of fever and rapid breathing is a common and important pediatric presentation. While the differential diagnosis is vast (Table 28.9), a serious underlying condition must always be considered, in particular sepsis (bacteremia or septicemia) and bacterial pneumonia.

Table 28.9   Differential diagnosis of the child with fever and increased respiratory rate

Serious infections
Bacteremia/septicemia
Bacterial pneumonia (with or without parapneumonic effusion)
Other focal bacterial infections (including meningitis, osteomyelitis, septic arthritis)
Less serious infections
Viral or *Mycoplasma* bronchopneumonia
Mild infections
Viral upper respiratory tract infection (URTI)
Viral bronchitis
Viral exanthema
Fever and increased respiratory rate with upper airways obstruction (stridor)
Viral laryngotracheobronchitis (viral 'croup')
Fever and increased respiratory rate with lower airways obstruction (wheeze)
Acute viral bronchiolitis (usually due to RSV)
Asthma triggered by intercurrent viral upper respiratory tract infection

Fortunately, these serious conditions are uncommon and most infants and young children presenting with fever and increased respiratory rate simply have a relatively minor viral upper respiratory tract infection. In this situation, the respiratory rate is only mildly elevated and not associated with any other obvious signs of increased work of breathing (such as intercostal and/or subcostal retractions).

Both the level of the fever and the degree of tachypnea are key indicators of a serious versus minor infection: the higher the level, the greater the likelihood of a serious bacterial infection. In addition, infants and young children with serious infections will have other features, both on history and physical examination, which will assist with the diagnosis. These include signs of marked increased work of breathing, and 'grunting' respirations with extensive bacterial pneumonia. Further, infants and young children with serious bacterial infections will look ill, with signs such as pallor, cyanosis, apathy and altered level of consciousness. On the other hand infants and young children with a viral acute respiratory infection will have a history and physical evidence of a viral/coryzal illness with mild fever, clear rhinorrhea, conjunctival injection, redness of the tympanic membranes, sore throat and dry cough.

Clearly, the source or focus of infection must be thoroughly sought, both when taking the history and when performing the physical examination, in children presenting with this combination of symptoms. Recent contact with other children suffering from a viral infection (including one of the viral exanthemata) is vital information. Symptoms of a viral upper respiratory tract infection, or symptoms which localize the inflammation to a specific area of the respiratory tract, need to be elicited. This includes: a barking cough and inspiratory stridor indicating viral laryngotracheobronchitis (croup); coryzal symptoms plus acute history of significant cough (acute viral bronchitis); coryzal symptoms with acute wheeze, cough and shortness of breath (acute viral bronchiolitis in infants; acute asthma in older children).

A major symptom and sign to look for in children with fever and tachypnea is wheezing. In infants this is most likely to be due to acute viral bronchiolitis (usually due to respiratory syncytial virus), and in older children to an episode of acute bronchospasm (asthma) triggered by an intercurrent viral respiratory tract infection. In both these situations wheeze will be present, either audible with the ear or with a stethoscope. Generally, there will also be hyperinflation of the thoracic cage, tachypnea and other signs of increased work of respiration. In infants with acute viral bronchiolitis, diffuse inspiratory crackles are generally audible throughout the chest plus the loud expiratory, musical wheezing.

Infants and children with viral or *Mycoplasma* bronchopneumonia generally have other coryzal symptoms and signs in the ear, nose and throat plus a marked cough, which is often the major complaint. By contrast bacterial pneumonia presents with high fever, 'grunting' respirations and tachypnea, but no cough, particularly in the early phases of the illness.

The infant and young children with bacterial sepsis will generally have high fever (over 38.5 °C), rapid respiratory rate and rapid pulse and will look ill. On close inspection some of these children may have localized features of serious infection such as meningitis, osteomyelitis, septic arthritis or endocarditis. Infants with a bacterial urinary tract infection will have very few localizing symptoms or signs apart from fever and mild elevation of respiratory rate.

In summary, there is a large differential diagnosis of the infant or young child presenting with a combination of fever and increased respiratory rate. This can range from a severe life-threatening illness to a trivial head cold. The latter is far more likely, and most will have only mildly elevated temperature and respiratory rate plus other symptoms and signs to indicate an intercurrent viral upper respiratory tract syndrome. On the other hand, a markedly elevated temperature and respiratory rate in a very sick child indicates a serious infection, particularly bacteremia/septicemia or bacterial pneumonia.

When in doubt, further investigations and/or a further period of observation are essential. These may include CXR, blood cultures, lumbar puncture and blood or urine for bacterial antigen testing.

In obviously sick infants and children, or those in whom a serious underlying bacterial infection is likely, appropriate antibiotics should be given while waiting for the results of the above testing.

COUGH AND FEVER

The presence of cough signifies irritation or stimulation of cough receptors in the upper or lower airways. This is most commonly secondary to inflammation from a viral infection of the upper or lower airways and will be accompanied by mild fever. Cough is also a feature of bronchial asthma, which is also often accompanied by fever, since the commonest trigger for an acute exacerbation in young children is an intercurrent viral upper respiratory tract infection.

Thus the combination of fever and cough suggests an infection somewhere in the respiratory tract and this is far more likely to be due to a virus rather than bacteria. Diffuse, mild inflammation is typical of viral infection, while focal, severe inflammation is typical of bacterial infection in the respiratory tract. Indeed, one of the major distinguishing features between streptococcal pharyngitis and a viral upper respiratory tract infection is the absence of cough and coryzal symptoms in streptococcal throat infections.

To determine the likely cause of cough and fever requires a comprehensive history and physical examination. Laboratory investigations may occasionally be required to further elucidate the cause.

If there is a past history of bronchial asthma, the fever and cough are almost certainly due to episodic asthma or 'wheezing associated respiratory infection' (WARI). If there is a past history of chronic bronchitis (frequent episodes of protracted cough with intercurrent viral acute respiratory infections) then it should be obvious from the history that the child is having a further episode of acute viral bronchitis.

Fever and cough due to an upper respiratory tract infection should be readily distinguishable by the coryzal symptoms of rhinorrhea, conjunctival injection and a dry cough but no increased work of breathing and no wheeze. While the child with viral laryngotracheobronchitis will have signs of a coryzal illness, the striking features will be the barking, 'croupy' quality of the cough and probable inspiratory stridor, particularly when the child is upset. When severe this inspiratory stridor will be associated with increased work of breathing (chest wall retractions, tracheal tug). Acute viral bronchitis is characterized by troublesome dry or wet cough in association with an acute respiratory infection. On auscultation there may be scattered coarse crackles (due to excessive airway secretions), which should clear following active coughing. Acute viral bronchiolitis is characterized by coryzal symptoms plus hyperinflation of the chest, loud wheezing, inspiratory crackles throughout both lung fields, and varying degrees of respiratory difficulty in addition to fever and cough. Viral and *Mycoplasma* bronchopneumonia will be characterized by coryzal symptoms, marked cough, increased work of breathing and widespread, scattered, inspiratory crackles.

A less common but important cause of cough and fever is foreign body inhalation, e.g. nuts and peanuts. Initially this is a dry cough, often with wheeze and difficulty breathing. If retained, the cough becomes loose and productive of purulent sputum. A child with a loose, productive cough and fever could also be suffering from chronic suppurative lung disease – bronchiectasis or chronic bronchitis. Most of these children will have some underlying problem (e.g. cystic fibrosis or immune deficiency).

In summary, fever and cough signify some inflammatory process in the airways. This can range from a relatively uncomplicated viral upper respiratory tract infection due to rhinovirus through to viral or *Mycoplasma* bronchopneumonia (Table 28.10). A major differential to consider is whether the fever and cough are due to an exacerbation of asthma in the child with underlying episodic asthma.

RHINITIS

Rhinitis implies inflammation of the nasal 'mucosa', and in children this is most commonly due to a viral upper respiratory tract infection. The

Table 28.10 Causes of cough and fever

Acute respiratory tract infections
    Viral upper respiratory tract infection (URTI)
    Acute viral bronchitis
    Acute viral laryngotracheobronchitis (viral croup)
    Acute viral bronchiolitis (infants)
    Acute viral bronchopneumonia
    Mycoplasma (bronchitis and bronchopneumonia)
Asthma syndromes
    Classical bronchial asthma
    Wheezing associated respiratory infection (WARI)
Less common causes
    Foreign body inhalation
    Suppurative lung disease (chronic bronchitis/bronchiectasis)

inflammation normally results in a combination of rhinorrhea and nasal obstruction. Sneezing is commonly associated with these symptoms.

The major differential diagnosis of rhinitis secondary to a viral upper respiratory tract infection is allergic rhinitis. In children allergic rhinitis is generally perennial rather than seasonal and is characterized by its persistence for weeks or months rather than the short term nasal symptoms of an acute viral infection. The symptoms of allergic rhinitis have a typical diurnal pattern (classically worse in the mornings) and there is absence of fever and other signs suggesting a viral upper respiratory tract infection. Nasal itch and sneezing are common as are clear rhinorrhea and nasal obstruction. There is often an associated allergic conjunctivitis which can simulate a viral rhino-conjunctivitis. The child with allergic rhinitis generally has other signs of clinical atopy, particularly atopic eczema or bronchial asthma.

Vasomotor rhinitis is uncommon in young children and typically causes sudden onset (and sudden cessation) of clear rhinorrhea – often for only hours – but with recurrent episodes.

Other rarer causes of rhinitis include:
- Foreign body – particularly small parts of toys and polystyrene beads. Causes unilateral nasal symptoms.
- Unusual infections (e.g. nasal diphtheria).

The distinction between acute viral rhinitis secondary to a viral infection and acute sinusitis is subtle and arbitrary. Most definitions base the distinction on duration of symptoms. Conventionally, acute sinusitis is the appropriate diagnosis if the nasal discharge is severe and persists for more than 10 days. These symptoms would generally be associated with cough and possibly bad breath.

Chronic sinusitis is arbitrarily defined as a persistent, mucopurulent nasal discharge for over 30 days. This is most commonly seen in children with underlying abnormalities of mucus, mucociliary clearance or immune function (e.g. cystic fibrosis, primary ciliary dyskinesia, agammaglobulinemia).

Drug therapy for rhinitis associated with a viral upper respiratory tract infection is generally not required. However, in small infants the nasal obstruction and rhinorrhea may interfere with feeding and saline drops followed by suctioning of the drops ('nasal lavage') may be helpful, particularly immediately prior to feeds. Acute sinusitis is generally viral although secondary bacterial infection may occur. While there is some uncertainty as to whether or not antibiotics are indicated in this situation, there is little doubt that the color of the nasal discharge changes promptly with administration of antibiotics, but such treatment is best reserved for those who are more severely affected by the symptoms. Chronic sinusitis should be treated with antibiotics and prolonged courses (three weeks) may be necessary.

Perennial allergic rhinitis in children warrants treatment, particularly if the symptoms are severe. The most effective treatment is regular nasal topical corticosteroid (e.g. budesonide nasal spray).

In summary, while there are many possible causes for rhinitis (Table 28.11), most commonly it is the result of either a respiratory virus or allergic rhinitis.

Table 28.11   Causes of rhinitis

Common
   Viral upper respiratory tract infection (acute viral nasopharyngitis
   – most commonly due to rhinovirus)
   Perennial allergic rhinitis
Uncommon
   Acute viral or bacterial sinusitis
   Vasomotor rhinitis
Rare
   Retained foreign body
   Uncommon infections (e.g. nasal diphtheria)

NOISY BREATHING

Audible noises of respiration are common in children. Clarification of the type of noise is critical with respect to identifying the most likely underlying cause. In general, noisy breathing signifies some obstruction to airflow, and the specific type of noise – especially which phase of respiration – can greatly assist in determining the anatomic site of the airflow obstruction.

The types of noises identifiable are listed below in Table 28.12, together with the phase of respiration in which they are most audible, and the usual anatomic site for the noise.

An important principle is: the noise is predominantly inspiratory when the obstruction is outside the thoracic cage (upper airways), and predominantly expiratory when the obstruction is inside the thorax (lower airways).

If a child has the noise when being examined then there is no difficulty determining its features. However, when the noise is from history alone this can create difficulties with respect to the terminology used by parents. In such instances, mimicking these noises will often assist with the accurate diagnosis. Alternatively, asking the parents to obtain tape recordings will enable clear identification of the type of noise.

There will generally be associated symptoms and signs with these noises, which will assist clinically in determining the exact site and

Table 28.12   Types of identifiable noises

Noise	Inspiration	Expiration	Site of obstruction
Snuffliness	+ +	±	Nasal
Snoring	+ +	±	Oronasopharynx
Stridor	+ + +		Extrathoracic trachea (subglottis/larynx)
Rattliness	+ +		Central tracheobronchial tree (trachea)
Wheeze		+ +	Small and medium sized intrathoracic airways
Grunting		+ + +	Alveoli

cause for the obstruction. For example, a child with acute onset inspiratory stridor and a barking cough in association with an URTI has acute viral 'croup' (laryngotracheobronchitis). On the other hand, a child with grunting respirations and high fever who looks toxic and unwell is probably suffering from acute (bacterial) pneumonia.

The causes of obstruction are numerous and are summarized in Table 28.13.

In summary, the child presenting with the problem of noisy breathing requires a comprehensive history and examination to determine the exact nature of the noise and to determine whether there are any associated symptoms or signs. By accurately determining the nature of the noisy breathing, the likely anatomical site of the obstruction can usually be determined, and this will greatly assist with the final diagnosis.

SUSPECTED MENINGITIS

Over the last five years, notified cases of bacterial meningitis have fallen to less than 1500 cases a year in England and Wales (Table 28.14). The mortality from these infections has also declined in recent years, but there is evidence that the long term consequences of meningitis are considerable, particularly when the disease occurs early in life.

ETIOLOGY AND PATHOPHYSIOLOGY OF BACTERIAL MENINGITIS

The commonest route of meningeal infection is from the bloodstream, so the spectrum of pathogens causing meningitis is similar to that seen in bacteremia and sepsis. The introduction of the *Haemophilus influenzae* type b (Hib) polysaccharide-conjugate vaccine into the UK vaccination program has had a dramatic effect.[43] The incidence of Hib meningitis has dropped from around 2500 cases per year to 44 per year, with *Neisseria meningitidis* now the commonest cause of community acquired bacterial meningitis in the UK, followed by *Streptococcus pneumoniae*. The relative importance of these pathogens varies considerably with age (Table 28.14) and the nature of the immunization programs in operation. In the neonatal period, group B streptococcus is the prominent meningeal pathogen, followed by Gram negative bacilli, *S. pneumoniae* and *Listeria monocytogenes*. In children older than 3 months and in young adults, the most frequent cause of bacterial meningitis is *N. meningitidis* followed by *S. pneumoniae*. Infants between 1 and 3 months old are susceptible to *N. meningitidis* and *S. pneumoniae*, as well as the neonatal pathogens. The propensity of neonates to get meningitis is in part due to their immunological immaturity. Older children with congenital or acquired deficiencies in complement, immunoglobulin production, lymphocytes, neutrophils or splenic function are at increased risk from meningitis, sometimes due to atypical pathogens. A rare but serious form of bacterial meningitis is caused by *Mycobacterium tuberculosis*. This organism can affect patients of all ages and should be considered in any atypical presentation of meningitis, particularly patients presenting with an insidious illness.[44]

Table 28.13   Causes of obstruction

	Causes of noise	
	Acute	Persistent
Snuffliness	Viral upper respiratory tract infection	Perennial allergic rhinitis
Snoring	Acute tonsillitis/upper respiratory tract infection	Chronic enlargement of tonsils and adenoids
Stridor	Viral croup	Congenital subglottic stenosis or other fixed upper airway malformations
Rattle	Acute viral bronchitis	Cerebral palsy/CNS disorders ('sputum retention')
Wheeze	Asthma	Chronic small airways obstruction (e.g. cystic fibrosis)
Grunt	Acute bacterial (lobar) pneumonia Hyaline membrane disease (neonate)	Chronic interstitial lung disease (e.g. pulmonary fibrosis)

Table 28.14 Statutory notifications of meningitis cases in 2000 and 2005 (data from Health Protection Agency)

	Year	1–11 months	1–4 years	5–9 years	10–14 years	15–24 years
Haemophilus influenzae	2005	11	15	3	2	3
	2000	5	10	1	1	2
Neisseria meningitidis	2005	163	121	42	26	92
	2000	231	220	105	86	219
Streptococcus pneumoniae	2005	63	32	10	7	5
	2000	53	27	4	9	14

Table header note: Age group spans the columns 1–11 months, 1–4 years, 5–9 years, 10–14 years, 15–24 years.

While meningitis often occurs in the context of systemic infections, it can also follow bacterial invasion from a contiguous focus of infection, such as the mastoids or paranasal sinuses, or from osteomyelitis of the skull. Skull fractures, craniospinal dermal sinuses, neurenteric or dermoid cysts, occult intranasal encephaloceles, or transethmoid meningoceles are also potential portals of entry for pathogens into the subarachnoid space.[45] The possibility of a cranial defect should be considered in children with recurrent meningitis. Neurosurgical procedures and the presence of ventriculoperitoneal shunts also provide routes for meningeal infection. In such cases, *Staphylococcus aureus* and coagulase negative staphylococci are more likely pathogens.

Bacterial invasion of the cerebrospinal fluid (CSF) is followed by an outpouring of inflammatory cells which cross the blood–brain barrier and enter the CSF. Inflammatory cytokines such as tumor necrosis factor and interleukins 1, 6 and 8 are central to the inflammatory response. These mediators increase adhesion molecule expression on endothelial cells and leukocytes, which act in concert to facilitate the migration of cells into the CSF. Antibodies to adhesion molecules limit leukocyte migration and the consequences of meningeal infection.[46] The meninges become inflamed, swollen and covered by fibrino-purulent exudate. The thickest exudate is usually at the base of the brain. This leads to obstruction of the exit foramina of the fourth ventricle or the subarachnoid basal cisterns, restricting the CSF circulation to produce hydrocephalus. The ependymal lining of the cerebral ventricles may also be a site of intense inflammation (ventriculitis), causing ventricular enlargement and subsequent subependymal gliosis. A combination of cerebral vasculitis, thrombosis, cerebral edema and raised intracranial pressure leads to globally reduced cerebral blood flow and focal ischemia. This results in neuronal injury and cerebral damage, manifest clinically as coma, seizures and focal neurological signs.

CLINICAL FEATURES

The fully developed clinical picture of acute meningitis in children is sufficiently characteristic to be recognized without difficulty. More than 80% of children will have fever, vomiting, severe headache and signs of meningeal irritation. However, in the early stages of disease, and in young children, the symptoms and signs are often nonspecific. Fever may be absent in up to 30% of individuals, and 20–30% do not have signs of meningism at presentation. Previous antibiotic therapy may also mask the significance of the presenting illness.[47]

Older children will often complain of headache or pain at the back of the neck, nausea and photophobia. The physical signs of meningeal irritation are neck stiffness and a positive Kernig test, which reflect inflammation of nerve roots of the spinal canal and adjacent sensory nerves. The most comfortable position for the patient is to lie with an extended neck and flexed hips and knees to reduce tension on the nerves emanating from the spinal cord. Neck stiffness can be detected by placing a palm of the hand on the supine child's occiput. Any attempt at flexing the child's neck will result in the lifting of the whole trunk. Kernig's sign is elicited with the child supine. The hip and knee joints are bent 90 degrees and then an attempt is made to extend the knee fully. In the presence of meningitis, there is resistance and severe pain as the sciatic

nerve is stretched. A positive Brudzinski sign is involuntary muscular contraction causing leg flexion upon passive flexion of the neck, but this is a less reliable sign of meningitis. Additional evidence of neurological involvement includes convulsions, which occur in 30% of children within 3 days of presentation, cranial nerve palsies (particularly III, IV, VI, and VII), delirium, drowsiness and coma.

In infants and toddlers, the symptoms are often those of a generalized illness. Irritability, lethargy, convulsions, refusal of feeds, vomiting, a high pitched cry and a bulging fontanelle should all alert the physician to the presence of meningitis. The 'typical' features of meningitis may be absent or difficult to interpret or elicit. When present they are often indicative of advanced disease.

Neisseria meningitidis is the commonest cause of bacterial meningitis in the UK (Table 28.14). More than 50% of patients infected with this organism will have a petechial rash, so a vigilant search for petechiae should be made in any child with features suggesting a diagnosis of meningitis. The whole skin surface should be carefully examined, since there may initially be only one or two petechiae. However it is also important to note that initially the rash of *N. meningitidis* may be maculopapular or urticarial in nature, and so an atypical rash should not be taken as evidence to exclude the diagnosis. In all age groups, the clinical manifestations of bacteremia and sepsis may be the earliest evidence of infection (see section on sepsis and meningococcal infection). If the condition can be picked up at this stage and treated appropriately, meningitis can be prevented.

DIAGNOSIS

If meningitis is suspected, the diagnosis should be confirmed by lumbar puncture and examination of CSF. Over the last 10 years, there has been a move away from performing diagnostic lumbar punctures (LP) in patients presenting with suspected meningitis, since it is frequently argued that an LP will not affect patient management and may be hazardous. However, an LP offers immediate confirmation of the diagnosis and allows appropriate treatment to be started, which may be particularly important in neonates and immunocompromised patients in whom the differential diagnosis is wide. Identifying the etiological agent and its antibiotic sensitivities may be crucial to administering the most appropriate antibiotics and providing important prognostic information.[47]

There are, however, specific and clear contraindications to LP in patients with meningitis.[48] These are:

1. signs of raised intracranial pressure with changing level of consciousness, focal neurological signs or severe mental impairment;
2. cardiovascular compromise with impaired peripheral perfusion or hypotension;
3. respiratory compromise with tachypnea, an abnormal breathing pattern or hypoxia;
4. thrombocytopenia or a coagulopathy.

An LP should also be avoided if it will result in a significant delay in treatment. The association between LP and cerebellar tonsillar herniation has not been shown to be causal, and has not been reported in the absence of the specific contraindications listed above.

Lumbar puncture should be performed in the third to fourth lumbar space using a needle with a stylet, since use of a needle alone has been associated with the development of implantation dermoid cysts. CSF should be collected for microscopy and culture, bacterial and viral polymerase chain reaction (PCR), latex agglutination tests for bacterial antigens, protein and glucose. Blood cultures may also identify the etiological agent if an LP is not performed or fails to establish the cause of meningitis.

Analysis of the CSF leukocyte count, glucose and protein can usually establish a positive diagnosis of meningitis, but normal results do not necessarily exclude meningitis. The absence of cells may indicate very early meningitis before the migration of leukocytes into the CSF. Very high white cell counts of up to 20 000/mm³ can be observed in bacterial meningitis, although the number of cells is usually less than 3000/mm³. There is a broad association between a predominance of polymorphonuclear leukocytes in the CSF and bacterial meningitis. However, lymphocytes may predominate in early or partially treated bacterial meningitis, in tuberculous meningitis and in neonates. In bacterial meningitis, CSF glucose is usually low with a CSF:blood ratio of less than 0.5, and protein is frequently raised to more than 0.4 g/L. Numerous studies have now shown that even after the administration of intravenous antibiotics, the diagnostic cellular and biochemical changes in the CSF may persist for at least 48 h. In the context of a negative Gram stain and CSF culture, the presence of bacterial antigens and PCR tests may prove invaluable for establishing a diagnosis of bacterial meningitis.

THE USE OF CT SCANS

Following the clinical diagnosis of bacterial meningitis, it has become common practice to arrange a computerized tomographic (CT) brain scan to exclude raised intracranial pressure prior to undertaking a lumbar puncture. This approach has three important drawbacks. First, raised intracranial pressure (ICP) is very common amongst children with meningitis and clinically significant raised ICP cannot be ruled out by brain CT. Second, it is hazardous to transport patients to a CT scanner before they have been adequately stabilized. Third, the inevitable delay in undertaking the CT scan requires that empirical antibiotics be given while awaiting the procedure, therefore impairing the diagnostic yield from a subsequent LP. Patients presenting with clinical signs of raised ICP are the minority, and these children should not undergo LP, regardless of their CT findings. CT scans can exclude lesions requiring neurosurgical intervention and identify conditions such as cerebral abscess or hydrocephalus requiring shunting. The diagnostic yield from a CT scan in children is, however, low and should not be allowed to compromise the procedures required for diagnosis and to initiate appropriate treatment.[47]

ANTIBIOTICS

Except in cases where the patient is well and the diagnosis very uncertain, antibiotics should be administered empirically while awaiting the result of the LP. The selection of the optimal antibiotic for the treatment of bacterial meningitis should be based on the following criteria: the spectrum of pathogens known to cause meningitis in different age groups (Table 28.14); the changing pattern of antimicrobial resistance;[49,50] the pharmacological properties of the antibiotics available and the results of therapeutic trials. In infants up to 3 months of age, a combination of ampicillin and cefotaxime is a logical choice, as cefotaxime provides cover for both neonatal and infant pathogens, and ampicillin is effective against *Listeria monocytogenes*. For the same reason, ampicillin should be included as part of empirical therapy for immunocompromised patients. Penicillin-resistant meningococci are emerging worldwide, as are chloramphenicol-resistant strains, but these have not yet resulted in treatment failures. Fortunately, almost all strains in the UK remain sensitive to the third generation cephalosporins.

In the USA and some countries in Europe including Spain, France and Romania, more than 25% of pneumococcal isolates are resistant to penicillin and this proportion exceeds 50% in South Africa. Penicillin-insensitive strains of pneumococci are more likely to be resistant to third generation cephalosporins, and there have been documented cases of microbiological failure in the treatment of pneumococcal meningitis with third generation cephalosporins. In the UK, the level of penicillin resistance is stable at less than 5%.[50] In most UK cases, penicillin resistance is low level and cephalosporin resistance is rare and so a third generation cephalosporin (cefotaxime or ceftriaxone) is adequate for most community acquired meningitis in children over 3 months. The routine use of vancomycin for community acquired meningitis is not justified in the UK at the present time. However, vancomycin should be added to the treatment regimen for any patient coming from an area where high levels of penicillin resistance are endemic. The addition of rifampicin to vancomycin or the administration of vancomycin intraventricularly has been recommended by some authorities.[51]

THE ROLE OF CORTICOSTEROIDS

It is now widely accepted that much of the cerebral damage which occurs in bacterial meningitis is not caused by the invading organism itself but by the host mediated inflammatory response.[52] While a number of adjunctive anti-inflammatory agents have been suggested, only corticosteroids have been extensively tested in clinical trials. Several studies have shown some improvement in morbidity (deafness or neurological deficit), although these studies were largely conducted in children with *Haemophilus influenzae* type b meningitis, and this approach requires administration of corticosteroids either before antibiotic administration or at the same time.[53] Fewer data are available in children with pneumococcal and meningococcal meningitis. However, a recent systematic review of 18 studies in children and adults supports the use of steroid administration as a means of reducing the mortality and morbidity associated with meningitis.[54] These data imply that, at least at the present time, concerns that limiting meningeal inflammation could actually delay sterilization of the CSF by agents such as vancomycin, since these antibiotics cross the blood–brain barrier poorly, have not been substantiated.

NEUROLOGICAL AND FLUID MANAGEMENT

Hyponatremia is frequently observed in patients with bacterial meningitis. While this is associated with elevated serum antidiuretic hormone (ADH), possibly suggesting inappropriate ADH secretion (SIADH), more recent studies indicate that SIADH is overdiagnosed and the patients are hypovolemic.[55] Treatment of suspected SIADH with fluid restriction could potentially compromise circulating volume and therefore cerebral blood flow. Circulatory shock should be treated aggressively, significant dehydration corrected carefully, fluid balance monitored frequently and maintenance fluids given with care.

Patients presenting with clinical signs of raised ICP require very careful fluid balance monitoring to help maintain adequate cerebral blood flow. Intubation and mechanical ventilation should be instituted early to facilitate oxygenation, allow adequate sedation and permit normalization of $PaCO_2$. Such patients should be nursed head up and central venous catheters should not be placed in the neck. Intravenous mannitol may be useful for managing acute changes in intracranial pressure, and anticonvulsants for control of fits.[47]

COMPLICATIONS

Convulsions occur in 20–30% of children, usually within 72 h of presentation. The onset of late or persistent fits is associated with a poor prognosis. Subdural collections of fluid are common, particularly during infancy. They are usually sterile and rarely require aspiration unless there is evidence of increasing ICP, the presence of focal neurological signs, convulsions or persistent fever due to subdural empyema. Cerebral abscesses are rare outside the neonatal period. More frequent causes of persistent fever include intercurrent viral infection, ongoing inflammation and drug fever. In the absence of a definitive microbiological etiology, the combination of persistent fever and poor clinical condition may indicate that the meningitis is due to organisms resistant to the prescribed antibiotic therapy. A repeat LP should then be performed.

The commonest long term complication of meningitis is sensorineural deafness. This appears to develop early in the course of the disease and may occur in spite of early recognition and appropriate treatment. All children should undergo audiological assessment after recovery from infection. The overall rate of permanent deafness following meningitis may be less than 5% but is higher in cases of pneumococcal meningitis than in meningococcal infections. However, reversible hearing loss is seen in many more children, with reports of up to a third of children showing some impairment during the early phase of infection. In a study of morbidity after an episode of meningitis in infancy, almost a fifth of patients had some degree of disability.[56] This figure is higher if subtle defects are included, such as behavioral problems, middle ear disease and squints. Morbidity was highest following neonatal meningitis and also after meningitis caused by *S. pneumoniae*, group B streptococcus and atypical pathogens.

PREVENTION

Conjugate vaccines against *H. influenzae* type b (Hib), *N. meningitidis* group C and *S. pneumoniae* are now routinely given in the UK as part of the primary course of immunization and as a booster in the second year of life. An effective vaccine against *N. meningitidis* group B is not yet available.

When a child presents with meningococcal or Hib meningitis, other family members and close contacts are at increased risk of infection. Rifampicin (rifampin) is currently recommended for contacts of meningococcal disease (four doses of 10 mg/kg per dose 12 hourly) and *H. influenzae* type b (20 mg/kg per dose daily for 4 days). Decisions on who should receive prophylaxis can be difficult, and advice should be sought from the Consultant in Communicable Disease Control.

SEPTIC SHOCK

Despite the vast array of potential pathogens, the human host is remarkably resistant to life-threatening infection. Most pathogens are restricted by host defenses to their primary sites of invasion, with minimal clinical consequences. These first line defense mechanisms successfully intercept invading organisms in the majority of cases. On occasion, however, microbial invasion of the bloodstream can and does occur, even in apparently immunocompetent children, with potentially devastating consequences. The sequence of events following successful entry of microbes or microbial products to the circulation is complex, and depends both upon the virulent properties of the offending microorganism and the host response. Initial microbial invasion may be clinically silent and indeed may resolve without antimicrobial therapy. If, however, bacterial proliferation ensues a systemic response is initiated in the host. This is referred to as the systemic inflammatory response syndrome (SIRS) and is defined by the presence of abnormalities in two or more of the following: temperature, heart rate, respiratory rate and white blood count, of which one must be temperature or white count. SIRS can follow any severe insult including infection, trauma, major surgery, burns or pancreatitis, but when SIRS occurs in the context of infection, the patient is described as *septic*.

The term *severe sepsis* can be used to describe a state characterized by hypoperfusion, hypotension and organ dysfunction, while the term *septic shock* is restricted to patients with persistent hypotension despite adequate fluid resuscitation and/or hypoperfusion even following adequate inotrope or pressor support.[57] In practice it can be difficult to divide patients neatly into these defined states, but the use of these terms serves to highlight the sequential nature of the events associated with microbial invasion, and will help in the evaluation of future clinical trials in septic patients.

MICROBIAL ETIOLOGY OF SEPSIS

In view of the multitude of potential pathogens with the capacity to cause disease, it is perhaps surprising that a very limited range of microorganisms is responsible for invasive infections in healthy children beyond the neonatal period. Three organisms predominate: *Streptococcus pneumoniae*, *Neisseria meningitidis* and *Haemophilus influenzae* type b.

The incidence of sepsis due to vaccine preventable organisms has been drastically reduced in countries with appropriate vaccination programs. However, even in these countries, otherwise healthy children who are not yet fully vaccinated, children in whom the vaccine has not provided adequate cover (vaccine failures), and children with infections caused by *N. meningitidis* group B continue to present with severe and life-threatening infections. Rarer causes of sepsis in healthy children include *Staphylococcus aureus*, group A, C and G streptococci and *Salmonella* spp., and these may be associated with wound and skin infections or a history of diarrhea respectively. In vulnerable patient groups other pathogens are implicated. In neonates, group B *Streptococcus*, *Escherichia coli*, other Gram negative bacteria, and *Listeria monocytogenes* are the usual causes of sepsis. In immunocompromised patients, Gram negative organisms such as *Pseudomonas aeruginosa*, and fungi may be responsible. Any patient with an indwelling catheter is particularly at risk of sepsis from coagulase negative staphylococci and enterococci as well as methicillin resistant *Staphylococcus aureus* (MRSA). With all of these organisms, the onset of bacteremia is a crucial event in the pathogenesis of sepsis, but invasion of the bloodstream is not necessary for bacteria to induce features of septic shock. Enterotoxins from staphylococci and streptococci are potent stimulators of T cell proliferation and activation, and can produce toxic shock syndromes even in patients with an apparently localized focus of infection. Some viruses, including herpes viruses, enteroviruses and adenoviruses, can produce diseases which may be indistinguishable clinically from bacterial sepsis, particularly in neonates and infants.

PATHOPHYSIOLOGY OF SEPSIS

Over the last three decades it has emerged that it is the host response to microbial invasion which is predominantly responsible for the clinical features of sepsis and septic shock. Lipopolysaccharides (LPS) from Gram negative bacteria, and a variety of other microbial products have the capacity to stimulate the production of mediators from many cells within the human host. Tumor necrosis factor, interleukin 1 and interleukin 6 are just a few of the many inflammatory mediators reported to be present at high levels in septic patients. It has now been established that families of pattern recognition receptors exist which are able to transduce cellular signals in response to microorganisms, including bacteria. One important family, the human Toll-like receptors (hTLR), consists of at least ten proteins, with hTLR4 acting as the principal mediator of LPS signaling, while other members of the family, such as hTLR1, hTLR2 and hTLR6, can mediate signals induced by lipoproteins of mycobacteria and Gram positive bacterial peptidoglycans. The cytokines and inflammatory mediators produced in response to microbial stimuli activate neutrophils, endothelial cells and monocytes and influence the function of vital organs, including the heart, liver, brain and kidneys. The net effect of excessive inflammatory activity is to cause the constellation of pathophysiological events seen in patients with sepsis and septic shock.

PRO- VERSUS ANTI-INFLAMMATORY MECHANISMS IN SEPSIS

The proinflammatory mediators produced in response to microbial invasion prime and activate cells to fight infection. However, the host also responds to proinflammatory stimuli by producing antagonists, known collectively as anti-inflammatory mediators. Interleukin 10 and soluble cytokine receptors or antagonists such as interleukin 1 receptor antagonist occur naturally and act to limit the effects of proinflammatory cytokines. The balance between pro- and anti-inflammatory mediators is probably more critical than the levels of either alone. Patients who survive the initial inflammatory insult, but who still require assisted ventilation and intravenous support, have high levels of anti-inflammatory mediators. These patients are resistant to further proinflammatory stimulation and may be more susceptible to nosocomial infections. Such patients may actually benefit from immune stimulation[58] to provoke the production of more inflammatory mediators, and the balance of pro- and anti-inflammation may prove crucial in therapeutic interventions. In the future, a clear characterization of the inflammatory status of septic patients may therefore be essential before adjuvant therapy is instituted (see below).

CLINICAL PRESENTATION AND DIAGNOSIS

The symptoms and signs of the initial phase of bacteremia are dependent upon the age and pre-existing health of the patient and the duration of the illness, as well as the causative organism. Bacteremia, with little inflammatory response, can be very difficult to diagnose clinically because of the overlap in clinical presentation with common viral illnesses. A number of clinical parameters have been examined to try to estimate the probability of bacterial rather than viral infection: children with a bacteremic illness are more likely to have a fever $> 39\,°C$ and a white blood cell count (WBC) $> 15 \times 10^9/L$ or $< 2.5 \times 10^9/L$. However, the specificity and sensitivity of these parameters for diagnosing bacteremia is low and does not greatly add to the physician's general assessment of the child's condition.[59] Therefore frequent reassessment of the patient may be necessary if impending severe sepsis is to be recognized at an early stage. Nonspecific signs, including lethargy, irritability, hypotonia, poor feeding, nausea and vomiting, may be the earliest features of impending severe sepsis. Fever is not invariably present and hypothermia may also occur, particularly in neonates and infants. Cardiovascular involvement with tachycardia or bradycardia, inadequate peripheral perfusion, prolonged capillary refill, cold extremities, peripheral edema, decreased urine output and evidence of shock may all be manifest as the systemic response to bacterial invasion progresses. Respiratory, gastrointestinal and neurological derangement may indicate systemic disease or involvement of these specific organs in the infectious process. A petechial rash may be indicative of meningococcal disease, and in staphylococcal and streptococcal toxin-mediated shock, erythroderma, conjunctival and mucosal erythema and edema are usually present.

In all patients with suspected sepsis, blood cultures should be taken. The success of this procedure is dependent upon adequate blood inoculation of the culture media. If only a small volume of blood is available for culture, this should be added to the aerobic bottle, as few of the causative organisms will be anaerobes. Samples from potential sources of infection should be collected where appropriate. These include indwelling catheters, urine microscopy and culture, diagnostic radiology and aspiration for intra-abdominal sepsis, and lower respiratory tract secretions in ventilated patients, preferably by bronchoalveolar lavage. A lumbar puncture should be considered in patients with suspected meningeal involvement but is contraindicated in the presence of shock, coagulopathy, reduced conscious level or focal neurological signs. Samples can also be analyzed by molecular microbiological techniques for bacteria, fungi and viruses, although these investigations are not always routinely available. In patients with suspected toxic shock syndrome, analysis of staphylococcal and streptococcal isolates for the presence of toxin production and of V beta T cell receptor repertoires may be instructive. WBCs, high or low, and markers of inflammation including C-reactive protein (CRP), procalcitonin and proinflammatory cytokine levels may be useful. However, none of these investigations is specific or diagnostic. Coagulation studies, hemoglobin, urea and electrolytes, glucose and liver function tests should be performed to help inform further management and guide fluid and electrolyte replacement and general support.

MANAGEMENT OF SEPSIS
Recognition

Most cases of sepsis begin with the invasion of the bloodstream by a limited number of microbes. As the organisms multiply, often logarithmically, the host response intensifies and the condition of the patient deteriorates. The chances of a favorable outcome are greatly enhanced by initiating treatment at the earliest possible stage, so the most important aspect of sepsis management is the earliest possible recognition of the condition. In view of the diagnostic difficulties described above, it is imperative that otherwise healthy children presenting with nonspecific features are observed carefully. Even if a health care professional considers the risk of impending sepsis to be low and the patient well enough to be at home, a detailed plan of management should be discussed with the family. The parents or guardians should have a clear understanding of the clinical features to observe and what actions to take if there is deterioration or failure to improve and a plan agreed for the clinician to review the child's condition. In patients at increased risk of bacteremia, such as neonates, immunocompromised children and children with neutropenia or sickle cell disease, there should be a low threshold for initiating antimicrobial therapy.

Antimicrobial therapy

The choice of antibiotics is dependent upon the most likely pathogens and the particular antibiotic resistance patterns of the community or hospital. In otherwise healthy children without an obvious source, a third generation cephalosporin such as cefotaxime or ceftriaxone is appropriate. The emergence of antibiotic resistance precludes penicillin as adequate initial therapy. In more vulnerable populations, other considerations apply. For example, in neonates, a third generation cephalosporin is frequently used together with ampicillin to treat *Listeria monocytogenes*, sometimes with the addition of an aminoglycoside for additional Gram negative bacterial cover.

Immunocompromised patients are vulnerable to infection with a wider spectrum of pathogens. Children with B cell and antibody deficiencies or with reduced or absent splenic function are at increased risk from encapsulated bacterial infections. Neutropenic patients are particularly susceptible to staphylococcal and Gram negative bacteria including pseudomonal infections. A combination of an antipseudomonal penicillin (e.g. piptazobactam) with an aminoglycoside (e.g. gentamicin) is usually prescribed for this population. However, a glycopeptide (e.g. vancomycin) and antifungal therapy may be required if initial therapy fails to control the infection. Patients with sickle cell disease are at risk of salmonella septicemia and may require treatment with ciprofloxacin. In patients with staphylococcal toxic shock syndrome, treatment with antistaphylococcal therapy is advisable, even though the total number of bacteria may be small. These are general guidelines, and advice about local antimicrobial prescribing policies should always be sought.

Subsequent management

The details of the emergency treatment of shock are covered in Chapter 36. Children will usually require transfer to a pediatric intensive care unit. Hypovolemia is invariably present due to fluid maldistribution, which occurs as a result of the release of vasoactive mediators by host inflammatory and endothelial cells. The loss of circulating volume is compounded by a loss of intravascular proteins and fluid due to endothelial dysfunction (capillary leak). Continuous monitoring of central venous pressure and urine output is required to guide fluid replacement. Large volumes of plasma or blood are normally required, and mechanical ventilation may be necessary to manage capillary leakage of fluid into the lungs.[60] The net effect of the host response to infection frequently leads to myocardial depression, necessitating the use of inotropic support. Severe peripheral vasodilatation compounds hypotension, and vasopressors may be required. Dysregulation of the coagulation and thrombotic pathways leads to widespread microvascular thrombosis and consumption of clotting factors. Treatment of disseminated intravascular coagulation (DIC) is largely symptomatic, with administration of fresh frozen plasma and platelets if bleeding occurs. While administration of antibiotics will prevent further bacterial proliferation, the concentration of microbial components such as LPS and outer membrane proteins may persist for some time. These will continue to cause inflammation and further deterioration in the patient's condition. Continuous reassessment and adjustment of supportive therapy is therefore required to optimize further management.

Adjuvant therapy

The recognition that much of the pathology seen in sepsis is due to host-derived mediators has led to the development of numerous antagonists to offending bacterial and host components. Initial attempts to reduce the inflammatory response in sepsis used steroids. However, high doses of methylprednisolone were found to be detrimental in sepsis, and as a result routine use of high dose steroids in sepsis was abandoned. More recent data have shown that physiological doses of glucocorticoids may shorten the duration of shock and improve survival rates.[61] More selective agents have been developed, including antagonists of tumor necrosis factor, interleukin 1, platelet activating factor and endotoxin. None of these has proved to be beneficial in large clinical trials. However, it is too early to discard these new forms of treatment, since a clearer understanding of the sequence of events in sepsis may identify subgroups of patients who might benefit from these interventions.

The use of high doses of intravenous immunoglobulin may be beneficial in toxic shock syndromes and may be useful in other septic populations.[62] There is also evidence that administration of activated protein C (APC) can reduce mortality in adults with sepsis-induced organ failure.[63] This suggests that downstream inflammatory pathways, such as the protein C anticoagulation pathway, critical in thrombosis and hemostasis, may present potential targets for future interventions. However, in a trial of APC in children, no beneficial effect was observed. Perhaps the most important recent development in critical illness concerns the modulation of endocrine pathways. The administration of growth hormone to critically ill adults was found to significantly increase mortality, whilst low doses of steroids and tight glycemic control appear to be advantageous.[64] The role of the endocrine axis in children with sepsis is still unclear but is currently under investigation.

CONGENITAL AND NEONATAL INFECTIONS

SPECIFIC INFECTIONS
Congenital rubella

The association between rubella infection during pregnancy and congenital cataracts in the newborn was first made by an Australian ophthalmologist, Norman Gregg, in 1941.[65] The introduction of effective rubella vaccination programs has made congenital rubella syndrome (CRS) an uncommon disorder in resource rich countries such as the UK. Falling vaccine coverage and immigration of nonvaccinated women was the likely cause of a small resurgence in the number of reported cases of CRS over the period 1996–2000.[66,67]

Both the risk of fetal infection and the risk of sequelae vary with the gestation when maternal infection occurs. Transmission of the virus to the fetus occurs in 90% in the first 11 weeks, 50% from 11 to 20 weeks' gestation, 37% from 20 to 35 weeks, and 100% during the last month of pregnancy.[68] However, the risk of serious sequelae to the fetus after confirmed maternal rubella infection is greatest in early pregnancy, being 90% if infected < 11 weeks, 30% at 12–20 weeks and none thereafter, aside from some mild growth retardation.[68] The majority of infants with congenital rubella disease result from primary maternal rubella infection, although maternal reinfection may rarely result in an infant with anomalies.[69]

Clinical manifestation

The common manifestations of congenital rubella infection are shown in Table 28.15. Important clinical manifestations are disorders of the eye (microphthalmia, cataract, congenital glaucoma, retinitis), congenital

Table 28.15 Clinical features of rubella, cytomegalovirus and toxoplasmosis

	Cytomegalovirus	Rubella	Toxoplasmosis
CNS			
Hydrocephaly	+	−	+++
Microcephaly	+	+++	−
Calcification	+++	+	++
Deafness	++	+++	++
Encephalitis	−	−	+
Eyes			
Microphthalmia	+	+	+++
Cataracts	−	++	+
Chorioretinitis*	+	+	+++
Intrauterine growth retardation	+	+++	+
Cardiac lesion	−	++	+
Purpuric rash	++	+++	−
Pneumonia	+++	++	++
Hepatosplenomegaly	++	+++	++++
Lymphadenopathy	−	−	+
Bony lesion	+	+++	−

*The choroidoretinitis caused by *Toxoplasma gondii* and *Treponema pallidum* has been confused with the Aicardi syndrome, in which the lesions are always bilateral, rarely peripheral, and lack pigments, in contrast to that due to these two organisms.
Infecting organisms are listed alphabetically and not in order of likelihood.

heart disease (patent ductus arteriosus, peripheral pulmonary artery stenosis), and neurological sequelae (mental retardation, behavioral disorders, meningoencephalitis, convulsions). There may also be intrauterine growth retardation, microcephaly, thrombocytopenia, hepatosplenomegaly, purpuric skin lesions, pneumonitis and linear bone lesions. Only 68% of infected infants show signs at birth and up to 20% of these may die in infancy. A number of manifestations, however, present much later in life. These include hearing loss 87%, congenital heart disease 46–60%, mental or psychomotor retardation 30–50%, cataract or glaucoma 30–40%, diabetes mellitus and thyroid dysfunction.

Diagnosis

Virus isolation, either from nasopharyngeal washing, urine or cerebrospinal fluid (CSF) is the most direct method of diagnosis, but may take many weeks. A positive rubella-specific immunoglobulin M (IgM) in a neonate and/or the detection of rubella RNA in urine or nasopharyngeal secretions by polymerase chain reaction (PCR) usually indicates recent postnatal or congenital infection, although false positive results do occur. A number of sensitive immunoassays are available for the detection of rubella-specific IgG. Rising or persistently stable levels of IgG from the newborn period to beyond 9 months of age confirm perinatal or congenital infection.

Management

There is no specific treatment for rubella infection. In countries where routine rubella vaccination has been used, the infection rate has been considerably reduced. Seronegative women of childbearing age should be offered vaccination either after a pregnancy test or immediately postpartum. Rubella immunization of 13-year-old girls, which started in the UK in 1970, reduced the incidence considerably and the use of the measles, mumps and rubella (MMR) vaccine in the UK from 1988 has made congenital rubella rare.[66] Most new reports of congenital rubella in the UK are of infants born to mothers who were themselves born abroad and came to the UK after the age of schoolgirl immunization. In 2004, the World Health Organization adopted a strategy to improve global control of rubella and CRS by 2010 by increasing vaccination coverage of women of childbearing age using the combined measles–rubella vaccine, and by improving surveillance for CRS.[70,71]

Cytomegalovirus (CMV)

Cytomegalovirus (CMV) infection is the most common congenital infection in Europe with a prevalence of 3–4 per 1000 births. CMV is a member of the herpes virus family and, as such, establishes a latent infection after the initial infection and reactivates, especially under states of altered cellular immunity. It is ubiquitous in the community, although not highly infectious. It may be transmitted transplacentally or through genital secretions, saliva, breast milk or blood transfusion.

About 50% of women of childbearing age in the UK remain susceptible to CMV infection and 1% of those susceptible at the beginning of pregnancy will have a primary infection during pregnancy. Like rubella, the greatest risk of fetal damage occurs after primary maternal infection. In about 50% of primary infections of the mother, the fetus will be infected, but only 10% of these infants will display symptoms at birth or through childhood. After a recurrent maternal CMV infection, there is a low risk of transmission to the infant (≤1%), with an equally low risk of sequelae.[72] However, some cases of infants with severe, symptomatic congenital CMV disease due to either maternal reinfection with a new CMV strain or reactivation of latent CMV infection during pregnancy have been reported.[73] Unlike rubella, fetal damage may follow primary infection or recurrent infection at any stage of pregnancy.

Clinical manifestations

The majority of infants with congenital CMV infection are asymptomatic. When symptomatic, the main clinical features are as shown in Table 28.16. The risk of neurological sequelae and intrauterine growth retardation in the fetus is greatest after infection in the first 20 weeks of pregnancy, but infants of mothers with pre-existing immunity to CMV can have clinical sequelae.[74] Such effects include microcephaly, chorioretinitis, mental retardation, sensorineural hearing loss and intracerebral periventricular calcification. Infection in the second half of pregnancy usually results in visceral disease such as hepatitis, purpura, hyperbilirubinemia and thrombocytopenia. Other effects include dental abnormalities and inguinal hernias. Pneumonitis is a common feature of postnatally acquired CMV infection, especially in the premature infant, but rarely follows true congenital infection. Those infants who have symptoms in the newborn period nearly always have subsequent handicap. The presence of microcephaly at birth is the strongest predictor of poor cognitive outcome in later life.[75] Of the infected infants who are asymptomatic at birth, up to 10% will have CMV-related problems by 3 years of age, the most common problem being sensorineural hearing loss.[76,77] High CMV viral blood load (10^4 viral DNA copies per 10^5 poly-morphonuclear leukocytes) in the newborn has recently been identified as a strong predictor for adverse long term clinical sequelae.[78]

Perinatal CMV infection

Many infants acquire CMV infection through breast-feeding or by contact with other infected secretions in the first weeks of life or, in hospitalized babies, through blood products. This usually results in an asymptomatic infection. The exception is premature infants, especially those with extremely low birth weight, or infants with cellular immunodeficiency in whom CMV infection may result in pneumonitis, hepatitis, thrombocytopenia, neutropenia and, uncommonly, gastroenteritis. In general, postnatal CMV infection does not result in long term sequelae, with the possible exception of babies less than 2000 g.[79]

Diagnosis

Diagnosis is based on isolation of the virus in throat washings or urine or by detection of CMV DNA in these specimens by PCR. Cultures must be obtained within the first 3 weeks of life to distinguish congenital CMV infection from perinatally acquired infection. Demonstration of CMV-specific IgM antibody in neonatal serum is also suggestive of congenital infection, but it can only be detected in about 70% of infected newborns. Later in infancy, in the absence of clinical signs suggestive of congenital infection, laboratory methods alone will not make the distinction between CMV acquired during intrauterine life and postnatal infection. Retrospective diagnosis of congenital CMV infection can be made by detection of CMV DNA in dried blood on the filter paper from newborn screening cards.

Treatment and prevention

Ganciclovir therapy may be used to treat some congenitally infected infants with life-threatening CMV-related organ disease or retinitis involving the macula. Work is in progress towards production of a vaccine. Intravenous ganciclovir has also been used in a series of small clinical trials to try to reduce the risk and extent of central nervous system damage after symptomatic congenital CMV infection.[80,81] However, no firm conclusions about the efficacy of this treatment could be drawn due to the small sample sizes, and until more efficacy data are available it is not routinely recommended. Some groups nevertheless recommend ganciclovir therapy for infants with signs of disseminated disease without severe hearing loss [≥ 100 dB by brainstem auditory evoked response (BAER)] due to the high risk of late progression,[82] and others prescribe prolonged therapy with oral valaganciclovir.[83] However, there is a lack of clinical trial data to support these opinions.

Table 28.16   Lesions that may be caused by prenatally acquired viral infections

Pathogen	Clinical sequelae
1. Coxsackie virus	Abortion, mild febrile disease, rash, meningitis, hepatitis, gastroenteritis, myocarditis, congenital heart disease and neurological deficits
2. Cytomegalovirus	Microcephaly, hydrocephaly, microphthalmia, retinopathy, cerebral calcification, deafness, psychomotor retardation, anemia, thrombocytopenia, hepatosplenomegaly, jaundice and encephalopathy
3. ECHO virus	Same as coxsackie virus
4. Hepatitis B virus	Low birth weight, asymptomatic hepatitis carrier, acute hepatitis, chronic hepatitis
5. Herpes simplex virus	Abortion, microcephaly, cerebral calcification, retinopathy, encephalitis, multiple organ involvement
6. Human immunodeficiency virus	Abortion, hydro/microcephaly, limb deformities, intrauterine growth retardation, failure to thrive, rash, hepatosplenomegaly, pneumonia
7. Influenza virus	Abortion
8. Measles virus	Abortion, congenital measles
9. Polio virus	Abortion, congenital poliomyelitis with paralysis
10. Rubella virus	Abortion, microcephaly, cataract, microphthalmia, congenital heart disease, deafness, low birth weight, hepatosplenomegaly, petechiae, osteitis
11. Vaccinia virus	Abortion, congenital vaccinia
12. Varicella-zoster virus	Abortion, limb, cerebral and skin malformation
	Stillbirth, low birth weight, chorioretinitis, congenital chickenpox, or disseminated neonatal varicella or zoster
13. Variola virus	Abortion, congenital variola

In alphabetical order and not in order of frequency or seriousness.

CMV is spread by intimate contact with infected secretions. Pregnant caregivers and hospital personnel should employ careful hand washing after exposure to the secretions of a CMV-infected infant. Passive immunotherapy with CMV hyperimmune globulin of women with primary CMV infection during early pregnancy has been shown in an open labeled phase I trial to be safe and possibly effective at reducing transmission to and sequelae in the offspring.[84] Results have yet to be confirmed in a randomized clinical trial.

Varicella–zoster (chickenpox)
Congenital infection
Maternal varicella-zoster infection during the first 20 weeks of pregnancy may result in spontaneous abortion or fetal death in utero, or in an embryopathy characterized by dermatomal skin scarring and limb hypoplasia. There may also be disorders of the central nervous system (microcephaly, cortical atrophy) and eyes (cataracts, chorioretinitis), of the gastrointestinal tract and of the genitourinary tract. It is hypothesized that the damage results from in utero reactivation of varicella-zoster virus (VZV) or disseminated fetal infection.

Maternal infection in the second half of pregnancy may result in an asymptomatic primary fetal infection followed by herpes zoster in the first years of life in about 1% of exposed infants. A large prospective study from the UK and Germany of the effects of maternal VZV infection in pregnancy estimated the overall risk of embryopathy during the first 20 weeks of pregnancy to be 1%, with the highest risk of transmission of 2% being in the period 13–20 weeks.[45] Occasional cases resulting from maternal infection at 23 weeks have been reported.[86] Administration of varicella-zoster immunoglobulin (V-ZIG) to the mother may modify the course of chickenpox, but it has not been shown to alter the risk of transmission to the fetus.[87]

Perinatal infection
Maternal varicella that occurs in the period 5 days before delivery to 2 days after delivery may result in life-threatening, disseminated VZV infection in the infant due to transplacental passage of the virus in the absence of maternal antibody. If the onset of maternal infection is more than 7 days prior to delivery, there is usually sufficient passive transfer of antibody unless the infant is less than 28 weeks' gestation. Administration of V-ZIG to the infant has been shown to prevent or modify the course of the illness in most cases. However, as a significant number of infants will develop systemic VZV despite the administration of V-ZIG,[88] all infants with perinatal VZV exposure should be monitored closely for systemic disease, with prompt initiation of intravenous aciclovir should vesicles appear. Hospitalized infants with chickenpox should be placed in respiratory and contact isolation until the lesions have crusted, but breast-feeding can continue.

Herpes simplex virus (HSV)
Neonatal HSV infection carries a high mortality if untreated. The incidence of disease ranges from 1:2500 live births in some parts of the USA[89] to 1:60000 live births in the UK.[90] In the past, up to 75% of cases of neonatal infection were due to HSV type 2 and the rest due to type 1. More recently, the proportion of cases due to neonatal HSV-1 infection is increasing in the UK and elsewhere around the world, possibly due to an increase in genital HSV-1 disease.[90] The infection is acquired from passage through an infected birth canal in 85% of cases, and is postnatally acquired from the oral lesions of an infected caregiver in 10–15% of cases. A true congenital syndrome is seen in < 5% of cases. The greatest risk for transmission (about 50%) is from a primary maternal infection when there has been insufficient time for seroconversion and transplacental transfer of antibody.[91] If a woman with a recurrent infection is shedding virus at delivery, the risk may be 5% or less. Cesarean delivery is not completely effective in preventing transmission to the infant.

Clinical manifestations
Neonatal HSV disease may manifest as lesions localized to the skin, eye or mouth (SEM), as encephalitis, as pneumonitis or as a disseminated multiorgan infection with or without central nervous system involvement.

The age of presentation varies with the category of disease. In general, neonatal HSV disease usually presents in the first 3 weeks of life, but it may manifest at any time from day 1 to 4 weeks of life. About 50% of cases now present as SEM disease, possibly due to better awareness of the condition. The typical vesicular, ulcerative lesion usually occurs on the presenting part. Up to 70% of SEM disease will spread to the central nervous system or elsewhere without treatment, but is rarely fatal. Infants with SEM disease have 10% long term morbidity, with higher rates seen if there are frequent cutaneous recurrences in early life.

The disseminated form typically commences at about 1 week of age with a shock-like syndrome in the absence of positive bacterial cultures with thrombocytopenia, disseminated intravascular coagulation, hepatitis, jaundice, and sometimes encephalitis and seizures. Skin lesions appear in 50% of these cases. Disseminated HSV infection may also present as an interstitial pneumonitis, usually presenting about day 3 of life. The mortality in this group is as high as 50% even with treatment, and over half of the survivors are left with long term sequelae (mental retardation, blindness, seizures, learning defects). The third group presents with central nervous system symptoms such as poor feeding, apnea, lethargy and seizures without visceral involvement, typically in the second to third week of life. It has been hypothesized that this group represents reactivation of an earlier asymptomatic infection. They have a 15% mortality, with severe long term central nervous system effects seen in 65%.[92]

Congenital infection
Intrauterine HSV infection may manifest as the presence of vesicles or scarring at birth, chorioretinitis, microphthalmia, microcephaly, hydranencephaly or cerebral atrophy on CT scan in the first week of life, organ calcification or organomegaly. The majority of reported cases are due to HSV-2. There is a high rate of early neonatal death and long term central nervous system sequelae.

Diagnosis
If neonatal HSV disease is suspected, viral swabs of skin vesicles, eyes, nasopharynx and rectum should be sent for HSV culture and immunofluorescence or HSV PCR, CSF collected for routine examination, HSV PCR and culture, blood sent for liver function tests, platelet count and coagulation screen, and empirical therapy with systemic intravenous aciclovir promptly commenced. A chest radiograph may be indicated if respiratory distress is present. Imaging of the head by ultrasound or CT scan should be performed. Serologic assays are usually not helpful in the acute diagnosis of neonatal HSV disease.

Treatment and prevention
Mothers with primary lesions should be delivered electively by Cesarean section while mothers with recurrent lesions, if they have a negative culture and do not have lesions or prodrome of infection, may be delivered vaginally. The use of invasive fetal monitoring and vacuum delivery should be avoided where possible in women with known genital HSV disease. Some suggest that the infant should be screened for infection by surface viral swabs at 48 h of life.

Aciclovir 60 mg/kg/d in three divided doses given intravenously should be commenced as soon as neonatal HSV disease is suspected. Many suggest it should be commenced empirically in the offspring of women with known primary genital HSV infection due to the high attack rate. The duration of therapy is 14 days for SEM disease and 21 days for all other categories or where a lumbar puncture could not be performed.[93] Topical therapy may be given in addition to systemic therapy for HSV eye disease under the direction of an ophthalmologist. The prognostic significance of persistence of HSV DNA at the end of therapy is currently under evaluation.

Prevention of neonatal HSV disease demands a vaccine to prevent maternal infection and/or reactivation. Recently a recombinant HSV type 2 glycoprotein subunit vaccine has been shown to be partly effective at reducing the risk of infection and development of clinical disease in women without prior immunity to HSV types 1 or 2.[94] Its efficacy is currently being evaluated in HSV-1 seronegative girls prior to the onset of sexual activity.[95] Other prevention strategies include the use of an oral antiviral in late pregnancy in women with primary HSV infection during pregnancy or in HSV-seropositive women with frequent clinical recurrences in the genital area.[96]

The shock-like syndrome associated with the disseminated form of neonatal HSV disease has been associated with signaling through Toll-like receptor (TLR)-2,[97] raising the possibility that future therapeutic strategies for this condition may target TLR signaling pathways.

PARASITIC INFECTIONS

Toxoplasmosis

Toxoplasmosis is a worldwide disease. In the UK between 20 and 40% of the population have been infected with this protozoan by adult life. The incidence of congenital toxoplasmosis in Europe is 1–10 in 10 000 newborns.[98,99]

Congenital toxoplasmosis infection usually occurs as a result of placental infection after a primary infection in a pregnant woman. Parasites form small focal lesions in the placenta, proliferate and are released as active forms into the fetal bloodstream. Rare cases of fetal transmission have been reported after preconception maternal infection in immunocompetent women,[100] presumably due to myometrial infection. It is generally accepted that women who bear a congenitally infected child do not have infected children in subsequent pregnancies, probably owing to persistence of immunity after the primary infection. Exceptions to this rule do occur, and it is suggested that the persistence of *Toxoplasma gondii* as cysts in the myometrium with liberation of active forms during pregnancy is one of the main infectious causes of repeated abortion in women. Congenital toxoplasmosis has been reported following reactivation in women with HIV infection, although it is a rare event as shown by a European Collaborative Study.[101]

The risk of transmission and the clinical outcome after maternal toxoplasmosis infection vary with the trimester of pregnancy. Recently, up-to-date risk estimates of maternal transmission of toxoplasmosis during pregnancy have come from a large study of women with confirmed infection who were referred to a toxoplasmosis reference laboratory in France.[98] Infection in early pregnancy carried a low risk of transmission; this rose to 6% by 13 weeks, thereafter rising sharply to 40% at 26 weeks, and 72% at 36 weeks. If a fetus is infected, the risk of developing clinical signs (and the severity of disease) is greatest the earlier in pregnancy the infection occurs, falling from 61% at 13 weeks, to 25% at 26 weeks, to 9% at 36 weeks.[98]

Clinical manifestations

Infection of the fetus with virulent strains early in pregnancy may produce fetal death and abortion; still later, severe fetal damage or stillbirth; and later still, a liveborn infant with stigmata of congenital toxoplasmosis. However, up to 70% of infants with congenital toxoplasmosis are asymptomatic at birth. The most common single presenting feature is chorioretinitis and both eyes are involved in 40% of cases. Other important clinical features are given in Table 28.15. They include hydrocephalus, intracranial calcification, hepatosplenomegaly, jaundice, thrombocytopenia and a maculopapular rash. Clinical sequelae of congenital infection, including visual disturbance, seizures and mental retardation, may not manifest until later in life. A recent long term follow-up study of visual sequelae from congenital toxoplasmosis infection has confirmed that late onset retinal lesions and relapse in existing visual lesions can occur many years after birth. The prognosis for patients with central nervous system involvement must be extremely guarded.

Diagnosis

This is usually based on *Toxoplasma* IgM and/or *Toxoplasma* IgA antibody test. The sensitivity of the IgM-ISAGA test is probably the highest. Persistently elevated *Toxoplasma* IgG beyond 12 months of life, and detection of *Toxoplasma* DNA by PCR in the placenta, neonatal blood or CSF may also be used to make the diagnosis. In the infant with suspected congenital toxoplasmosis, ophthalmological examination, hearing assessment and central nervous system examination and imaging should also be performed.

Treatment

Infants diagnosed with symptomatic or asymptomatic congenital toxoplasmosis infection should be treated to reduce the incidence of long term sequelae such as chorioretinitis. Two synergistic antimicrobials, either sulfadimidine or sulfadiazine together with pyrimethamine, are used in various combinations. Prolonged treatment for up 12 months is required to reduce the risk of late reactivation in the eye.[102] Corticosteroids should be used in the presence of chorioretinitis or raised CSF protein. Many advise treatment of pregnant women with primary toxoplasmosis. A recent systematic review suggests that there are still insufficient data on whether this treatment is effective in preventing neonatal infection.[103]

Pregnant women should be educated to avoid ingestion of *Toxoplasma* cysts by adequate cooking of meat, washing of garden produce, and washing hands after contact with soil.

ENTEROVIRUSES (NON-POLIO)

Intrauterine, perinatal and postnatal transmission of enteroviruses [coxsackie viruses group A and B, enteric cytopathogenic human orphan (ECHO) viruses, enteroviruses 68–71] has been documented, although there are no data available on the risks of transmission to the fetus or of sequelae should this occur. While maternal enterovirus infection during pregnancy has not been conclusively proven to cause an embryopathy, there have been links between some specific maternal enteroviral infections and anomalies in the infant (coxsackie B virus infection with urogenital anomalies, coxsackie B3 and B4 viruses with cardiac anomalies, coxsackie A9 with digestive anomalies).

Perinatal enteroviral infections generally cause asymptomatic infection or mild, nonspecific illness, particularly if the baby acquires infection 'horizontally' from other babies. However, if a woman is infected just before or after delivery, severe disease may develop in the 'vertically' infected newborn, in the first week after birth. The mother may present with severe abdominal pain mimicking abruption, or with respiratory or gastrointestinal symptoms. The baby may present with one or more of the following: a sepsis-like syndrome [fever or hypothermia, anorexia, vomiting, lethargy, disseminated intravascular coagulation (DIC)], gastrointestinal (vomiting, diarrhea, fulminant hepatitis, pancreatitis), neurological (aseptic meningitis, encephalitis or paralysis), respiratory (pneumonitis, pharyngitis, laryngotracheobronchitis), skin or mucosal manifestations (erythematous, maculopapular rash, herpangina, hemorrhagic conjunctivitis) or cardiac disease (myocarditis, pericarditis). Some specific enteroviruses are associated with particular syndromes (see Enteroviruses). Severe ECHO virus infections are more likely to cause hepatitis with massive hepatic necrosis, DIC and death, while coxsackie viruses are more likely to cause myocarditis and meningitis. Neonatal outbreaks of enterovirus 71 (EV 71) have recently been associated with neurological manifestations such as encephalitis, Guillain–Barré syndrome and neurogenic pulmonary edema.[104,105]

Diagnosis

Enteroviruses may be cultured from the nasopharynx, throat swab or feces. Serology is rarely helpful due to poor sensitivity. Detection of enterovirus nucleic acid in the CSF by PCR can be useful in the diagnosis of enteroviral meningitis.

Treatment

The antiviral agent pleconaril has been shown to have in vitro activity against a number of enteroviruses, but not EV 71.[106] In a small case series, treatment of severe neonatal enterovirus infection with oral pleconaril was associated with both virological and clinical improvement, but the sample size was too small to determine if this outcome was significant. Intravenous immunoglobulin has also been used to treat life-threatening disease, but its efficacy is unproven for this use.

HOSPITAL INFECTION CONTROL

Nosocomial infections are defined as infections acquired by hospitalized patients which were not present or incubating at the time of their hospital admission.[107] Infection control developed as a formal discipline during the 1950s and 1960s primarily as a response to nosocomial staphylococcal infections. Today infection control, enhanced by the application of epidemiological methods and the use of statistical analysis, has a major role in identifying and analyzing adverse outcomes in the health care setting. The central role of an infection control program is to reduce the risk of nosocomial infection with resulting protection of patients, health care workers, students and visitors.

All hospitals should have in place a multidisciplinary infection control committee with members who are interested and knowledgeable in infection and infection control and represent areas of the hospital where infection is either a potential problem or are involved in controlling these infections. The infection control committee must have the delegated authority of the hospital executive to efficiently and tactfully implement actions to control infection. It is recommended that the committee should consist of a medical microbiologist, medical virologist, infection control practitioner and an infectious disease physician and, in addition, personnel from medical and nursing and administration as well as pharmacy, operating theaters, housekeeping, engineering and maintenance. Ideally the chair of the committee should have expertise in hospital epidemiology and infection control.

Nosocomial infections are predominantly transmitted via contact, primarily by the contaminated hands of health care workers who have touched a colonized patient or something in the patient's environment. Hand washing with soap and water remains the single most important method in the prevention of nosocomial infections, but numerous studies have shown that hand washing compliance by health care workers is poor and often less than 50%. To improve the situation, there has been a recent increase in use of alcohol-based hand antiseptics. The application of these alcohol-based hand antiseptics, a process called hand hygiene, kills bacteria (except *Clostridium difficile*) very rapidly. Hand hygiene takes much less time than traditional hand washing and is gentler on the skin of the hands than repeated use of soap and water. In addition, hand lotions and moisturizers should be available to health care workers to decrease skin irritation which may result from frequent hand washing and hand hygiene.[108]

Isolation of patients is done to prevent the spread of microorganisms from infected or colonized patients to other patients or health care workers, thus interrupting transmission. The current isolation guidelines are based on our understanding of the mechanisms of disease transmission. There is essentially a two-tiered approach to isolation. The first is the use of **standard precautions**, the basis of infection control, which applies to all patients. The second approach is **transmission-based precautions**, contact, droplet and aerosol, which apply to patients with documented or suspected infections (see Table 28.17).

Standard precautions involve hand washing before patient contact and after leaving the patient's environment. In addition, personal protective equipment. masks, gowns, gloves and eye protection, provides a barrier to reduce the opportunities for transmission of infectious agents if there is contact with body fluids. A fluid resistant gown or apron made with impervious material, fluid repellent mask or face shield and protective eyeware should be worn when performing any procedure where there is the likelihood of splashing or spreading of blood or other body substances.[109] Gloves are worn as a barrier to protect the health care worker's hands from contamination and prevent the transfer of microorganisms. The type of gloves selected should be appropriate to the type of risk of the procedure. Sterile gloves are worn if the procedure involves contact with tissues that would be sterile under normal circumstances. Medical examination gloves, which are clean but not sterile, are used in all procedures that may involve direct skin or mucous membrane contact with blood or fluids capable of transmitting blood-borne pathogens. General purpose gloves are used for housekeeping activities and cleaning instruments. The gloves must be changed and discarded as soon as they are torn or punctured, after contact with an individual is completed and before care is

provided to another individual or when performing separate procedures on the same patient where there is a risk of transmitting infection from one part of the body to the other. It should be emphasized that hands must be washed and cleaned after the removal and disposal of gloves.

Health care workers are susceptible to infectious diseases and may therefore be infected by, or transmit infection to, patients. It is therefore strongly recommended that health care workers working in clinical areas be protected against those infectious diseases where vaccination is possible. It is recommended that health care workers be vaccinated against diphtheria, tetanus, pertussis, measles, mumps, rubella, varicella, influenza and hepatitis B.[109] Other vaccinations such as meningococcal, typhoid and hepatitis A virus vaccines may be indicated in special circumstances.[110]

The potential transmission of blood-borne diseases is greatest where a needle, scalpel blade or other sharp instrument is used. All health care workers are responsible for the management and disposal of the sharps they have used and should take care to ensure they are disposed of in a safe manner. Particular care should be taken in removing disposable scalpel blades from scalpel handles. In addition, needles should not be removed from disposable syringes and should not be purposefully bent or broken. Needles should not be re-sheathed after use, if possible. All sharps should be disposed of immediately after use into a sharps container which is puncture resistant and waterproof.[111]

It is generally agreed that antimicrobial resistance is driven by antibiotic use, and excessive and unnecessary use of antimicrobials can be expected to increase the prevalence of resistant microorganisms. Infection

Table 28.17 Isolation and types of precautions

Isolation precautions	Requirements	Examples of infections
Standard	Hand washing before and after patient contact Personal protective equipment (PPE): Gloves, gown and mask should be worn by staff when touching or handling blood or body substances Hands must be washed before attending patients and after removal of gloves	All patients require standard precautions
Contact	Standard precautions plus: Single room if possible and cohorting of patients with like illness if possible	Respiratory syncytial virus Rotavirus Impetigo Herpes zoster (shingles) Hepatitis A Methicillin-resistant *S. aureus* (MRSA) Extended-spectrum beta-lactamase (ESBL) positive Enterobacteriaceae Carbapenem-resistant *Acinetobacter baumannii*
Droplet	Contact precautions plus: Use of a mask if within 1 meter of the patient The room door must remain closed	Influenza virus Adenovirus *N. meningitidis* (invasive) *B. pertussis*
Airborne	Droplet precautions plus: Single negative pressure room with 6–12 air changes per hour	Measles Chickenpox Tuberculosis

of patients with multiresistant organisms leads to increased morbidity and mortality as well as increased financial costs. All health care institutions need to develop policies for the control of antimicrobial use by developing guidelines and authorization for their use in specific situations. Advice from the medical microbiologist or infectious diseases physician may assist general clinicians in more appropriate selection of antimicrobial agents.[112]

Routine surveillance for selected pathogens may be a method to assess the efficacy of infection control policy and procedures and determine if an outbreak occurs. A nosocomial infection outbreak may be described as an epidemic, or an increase above normal of the expected level of an infection in the clinical setting. The main goal of managing an outbreak is to prevent a further increase in the incidence of health care associated infection by identifying factors which may have contributed to the outbreak. This also allows for the development and implementation of measures to prevent future outbreaks. General management of an outbreak involves first determining a case definition and, second, confirming an increase in cases by the infectious agent above the background rate. It is then necessary to collect information regarding cases as descriptive epidemiology to determine if there are any recognized modes of transmission.[113] Implementation of appropriate infection control measures as described in Table 28.17 should be undertaken to contain the outbreak.

Managing infection control in a pediatric hospital presents some unique challenges. Young children usually have poor personal hygiene and require significant adult supervision to ensure this practice. They are also mobile and quite impulsive and may require isolation to prevent contact spread of infecting organisms to other patients. Isolation of small children can often distress them and it is essential to provide adequate supervision for their safety and suitable age-related activities to relieve their distress.

BACTERIAL INFECTIONS

THE USE OF THE BACTERIOLOGY LABORATORY BY THE PEDIATRICIAN

A proficient and well managed microbiology laboratory is essential for any health care institution.[114] Pivotal to the function of the microbiology laboratory is excellent communication between the physician and the laboratory personnel. After considering the clinical and epidemiological circumstances of the patient infection, the physician must collect appropriate samples for culture. Ideally specimens should be obtained directly from the site of infection before commencement of antibiotic therapy. However, this may not always be possible in patients who are critically ill, when antimicrobial therapy may need to start immediately. It is critical that all specimens submitted to the laboratory be correctly collected, labeled and transported as well as being of sufficient quality and quantity for adequate microbiological testing. They should be submitted promptly to the laboratory along with all relevant clinical and epidemiological data to assist the laboratory in selection of appropriate testing protocols.

DIRECT MICROSCOPY

Gram stain is one of the most useful and rapid diagnostic tests offered by the microbiology laboratory. It can be performed on exudates, tissue smears, fluids and aspirates to detect bacteria and fungal elements. In addition to bacteria, the presence and type of inflammatory cells is also detected. Information about bacterial morphology, i.e. cocci or rods, and the staining appearance, Gram positive or Gram negative, can give important preliminary information about the possible genus of the infecting microorganism and thus guide empiric antimicrobial therapy. If infection with mycobacteria or *Nocardia* spp. is suspected, the acid-fast or modified acid-fast stains respectively can be performed to detect these microorganisms.

BLOODSTREAM INFECTIONS

Blood cultures are among the most important specimens processed by the microbiology laboratory. Bloodstream infections can be considered to be transient, intermittent or continuous, and diagnosis of a bloodstream infection is very important in managing sick patients.

An example of transient bacteremia is that which occurs following cleaning one's teeth; transient bacteremia is rarely of clinical significance. An intermittent bacteremia occurs in patients who have serious bacterial infections such as pneumonia, urinary tract infections or osteomyelitis, where organisms may be isolated from the bloodstream but this is not uniformly the case. Continuous bacteremia occurs in patients who have infection within the vascular space and this includes patients with bacterial endocarditis or septic thrombophlebitis.

Because diagnosis of a bloodstream infection may be critical for patient care, it is essential that these specimens are collected correctly. Optimal collection of a blood culture starts with proper skin preparation. The skin must first be cleaned with 70% alcohol followed by tincture of iodine for 1 min or alternatively povidone–iodine for 2 min. It is important to allow these disinfectants to dry as killing bacteria takes time. Alcohol should not be used as a second antiseptic agent when an iodophor is used as it may inactivate these compounds. It is also recommended to clean the septum of the blood culture bottle with 70% alcohol and allow this to dry before injecting blood. The blood must be injected without changing needles.

It is important to take the volume of blood which is recommended for the blood culture system being used. Optimal blood volume enhances recovery of agents as blood is an important component of the culture media itself. The maximum amount of blood that can be taken from a child will depend on the weight and the clinical status of the child and it is usual for 1–3 ml to be obtained from a child younger than 6 years, whereas the neonate may only be able to afford 0.5–1 ml. When collecting blood cultures from children it is advisable to use a pediatric blood culture system which is optimized to function with much smaller volumes than adult blood culture systems. Addition of extra blood can often lead to a false positive signal due to blood cell metabolism, as modern automatic blood culture systems detect carbon dioxide production, and additional blood does not enhance bacterial detection. Blood culture media also contain an anticoagulant, sodium polyanethole sulfonate (SPS), which in addition to its anticoagulant action has an anticomplement and antiphagocytic effect that prevents intracellular killing of microorganisms by neutrophils following injection of the blood into the culture bottle and thus enhances sensitivity. However, SPS may inhibit recovery of organisms such as *Neisseria gonorrhoeae*, *Neisseria meningitidis*, *Gardnerella vaginalis*, *Streptobacillus moniliformis* and *Peptostreptococcus anaerobius*. Ideally blood cultures should be obtained before the start of antibiotic therapy to prevent inhibition of microorganism growth.

More recently, bacteremias have been associated with the increased use of indwelling intravenous catheters for a variety of vascular access needs.[115] Where the use of indwelling catheters is common, institutions have seen an increase in organisms such as coagulase negative staphylococci, corynebacteria bacilli, yeasts and a variety of uncommon but opportunistic Gram negative rods. When collecting blood cultures through an indwelling catheter, it is strongly recommended that blood cultures are collected simultaneously from a peripheral noncannulated site, to determine if a positive culture represents true bacteremia or infection of the central venous line. While it is recommended not to take blood cultures through central venous lines, this practice is usually quite common because of the ease of drawing blood through these catheters with little discomfort to the patient. Identification of a contaminated catheter may result in treating patients with antibiotics for a period of time, possibly preventing more serious systemic infection and also obviating the need to remove the catheter.

Blood cultures are usually incubated for 5–7 days before being declared negative. The length of culture may be extended in specific situations, for example when fastidious organisms are anticipated as in subacute bacterial endocarditis or in prolonged fever of unknown origin.

URINARY TRACT INFECTIONS

The commonest site of clinically significant bacterial infection in infants and children is the urinary tract. Urinary tract infections may occur within the renal parenchyma, in the tubules or pelvis, or at any point along the ureters, urinary bladder or urethra. Studies relating clinical infection to the number of bacteria in a voided urine specimen demonstrated that at least 100 000 variable bacteria on culture per milliliter of urine correlated strongly with infection in the upper urinary tract. Most urinary tract pathogens grow easily and quickly and include *Escherichia* spp., *Klebsiella* spp., *Enterobacter* spp., *Proteus* spp., *Pseudomonas* spp., *Enterococcus* spp. and *Staphylococcus* spp. Bacteria that are generally considered contaminants and disregarded include lactobacilli, diphtheroids, non-enterococcal alpha-hemolytic streptococci and coagulase negative staphylococci, other than *Staphylococcus saprophyticus* which is a common cause of urinary tract infection in pubertal girls and young women.

Yeasts, particularly *Candida* spp., may cause urinary tract infections. Determination of true urinary tract infection due to the yeast is more complex than with bacteria as there is no correlation with colony number and formal diagnosis may require an invasively obtained specimen, e.g. catheterization of the bladder, to avoid genital colonization which may contaminate the culture. Urine specimen may on occasions be used to detect *Mycobacteria* spp. and leptospira.

In addition to culture information, with identification of the bacterium and provision of antibiotic sensitivity results, the cell count per high power field is also helpful in determining the significance of results. The presence of a high white blood cell count, greater than 100 per high power field, indicates the presence of a significant inflammatory reaction occurring within the upper urinary tract. Where there is sterile pyuria, consideration must be given to whether the patient has already received an antibiotic rendering the sample sterile or whether there is some other non-infectious inflammatory lesion of the upper urinary tract. Some laboratories will also test the urine to see if it contains antibacterial activity, indicating the presence of antibiotic in the urine and thus warning the clinician of possible false negative results.

The presence of greater than 10 epithelial cells per high power field in the urine specimen is indication of significant contamination from the terminal urethra or vulva, so culture results need to be interpreted with great caution. Collection of the urine specimen should be done so as to minimize possible contamination by external colonizing bacteria in the urogenital tract. Suprapubic bladder aspiration of urine is the procedure least likely to result in contaminated urine. Alternatively, urine obtained by insertion of a catheter through the urethra into the bladder, collection of the urine specimen and removal of the catheter is also much less likely to be contaminated than voided specimens. If a voided specimen is to be collected, careful cleaning of the urethral meatus with sterile water in both males and females is strongly recommended prior to collection of a mid-stream urine specimen. It is desirable to ask the patient to void a small volume first (about 5 ml) and then collect the next urine passed, a mid-stream urine specimen. The initial voiding helps clean any colonizing bacteria from the terminal urethra prior to collection of the specimen for culture.

RESPIRATORY TRACT INFECTION

Respiratory tract infections can be divided into upper respiratory and lower respiratory. Common upper respiratory tract specimens include throat swabs and nasopharyngeal swabs or aspirates. Aspirates from sinuses or the middle ear are submitted only occasionally, because they are difficult to collect and empiric therapy without culture is usually effective. Throat swabs are cultured only for group A streptococci (*Streptococcus pyogenes*) unless there is a specific request to look for other agents.[116] Group C and group G beta-hemolytic streptococci can also cause throat infection, but there is no association with rheumatic fever or acute post-streptococcal glomerulonephritis. If diphtheria (*Corynebacterium diphtheriae*) or whooping cough (*Bordetella pertussis*) is suspected, the laboratory should be contacted so that the specimens are collected in the correct way and cultured on appropriate media for detection of these organisms.

Expectorated sputum is the most common specimen for diagnosis of lower respiratory tract infections (primarily pneumonia). In addition to sputum culture, more invasive methods for collection of specimens from the lower respiratory tract include bronchial washes, bronchial brushes, transbronchial biopsy and bronchoalveolar lavage. In difficult and serious clinical situations a surgical open lung biopsy may be indicated.[117]

Microbiology laboratories routinely use screening microscopy guidelines to reject sputum specimens of poor quality and thereby minimize unnecessary and potentially misleading culture results. The quality of the specimen is assessed by the number of squamous epithelial cells present per high power field with numbers exceeding 25 per low power field indicating that the specimen is heavily contaminated with saliva (oropharyngeal contamination) and unlikely to produce reliable results. The presence of polymorphonuclear leukocytes indicates a sputum specimen usually of apparent good quality. These criteria are not suitable and have not been validated for rejection of specimens where *Legionella* spp., fungi or *Mycobacteria* spp. are being cultured. The range of microorganisms that can cause lower respiratory tract infections is very diverse and it is important to provide an appropriate history to the laboratory so that testing can be targeted to the most relevant causes. Lower respiratory tract infection may be community acquired or nosocomial and other relevant clinical information including the type of infiltration seen on chest X-ray, the immunological status of the patient, any underlying diseases such as cystic fibrosis, a history of exposure to tuberculosis or travel, occupational or other exposures may be very helpful to the laboratory in identifying the causative organism.

CENTRAL NERVOUS SYSTEM INFECTION

Cerebrospinal fluid (CSF) must be transported to the laboratory promptly, because fastidious organisms such as *Neisseria meningitidis* may become nonviable if the specimen cools. In addition, cells in the specimen begin to degenerate and are difficult to identify morphologically in specimens greater than 6 h old.

It is customary to collect at least three tubes of CSF to send to the laboratory and it is important that a sufficient quantity is collected for all testing that is requested. In addition to culture, all CSF specimens are examined for cell count including red cells and white cells, with the white cells differentiated into polymorph lymphocytes and monocytes, as well as determining the biochemical parameters of protein and glucose concentration.[118]

Gram stains must be performed on all spinal fluids and any microorganism seen immediately reported to the responsible clinician as this may be of critical assistance in managing the patient and optimizing antibacterial coverage. Bacterial antigen tests for *Neisseria meningitidis*, *Streptococcus pneumoniae*, *Haemophilus influenzae* type b, group B streptococcus (*Streptococcus agalactiae*) and *Escherichia coli* are not routinely performed by many laboratories as the sensitivity of these tests does not exceed that of Gram stains. More recently, polymerase chain reaction (PCR) testing for *Neisseria meningitidis* and *Streptococcus pneumoniae* has become available, and these tests have been particularly helpful in the early management of cases of acute bacterial meningitis, especially when antibiotics have been given before taking cultures.[119] However, culture remains essential as the infecting organism can be tested for antibiotic susceptibility to guide therapy.

In addition to bacterial cultures, cultures for mycobacteria and fungi may also be indicated in specific clinical situations. However, cultures for both these types of organisms require reasonable volumes of CSF, at least 2 ml per sample and preferably 5–10 ml.

DIARRHEAL DISEASES

Acute diarrhea can be caused by a broad range of microorganisms including bacteria, viruses and parasites. Ideally stool specimens are preferred to rectal swabs and should be transported to the laboratory promptly. Most laboratories will reject a stool specimen which is not diarrheal, i.e. the specimen must take up the shape of the container, unless one is specifically looking for *Salmonella* spp. carriage. Most laboratories routinely culture for *Salmonella*, *Shigella* and *Campylobacter*. In addition, white and red cells are often looked for by direct microscopy as an indication of colitis. It is important to provide a good history to complement the specimen, such as any history of travel, ingestion of seafood or recent antibiotic therapy, and it is necessary to inform the laboratory if the clinician is looking for *Vibrio* spp., *Aeromonas* spp., *Plesiomonas* spp., *Yersinia* spp. or enterohemorrhagic *Escherichia coli*, as specific techniques in the laboratory will be needed to detect these organisms.[120] Parasites can be a common cause of diarrhea in young children, including *Cryptosporidium* and *Giardia*, and microscopy or antigen detection is required to detect these.

GENITAL TRACT INFECTIONS

Genital specimens are usually collected on pediatric patients when looking for evidence of sexually transmitted disease following alleged sexual assault and child abuse. The genital tract contains many nosocomial organisms including coagulase negative staphylococci, lactobacilli, corynebacteria, streptococci, anaerobes and yeasts. Some genital tract infections not associated with sexually transmitted disease may be caused by endogenous bacteria, for example *Gardnerella vaginalis* or group B streptococci or rarely *Staphylococcus aureus*.

The common sexually transmitted diseases which need investigation are *Neisseria gonorrhoeae*, *Chlamydia trachomatis* and *Treponema pallidum* (syphilis). Both gonorrhea and chlamydia can be confirmed by culture. It is important to ensure that the cultures are collected with the correct type of swabs, as both organisms are extremely fastidious and the method of specimen collection and transport to the laboratory are critical. More recently, detection of these microorganisms using PCR on first void urine specimen has proved both sensitive and specific as well as having increased patient acceptance. It should be noted that PCR for gonorrhea should not be performed on any other specimen other than the urogenital specimens as there is a high rate of false positive results if eye or throat specimens are collected, due to cross-reaction with nonpathogenic nosocomial *Neisseria* spp. It is important to have culture evidence if at all possible as antibiotic susceptibility testing can be done for gonorrhea and these results are more reliable if legal proceedings arise from the case. Syphilis can be detected by dark field examination of exudate from any ulcerative lesion, but is more commonly diagnosed serologically.

ANTIMICROBIAL SUSCEPTIBILITY TESTING

Antimicrobial susceptibility testing is advisable for presumed pathogens where response to antimicrobial agents is not predicted from identification alone. It is becoming increasingly needed with dissemination of resistance genes amongst bacteria. The aim of antimicrobial susceptibility testing is to demonstrate that in vitro growth inhibition of an infecting microorganism by a specific antimicrobial agent correlates with clinical response to that agent. Most testing is performed to detect the minimal inhibitory concentration (MIC), which is the lowest concentration of a specific antimicrobial agent that prevents visible growth of the test organism. Minimal bacterial concentration (MBC) is the lowest concentration of a specific antimicrobial agent that kills most (greater than 99.9%) of the inoculum of the organism and is rarely performed except under specialized circumstances. The more common and nonfastidious organisms can be tested. There need to be adequate data substantiating the clinical response of a species, and a minimal inhibitory concentration (MIC) for that agent, to provide interpretive data. There are many organisms for which these data are not available, examples being *Bacillus* species other than *Bacillus anthracis*, *Corynebacterium* spp. and many fastidious or unusual species, e.g. *Eikenella*, *Capnocytophaga*, *Leuconostoc*. It is also important to know that there are some specific organism–antimicrobial agent combinations where results are not reported because in vitro data are often misleading.

PRINCIPLES OF ANTIMICROBIAL THERAPY

Antimicrobial therapy is indicated when there is clinical or culture evidence of an infection and the use of an antimicrobial agent would be expected to significantly shorten the duration of illness or lower the incidence of complications. However, not all bacterial infections need specific antimicrobial treatment, including minor skin infections and some gastrointestinal infections, e.g. *Salmonella* spp., where host defense mechanisms usually effect cure.

INITIAL MICROBIOLOGICAL EVALUATION

Patients in whom an infectious illness is suspected should always be investigated to establish a microbiological diagnosis as this will aid ongoing therapeutic decisions. Initial microscopic examination of a Gram stained specimen from a sterile site often shows excellent correlation with the cause of the infection. However, if the specimen must pass through an area which is normally colonized with commensal bacteria, such as wound cultures or the mouth with sputum specimens, then the Gram stain should be evaluated carefully. In these situations, the bacterial culture report should be interpreted cautiously and contamination with commensal bacterial flora and the pathogenic potential of the isolated organism carefully considered. With sputum specimens, the presence of many polymorphs compared to epithelial cells on Gram stain and microscopy can be used to quality control the specimen, with predominance of polymorphs supporting purulent sputum while predominance of epithelial cells indicates heavy salivary contamination and probable invalid and contaminated culture results.

When there are clinical signs suggestive of a systemic infection, blood cultures should always be collected. Positive cultures from normally sterile fluid such as blood, CSF, pleural and synovial fluid should always be considered accurate, unless there is strong evidence to suggest otherwise. Bacteria such as *Neisseria meningitidis* and *Streptococcus pneumoniae* growing on cultures from sterile sites are never contaminants and the *Enterobacteriaceae* are rarely contaminants. However, when normal skin flora, such as alpha-hemolytic streptococci, *Propionibacterium acnes* or coagulase negative staphylococci are isolated, their significance and the clinical picture must be carefully reviewed to decide whether the isolated bacteria are indeed pathogens.

CHOICE OF ANTIBACTERIAL AGENT

The optimal antibiotic for treating a bacterial infection is one with action against the infecting agents, the narrowest possible spectrum of antibacterial activity, the fewest side-effects and the lowest toxicity.

The microbiology laboratory reports bacteria as susceptible or resistant to a particular antibacterial agent, depending on the amount of antibiotic that corresponds to achievable serum concentrations with standard dosage and schedule. Many infections occur at sites other than the bloodstream where there may be issues of antibiotic penetration (e.g. the CSF) or activity (e.g. aminoglycoside activity is decreased in pus). The antibiotic should be administered in a dose, at a dose interval and by a route that achieves an antibacterial level at the site of infection at least equal to, or preferably several times higher than, the level of that agent required to inhibit bacterial growth in vitro.

The choice of an empiric antibiotic agent for a suspected or proven infection is based upon (1) the site(s) of infection, (2) those bacteria that are most likely to cause that particular infection, (3) the bacteria presumptively identified by Gram stain of a specimen from the infected site, (4) the predicted susceptibility of the organism to the antibiotic, (5) the pharmacological properties of the antibiotic, and (6) the cost.

TREATMENT WITH MORE THAN ONE ANTIBIOTIC

The indications for using more than one antibiotic in the treatment of an infection are: (1) to treat infection due to more than one microorganism if they are not susceptible to the same drug; (2) to treat empirically a life-threatening infection where the causative bacterium is unknown and broad spectrum coverage of potential infecting bacteria must be achieved immediately; (3) to treat difficult organisms or infections for which synergy of an agent has been demonstrated or is postulated, e.g. enterococcal endocarditis; (4) to prevent the emergence of resistance during treatment.

DURATION OF ANTIMICROBIAL THERAPY

The appropriate duration of an antibacterial treatment course is defined as the shortest period necessary to prevent bacteriological or clinical relapse, i.e. produce a cure. The duration of treatment for a bacterial infection depends on the site and extent of the infection, the bacterium and the host response. The duration of treatment for cure has been reliably established for some infections, e.g. streptococcal pharyngitis, but it has not been established for many others. Response to therapy in patients with infections is best monitored clinically rather than bacteriologically. Repeat cultures are usually unnecessary and not helpful in the patient who has a good clinical response.

FAILURE OF ANTIMICROBIAL THERAPY

Failure of antibiotic therapy is defined as detection of bacteria beyond the expected time of clearance, usually accompanied by clinical failure of response to therapy. It is self-evident that antibiotics cannot be expected to cure a nonbacterial disease. If there is a failure of therapy with antibiotic therapy then details of the regimen should be examined, such as the susceptibility of the bacterium, dosage, route of administration, dosage interval and penetration into the site of infection. When there is an abscess, drainage is often far more effective than antibiotic treatment in resolving the infection. Common reasons for antibiotic treatment failure are: (1) failure of the patient to take medication as directed; (2) deficiency in host defense mechanisms including poor nutritional status; (3) inability to clear respiratory or other secretions; and (4) poor penetration of the antibiotic to the site of infection, e.g. poor tissue perfusion. The development of antibiotic resistance by an initially susceptible bacterium during treatment occurs but is uncommon.

ANTIBACTERIAL PROPHYLAXIS

Antibiotic prophylaxis is the use of an antibacterial agent to prevent infection and is most efficacious when attempting to prevent infection for a relatively brief period. The administration of antibiotics to prevent postoperative wound infection is now well established. The risk of contamination of the wound occurs at the beginning of the operation, so if prophylaxis is to be effective the antibiotic must be administered immediately prior to the operation to maintain high effective blood and tissue levels throughout the procedure. The use of prophylactic antibiotics has resulted in a significant decrease in the incidence of infections in procedures involving areas that are heavily contaminated with bacteria, such as the head and neck, and in gynecological and colonic surgery. Factors that predispose to contamination in surgery are long operations and the placement of prosthetic devices. Preventing infection of a prosthesis can be achieved with a short duration of therapy, up to 12 h. However, in specific situations such as cardiac surgery or placement of orthopaedic prostheses, prophylactic antibiotics are frequently continued for 2 days.

CLINICAL PHARMACOLOGY OF ANTIMICROBIAL AGENTS

Absorption

Many antimicrobial agents are well absorbed after oral administration while others are very poorly absorbed, e.g. vancomycin and aminoglycosides are very rapidly degraded in the intestinal tract so they must be administered parenterally to treat systemic infections. With few exceptions, oral administration of antibiotics results in lower serum concentrations of antibiotics than when using identical parenteral dosing, exceptions being metronidazole and chloramphenicol.

Serum concentrations achieved by the usual oral doses of agents such as ampicillin, first generation cephalosporins and tetracycline are generally not high enough to inhibit Gram negative enteric bacteria susceptible to these drugs. However, they may be used in urinary tract infection, because they are concentrated in the urine. In hospitalized patients with severe infection, antimicrobial therapy is generally administered parenterally to ensure adequate levels.

Distribution

After administration and absorption, antimicrobial agents are bound to plasma proteins to varying degrees. The time of serum decline relates to excretion and inactivation and is measured as serum half-life, i.e. the time required for a 50% decrease in serum concentration, which is a measure of the duration of the pharmacological effect. Serum half-life is an important determinant of a dosage schedule, in both normal patients and those in whom the half-life is prolonged because of decreased drug excretion or metabolism.

The initial rise in serum concentration after drug administration is followed by a decrease as the drug is distributed to body tissues. The tissue concentration of antibiotic depends on the degree of protein binding, the concentration gradient from serum to tissue, and the drug diffusibility. Most antibiotics penetrate well into pleural, peritoneal, pericardial and synovial fluid. Penetration into brain, CSF, eye and placenta is more variable. In general, penetration of antibiotics into body compartments increases with the presence of inflammation, e.g. penicillin penetrates into the CSF much more easily in an inflammatory state.[121]

Inactivation and excretion

There are several mechanisms of excretion and inactivation of antimicrobial agents, which include excretion by the bowel, removal by the kidney, inactivation by the liver, or inactivation by other unknown means. Antimicrobial agents may be inactivated by more than one mechanism.

Renal excretion is the major means of clearance of most antimicrobials, exceptions being chloramphenicol, erythromycin, clindamycin, doxycycline, ceftazidime and metronidazole. Renal failure results in accumulation of antimicrobials normally excreted by the kidney and dosage changes are essential for such agents as aminoglycosides and glycopeptides which have a low therapeutic-to-toxicity ratio and a single means of excretion or inactivation.

MECHANISM OF RESISTANCE

Bacteria acquire resistance to antibiotics most commonly by one of three main mechanisms:

1. Inability to reach the site of action due to decreased cell wall permeability or increased action of efflux pumps. Examples of this type of mechanism occur in *Pseudomonas* spp. and *Enterobacteriaceae* as a mechanism of resistance to aminoglycosides.
2. Alteration in the antimicrobial target. An example is alteration in the penicillin-binding protein 2 in staphylococci to PBP-2a encoded by the mec A gene, which renders all beta-lactam antibiotics, including the penicillinase-resistant penicillins, inactive, i.e. MRSA.[122]
3. Production of an enzyme that inactivates the antibiotic. Examples are beta-lactamases, which cleave the beta-lactam ring and render these antibiotics inactive.[123] Beta-lactamases have co-evolved with the increased use of beta-lactam antibiotics over the last 50 years, and are a major mechanism of defense by Gram negative bacteria against beta-lactam antibiotics. The introduction of penicillin saw a very rapid increase in prevalence of beta-lactamase production by staphylococci which inactivate penicillin but not penicillinase-resistant penicillins (see below) which are stable and therefore remain active.[122] Beta-lactamases have spread to organisms which previously did not have them, including *Haemophilus influenzae* and *Neisseria gonorrhoeae*.

Hundreds of beta-lactamases have been described and can be assigned to one of four groups, A to D. Class A beta-lactamases are usually plasmid-mediated and can spread easily between bacteria of different genera. They occur commonly in *E. coli* and other *Enterobacteriaceae*. More recently, mutants have emerged with an 'extended spectrum', which can attack not only penicillins but many of the first, second and third generation cephalosporins, called extended-spectrum beta-lactamases or ESBLs.[124-126] The class A beta-lactamases can be inhibited by beta-lactamase inhibitors such as clavulanic acid (see below). On the other hand, class C beta-lactamases, which have a broader spectrum than class A enzymes and mediate resistance to penicillins and most cephalosporins, are chromosomal, intrinsically produce a beta-lactamase, and are confined to specific bacterial species such as *Enterobacter* spp., *Serratia marcescens*, *Citrobacter freundii*, *Acinetobacter* spp., *Aeromonas* spp., indole positive *Proteus* spp. and *Morganella morganii*, often referred to as the ESCAAPM group. The class C beta-lactamases cannot be inhibited by clavulanic acid. Both class A and class C beta-lactamases inactivate penicillins and cephalosporins but do not inactivate carbapenems. However, more recently, metallobeta-lactamases, which are usually class B and inactivate all beta-lactams including carbapenems, have become more prevalent by spreading on plasmids among Gram negative bacteria.[123]

Aminoglycosides, which are very potent bactericidal antibiotics with a broad range of activity especially against Gram negative bacteria, can induce enzymes which catalyze phosphorylation, acetylation or adenylation of this class of antibiotics causing covalent modifications leading to poor ribosomal binding resulting in high-level resistance to these agents.[127]

CLASSES OF ANTIMICROBIAL AGENTS

Beta-lactams

The antimicrobial agents of most value in treating infants and children are the beta-lactams, including penicillins, cephalosporins, monobactams and carbapenems, which have in common a beta-lactam ring.

The bacterial targets of beta-lactam antibiotics are penicillin binding proteins (PBPs), which are vital for bacterial cell division, shape and structural integrity. The exact mechanism of action of beta-lactams remains elusive. Recent evidence suggests it is a complex process involving both inhibition of cell wall synthesis and activation of endogenous autolytic systems. Their action is usually bactericidal. Some bacteria have a deficiency in this system of autolytic enzymes that results in inhibition but not killing of the bacteria by the beta-lactam. This phenomenon is called tolerance and is demonstrated, in vitro, by a minimal inhibitory concentration (MIC) in the susceptible range but a minimal bacterial concentration (MBC):MIC ratio of 32 or greater.

The nature of the bactericidal activity of beta-lactam has been described as time-dependent killing. The important determinant of bactericidal activity for beta-lactams is the length of time during the dosing interval that the concentration of the antibiotic exceeds the MIC of the infecting microorganism. Bactericidal activity is thought to be greatest when the concentration of the beta-lactam antibiotic at the site of infection is 4–10 times greater than the MIC of the infecting microorganism. The rapidity and extent of bacterial killing are not increased when concentrations exceed this ratio.

Resistance to beta-lactam antibiotics is either by production of a beta-lactamase or by alterations in the PBPs.

Penicillin

The penicillins can be classified into four groups based on their antimicrobial activity. There are some overlaps in activity. The four groups are the natural penicillins, the amino-penicillins, the penicillinase-resistant penicillins and the extended-spectrum penicillins. The mechanism by which most bacteria have acquired resistance to penicillins G is beta-lactamase production. Resistance to penicillin by *Streptococcus pyogenes* (group A streptococcus) and *Streptococcus agalactiae* (group B streptococcus) has not emerged. Resistance caused by altered PBPs occurs less commonly, but the increasing resistance of *Streptococcus pneumoniae* to penicillin is a result of altered PBPs.

1. *Aqueous penicillin G* produces high peak concentrations of antibacterial activity in the serum within 30 min of administration. The drug is rapidly excreted by the kidneys resulting in low serum concentrations within 2–4 h. When treating severe disease such as meningitis, pneumonia or endocarditis, penicillin G should be administered usually every 4 h until the infection has been cured.
2. *Procaine penicillin G* given intramuscularly produces serum levels of approximately 10–30% of those of aqueous penicillin, but the activity persists in serum for as long as 4 h. IM procaine penicillin is very painful and can cause injection site abscesses. It is only recommended for short term treatment of children with mild to moderate disease when IV access cannot be achieved.
3. *Benzathine penicillin G* is given intramuscularly as a depot preparation that provides for low continuous concentrations approximately 1–2% of those achieved by the aqueous penicillin G. Penicillin is detectable in the serum for 3 weeks or more following injection. Benzathine penicillin G can be used for the treatment of group A streptococcal pharyngitis, impetigo or prophylaxis of streptococcal infections in children who have rheumatic carditis, although pain at the injection site is a major deterrent to the use of this antibiotic.
4. *Phenoxymethylpenicillin* (oral penicillin or penicillin V) is well absorbed from the gastrointestinal tract with peak concentrations in serum approximately 40% of that of the same dose of aqueous penicillin G. Oral penicillin is satisfactory for treating mild to moderate infections with susceptible organisms.

All penicillins are excreted by both glomerular filtration and tubular secretion. Concomitant use of probenecid, a drug that blocks tubular secretion of organic acids, can produce higher peaks and more sustained serum concentrations resulting in greater antimicrobial activity. Dosages and dosing intervals will need adjustment when penicillins are administered to persons with decreased renal function.

Penicillinase-resistant penicillin

Penicillinase-resistant penicillins are the drug of choice for the initial management of patients with suspected staphylococcal disease, as most strains of *S. aureus* produce a beta-lactamase, penicillinase. Common penicillinase-resistant penicillins are cloxacillin, dicloxacillin, flucloxacillin, oxacillin and nafcillin. These agents are active against streptococci and can be used for treatment of infections commonly caused by both staphylococci and streptococci, e.g. impetigo. However, as these agents are less active than penicillin G against streptococci, penicillin G should be used if streptococci alone are isolated from culture. It should be noted that penicillinase-resistant penicillins have no activity against Gram negative bacteria or enterococci.

Disease caused by methicillin-resistant *Staphylococcus aureus* (MRSA) was reported shortly after the introduction of methicillin in the 1960s. Methicillin resistance is caused by alterations in PBP-2 rather than by production of a beta-lactamase, so MRSA is resistant to all currently available beta-lactam agents including penicillins, cephalosporins and carbapenems.

Coagulase-negative staphylococci, most commonly *Staphylococcus epidermidis*, a skin commensal, may be a pathogen in neonates or cause infections of prosthetic devices such as heart valves, CSF shunts and intravenous lines. Many strains of coagulase-negative staphylococci produce beta-lactamase and have altered PBPs making them methicillin resistant. Vancomycin is the drug of choice for diseases known to be caused by MRSA or methicillin-resistant *Staphylococcus epidermidis* (MRSE).

Amino-penicillin

The amino-penicillins include ampicillin and amoxicillin which have extended activity compared with penicillin, with activity against some Gram negative organisms, including *H. influenzae*, *E. coli*, *Proteus mirabilis*, *Salmonella* spp. and *Shigella* spp. The amino-penicillins can also retain activity against penicillin-susceptible Gram positive bacteria. Amino-penicillins are the drug of choice for treatment of infections caused by *Listeria monocytogenes* and the enterococci. These drugs are used frequently in the treatment of susceptible pathogens causing (1) lower respiratory tract infection, (2) acute otitis media, (3) urinary tract infections, and (4) acute diarrheal disease when therapy is indicated. It should be noted that amoxicillin is significantly less effective than ampicillin for the treatment of shigellosis. Ampicillin is associated more frequently with diarrhea than amoxicillin.

Extended-spectrum penicillins

Extended-spectrum penicillins are semisynthetic derivatives of ampicillin and have better activity against Gram negative bacteria because of high affinity for PBPs and greater penetration to the Gram negative outer membrane. The carboxypenicillins include carbenicillin and ticarcillin while the ureidopencillins include piperacillin and mezlocillin. These extended-spectrum penicillins have activity against *Pseudomonas aeruginosa* but are significantly less active against Gram positive cocci than ampicillin.

Extended-spectrum penicillins (often combined with an aminoglycoside) have been used for the treatment of intra-abdominal and upper urinary tract infections as well as for sepsis in neutropenic patients. They are only available as parenteral formulations.

Beta-lactamase inhibitor/beta-lactam combinations

Beta-lactamase inhibitors, such as clavulanic acid, sulbactam and tazobactam, are compounds that have weak intrinsic antibacterial activity but bind irreversibly to many beta-lactamases rendering the beta-lactamases inactive. Beta-lactamase inhibitors are combined in a fixed ratio with a beta-lactam antibiotic, e.g. amoxicillin/clavulanic acid or piperacillin/tazobactam. The spectrum of activity of the combination is determined primarily by the spectrum of activity of the beta-lactam. The main indication for use of these combination antimicrobial agents is the treatment of infections caused by susceptible beta-lactamase producing pathogens.

Ampicillin/sulbactam or amoxicillin/clavulanic acid can be used to treat beta-lactamase producing strands of *Staphylococcus aureus* (but not methicillin-resistant *Staphylococcus aureus*), *Haemophilus influenzae*, *Moraxella catarrhalis*, *Neisseria gonorrhoeae*, *Escherichia coli*, some *Proteus* spp., *Klebsiella* spp. and some anaerobic bacteria including *Bacteroides fragilis*.

Adverse effects and allergies of penicillins

The penicillins have very little dose-related toxicity. Adverse reactions include electrolyte disturbance of sodium and potassium, gastrointestinal problems with diarrhea, and hematological changes with hemolysis, neutropenia or platelet dysfunction. Drug-induced hepatitis can occur determined by elevated aspartate aminotransferase (AST), neurological abnormalities are rare and include seizures, while renal problems can occur with interstitial nephritis.

Allergy, however, is an important factor and can occur quite frequently with penicillin compounds.[128] The penicillin are haptens, low molecular weight compounds too small to induce an immune response but which bind to host proteins and are highly immunogenic. The four types of immune-mediated reactions that can occur after the administration of penicillins are: (1) immediate hypersensitivity (IgE mediated); (2) cytotoxic antibody reactions; (3) immune complex reactions (Arthus reactions); and (4) delayed cell-mediated hypersensitivity. It is estimated that serious immediate reactions will occur in 2 of every 10 000 cases and fatal reactions in 1 in 100 000 treatment cases of penicillin administration. Identifying patients who will have a significant reaction to penicillin remains difficult. At present, physicians must rely on the patient's history of reactions after administration of penicillin to identify those likely to be allergic and avoid administration of penicillin in these patients for anything other than very serious infections, e.g. endocarditis, where desensitization may be necessary. All penicillins are cross-reactive with regards to sensitization, and allergy to one implies sensitization to all, although this cross-sensitivity is less than 100%.

Cephalosporins

The cephalosporins have a very broad range of activity which includes Gram positive, Gram negative and anaerobic bacteria. Cephalosporins are categorized as first, second, third and fourth generation depending on their pattern of in vitro activity. Cephalosporins have no activity against enterococci or methicillin-resistant staphylococci.

First generation cephalosporins. The first generation cephalosporins are effective against Gram positive cocci including beta-lactamase producing *Staphylococcus aureus*. They have variable activity against Gram negative enteric bacilli, such as *Escherichia coli*, *Proteus mirabilis* and *Klebsiella* species, with minimal if any activity against *Haemophilus influenzae* and *Moraxella catarrhalis* and are inadequate against penicillin-sensitive *Streptococcus pneumoniae*. They should therefore not be used for treatment for respiratory tract infection.

Second generation cephalosporins. The second generation cephalosporins in common use are cefuroxime and cefaclor. When compared with the first generation cephalosporins, second generation cephalosporins have similar or somewhat less activity against Gram positive cocci with better activity against *Haemophilus influenzae*, *Moraxella catarrhalis*, *Neisseria meningitidis* and *Neisseria gonorrhoeae* and some members of the *Enterobacteriaceae*.

Third generation cephalosporins. The common parenteral third generation cephalosporins used in children are cefotaxime, ceftriaxone and ceftazidime. There are oral third generation cephalosporins and cefixime is the most commonly used. Third generation cephalosporins are very potent against Gram negative and enteric bacteria and have excellent activity against *Haemophilus influenzae*, *Moraxella catarrhalis*, *Neisseria gonorrhoeae* and *Neisseria meningitidis*, group A streptococci and penicillin-susceptible pneumococci. They have relatively poor activity against staphylococci. Ceftazidime is the only third generation cephalosporin used in children with activity against *Pseudomonas aeruginosa*. The increasing prevalence of extended-spectrum beta-lactamases (ESBL) in the *Enterobacteriaceae* is increasing the prevalence of resistance to these agents. The parenteral third generation cephalosporins achieve high levels in the serum and adequate concentration in CSF.

Fourth generation cephalosporins. The fourth generation cephalosporin, cefepime, exhibits very rapid entry into the bacterial cell and stability against a range of beta-lactamases as well as increased binding affinity to multiple PBPs. These factors explain cefepime's expanded spectrum of activity and improved efficacy against Gram negative pathogens compared with third generation cephalosporins.[129]

Adverse reactions. The safety profile of cephalosporins is similar to penicillins with hypersensitivity reactions being the most frequent.

Monobactams

Aztreonam is the prototype monobactam. It has aerobic Gram negative antibacterial activity similar to that of ceftazidime but has no significant Gram positive activity.

Carbapenems

The carbapenem class of antimicrobial agents exhibits the broadest spectrum of activity of all beta-lactam antibiotics. They include imipenem-cilastatin and meropenem and have activity against most clinically significant Gram positive and Gram negative pathogens including anaerobic organisms.

The glycopeptides

The glycopeptides, vancomycin and teicoplanin, exhibit time-dependent bactericidal activity against most clinically significant Gram positive bacteria except that they are only bacteriostatic for enterococci. The glycopeptides interfere with the development of the peptidoglycan cell wall at a site of action distinct from that of beta-lactams, so there is no cross-resistance or competitive inhibition between these drug classes.

Vancomycin is not metabolized significantly and is excreted by glomerular filtration. In patients with severe renal failure the half-life may extend 7 or more days, and furthermore vancomycin is not removed effectively by either peritoneal or hemodialysis. The dosing interval needs to be adjusted when using vancomycin in patients with impaired renal function.[130]

Adverse effects. Ototoxicity and nephrotoxicity have been considered serious adverse effects of vancomycin therapy in the past, but these serious events are much less frequent than previously thought. Infusion-related side-effects are the most common side-effect seen with vancomycin with the rapid onset of a widespread erythematous rash. This can usually be managed by slowing the infusion rate or premedicating the patient with antihistamines.

Aminoglycosides

The aminoglycosides, gentamicin, tobramycin and amikacin, demonstrate rapid concentration-dependent bactericidal activity with a post-antibiotic effect, i.e. killing of bacteria continues in the absence of any detectable serum antibiotic.[131] The higher the peak concentration of the aminoglycoside, the longer the duration of the post-antibiotic effect. The mechanism of the bactericidal action is binding to the bacterial ribosome and interfering with bacterial protein synthesis by inducing translational errors. The uptake of aminoglycosides by bacteria can be facilitated by concomitant therapy with a cell wall-active antibiotic such as vancomycin or a beta-lactam. Aminoglycosides have activity against a range of facultative aerobic bacteria, but their activity is reduced in infections at sites with reduced oxygen tension, e.g. abscesses. Anaerobic bacteria and fermentative bacteria such as streptococci are inherently resistant to aminoglycosides. Aminoglycosides penetrate the blood–brain barrier very poorly in the absence of inflammation and thus are not very successful in the treatment of Gram negative meningitis. Aminoglycosides are not metabolized after parenteral administration and are excreted unchanged in the kidney by glomerular filtration.

Resistance to aminoglycosides can evolve in a number of ways: (1) alteration in the bacterial target affecting binding; (2) decreased cell permeability making it more difficult for the drug to reach the ribosomal target; and (3) breakdown of the drug by bacterial enzymes.

The major use of aminoglycosides in children is for serious infections caused by Gram negative enteric infections, neonatal sepsis, sepsis in a child with immunodeficiency, especially neutropenia, abdominal and systemic infections associated with fecal contamination of the peritoneum, and complicated urinary tract infections.

Adverse effects. All aminoglycosides can damage the proximal renal tubules, the cochlea, the vestibular apparatus or a combination of these, and rarely can cause neuromuscular blockade. To avoid toxicity and ensure therapeutic levels, the concentration of aminoglycoside in serum should be monitored in all patients.

Macrolides

The macrolides, erythromycin, clarithromycin and azithromycin, have similar antibacterial spectra, mechanism of action and mechanism of resistance but they differ in their pharmacokinetic characteristics. They all bind reversibly to the 23S component of the 50S ribosomal subunit and inhibit protein synthesis. The macrolides are bacteriostatic but clarithromycin and azithromycin are bactericidal against *Streptococcus pyogenes*, *Streptococcus pneumoniae* and *Haemophilus influenzae*.

The newer macrolides have a spectrum of activity similar to that of erythromycin, but clarithromycin has greater activity against *Moraxella catarrhalis*, *Haemophilus influenzae*, *Mycoplasma pneumoniae*, *Chlamydophila pneumoniae*, *Chlamydia trachomatis*, *Legionella pneumophila*, *Ureaplasma urealyticum* and *Neisseria gonorrhoeae*. Clarithromycin also has activity against organisms that are resistant to erythromycin, including *Toxoplasma gondii*, *Mycobacterium leprae*, *Mycobacterium chelonae* and *Mycobacterium avium-intracellulare* (MAC).

Azithromycin is effective in vitro against a diverse group of microorganisms including *Bordetella pertussis*, *Legionella pneumophila*, *Corynebacterium diphtheriae*, spirochetes including *Treponema pallidum*, the mycoplasmas (except *M. hominis*), chlamydiae, and aerobic and anaerobic Gram positive cocci.[132] Azithromycin is highly active against *Campylobacter jejuni*. When compared with erythromycin, azithromycin has less activity against Gram positive bacteria and greater activity against Gram negative bacteria including some *Enterobacteriaceae* such as *Shigella* and *Salmonella* species.

Adverse effects These include local gastrointestinal irritation with nausea, vomiting and abdominal pain. Cholestatic hepatitis occurs rarely but is a serious reaction requiring cessation of therapy. Erythromycin has been associated with infantile hypertrophic pyloric stenosis.

Miscellaneous antibacterial agents
Clindamycin

Clindamycin is a semisynthetic derivative of lincomycin and has much better oral absorption and greater antimicrobial activity. It has action against Gram positive bacteria as well as Gram positive and Gram negative anaerobes including *B. fragilis*. Clindamycin penetrates well into most tissues including bone but has poor penetration into the CNS. It is inactivated in the liver and excreted in bile with very little renal excretion. It is useful in the treatment of staphylococcal infections in penicillin-allergic individuals and MRSA.

Adverse effects. Clindamycin can often cause diarrhea and less commonly the more serious *Clostridium difficile* associated pseudomembranous colitis. The occurrence of pseudomembranous colitis is a strong indication to cease this agent. Clindamycin is also associated with allergic reactions and rashes and rarely causes erythema multiforme and anaphylaxis.

Trimethoprim–sulfamethoxazole (co-trimoxazole)

Trimethoprim is active against many Gram positive and Gram negative bacteria, except *Pseudomonas aeruginosa*. Trimethoprim is often combined with sulfamethoxazole because the two drugs act synergistically. The drug is widely distributed in tissues including the CNS, and a significant amount is excreted unchanged in the urine giving high concentrations which makes it useful for treating urinary tract infections. Trimethoprim–sulfamethoxazole also has activity against *Haemophilus influenzae* and *Pneumocystis carinii*.

Adverse effects. The most common side-effects are nausea, vomiting, diarrhea and hypersensitivity reactions. Prolonged administration may be associated with a megaloblastic bone marrow or leukopenia; thrombocytopenia and anemia may also occur.

A discussion of the mechanisms of action, clinical indications and modes of resistance of antiviral agents and antifungal agents is beyond the scope of this chapter. The reader is referred to other publications for this information.[133-135]

Management of infections is complex. The clinician needs a good understanding of infectious clinical syndromes, likely pathogens, antimicrobial resistance patterns, and knowledge of antimicrobial agents, their spectrum of activity, penetration to the site of likely infection and possible adverse effects, to effectively and safely treat common childhood illnesses.

BACTERIAL INFECTIONS: BOTULISM

The name botulism derives from the Latin *botulus* for sausage, and was coined following an outbreak in Germany in 1793 in which 13 people who shared a large sausage became ill and 6 died.

Classical botulism is a paralytic disease caused by ingestion or absorption of one or more preformed neurotoxins produced by the soil organism, *Clostridium botulinum*. Cases occur singly or in small clusters following consumption of home-canned or prepared foods in which the heat-resistant spores of *C. botulinum* have germinated under anaerobic conditions. Canned or bottled foods, especially soil-contaminated vegetables, smoked fish and continental sausage, are classic food vehicles. High temperatures are required to inactivate spores. If toxin production does occur, poisoning can be avoided by adequate cooking or reheating of the food, because the toxin is inactivated by moderate heat. Raw fish or fish products are also potential sources of botulinum toxin.

Infant botulism is a different condition from the botulism due to preformed toxin. Infant botulism results from multiplication of *C. botulinum* in the baby's intestine, and causes an indolent presentation. The median age of onset is 2 months, with a range of less than 3 weeks to

12 months.[136–138] Infant botulism is more common in babies living in rural areas or on a farm: in Australia cases occur when it is hot, dry and windy and spores may blow into the baby's mouth or into the water supply.[136] There is a particular association with babies whose pacifiers were dipped in honey, although only 11 of 68 US babies reported with infant botulism had honey exposure.[137,138] Corn syrup ingestion (20 of the 68 babies) and breast-feeding were other risk factors. Breast milk is thought to generate favorable conditions for germination of spores.

CLINICAL FEATURES AND DIAGNOSIS
Classic botulism
Typically, after an interval of 12–36 h, patients present acutely with malaise, nausea, vomiting, dizziness, weakness and dry mouth. After hours or days cranial nerve palsies develop, causing ptosis, blurred vision, diplopia, dysphagia and dysarthria. Paralysis may progress over a period of hours or days to involve many muscle groups and the patient may require respiratory support. Recovery occurs over weeks to months.

Infantile botulism
This is characterized by an insidious onset of severe, progressive hypotonia, poor suck, constipation and bilateral ptosis. The pupils are often dilated and there may also be pooling of oral secretions, reduced facial movements and ophthalmoplegia. The gag reflex is often weak. Peripheral tendon reflexes are normal or diminished, but not usually absent. Paralysis may progress to involve the respiratory muscles and the infant may require respiratory support.[138]

The differential diagnosis includes spinal muscular atrophy (absent reflexes, fasciculations), myotonic dystrophy [myotonia, electromyogram (EMG) pattern], wild-type or vaccine-associated paralytic poliomyelitis (asymmetric paralysis, CSF pleocytosis) and Guillain–Barré syndrome (ascending paralysis, raised CSF protein). The EMG in infant botulism shows denervation. The diagnosis is primarily based on clinical findings and EMG, and can be supported by detecting *C. botulinum* toxin in stools (by PCR or animal inoculation) and/or by growing *C. botulinum* from stool culture. An association between infant botulism and sudden infant death syndrome (SIDS) has been proposed but is unproven.

TREATMENT
Infant botulism is managed by protecting the airway and using artificial ventilation if required. Babies who require artificial ventilation recover after 3–4 weeks. With proper supportive care the outcome is excellent, with complete recovery the rule.

Tracheostomy prolongs hospitalization.[138] Nasogastric tube feeds are usually well tolerated. Antibiotics such as penicillin do not speed recovery and gentamicin may exacerbate neuromuscular problems. Antibiotics are only indicated for complications such as pneumonia. Botulism antitoxin, harvested from hyperimmune adults (hBIG) and available only to investigators in the USA, halves the mean time to resolution of symptoms in infant botulism.[139,140] Equine antitoxin made in horses (eBIG) has long been used in the treatment of adult botulism but has not been shown to be effective in infant botulism.[141] A new intravenous botulinum immunoglobulin, produced in the USA, reduced the duration of mechanical ventilation and hospitalization significantly in infant botulism.[142]

In older children, circulating toxin needs to be neutralized with antitoxin, in the form of botulinum immune globulin, as soon as possible. This has no effect on bound toxin but it is always indicated as toxin may circulate for days. The remainder of the care is supportive of respiration, as for infant botulism.

BACTERIAL INFECTIONS: BRUCELLOSIS; UNDULANT FEVER
Brucellosis is usually caused by one of three organisms: *Brucella abortus*, *Brucella melitensis* or *Brucella suis*. All three are primarily diseases of domesticated animals (cattle, goats and pigs, respectively). The clinical picture ranges from clinically asymptomatic infection via acute brucellosis (with septicemic manifestations) to chronic brucellosis.

EPIDEMIOLOGY
Human brucellosis is mostly a disease of those who come into contact with infected animals in rural areas. Spread of infection from animal to animal occurs readily and the resulting illness is often chronic with long term excretion of the organism. Infection is transmitted to humans by infected milk or milk products and, less frequently, by direct contact or entry through skin. Person-to-person spread rarely occurs. Elimination of brucellosis in animal populations (by vaccination or slaughter policies) will eliminate new infections in humans. World Health Organization sources estimate that there are 500 000 cases worldwide each year (childhood infections accounting for less than 10% of cases). In the UK there are about 20 patients each year, most with disease caused by imported *B. melitensis* infection or laboratory accident. The low incidence of brucellosis in children which results from milk-borne infection is unexpected and some have suggested that environmental exposure may be more relevant.

PATHOLOGY
Acute brucellosis is a septicemic illness, with seeding of organisms in the body, which may become apparent immediately or later after the systemic features have resolved. There is widespread reticuloendothelial system hyperplasia and focal manifestations may occur in many organs, particularly in the liver or spleen. Chronic brucellosis may follow acute brucellosis or begin insidiously. In chronic brucellosis the organisms usually remain intracellularly where they are relatively protected against host defenses and antibiotics.

B. melitensis often produces more invasive manifestations and debility than *B. abortus*, an important point to realize when generalizing about brucellosis. Those with low gastric acid levels are thought to be at particular risk of infection.

CLINICAL FEATURES
The incubation period of acute brucellosis is from a few days to a month.

With acute brucellosis symptoms develop rapidly with high fever, rigors, arthralgia and profuse sweating: patients often feel much more ill than signs suggest but recovery follows in most. Fever has no particular pattern. Weight loss and secondary anemia may develop. If the patient does not recover then a state of chronic brucellosis ensues with vague irritability, malaise, fatigue, musculoskeletal aches and pains, headaches and depression. Fever may be intermittent, occurring every few weeks – hence the name 'undulant fever'.

Although chronic brucellosis is rarely life threatening the morbidity may be significant.

With both acute and chronic brucellosis suggestive signs may be prominent or absent, constituting a pyrexia of unknown origin. There may be hepatomegaly, splenomegaly or lymph node enlargement. Particularly with *B. melitensis* infection lymph nodes may suppurate and osteomyelitis or arthritis may develop.

Other rare, but potentially life-threatening manifestations include meningitis, endocarditis, peritonitis and encephalitis.

DIAGNOSIS AND DIFFERENTIAL DIAGNOSIS
Clinical diagnosis may be easy in areas where animal infection is endemic. In non-endemic areas clinical diagnosis may be difficult unless it is realized that patients have visited endemic areas or ingested milk products from endemic areas.

In acute brucellosis blood cultures may be positive, but the organisms are difficult to culture and cultures may take up to 2 weeks to become positive. Agglutination tests to detect IgM and IgG antibodies may be helpful but may be positive in asymptomatically infected patients in endemic areas. Nevertheless increasing titers are almost certainly diagnostic. Agglutination titers of greater than 1:160 in a patient with appropriate clinical features are very suggestive.

In chronic brucellosis blood cultures are rarely positive and bone marrow culture or, less often, liver or splenic biopsy culture may be necessary. If there is renal involvement urine cultures may be positive. Biopsy shows noncaseating granulomas.

If available, the presence of *Brucella*-specific IgM is diagnostic of acute brucellosis or of chronic brucellosis in an acute relapse, whilst *Brucella*-specific IgG indicates infection at some stage. Lymphocytosis with neutropenia may be found.

The differential diagnosis of acute brucellosis includes malaria, salmonellosis (including typhoid fever), tuberculosis, tularemia, rheumatic fever, infective endocarditis, Q fever, leptospirosis and non-infective conditions. If malaise and debility predominate, depression enters the differential diagnosis, as well as being a complication in its own right.

TREATMENT[143]

In acute brucellosis antibiotic treatment probably shortens the illness and reduces the risk of progression to chronic brucellosis. Opinions differ as to the optimal treatment: comparison of treatment results of *B. abortus* and *B. melitensis* infection is not necessarily valid. Most studies of children with brucellosis deal with children with *B. melitensis* infection. Regimens advocated include (either alone or in combination) co-trimoxazole, rifampicin or streptomycin. In chronic brucellosis suppression of intracellular infection may be attempted in the hope that the host's immunity will eventually eliminate or contain infection. Regimens advocated include protracted courses of the antibiotics used in acute brucellosis. Tetracyclines are useful but obviously cannot be used in children unless there is no alternative.

Single agent treatment carries a relapse rate of 5–40%, thought to be caused by inadequate killing rather than development of resistance.

Antipyretics, analgesics and antidepressant treatment may be indicated. Vaccination of humans with the live attenuated organisms used in animals is not practicable and would certainly make subsequent interpretation of serological tests very difficult.

BACTERIAL INFECTIONS: CHOLERA

Cholera is an acute bacterial enteric disease characterized in its severe form by sudden onset, profuse, painless, watery stools, occasional vomiting, and, in untreated cases, rapid dehydration, acidosis, hypoglycemia and circulatory collapse. Cholera is caused by infection with toxin-producing strains of *Vibrio cholerae*: 01 (includes two biotypes – classical and El Tor) and 0139 (non-01). The clinical picture is similar, because the organisms elaborate a similar enterotoxin that is critical in the pathogenesis. In any single epidemic, one particular biotype tends to be dominant.

EPIDEMIOLOGY

From the nineteenth century, pandemic cholera has spread repeatedly from the Gangetic delta of India to most of the world. Since 1961, *V. cholerae* of the El Tor biotype has spread through most of Asia into Eastern Europe, Africa and Latin America, assuming a worldwide distribution in resource limited countries. Sporadic imported cases occur among returning travelers or immigrants to high-income countries. Humans are the main reservoir of infection, but other environmental reservoirs such as small crustaceans exist in brackish water or estuaries. Outbreaks occur as a result of ingestion of infected water due to poor sanitation and hygiene and occasionally as a result of ingestion of infected food, especially shellfish.

The arrival of cholera in a region may be heralded by an epidemic of severe disease among all age groups: the presentation of large numbers of adults (as well as children) with severe dehydrating diarrhea should alert to the possibility of a cholera epidemic. The initial outbreak may be explosive due to the short incubation period (1–5 days) and the ease of fecal–oral transmission in areas where standards of environmental sanitation and personal hygiene are low. Cholera may then become endemic, causing disease mainly in young children of less than 5 years. This is particularly likely with the El Tor biotype, which has a longer carrier period (up to 2–4 weeks) than classical, a longer viability in water and a higher infection:case ratio. El Tor cholera has largely replaced classical cholera as the major pathogen of public health importance worldwide. *V. cholerae* 0139 has been a cause of severe outbreaks in the Bay of Bengal region since 1992.

ORGANISM AND PATHOPHYSIOLOGY

V. cholerae are Gram negative curved rods measuring $1.5–3.0\,\mu m \times 0.5\,\mu m$. In culture, they may assume other forms such as spiral shapes. They possess somatic (O) antigens and flagellar (H) antigens that may be used to distinguish serological strains such as Ogawa, Inaba and Hikojima. In hanging-drop preparations, they are highly motile. Diarrhea is mediated via an enterotoxin that consists of A and B subunits. The B subunit binds the toxin to surface receptors on the enterocyte and activates arachidonic acid metabolism. Once binding has occurred, the A subunit activates the enzyme adenylate cyclase to produce cyclic adenosine monophosphate (cAMP) which inhibits the absorption of sodium chloride and water. cAMP also stimulates secretion of sodium chloride and bicarbonate from the crypt epithelial cells. The excessive intestinal secretions accumulate in the intestinal lumen and are then expelled in the diarrheal stools. The severity of disease depends on the size of the infecting dose, and the organism is easily destroyed by gastric acid. Most patients with cholera are infected with large inocula of the organism or have relative achlorhydria. Breast-feeding is protective.

The electrolyte content of stools of patients with adult cholera, cholera in children and diarrhea due to other organisms is summarized in Table 28.18. Generally, stool osmolarity in pediatric cholera is isotonic with plasma. The stool sodium content of children with cholera is intermediate (~100 millimoles/litre) between that found in childhood diarrhea due to other organisms such as rotavirus (~30 mmol/L) or *Shigella* (~60 mmol/L) and that found in adult cholera (130–150 mmol/L). Stool potassium is higher in pediatric cholera (~30 mmol/L) compared to adult cholera (~15 mmol/L) and bicarbonate losses (~45 mmol/L) are also high. Cholera does not invade the gut mucosa, but colicky abdominal pain and ileus can occur due to electrolyte disturbances such as hypokalemia and hypocalcemia with acidosis.

CLINICAL FEATURES

The majority of infections with *V. cholerae* are asymptomatic or mild and clinically indistinguishable from other causes of acute watery diarrhea. The typical presentation of severe disease is of acute frequent diarrhea with copious, odorless, virtually colorless (described as 'rice-water') stools. Vomiting is common but fever is unusual. A similar presentation can occur in infants with rotavirus gastroenteritis. In older age groups, the presentation of acute diarrhea among a family group may be confused with food poisoning but severe vomiting which precedes diarrhea and marked abdominal pain are characteristics of food poisoning that are unusual with cholera.

Table 28.18   Relative electrolyte constituents of stools

	Sodium	Potassium	Chloride	Bicarbonate
Cholera in adults	+++	+	+++	+++
Cholera in children	++	++	++	++
Noncholera infantile diarrhea	+	++	+	+

The main clinical features of cholera are those due to severe water and electrolyte loss. Dehydration is commonly isotonic or hypotonic with typical sunken eyes, reduced skin turgor, thirst and dry mucous membranes. Hypovolemic shock may occur within hours of onset. Hypoglycemia is not uncommon and, along with acidosis and hypovolemic shock, leads to deterioration in level of consciousness and occasional convulsions. Hypokalemia and hypocalcemia may also develop and cause colicky abdominal pain, paralytic ileus, muscle cramps and arrhythmias. In severe untreated cases, death may occur within a few hours, and the case-fatality rate may exceed 50%. With proper treatment, the mortality is < 1%.

DIAGNOSIS

Infection with *V. cholerae* is confirmed microbiologically by culture of stools or rectal swabs. Isolates should be serogrouped, and tested for toxin production and antibiotic susceptibility. If laboratory facilities are not nearby, specimens should be transported in special medium such as Cary-Blair transport medium.[144] Traditional culture techniques usually take over 48 h to complete. For clinical purposes, a quick, presumptive diagnosis can be made by dark field or phase microscopic examination of wet preparation showing the vibrios moving like 'shooting stars' and inhibited by serotype-specific antiserum. Rapid dipstick tests that could be used by non-laboratory trained health workers show promise.[145] Earlier confirmation of a cholera outbreak could reduce the case-fatality rate, usually highest at the beginning of an outbreak, and lead to earlier implementation of infection control measures.

MANAGEMENT

The basis of therapy is replacement of water and electrolyte losses from the stool. In cases with no dehydration or mild dehydration, oral solutions will suffice but ongoing review is important. The World Health Organization oral rehydration solution (WHO-ORS) was developed for cholera management and the electrolyte content is appropriate replacement for the above mentioned stool losses. Absorption is dependent on the glucose-facilitated membrane transport of sodium. Other more complex substrates with a lower osmolality such as in cereal-based ORS (e.g. rice-based) are more effective at reducing fluid losses in children with acute watery diarrhea.[146] Stool sodium content is higher in cholera than in noncholera diarrhea, yet a meta-analysis[147] concluded that reduced osmolarity ORS (sodium 75 mEq/L, glucose 75 mmol/L, osmolarity 245 mmol/L) is safe and at least as effective as WHO-ORS (sodium 90 mEq/L, glucose 111 mmol/L, osmolarity 311 mmol/L). The WHO now recommends low osmolarity ORS and zinc supplementation for all children with acute watery diarrhea.[148]

Patients with moderate dehydration have a fluid deficit of between 5 and 10% with decreased skin turgor, thirst, sunken eyes and tachycardia but an intact sensorium. Rehydration and maintenance may be oral or intravenous. Those with severe dehydration, with fluid deficits of more than 10%, will show all the above signs together with peripheral cyanosis, drowsiness or coma, and weak or absent peripheral pulses. Such patients require rapid rehydration with intravenous (or intraosseous) fluids. Ringer's lactate is the most appropriate, widely available intravenous fluid for rehydration but normal saline can also be used. Provision must be made for ongoing stool losses and frequent review of fluid management is essential. Electrolytes and blood sugar should be assessed at intervals to guide ongoing therapy. Potassium will need to be added (at least 20 mmol/L) if normal saline is used during the maintenance phase.

Antibiotics can shorten the duration of diarrhea, reduce fluid losses and requirements and reduce vibrio excretion. Alternatives include doxycycline, erythromycin, azithromycin or ciprofloxacin. Antibiotic-resistant strains are increasingly common, and treatment protocols should be guided by in vitro susceptibility testing. Chemoprophylaxis for contacts has never succeeded in markedly limiting spread but is justified for close household contacts of an index case or if the outbreak is in a closed group, e.g. aboard ship. Mass chemoprophylaxis of whole communities is never indicated and encourages antibiotic resistance.

CONTROL AND PREVENTION

During an outbreak, a coordinated response is important.[144] An emergency treatment center should be established that is accessible to the community and appropriately supplied and staffed. Standardized treatment regimens and frequent review are essential for effective therapy. Early case-finding and management of household contacts should be organized. Educate the population at risk concerning the need to seek appropriate treatment without delay. Initiate a thorough investigation designed to find the vehicle and circumstances of transmission (time, place, persons). Support with laboratory examination of implicated water or food sources and sewage, and plan control measures accordingly. It may be necessary to educate the community by dissemination of important, factual information relating to water safety, food preparation and human waste disposal, and to obtain public support for control activities. Adopt emergency measures to ensure a safe water supply. Chlorinate public water supplies and chlorinate or boil water used for drinking, cooking and washing dishes and food containers. Provide appropriate safe facilities for sewage disposal.

Cholera will ultimately be brought under control only when water supplies, sanitation and hygienic practices attain such a level that fecal–oral transmission of *V. cholerae* becomes an improbable event. Active immunization with a cheap, oral killed whole-cell vaccine that provides a moderate level of protection is gaining recognition as an effective control strategy.[149,150] Indirect herd protection to nonvaccinated neighbors improves effectiveness[151] and the vaccine may provide protection for 3–5 years.[152]

BACTERIAL INFECTIONS: DIPHTHERIA

Diphtheria is an acute infectious disease caused by exotoxin-producing *Corynebacterium diphtheriae*. Although local disease at the primary site of infection, usually the respiratory tract, may be severe, the most significant clinical manifestations are often those at distant sites following systemic absorption and dissemination of the extremely potent diphtheria toxin. Having been one of the leading causes of pediatric mortality in Europe and the USA in the early twentieth century, a combination of improved social welfare and the introduction of mass immunization programs resulted in a dramatic decline in the incidence of diphtheria in resource rich countries by the 1980s (Table 28.19). However, a major resurgence occurred in the newly independent states of the former Soviet Union during the 1990s,[153] emphasizing the potential for rapid re-emergence of the disease in situations where overcrowding, lack of basic infrastructure, natural disasters and/or social unrest disrupt immunization programs and increase exposure to the organism.[154] Nowadays, diphtheria is encountered most frequently among children in South and Southeast Asia, where it remains endemic. Worldwide, more than 5000 deaths from the disease were reported in 2002.[155] Imported cases continue to occur in Europe, particularly among inadequately vaccinated travelers to or from the Indian subcontinent.[156–158]

Table 28.19 Diphtheria – England and Wales

	Cases	Deaths
1920	69 481	5648
1930	74 043	3497
1940	44 281	2480
1950	962	49
1960	49	5
1970	22	3
1980	5	0

BACTERIOLOGY AND PATHOGENESIS

Corynebacterium diphtheriae is a nonmotile unencapsulated nonsporulating Gram positive bacillus. It grows readily on ordinary nutrient agar but is more easily identified by early growth on the nutritionally inadequate Loeffler's medium or on blood tellurite agar, on which growth of other throat organisms is inhibited. Conventionally, three biotypes (gravis, intermedius and mitis) are recognized on the basis of differences in colonial morphology, fermentation reactions and hemolytic potential. Toxin production, the major virulence factor of *C. diphtheriae*, depends on the presence of a lysogenic phage carrying the tox structural gene and is not related to biotype. Highly toxic strains may carry two or three tox+ genes inserted into the genome. Strains lacking the phage do not produce toxin, although conversion to toxigenicity by transfer of a tox+phage can occur. An immunoprecipitation assay was traditionally used to demonstrate toxigenicity of individual strains, but both PCR for the gene and rapid enzyme immunoassays for the toxin are now available.[159-161]

In the absence of toxin production, *C. diphtheriae* is not particularly invasive, usually remaining in the superficial layers of the respiratory mucosa and inducing only a mild inflammatory reaction. The toxin, a 58 kDa polypeptide, consists of two fragments; fragment B binds to specific receptors on susceptible cells allowing fragment A to enter the cell and catalyze the inactivation of elongation factor 2, thereby inhibiting protein synthesis and leading to cell death.[162] At the site of infection, local toxin production induces tissue necrosis and the formation of a dense, necrotic mass of fibrin, leukocytes, dead epithelial cells and organisms, closely adherent to the underlying mucosa (Fig. 28.18). Attempts to remove this 'pseudomembrane' often result in bleeding from the edematous submucosal layers. Systemically absorbed toxin can affect all organs in the body, but the major clinical consequences generally involve the heart, kidneys and nervous system. Renal involvement is seen in persons with massive toxin absorption, most of whom die within the first week of illness. In contrast there is often a latent period before cardiac and neurological complications become apparent. The severity of these late complications usually reflects the severity of the initial infection and the extent of the membrane.

Reports of endocarditis and osteomyelitis caused by invasive nontoxigenic strains indicate that other virulence factors may exist.[163,164] A related microorganism, *Corynebacterium ulcerans*, is also able to produce diphtheria toxin and has occasionally been isolated from patients with otherwise classical diphtheria, as well as from individuals with milder symptoms.[165,166]

CLINICAL MANIFESTATIONS

Acute disease

The incubation period is typically between 2 and 5 days. The clinical manifestations depend on the site of the primary infection, the immunization status of the host, and the degree to which systemic absorption of toxin has occurred. The disease is conveniently classified into several clinical phenotypes according to the site of primary infection.

Nasal diphtheria is characterized by a serosanguinous or seropurulent nasal discharge associated with a subtle membrane inside the nostrils, and sometimes excoriation of the external nares and upper lip.

If the infection is limited to the anterior nares, the acute illness is often mild, absorption of toxin is limited and systemic complications rare.

Faucial diphtheria is usually a more severe presentation. Anorexia, malaise, sore throat and low grade fever are followed after one or two days by the development of membrane, typically on one or both tonsils, extending variously up to the uvula and soft palate or down to the larynx and trachea and compromising the patency of the airway. Local soft tissue edema and lymphadenitis give rise to the 'bull-neck' appearance seen in severe cases (Fig. 28.19). The extent of the membrane correlates with the severity of the bull-neck, the degree of airway obstruction and the signs of acute systemic toxicity. In very severe cases massive toxin absorption occurs resulting in cardiac and respiratory collapse, renal failure and death within a few days. However, with appropriate treatment and good supportive care the membrane sloughs off after 5–7 days and the patient recovers from the local infection, although remaining at risk of the delayed toxin-mediated problems.

Laryngeal involvement generally represents downward extension of the membrane from the pharynx and is correspondingly severe. In some cases the membrane extends to involve the whole of the tracheo-bronchial tree and death is virtually inevitable. Occasionally, however, isolated laryngeal disease occurs and the membrane is limited to the larynx alone; hoarseness, a brassy cough, and rapidly progressive stridor and respiratory distress develop after a short prodromal illness. Relief of the airway obstruction by emergency tracheostomy provides dramatic relief and late complications are unusual as absorption of toxin tends to be limited in such cases.

Cutaneous, ocular, aural and genital diphtheria may all occur, but are rarely associated with significant toxin-mediated disease. The indolent ulcers of cutaneous diphtheria are common in the tropics and may serve as a reservoir for the organism, whilst at the same time inducing good immunity in the host. Cutaneous diphtheria is also seen among alcoholics, the indigent and the homeless in resource rich countries.[167,168]

Late complications

Characteristically cardiac complications become evident during the second, or occasionally third, weeks of illness and are often insidious in onset. ECG abnormalities such as subtle ST–T wave changes, increased rates of ectopy and/or first-degree heart block are detectable in many patients, but clinical dysfunction is apparent in only 10–25%.[169-171] In these patients, the initial ECG abnormalities tend to progress to more complex conduction abnormalities, notably complete heart block, as clinical myocarditis develops. Findings at this stage include profound bradycardia, diminished heart sounds, a gallop rhythm, and varying degrees of congestive failure. A hypotensive low output state is a very poor prognostic sign, usually associated with major conduction disturbances, and suggests extensive myocardial damage. Ventricular and supraventricular tachyarrhythmias may also occur and are often fatal.

Neurological complications occur in around 10–20% of patients overall. Bulbar involvement is sometimes seen during the first or second week, although minor dysfunction can be difficult to identify in children during the acute stage. In general neurological symptoms are identified later, usually arising between the third and eighth weeks of illness. In some cases there may be a biphasic course with initial partial recovery

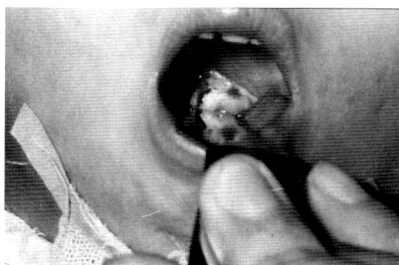

Fig. 28.18 Typical 'pseudomembrane' in a child with faucial diphtheria.

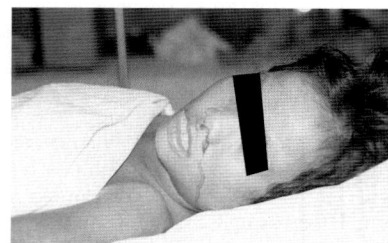

Fig. 28.19 Severe diphtheria showing brawny erythematous swelling of the neck (bull-neck) and serosanguinous nasal discharge.

from early bulbar symptoms, followed by late secondary deterioration with bulbar and peripheral manifestations.[172] The early symptoms are likely due to local effects of toxin on the nerve endings in bulbar muscles, while the later effects reflect systemic absorption and dispersion of the toxin. The neurological manifestations are typically bilateral and motor rather than sensory, and electrophysiological studies indicate an underlying demyelinating process. Difficulty in swallowing with nasal regurgitation due to palatal paralysis is often the first symptom, followed by ocular and other cranial nerve palsies, and later a peripheral polyneuropathy similar to but usually more severe than Guillain–Barré syndrome.[173] If diaphragmatic or respiratory muscle paralysis occurs, the course may be severe and prolonged.

DIAGNOSIS

The diagnosis of diphtheria should be made on the basis of clinical findings, without waiting for laboratory confirmation, since any delay in treatment may have serious consequences. Definitive diagnosis relies upon isolation of the organism; swabs should be obtained urgently and the microbiology service informed of the possibility of diphtheria so that appropriate cultures can be set up and tests for toxigenicity performed.

Differential diagnoses include infectious mononucleosis, herpetic tonsillitis, Vincent's angina, streptococcal pharyngitis and blood dyscrasias. In resource rich countries where diphtheria is a rarity it may easily be missed, and a high index of suspicion is required, particularly in patients without adequate immunization cover and in those who have recently visited an area endemic for diphtheria.

MANAGEMENT

Neutralization of free toxin with diphtheria antitoxin is the most important aspect of management. The antitoxin is only effective before the toxin enters cells so prompt administration is critical. Empirical dosage recommendations are given in Table 28.20.[174] As the antiserum is raised in horses, after preliminary sensitivity testing with 0.1 ml of a 1:1000 dilution of antitoxin, a single dose should be given to try to avoid sensitization. Facilities for resuscitation must be available, even in the absence of a reaction to the test dose.

Antibiotic therapy should be given to eliminate the organism and prevent spread, with penicillin probably the antibiotic of choice. Erythromycin may be more effective at preventing carriage but some resistant clinical isolates have been identified.[175] Parenteral treatment (benzylpenicillin 25 000–50 000 units/kg/d, or erythromycin 40–50 mg/kg/d for those with a history of penicillin allergy) should be started immediately, changing to oral therapy as the patient improves. Treatment should be continued for 10–14 days and the patient should be barrier nursed until eradication of the organism has been confirmed by culture of appropriate swabs. The disease is notifiable and all suspected cases should be reported immediately to the relevant authority so that measures can be taken to minimize the likelihood of spread.

Good supportive care is also critical. Emergency tracheostomy may be lifesaving in children with severe airway obstruction. However, endotracheal intubation should be avoided unless absolutely necessary in case part of the membrane becomes dislodged and obstructs the lower airways. Ventilatory support is not usually required except in those with extensive pulmonary involvement or those with respiratory failure due to neurological dysfunction. A short course of corticosteroids is often given to patients with 'bull-neck' or upper airway obstruction in order to reduce local edema.

Patients recovering from moderate to severe local disease should be kept on strict bed rest for a minimum of 2 weeks until cardiac involvement has been excluded. Careful clinical examination and regular ECG and echocardiographic monitoring allow early detection of conduction disturbances and impending myocarditis.[176] Patients who develop mild to moderate cardiac failure but maintain normal blood pressure can usually be managed successfully with bed rest, oxygen, diuretics and ACE inhibitors. However, recovery may take many weeks and occasional patients are left with permanent conduction abnormalities. Steroids have not been shown to be of benefit for treatment or prevention of myocarditis, although the number of patients involved in formal research studies has been limited.[177]

The prognosis for patients developing severe conduction disturbances depends largely on the severity of the overall myocardial involvement. Profound bradyarrhythmias are usually associated with major heart muscle disease; if a low output state with hypotension and renal compromise develops, the response to cardiac pacing and/or inotropic agents is poor and the outlook is bleak.[178] Cardiac pacing may be helpful in those with significant conduction abnormalities in whom a reasonable stroke volume is maintained.[179] However, in some such cases the conduction disturbance resolves without intervention after a few days.

Later still, patients with severe neurological involvement may require assisted ventilation and nutritional support for prolonged periods, together with physiotherapy, treatment for nosocomial infections as they arise, and eventually rehabilitation.

PROGNOSIS

Before the introduction of antitoxin, antibiotics and routine immunization, the prognosis was grave, with mortality rates of 30–50%. Currently mortality rates of around 5–10% are usual,[180] with the majority of deaths in those with overwhelming disease at presentation or those who develop myocarditis. If antitoxin is administered within the first 72 h severe disease and death are rare.

PREVENTION

Humans are the only known reservoir for *C. diphtheriae*. The principal modes of spread are by respiratory droplets from acute cases or asymptomatic carriers, or by direct contact with infected skin lesions. Immunization with diphtheria toxoid (formalin inactivated toxin) is very effective at protecting against the effects of the toxin, but does not prevent infection with the organism. Before the vaccine era diphtheria was predominantly a disease of the young and most people acquired natural life-long immunity through repeated exposure to the organism during childhood. Vaccine induced immunity wanes gradually over time, however, and during the recent resurgence of diphtheria in the former Soviet Union many adults acquired the disease and mortality was high in this group.[181]

The standard schedule for routine immunization should include a minimum of 3 doses of the triple vaccine (DTP) early in the first year of life, with a DTP booster at school entry, and a further booster at school

Table 28.20   Dosage of antitoxin recommended for various types of diphtheria

Type of diphtheria	Dosage (units)	Route
Nasal	10 000–20 000	Intramuscular
Tonsillar	15 000–25 000	Intramuscular or intravenous
Pharyngeal or laryngeal	20 000–40 000	Intramuscular or intravenous
Combined types or delayed diagnosis	40 000–60 000	Intravenous
Severe diphtheria, e.g. with extensive membrane and/or severe edema (bull-neck diphtheria)	40 000–100 000	Intravenous or part intravenous and part intramuscular

leaving using the low dose adult vaccine (usually as Td). Supplementary boosters should be given to high-risk groups including health care workers, travelers to endemic areas, alcoholics and the homeless, and periodic boosters for the general population may become routine in the future. Patients suffering from diphtheria should receive active immunization after recovery, since clinical disease may not induce adequate antitoxin levels.

BACTERIAL INFECTIONS: *ESCHERICHIA COLI*

Escherichia coli was first described by Theodore Escherich in 1885. It is a Gram negative, non-spore-forming, fimbriate bacillus which is motile by means of flagella (Fig. 28.20). Although *E. coli* is responsible for the vast majority of human infections there are four other species in the genus, *E. blattae, E. vulneris, E. fergusonii* and *E. hermannii. E. blattae* is an intestinal commensal of cockroaches and does not cause human infection, but the other three have been described as rare opportunists. In contrast *E. coli* is a major pathogen, both primary (Table 28.21) and opportunist. It is also the major aerobic Gram negative rod found in the human (and other animals) gastrointestinal tract at a concentration of approximately 10^8 colony forming units (cfu) per gram. It can be found in soil and water, but this is invariably a result of fecal contamination.

The complete genome sequences of both *E. coli* K12 (a nonpathogenic laboratory strain) and *E. coli* O157 are available.[182,183] *E. coli* K12 encodes some 4405 genes on a large circular chromosome of 4639 kilobase pairs. *E. coli* O157, which causes hemorrhagic colitis and hemolytic uremic syndrome (HUS), has a larger genome with 1387 new genes encoded in clusters or islands not found in *E. coli* K12. *E. coli* K12 and *E. coli* O157 share a common backbone but diverged some 4.5 million years ago.[184] Most of the differences result from acquisition of islands of genes. These islands encode pathogenicity determinants (pathogenicity islands),

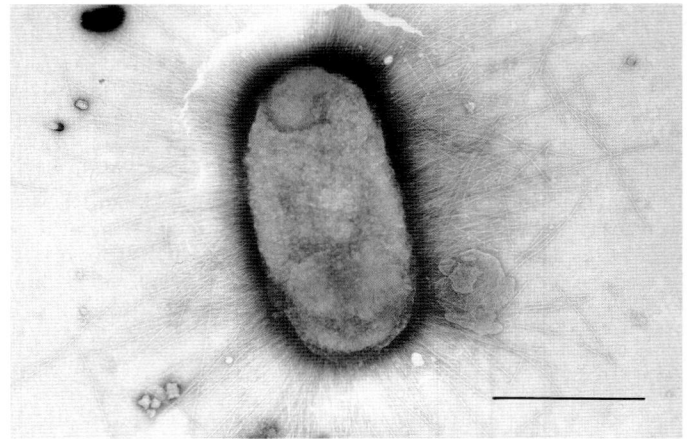

Fig. 28.20 Negative stain electron micrograph of *Escherichia coli* showing numerous fimbriae.

metabolic functions (metabolic islands) and several pro-phages (bacterial viruses whose genome has been incorporated into the bacterial chromosome). Other pathogenic *E. coli* such as enteropathogenic *E. coli* (EPEC), uropathogenic P-fimbriate *E. coli* (PFEC) and the neonatal pathogen *E. coli* K1 also encode different pathogenicity islands in their genomes.

EPIDEMIOLOGY

E. coli is subdivided into a large number of serotypes based on O- or somatic (on lipopolysaccharide on the outer membrane of the bacterium) antigens, H- or flagellar antigens and K- or capsular antigens. There are

Table 28.21 *Escherichia coli* as a primary pathogen

	Serogroups	Pathogenicity determinants	Infection sites	Disease associations
Gastrointestinal tract				
Enterotoxigenic *E. coli* (ETEC)	O6, O8, O5, O20, O25, O128, O139, O148, O153, O159	CFA (pili), heat labile (LT) and heat stable (ST) toxins	Small bowel	Secretory diarrhea in travelers and children in resource limited countries
Enteroinvasive *E. coli* (EIEC)	O28, O29, O124, O136, O143	*Ipa* pathogenicity island on plasmid *ial*, adhesin	Large bowel	Mild dysentery in children in resource limited countries
Enteropathogenic *E. coli* (EPEC)	O55, O86, O111, O119, O125, O126, O127, O128, O142	Locus of enterocyte effacement pathogenicity island (LEE), *tir, eae*	Small and large bowel	Acute and chronic diarrhea in neonates and infants in resource limited countries
Enterohemorrhagic *E. coli* (EHEC)	O26, O111, O128, O157	*eae*A, *eae*B, shigatoxins 1 & 2	Large bowel	Hemorrhagic colitis, hemolytic uremic syndrome, encephalopathy
Enteroaggregative *E. coli* (EaggEC)	O44, O111, O121 but most are nongroupable	Adhesin, EAST-1	Small and large bowel	Acute and chronic diarrhea in children and travelers
Diffuse adhering *E. coli* (DAEC)	O75 but most are nongroupable	Adhesins	Unknown	Perhaps a cause of diarrheal disease
Urinary tract				
P-fimbriate *E. coli* (PFEC)	O1, O2, O3, K1	P-fimbriae (adhesions) encoded on a pathogenicity island	Urinary tract, septicemia	Cystitis, pyelonephritis
S-fimbriate *E. coli* (SFEC)	O1, O2, O3	S-fimbriae (adhesins)	Urinary tract, septicemia	Cystitis, pyelonephritis
Neonatal meningitis and bacteremia				
E. coli K1	O1, O2, O3, K1	K1 capsule plus pathogenicity island function unclear	Urinary tract, meninges, septicemia	Urinary tract infection, meningitis, septicemia

167 different O-serogroups and at least 82 K-antigens.[185] Serogrouping is of importance not just for epidemiological purposes but also delineation of pathogenicity. However, a number of molecular biological techniques provide more accurate epidemiological and pathogenicity related markers. These include techniques for whole genome analysis such as pulsed field gel electrophoresis (PFGE) of macrorestricted chromosomal DNA,[186] analysis of housekeeping genes (multilocus sequence testing; MLST) or of insertion sequence distribution (eubacterial repetitive intergenic consensus sequences; ERICS). E. coli can also be divided into four main phylogenetic groups by analysis of two genes (chuA, yjaA) and an anonymous DNA fragment.[187] Most virulent extra-intestinal strains belong to group B2 and to a lesser extent group D, whereas most commensal strains are in group A.

E. coli is part of the normal flora of most mammalian species. For example, E. coli O157 is excreted asymptomatically by cattle but can be transferred to humans as a 'food-poisoning' to cause hemorrhagic colitis, HUS and encephalopathy. The uropathogenic PFEC and the neonatal pathogen E. coli K1 colonize the gastrointestinal tract[188] thence reaching their infective sites by ascending the urinary tract and by hematogenous spread respectively. In addition the commensal E. coli that do not possess defined pathogenicity determinants are important opportunist pathogens, for example after gastrointestinal surgery or in patients with indwelling urinary catheters. Finally the commensal E. coli are an important reservoir of antibiotic resistance genes that can be transferred to more pathogenic bacteria.[189]

Enteropathogens

Enterotoxigenic E. coli (ETEC) are solely human pathogens, although similar bacteria can cause diarrheal disease in domestic animals. They cause up to 25% of cases of diarrheal disease in children in resource limited countries and are a major cause of traveler's diarrhea (c. 80% of cases). Infection is usually acquired via food or water contaminated with human excreta. The infective dose is high (c. 10^7 cfu). Enteroinvasive E. coli (EIEC) are a minor cause of diarrheal disease, in most surveys being responsible for less than 5% of cases in children in the tropics. Enteropathogenic E. coli (EPEC) were responsible for epidemics of infantile diarrhea in the UK and the USA in the 1940s and 1950s but are now found predominantly in neonates and infants in resource limited countries (in one study causing 11% of cases of infantile diarrhea). The infective dose is low (< 10^4 cfu) so direct person-to-person spread is also possible.

Enterohemorrhagic E. coli (EHEC) are most often acquired as food poisoning, but since the infective dose is low (< 10^2 cfu), person-to-person spread in households and hospitals has been described. Enteroaggregative E. coli (EaggEC) are the most recently described group and are responsible for cases of acute and chronic diarrhea in children and traveler's diarrhea. They are particularly associated with chronic diarrhea in children in resource limited countries. The infective dose is unknown. It is still unclear what role diffuse adhering E. coli (DAEC) play in diarrheal disease and little is known of their epidemiology.

Uropathogens

Most E. coli causing urinary tract infection fall into serogroups O1, O2, O4, O6 and O75, have thick capsules and express adhesins. Of particular importance are PFEC which bind to the P-blood group receptor. They colonize the intestine and, in females, the vagina, perineum and anterior urethra. From there they ascend to produce cystitis and pyelonephritis.

Neonatal sepsis

E. coli K1 is responsible for 40% of the cases of neonatal bacteremia and 75% of the cases of neonatal meningitis that are due to E. coli. The incidence rate of E. coli neonatal meningitis in the USA is 1 case per 1000 live births. Infection is acquired from mother-to-baby at birth or baby-to-baby and staff-to-baby in neonatal intensive care units. Approximately 50% of women of childbearing age have intestinal carriage of E. coli K1 and 70% of neonates born to carrier mothers will acquire carriage. The colonization to disease ratio is approximately 200–300 to 1.

PATHOGENESIS

Enteropathogens

ETEC cause a non-inflammatory, secretory, small intestinal diarrhea. To do this they must colonize the upper small intestine by adhering to enterocytes using fimbriae (protein spikes) termed colonization factor antigens (CFA) in human ETECs. In addition they secrete one or both of heat labile (LT) and heat stable (ST) toxins. The LTs (I and II) are subunit toxins. They consist of five (toxophore) B subunits that carry and bind the toxin to ganglioside receptors on the enterocyte surface and one A (toxin) subunit. The A subunit is activated by cleavage to A1 which activates adenosine diphosphate (ADP) ribosylation of a regulatory subunit of adenyl cyclase. This results in activation of adenyl cyclase and raised intra-enterocyte concentrations of cyclic adenosine monophosphate (AMP). This results in fluid and electrolyte secretion into the small intestinal lumen, and thus a voluminous watery diarrhea. LTI is very similar to cholera toxin. ST (a and b) are smaller (16–18 amino acids) and activate guanylate cyclase by mimicking guanylin, the endogenous modulator of cyclic guanosine monophosphate (GMP) signaling. How raised intracellular cyclic GMP levels induce diarrhea is unclear. EIEC cause colitis and an inflammatory diarrhea. They have similarity with Shigella spp. in that similar pathogenicity genes (on a pathogenicity island) are encoded as large plasmids in both genera. They attach to and invade colonic enterocytes (Fig. 28.21). They can then migrate laterally from colonocyte to colonocyte. How this causes colonocyte death, loss of mucous membrane integrity and an inflammatory response is unclear, but the initial stages might involve induction of colonocyte apoptosis.

EPEC produce specific ultrastructural lesions on the enterocyte surface, termed attaching effacement, in which there is very close intimate attachment of the bacteria to the enterocyte surface with local loss of the microvilli (brush border) (Fig. 28.22). Although this lesion can be detected throughout the gastrointestinal tract it is the effect on the small intestine that is most important. EPEC initially adhere to the enterocyte surface by means of bundle forming pili. This then activates a chromosomal pathogenicity island called the locus of enterocyte effacement (LEE) which assembles a type III secretion system. Through this, the bacterium injects effector molecules into the enterocyte. One is Tir (transferable intimin receptor) which inserts into the enterocyte membrane and acts as a receptor for a molecule (intimin) on the bacterial surface thus promoting intimate attachment of the bacterium to the enterocyte. Other effectors cause damage to the microfilaments of the terminal web causing loss of the microvilli (termed effacement). This causes a great loss of surface area for absorption and of the brush border disaccharidases sucrase, maltase and lactase, and leads to malabsorption and an osmotic diarrhea.

EHEC such as E. coli O157 have a pathogenicity island very similar to the EPEC LEE but their attaching effacement is confined to the

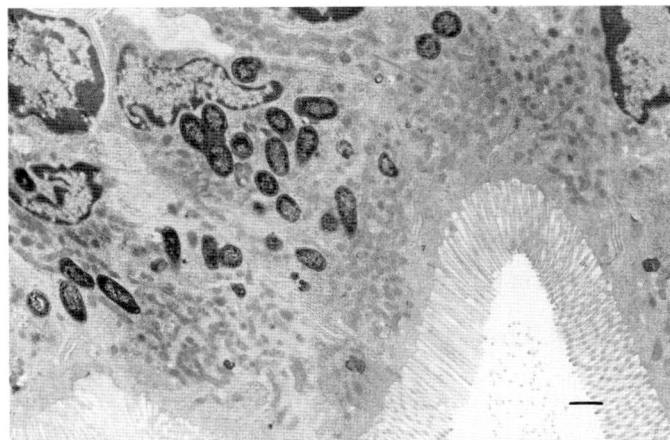

Fig. 28.21   Thin section electron micrograph of colonic enterocytes with numerous enteroinvasive Escherichia coli in the cytoplasm.

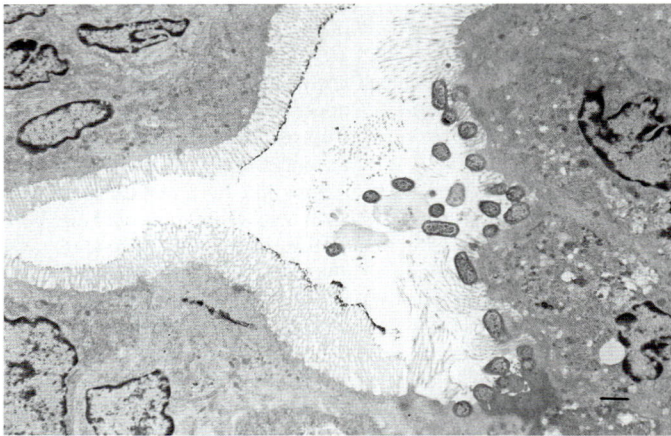

Fig. 28.22 Thin section electron micrograph showing enteropathogenic *Escherichia coli* closely adherent to duodenal enterocytes with loss of microvilli (attaching effacement).

terminal ileum and colon. In addition they elaborate Shiga toxins (ST) 1 and/or 2 (previously known as verocytoxins). These are subunit toxins with five B (toxophore) units and one A (toxin) unit. The B units carry, protect, and bind the A subunit to the enterocyte utilizing a globoside glycolipid receptor. The A subunit inhibits protein synthesis and is one of the most potent toxins known. ST-1 is identical to Shiga toxin and both it and ST-2 are encoded on promiscuous bacteriophages. This means that these toxin genes are widely distributed in enteric bacteria, but in order to produce disease, *E. coli* must have both LEE and ST. ST kills colonocytes causing hemorrhagic colitis. If ST enters the circulation it binds to receptors on endothelial cells, in particular in the renal vasculature. This causes fibrin deposition, cell swelling and narrowing of the lumen of the vessel, and results in a microangiopathic hemolytic uremia or HUS.

EaggEC are so called because they produce a 'stacked brick' appearance when adherent to cells in culture and each other. They adhere to both small and large intestinal mucosa by means of plasmid-encoded fimbriae (AAF/I, AAF/II). They elaborate toxins including EaggEC heat stable toxin-1 (EAST-1) which resembles ETEC ST and a plasmid encoded toxin (Pet) which induces mucin release, exfoliation of cells and crypt abscesses. Recently it has been shown that a novel flagellin from EaggEC induces the release of the inflammatory chemokine IL-8 from intestinal epithelial cells.

PFEC have two pathogenicity islands in their genome which encode expression of fimbriae with a receptor binding molecule at their tip which recognizes the P-blood group antigen. This is a glycolipid with terminal digalactose residues and is expressed on most tissues including the epithelium of the urinary tract. Thus the bacteria are able to adhere and resist the flushing action of urine. How they induce inflammation is less clear but probably involves induction of cytokine and chemokine release.

E. coli K1 produces a thick capsule that allows it to evade the killing effects of neutrophils and complement. It, like the group B meningococcal capsule, is a homopolymer of N-acetyl neuraminic acid which is a self-antigen being expressed on neuronal tissue in particular. Further pathogenicity determinants are gradually being uncovered.

CLINICAL FEATURES

The clinical features associated with enteropathic *E. coli* are outlined in Table 28.21. For a more detailed description of this and of urinary tract infections and neonatal sepsis, see the appropriate sections.

DIAGNOSIS AND DIFFERENTIAL DIAGNOSIS
Enteropathogens

For definitive diagnosis, *E. coli* must be isolated from fecal samples. Although O-serogrouping was the method originally used to describe the different pathogenic types it is of little value except in outbreaks. For specific diagnosis, the pathogenicity genes or their products must be detected. This is most conveniently done by polymerase chain reaction (PCR) and a number of multiplex PCR systems have been described although none is commercially available.

Uropathogens and neonatal sepsis

Standard microbiological procedures are used to isolate *E. coli* from urine, blood or CSF. It is possible to demonstrate PFEC or *E. coli* K1 using specific antisera, although this is not entirely necessary.

TREATMENT, PROGNOSIS AND PREVENTION
Enteropathogens

In general, diarrheal disease should be managed by assessment of dehydration and appropriate rehydration. Antimicrobial therapy is not normally indicated and in some cases, for example with *E. coli* O157, might be harmful. However, some infections with EPEC and EaggEC can produce persistent diarrhea and in such cases antimicrobial chemotherapy directed by in vitro sensitivity testing is appropriate.

The prognosis is good with full recovery without antibiotic therapy in most cases. There are no vaccines currently available, so good hygiene and recognition of risk are the mainstay of infection prevention both in hospital and the community.

Uropathogens

For uncomplicated infections, short course (3–5 days) antimicrobial chemotherapy will suffice. If complicated by pyelonephritis or septicemia, longer duration of treatment will be needed. For prognosis, prevention and follow-up, see the appropriate section on urinary tract infection.

Neonatal sepsis

For pre-emptive, empiric therapy, see the section on neonatal sepsis. This will need to be modified in the light of the local antimicrobial susceptibility patterns. No vaccine is available, especially since the K1 capsule is a self-antigen.

BACTERIAL INFECTIONS: *HAEMOPHILUS INFLUENZAE*

GENERAL FEATURES AND EPIDEMIOLOGY

Haemophilus influenzae was first reported by Pfeiffer in 1892. A small Gram negative bacterium, it may be encapsulated or non-encapsulated (nontypable). In 1931 Pitmann[190] described six antigenically distinct capsular types, designated a to f. The possession of the capsule is an important virulence determinant and it is *H. influenzae* of capsular serotype b (Hib) that stands out as the most virulent strain, responsible for the great majority of invasive *Haemophilus* infections. Prior to the widespread use of effective vaccines against Hib, it was the major cause of bacterial meningitis and the predominant cause of epiglottitis in young children. In the Oxford region between 1985 and 1990 for example, the incidence of all invasive Hib disease was 36 cases/100 000 children < 5 years old.[191] Table 28.22 summarizes several characteristics relating to carriage and pathogenicity.

H. influenzae is among the bacteria normally found in the human pharynx and also colonizes the mucosae of the conjunctiva and genital tracts. Spread from one individual to another occurs by airborne droplets or by direct transfer of secretions. Exposure begins during or immediately after birth so that from infancy onwards, carriage of one or more strains for periods lasting from days to months is common. The presence of *H. influenzae* in cultures obtained from the upper (but not the lower) respiratory tract is therefore a common and normal finding. In about 3–5% of individuals, the organisms are encapsulated, most often with the serotype b antigen (in an unvaccinated population). Following widespread vaccination, however, carriage of type b strains has declined. In general, carriers of *H. influenzae*, whether colonized

Table 28.22 Carriage and pathogenicity of *Haemophilus influenzae*

Strains	Common upper respiratory tract carriage rates	Principal manifestation of pathogenicity
Non-encapsulated (nontypable)	50–80%	Exacerbations of chronic bronchitis, otitis media, sinusitis, conjunctivitis, lower respiratory tract infections Bacteremic infections rare
Encapsulated, type	2–4% b (pre-vaccine)	Meningitis, epiglottitis, pneumonia and empyema, septic arthritis, cellulitis, osteomyelitis, pericarditis, bacteremia
Encapsulated, types a and c through f	1–2%	Rarely incriminated as pathogens. May cause bacteremia and meningitis

with encapsulated or nontypable organisms, remain healthy, but occasionally disease occurs. Two contrasting patterns of *H. influenzae* disease can be identified. The more serious in its consequences is invasive infections such as meningitis, septic arthritis, epiglottitis and cellulitis; these infections typically occur in young children, are associated with bacteremia and are caused by encapsulated type b strains. The second category includes less serious, but numerically more common infections that occur as a result of contiguous spread of *H. influenzae* within the respiratory tract. *H. influenzae* is a common cause of otitis media (accounting for 23% of bacteria isolated by tympanocentesis),[192] sinusitis, conjunctivitis and lower respiratory tract infection. These infections are usually, but not invariably, caused by nontypable strains. These generalizations are not hard and fast; nontypable strains are a cause of neonatal sepsis, as well as sepsis and meningitis in infants and children.[193] They are a common cause of severe, acute lower respiratory tract infections (often accompanied by bacteremia) among young children living in resource limited countries[194] and are responsible for about 50% of all *H. influenzae* causing invasive disease in adults.[195] Epiglottitis, however, appears to be a syndrome associated overwhelmingly with serotype b. Brazilian purpuric fever is a rare disease caused by a nontypable *H. influenzae*, biotype *aegyptius*. This occurs in young children who present initially with a conjunctivitis and go on to develop a serious, potentially fatal form of septicemia which can mimic meningococcemia.

PATHOGENESIS

The host and microbial determinants of colonization by *H. influenzae* are poorly understood. In animal experiments infection is potentiated by viruses such as influenza. Adhesins facilitate attachment to mucus and to human epithelial cells and there are cell wall components that inhibit the normal ciliary function of respiratory tract epithelium. The primacy of type b capsule as a crucial factor in the pathogenesis of invasive disease has been well established. Lipopolysaccharide is also important in facilitating bloodstream survival and blood–brain barrier damage in experimental infections. In rat and primate models of *H. influenzae* type b meningitis, organisms were found to invade the submucosa of the nasopharynx and to reach the meninges as a result of bacteremia rather than by direct penetration of contiguous structures such as the cribriform plate or the inner ear. The occurrence of meningitis correlated strikingly with the duration and intensity of bacteremia; experimental manipulation of the host factors that decrease the efficiency of intravascular clearance (e.g. splenectomy) increased the incidence of meningitis.[196]

IMMUNITY

Among the host factors governing susceptibility to invasive type b infection, the role of serum antibodies to polyribosyl-ribitol phosphate (PRP), the type b capsular antigen, has been shown to be critical. Serum anti-PRP antibodies in conjunction with complement-mediated bactericidal and opsonic activity mediate protective immunity against systemic infections in humans. The sera of newborns and young infants (up until about 3 months old) generally have sufficient amounts of passively acquired antibody to afford protection. Thereafter, the natural decline of these maternally derived antibodies is followed by a period lasting until the age of 2–4 years when the levels of antibody are inadequate to provide protection. The delay in the acquisition of serum anti-PRP antibodies is characteristic of children less than 2 years old and is a major reason for the high attack rates of *H. influenzae* b invasive disease in early infancy. Although some infants may be exposed to type b *H. influenzae* through nasopharyngeal carriage, the antigenic stimulus for these antibodies may also be different commensal bacteria or ingested foods, which immunize through their cross-reacting antigens.

In an infant rat colonization model, anti-PRP antibodies given intranasally are able to prevent nasopharyngeal colonization by Hib. The same effect is seen when these antibodies are given intraperitoneally and a minimum effective serum level can be defined.[197] If it is assumed that anti-PRP antibodies function in a similar manner on the oropharyngeal mucosa of human children, both serum-derived IgG and locally produced IgA may reduce Hib carriage and thereby protect against invasive disease. A clinical study has correlated protection against carriage of *H. influenzae* b in infants with vaccine-induced serum anti-PRP IgG antibodies of greater than or equal to 5 mcg/ml.[198]

CLINICAL FEATURES

Meningitis is the most serious manifestation of invasive infection due to *H. influenzae* b. Antecedent symptoms of upper respiratory infection are common. The most common signs are fever and altered behavior – including poor feeding, vomiting, irritability and drowsiness. Thus, none of these clinical features distinguishes the child with *H. influenzae* meningitis from several other infectious diseases or other forms of meningitis. In particular, young infants have few specific signs; nuchal rigidity and a bulging fontanelle are typical, but often absent, early in the course of established meningeal infection. Seizures, cranial nerve involvement and coma may develop as the disease progresses and the effects of raised intracranial pressure, cerebral edema and vasculitis prevail. Subdural effusions are common but these very rarely require specific management and are usually sterile. Overall mortality for *H. influenzae* meningitis is less than 5% in resource rich countries but significantly higher, ranging from 22 to 40%, in resource limited countries. Sequelae occur in 15–30% of those who survive; the commonest complication is sensorineural deafness.

Acute respiratory obstruction caused by involvement of the supraglottic tissue by *H. influenzae* b (epiglottitis) is a potentially lethal disease of characteristically rapid onset. Typically, the child is aged 2–7 years and presents with sore throat, fever, dyspnea and dysphagia (causing pharyngeal pooling and then oral drooling of secretions). The child is restless and anxious and often adopts a characteristic posture in which the neck is extended and the chin is protruded in order to minimize airway obstruction. Abrupt deterioration leading to death within a few hours may occur if adequate treatment is not provided. The characteristic findings are supralaryngeal. The epiglottis is red and swollen and resembles a red cherry at the base of the tongue. Although an abrupt death is usually the result of acute airway obstruction, sudden collapse may result from less well defined mechanisms associated with acute toxemia. It should be emphasized that examination of the pharynx of a child in whom acute epiglottitis is suspected should only be attempted under conditions in which the airway can be secured immediately, otherwise the examination may precipitate respiratory arrest.

Invasive disease due to non-type-b encapsulated and nontypable *H. influenzae* is rarer but may present in a similar fashion. Presentation may also be similar in the rare group of children who develop invasive disease with *H. influenzae* b despite vaccination, 'vaccine failures'. In both groups, predisposing host factors such as immunodeficiency should be sought.[193,199]

Confirmation of the clinical impression of invasive *H. influenzae* infection depends upon cultures of normally sterile fluids (e.g. CSF, blood, pleural or synovial fluid). Positive nasopharyngeal cultures are not helpful since carriage is common among healthy persons. Needle aspiration of the middle ear (tympanocentesis), sinuses, the margins of an area of cellulitis or lung may occasionally prove helpful in selected cases, especially in a very sick child in whom no diagnosis has been established. Whenever practical, the results of Gram stain should be sought immediately; in up to 70% of cases of meningitis, CSF smears show the typical pleomorphic, Gram negative coccobacilli. Detection of capsular antigen in serum, CSF or concentrated urine by immunoassay (e.g. latex agglutination) may be useful, especially in children who have received prior antibiotic treatment. This test should be interpreted with caution, however, in those who have recently received Hib vaccine, as a false positive result is possible.

TREATMENT

Severe infections due to *H. influenzae* should be treated with parenteral third generation cephalosporins, for example cefotaxime or ceftriaxone. Ampicillin resistance has emerged among both encapsulated and nontypable strains (in the range of 10–30% for European and USA strains). Resistance is almost always mediated by beta-lactamases. This has particular relevance to the antibiotic management of less severe infections, such as otitis media and sinusitis. Although ampicillin/amoxicillin remains the antibiotic of choice, others such as amoxicillin–clavulanate or macrolides have become alternative first- and second-line choices.

The use of dexamethasone as adjunctive therapy in Hib meningitis can result in a reduction in sensorineural deafness.[200] Early administration, close to or even prior to the first dose of antibiotic, is preferable. Elective intubation and antibiotics are usually mandatory in cases of epiglottitis.

PREVENTION

Active immunization

The first generation of vaccines against Hib consisted of the purified type b polysaccharide. A trial in 1974 in Finland demonstrated efficacy in children older than 18 months of age but not in younger infants.[201] This led to the development of a second generation of vaccines in which the immunogenicity of PRP is enhanced by covalent linkage of the capsular polysaccharide or oligosaccharides to protein to form conjugate vaccines. Conjugate vaccines elicit significantly enhanced antibody responses when compared to PRP and, in contrast to the latter, are found to prime for a secondary antibody response. Clinical trials and national surveillance have confirmed their efficacy in infancy.[202] An unexpected outcome has been a reduction in Hib colonization of the upper respiratory tract and this has contributed to the near elimination of Hib disease in countries where immunization has become routine. Unfortunately, on a global scale too few countries have had the resources to use this vaccine for routine immunization. Experience from The Gambia[203] and Kenya[204] suggests that a dramatic effect on disease rates can be expected when vaccination is eventually implemented in all resource limited countries.

Children and adults who have an increased risk of invasive disease, e.g. those without spleens or with malignancy, should also receive *H. influenzae* b conjugate vaccines. These vaccines are safe and, in general, protective antibody responses are seen.

The burden of disease due to nontypable *H. influenzae* strains is also recognized and its prevention through vaccination is desirable. A recent study with an 11-valent pneumococcal polysaccharide–protein conjugate vaccine, in which the protein is protein D, a highly conserved cell surface lipoprotein of *H. influenzae*, has, for the first time, demonstrated efficacy against otitis media due to *H. influenzae*.[205]

Chemoprophylaxis

Young unimmunized or partially immunized children living in the same household as a case of invasive *H. influenzae* b disease are likely to be at significantly increased risk of secondary disease. In the pre-vaccine era secondary attack rates in household contacts were estimated to be 2–4% and in 'day-care centers' up to 1.3%. It is plausible that antibiotic prophylaxis could decrease this secondary attack rate. Rifampicin (20 mg/kg, maximum dose 600 mg/d), given orally once daily for 4 days, is effective in eradicating nasopharyngeal carriage. Treatment of household contacts (children and adults) where there are susceptible children less than 4 years old should be considered, as should treatment of such children in nurseries who are contacts of a case. The course of Hib vaccines should also be completed. The index case should also receive rifampicin prior to discharge unless he or she has been treated with a third generation cephalosporin.

BACTERIAL INFECTIONS: LEPROSY

EPIDEMIOLOGY

Worldwide, 4 million individuals have or are disabled by leprosy. The incidence, however, remains stable at around 450 000 new cases annually with high rates of childhood cases. India dominates the global picture with 67% of the global caseload. Few childhood cases are seen in Europe and North America, but in India childhood cases comprise at least 17% of the new case detection. In the UK, all new leprosy cases acquired their infection abroad. Average incubation times of 2–5 years and 8–12 years have been calculated for tuberculoid and lepromatous cases respectively. Age, sex, household contact and BCG vaccination are important determinants of leprosy risk. Leprosy incidence reaches a peak at age 10–11 years, and equal numbers of male and female cases are seen until puberty, after which there is an excess of male cases. Improved socioeconomic conditions, extended schooling and good housing reduce the risk of leprosy. HIV infection is not a risk factor for leprosy but may worsen leprosy nerve damage, and leprosy has been reported presenting as an immune reconstitution syndrome in adults treated for HIV.

MICROBIOLOGY AND PATHOLOGY

Leprosy is caused by *Mycobacterium leprae*, an acid-fast, intracellular organism that has the longest doubling time of all known bacteria (12 days) and cannot be cultivated on artificial media. *M. leprae* is a hardy organism, retaining viability for 5 months drying in the shade. The optimum temperature for growth is 27–30 °C, which corresponds with the clinical observation of maximal *M. leprae* growth at cool superficial sites (skin, nasal mucosa and peripheral nerves). The *M. leprae* 3.27 Mb genome has been sequenced. Less than half the genome contains functional genes: 165 genes are unique to *M. leprae*, but functions can be attributed to only 29. *M. leprae* has lost many genes for carbon catabolism and many carbon sources (e.g. acetate and galactose) are unavailable to it. The genome sequence is opening new possibilities for understanding the biological uniqueness of *M. leprae*.

Untreated lepromatous patients sneeze organisms into the environment. In Indonesia and Ethiopia, *M. leprae* DNA has been detected in nasal swabs in up to 5% of the population. After entry via the nose, *M. leprae* is inhaled, multiplies on the inferior turbinates and then has a brief bacteremic phase before binding to Schwann cells and macrophages. The skin is unimportant in leprosy transmission. Bacilli are not excreted by the skin and are rarely found in the epidermis. Untreated lepromatous leprosy mothers excrete *M. leprae* in their breast milk, but treatment renders the bacteria nonviable.

PATHOLOGY

There are four important aspects to the pathogenesis of leprosy: bacterial load, the host immune response, the nerve damage and immune-mediated reactions. Schwann cells and skin macrophages are infected early with granuloma formation. In established infection the host immune response determines not only the histological picture but also the clinical features of disease and the prognosis. The Ridley–Jopling spectrum describes the range of responses with tuberculoid and lepromatous poles. At the tuberculoid (TT) pole there is well-expressed cell-mediated immunity and delayed hypersensitivity control of bacillary multiplication, with formation of epithelioid cell granulomas. In the lepromatous (LL) form there is cellular anergy towards *M. leprae*, with abundant bacillary multiplication and unactivated macrophages. Between these two poles is a continuum, varying from the patient with moderate cell-mediated immunity (borderline tuberculoid, BT) through borderline (BB) to the patient with little cellular response, borderline lepromatous (BL).

Nerve damage occurs in small dermal nerves in skin lesions and peripheral nerve trunks. Acute immune-mediated reactions are serious complications because they cause nerve damage. Reversal reactions (type 1) are episodes of delayed hypersensitivity occurring at sites of localization of *M. leprae* antigens. Erythema nodosum leprosum (ENL) (type 2) reactions are due to immune complex deposition.

CLINICAL FEATURES

Patients commonly present with skin lesions, weakness or numbness due to a peripheral nerve lesion, or a burn or ulcer in an anesthetic hand or foot. Borderline patients may present with nerve pain, sudden palsy, multiple new skin lesions or pain in the eye. Childhood cases are frequently detected in school surveys or as household contacts of adult leprosy patients. In an Indian study based on a survey area, 30% of cases had a household contact with leprosy, usually a parent or grandparent.[206]

Cardinal signs
- Typical skin lesions, which are anesthetic at the tuberculoid end of the spectrum
- Thickened peripheral nerves
- Acid-fast bacilli on skin smears or biopsy.

Presenting symptoms
Early lesions
Indeterminate lesions are slightly hypopigmented or erythematous macules, a few centimeters in diameter, with poorly defined margins. Hair growth and nerve function are unimpaired. The indeterminate phase may last for months or years before resolving or developing into one of the determinate types of leprosy.

Skin
The commonest skin lesions are macules or plaques; more rarely papules and nodules are seen.

Anesthesia
Anesthesia may occur in skin lesions when dermal nerves are involved or in the distribution of a large peripheral nerve. In skin lesions, the small dermal sensory and autonomic nerve fibers supplying dermal and subcutaneous structures are damaged causing local sensory loss and loss of sweating within that area.

Peripheral neuropathy
Peripheral nerve trunks are vulnerable at sites where they are superficial or are in fibro-osseous tunnels. Damage to peripheral nerve trunks produces characteristic signs with dermatomal sensory loss and dysfunction of muscles supplied by that peripheral nerve. The sites of predilection for peripheral nerve involvement are ulnar (at the elbow), median (at the wrist), radial, radial cutaneous (at the wrist), common peroneal (at the knee), posterior tibial and sural nerves (at the ankle), facial nerve (on the zygomatic arch), and great auricular in the posterior triangle of the neck.

The leprosy spectrum
Classifying patients according to the Ridley–Jopling scale is clinically useful. Table 28.23 gives the skin and nerve features of disease across the spectrum. There is also a simpler field classification of paucibacillary/multibacillary (Table 28.24) which guides the length of treatment. BB disease is unstable, and BT leprosy may be associated with rapid, severe nerve damage. BL patients are at risk of both reversal and ENL reactions.

LL has an insidious onset. The earliest lesions are ill defined with shiny erythematous macules. Gradually the skin becomes infiltrated and thickened and nodules develop; facial skin thickening causes the characteristic leonine facies. Dermal nerves are destroyed and sensory loss develops in a glove and stocking distribution. Sweating is lost. Damage to peripheral nerves is symmetrical and occurs late in disease. Testicular atrophy results from diffuse infiltration and the acute orchitis that occurs with ENL reactions.

Most studies in childhood report all types of leprosy; incidence rates and proportion of lepromatous cases increase with age. Few children present under the age of 5 years.

Eye
Eye damage results from both nerve damage and bacillary invasion. Lagophthalmos results from paresis of the orbicularis oculi due to involvement of the facial (7th) nerve. Damage to the ophthalmic branch of the trigeminal (5th) nerve causes anesthesia of the cornea putting it at risk of ulceration. Invasion of the iris and ciliary body makes them extremely susceptible to reactions.

DIAGNOSIS

Leprosy should be considered as a possible diagnosis in anyone with peripheral nerve or skin lesions who has lived in a leprosy endemic area. The diagnosis is clinical and based on finding a cardinal sign of leprosy, supported by the finding of acid-fast bacilli on slit skin smears. Where resources permit, histological examination of a skin or nerve biopsy

Table 28.23 Major clinical features of the disease spectrum in leprosy

Classification	TT	BT	BB	BL	LL
Skin					
Infiltrated lesions	Defined plaques Healing centers	Irregular plaques Partially raised edges	Polymorphic Punched out centers	Papules, nodules	Diffuse thickening
Macular lesions	Single, small	Several, any size	Multiple, all sizes Geographic	Innumerable, small	Innumerable, confluent
Nerve					
Peripheral nerve	Solitary, enlarged nerves	Several nerves Asymmetrical	Many nerves Asymmetrical	Late neural thickening Asymmetrical anesthesia and paresis	Slow, symmetrical loss Glove and stocking anesthesia
Microbiology					
Bacterial index (0–6)	0–1	0–2	2–3	1–4	4–6

BB, borderline; BL, borderline lepromatous; BT, borderline tuberculoid; LL, lepromatous leprosy; TT, tuberculoid.

Table 28.24   Modified WHO recommended multidrug therapy regimens

| Type of leprosy | Drug treatment | | Duration of treatment |
	Monthly supervised	Daily self-administered	
Paucibacillary	Rifampicin 450 mg (or 10 mg/kg)	Dapsone 50 mg (or 1 mg/kg)	6 months
Multibacillary (MB)	Rifampicin 450 mg (or 10 mg/kg) Clofazimine 150 mg (or 3 mg/kg)	Clofazimine 50 mg (or 1.5 mg/kg) alternate days Dapsone 50 mg (or 1 mg/kg)	24 months
Paucibacillary single lesion	Rifampicin 450 mg, ofloxacin 200 mg, minocycline 50 mg (supplied in a single blister pack)		Single dose

WHO classification for field use when slit skin smears are not available:
- paucibacillary single lesion leprosy (one skin lesion);
- paucibacillary (2–5 skin lesions);
- multibacillary (more than five skin lesions).

In this field classification WHO recommends treatment of MB patients for 12 months only.

is ideal for accurate classification. Serological and polymerase chain reaction based diagnostic tests are not yet clinically useful.

Skin examination

The whole body should be inspected in a good light, otherwise lesions may be missed, particularly on the buttocks in borderline disease. Skin lesions should be tested for anesthesia.

Neurological examination

The peripheral nerves should be palpated systematically looking for enlargement and tenderness. Nerve function should be assessed by testing the small muscles of the hands and feet. Sensation on the hands and feet can be assessed and monitored using Semmes Weinsteinmonofilaments. These are now widely used in leprosy and diabetic clinics.

Slit skin smears

These should be undertaken from suspect lesions and standard sites (earlobes, arms and buttocks). Slit skin smears should be read by experienced technicians.

Outside leprosy endemic areas doctors frequently fail to consider the diagnosis of leprosy. Diagnosis had been delayed in over 80% of new patients seen between 1995 and 1999 at The Hospital for Tropical Diseases, London.[207] Patients had been misdiagnosed by dermatologists, neurologists, orthopedic surgeons and rheumatologists. A common problem was failure to consider leprosy as a cause of peripheral neuropathy in patients from leprosy endemic countries. These delays had serious consequences for patients, with over half of them having nerve damage and disability.

DIFFERENTIAL DIAGNOSIS

Skin

The variety of leprosy skin lesions means that many skin conditions need to be included in the differential diagnosis. In suspected tuberculoid lesions the presence of lesional anesthesia is crucial in differentiating leprosy from fungal infections, vitiligo, vitamin A deficiency and eczema. Single facial patches in children may be difficult to test for anesthesia and one may have to observe a lesion over some months. In lepromatous disease the presence of acid-fast bacilli in smears differentiates leprosy nodules from onchocerciasis and post kala-azar dermal leishmaniasis.

Nerves

Peripheral nerve thickening is rarely seen except in leprosy. Hereditary sensory motor neuropathy type III is also associated with palpable peripheral nerve hypertrophy.

TREATMENT

The treatment of leprosy has six main components: chemotherapy, monitoring and treating nerve damage, management of reactions and neuritis, patient education, prevention of disability and social and psychological support.

Chemotherapy

All children with leprosy should be given an appropriate multidrug combination. The first line anti-leprosy drugs are rifampicin, dapsone and clofazimine. Table 28.24 shows the drug combinations, doses and duration of treatment.

Rifampicin

Rifampicin is a potent bactericidal drug for *M. leprae*. Because *M. leprae* resistance to rifampicin can develop as a one-step process, rifampicin should always be given in combination with other anti-leprotics. Parents and children should be warned that their urine, sweat and tears will be red for 48 h after taking rifampicin.

Dapsone (DDS)

Dapsone (4,4-diaminodiphenylsulfone) is only weakly bactericidal. It commonly causes mild hemolysis but rarely anemia. Glucose-6-phosphate dehydrogenase deficiency is rarely a problem.

Clofazimine

Clofazimine has a weakly bactericidal action. It also has an anti-inflammatory effect, which has reduced the incidence of ENL reactions. Skin discoloration is the most troublesome side-effect, ranging from red to purple-black. The pigmentation usually fades slowly after stopping clofazimine. Clofazimine also produces a characteristic ichthyosis on the shins and forearms.

More than 14 million patients have been treated successfully with multiple drug treatment (MDT). Clinical improvement is rapid, toxicity rare, and duration of treatment is shortened. Monthly supervision of the rifampicin component has been crucial to success. The three drugs used for MDT are donated by Novartis free of charge for distribution in blister packs (pediatric and adult). At the end of 6 months' treatment of borderline disease there may still be signs of inflammation, which should not be mistaken for active infection. The distinction between relapse and reaction may be difficult. WHO studies have reported a cumulative relapse rate of 1.07% for paucibacillary leprosy and 0.77% for multibacillary leprosy at 9 years after completion of MDT. *M. leprae* is such a slow-growing organism that relapse only occurs after many years. Patients with a high initial bacterial load may be at greater risk of relapse and so require treatment until skin-smear negative.

Short course chemotherapy regimens have been tested for pauci-bacillary (PB) leprosy using either rifampicin in weekly doses or single dose chemotherapy using a combination of currently used drugs. So far all of these regimens have had higher relapse rates than the current WHO PB regimen. The fluoroquinolones (pefloxacin and ofloxacin) and the macrolide minocycline are all highly active against *M. leprae*, but because of cost are rarely used in field programs. A single dose of triple drug combination (rifampicin, ofloxacin and minocycline) has been tested in India for patients with single skin lesions and produced marked clinical improvement at 18 months in 52% of patients. Although the study had major flaws, and single dose treatment is less effective than the conventional 6-month treatment for PB leprosy, it is an operationally attractive field regimen.

Monitoring and treating nerve damage

Nerve damage may occur before diagnosis, or during and after MDT. It may occur during a reaction or without overt signs of nerve inflammation (silent neuropathy). About 30% of newly diagnosed patients have nerve damage and at least 25% of multibacillary patients develop nerve damage during treatment. Children are at the same risk as adults of developing nerve damage and having reactions. Monitoring sensation and muscle power in a child's hands, feet and eyes should be part of the routine follow-up so that new nerve damage is detected early. Any new damage should be treated with a course of oral steroids, starting with prednisolone 0.5 mg/kg/d and reducing by 0.1 mg/d each month. Response rates vary depending on the severity of initial damage, but even when promptly treated, nerve damage will only improve in 60% of cases.

Management of reactions and neuritis

Reversal (type 1) reactions

Reversal reactions manifest clinically with erythema and edema of skin lesions and tender, painful peripheral nerves. Loss of nerve function may be dramatic and foot drop can occur overnight. Awareness of the early symptoms of reversal reactions by both patient and physician is important, because, if left untreated, severe nerve damage may develop. The peak time for reversal reactions is in the first 2 months of treatment. The treatment of reactions is aimed at controlling acute inflammation, easing pain, reversing nerve damage and reassuring the patient. MDT should be continued. If there is any evidence of neuritis (nerve tenderness, new anesthesia and/or motor loss) corticosteroid treatment should be started using the regimen given above.

Erythema nodosum leprosum type 2 (ENL) reactions

This complication affects only BL and LL patients and presents with crops of small, pink, tender skin lesions on the face and the extensor surfaces of the limbs. In a cohort study from Hyderabad, India, 31% of children with BL/LL disease developed ENL.[208] The patient is usually unwell with malaise and fever. Other accompanying signs are acute iritis and episcleritis, lymphadenitis, orchitis, bone pain, dactylitis, arthritis and proteinuria. This is a difficult condition to treat and frequently requires treatment with high dose steroids (1 mg/kg daily, tapered down rapidly) or thalidomide. Since ENL frequently recurs, steroid dependency can easily develop. Thalidomide (5 mg/kg daily) is superior to steroids in controlling ENL and is the drug of choice for young men with severe ENL. Unfortunately thalidomide is unavailable in several leprosy endemic countries despite its undoubted value. Clofazimine has a useful anti-inflammatory effect in ENL and can be used at 3 mg/kg daily for several months.[209] Acute iridocyclitis is treated with 4-hourly instillation of 1% hydrocortisone eye drops and 1% atropine drops twice daily.

Neuritis

Silent neuritis should be treated similarly to reversal reaction (see above). In the Hyderabad study 24% children developed neuritis.[208]

Patient education

Patients and their parents deserve a clear explanation of the etiology, diagnosis and prognosis of leprosy. It should be emphasized that the infection is curable provided that they comply with the antibiotic regimen. It is important to stress that deformity is not an inevitable disease endpoint. It may be helpful to ask parents and older patients about their views of leprosy as there are many myths about leprosy, which can be dispelled. Lepromatous patients become non-infectious within 72 h of starting antibiotics. Patients and their families should be encouraged to lead a normal life and be reassured that family activities such as eating together, sharing baths and bed linen pose no risks to other family members. It should be emphasized that leprosy is not transmitted sexually nor is it hereditary.

Prevention of disability

It is vital in preventing disability to create patient self-awareness so that damage is minimized. In a study from south India, 33% of children presenting to a referral center had visible deformities.[210] The child with an anesthetic hand or foot needs to understand the importance of daily self-care, especially protection when doing potentially dangerous tasks and regular inspection for trauma. For each patient it is helpful to identify potentially dangerous situations, such as cooking, radiators and hot food. Soaking dry hands and feet followed by rubbing with oil keeps the skin moist and supple.

An anesthetic foot needs the protection of an appropriate shoe. For anesthesia alone, a well-fitting 'trainer' with a firm sole and shock-absorbing inner will provide adequate protection. Once there is deformity, such as clawing, special shoes must be made to ensure protection of pressure points and even weight distribution.

Children should be taught to work out why an injury occurred so that the risk can be avoided in future. Plantar ulceration occurs secondary to increased pressure over bony prominences. Ulceration is treated by rest. In leprosy, ulcers heal if they are protected from weightbearing. No weightbearing is permitted until the ulcer has healed. Appropriate footwear should be provided to prevent recurrence.

Physiotherapy exercises should be taught to maximize function of weak muscles and prevent contractures. Contractures of hands and feet, foot drop, lagophthalmos, entropion and ectropion are amenable to surgery.

Social, psychological and economic rehabilitation

The social and cultural backgrounds of the patient determine the nature of many of the problems that may be encountered. The family may have difficulty in coming to terms with leprosy. The community may reject the patient. Education, confidence from family, friends and doctor, and plastic surgery to correct stigmatizing deformity all have a role to play.

PROPHYLAXIS

In non-endemic areas it is very unusual to see leprosy in contacts of leprosy patients. The last case of secondary transmission in the UK was reported in 1923. Household contacts of new patients should be examined for clinical signs of leprosy and advised to report any new skin lesions promptly and to tell their physicians that they have had contact with a known case of leprosy. In the UK, BCG vaccination is given to contacts under the age of 12; chemoprophylaxis is reserved for children under 10 years who are household contacts of lepromatous cases. They are given prophylaxis with rifampicin 15 mg/kg body weight given monthly for 6 months.[211] BCG gives variable protection, ranging from 80% in Uganda to 20% in Burma. In trials in Malawi and Venezuela, adding killed *M. leprae* to BCG did not enhance protection.

BACTERIAL INFECTIONS: LEPTOSPIROSIS

Leptospirosis is a worldwide zoonosis transmitted to humans by infected urine of a wide range of domestic and wild animals: often the causative spirochetes are excreted asymptomatically for long periods of time.

Adults usually acquire infection because of occupational exposure: children may acquire infection by playing in areas contaminated with animal urine or by playing with the animals themselves.

PATHOLOGY

In the UK and USA the common serotypes of the genus *Leptospira* include *Leptospira icterohaemorrhagiae* (commonly acquired from rat's urine), *Leptospira canicola* (commonly acquired from dog's urine), *Leptospira pomona* (commonly acquired from pig's urine), *Leptospira hebdomadis* and *Leptospira ballum*. Correlation of named serotypes with specific syndromes is impossible because of the variability of illness produced by each serotype.

Leptospires gain entry to humans via ingestion, mucous membranes, skin abrasions or the conjunctivae. After entry, the organisms affect capillary epithelium and may cause capillary damage, hypoxia and hemorrhage into various organs. Liver damage may cause jaundice (although hemolysis may also play a part), renal damage may cause renal failure, central nervous system damage meningitis and encephalitis, and skeletal muscle involvement muscle pain. Blood clotting parameters are often not disordered enough to account for the hemorrhagic tendency. Illnesses may be biphasic with initial symptoms caused by leptospiremia and later symptoms by host immune responses.

CLINICAL FEATURES

The incubation period is probably from a few days to just under 3 weeks.

The clinical manifestations range through asymptomatic infection to multisystem disease. With clinical disease there is usually an abrupt onset of fever with several possible accompaniments:

1. muscular pains;
2. marked constitutional upset and hemorrhagic manifestations;
3. nephritic features usually without associated hypertension;
4. jaundice with or without hemorrhages;
5. jaundice with leukocytosis or a raised erythrocyte sedimentation rate (leukocytosis and a raised sedimentation rate are unusual in viral hepatitis);
6. meningitis with injected or hemorrhagic conjunctivae, or a lymphocytic meningitis with normal biochemical parameters: this syndrome is typically associated with *L. canicola* infection;
7. persistent fever lasting up to 3 or 4 weeks, perhaps without other signs;
8. jaundice with nephritis – Weil syndrome, usually caused by *L. icterohaemorrhagiae* infection in which renal failure is a common cause of death (in contrast most patients with viral hepatitis have a low or normal blood urea and present with gradual-onset malaise and fever which usually remits once jaundice is apparent).

DIAGNOSIS AND DIFFERENTIAL DIAGNOSIS

Blood cultures may be positive in early illness, but some *Leptospira* resist standard culture and the diagnosis has to be confirmed by dark ground microscopy or by serology. Usually reactive antibody becomes detectable after the first week of illness. Agglutination and complement fixation tests are often used. If there is a meningitic clinical picture the CSF is usually lymphocytic; the CSF biochemistry is often normal and CSF culture may be positive. Urine culture or dark ground microscopy may be positive once infection is established, and may remain positive for several weeks.

The differential diagnosis is very wide: if a zoonosis is suspected, Q fever and brucellosis are major contenders.

TREATMENT

Eradication of noncommercial animals (such as rats) or reducing potential exposure to animal urine is ideal. *Leptospira* are sensitive to penicillin, tetracyclines (which are contraindicated in renal failure and which, depending on the severity of illness, are contraindicated in children) and erythromycin. Usually high doses are given for 10 days. Early treatment is essential as antibiotics will do little to alleviate the immune-mediated elements of the illness. Isolation of patients

is unnecessary as person-to-person spread is unlikely. Despite serious dysfunction of infected organs in acute illness, recovery is usually complete in survivors.

LYME DISEASE

Lyme disease is a seasonal non-occupational bacterial zoonosis which is distributed throughout the temperate zones of the world.[212] It was first recognized in 1975 because of a geographic clustering of children with arthritis in Lyme, Connecticut.[213] It is now recognized that the causative agent is an arthropod-borne spirochete called *Borrelia burgdorferi* which is transmitted by the hard tick *Ixodes dammini* or related ixodid ticks depending on the geographical distribution, e.g. *Ixodes ricinus* is predominant in Europe.[214] The tick, which has a wide range of hosts (deer, cattle, sheep, mice, squirrels, dogs), appears to prefer the white-footed mouse and white-tailed deer. Birds are now also recognized as reservoirs.

The anatomical location of tick bites appears important. Patients bitten on the head and neck had significantly more neurological manifestations, perhaps explaining the higher frequency of neuroborreliosis among children compared with adults.[215]

The illness is a multisystem disorder, which consists of a prodromal febrile illness with the characteristic rash of erythema chronicum migrans (ECM) and associated symptoms. Without antibiotic treatment a substantial number of patients will go on to cardiac, neurological and rheumatological sequelae. However, progression from early to late stage is not inevitable, even in the absence of antibiotic treatment. 'Incomplete' cases with minimal or absent rash can occur, and patients may have aseptic meningitis, facial palsy, carditis or arthritis as the first sign of disease.

ETIOLOGY AND VECTOR

In 1982 a previously unrecognized spirochete was isolated from *I. dammini* ticks that had been collected from Shelter Island, New York. This discovery was followed in 1983 by the successful culture of the spirochete named *B. burgdorferi* from patients with Lyme disease.

The main vector species are *I. ricinus* in Europe and the *I. scapularis* group in North America.[216] The life cycle of the tick consists of larval, nymphal and adult stages. The larvae and nymphs primarily feed on rodents such as the white-footed mouse, the natural reservoir for *I. dammini*. The adults usually feed on large mammals like deer, sheep and horses. Furthermore, the growth of the vector population is promoted by deer and fails to occur in their absence. The nymphal stage, whose peak questing period is May through July, is primarily responsible for transmission of disease. As these immature ticks feed aggressively on more animal species they facilitate rapid transmission of the organisms and often escape detection by the human host because they remain very small, even after a feed.

EPIDEMIOLOGY

Lyme disease is the most common vector-borne disease among children with more cases in children than in adults. However, there is substantial regional variation in the incidence of Lyme disease although most cases appear to occur during the summer months. The estimated incidence in the USA in 1992 was 3.9 per 100 000 population with Connecticut having the highest incidence (53.6/100 000). These figures are undoubtedly underestimates as only a small proportion of cases are reported. In the UK, for example, the incidence of Lyme disease is not well documented although experience suggests that serious disease is not common. Children between the ages of 5 and 10 years appear to be at highest risk in endemic areas.

PATHOGENESIS

In early Lyme disease the spirochete is injected into the bloodstream or skin through tick saliva. It may also be deposited in fecal material on the skin, and from there the organism may invade the skin or blood. Following an incubation period of 3–32 days the organism migrates outwards in the skin to produce the classical immune-mediated lesion of ECM. It may also spread to the lymphatics or disseminate in the blood or organs such as the brain, heart or joints or to other sites to produce the secondary lesions of late stage disease. The propensity to produce damage of a specific target organ appears to be determined by a number of factors including genospecies of *Borrelia* isolate as well as host factors such as human leukocyte antigen (HLA) phenotype. For example, *B. afzelii* is more common in patients with mainly dermatological manifestations, whereas *B. garinii* is more often associated with neurological complications. Furthermore, arthritis, which is a more common presentation of early or late Lyme disease in Europe as opposed to ECM in North America, is more commonly seen in patients with HLA-DR4 and -DR2.[217] There is also some evidence that patients with severe and prolonged illness, especially neurological or joint disease, have an increased frequency of the B cell alloantigen HLA-DR2.[218]

CLINICAL CHARACTERISTICS

Like other spirochetal infections the illness can occur in distinct stages which may overlap or occur alone without recalling earlier features.

Early manifestations[219]

Up to one third of patients remember a tick bite which often leaves a nonspecific small red macule or papule. About 1 week later this area expands to the pathognomonic warm, painless, erythematous, annular lesion called ECM which reaches a maximum diameter of 15 cm (larger areas up to 70 cm have been reported) and usually has a bright red outer border. In the largest community-based prospective study reported in children, 89% of those studied presented with a single or multiple lesions of ECM.[220]

This lesion, which resolves within 4 weeks without therapy, can occur at any site although the thigh, groin and axilla are particularly common. Concomitant signs and symptoms include high fever (particularly in children), malaise, regional lymphadenopathy, meningism, myalgia and migratory arthralgias. Most of the early clinical features are characteristically intermittent and fluctuating during a period of several weeks, before spontaneous resolution occurs. About 10% of patients have features suggestive of anicteric hepatitis. Cellulitis secondary to an infected insect bite is a common misdiagnosis.

Two uncommon skin lesions, acrodermatitis chronica atrophicans and lymphadenosis benigna cutis, which are rare both in children and in North America, are regarded as specific late skin manifestations in Lyme disease.[221]

Late manifestations

These manifestations occur some weeks to months after the initial infection and the clinical features are dependent on the organ affected and the severity of damage.

In about 10–40% of patients, frank *neurological abnormalities* usually occur weeks to months after infection. The classical triad of early neurological disease includes a lymphocytic meningitis, cranial neuropathy and radiculoneuritis. Neuroborreliosis in children most commonly presents as mild encephalopathy, lymphocytic meningitis and cranial neuropathy.[222] Radiculopathy, particularly in European children, and peripheral neuropathy, both of which occur late in the disease, are rare in children. Typically patients develop a fluctuating lymphocytic meningitis about 4 weeks after the onset of ECM often with superimposed cranial (especially facial) neuritis. Patients will have a CSF lymphocytic pleocytosis. Other less common neurological complications include ataxia, spastic paraparesis due to an acute myelitis, hemiparesis, optic neuritis, hydrocephalus, Guillain–Barré syndrome and a pseudotumor cerebri-like syndrome.

Cardiac disease, which is relatively uncommon in children, occurs roughly 5 weeks after the tick bite. The disease spectrum includes myopericarditis, cardiomegaly, left ventricular dysfunction and especially fluctuating degrees of atrioventricular block, which may progress to complete heart block. The latter may require temporary pacing. The duration of cardiac involvement is usually brief (3 days to 6 weeks) and self-limiting. The clinical features show similarities to rheumatic fever although valvular involvement has not been reported.

Arthritis is a common late sequela of Lyme disease occurring in up to 60% of patients within a few weeks to 2 years after the onset of illness; 20–40% of patients do not remember having ECM. The spectrum of Lyme arthritis ranges from subjective joint pains which are often migratory, to intermittent attacks of arthritis to chronic erosive disease (10%).[223] The commonest pattern of joint involvement is an acute asymmetric mono- or oligoarticular arthritis primarily affecting the large joints. Most commonly (> 90%) involved is the knee joint and the child typically presents with subacute effusion of the knee. The attacks of arthritis typically last for a few weeks to months and recur intermittently over several years. Fatigue is the commonest associated non-articular symptom, whereas fever or other systemic symptoms are unusual.

Numerous other rare manifestations have been associated with Lyme disease. These include ophthalmic complications (conjunctivitis, episcleritis, photophobia, uveitis), hepatitis, hepatosplenomegaly and testicular swelling. There is no clear evidence that *B. burgdorferi* causes congenital disease, although the existence of this rare syndrome cannot be ruled out.[224] Furthermore, transmission of Lyme disease in breast milk has not been documented.

DIAGNOSIS

The diagnosis is not always easy, given that symptoms may be nonspecific and serology may be misleading.[225] The hallmark for confirming the diagnosis is to obtain appropriate fluid or tissue for culture. Such tests are unlikely to be of value in everyday clinical practice and future diagnostic tests such as polymerase chain reaction (PCR) have not yet been adequately tested. Therefore, the diagnostic tests used most frequently are serological and detect antibodies against *B. burgdorferi*. The most commonly used of these tests, which is now widely available as a pre-packed commercial kit, is the enzyme linked immunosorbent assay (ELISA). Unfortunately, this test yields many false positive reactions with other spirochetal infections, connective tissue diseases and certain viral infections.[224] There is also cross-reactivity with antigens of spirochetes belonging to the normal flora. The immunoblotting technique currently offers the best means of validating a positive or equivocal ELISA in a patient with a low likelihood of Lyme, although this test is not widely available and its proper interpretation is as yet unclear.[226]

Currently the diagnosis of early Lyme disease, especially in the presence of skin lesions, is made on clinical and epidemiological grounds since serology (*B. burgdorferi* IgM) does not usually become positive until 3–6 weeks after the onset of the erythema migrans. Also, the antibody response may be aborted in patients with early Lyme who are treated promptly with an effective antimicrobial agent. The specific IgG antibody rises slowly and may not reach a level of diagnostic significance in early disease. It usually peaks months or years later, often when arthritis is present, and can persist for many years despite adequate treatment or cure. Furthermore, a substantial proportion of people who become infected by *B. burgdorferi* never have a clinical illness but have positive serology. Serological testing is not necessary for diagnosing typical ECM but is helpful in untreated atypical skin lesions, patients with acute meningitis, neuropathies and arthritis due to Lyme. The negative and positive predictive values of currently available serological tests are very much dependent on the pretest likelihood that a patient has Lyme disease. For example, a patient with ECM who lives in an endemic area has a very high probability of having Lyme even if the serological test is negative. Conversely, a patient with vague nonspecific symptoms with a positive test is unlikely to have Lyme despite positive serology. Therefore, serological tests should not be used on patients with nonspecific symptoms but clinicians should order serological tests for Lyme disease in selected groups such as those with clinical findings suggestive of Lyme or in highly prevalent areas so that the predictive value of the test is high.[224]

Notably the predictive value of positive serology in patients with erythema chronicum migrans as a single manifestation of Lyme disease is low.[227]

Patients reported to have Lyme disease who did not meet the United States Centers for Disease Control and Prevention (CDC) case definitions had increased symptoms and worsening quality of life indices, the implication being that such patients did not have Lyme disease.[228] A consensus paper noted that the risks of intravenous antibiotics in patients with nonspecific complaints outweighed potential benefits.[229]

The differential diagnosis is wide but includes other tick-borne diseases including ehrlichiosis and babesiosis.

TREATMENT

Since no clinical trials of treatment have been performed in children the recommendations for treatment have been extrapolated from adult studies.[230,231] Doxycycline 2.5 mg/kg (max 100 mg) orally, 12-hourly for 14–21 days is the oral antibiotic of choice for children 8 years or older. For younger children, amoxicillin 25 mg/kg orally, 12-hourly for 14–21 days, is recommended. Ceftriaxone 75–100 mg/kg, IM, once daily is recommended for persistent or recurrent arthritis and either ceftriaxone or benzylpenicillin 50 000 U/kg IV, 4-hourly for carditis, meningitis or encephalitis. Lyme disease will respond well to antibiotic therapy if treated early, shortening the duration of illness and reducing the incidence of complications. The long term prognosis for this group as well as those treated for late Lyme disease is excellent.

PREVENTION

Acquisition of Lyme borreliosis can be reduced by simple practical methods such as wearing long trousers, tucking trousers into socks, wearing boots, promptly removing any attached ticks and impregnating clothes with DEET or permethrin. A vaccine is currently under development.

BACTERIAL INFECTIONS: MENINGOCOCCEMIA

Despite the recent introduction of an effective vaccine against group C organisms in the UK, *Neisseria meningitidis* is still the most frequent cause of septicemia in childhood, and affects otherwise healthy children of all ages after the neonatal period. In the UK, there are over 1200 microbiologically confirmed cases a year (Statutory Notifications of Infections Diseases 1995–2006)[232] and probably double that number diagnosed on clinical grounds alone. About 50% will have meningitis. In the last decade, wider public awareness, better diagnosis and intensive care have improved the outcome, but mortality is still between 5 and 10%.

N. meningitidis is a Gram negative diplococcus which is surrounded by an outer polysaccharide capsule, an outer membrane and an underlying peptidoglycan layer. Pili or fimbriae extend through the capsule and are thought to play a role in the attachment to epithelial cells within the nasopharynx. Between 2 and 10% of the general population are colonized, but carriage rates may be much higher in outbreaks. The precise relationship between carriage and invasive disease remains unclear. Spread is predominantly by respiratory droplets from close contacts.

In Western Europe, the group B organism is still the most commonly isolated strain but is closely followed by group C organisms. In the UK, the introduction of a group C conjugate vaccine has reduced the rate of group C infections in the younger age group dramatically. Group A organisms have been responsible for large epidemics, particularly in sub-Saharan Africa, and another serogroup, W135, has caused a number of infections in pilgrims returning from the Hajj.

In spite of high colonization rates, only a relatively small number of colonized individuals develop invasive disease. Progression from nasal carriage to bacteremia is thought to be influenced by both bacterial and host factors. Certain bacterial properties, such as the presence of a capsule, pili and lipopolysaccharide (LPS) structure are known to be associated with invasive disease. There are also some data to indicate that smoking, respiratory tract infections and mucosal injury may aid colonization. However, the most important host factor predisposing individuals to this infection is the presence of defects within the complement cascade. Deficiencies of terminal complement components C5–C9, properdin and mannose-binding lectin all lead to an increased incidence of disease, and sometimes recurrent disease.

Having gained access to the circulation, bacterial components including LPS cause a host inflammatory response with the release of pro-inflammatory mediators such as tumor necrosis factor, IL-1, IL-6 and IL-8. These cytokines influence a number of cellular and non-cellular functions including neutrophil, monocyte and endothelial cell activation, thrombotic and hemostatic pathway imbalance and complement activation. In addition, the organism can bind to vascular endothelial cells inducing adhesion molecule expression, with consequent leukocyte attachment and migration. Uninterrupted, this intense inflammatory process leads to tissue injury and ultimately to multiple organ failure and death.[233]

CLINICAL FINDINGS

There are two major clinical presentations of meningococcal disease: meningitis and septicemia. A proportion of patients will have evidence of sepsis and meningitis. Once in the bloodstream, however, *N. meningitidis* can localize to other sites including joints, bones, eyes and heart. Most deaths occur in the predominantly septicemic form of the disease. The presence of meningitis is a good prognostic indicator, and may indicate that host defenses have contained the infection long enough for the bacteria to invade the blood–brain barrier. Sepsis commonly presents with nonspecific symptoms of fever, vomiting, abdominal pain and muscle aches. These patients may also have a characteristic rash, which can occur anywhere and may be purpuric or morbilliform (Fig. 28.17). The extent of the inflammatory response will influence other signs of sepsis or septic shock. In the early stages, fever, tachycardia and tachypnea may be present with the rash. Later, signs of shock develop, with poor peripheral perfusion, hypotension and oliguria. These are generally accompanied by an extensive purpuric rash and evidence of disseminated intravascular coagulopathy (DIC) (Fig. 28.16). Recent evidence indicates that polymorphisms within the cytokine and hemostatic/thrombotic pathways can influence the severity of this disease. Hemorrhage into internal organs may occur. Classically, this involves the adrenal glands in the Waterhouse–Friderichsen syndrome. In those who recover, skin necrosis or vascular occlusion may cause the loss of an extremity, though most small lesions heal with minimal scarring.

The predominantly meningitic form of the disease presents with symptoms and signs of meningitis with fever, vomiting, headache and neck stiffness. Patients with meningitis may develop convulsions, focal neurological signs, a depressed level of consciousness, coma and death due to raised intracranial pressure (see Suspected meningitis). As the organism gains access to the central nervous system (CNS) from the blood, the petechial rash may be present and helpful in the diagnosis.

Arthritis, pericarditis and pleural effusions may occur as autoimmune phenomena 5–10 days after the acute infection. This is due to immune complex formation and is self-limiting, although a large pericardial effusion may cause cardiac tamponade. A rare chronic form of meningococcal sepsis can occur and is characterized by anorexia, weight loss, fever, arthralgia or arthritis and skin rash; erythema nodosum or bacterial endocarditis may also occur.

In the differential diagnosis, other bacterial and viral infections which cause purpura must be considered. Anaphylactoid purpura and idiopathic thrombocytopenic purpura may cause similar purpuric rashes. A morbilliform rash may be confused with a drug eruption or a number of viral infections including measles. Subacute or chronic meningococcemia presents a greater challenge. The differential diagnosis includes the many causes of arthritis and fever in children. However, a petechial rash in a febrile child should be considered as suggestive of meningococcal disease until proved otherwise.

LABORATORY INVESTIGATION

The diagnosis is established by recovery of *N. meningitidis* from the blood, petechial lesions or the CSF, but lumbar puncture is contraindicated in the presence of shock, coagulopathy, reduced conscious level or focal neurological signs. The practice of giving penicillin before hospital admission to patients in whom meningococcal infection is suspected, which has saved lives, has also decreased successful culture of the organism. In these situations, meningococcal DNA may still be detected by polymerase chain reaction (PCR) in blood and CSF. Serology may confirm the clinical diagnosis retrospectively. The complete blood count may show a polymorphonuclear leukocytosis. Neutropenia is invariably present in severe disease, however, and indicates a poor prognosis (see below). There is usually also evidence of DIC with thrombocytopenia, a coagulopathy and intravascular fibrin and thrombosis within dermal vessels. The importance of platelets and neutrophils in this disease is highlighted in a number of studies, which show that reduced circulating numbers of both cell types is correlated with a worse outcome.

TREATMENT

The most important aspect of meningococcal disease management is recognition. Recent work has shown that the classical signs of meningococcal disease with rash and meningism occur relatively late, 13–22 h after onset of illness. Early signs of disease include leg pains, cold hands and feet and pallor or mottling.[234] It is essential for the disease to be recognized early because, as with other forms of bacterial sepsis, bacterial load is critical, with higher bacterial concentrations leading to a more severe inflammatory response and organ dysfunction.[235] In patients with little capacity to limit bacterial growth within blood, a single bacterium may proliferate to more than a million organisms in under 8 h. Most deaths occur in patients with a bacterial load of more than a million organisms/ml. Early intervention with antibiotics will rapidly arrest bacterial growth and reduce levels of circulating LPS and other bacterial components. A third generation cephalosporin, such as cefotaxime or ceftriaxone, has become the standard therapy for the initial treatment of suspected meningococcal disease. Once the organism is isolated and sensitivity determined, penicillin can be used in the majority of cases. It is recommended that family doctors who see a patient with suspected meningococcal infection in the home give a dose of intramuscular penicillin immediately. Some recent data suggest that this course of action is associated with a higher mortality, but this is probably because primary care physicians administer penicillin to the sickest children.

In shocked children, vigorous resuscitation is required. Volume expansion with plasma and/or 4.5% albumin (20 ml/kg and repeat as required) is the crucial first step. Emergency transfer to the regional intensive care unit is usually advisable as inotropic and vasopressor agents, artificial ventilation and hematological support are frequently required (see section on sepsis). In very severe disease, extracorporeal membrane oxygenation may be life saving.

New therapies, which alter the immune response or inflammatory cascade, are under investigation at present, but no such agents have been shown to be effective to date. However, as in other forms of sepsis (see section on sepsis), corticosteroids, endotoxin and inflammatory modulation, activated protein C administration and endocrine manipulation may prove beneficial in the future.

PROPHYLAXIS

Prophylaxis against invasive disease should be given to the family and close contacts of the patient. Rifampicin, given in 4 doses over 2 days, has been shown to be effective in clearing the organism. A single injection of ceftriaxone, or an oral dose of ciprofloxacin, are appropriate alternatives.

In the UK, a conjugate meningococcal C vaccine has now been introduced with evidence of a marked decline in this organism in vaccinated individuals. Polysaccharide vaccines are available for *N. meningitidis* groups A, C, Y and W135 for patients traveling to endemic areas. Trials continue on vaccines against *N. meningitidis* group B.

PROGNOSIS

The mortality from acute meningococcemia remains high at between 5 and 10%, most deaths occurring in patients with very high bacterial loads. Early recognition is the key to improved outcome. Survivors may suffer extensive tissue injury, sometimes requiring amputation and/or skin grafting. A number of prognostic scores have been developed, the most frequently quoted being the Glasgow meningococcal septicemia prognostic score. This is predominantly based upon clinical parameters such as blood pressure and coma, but as supportive care has improved, this score may no longer accurately identify patients at greatest risk of mortality. Other scores have now been developed which revolve around hematological parameters, and a simple score based on the product of the initial platelet and neutrophil count has been shown to be a better prognostic guide to mortality. This score may help to identify those patients at whom novel therapeutic agents should be targeted.[236]

BACTERIAL INFECTIONS: *MYCOBACTERIUM TUBERCULOSIS*

In technically advanced countries, morbidity and mortality from tuberculosis have declined progressively over the decades. This is associated with improved living conditions and medical care, particularly case finding and chemotherapy. However, it is still an important problem, especially in immigrant and minority groups. In some resource limited countries, the case rate has hardly changed and any decline is offset by an increase in population.

The majority of children infected by *M. tuberculosis* are asymptomatic. However, in a small number, especially young children, the disease is serious or fatal, due to meningitis or disseminated disease, and survivors may be left with sequelae such as cerebral palsy, mental retardation or chronic lung or bone and joint disease.

MICROBIOLOGY

The 'tubercle bacillus' was first described by Robert Koch in 1882 and is now called *Mycobacterium tuberculosis*. Mycobacteria derive their name from their mold-like appearance on culture. One of their unique characteristics is a highly complex, lipid-rich cell wall which protects the bacillus from digestion by the lysosomal enzymes of macrophages and which, when stained, resists decolorization by acid alcohol. Like *Mycobacterium leprae*, but different from other mycobacteria, *M. tuberculosis* is an obligate parasite with total dependence on the living host.

The two major species of mycobacteria infecting man are *M. tuberculosis* and *M. bovis*. *M. bovis* differs from the other types in its resistance to pyrazinamide. *M. tuberculosis* is aerophilic but *M. bovis* is micro-aerophilic (prefers reduced oxygen tension). Within the host, mycobacteria may lie dormant for many years.

M. tuberculosis is cultured on Lowenstein–Jensen medium and is slow growing, taking an average time of 21 days, and occasionally 1–2 months or longer. Growth of *M. tuberculosis* may be detected in 7–10 days using liquid culture media, e.g. the BACTEC radiometric or Roche biphasic systems.

There are two major methods for direct identification in specimens: Ziehl–Neelsen stain and fluorescence microscopy with auramine–rhodamine stain. The latter is the more rapid, more sensitive and more specific.

A number of serological tests have been developed using purified protein derivatives of *M. tuberculosis* in enzyme linked immunosorbent assay (ELISA) or solid-phase radioimmunoassays. However, many lack sensitivity and specificity, especially for culture-negative cases, and thus are not used for routine laboratory diagnosis.[237] Tests for antigen in CSF are useful, but not routinely available. Gene probes can identify mycobacteria rapidly once they have grown in culture. In adults, nucleic acid amplification (NAA) has sensitivity > 90% and specificity 98% for smear positive respiratory specimens, but only 50–70% sensitivity for smear negative specimens.[238] Sensitivity for nonrespiratory specimens, particularly CSF, is lower than for respiratory specimens. This is partly due to inhibitors especially in pleural, ascitic and CSF specimens. There are few studies in children and they are limited by numbers of confirmed or probable cases of tuberculosis.[239,240] Sensitivities for polymerase chain reaction (PCR) in gastric aspirates in children with confirmed or clinical pulmonary tuberculosis vary from 40 to 80% and generally are higher than culture. Sensitivity is increased by testing multiple samples. Specificity is reported to be 94–100%, although PCR may be positive in a third of children with tuberculous infection only. Sensitivities are no higher in bronchoalveolar lavage (BAL) than in gastric aspirates. PCR can differentiate between *M. tuberculosis* and environmental mycobacteria and PCR methods are available to detect rifampicin resistance. DNA fingerprinting is a valuable tool in studying transmission of tuberculosis.

EPIDEMIOLOGY

In studies of tuberculosis, differentiation has to be made between tuberculous infection (as evidenced by a positive tuberculin test) and disease. In tuberculous disease there is clinical, radiological or bacteriological evidence of infection. The great majority of infected people remain asymptomatic. In England and Wales in 1949–1950, a national survey showed that nearly half of 14-year-old children were tuberculin positive. Today, less than 1% of 11–13-year-old children are tuberculin positive at routine school examination.

Three quarters of tuberculosis cases occur in resource limited countries where 0.2–1% of the population are expectorating the tubercle bacillus. A rise in case rates in adults and children has been observed in countries with a high prevalence of HIV infection, especially sub-Saharan Africa.[241]

In technically advanced countries, with a low prevalence of smear positive cases, the infection rate in children will be low and the majority of adults with tuberculosis will have endogenous reactivation. Conversely, in resource limited countries, the high prevalence of smear positive cases will result in a significant proportion of children and young adults developing primary tuberculosis, and exogenous reinfection in older adults will be common. Children under 14 years may comprise up to 20% of case load in the Indian subcontinent, 39% in South Africa and 5% in the United States.[241,242]

National surveys for England and Wales for the periods 1978–1979, 1983, 1988, 1993 and 1998 found 747 (estimate based on 6 month survey), 452, 308, 408 and 364 newly notified children under 15 years respectively.[243] In 1998, rates (per 100 000) for children were highest for black African (70.6) and Indian subcontinent (23.1) compared to black Caribbean (9.0) and white (1.1) groups. Although rates for the Chinese group were high (82.1), cases were low (14).

The decline in the incidence of tuberculosis began in Europe before the introduction of BCG and chemotherapy. In the decade 1979–1988 there was an average reduction in notification rates in England of 7.2% per year. However, since 1988 there has been a 21% rise in notifications, with the highest increase in the London area. In the 1998 survey, 49% of children with tuberculosis were resident in London, 44% of whom were born abroad, compared to 10% resident elsewhere.[243] There has also been a rise in notifications in parts of Europe and the USA. Factors associated with the rise in notifications in the USA since 1987 include HIV infection, homelessness, immigration and decline in resources for tuberculosis control. The increase is focal, mainly confined to inner cities, and 80% of childhood cases are in minority ethnic groups. Multidrug resistance is a major problem. However, with increased support for tuberculosis control, the rise in cases has reversed. In the period 1993–2003 the incidence decreased by 44%.[244]

Most cases of tuberculosis are caused by *M. tuberculosis*. *M. bovis*, which was an important cause of tuberculosis of the gastrointestinal tract, lymph nodes and bones, has virtually disappeared from technically advanced countries through eradication of tuberculosis in cattle and pasteurization of milk. In the UK before 1950, *M. bovis* was the cause of 33% of childhood and 10% of adult extrapulmonary disease.

However, there has been a recent increase in tuberculosis in cattle which is considered to be related to infection in badgers.[245] *M. bovis* infection is also an uncommon cause of tuberculosis in resource limited countries, except in communities where large amounts of raw milk are consumed, when it commonly presents with cervical adenitis. In the UK, it is still isolated from reactivated lesions in approximately 1% of adults.[245] *M. bovis* is resistant to pyrazinamide.

PATHOLOGY

The pathology of tuberculosis has been described by Miller.[246] The first response to the presence of the tubercle bacilli at the point of entry and in the regional nodes is a serous exudate. Neutrophils accumulate, then macrophages which ingest the bacilli and may be transformed into epithelioid cells, which contain more effective digestive enzymes in their lysosomes. Fusion of either macrophages or epithelioid cells forms characteristic multinucleate giant cells. Death of cells in the center of the tubercle (granuloma) results in caseation necrosis. Lymphocytes form a zone around the tubercle and are particularly apparent during the second month of infection, which coincides with the development of tuberculin sensitivity. Healing takes place with the deposition of collagen fibrils by fibroblasts, which wall off the caseous area from healthy tissue. After 12 months or more, calcification may be seen, which remains for years but may be completely reabsorbed. It usually has a stippled appearance. Alternatively, healing may not occur, or the tubercle-containing dormant bacilli may reactivate after months or years. Extensive necrosis with caseation and liquefaction may develop. Liquefaction allows bacilli to survive, inhibits macrophage and lymphocyte function because of lack of oxygen, and prevents drug penetration. Activity and healing of the lesion may occur concurrently.

IMMUNOLOGY

The main defense against infection by the tubercle bacillus is cell mediated. The role of B cells is unclear.

Tubercle bacilli are readily ingested, but are not killed by macrophages, in which they multiply. Toxic substances and other properties in the lipid-thick cell wall protect the bacillus against lysosomal enzymes. CD4 T lymphocytes (T helper cells), when sensitized by tubercle bacilli, produce cytokines which activate macrophages and CD8 cytotoxic T lymphocytes (CTL). CTLs lyse cells containing mycobacteria and enable macrophages to kill their ingested bacilli. The positive effect of T helper cells may be countered by suppressor activity. In advanced disease or in the presence of a large bacterial load these suppressor effects may predominate, which may explain the anergy commonly seen in these children.

Defense against tuberculosis has two major components: (1) cell-mediated immunity (CMI) controls the infection by activating macrophages which enables them to kill ingested mycobacteria, and (2) delayed type hypersensitivity (DTH) is active when the bacillary antigens reach high levels.[247] DTH is responsible for the tissue damage and caseation necrosis characteristic of post-primary tuberculous disease. There is no correlation between the degree of hypersensitivity and resistance to tuberculosis. The balance between hypersensitivity and resistance will influence the manifestation of tuberculosis, i.e. the former will be associated with clinical and radiological signs of the disease, whereas with the latter there will be a paucity of signs. Improved knowledge of T helper cells has enhanced understanding of the above mechanisms.[248] Three types of T helper cells are recognized: T_H0 (naive cells), T_H1 and T_H2. T_H0 cells differentiate into T_H1 cells or T_H2 cells. T_H1 lymphocytes secrete IL-2, interferon-gamma (IFN-gamma) and lymphotoxin-alpha and stimulate type 1 immunity, which is pro-inflammatory and characterized by phagocytic activity and DTH. IFN-gamma and lymphotoxin-alpha promote secretion of pro-inflammatory cytokines such as tumor necrosis factor-alpha (TNF-alpha). T_H2 cells secrete interleukins such as IL-4 and IL-5, which promote eosinophils and IgE and stimulate a more allergic type 2 immune response. The immunological reactions to tuberculosis are not as clearcut in humans as in mice (in which most experimental work has been undertaken), nor as in leprosy. It would seem, however, that in humans a type 1 response is important in protective inflammation and mounting a DTH response, and a switch to a type 2 response is associated with the period of healing and granuloma organization. High or prolonged type 1 activity may result in excessive DTH reactions and tissue destruction, associated with raised IFN-gamma and TNF-alpha levels. Conversely, failure to control infection, as in immunocompromised patients, is associated with increased type 2 activity. It is suggested that, in humans, excessive tissue destruction may relate to mixed T_H1/T_H2 response whereby a factor produced by type 2 cells makes tissues very sensitive to TNF-alpha.[249] Other important factors include transforming growth factor beta (TGF-beta) produced by mononuclear phagocytes, which may have negative effects on T_H1 activity and 1,25 $(OH)_2$ vitamin D_3 which appears important for action of macrophages in controlling intracellular mycobacterial replication.

A number of primary factors influence the outcome of the immune response, including the number of inhaled bacilli, their virulence and the immune response by the host. These are affected by secondary factors, e.g. age of the patient, infections such as measles, malnutrition, malignancy and immunodeficiency states. Children under 5 years and adolescents (especially females) are at higher risk of developing tuberculous disease.

PATHOGENESIS

The first infection by tubercle bacillus occurs most commonly by inhalation through the lungs, less often by ingestion through the alimentary tract (tonsils and ileum), and rarely by infection of an open wound on the skin. Infection of the mouth, skin and eyes may result from exposure to a dental surgeon with pulmonary tuberculosis. Enlargement of the regional lymph nodes provides an indication of the site of primary focus.

Primary infection

The primary focus in the lung is usually single and situated just under the pleura (Ghon focus) in a well-ventilated part of the lung. Bacilli multiply at the primary focus and in the regional lymph nodes. The primary focus and nodes form the primary complex. In most cases there is hematogenous and lymphatic dissemination throughout the body and to other parts of the lungs. Certain organs favor survival of the bacilli and these may later be affected by disease, e.g. apical and subapical regions of the lungs (Simon focus), where there is a higher oxygen tension, renal parenchyma, epiphyseal lines of bones, cerebral cortex and regional nodes. At about 4–8 weeks, acquired immunity develops and usually contains the infection; sensitivity to tuberculoprotein develops simultaneously. Bacilli stop multiplying and, in the great majority of cases, die or remain dormant indefinitely within the healing tubercle or macrophages. Tubercles, especially if large and apical or subapical, may reactivate at any time in life, if the balance between the organism and the host defense is upset.

In children, the primary focus in the lung is usually small or invisible on chest X-ray, but the regional nodes are enlarged and prominent. In contrast, regional nodes are usually not prominent in primary infection in adults.

The initial infection is usually asymptomatic. Occasionally a short period of fever and malaise may have been noted. Erythema nodosum may appear within a few weeks of the primary infection, coinciding with tuberculin conversion. It is an allergic hypersensitivity reaction, which may be associated with high levels of circulating immune complexes. Phlyctenular conjunctivitis is another, though rare, manifestation of hypersensitivity.

If the infecting load of bacilli is large or the host defense inadequate there may be (Fig. 28.23):

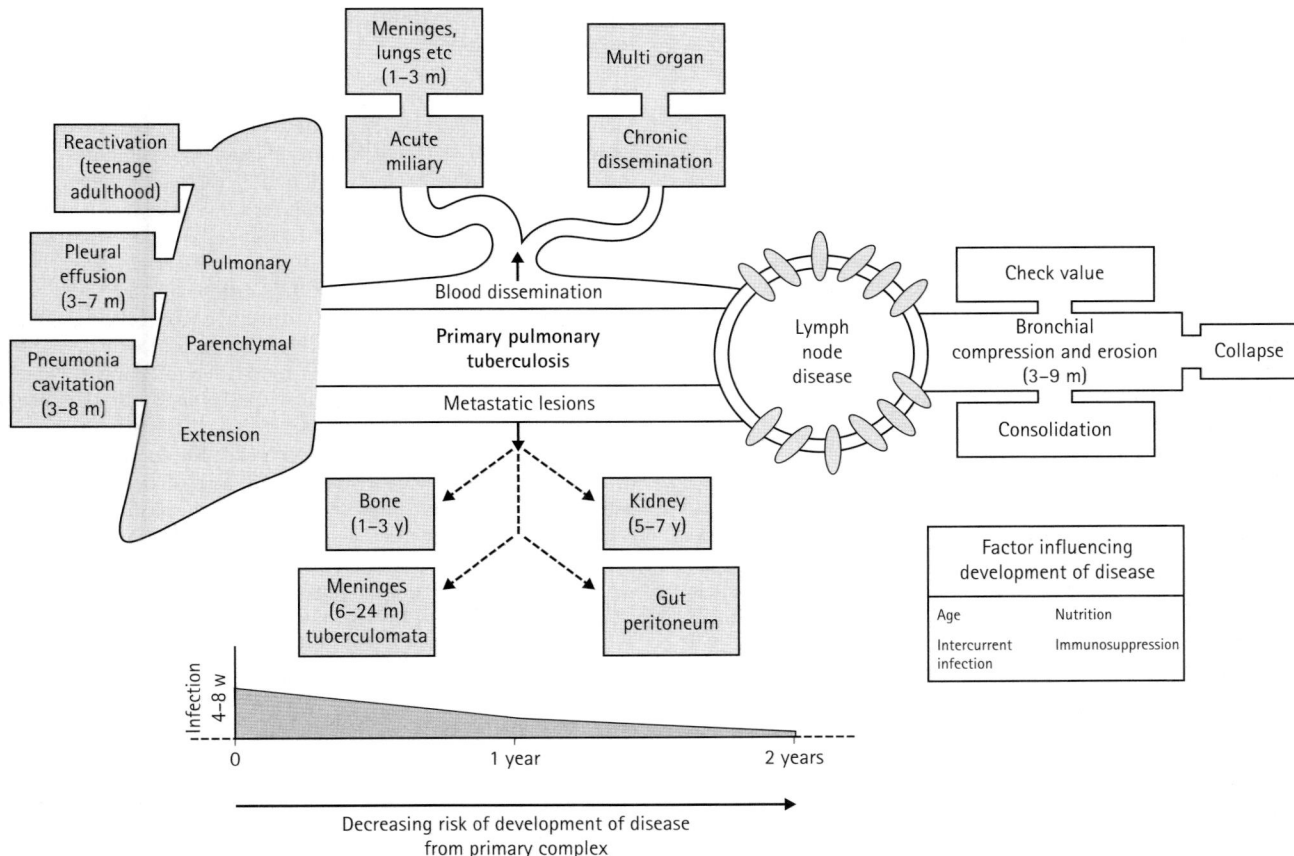

Fig. 28.23 Complications of primary pulmonary tuberculosis. Approximate interval between establishment of primary complex and development of complications in parentheses.

1. extension of the lung focus;
2. softening of the regional nodes;
3. extension of foci in other parts of the body;
4. hematogenous spread with dissemination of bacilli throughout the body (miliary tuberculosis), or chronic low grade dissemination (cryptogenic tuberculosis).

In a newly infected person the risk of developing tuberculous disease is highest in the first 2 years following a primary infection (especially in the first year). The risk is greater in infants and young children and those with malnutrition or immunosuppression. Infants have a risk of 40% or more of developing disease compared with 5% for adults. Pulmonary disease, miliary tuberculosis and meningitis are usually manifest within 1 year of infection, especially in young children, whereas bone disease presents later (within 3 years), and renal disease usually much later (over 5–7 years).

Post-primary tuberculosis

Post-primary tuberculosis occurs when a person who has previously had tuberculosis develops active disease. Post-primary tuberculosis can develop from endogenous reactivation of a primary lesion, from exogenous reinfection or both. Though sometimes termed 'adult'-type pulmonary tuberculosis, it may be seen in children.[246] It is characterized by strong resistance, which keeps the disease localized to the affected organ, and an active hypersensitivity state, which results in extensive tissue destruction and necrosis. The tubercle bacillus may have reached the area through blood spread following primary infection or via the airways in exogenous reinfection. For the latter, as the apices are not well ventilated, multiple exposure will usually be necessary.[250] It affects particularly the apical regions of the lungs, where the oxygen tension is higher. There is widespread caseation necrosis, liquefaction with cavity formation and healing by fibrosis.

TUBERCULIN SENSITIVITY

The intradermal tuberculin test using old tuberculin was described by Charles Mantoux in 1908. A positive response results in induration within 72 h, associated with migration of activated lymphocytes and macrophages to the site of injection.

Purified protein derivative (PPD)-S 5 IU is the standard strength in many countries. PPD RT 23 Statens Serum Institute (SSI), Copenhagen is administered at a strength of 2 tuberculin units (TU). Induration of ≥6 mm with RT 23 is regarded as positive. Because the active principle of RT 23 adheres to glass walls of containers, Tween 80 is added to reduce absorption. This multiplies the strength by a factor of 4–5. Weaker and stronger products are available. In phlyctenular conjunctivitis or tuberculosis of the eye it is suggested to use a weaker strength initially as a stronger solution may result in a severe eye reaction. Stronger solutions, e.g. 10 TU, are rarely indicated as they may give false positive reactions with environmental mycobacterial infections.

Technique of tuberculin test

The skin is cleaned and dried, and the injection given *intradermally* into the upper third of the flexor surface of the forearm (Mantoux test) with a 1 ml syringe and a small needle (short bevel gauge 25–26) producing a wheal of at least 5 mm (see BCG technique). The result should be read at 48–72 h, but a valid result may be obtained at up to 96 h. In strongly tuberculin positive subjects, a wheal may appear within 24 h. Rarely, lymphangitis or a systemic reaction may develop following the tuberculin test. If necrosis and ulceration develop, local hydrocortisone ointment may relieve the discomfort.

Interpretation

The transverse diameter of induration is measured. In older children and adults, an indurated wheal of 5 mm or less is regarded as negative, 6–9 mm is likely to be associated with infection by environmental mycobacteria, and 10 mm or greater is indicative of infection by *M. tuberculosis*, unless the person has received BCG recently. In infants and young children with clinical evidence suggestive of tuberculosis, those with malnutrition or immunosuppression or in close contact with a case, an intermediate reaction of 6–9 mm should be considered positive. After BCG, the tuberculin response is usually less than 15 mm. A tuberculin reaction of 15 mm or greater in any child is suggestive of sensitivity to *M. tuberculosis*. Where there is doubt about interpretation of the tuberculin reaction, an IFN-gamma assay should be undertaken.

A negative or weak response in the presence of tuberculosis may occur in the following conditions: 6–10 weeks after onset of infection, but before tuberculin sensitivity has developed; malnutrition; miliary or overwhelming tuberculosis; nonrespiratory disease, especially tuberculous meningitis; tuberculosis in infants less than 6 weeks of age; recent viral infections such as measles and glandular fever, or whooping cough; recent immunization (within 6 weeks) against measles, mumps and rubella; immunosuppressive diseases including HIV, malignancy, and other debilitating diseases; and current treatment with immunosuppressive agents (including corticosteroids). In resource limited countries the tuberculin test is often negative in children with tuberculosis, probably owing to immunosuppression due to malnutrition, HIV infection and/or overwhelming disease.

When the tuberculin test is negative in children with tuberculosis due to malnutrition, overwhelming infection or other causes, if it is repeated some months after treatment when the general condition of the patient has improved, it will usually be positive. However, a small proportion of children with culture-proven tuberculosis (perhaps 5%) are consistently negative, despite the absence of adverse factors such as malnutrition, overwhelming tuberculosis or other infections.[251] In children infected by *M. tuberculosis* (and those given BCG), tuberculin sensitivity may revert to negative over some years, particularly in those in whom there was not a strong initial reaction or who have had prompt treatment. This does not necessarily imply that they are not protected from reinfection. Repeated administration of tuberculin in subjects sensitized by BCG or tuberculosis may enhance tuberculin sensitivity (booster phenomenon).

Multiple puncture techniques

Multiple puncture tests such as the Heaf test are used to screen large numbers of children. Other tests include the Tine and Imotest. The Heaf test is the most reliable, but all doubtful reactions following multiple puncture techniques should be confirmed by a Mantoux test. The Heaf test was discontinued in the UK in 2005.

Interferon-gamma assays

IFN-gamma assays are based on antigens encoded by genes located within the region of difference 1 (RD1) of the *M. tuberculosis* genome, e.g. early secretory antigenic target 6 (ESAT6) and culture filtrate protein 10 (CFP10). Neither ESAT6 nor CFP10 is present in BCG strains or in most environmental mycobacteria.

Presently there are two commercial IFN-gamma assays, the QuantiFERON-TB Gold and T SPOT-TB assays. Both measure IFN-gamma released from T cells sensitized when they are exposed to ESAT6 and/or CFP10. The former is an ELISA and the latter an enzyme-linked immunospot (ELISPOT) assay. IFN-gamma assays have similar or higher sensitivity than the tuberculin test.[252] A study in South African children which included those with HIV infection and severe malnutrition found that the ELISPOT had a higher sensitivity than the tuberculin test.[253]

The main advantage of IFN-gamma assays over the tuberculin test is the higher specificity due to lack of cross-reactivity with BCG and environmental mycobacteria and likely higher sensitivity in children with HIV infection and malnutrition.

BCG VACCINATION

BCG vaccine is an attenuated bovine strain of mycobacteria introduced by Calmette and Guérin in France in 1921 and originally given orally. It was first used in Sweden in 1927 and in England in 1948.

After intradermal injection of BCG, there is dissemination of small numbers of bacilli to internal organs, particularly the liver and lungs, where granulomata develop. BCG sensitizes individuals so that when they are infected by *M. tuberculosis* multiplication of bacteria is curtailed and a granuloma develops quickly which walls off the infection. Systemic hematogenous dissemination is reduced, as also is secondary infection of the lung either from local extension of lesions or seeding from the blood. BCG vaccination does not prevent tuberculous infection; it particularly reduces the risk of meningitis and disseminated disease (and death), and, to a lesser extent, pulmonary disease.

Indications

In the UK, BCG vaccination is recommended for the following groups:[254]

1. all neonates and infants (0–12 months) living in areas where the incidence of tuberculosis is greater than 40 per 100 000;
2. neonates, infants and children under 16 years with a parent or grandparent born in a country with an incidence of tuberculosis greater than 40 per 100 000;
3. previously unvaccinated new immigrants aged under 35 years who were born in, or lived for more than 3 months in a country with an incidence of tuberculosis greater than 40 per 100 000;
4. contacts of those with respiratory tuberculosis;
5. individuals at occupational risk aged under 35 years including health care workers and laboratory staff who are likely to have contact with patients, clinical materials or derived isolates, veterinary and other staff who handle animal species susceptible to tuberculosis, and staff working directly with prisoners, in care homes for the elderly, or in hostels or facilities for the homeless or refugees;
6. individuals aged under 35 years intending to live or work with local people for more than 1 month in a country with an incidence of tuberculosis greater than 40 per 100 000.

Contraindications

BCG vaccination is contraindicated in patients with immunosuppressive disorders or malignancy, those receiving corticosteroids or immunosuppressive treatment, and in generalized infective conditions. If eczema exists, vaccination should be given in an area free from skin lesions. An interval of 3 weeks should be allowed between administration of BCG vaccine and other live vaccines, with the exception of oral polio vaccine. BCG vaccination is not given to tuberculin positive subjects

The recommendations for BCG vaccination of infants born to mothers infected by HIV vary according to the prevalence of tuberculosis. In industrialized countries, BCG is contraindicated in infants suspected of HIV infection. In countries where both HIV infection and tuberculosis are endemic, routine BCG immunization of newborns is recommended. However, in resource limited countries where neonatal BCG is routine, a small proportion of recipients with perinatal HIV infection or congenital immunodeficiency syndromes will develop distant or disseminated disease with a high mortality.[255,256]

Technique

BCG is given to subjects whose tuberculin reaction is < 6 mm. Re-vaccination is unnecessary for people with a definite BCG scar, even if the tuberculin test is negative. A pre-vaccination tuberculin test is not required in children < 6 years old unless they have stayed > 1 month in a country with an incidence of tuberculosis > 40 per 100 000 or had contact with a person with tuberculosis.

BCG vaccine is injected intradermally, usually into the left upper arm at the insertion of the deltoid muscle: 0.1 ml is given with a 1 ml syringe and a short bevelled needle gauge 25–26 (as per Mantoux test). It is advised that neonates and infants < 12 months are given 0.05 ml because of the increased risk of local lymphadenopathy. Proper technique is essential. The needle should be inserted, bevel upwards, into the superficial layers of the dermis (almost parallel with the surface) for about 3 mm and a wheal of at least 5–7 mm produced. If resistance is not felt during injecting, the needle has been inserted too far (or the fluid

has leaked externally) and it should be withdrawn. Injecting the vaccine subcutaneously may result in an abscess or large ulcer. Normally a small papule develops at the site of vaccination within 2–6 weeks. Sometimes it may ulcerate and discharge but it usually heals after about 2–3 months, leaving a small scar (for management see Complications).

Accelerated BCG reaction

If BCG vaccine is given to persons infected by tuberculosis or who have received BCG previously, an accelerated reaction may result: a papule appears within 24–48 h, a pustule by 5–7 days, and a scab by 2 weeks. In malnourished children with tuberculosis, the tuberculin test is often negative, but there may be an accelerated reaction to BCG which could potentially be used as a diagnostic test for tuberculosis. A papule of 5 mm or more appearing by the third day is regarded as positive. BCG is considered to be equivalent to 20–50 TU PPD. Because of the risk that a malnourished child has HIV infection, this practice is now not recommended.

Complications

If > 1% of recipients develop an adverse local reaction to BCG, this usually indicates incorrect dosage or bad technique. The commonest complication is the development of a local abscess or large ulcer. Unless there is superinfection with a pyogenic organism, the abscess is non-tender and the child afebrile. Swelling of local lymph nodes with or without sinus formation is more likely in young infants. These complications usually result from an inadvertent subcutaneous injection.

Nonfluctuant enlarged nodes should be left untreated. Abscesses should be aspirated. If repeated aspiration of fluctuant nodes does not result in resolution they may be excised. Discharging ulcers should be cleaned with an antiseptic two or three times a day, left uncovered as much as possible, and, when necessary, a non-adherent dressing should be used. For ulcers that do not respond to these methods, isoniazid 6 mg/kg/d for 6 weeks usually results in healing. Hypertrophic or keloid scars may develop at the site of vaccination, especially if given at sites other than insertion of the deltoid. Excision is not always successful. Local injection of triamcinolone at monthly intervals for 3–4 doses may result in atrophy.

Other rare complications of BCG vaccination include anaphylactic reactions, satellite lesions, bone lesions, meningitis or overwhelming infection. The latter usually occurs in immunodeficient infants (see above under Contraindications and HIV infection).[257] Focal lesions such as osteitis may occur in apparently immunocompetent infants and in some cases have been associated with increased potency of the vaccine.[258] Osteitis may develop 6–9 months to some years after vaccination. In HIV-infected infants, enlarged lymph nodes (usually ipsilateral to BCG injection) with sinus formation may develop months to years after the vaccination has apparently healed, coinciding with the onset of immunosuppression or administration of antiretroviral therapy.[256]

Efficacy

The effectiveness of BCG in preventing tuberculosis, particularly meningitis and disseminated disease, has been demonstrated in a number of prospective trials and case control studies.[259–261] It also provides some protection against leprosy and Buruli ulcer. Protection persists for up to 10 years. However, results of studies vary between different communities and are influenced by factors such as the prevalence of and exposure to tuberculosis, distance from the equator, the prevalence of environmental mycobacteria, the administration and potency of the vaccine, and the age and nutritional status of the population.[262]

Schoolchildren in the UK vaccinated at around 13 years have demonstrated a consistent level of protection of about 75%, persisting for 15 years.[263]

Two controlled trials of BCG in the newborn, one in North American Indians living in Saskatchewan, the other in Chicago, have shown 75–80% protection, and some case control studies have also demonstrated over 70% protection.[259,261]

In the northern hemisphere, BCG continues to provide substantial protection against tuberculosis overall and up to 80% for meningitis and disseminated disease.

Tuberculin sensitivity after BCG vaccination

When the technique and potency of vaccine is adequate, most vaccinated infants will have a scar and >90% will be tuberculin positive (≥6 mm). Low grade tuberculin sensitivity will remain in most children for at least 5–12 years.[264,265] Preterm infants and those with severe intrauterine growth retardation may have a reduced response to BCG vaccination, possibly due to impaired cell-mediated immunity. Scars are less likely to persist in infants vaccinated in the neonatal period.

In resource limited countries, tuberculin sensitivity following neonatal BCG wanes considerably over the first few years. After 2–3 years most children will be tuberculin negative or have low sensitivity.[266] Thus neonatal BCG should not affect the interpretation of the tuberculin test in these areas. In children recently vaccinated with BCG, who are in contact with a smear positive case of tuberculosis, a Mantoux reaction of ≥15 mm should be interpreted as likely infection by M. tuberculosis. Repeat BCG vaccination is associated with larger tuberculin reactions. An IFN-gamma assay should help in identifying a false positive tuberculin test.

New vaccines

Vaccines are required which are more effective in preventing exogenous reinfection, especially in adolescents and adults, in people already infected by environmental mycobacteria and in those who have received conventional BCG. Candidate vaccines include live attenuated vaccines comprising BCG or M. tuberculosis subunit vaccines and fusion proteins formulated in various adjuvants.[267] Phase 1 trials have been completed for some and phase 2 trials are in progress or planned.

PREVENTION AND CONTACT TRACING

In the UK today, the majority of children in whom tuberculosis is diagnosed are detected through contact tracing of smear positive cases of tuberculosis. Children with primary tuberculosis (as opposed to adolescents with cavitary disease) and patients with nonrespiratory tuberculosis are rarely infectious. However, children with tuberculosis and their visitors should be segregated from the rest of the ward until family and visitors have been screened. Smear positive adults who receive drug regimens which include rifampicin usually have a negative sputum culture within 2 weeks.

Procedures for control and prevention of tuberculosis in the UK have been outlined.[268] When a case of tuberculosis is diagnosed, household contacts should be screened. Children and young adults should have a tuberculin test and, when positive, a chest X-ray. Older adults and those who have received BCG vaccination should have a chest X-ray. If the tuberculin test is negative, it should be repeated after 6 weeks as the first test may have been done too early in the course of infection. Tuberculin negative subjects should be offered BCG. Tuberculin positive subjects with a normal chest X-ray should be given chemoprophylaxis (see below).

Young children are usually infected in the home. For older children it may be necessary to search outside the home, e.g. staff at school, a swimming pool attendant or a youth leader. In tuberculosis of the face or gums, the possibility of infection by a dentist should be considered.

Chemoprophylaxis and follow-up of contacts

This section outlines the recommendations for chemoprophylaxis of contacts of a known case of tuberculosis.

Chemoprophylaxis is indicated for tuberculin positive children (≥10 mm) or those with a positive IFN-gamma assay with a normal chest X-ray, who have not had BCG. It should be considered in those with ≥15 mm who have received BCG. Guidelines for children < 2 years in close contact with smear positive pulmonary disease are as follows:

1. *No prior BCG*: give chemoprophylaxis irrespective of tuberculin test. Repeat tuberculin test after 6 weeks: if negative, stop chemoprophylaxis and give BCG; if positive (and chest X-ray excludes disease) give full chemoprophylaxis.
2. *Prior BCG*: if tuberculin test is strongly positive (≥15 mm) give chemoprophylaxis. If tuberculin test is weak (≤10 mm), repeat in 6 weeks. If there is no change, no further action is required. If size of reaction increases (and chest X-ray excludes disease), give full chemoprophylaxis. Routine follow-up chest X-rays are only required for those who are eligible for, but did not receive, chemoprophylaxis.

For chemoprophylaxis, isoniazid (INH) plus rifampicin (RIF) should be given for 3 months, or INH only 6 mg/kg/d should be given for 6 months. In young infants exposed to smear positive patients, or in contacts at any age when the source is suspected to harbor INH-resistant M. tuberculosis, RIF may be added to INH and the combination given for 4–6 months. If INH resistance is confirmed, RIF alone may be given for 6 months.[268,269]

CLINICAL FORMS OF TUBERCULOSIS

The commonest presentation of tuberculosis is respiratory disease, followed by involvement of lymph nodes.[243] In resource limited countries, extrapulmonary disease accounts for 35–40% of tuberculosis, compared to around 20% in the USA.[241] It is important to remember that tuberculosis can infect virtually any part of the body. Figure. 28.23 shows an outline and a time scale of some of the complications of primary tuberculosis.

Intrathoracic tuberculosis

Primary pulmonary tuberculosis

The primary complex consists of a focal lesion usually 1–2 cm in diameter which may be found in any part of the lung, and enlarged hilar nodes or, in heavier infections, paratracheal nodes. Lymph node enlargement is particularly prominent in infants and young children (Figs. 28.24b and 28.25a). The primary complex is usually asymptomatic and discovered during contact tracing or a routine tuberculin test. Often the primary focus has resolved or is not visible and the diagnosis is based on enlarged regional nodes. Calcification of the focus and, more often, the nodes may occur after about 12 months, generally within 2–3 years of the infection, and remains an indication of previous infection. Calcification usually indicates healing of the tuberculous process, but healing and progression of the disease may continue concurrently. In many cases the calcium slowly resolves leaving clear lung fields, which explains the common finding in adults where the tuberculin test is positive and the chest X-ray normal.

In older children and adolescents, the lung component is more prominent and commonly presents as an enlarging upper lobe infiltrate and cavitation, usually without lymph node enlargement, and is indistinguishable from postprimary tuberculosis. Pleural effusion is more common at this age.

Progression of primary tuberculosis

Progression of primary tuberculosis may result from extension of the pulmonary focus (progressive primary tuberculosis) or, more commonly, softening of regional lymph nodes. Extension of the pulmonary focus may cause bronchopneumonia or rupture into the pleura resulting in pleural effusion. Tuberculous empyema may result from rupture of caseous material into the pleural space, which may be complicated by pneumothorax (pyopneumothorax). Evacuation of caseous material into a bronchus may result in the appearance of a cavity. Cavities in primary pulmonary tuberculosis are not uncommon in malnourished and debilitated infants with progressive primary tuberculosis (Fig. 28.24b).

Complications from enlargement or softening of regional nodes have a variety of manifestations. The bronchus may be compressed externally; more likely, the wall is eroded and caseous material either partly or completely blocks the lumen (endobronchial tuberculosis); or rupture

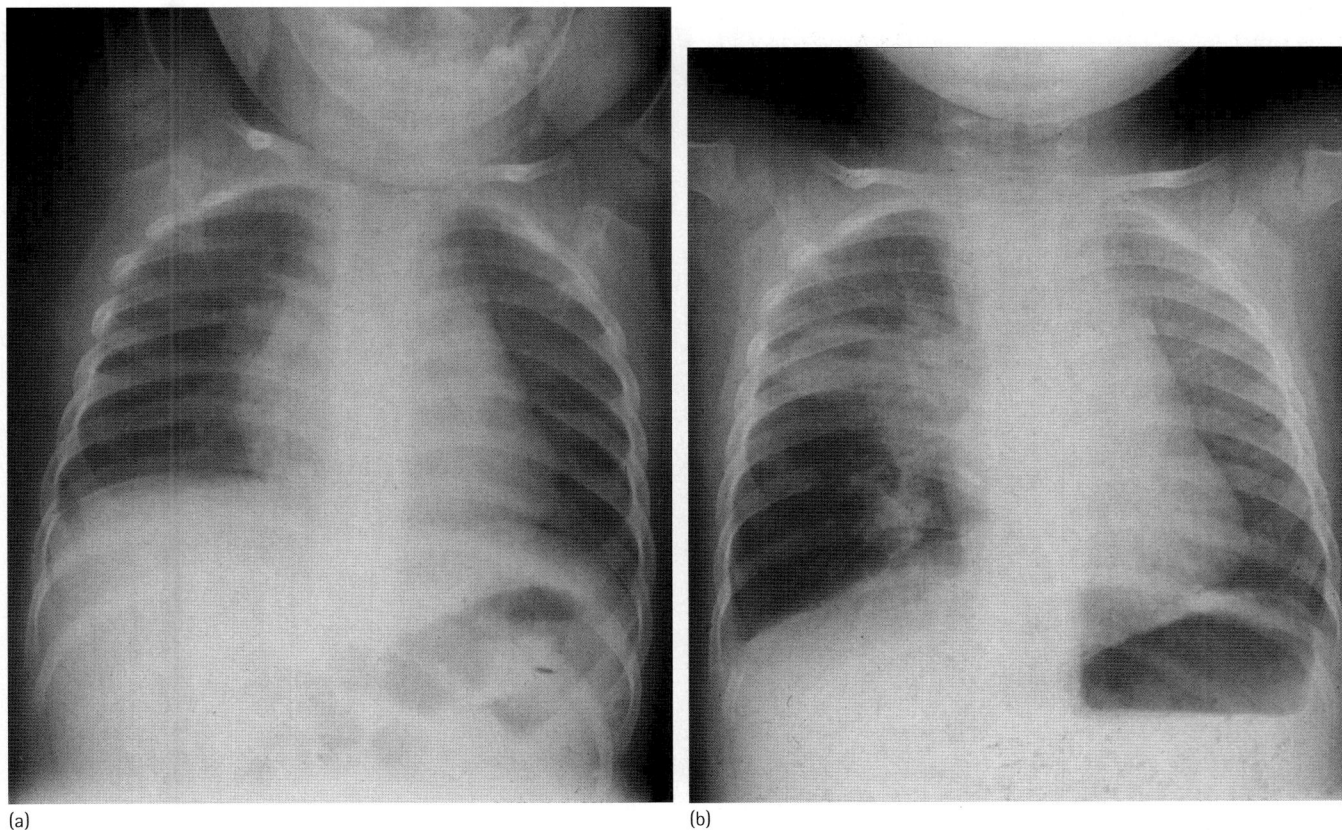

(a)   (b)

Fig. 28.24 (a) A 2½-year-old asymptomatic girl with a strongly positive tuberculin test was in contact with a smear positive case of tuberculosis. Chest X-ray shows a nonspecific opacity in the right upper zone. (b) She was put on chemoprophylaxis with isoniazid plus rifampicin but did not comply with treatment. Chest X-ray taken 2 months later shows an enlarged right mediastinal node with compression of the trachea, collapse/consolidation in all three zones of the right lung, a cavity in the upper lobe and hyperinflation of the right lower lobe. She now had symptoms – cough, stridor and wheeze. This case demonstrates progression of untreated primary tuberculosis.

of the wall results in bronchopneumonia. Partial obstruction may result in a ball-valve effect with lobar emphysema (Fig. 28.24b). This is often transient, because either the bronchus blocks completely or the material is coughed up with clearing of the obstruction.[270] More commonly, there is *segmental* collapse with or without consolidation. Rupture of caseous material into the bronchus may result in a predominantly allergic response with exudation, or, if there are a large number of bacteria present, a progressive tuberculous bronchopneumonia. The former may be associated with marked changes on chest X-ray but which clear spontaneously, whereas the latter, which is more often seen in debilitated children, may prove fatal if not treated. Spread of infected material into both main bronchi may result in bilateral bronchopneumonia.

Rarely, a caseous node may rupture into the trachea, resulting in bilateral obstructive emphysema or asphyxia, into the esophagus resulting in a fistula or the development of an esophageal pouch, or into the pericardium. Other complications from enlarged nodes include superior vena cava obstruction and recurrent laryngeal or phrenic nerve compression.

There may be nonspecific symptoms of irregular fever, anorexia and weight loss. In severe or long-standing cases, the child may be severely wasted. Compression of the bronchi may result in a spasmodic cough simulating whooping cough. When there is obstructive emphysema, the symptoms may be mistaken for asthma, though clinical examination will usually demonstrate signs of mediastinal shift. In long-standing cases, the child may present with clubbing of the fingers and bronchiectasis.

Adolescent tuberculosis

In adolescents, infection is usually in the upper lobes or the superior segments of the lower lobes, and is usually confined to the lungs with no hematogenous spread. In some cases it results from reactivation of a former primary lesion (post-primary tuberculosis) and, though usually associated with adults, this may occur in children and adolescents (Fig. 28.25a, b). Evidence of a previous primary pulmonary complex may be detected.[270] In other cases it is a primary exogenous infection. Common symptoms include a productive cough, especially in the morning, and there may be hemoptysis, fever, night sweats, malaise and weight loss.

Chest X-ray may show a variety of lesions including nodular or patchy shadows, cavities and various stages of healing with fibrosis and calcification. Both lungs may be affected and there may be a pleural effusion.

Diagnosis

The diagnosis of primary pulmonary tuberculosis is based on a positive tuberculin test (10 mm) and/or a positive IFN-gamma assay and enlarged nodes on chest X-ray with or without a pulmonary infiltrate. History of contact provides strong support. Enlarged lymph nodes may not be easily demonstrated; a lateral chest X-ray may be helpful. Persistent pulmonary infiltrate(s) in the presence of a positive tuberculin test is highly suggestive of tuberculosis.

Chest X-ray usually shows enlarged nodes with opacities more often in the right than left lung, due to collapse and/or consolidation. Bilateral disease may be seen in 25% of cases. In progressive disease, cavities may be seen. Lymph nodes may be detected on CT scan in children with normal chest X-rays.[271] The tuberculin test may be negative in debilitated children. This is a common problem in resource limited countries where, in the absence of facilities for mycobacterial culture, the diagnosis is often based on the response to a trial of chemotherapy.

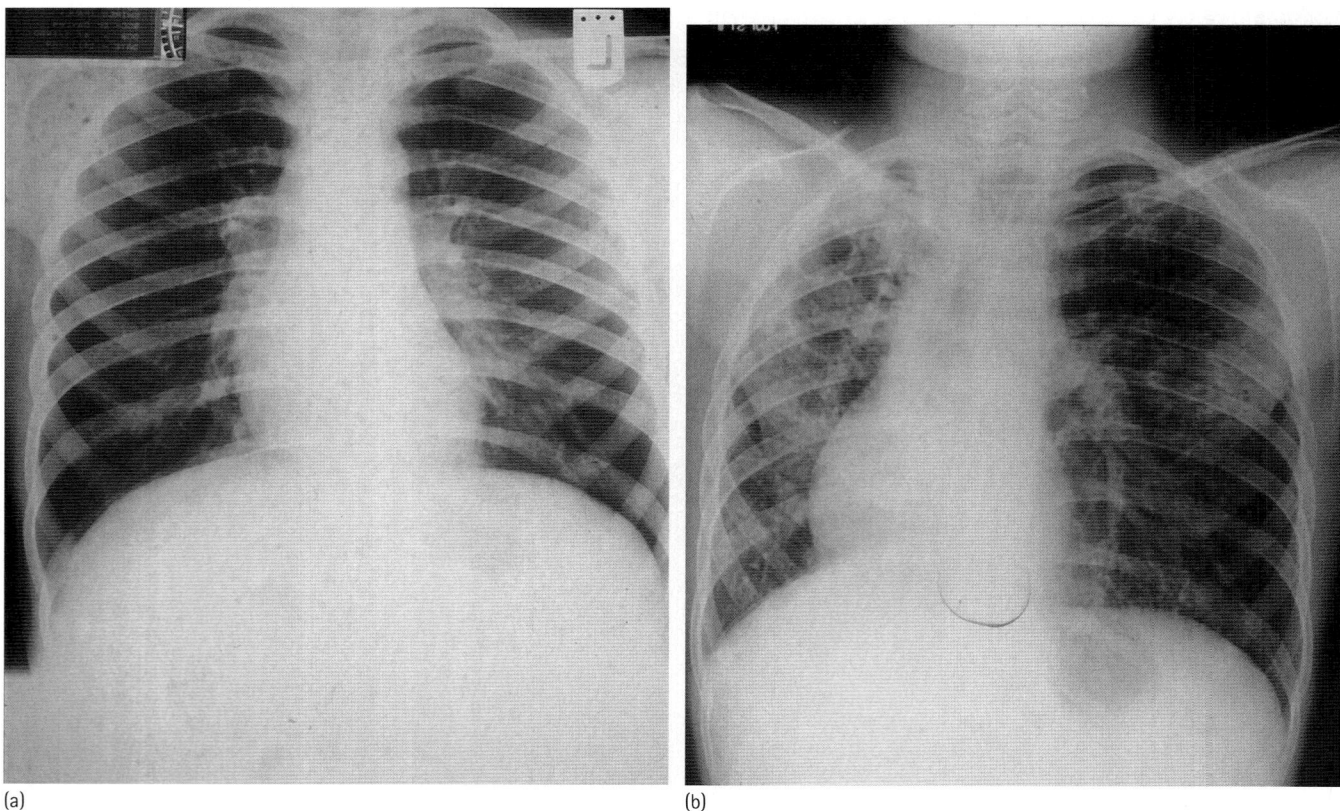

(a)   (b)

Fig. 28.25   (a) An 8-year-old boy was in contact with his grandmother who had smear-positive tuberculosis. His tuberculin test was negative. Although the chest X-ray shows an enlarged right hilar node it was regarded as normal and he did not receive chemoprophylaxis. He was given BCG and developed an accelerated reaction to it. (b) Four years later he presented with a cough for 6 months, dyspnea and weight loss. Chest X-ray shows loss of volume of the right lung with multiple cavities and fibrosis in the right upper lobe and a cavity in the left apex and left mid zone and a miliary pattern. Sputum smear was strongly positive for acid-fast bacilli. This is an example of post-primary tuberculosis. (Fig. 28.25b Reproduced with permission from the *Journal of Medical Microbiology* 1996; 44:7, Fig 1.)

In older children with post-primary or adult type tuberculosis, diagnosis is made by smear and culture of sputum. For younger children, if sensitivities of the contact are not available or diagnosis is unclear, three early morning gastric aspirations should be undertaken while the child is recumbent and has been fasted overnight. If the gastric aspirate (usually 5–10 ml) is very small or the tube is blocked, sterile water (< 20 ml) may be injected and after a few minutes aspirated. If there is delay in transporting the specimen to the laboratory, the acid should be neutralized (pH 7.0) by adding approximately 3 ml of sodium bicarbonate (100 mg/ml). Smear is seldom positive on gastric aspirates in industrialized countries and in some cases it may be due to environmental mycobacteria. However, in resource limited countries where the infective load of *M. tuberculosis* may be high, 10–15% of patients may have a positive smear. Culture is positive in no more than 30–50% of cases.[272] It is more likely to be positive in infants (75%) and those with extensive parenchymal disease.[273] However, it may be positive in children with only enlarged intrathoracic nodes and rarely in those with normal chest X-ray. Gastric aspiration undertaken in an ambulatory clinic has generally lower sensitivity for culture than when taken in the early morning.

Alternative methods to obtain sputum include induced sputum, laryngeal swab and nasopharyngeal aspirate.[274] Laryngeal swabs or nasopharyngeal aspirates are useful for ambulatory clinics and when gastric aspiration is not possible.[275–277] Induced sputum is increasingly used for diagnosis of tuberculosis and may be undertaken in infants, or in adolescents without productive sputum.[278,279] Culture of respiratory secretions obtained through induced sputum, laryngeal swab or nasopharyngeal aspirate is less sensitive (25–30%) than gastric aspirate (30–50%).[276–279] Bronchoscopy is no more sensitive for culture

of *M. tuberculosis* than gastric aspiration.[280,281] If diagnosis is important for management, biopsy of enlarged lymph nodes should be considered.

The blood count usually shows a normal white cell count. A raised ESR is associated with activity of the disease but otherwise has no diagnostic value.

A *pleural effusion* is due to an allergic response to the mycobacteria and thus the tuberculin test is usually strongly positive, except in very debilitated children. If large, or required for diagnostic purposes, it should be aspirated. The fluid is usually clear and straw-colored, but may be opalescent if there is a high cell count. Lymphocytes will be seen on microscopy, but early in the disease neutrophils may also be present. The protein content will be raised, > 40 g/L, and the glucose low, < 1.7 mmol/L. Mycobacteria are often not detected on direct smear, but in about half the cases they may be cultured, especially if a large volume of fluid is centrifuged. Mycobacteria are more likely to be cultured from an empyema. Pleural biopsy may also be taken for histology.

Management

Uncomplicated primary infection usually heals without treatment. The main purpose of chemotherapy is to prevent hematogenous spread and progression of disease, which is more likely in young, debilitated or malnourished children. Segmental collapse may occur despite chemotherapy, but tuberculous bronchopneumonia or pleural effusion is usually prevented. Radiological changes resolve slowly and 50% of children may still have evidence of the primary complex after 18 months. Lymph nodes may enlarge during chemotherapy, but there is usually no necessity to prolong therapy because of this.

Standard three-drug chemotherapy is isoniazid (INH), rifampicin (RIF) and pyrazinamide (PZA) for 2 months followed by INH and RIF for 4 months. Ethambutol (EMB) is added if drug resistance is suspected or burden of infection is high. If PZA is not given, INH + RIF should be given for 9 months. For alternative regimens see section on Chemotherapy. For hilar lymphadenopathy alone a three-drug regimen followed by INH + RIF for just 2 months or INH + RIF for 6 months may be adequate.[282]

Bronchial obstruction. Incomplete bronchial obstruction with air trapping and the development of *obstructive emphysema* may respond to corticosteroids (see Management). However, the transient nature of this lesion should be remembered, i.e. it may resolve or the bronchus may become completely obstructed. Complete obstruction will result in absorption collapse, and bronchoscopy should be performed to exclude other pathology, such as foreign body, and to suck out as much of the caseous material in the bronchial lumen as possible. Unfortunately, the obstruction may be difficult to visualize, especially in young infants.

Pleural effusion. The infective load in pleural effusion is low and responds quickly to treatment. The addition of corticosteroids may enhance the absorption of fluid but long term benefit regarding reduction of pleural thickening and adhesions has not been demonstrated.[283] In the presence of empyema, surgical drainage may be required.

Pericarditis

M. tuberculosis may reach the pericardium by lymphatic extension from mediastinal lymph nodes, direct extension from caseous lung tissue or lymph nodes, or from hematogenous spread. It is more common in resource limited countries.[284] A loud pericardial rub may be heard in dry pericarditis. Occasionally, there is a large effusion, which may cause tamponade. An effusion will be detected by echocardiography. Pericardial aspirate is often blood-stained, and polymorphonuclear leukocytes may be seen in the early stages, after which lymphocytes predominate. *M. tuberculosis* may be cultured in over half the cases, and in up to 75% using double strength Kirchner culture medium. Diagnosis may also be made by culture and histology of a pericardial biopsy. Constrictive pericarditis may ensue in spite of treatment.

Standard antituberculous treatment is given. Open drainage may prevent subsequent requirement for pericardial aspiration. Corticosteroids may enhance the rate of improvement and reduce the requirement for aspiration, but seem not to reduce the need for pericardectomy.[285,286]

Extrathoracic tuberculosis

Nonrespiratory disease usually results from hematogenous spread. Virtually any organ may be affected. Some of the common types are described below. Tuberculosis may also affect the larynx, middle ear and mastoid bones. Middle ear disease may be associated with HIV infection. Virtually any part of the eye may be infected and tuberculosis should be remembered as a cause of an orbital mass. Tuberculosis of the skin may result from primary inoculation, from hematogenous dissemination, or from a cold abscess in an underlying structure.

Lymph node tuberculosis

Superficial lymph node tuberculosis commonly occurs in the cervical or supraclavicular, and, less often, the axillary or inguinal regions. As in primary tuberculosis of the lungs, the regional nodes enlarge in response to a focus. Less commonly, enlargement of a number of superficial lymph nodes results from hematogenous spread. The focus may be the tonsils, gums, lungs or elsewhere. In cervical adenitis, the commonest focus is the upper lung fields. Enlarged axillary or inguinal nodes may be due to disseminated disease or infection of the skin. In the UK, in the majority of cases of white children with histological evidence of mycobacterial infection of the cervical glands, it is associated with environmental mycobacteria such as *M. avium-intracellulare*. *M. tuberculosis* is more common in immigrant children.

Initially the nodes are discrete, mobile and non-tender, later becoming matted together. Without treatment, softening of nodes usually develops within 6 months of infection, and nodes may discharge forming a sinus or track along the fascial planes. Swelling and softening may occur in up to a third of patients during treatment or even years after the node is calcified and apparently healed. This phenomenon of paradoxical enlargement may be due to hypersensitivity to tuberculoprotein, released at intervals from the lesion, and does not usually indicate active infection.

The tuberculin test is usually positive and a chest X-ray should be taken to exclude pulmonary tuberculosis. Calcification within the node may be detected radiologically. Ultrasound or MRI is helpful in confirming that the lesion is a lymph node and in detection of caseous necrosis. Fine needle aspiration for smear and culture, or preferably excision biopsy, will usually confirm the diagnosis. All specimens, either from biopsy or aspiration, should be cultured as it is important to ascertain whether the infection is caused by *M. tuberculosis* or environmental mycobacteria. However, culture may be positive in only two thirds of cases. The main differential diagnosis is from a cervical pyogenic abscess. Local viral or streptococcal infection of the tonsils may cause enlargement of existing tuberculous nodes. Other differential diagnoses include glandular fever, HIV infection, cat-scratch disease, malignancy or an infected branchial or thyroglossal cyst and, in HIV endemic regions of sub-Saharan Africa, Kaposi sarcoma.

Treatment with standard chemotherapy is adequate. If softening of the node occurs, it may be aspirated. If excision is necessary, the primary node should be removed intact, or, if not feasible, as much of the caseous material as possible.[246] Cold abscesses are frequently of the 'collar stud' variety, and will recur if the abscess in the deep fascia is not adequately drained.

Disseminated tuberculosis

Hematogenous dissemination of small numbers of bacilli probably occurs in the majority of children with primary uncomplicated tuberculosis. In resource limited countries, a liver biopsy for an unconnected disease may show tuberculous granulomata in children not known to have had tuberculosis. These rarely become symptomatic. Massive hematogenous spread is referred to as acute miliary tuberculosis and if untreated is usually rapidly fatal. It may be associated with caseous necrosis involving a blood vessel or inadequate immunological response to the infection. It may be found at autopsy without being evident on chest X-ray. A more chronic form, cryptogenic disseminated, also occurs. In both forms, disease may develop in virtually any organ of the body.

Acute miliary tuberculosis. Acute miliary tuberculosis (miliary means 'millet seed') is most common in young children and usually occurs within a year of the primary infection. The most important complication is meningitis. The onset is usually insidious. Presenting signs include pyrexia, dyspnea, anemia, hepatosplenomegaly and lymphadenopathy.[287] Anorexia and weight loss are common and variable degrees of malnutrition will be evident depending on the length of the illness. The lungs show a 'snowstorm' picture on chest X-ray. Rarely, respiratory failure with adult respiratory distress syndrome may develop. Choroid tubercles are pathognomonic of the disease. Cutaneous lesions include macules, papules, purpura and papulonecrotic tuberculides.

Except in the early stages, the diagnosis will usually be evident from a chest X-ray. Miliary disease may be detected on CT scan when the chest X-ray is normal. There may also be lobar infiltrates and hilar lymphadenopathy. The tuberculin test may be weak or negative in the early stages or if the child has severe debility. A lumbar puncture is essential in all cases to exclude meningitis. Bacteriological confirmation will be obtained in the majority of children, particularly from culture of gastric contents, and also CSF and urine. In difficult cases the diagnosis is sometimes made on liver, lung or marrow biopsy.

Acute miliary disease usually responds promptly to chemotherapy. Most deaths are related to meningitis and/or late diagnosis. A short course of corticosteroids will speed the resolution of symptoms, especially if there is alveolar capillary block. Standard chemotherapy is adequate. Prolonged (9 months) therapy may be required in complicated cases or meningitis.

Chronic disseminated (cryptic) tuberculosis. In chronic disseminated tuberculosis, small numbers of bacilli seed the bloodstream at intervals and produce metastatic foci in organs throughout the body. Apart from the lung lesions, there is usually generalized lymphadenopathy and often hepatosplenomegaly, and involvement of the pleural, pericardial and peritoneal cavities, bones and kidneys may occur. There may be multiple bone involvement with dactylitis or involvement of the skin with papulonecrotic tuberculides. In some cases the chest X-ray is normal and the primary site is unknown. A variety of hematological abnormalities may be seen, e.g. pancytopenia, or leukemoid reactions, which suggest leukemia or a lymphoma. The tuberculin test may be negative. Bone marrow biopsy may show necrotic foci with little cellular reaction but teeming with mycobacteria.

Treatment is similar to that of acute miliary disease. Corticosteroids may be of benefit in debilitated children.

Tuberculosis of the central nervous system

Tuberculosis of the central nervous system may have a variety of manifestations.[288] There may be generalized inflammation affecting brain and spinal cord; less commonly, single or multiple tuberculomata enlarge and present as an intracranial space-occupying lesion or rarely tuberculous disease may be confined to the spine.

Tuberculous meningitis. Tuberculous meningitis is most common in children under 5 years of age, often occurring within 6 months and usually within 2 years of primary infection, but it may occur at any age. It results from rupture of one or more tubercles (Rich focus) into the subarachnoid space. The tubercle(s) is commonly situated in the sub-cortex of the brain, and less often in the meninges or spinal cord. Characteristically, the severe inflammatory response results in a thick gelatinous exudate and adhesions around the base of the brain with hydrocephalus and spinal block. Involvement of cranial nerves may result in single or multiple palsies. Arteritis may cause thrombosis and infarction of nervous tissue with permanent damage. Occasionally there is little exudate and the illness is termed *serous meningitis*. Spontaneous recovery without treatment has been described in some of the latter cases.

Symptoms develop over some weeks and may be grouped into stages, which give a guide to prognosis. Initially, the symptoms are nonspecific and include irritability, malaise, anorexia, vomiting, constipation and low grade fever. Unless the child is a contact of tuberculosis or there is a high index of suspicion, the diagnosis is rarely made at this stage. Within a few weeks specific features in addition to the above become apparent: there is headache, disorientation, meningism, focal neurological signs, such as cranial nerve palsy, hemiplegia or visual defect, and seizures may develop. In young infants the fontanelle may be distended. Fundoscopy may demonstrate choroid tubercles, especially when there is miliary disease, papilledema or the development of optic atrophy. The third and often terminal stage is manifest by coma, a posture of decerebrate rigidity, dilated pupils, and the child is usually wasted.

Diagnosis. The diagnosis is based on CSF findings with or without a positive tuberculin test. There may be radiological evidence of pulmonary disease, or clinical evidence of disease elsewhere in the body. The tuberculin test may be negative in over a third of cases, especially in the advanced stages when there is wasting.

The CSF is clear, unless there is a high cell count, when it may appear turbid. The cell count is usually less than 500/mm³ and mainly lymphocytic, except in the very early stages when neutrophils may predominate. Neutrophils may also increase after commencement of chemotherapy. The protein is usually raised (0.8–4 g/L) and in spinal block may be > 10 g/L, and the CSF is xanthochromic. The glucose is usually low. However, it should be remembered that the first lumbar puncture may be normal, that the cell count, protein and glucose levels may fluctuate from day to day, and that the cell count and protein may be lower in ventricular than in spinal fluid.[289] The chance of detecting tubercle bacilli microscopically is higher if a large amount of CSF is obtained and centrifuged; the success rate claimed varies from 30 to 90% depending on the volume of CSF and the care taken in examining the fluid. Brain imaging will be abnormal in 75–100% of cases; usually there is hydrocephalus, parenchymal disease and basilar meningitis. Tuberculomata may be detected on initial brain scans or appear later. If raised intracranial pressure is suspected, CSF should be taken off slowly with a fine needle or from the ventricles. The CSF should always be cultured for mycobacteria, but is positive in less than half the cases. It may be possible to detect tubercle bacilli after chemotherapy has commenced. Occasionally, tuberculous meningitis may be complicated by pyogenic meningitis. Studies of tuberculous meningitis, mainly in adults, have demonstrated sensitivities and specificities for PCR in CSF ranging from 33 to 100% and 88 to 100%, respectively, and generally higher sensitivity than culture.[238]

Spinal tuberculosis. Spinal tuberculosis is usually secondary to downward extension of the tuberculous process, and usually occurs during treatment of tuberculous meningitis. There is pain and stiffness in the spine at the level of the lesion and symptoms are related to involvement of the spine or nerve roots. The CSF protein is high and there is evidence of a spinal block, which can be confirmed by MRI scan or a myelogram.

Rarely, diffuse tuberculous spinal subarachnoiditis may occur as a result of extension of a primary focus in the spine. It presents as a subacute, transverse or ascending myelitis with upper and lower motor neurone signs and may be mistaken for other causes of cord compression and polyneuritis.

Tuberculoma. A tuberculoma is a tuberculous focus, which enlarges within brain tissue. It may be single or multiple. It may give rise to signs of raised intracranial pressure or a hemiplegia, or cranial nerve palsy if in the brainstem. A skull X-ray may show calcification. CT scan usually shows a hypodense mass and ring enhancement with contrast. MRI scan is more sensitive for detecting tuberculomas, infarcts and spinal lesions. Tuberculomas may expand weeks to months after commencing treatment for meningitis or pulmonary tuberculosis and result in raised intracranial pressure sometimes requiring surgical decompression.[290,291] This phenomenon of paradoxical enlargement may be a hypersensitivity response (as in cervical lymphadenitis).

Management. The key to success in treating tuberculous meningitis is early diagnosis and immediate treatment. If there is doubt, antituberculous chemotherapy should be commenced, along with conventional antimicrobials for bacterial meningitis if necessary.

Optimal chemotherapy is a combination of drugs with good penetration into the CSF and low toxicity. Standard chemotherapy is INH (15–20 mg/kg) and RIF (15–20 mg/kg) given for 9–12 months, with the addition of PZA (40 mg/kg) for the first 2 months of treatment. If drug resistance is suspected, ethionamide or protionamide 20 mg/kg, or ethambutol (EMB) [or streptomycin (SM)] should be added. A 6-month course may be adequate in most cases.[292,293]

A study of 99 children in Cape Town, of whom 96% had stage II or III, treated for 6 months with INH 20 mg/kg, RIF 20 mg/kg, PZA 40 mg/kg and ethionamide 20 mg/kg, had a satisfactory outcome, with only one probable relapse.[293]

Drugs cross the blood–brain barrier more readily in the first 2–3 months of the disease when the meninges are inflamed. INH and PZA achieve high levels in the CSF, even when meninges are not inflamed. Ethionamide has adequate, RIF and EMB moderate to poor and SM poor penetration across the meninges.[294–296] Ethionamide is useful for isoniazid-resistant *M. tuberculosis*. In children who are vomiting, INH, RIF and SM can be given parenterally and other drugs by nasogastric tube. Controlled trials on the value of corticosteroids in tuberculous meningitis have demonstrated benefit especially in stage II and III disease.[295,297–299] The rationale is based on their ability to reduce the inflammatory exudate and thus prevent the development of adhesions which result in internal hydrocephalus and basilar arachnoiditis. In South Africa, 141 children with stage II–III disease were randomized to receive prednisolone 4 mg/kg or placebo for 1 month.[298] The prednisolone treated group had a reduced mortality in stage III, a better cognitive function in survivors and a reduction in size of existing, and development of new, tuberculomas. Dexamethasone 0.6 mg/kg/day or prednisolone 4 mg/kg/day may be given for 2–3 weeks then tailed off over 2–3 months. A higher dose of corticosteroids was used in the South African study because of theoretical concerns about interaction with rifampicin, but others have used a more conventional dose of prednisolone to equal effect.

Serial brain imaging will detect cerebral edema and the presence or development of hydrocephalus or tuberculomas. In the presence of cerebral edema, controlled ventilation (with monitoring of intracranial pressure if necessary) may be indicated. Obstructive hydrocephalus is common and is not always clinically evident. If it is symptomatic, it should be treated by a ventriculo-peritoneal shunt. In the initial stages, before the drugs have controlled the infection, the shunt may be exteriorized.

Spinal arachnoiditis with a CSF block may develop during treatment. If not improved by corticosteroids, release of pressure by surgery may be necessary.

Tuberculomas are treated on similar lines to meningitis. Most of the small and medium-sized lesions resolve completely with chemotherapy. Rarely, large lesions and those not responding to chemotherapy may require excision. Enlargement during treatment of pulmonary or tuberculous meningitis can cause raised intracranial pressure or cranial nerve palsies. Corticosteroids should be tried and, failing this, a ventriculo-peritoneal shunt may be necessary. Most patients with unresolved tuberculomas have been given prolonged antituberculous therapy, e.g. 12–18 months or more. In some cases of meningitis, a second course of corticosteroids may be indicated for treatment of tuberculomas.

Prognosis. The prognosis for meningitis is related to age of the child (young children have a worse prognosis) and the stage of the disease at which therapy is commenced. The stages have been classified as follows:

Stage I: consciousness undisturbed; no, or only mild and focal, neurological signs.

Stage II: consciousness disturbed, but patient not comatosed or delirious. Mild or moderate neurological signs, such as paraparesis, hemiparesis, and cranial nerve palsies, may be present.

Stage III: patient comatose or delirious with mild, moderate or severe neurological signs.
In a study of 199 children in Hong Kong, complete recovery occurred as follows: stage I 96%, stage II 78% and stage III 21%. Of children in stage III, 17% died as opposed to 1% in stage II.[300] Resolution of neurological disability may continue for many months after commencement of therapy.

Abdominal tuberculosis

Abdominal tuberculosis usually results from swallowed sputum or *M. bovis*-infected milk, but may be associated with extension from thoracic nodes or hematogenous dissemination, or may be an extension of pelvic tuberculosis post menarche. The primary focus is usually in the terminal ileum. Symptoms of disease in children are usually due to enlargement or softening of regional mesenteric nodes and/or involvement of the peritoneum. In adults with cavitatory pulmonary disease, there may be a chronic enteritis and fistulo in ano resembling Crohn's disease or other inflammatory bowel disease.

Common symptoms are abdominal pain, fever, weight loss and abdominal swelling or there may be symptoms of intestinal obstruction. Enlarged mesenteric lymph nodes or a mass associated with adhesions of the omentum and intestines may be palpated, usually on the right side of the abdomen.

Peritonitis may be the dominant condition and is often unassociated with demonstrable pulmonary disease. It may result from extension of a mesenteric node or hematogenous spread. In the latter situation, rarely there may be a polyserositis with involvement of the pleura and pericardium. The ascitic fluid has a predominance of lymphocytes and a protein concentration above 25 g/L (usually lower than in a tuberculous pleural exudate). Mycobacteria are not often identified and the culture may be positive in only a quarter of cases.

Diagnosis is made on the basis of a positive tuberculin test, peritoneal aspiration and bacteriological and histological examination of specimens obtained by laparoscopy, endoscopy, or at laparotomy.

Ultrasonography and CT scan are useful for diagnosis and guidance for needle aspiration. Calcification may be detected on abdominal X-ray.

Treatment is by standard chemotherapy.

Tuberculosis of bones and joints

Tuberculosis of bones and joints results from hematogenous spread, usually affecting a single or a few joints within 6–36 months of primary infection. The spine is affected in over half the cases (Pott disease), followed by the knee, hip and ankle. In chronic disseminated tuberculosis, multiple large or small joints may be affected, with or without associated abscesses, or there may be dactylitis of one or both hands. Sometimes punched out cystic lesions are seen with few inflammatory changes affecting surrounding tissue. Lesions confined to the skull may resemble eosinophilic granuloma of bone, or, if associated with miliary disease, the systemic form of Langerhans' cell histiocytosis.

Infection usually starts in the well-vascularized metaphyses near the epiphyseal line of long bones, or, less commonly, in the synovium of the joint. Typically there is minimal periosteal reaction or new bone formation. Progression of the disease may result in destruction of the joint, and/or abscess or sinus formation. The cold abscess may track a considerable distance from the primary focus. For example, a cold abscess from the cervical vertebrae may present as a retropharyngeal mass or, from the lumbar vertebrae, as a psoas abscess pointing in the groin.

Treatment is standard 6-month chemotherapy. However, if evacuation of necrotic sequestrum and abscesses is not adequate, drug penetration might be impaired and a longer course (9–12 months) necessary.[301] Ambulatory chemotherapy without surgery has been found the most satisfactory treatment for spinal disease in resource limited countries. Acute cord compression may respond to chemotherapy alone, but if the necessary technical expertise is available, early spinal decompression is the treatment of choice. A bone graft may be necessary in cases of extensive destruction of vertebrae or weightbearing bones, such as the neck of the femur.

Genitourinary tuberculosis

Tuberculosis of the kidneys is uncommon in children as it usually presents 5–7 years or more after the primary infection, although it may occur sooner. The first symptom is dysuria and typically there is a sterile pyuria with or without red cells. There may not be any symptoms and even in advanced disease there may be very few leukocytes in the urine. Culture of urine for mycobacteria is usually positive.

Glomerulonephritis with immune complex disease complicating miliary tuberculosis has been described, and may be found to be more common if actively sought.[302]

Tuberculous epididymitis is seen in young boys and epididymo-orchitis in older boys.[246] The development of a cold abscess may be the first manifestation of disease. In girls, tuberculosis of the uterus or Fallopian tubes occurs after the onset of puberty and may be complicated by peritonitis.

Tuberculosis of the kidneys and genital tracts should be treated by standard chemotherapy.

Management during pregnancy and of the newborn

Active tuberculosis during pregnancy is associated with infection of the placenta in approximately half the cases; congenital tuberculosis is rare. The main considerations are of the mother during pregnancy and management of the infant at birth.

The only commonly used drug absolutely contraindicated during pregnancy is SM because of its ototoxic effect on the fetus. INH and RIF are given for 6 months and PZA is added during the first 2 months of treatment. Pyridoxine supplements should be given with INH because of increased requirements during pregnancy.

At birth, if the mother has completed treatment or has inactive disease, the infant is given BCG. If she has active disease and/or is receiving treatment, the infant is given INH 6 mg/kg/d for 3 months and is then given a tuberculin test (and a chest X-ray if necessary). If these are negative INH may be stopped (presuming the mother is not infectious) and BCG given. If respiratory symptoms develop a chest X-ray should be taken. Where it is doubtful that the mother will comply with treatment, BCG may be given at birth and the infant also given INH for 3–6 months. The extent to which INH may interfere with BCG vaccination is not clear, but is probably small.[303] It is not necessary to use isoniazid-resistant BCG.

If the tuberculin test is positive (> 5 mm), full investigation for tuberculosis should be undertaken. If no clinical or bacteriological evidence of disease is detected, INH should be continued for a total of 6 months. If disease is detected, full treatment as for congenital infection should be given.

Unless the mother has multidrug resistant tuberculosis she should not be separated from her child and should continue breast-feeding, once both are on appropriate chemotherapy. Small amounts of antituberculous drugs are excreted in breast milk, but they are not harmful to the infant. Consideration should be given to testing mother and infant for HIV infection.

Perinatal tuberculosis

Perinatal tuberculosis is uncommon, although increasing numbers are reported in areas where HIV/tuberculosis coinfection of women has risen.[304] Whether the infection is contracted before birth (congenital) or in the neonatal period is probably only of epidemiological significance. There are three possible routes for congenital infection:

1. transplacental, when the primary infection will be in the liver, or it may possibly bypass the liver through the ductus venosus and be detected in the lungs;
2. aspiration of infected amniotic fluid or infected material in the genital tract, when the lungs will be infected;
3. ingestion, when presumably the liver will be infected.

Symptoms of congenital infection may occur from birth up to 2 months of age with the majority presenting within 2–5 weeks. In neonatal infection, onset of symptoms is later (1–2 months). Common clinical features are respiratory distress, fever, hepatosplenomegaly, lymphadenopathy, poor feeding, and failure to thrive. There may also be skin lesions, ear discharge, jaundice and, in late diagnosed cases, meningitis. The tuberculin test is usually negative but may become positive 6 weeks or more after birth. An IFN-gamma assay may help in assessing whether the baby is infected. Chest X-ray may show bronchopneumonia, sometimes resembling staphylococcal pneumonia, or miliary changes but may not be abnormal in the early stages. Mycobacteria are often isolated from gastric aspirates, tracheal aspirates or ear discharge. The diagnosis may also be made from CSF, or liver, lung or lymph node biopsy. PCR should be undertaken on all specimens. Placental histology or endometrial curettage may confirm a prenatal source of infection. The mortality is high in overwhelming or late-diagnosed cases and preterm infants. Other bacterial or viral infections may be superimposed.

Treatment is with standard chemotherapy. If drug resistance is suspected, SM or kanamycin should be added for the first 2 months and then replaced by ethambutol. Duration of chemotherapy should be 9 months. There are no studies on the efficacy of chemotherapy for the newborn.

HIV infection

In industrial countries, tuberculosis/HIV coinfection is not a major problem.[305] In sub-Saharan Africa, in contrast, there has been a marked increase in frequency of children treated for respiratory tuberculosis since the mid-1980s, and 60–70% of cases may be HIV seropositive. Because of confounding factors, including the high prevalence of HIV infection in mothers and of tuberculosis in the household, difficulty in confirming both HIV infection in infants and tuberculosis generally, and confusion with HIV-related pulmonary disease, the true incidence of tuberculosis/HIV coinfection is unknown.[306] What is clear is that in HIV-infected children not receiving antiretroviral therapy the cure rate for tuberculosis is reduced, there is a higher rate of both relapse and reinfection, and mortality is increased.[306–308] For most cases there is no difference in the radiological features between HIV-infected and

non-infected children with tuberculosis, except possibly a tendency for increased frequency of disseminated disease in the more immunosuppressed. Coinfection with systemic environmental mycobacteria is also a feature in the latter group. In children presenting with tuberculosis and HIV-related pulmonary disease with bilateral reticulo-nodular changes, hilar lymphadenopathy and finger clubbing, the diagnosis of tuberculosis has to depend on methods other than radiology such as contact history, tuberculin test and culture of *M. tuberculosis*. Although the tuberculin test is often negative, it should always be undertaken as it is positive in a proportion of HIV-infected children.

Because of reports of slow eradication of *M. tuberculosis* and/or relapse, at least 9 months of chemotherapy is advised.[308] For HIV-infected children with a positive tuberculin test and no evidence of tuberculosis, 12 months of INH chemoprophylaxis is advised.[309] In HIV-endemic areas, SM should be avoided because of risks from unsterilized needles. Thiacetazone may cause severe skin reactions in HIV-infected children and is contraindicated.

The interaction of rifampicin with non-nucleoside reverse transcriptase inhibitors, nevirapine and efavirenz, and with protease inhibitors is a problem. Also an immune reconstitution inflammatory syndrome may occur, usually within 6 weeks of commencing antiretroviral therapy, comprising fever, lymphadenopathy and worsening of the chest X-ray.

General principles of chemotherapy

A 6 month short-course therapy is standard for respiratory and most nonrespiratory disease.[268,282,310,311] There are still differences of opinion regarding dosage of drugs, especially INH, and the management of meningitis, bone or joint disease, HIV infection and drug resistance. Duration of therapy need not exceed 1 year, except in unusual circumstances such as drug resistance or noncompliance. Intermittent therapy is useful where compliance may be in doubt and is cheaper, although probably only of practical value in areas where supervision is possible. Drugs are usually given twice- or thrice-weekly. Directly observed therapy (DOT) is indicated where there is poor compliance.[312]

Different drugs are effective (in order of efficacy) in:

1. killing actively dividing bacilli, e.g. in open cavities – INH, RIF, SM;
2. killing dormant, intermittently or nondividing bacilli, e.g. in closed caseous lesions – RIF, INH; or within macrophages – PZA, RIF, INH;
3. suppressing drug-resistant mutants – INH, RIF.

PZA is particularly active against bacteria inhibited by an acid environment (e.g. within macrophages and in areas of acute inflammation). Killing actively dividing bacilli and clearing the sputum of live infective bacilli can be accomplished rapidly but for cure or 'sterilization' a prolonged course of treatment is necessary to eradicate dormant and intracellular bacilli. Failure to do this may result in relapse. Mycobacteria may survive for years in a dormant state when metabolism is inhibited by low oxygen tension or low pH.

The most commonly used drugs are bactericidal, e.g. INH (the most potent), RIF, PZA, SM. INH can kill up to 90% of the bacillary population during the first few days of chemotherapy. Bacteriostatic drugs may be used along with bactericidal drugs to prevent emergence of resistance to the bactericidal drugs, e.g. EMB (bactericidal in large doses), ethionamide, thiacetazone and p-aminosalicylic acid (PAS).

The *standard regimen*, used for most types of tuberculosis, is INH + RIF for 6 months, with addition of PZA for the first 2 months. EMB is advised as a fourth drug for the first 2 months if drug resistance is a possibility or there is a high burden of organisms. A longer duration of 9–12 months is advised for some types of disease as indicated in the respective sections. Other schedules are shown in Table 28.25. Caution is advised for EMB in children < 5 years old, because they are too young to report symptoms of optic neuritis, although it is unlikely that problems would arise at a dose of 15 mg/kg.[269] Visual testing should be undertaken where possible. In Table 28.26, the drug dosage and common side-effects are shown. The doses for INH (6 mg/kg) and RIF are minimal and they should be rounded up rather than down. Higher doses, 15–20 mg/kg, are advised for serious forms of tuberculosis such

Table 28.25 Drug regimens

Regimen	Duration
Standard daily	
HRZ(E)[a]: 2 months, then HR: 4 months	6 months
HR: 9 months	9 months
HRZ: 2 months, then HR: 2 months	4 months[b]
Intermittent thrice weekly	
HRZ: 2 months, then HR thrice weekly: 4 months	6 months
Alternative less potent daily:[c]	
HRZ(E): 2 months, then HE: 6 months	8 months

[a] Add E if drug resistance is suspected or burden of organisms is high.
[b] For hilar lymphadenopathy alone.
[c] Resource limited countries.
H, isoniazid; R, rifampicin; Z, pyrazinamide; E, ethambutol.

as meningitis. Adverse reactions are reported in approximately 1–2% of patients.[313] They are less common in children and usually apparent within 6–8 weeks of starting treatment. Peripheral neuropathy as a complication of INH is rare in children. Slow acetylators are at increased risk and pyridoxine will prevent it. Pyridoxine 10 mg is indicated only for children on meat- or milk-deficient diets, breast-feeding infants, malnourished children, and during pregnancy. Higher doses may interfere with the activity of INH.

The main complication is hepatic toxicity.[314] Transient elevation of transaminases occurs in 7–17% of children taking INH, is dose-related and is more likely if RIF is also given. There are case reports of hepatocellular toxicity and death from INH therapy in children.[313] There is no need to monitor serum transaminases unless there is pre-existing liver disease or high doses of these drugs are administered, e.g. in meningitis. Parents should be asked to report persistent nausea, vomiting, malaise and especially jaundice. Children who are rapid acetylators do not have an increased risk of hepatitis when exposed to INH.

Cutaneous reactions, if mild, may not require cessation of treatment, but generalized hypersensitivity will. If toxicity occurs, all drugs should be stopped and reintroduced sequentially in the order INH, RIF and PZA in a small dose (approximately a quarter of the full dose) the first day, increasing to full dose over the next 2–3 days.[314]

Corticosteroids reduce the host's inflammatory response, which may contribute to tissue damage. However, there is only strong evidence of benefit in tuberculous meningitis, although they are sometimes used with less evidence in spinal block, obstruction of bronchi by lymph nodes, miliary disease with alveolar capillary block, pleural effusion and pericarditis.[315] Prednisolone 1.5–2 mg/kg/d is given for 2 weeks and gradually tailed off over 6 weeks. Higher doses are given by some for meningitis.[298]

In children, knowledge of drug resistance is usually obtained from culture and sensitivity of the contact. If drug resistance is suspected or is likely, four bactericidal drugs, e.g. INH, RIF, PZA and EMB, should be given. If possible, SM should be avoided because of the trauma of daily injections. In drug resistance, at *least two drugs* to which the mycobacteria are susceptible should be given. For INH resistance RIF, PZA and EMB are given for a 9–12 month course. For multiple drug resistance, e.g. to INH, RIF and SM, four or more drugs are required initially and treatment should continue for 12–24 months.[269,310] Depending on sensitivities, PZA and EMB are given with three or more second line drugs, e.g. ethionamide, ciprofloxacin, cycloserine or parenterally administered drugs, e.g. kanamycin, amikacin or capreomycin. DOT should be considered.

Patients should be seen monthly for the first 2–3 months to make sure of compliance and to monitor any problems with drugs. Chest X-ray should be repeated at 1–2 months, at the end of therapy, and 3 or more months later. Resolution of pulmonary infiltrates may take over a year and lymphadenopathy (intra- or extra-thoracic) 2–3 years. If adequate chemotherapy has been given, there is no need to prolong treatment; if

relapse occurs or the patient stops treatment for a period, the same standard drug regimen should be given, preferably for 9 months' duration. If in doubt about activity of a pulmonary lesion, gastric aspirates or sputum should be obtained for microscopy and culture. Chest X-rays should be repeated every 6–12 months after cessation of therapy until stable.

Children with primary tuberculosis are rarely infectious and sputum is usually non-infectious after 2–3 weeks of chemotherapy and so they may return to school after this period.

BACTERIAL INFECTIONS: MYCOBACTERIA – ENVIRONMENTAL

Mycobacteria may be divided into those associated with tuberculosis and leprosy and those causing disease associated with the environment, also referred to as nontuberculous, or atypical mycobacteria. The former (including *Mycobacterium leprae*) are highly infectious and are passed from person to person. Environmental mycobacteria, of which there are over 50 species, exist principally as harmless saprophytes in water, soil and vegetation, and also as pathogens in animals such as birds, reptiles and fish. Person-to-person transmission is extremely rare. Environmental mycobacteria generally prefer warm climates and the geographical distribution of the different species is quite variable. Water (fresh or salt) is probably a major vector, e.g. drinking, washing or aquatic sports, or by inhalation of aerosols.[316] The main portals of entry are probably through the skin or mucosa, and by inhalation or ingestion.

DIAGNOSIS

Environmental mycobacteria may be detected as commensals in sputum or gastric aspirates, swabs from wounds or abscesses, or in inadequately sterilized sputum pots. More definite proof of their pathogenicity is obtained when they are derived from a closed lesion, e.g. by aspiration or resection, or the same strain of mycobacteria is repeatedly isolated. Differentiation between mycobacteria is by their cultural characteristics or by PCR. Histologically, it is usually not possible to differentiate lesions from the granulomata of tuberculosis, although nontuberculous infection is more likely to show 'nonspecific' inflammation with less prominent caseation. Variable numbers of acid-fast bacilli may be seen.

There may be a moderate reaction to the tuberculin test (purified protein derivative, PPD-S), approximately 3–25 mm, or no reaction.[317] Differential intradermal tests with antigens prepared from specific environmental mycobacteria, e.g. *Mycobacterium avium*, *M. intracellulare*, *M. malmoense*, *M. scrofulaceum* or *M. kansasii*, are more likely to produce a larger reaction than that with PPD-S.

The commonest clinical problem due to infection by environmental mycobacteria in children is cervical adenitis. Other conditions include cutaneous infections, rarely pulmonary or otolaryngeal disease, osteitis, disseminated disease and meningitis.[318,319] In adolescents and adults, infection in the presence of pre-existing pulmonary disease (including cystic fibrosis) is the commonest association.

LYMPHADENITIS

There appears to be a relative if not an absolute increase in incidence of lymphadenitis due to environmental mycobacteria in areas of the world where tuberculosis is now rare, which may be partly due to decline in neonatal BCG vaccination.[320] However, it also occurs in resource limited countries but is under-reported due to lack of facilities to identify environmental mycobacteria.[321] A defect in the type 1 cytokine pathway could be a factor in some cases.[322] Disease usually presents in children aged between 1 and 5 years, and is usually unilateral and cervical. The submandibular group of nodes is most often infected, followed by tonsillar, pre-auricular and anterior cervical groups. Infection of axillary, inguinal and epitrochlear nodes has been described. The area of entry is rarely identified, although occasionally a lesion on the tonsil

Table 28.26 Recommended drugs for tuberculosis

Drug	Daily dose			Thrice weekly dose			Side-effects
	Children	Adolescents		Children	Adolescents		
		<50 kg	>50 kg		<50 kg	>50 kg	
Isoniazid (INH)	6 mg/kg p.o., i.m., i.v. 15–20 mg/kg (meningitis)	300 mg	300 mg	15 mg/kg (max 900 mg)	15 mg/kg	Max 900 mg	Hepatic enzyme elevation, hepatitis, peripheral neuropathy, hypersensitivity
Rifampicin (RIF)	10 mg/kg p.o., i.v. 15–20 mg/kg (meningitis)	450 mg	600 mg	15 mg/kg (max 600 mg)	15 mg/kg	Max 900 mg	Orange discoloration of secretions and urine (also contact lens), nausea, vomiting, hepatitis, febrile reactions, thrombocytopenia
Pyrazinamide (PZA)	30–35 mg/kg p.o. 40 mg/kg (meningitis)	1.5 g	2.0 g	50 mg/kg	2.0 g	2.5 g	Hepatotoxicity, hyperuricemia, arthralgia, gastrointestinal upset, skin rash
Ethambutol (EMB)	15–20 mg/kg p.o.*	15 mg/kg (max 2.5 g)	15 mg/kg (max 2.5 g)	30 mg/kg	30 mg/kg	Max 2.5 g	Optic neuritis, skin rash
Streptomycin (SM)	15–20 mg/kg i.m.	750 mg	1.0 g	15–20 mg/kg	750 mg	1.0 g	Ototoxicity, nephrotoxicity
Thiacetazone	4 mg/kg p.o.	150 mg	150 mg	Not recommended	Not recommended	Not recommended	Gastrointestinal disturbance, vertigo, visual disturbance, hepatitis, agranulocytosis, exfoliative dermatitis in HIV infection
Ethionamide/ protionamide	15–20 mg/kg p.o. (divided doses)	750 mg	1.0 g	Not recommended	Not recommended	Not recommended	Gastrointestinal disturbance, hepatotoxicity, allergic reactions

*In children <5 years old, give 15 mg/kg.

or buccal mucosa is seen. Enlargement of pre-auricular nodes suggests that the eye might be a portal of entry in some cases. Enlargement of nodes occurs over weeks to months. The overlying skin becomes erythematous or purple prior to discharge of the abscess, but is not usually warm unless secondarily infected. It is commonly mistaken for a pyogenic cervical abscess. A sinus may develop and later calcification may occur. Some nodes probably settle spontaneously. Infection by environmental mycobacteria should be considered when a submandibular or pre-auricular node enlarges in a young child from a background of low tuberculous endemicity, in the presence of a normal chest X-ray and a negative or low grade sensitivity to PPD.

The treatment of choice is excision biopsy of the primary group of involved nodes.[317,318,323] Often the lesion is incised when mistaken for a cervical abscess, or it has discharged spontaneously. In these circumstances, as much necrotic material as possible should be removed and later, if necessary, the primary node excised. Fine needle aspiration is helpful for diagnosis, but mycobacterial culture or PCR is required for confirmation.

Chemotherapy is not usually indicated as the disease is local and the usual mycobacteria causing disease, e.g. *M. avium* complex (MAC) and *M. malmoense*, are commonly resistant to standard tuberculosis chemotherapy. However, if surgery is difficult, e.g. involvement of the parotid gland or closeness of the lesion to the facial nerve, limited incision and curettage may be undertaken and, if healing is slow, antimycobacterial therapy commenced. A suggested drug regimen is azithromycin (10 mg/kg) or clarithromycin plus rifabutin (6 mg/kg) daily for 6 months.[317] Occasionally, longer or repeat treatment is required. Azithromycin has the advantage of once daily treatment and high tissue concentration. There are no controlled trials on the value of single versus combined drugs or duration of therapy. Recurrence of disease in another site sometimes occurs and should be treated as usual.

OTOLARYNGEAL DISEASE

Chronic infection of the middle ear associated with tympanotomy tubes and chronic mastoiditis due to colonization by, particularly, rapidly growing mycobacteria, e.g. *Mycobacterium abscessus* and *Mycobacterium chelonei*, has been described. Debridement with removal of all diseased tissue and in the case of chronic mastoiditis securing maximum ventilation of the cavity is essential. Chemotherapy with appropriate drugs is given for 6 months. Treatment for *M. abscessus* and *M. chelonei* includes parenteral therapy with amikacin and cefoxitin or imipenem for a few weeks, followed by oral clarithromycin and/or ciprofloxacin, depending on sensitivities.[319,324]

SOFT TISSUE INFECTION

The most common soft tissue infections are 'swimming pool granuloma' and 'fish tank granuloma', both caused by *M. marinum*. Local abscesses may follow infection by *M. fortuitum* or *M. chelonei* at injection sites, trauma or surgery, and often present 3–4 weeks after infection, although the incubation period may be much longer in deep infections. Regional nodes are not usually enlarged. Mycobacteria can usually be detected in the lesions. Management comprises debridement of diseased tissue, with chemotherapy reserved for extensive or deep-seated disease.

'Swimming pool granuloma' commonly affects children bathing in infected water on areas of abrasion such as the knees or elbows. Papules, which may ulcerate, appear on the affected areas; scab formation follows. Spontaneous healing occurs within a few months. If drug therapy is required, a single agent such as co-trimoxazole, clarithromycin, ciprofloxacin, or, for more severe infections, dual therapy with rifampicin plus ethambutol, is given for 3–6 months.

Buruli ulcer derives its name from a district in northern Uganda and is known as Bairnsdale ulcer in Australia where the causative agent (*M. ulcerans*) was originally identified. *M. ulcerans* produces a potent toxin, mycolactone.[325] It occurs in localized places in a number of tropical rain forest areas around swamps and river banks. It is transmitted through minor skin injury after contact with water, soil or vegetation contaminated probably by water bugs.[325] It starts as a subcutaneous nodule, often on a leg or arm, ulcerates and gradually progresses to a large ulcer with deep, undermined edges. Satellite nodules or ulcers may be present. Perhaps a third of small lesions heal spontaneously. Diagnosis is by detection of acid-fast bacilli, culture, histology and PCR (98–100% sensitivity).[325] Treatment of large ulcers requires wide excision, cleansing with antiseptic such as 0.5% silver nitrate, and immediate skin grafting. Application of heat to maintain the temperature of the ulcer above 40 °C, which inhibits growth of *M. ulcerans*, may be successful, though not practical in resource limited countries. Chemotherapy is given along with surgery to assist healing. A suggested regimen is rifampicin plus streptomycin for at least 2 months. BCG may give some protection.

PULMONARY DISEASE

Pulmonary disease due to environmental mycobacteria is rare in immunocompetent children. It presents similarly to pulmonary tuberculosis: primary complex, bronchial obstruction, bronchopneumonia or primary progressive disease.[326] The majority of cases are caused by MAC, less often by *M. kansasii* and, in some cases, by other mycobacteria such as *M. fortuitum*. Obstruction of a bronchus should be resected either at bronchoscopy or thoracotomy. Prolonged chemotherapy may be required.

In about 13% of patients with cystic fibrosis, environmental mycobacteria may be recovered from respiratory tract specimens.[327] The decision to treat with chemotherapy depends on a number of indications including: recovery of mycobacteria on serial specimens, reduction in lung function not responding to standard management, changes on chest X-ray compatible with superinfection, and response to chemotherapy for mycobacteria. Choice of chemotherapy depends on species of mycobacteria. Drugs may need to be continued for up to 2 years.[328]

DISSEMINATED AND EXTRAPULMONARY DISEASE

Disseminated disease is usually associated with severe immunological defects, congenital or AIDS. When bone disease occurs, it is usually disseminated osteomyelitis, but can rarely be multifocal osteomyelitis without an apparent underlying immunodeficiency. Infection of the meninges may also occur. A variety of inherited defects in the IL-12 dependent gamma interferon (IFN-gamma) output pathway are recognized, which increase susceptibility to mycobacteria (especially environmental mycobacteria and BCG) and to Salmonella.[329] Some patients respond to IFN-gamma therapy.

In HIV infection, disseminated disease due to MAC is usually seen in older children with a low CD4 count and advanced disease. Trials are in progress regarding optimal chemotherapy. A suggested regimen is clarithromycin, ethambutol and rifabutin.[330] Other drugs include clofazimine, rifampicin, ciprofloxacin or amikacin.[324,328]

DRUG THERAPY

Drugs appropriate for environmental mycobacteria are outlined in Table 28.27. In vitro drug sensitivities may not predict clinical response. Duration of treatment and synergy between drug combinations are important factors. In general, neither isoniazid nor pyrazinamide is useful for environmental mycobacteria. Experience with many of the newer drugs is limited in children and it is important to be aware of side-effects, particularly when used in combination, e.g. plasma levels of rifabutin may be increased by clarithromycin and fluconazole with a risk of uveitis.

PERTUSSIS (WHOOPING COUGH)

Although theoretically vaccine-preventable, pertussis continues to be a significant health problem throughout the world. There are a number of reasons for this including:

Table 28.27 Suggested antimicrobials for treating environmental mycobacterial infection

Organism	Drugs
M. avium-intracellulare and M. scrofulaceum (MAIS complex) M. malmoense	Azithromycin/clarithromycin, rifabutin/ rifampicin, ethambutol, ciprofloxacin, clofazimine, amikacin
M. kansasii	Rifampicin, ethambutol, ciprofloxacin, clarithromycin
M. marinum	Rifampicin, ethambutol, clarithromycin, TMP-SMZ, ciprofloxacin
M. fortuitum M. chelonei M. abscessus	Amikacin, cefoxitin, clofazimine, clarithromycin, ciprofloxacin, imipenem

TMP-SMZ, trimethoprim–sulfamethoxazole.

- Immunization rates are low in some countries.
- The vaccine is not 100% effective and the immunity is transient.
- Because of potential adverse effects of the vaccine in older children and adults, booster vaccinations have rarely been given beyond the age of 5–6 years, although this is changing.
- Because of the transient nature of the immunity, many adults are non-immune and are now the major source of infection, particularly to pre-vaccinated or incompletely vaccinated infants.
- Because of perceived major adverse events from pertussis vaccine, many parents and medical practitioners are wary about giving this vaccine. Further, they will often give an incomplete course of pertussis vaccination if there have been any (even minor) adverse events from earlier vaccinations.
- Infants are born with no passive immunity to pertussis. The non-immune status of neonates means they are highly vulnerable to this disease until vaccination is complete (generally at 6 months). Unfortunately, this is also the age group where the disease is most deadly.

PATHOGENESIS

Pertussis is a bacterial infection due to a Gram negative coccobacillus, *Bordetella pertussis*. Although this organism is sensitive to antibiotics (particularly macrolides), once the paroxysmal cough is established, antibiotics have little or no effect on the clinical course of the illness, except to render that patient non-infectious to others. Thus, recognition and treatment of index patients to prevent further spread is an important public health measure.

It is ideal if pertussis is diagnosed *before* the development of the paroxysmal coughing phase, as antibiotics in this initial stage of the illness can reduce the severity of the clinical illness. Although recognition in the pre-paroxysmal phase is difficult, diagnosis of index cases and treatment of any household contacts with any respiratory symptoms (particularly young children) with the appropriate antibiotics is warranted. Indeed, in a young unimmunized infant (less than 6 months), contact with a known pertussis case is an absolute indication for immediate prophylactic antibiotics.

SPREAD

Droplet or aerosol spread is usual, and indirect spread (e.g. via fomites) is unlikely. The disease is highly infectious and over 80% of unvaccinated household contacts of a known case will develop the clinical illness.

CLINICAL FEATURES

There are several distinct phases of this illness (see Table 28.28). The initial early 'catarrhal' phase consists of upper respiratory tract symptoms and a nonspecific dry cough. This phase lasts for 7–10 days and is abruptly followed by the paroxysmal cough phase. During the early paroxysmal phase, there are violent spasms of uncontrollable cough with facial flushing. These spasms of cough can persist for several minutes and are classically followed by an inspiratory 'whoop'. Infants often vomit and may develop apnea and cyanosis with these coughing spasms, and a 'whoop' is often absent in this age group. This phase of the illness can persist for up to 3 months.

Between coughing spasms, children are strikingly well. Thus, pertussis is generally diagnosed on the basis of the history, unless a spasm is directly observed. The number of spasms per day is highly variable and generally peaks within the first 2–3 weeks of the illness, before a very gradual reduction in the frequency and severity of spasms.

In adolescents and adults the disease is highly modified, presumably reflecting their partial immune status. Thus, any adult with a troublesome cough which has persisted for 2–3 weeks should be suspected of having whooping cough. Epidemiological studies have repeatedly shown that adults are the major reservoir of *B. pertussis* infection, particularly of young unvaccinated or incompletely vaccinated infants.

CASE DEFINITION

The current World Health Organization case definition is as follows: *B. pertussis infection* should be suspected if there is severe cough for greater than or equal to *2 weeks* (i.e. 'probable' pertussis). If *one* of the following are present *in addition* to the above, the child should be notified and treated:
- Prolonged cough followed by apnea or cyanosis, and in the older child paroxysm followed by vomiting, inspiratory whoop or the presence of subconjunctival hemorrhages;
- exposure to suspected case in the previous 3 weeks;
- epidemic whooping cough in the area;
- a lymphocytosis of 15 000/mm³ or greater.

LABORATORY DIAGNOSIS

Confirmation of the diagnosis is an issue. While a positive culture is the gold standard, this lacks sensitivity and false negatives are common. Standardization of other laboratory methods, including PCR and serology, is required to firmly establish their role in diagnosis. Detection of *B. pertussis* by culture or PCR is used for infants and young children who do not mount a good serological response, while serology is more useful in older children and adults. The USA Centers for Disease Control suggest the following as a guide:
- during the first 7 weeks of the cough: culture and PCR;
- cough for 3–4 weeks: PCR and serology;
- cough for more than 4 weeks: serology only.

Table 28.28 Natural history of pertussis

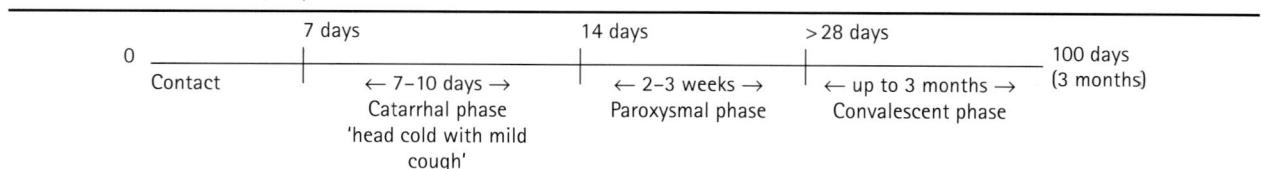

	7 days	14 days	>28 days	
0				100 days (3 months)
Contact	← 7–10 days → Catarrhal phase 'head cold with mild cough'	← 2–3 weeks → Paroxysmal phase	← up to 3 months → Convalescent phase	

EPIDEMIOLOGY

The disease is endemic in most resource rich countries despite widespread immunization programs. In addition to the endemic cases, there are frequent epidemic peaks, which classically occur every 2–5 years. The endemic nature of this disease presumably reflects the large reservoir of adults who develop a modified illness and infect infants and young children. The true incidence of pertussis is difficult to determine because of the problems with accurate clinical diagnosis, the low sensitivity of microbiology, and uncertainty concerning PCR and serological testing methods. As well as lack of recognition, there is almost certainly under-reporting of the condition in resource rich countries.

MORTALITY/MORBIDITY

The estimated annual burden of disease, as reported by the World Health Organization, is 200 million–400 million infections worldwide, causing 200 000–300 000 deaths.

The quoted mortality in resource rich countries for this disease is approximately 0.3%, and is slightly higher in infants < 6 months old (0.5%). Major complications resulting in prolonged morbidity include hypoxic encephalopathy and subsequent brain damage. Most of the morbidity and virtually all of the mortality is in infants < 6 months of age.

VACCINATION

Until recently, the standard vaccine used was a whole cell pertussis vaccine, which unfortunately had a reputation for being both relatively ineffective and potentially harmful. As a consequence, vaccination rates for pertussis often fluctuated and most countries observed major increases in the rates of pertussis when vaccine uptake fell or was low.

Because of the widespread perception of a poor risk:benefit ratio with pertussis vaccine, complete coverage of children < 5 years of age fell to < 50% in the UK in the late 1980s, and was associated with major epidemics.

The introduction of acellular vaccines, with high quality studies showing excellent effectiveness and low adverse event rates, has dramatically altered the situation.[331] Most resource rich countries have replaced whole cell vaccine with acellular vaccine, with increased coverage of complete vaccination in young children. However, to control B. pertussis infection will require repeated booster vaccinations in adolescents and adults. The introduction of the acellular vaccine, which can be safely given to adolescents and adults, means that eradication is now a real prospect.

VACCINE EFFICACY

The published data on vaccine effectiveness have been quite variable. For the whole cell vaccine efficacy varied from approximately 35 to 98%. While the whole cell vaccine offered protection against more severe disease, it did not confer long term immunity. Recent studies show that the efficacy of the acellular vaccine has ranged from 85 to 90%, with a much lower incidence of adverse events.

TREATMENT

In the paroxysmal phase, antibiotics are indicated to prevent the spread of infection. However antibiotics have little or no impact on the child's coughing illness. Although the usual antibiotic is erythromycin for 7–10 days, newer macrolides (e.g. azithromycin) are equally effective and better tolerated.

In young infants with severe and frequent spasms, admission to hospital and close observation is essential. Treatment revolves around experienced, high quality pediatric nursing care. This includes: avoidance of provoking spasms; close observation and treatment of spasms (with oxygen if necessary); minimal handling; and for uncontrollable life-threatening spasms – endotracheal intubation and mechanical ventilation.

BACTERIAL INFECTIONS: *PNEUMOCOCCUS*

Pneumococcus (*Streptococcus pneumoniae*) is a common cause of serious disease in children, particularly otitis media, pneumonia and meningitis. It is also a frequent cause of occult bacteremia.[332] S. pneumoniae are Gram positive oval cocci. They cause beta hemolysis (a green zone around the colony) on blood agar, and occur in pairs (diplococci) or short chains. Pneumococci can be characterized serologically by the capsular polysaccharides or by molecular biological techniques. More than 90 pneumococcal serotypes have been characterized but only a small number are responsible for the majority of serious, invasive infection.

EPIDEMIOLOGY

Approximately 50% of healthy children and 8% of adults[333] carry S. pneumoniae in the upper respiratory tract and it is thought that spread is mainly by healthy carriers although patient-to-patient and patient-to-doctor transfer has been documented. Children under 2 years have the highest rate of carriage, but why some infants develop disease whereas others remain unaffected is unknown. In resource limited countries, a high proportion of lower respiratory infection in young children is due to S. pneumoniae, and pneumococcal meningitis is associated with a high mortality (30–35%). Globally, S. pneumoniae is thought to cause over 1 million deaths in children under the age of 5 years.[334] The 'pneumonia season' in late winter and early spring has been attributed to indoor crowding and damage to respiratory mucosal defenses by recent virus infections.

From the nasopharynx, S. pneumoniae may reach the lungs or through impaired respiratory mucosa spread to the middle ear or meninges. Bacteremic spread to a variety of sites may occur, notably the joints.[335]

Antibiotics have reduced the severity and mortality of pneumococcal disease but have had little influence on disease incidence. Despite timely administration of appropriate antimicrobial therapy, infants with pneumococcal meningitis remain at considerable risk from neurological sequelae and the pneumococcus is more likely to cause permanent deafness than either the meningococcus or *Haemophilus influenzae*. Recurrent pneumococcal meningitis is occasionally seen when CSF leakage complicates skull fracture. Children with an absent or nonfunctioning spleen, impaired antibody production and HIV infection are at particular risk of serious pneumococcal infection.

DIAGNOSIS

In pneumococcal pneumonia there is usually tachypnea with grunting, inspiratory retractions, nasal flaring and cyanosis, but physical examination of the chest may be unhelpful and the radiological changes surprisingly few in the early stages of illness. Blood and CSF cultures are helpful in diagnosis. In bacteremic disease, the white blood cell count is often elevated to over 20×10^9/L. Recovery of the pneumococcus from the upper respiratory tract is unhelpful because of the frequency of the carrier state. Pneumococcal antigen detection in CSF, pleural fluid, serum and urine may be useful for rapid diagnosis, especially in children who have received antibiotics prior to culture.

TREATMENT

A worrying trend is the increasing antimicrobial resistance among S. pneumoniae worldwide.[336] There is regional variation in the incidence of resistant organisms and risk factors include recent antimicrobial use. Penicillin remains the drug of choice for infections with penicillin-sensitive organisms and high drug levels may overcome drug resistance if they exceed the minimum inhibitory concentration (MIC) of the organism. It may not be possible, however, to achieve adequate CSF levels, and pneumococcal meningitis due to resistant organisms should not be treated with penicillin. Multiply drug resistant pneumococci can also be resistant to ceftriaxone and cefotaxime so, whilst awaiting sensitivity results, vancomycin use is recommended (usually in combination with ceftriaxone) if there is a strong clinical suspicion of multiply resistant organisms.

PREVENTION
Pneumococcal vaccine

Although pneumococcal vaccines have been available for many years they have had, until recently, limited efficacy in children under 2 years and their use was therefore targeted towards older children with risk factors such as splenectomy.

The older pneumococcal polysaccharide vaccines (PPV) are manufactured using 23 (23-valent) pneumococcal serotypes, do not stimulate T cells, do not induce a boostable memory response and are ineffective in children under 2 years of age.[337]

The pneumococcal conjugate vaccine (PCV) is manufactured by conjugating carrier proteins to capsular polysaccharides from the seven (7 or hepta-valent) or nine (9-valent) commonest pneumococcal serotypes responsible for 80% of invasive disease. These vaccines are T cell dependent and thus are immunogenic in infancy and induce memory so that the immunological response is boostable.[337]

A pivotal, randomized controlled trial of heptavalent PCV in more than 18000 children given from 2 months of age showed 97.4% protection against invasive pneumococcal disease.[338]

PCV was introduced for routine use in infants and toddlers in the USA in 2000 and since then significant reductions in invasive pneumococcal disease have been seen in vaccinated children.[339-342] Hospitalization rates for all-cause pneumonia in children less than 2 years (the target population) have declined by 39%[343] but the introduction of the vaccine has also been linked with reduced invasive pneumococcal disease in young infants and adults suggesting changes in pneumococcal carriage rates, transmission and herd immunity.[339,344,345] The vaccine also appears effective in children with chronic diseases[342] including HIV infection.[340,346]

PCV was introduced into the UK childhood immunization program in the autumn of 2006 and offered to children age 2, 4 and 13 months (http://www.immunisation.nhs.uk).

PPV is recommended as an additional strategy for children aged 2 years or older in whom pneumococcal infection is likely to be more common and/or dangerous:

- asplenia or severe dysfunction of the spleen, e.g. homozygous sickle cell disease and celiac syndrome;
- chronic renal disease or nephrotic syndrome;
- immunodeficiency or immunosuppression from disease or treatment (including HIV infection;)
- chronic heart, lung or liver disease;
- diabetes mellitus;
- cochlear implants
- history of invasive pneumococcal disease
- presence of CSF shunt or other condition with risk of CSF leak

Note: Where possible, the vaccine should be given 4–6 weeks (but at least 2 weeks) before splenectomy and before courses of chemotherapy, together with advice about the risk of pneumococcal infection. If this is not possible, as for splenectomy following trauma, the vaccine should be given as soon as possible after recovery and before discharge from hospital. If not given before chemotherapy and/or radiotherapy its use should be delayed for at least 6 months after completion of treatment.

Chemoprophylaxis

An alternative for children with functional or anatomical asplenia, for those receiving immunosuppressive therapy, or for infants under 2 years, is to give them continuous antibiotic prophylaxis, e.g. phenoxymethyl penicillin.[347]

EDUCATION

Patients at risk (or their parents) need to be educated about the risks and the importance of seeking medical help at the onset of illness.

A MedicAlert bracelet should be used. A patient card and information sheet for asplenic or hyposplenic patients is available from: Department of Health, PO Box 410, Wetherby LS23 7LL.

BACTERIAL INFECTIONS: PSEUDOMONAS

PSEUDOMONAS AERUGINOSA

Pseudomonas aeruginosa is an important nosocomial pathogen with innate resistance to many antimicrobial agents and disinfectants. The bacterium grows readily in moist environments including ventilator and incubator humidification systems. Known to pediatricians as a cause of life-limiting respiratory infection in cystic fibrosis, P. aeruginosa can infect virtually any part of the body. Infection is usually associated with congenital or acquired immunodeficiency, prematurity, neutropenia or white cell dysfunction, malignant disease and its treatment, transplantation, prolonged instrumentation of body cavities (e.g. tracheostomy, ventricular drainage, bladder catheterization, venous catheterization, peritoneal dialysis) and following puncture wounds. P. aeruginosa infections are generally restricted to immunocompromised patients, but severe infections may occur in healthy children and require prompt diagnosis and treatment. The most important P. aeruginosa infections in pediatric patients include:

Septicemia

P. aeruginosa is an important cause of septicemia in oncology and neonatal units. However, anti-pseudomonas activity is not usually included in antibiotic protocols to cover presumed sepsis in children with no previous medical disorders. Even when appropriate antibiotic therapy is given, mortality is high. The characteristic necrotic skin lesion, known as ecthyma gangrenosum, is a typical feature of P. aeruginosa septicemia and may be useful in diagnosis.

Meningitis

P. aeruginosa meningitis is seen mainly in premature babies and in patients with ventricular drainage catheters or those undergoing intrathecal therapy. It calls for immediate intravenous therapy with a suitable antibiotic, guided by the results of antibiotic sensitivities.

Ear infection

P. aeruginosa is commonly cultured from chronically infected ears (otitis externa) and mastoids, particularly in regular swimmers (swimmers' ear). Occasionally an aggressive and painful infection is produced which is difficult to eradicate and may require surgery.

Eye infections

P. aeruginosa is an important cause of pediatric keratitis following corneal trauma, or secondary to immunosuppression or prematurity. The response to apparently appropriate systemic and topical antibiotic therapy is often disappointing and keratoplasty may be necessary. P. aeruginosa also causes orbital cellulitis.

Urinary tract infection

Urinary tract infection usually follows long term catheterization, but also occurs when chronic infection has impaired local tissue viability. The organism is a common commensal under the prepuce, and this should be suspected as the source of unexpected Pseudomonas bacteriuria.

Respiratory infections

P. aeruginosa pneumonia occurs in the presence of the predisposing factors outlined earlier or following prolonged treatment of other bronchopulmonary infections. Chronic airway infections with mucoid variants of P. aeruginosa and repeated debilitating exacerbations are a major cause of morbidity and mortality in individuals with cystic fibrosis.

Osteomyelitis

Pseudomonas osteomyelitis is particularly associated with penetrating injuries to the foot through sports shoes such as from stepping on a nail ('sneaker osteomyelitis'). In this setting or when osteomyelitis fails to respond to antibiotic therapy directed against *Staphylococcus aureus*, *Pseudomonas* should be considered. It is not always possible to isolate the organism from blood cultures, and antibiotic therapy may have to be broadened blindly.

Skin infections

Pseudomonas skin infections are seen where the skin of the foot has become macerated from prolonged immersion or the wearing of rubber footwear. Ecthyma gangrenosum, an aggressive skin infection usually arising in children with one of the predisposing factors already mentioned, produces necrotic ulcerative lesions involving particularly the anogenital and axillary areas, and can be rapidly fatal.[348]

Management of *Pseudomonas aeruginosa* infections

Treatment of *P. aeruginosa* infections can be difficult if not diagnosed early. The choice of antibiotic therapy should depend on the laboratory sensitivity of the isolate.[349] Many strains are sensitive to broad spectrum penicillins such as ticarcillin, aminoglycosides such as gentamicin, and anti-pseudomonal beta-lactams such as ceftazidime, all of which must be given parentally and usually in combination. Safety concerns over the use of quinolones in pediatric patients have reduced, and agents such as ciprofloxacin can be given orally.

BURKHOLDERIA (PSEUDOMONAS) CEPACIA COMPLEX

Pseudomonas cepacia, now classified as a group of closely related species known as the *Burkholderia cepacia* complex, are important pulmonary and transmissible pathogens in children with cystic fibrosis or chronic granulomatous disease.[350] Outbreaks of nosocomial infection in intensive care units can also occur and usually be traced to contaminated solutions, including disinfectants. In individuals with cystic fibrosis, the *B. cepacia* complex can be aggressive pathogens producing a rapidly fatal necrotizing pneumonia, known as 'cepacia syndrome'.

B. cepacia complex species are intrinsically resistant to many antibiotics but may be sensitive to antibiotic combinations containing two or three agents. Of the newer antibiotics, meropenem is the most active agent.

BURKHOLDERIA (PSEUDOMONAS) PSEUDOMALLEI

Burkholderia pseudomallei causes melioidosis, is spread mainly by contaminated monsoon waters and is endemic in tropical areas of southeast Asia and Australia. Pediatric pneumonia is an important feature of melioidosis, but it may also present with multiple metastatic abscesses and 'imitate' other infections. Melioidosis has a high mortality and responds better to intravenous ceftazidime than to conventional therapy with tetracyclines and chloramphenicol.[351]

OTHER *PSEUDOMONAS* SPECIES

Numerous species of *Pseudomonas* (e.g. *P. fluorescens* and *P. putida*), some renamed (e.g. *Stenotrophomonas maltophilia* and *Ralstonia pickettii*), are recovered from time to time from clinical microbiology specimens, particularly from immunocompromised or otherwise vulnerable patients.

PREVENTION OF NOSOCOMIAL *PSEUDOMONAS* INFECTIONS

In the management of *Pseudomonas* infections, prevention is easier than cure. Thorough drying (and preferably sterilizing) of equipment after cleaning, and scrupulous attention to the manufacturer's instructions for the storage and use of antiseptic solutions are important in curtailing outbreaks of nosocomial infection.

BACTERIAL INFECTIONS: RELAPSING FEVER

Relapsing fever is a disease caused by *Borrelia* species. It is characterized by sudden onset of fever with recurrent episodes of fever. There are two types of relapsing fever (RF): epidemic or louse-borne relapsing fever (LBRF) and endemic or tick-borne relapsing fever (TBRF).

EPIDEMIOLOGY

Relapsing fever has a worldwide distribution, though epidemic RF is prevalent in East Africa, particularly Ethiopia and the Sudan. LBRF epidemics usually follow massive movement of people or disasters such as famine, flooding and earthquake.[352,353] Disaster situations cause overcrowding and lapses in personal and domestic hygiene. The seasonality of TBRF infection varies depending on the behavior of the ticks, whereas LBRF peaks in the rainy season, when people tend to crowd. RF affects both sexes equally in children. Infants account for less than 5% of cases.[354]

ETIOLOGY

LBRF is caused by *B. recurrentis*, while TBRF is caused by various *Borrelia* species in different areas, including *B. duttoni* (East Africa), *B. hispanica* (Spain), *B. persica* (Asia), *B. hermsii* and *B. turicatae* (North America).

PATHOGENESIS

LBRF is transmitted from person to person by body lice. Man is the only reservoir for *B. recurrentis*. The lice prefer normal body temperature to higher temperatures, so lice leave febrile patients and infect afebrile ones.[355] Lice acquire *Borrelia* while feeding on the blood of an infected person. The ingested *Borrelia* enter the mid-gut of the louse. From the mid-gut, the *Borrelia* penetrate the gut wall, enter the hemolymph, and multiply in the body cavity. They do not reach the salivary glands or the ovaries. Human beings are infected when the infected lice are crushed on the skin and *Borrelia* enter the human body through the skin abrasions or intact skin. The louse can remain infective throughout its life span.

Ticks of the genus *Ornithodoros* are important vectors for the transmission of TBRF. Ticks inhabit rodent burrows, earthen floors and crevices of houses. Ticks get infected while feeding on infected animals, especially rodents. Within a few days the spirochetes enter the salivary glands, coxal glands, central ganglion and Malpighian tubules. Infected ticks transmit *Borrelia* to human beings through bites. An infected tick can transmit *Borrelia* to its offspring, which can also transmit to human beings.

In both types of RF spirochetemia occurs and the spirochetes can be detected in the blood of the patient. The characteristic recurrence of symptoms in RF is due to antigenic changes that result in new clones, and during relapse new antibodies are formed. An important clinical characteristic of RF is a Jarisch–Herxheimer (JHR) reaction following destruction of the spirochetes in the course of the disease or treatment. The cause is unclear, although JHR is associated with raised levels of tumor necrosis factor alpha (TNF-alpha), IL-6 and IL-8.[356,357]

CLINICAL FEATURES

The incubation period for both LBRF and TBRF is about 7 days, range 4–18 days. The clinical manifestations may be indistinguishable from the common tropical febrile illnesses such as malaria, typhus fever and typhoid fever. Concomitant infection with typhus is not uncommon in LBRF as both are transmitted by lice.

The onset of RF is characterized by sudden onset of high grade fever, shaking chills, dry cough, abdominal pain and headache accompanied by joint pain, back pain, neck pain and myalgia. Some patients have neck stiffness. Hepatomegaly with hepatic tenderness is common and about a third of patients have splenomegaly. Jaundice with dark-colored urine is occasionally seen, with or without hepatic abnormalities. Hemorrhagic manifestations can include petechial rash, epistaxis and/or hematuria. Neurological abnormalities in TBRF include peripheral neuritis and focal neurological deficits, while patients with severe RF of either type may develop confusion and altered consciousness. Severe cases may develop pneumonia and myocarditis. Myocarditis is usually the cause of death in RF, especially during JHR.

In untreated cases, symptoms disappear in about a week, but tend to recur after 7 or more days. With each relapse the symptoms are milder and shorter in duration. In LBRF the usual number of relapses is 1–2, but for TBRF it is 3 or more.

JHR occurs within a few hours of starting antibiotics in about a third of children and severity varies.[358] JHR has two phases: the chill phase and the flush phase.[359] The chill phase, which begins about an hour after administration of an antibiotic and lasts for 10–30 minutes, causes a rise in heart rate, arterial blood pressure and breathing rate, rigors and anxiety. This is followed by the flush phase, in which the temperature and arterial blood pressure drop and the patient becomes diaphoretic and may become shocked.

DIAGNOSIS

Diagnosis is based on the identification of *Borrelia* in blood films taken during the febrile period and stained with Wright or Giemsa stains. Detection of spirochetes can be enhanced by staining fixed smears with acridine orange and by dark-field or phase-contrast microscopy of wet-mount preparations. *Borrelia* can be cultivated by inoculation of rodents or in artificial medium. The role of serology in the diagnosis of RF is not well established. The leukocyte count may be normal or elevated, but is low in JHR. The platelet count is often low. Urinalysis often reveals increased leukocytes, red blood cells (RBC) and RBC casts. Blood urea nitrogen is elevated until patients are rehydrated and urine output is increased. Liver transaminases and bilirubin levels may be elevated. Cerebrospinal fluid analysis may reveal pleocytosis in a few patients, but CSF culture is negative.[358]

TREATMENT

The aim of treatment is to clear spirochetes from blood and tissues and to prevent or control JHR. A wide range of antibiotics is effective. A single dose of an antibiotic often clears the organism from the blood, but it is recommended to continue antibiotics for a couple of days to prevent relapses. Fast destruction of the spirochetes with antibiotics such as tetracycline increases the severity of JHR. Hence, it is recommended to start treatment with less intense destruction of the organisms by using penicillin followed by tetracycline for LBRF. A single dose of benzylpenicillin 400 000 units is given intramuscularly, followed by tetracycline 50 mg/kg/d in 4 divided doses for 2 days for children > 8 years old. Erythromycin or chloramphenicol is an alternative for children less than 9 years old, for whom tetracycline is contraindicated. Penicillin does not eradicate spirochetes from the blood in some patients,[354,360] probably due to poor penetration of penicillin across the blood–brain barrier to clear spirochetes persisting in the cerebral vessels. For TBRF, a 7–10 day course of penicillin is recommended.

It is important to be vigilant for the occurrence of JHR by monitoring vital signs. Keep an IV line open with normal saline to combat shock in case it occurs during JHR. Meptazinol has been claimed to be effective in diminishing the JHR.[361] Recent studies have shown that JHR is associated with increased levels of TNF-alpha, IL-6 and IL-8; when anti-TNFalpha-Fab was given 30 minutes before penicillin, plasma levels of IL-6 and IL-8 were reduced and the incidence of JHR decreased.[356,357] However, the place of antibodies against TNF-alpha in the treatment of JHR has not been well established.

PREVENTION

The most important measure is avoidance of lice and ticks. Improvement in personal and domestic hygiene is an important step to prevent breeding of vectors. Insecticides should be used to delouse the body, clothing and dwellings. In epidemics early case identification and treatment will decrease the size of the human reservoir in LBRF.

PROGNOSIS

In adults, the case fatality rate of LBRF is 3–4% among treated patients[359] and may be as high as 40% among the untreated.[361] In TBRF, the case fatality rate in children admitted to hospital is 8.8% in Tanzania.[362] Among hospital admitted children with LBRF, the case fatality rate is <2%.[354,358] In LBRF, death is associated with adulthood, delay in consultation and presence of vomiting.[363,364]

BACTERIAL INFECTIONS: SALMONELLOSIS

Salmonellosis is caused by nontyphoidal salmonellae (NTS) which are important causes of infection and disease in children worldwide. A relatively large dose (more than 10^5 colony-forming units) of *Salmonella* is usually required to cause infection. Neonates and young infants are at particular risk of infection because of relative achlorhydria and frequent milk feeds that increase gastric pH and because of lack of acquired immunity.

There are important differences between resource rich and resource limited countries regarding epidemiology and clinical presentation of salmonellosis.[365] In industrialized countries, NTS infection is usually food-borne, causing acute gastroenteritis, but extraintestinal disease is rare.[366] In the UK, most reported cases of food poisoning are due to *Salmonella*. These outbreaks are associated with infections contracted abroad and with infected food, especially from poultry, cattle and pigs. Infection may occur from unhygienic handling or inadequate cooking of food, especially of infected frozen meat that has not been allowed to thaw fully or of refrigerated eggs. Intensive farming methods with the addition of antibiotics to feeds have increased the frequency of infected food and added to the growing problem of multidrug resistant *Salmonella*. Intrafamilial spread and spread through institutions is common, and outbreaks at restaurants, parties and picnics are frequently reported. Pet reptiles are also occasional household sources of infection.

In resource limited countries NTS are also an important cause of invasive extraintestinal disease, particularly in tropical Africa during the rainy season.[367] Intensive rearing of food animals is uncommon in this context, but many children live in crowded conditions with poor sanitation and contaminated water sources. Human-to-human infection by chronic carriers and water-borne salmonellosis in sewage are more likely methods of spread in the community. Nosocomial infection is also relatively common.

PATHOGENESIS

The sites of invasion by salmonellae are usually the ileum and/or the colon. The bacilli can penetrate the mucosa to the lamina propria of the ileum without producing obvious damage to cells and invoke a mainly neutrophil response (as opposed to *S. typhi* which produces a monocytic response). Infection of the ileum results in a watery diarrhea, secretory in nature. Less commonly, invasion of the colon may produce a dysentery-type illness.

Under certain conditions there may be bloodstream invasion, resulting in septicemia or focal infection such as meningitis, osteomyelitis, septic arthritis or empyema. Risk factors for invasive disease include young age, malnutrition, and immunodeficiency including HIV infection. In tropical Africa, an association of invasive NTS disease with malaria and anemia has been reported. Conditions such as hypochlorhydria, hemoglobinopathies especially sickle cell disease, schistosomiasis and malignancy also increase risk of invasive disease.

In sickle cell disease, infarction of the gut may allow salmonellae access to the bloodstream, from where they may invade infarcted areas of bone resulting in osteomyelitis. Also, the impaired opsonization and phagocytic activity in sickle cell disease exacerbates the infection. People with schistosomiasis may harbor salmonellae within the worm or perhaps the granuloma, which protects them from the body's immune system. There may be prolonged or intermittent fever with joint pains and malaise. Treatment should include appropriate chemotherapy for schistosomiasis and *Salmonella*.

CLINICAL FEATURES

The incubation period of *Salmonella* enteritis is 12–48 h. Symptoms in essentially healthy individuals include nausea, vomiting, abdominal pains and diarrhea. In mild cases there may only be diarrhea. The diarrhea may be secretory in nature, with frequent high volume, watery stools resulting in hypotonic dehydration. Alternatively, the presence of blood and mucus may indicate colitis. In severe cases, toxic megacolon and perforation can occur.[367] Fever is common and occasionally there may be an enteric fever-type illness. A reactive arthritis may occur and is associated with HLA-B27 histocompatibility antigens. Symptoms usually settle after 5–7 days but loose stools may continue for several weeks.

In infants < 1 year old, especially neonates and infants < 3 months, septicemia with metastatic infections can occur. In systemic salmonellosis, gastrointestinal symptoms may not be prominent and the infection may be diagnosed only by blood culture. Serious consequences of blood invasion in young infants are meningitis, osteomyelitis and failure to thrive. In older infants and children, bacteremia is usually associated with fever or toxemia, but infants < 3 months old may be afebrile.

Studies in sub-Saharan African children have shown that invasive NTS disease is also common in children > 1 year old and is associated with a high mortality.[367,368] The presentation is often a nonspecific febrile illness or with cough, dyspnea or diarrhea. Associated clinical features are anemia, hepatosplenomegaly, malnutrition and malaria parasitemia. Other common presentations of extraintestinal disease include meningitis and septic arthritis.[367] Mortality is reported as 25% for NTS bacteremia and over 50% for NTS meningitis. In contrast, *Salmonella typhi* is the commonest blood isolate in under-5s in the Indian subcontinent, while NTS is relatively uncommon.[369]

DIAGNOSIS

Salmonella culture is more likely from feces than from a rectal swab. In suspected cases, repeat culture may be necessary as excretion of the organisms may be intermittent. Leukocytes are often seen, and red blood cells and mucus may be present. In *Salmonella* colitis, endoscopy may demonstrate a swollen edematous mucosa with mucus and areas of hemorrhage suggesting ulcerative colitis.

In invasive disease, blood, CSF, urine culture and culture of metastatic lesions such as bone will confirm the diagnosis. Blood culture is advised in infants < 3 months of age and immunocompromised children with *Salmonella*-positive stools, irrespective of whether or not there are symptoms of bacteremia. NTS are not fastidious organisms and are usually readily cultured.

MANAGEMENT

In cases of secretory diarrhea, rehydration and fluid maintenance alone may be necessary. Antibiotics are not indicated for otherwise healthy children with acute NTS gastroenteritis because they do not alter the course of the disease but may prolong excretion in stools and encourage development of multidrug resistance.[370,371] Resistance of NTS to antibiotics relates to their ability to acquire drug resistance from other bacteria in the gut through plasmids and transposons.

Antibiotics are indicated for children with invasive disease. Current preferred first choice is a third generation cephalosporin, cefotaxime or ceftriaxone, or one of the fluoroquinolones, e.g. ciprofloxacin, but multidrug resistance is increasingly common.[366] Treatment for NTS bacteremia should be given for at least 7 days, but longer courses are required for meningitis, osteomyelitis or for children with HIV/AIDS who are at particular risk of relapse after cessation of antibiotics. The advantages of fluoroquinolones are excellent efficacy and tissue penetration with either parenteral or oral administration, and eradication of intestinal carriage.

Antibiotics are indicated in suspected *Salmonella* enteritis, pending blood culture results, for infants < 3 months of age (particularly febrile infants and neonates), and for immunocompromised children.[372] In prolonged illness, with failure to thrive or in immunocompromised children, intravenous feeding should also be considered before significant weight loss has occurred.

Persistent excretion of *Salmonella* may occur for weeks or some months, especially in young infants. No action is necessary, except for advice regarding hygiene, e.g. when changing nappies and washing the hands of young children. No restriction of activities is necessary, if stools are normal.

TYPHOID FEVER

In England and Wales, from 1996 to 2006, there were on average 182 reports of *S. typhi*, 177 of *S. paratyphi* A, and 22 reports of *S. paratyphi* B infection per annum, over two thirds of which were contracted abroad, particularly in the Indian subcontinent.[373] *S. paratyphi* C was rare. There has been a recent increase in *S. paratyphi* A consistent with the increase reported in parts of Asia.[374,375] In many resource limited countries, where hygiene and sanitation are poor, typhoid fever is endemic and constitutes a major health problem.[374] It is considered that up to 80% of infections are mild or subclinical and thus hospital statistics grossly underestimate the prevalence. The classical features of typhoid fever are mainly found in school-age children and young adults. When *S. typhi* is isolated from young children the presentation is often atypical.[376]

S. typhi only infects humans. Subjects are infectious during the acute phase of the disease and when chronic infection of the biliary system, especially the gallbladder, occurs, persistent excretion of the bacteria in feces results. In patients with structural abnormalities of the urinary tract, such as those resulting from *Schistosoma haematobium* infection, there may be prolonged excretion of *S. typhi*.

Epidemiology

In technically advanced countries, typhoid fever is usually caused by contamination of food by a carrier. *S. typhi* can survive for long periods in food and can withstand freezing and drying. Outbreaks may occur from infected milk and ice cream, and in institutions a wide variety of foods have been infected when a carrier is involved with preparation. Oysters and shellfish cultivated in contaminated sewage may be infected. In resource limited countries, flies and insects may transmit infection and a contaminated water supply may be the source of an outbreak. Contaminated ice may also be a cause. The infective dose is much smaller than in nontyphoidal salmonellosis.

Pathogenesis and pathology

After ingestion, the bacilli invade mainly the upper bowel, with minimal inflammation, and pass to the local lymphatics where they are taken up by macrophages. Their easy access through the bowel may be explained by the ability of *S. typhi* to invade the gut without stimulating an acute inflammatory response or recruitment of neutrophils. If the macrophages have not been sensitized by a previous infection they are unable to kill the bacteria, which are then transported within the macrophages to the thoracic duct and thus to the reticuloendothelial system where the uncontained bacilli proliferate in the bone marrow, lymphoid tissue, liver and spleen. At this stage, marrow and blood culture will be positive. The degree of infection depends on the dose and virulence of the organism, the protective effects of gastric juice, and the host's immune response.

Proliferation of bacilli, which is enhanced by bile, continues in the bile ducts and especially the gallbladder, from where large loads of bacteria pass into the gut and may be cultured from a duodenal aspirate. The organisms are taken up by macrophages in Peyer's patches, particularly those in the ileum. By now, the macrophages have been activated by sensitized lymphocytes and an inflammatory reaction takes place. This results in swelling, necrosis and ulceration of Peyer's patches, which in most cases heal uneventfully. However, erosion of blood vessels may cause intestinal hemorrhage, and extension of the necrosis through the bowel wall may result in perforation. At this stage, which is usually 2–3 weeks after the initial infection, most of the bacteria are intracellular and so blood culture is less often positive, but continuous proliferation in the gallbladder results in shedding of large numbers of bacilli into the gut and stool culture becomes positive. Infection of urine reflects the bacteremia, and a quarter to one third of patients may excrete S. typhi during the illness.

Within the body, reaction to the infection continues. Many tissues are affected including the liver, spleen, kidney, heart and lungs. Typhoid nodules, which are foci of macrophages and lymphocytes, can be detected in a number of organs. Cloudy swelling of the liver and kidney occurs and the enlarged spleen is packed with proliferating cells in the sinusoids and pulp. Toxemia is the most likely cause of organ dysfunction, as signs of inflammation are patchy, and is also probably responsible for the mental confusion. Glomerulonephritis and renal failure may occur and are, in some cases, due to immune complex disease.

Rarely, local suppurative infections may develop in bone, joints, lung, kidney and meninges. S. typhi osteomyelitis is commonly associated with sickle cell disease.

Clinical features

The incubation period is around 10–14 days and shorter in those receiving a high infecting dose of the organism. During the first week of illness there are vague influenza-like symptoms, namely fever, malaise, aches and pains and headache. Persistence of fever for over a week should alert one to the diagnosis. At this stage, common symptoms are headache, drowsiness, anorexia, vomiting, abdominal pain, diarrhea and cough; constipation may be a symptom in older children. On examination the temperature is often 39–40 °C and may have a 'swinging' septicemic pattern. Occasionally, the temperature may be normal in moribund children and rise after resuscitation. Signs of toxemia and confusion are common. The respiration rate is often raised and nonlocalized wheeze and crackles may be heard in the chest. The pulse rate is raised and may be weak in late-diagnosed cases. A bradycardia relative to the level of temperature, seen in some adults, is usually not present in young children. Signs of heart failure may be present, especially if there is anemia and/or myocarditis. The abdomen is mild to moderately distended with vague nonlocalized tenderness. The spleen is enlarged in 20–30% of cases and the liver in a similar proportion. Rates of hepatosplenomegaly vary geographically and according to the duration of the disease. Meningism may be detected. Rose spots, which are pink macules that fade on pressure, may be seen, especially on the trunk. S. typhi may be cultured from them. They may appear in successive crops lasting 2–3 days. They have rarely been reported in children with dark skin.

In uncomplicated cases, treatment results in symptomatic improvement within 2 days and the temperature is usually normal within the week. The physical signs resolve in 2–4 weeks but the child may not regain full strength for 1–2 months.

S. typhi infection during pregnancy may cause abortion. Though transplacental infection occurs, perinatal infection is commonly due to infection during parturition.

In infants and young children, infection by S. typhi may present as a rapid septicemic-type illness with respiratory signs, seizures and meningism. Conversely, presentation may be milder in some infants compared to older children.[376]

In resource limited countries, the presence of nutritional anemia and malnutrition and diseases such as malaria, tuberculosis, sickle cell disease, schistosomiasis and leishmaniasis may complicate the diagnosis. In these diseases, splenomegaly is a common feature. The tendency to anemia in typhoid, which is commonly due to marrow depression, may be exacerbated by the above diseases, and also by glucose-6-phosphate dehydrogenase deficiency and the thalassemias.

The association between Salmonella infections and sickle cell disease and schistosomiasis is described in the section Salmonellosis.

Complications

Perforation of the gut is one of the major complications. It appears to be less common in young children. It is most common in the second to third week of the illness but may occur at any time. If it is observed in hospital, it is often associated with sudden deterioration, hypotension, tachycardia and abdominal rigidity. Sometimes perforation is less dramatic and presents more as an ileus. Occasionally air is detected under the diaphragm in a child who is not particularly sick. Presumably, the perforation, being small, has sealed off spontaneously. Intestinal hemorrhage may accompany or occur independently of perforation. Other complications include pneumonia, myocarditis, heart failure, glomerulonephritis, renal failure, hepatitis, focal or generalized central nervous system disorders and meningitis. The association between septic osteitis and sickle cell disease has already been mentioned.

Diagnosis

Blood culture is positive in 70–80% of cases in the first 7–10 days of the illness and in about half this number in the following 2–3 weeks and may still be positive after some weeks of illness. However, prior antibiotics may affect sensitivity, as may the volume of blood taken. For school-children 10–15 ml, and for preschool children 2–4 ml are required to achieve optimal isolation rates.[374] Culture of marrow is more often positive than blood, and both may remain positive despite previous or current antibiotic therapy. Early on, stool culture may be positive in 50% of cases and later in the disease in over 70%. Urine culture may be positive in 25–30% of cases. Thus, the combination of blood, stool and urine cultures should diagnose most untreated cases. Leukocytes, predominantly mononuclear, are usually detected in the stool and there is often some proteinuria.

In resource limited countries where routine blood cultures may not be available the Widal test is commonly relied upon for diagnosis; however, it lacks sensitivity and specificity.[374,375] A high titer of O antibody (> 1:160) or four-fold rise in titer in a child in a non-endemic area who has not had a recent typhoid vaccination (within 1 year) is highly suggestive of typhoid fever. In endemic areas, H antibodies may be raised from previous infections and vaccination also results in a sustained raised H titer. Also, in endemic areas an anamnestic response of O antibody to nontyphoid illnesses may necessitate having a higher diagnostic level during the first week of illness. Conversely, O antibodies may fail to develop and, if present, fail to rise in confirmed typhoid fever. In tropical countries, immunosuppression by malaria may be a factor. Persistence of Vi antibodies may be used as evidence of carrier status, but they may be raised (> 1:5) in only 70% of cases. A number of rapid diagnostic tests are being evaluated. These include tests to detect IgM antibodies against specific S. typhi antigens, e.g. Typhidot-M®. Tubex®, a dipstick test and nested PCR.[374,375]

Anemia is common and the white cell count is usually normal or low. There may be neutrophilia in young infants or when bowel perforation or a pyogenic abscess is present. There is usually a decrease in eosinophil count. Thrombocytopenia may be detected, especially in severe cases. The serum bilirubin is usually normal unless there is a hemolytic anemia, but serum transaminases are often raised. Hyponatremia is common.

Management

Correction and maintenance of fluid and electrolyte balance is important. Blood transfusion may be necessary. Care regarding overhydration is necessary in the presence of anemia, heart failure, nephritis and/or renal failure.

When the organism is known to be sensitive there is little to choose between chloramphenicol, co-trimoxazole and amoxicillin. Unfortunately, because of multidrug resistance (MDR) alternatives are usually required such as fluoroquinolones (ciprofloxacin or ofloxacin), third generation cephalosporins (ceftriaxone or cefotaxime) and for uncomplicated cases, azithromycin.[374,375,377] However, there are increasing reports of *S. typhi* with reduced susceptibility to fluoroquinolones but fortunately full resistance and resistance to cephalosporins is still rare. Nalidixic acid resistance is commonly used as a marker for resistance to fluoroquinolones but some organisms with reduced susceptibility to fluoroquinolones may be susceptible to nalidixic acid.[378] Also, presumably because of less use of first line drugs in Asia there has been a recent rise in reports of *S. typhi* with sensitivity to chloramphenicol.[374,375] In sub-Saharan Africa, where resistance is generally lower, in many areas chloramphenicol remains the standard drug.

In industrialized countries where most cases of typhoid fever have been contracted abroad, until full sensitivity results are available it should be presumed that *S. typhi* will be multidrug resistant and some cases will have reduced susceptibility to fluoroquinolones. Ceftriaxone 60–80 mg/kg once daily for 7–14 days or until 3 days after defervescence is effective. Fluoroquinolones have the advantage of better tissue penetration, oral administration and eradication of the carrier stage. Relapse rates may be lower than with third generation cephalosporins. If sensitive, ciprofloxacin 25 mg/kg/d intravenously, followed by 30 mg/kg/d orally, is given for 7–14 days. Fluoroquinolones are not licensed for routine use in children, owing to concerns regarding arthropathic effects on weight-bearing joints in juvenile animals. However, short courses of fluoroquinolones appear safe.[379] For MDR isolates with reduced susceptibility to fluoroquinolones, azithromycin (10 mg/kg/d) given for 7–10 days is an alternative.[377] Cefixime (20 mg/kg/d) is also used but may not be effective in treating MDR.[374] In areas where chloramphenicol is still sensitive it is given in a dose of 50–75 mg/kg/d. Therapy needs to be continued for a minimum of 14 days; 21 days significantly reduces the relapse rate. When fever subsides the dose may be reduced to 30 mg/kg.

Corticosteroids may be beneficial in severe cases. A controlled trial of dexamethasone, 3 mg/kg followed by 1 mg/kg every 6 h for 48 h in severely ill patients, produced a significant reduction in mortality.[379] Perforation should be managed surgically, after full resuscitation with correction of electrolyte and fluid imbalance, and blood transfusion if necessary.[380] Procedures will vary according to circumstances and include simple oversewing of the perforation, or resection, especially in those with multiple perforations. Additional antibiotics to cover Gram negative organisms and anaerobes such as gentamicin and metronidazole should be given.

For clearance of infection, three consecutive stools should be cultured at weekly intervals after chemotherapy ceases. With adequate chemotherapy relapse is uncommon. Children may return to school when symptom free; stools do not have to be culture negative. Preschool children and children unable to practice normal hygiene may need to be excluded until clear of infection. Carriage of *S. typhi* for over 3 months indicates that the child may have become a chronic carrier, but this is uncommon in children. It may be associated with defective cell-mediated immunity to *Salmonella*. Ciprofloxacin or another fluoroquinolone should be given for relapse or chronic carriage.

Prognosis

In the pre-antibiotic era, the mortality rate for typhoid fever for all ages was around 7–20% and in technically advanced countries is now <0.5%. In resource limited countries, the overall mortality in children shows marked geographical variation. This may depend on age and stage of disease on admission, prior administration of antimicrobials, bacterial resistance and management.

Prevention

Care should be taken in the handling of stools of infected children and attention paid to hygiene, particularly hand washing. Supervision of young and handicapped children is important.

There are two vaccines available for general use: parenteral Vi capsular polysaccharide and oral live attenuated vaccines which use the Ty21a strain. They provide approximately 50–70% protection.[381] A single dose of Vi polysaccharide vaccine is given by intramuscular injection and side-effects are usually only local and mild. There may be a suboptimal response in children under 2 years (vaccination is not recommended under 12 months). A booster dose is required about every 3 years. The Ty21a vaccine is given for three to four doses on alternate days. At present it is not recommended for children under 6 years. In unexposed children, reinforcement courses need to be given every year and every 3 years where there is repeated exposure.

The development of a Vi conjugate vaccine has the potential for mass immunization of infants and children in low income countries.[382]

PARATYPHOID FEVER

Paratyphoid fever, due to *S. paratyphi*, is similar to typhoid fever, but is usually milder with a shorter period of fever and a lower frequency of complications and mortality. The incubation period is often shorter and diarrhea is more common. However, in neonates and young infants complications and mortality may be high. It should be managed along the same lines as typhoid fever.

BACTERIAL INFECTIONS: *SHIGELLA* (BACILLARY DYSENTERY)

Shigella is a global infection that is notorious for disseminating rapidly in settings where there is crowding, inadequate sanitation and insufficient supply of clean water. The spectrum of symptoms ranges from mild watery diarrhea to fulminant bacillary dysentery, characterized by bloody stools, fever, prostration, cramps and tenesmus. The bacillus was first described by Kiyoshi Shiga in Japan in 1898. The organism he described was *Shigella dysenteriae* type 1, also known as the *Shiga bacillus*, the most virulent of all the shigellae.

Shigellae are nonmotile, Gram negative, non-lactose-fermenting rods belonging to the family *Enterobacteriaceae*. The genus *Shigella* is subdivided into four groups, or species: *Shigella dysenteriae* (12 serotypes), *Shigella flexneri* (15 serotypes and subtypes), *Shigella boydii* (18 serotypes) and *Shigella sonnei* (a single serotype). The most common serogroup of *Shigella* circulating in a community appears to be related to the level of industrialization. *S. flexneri* predominates in resource limited countries (~60% of isolates), with *S. sonnei* being the next most common (~15%).[383] In industrialized countries, *S. sonnei* is the most common serogroup (~77%).[383]

EPIDEMIOLOGY

The major mode of transmission is by fecal–oral contact, and a low infectious inoculum (as few as 10 organisms) renders *Shigella* highly contagious for humans, the only natural host. Persons symptomatic with diarrhea are primarily responsible for transmission. The majority of infections are due to endemic shigellosis which primarily affects children 1–4 years of age. Endemic strains of *Shigella* cause approximately 10% of all diarrheal episodes in resource limited countries and contribute disproportionately compared to other enteric pathogens to adverse outcomes such as persistent diarrhea, malnutrition, and even death. In contrast, *Shigella* causes fewer than 5% of diarrhea episodes among young children in industrialized countries where it generally has a benign outcome. *Shigella* is an important etiologic agent of diarrhea among residents of industrialized countries (including military personnel) who travel to less developed regions of the world and tends to produce a more disabling illness than other etiologic agents.

Outbreaks of shigellosis occur in settings where suboptimal hygiene allows fecal–oral transmission, such as children attending day care and persons residing in custodial institutions. Outbreaks in the child care setting often result in high attack rates (33–73%) and secondary cases in many families. Outbreaks which involve contaminated food and water in addition to direct contact can be quite extensive, involving thousands of people over a brief period of time. When feces are improperly disposed of, flies may transmit infection. In such settings, the simple introduction of fly-traps can effectively diminish the incidence of shigellosis.

One serotype of *S. dysenteriae* (type 1) is uniquely capable of pandemic spread. During the twentieth century, pandemics of *S. dysenteriae* type 1 appeared in Central America, south and south-east Asia and sub-Saharan Africa, primarily affecting populations in areas of political upheaval and natural disaster. Typically these strains are resistant to multiple antibiotics and induce high attack rates and case fatality in all age groups. A tragic example of the potential for devastation occurred among Rwandan refugees who fled into Zaire in 1994. During the first month alone, approximately 20 000 persons died from dysentery caused by a strain of *S. dysenteriae* type 1 that was resistant to all of the commonly used antibiotics.[384]

PATHOGENESIS AND PATHOLOGY

After oral inoculation, *Shigella* passes to the terminal ileum and colon where it invades and proliferates within enterocytes, produces cell death, incites an inflammatory reaction and induces intestinal fluid secretion. The ensuing cellular destruction and inflammation result in mucosal ulceration and microabscesses. Two *Shigella* enterotoxins (ShETs), designated ShET1 and ShET2, have been incriminated as mediators of the watery diarrhea seen early in the course and may possess other virulence properties. *S. dysenteriae* 1 uniquely produces the highly potent cytotoxin called Shiga toxin which has been implicated in hemolytic uremic syndrome (HUS). The Shiga toxin produced by *S. dysenteriae* 1 has genetic and functional homologies to the Shiga toxins produced by the enterohemorrhagic *Escherichia coli*, and both can cause HUS.

IMMUNITY

Exposure to wild-type *Shigella* infection confers immunity, at least to the same serotype. This immunity is associated with serum antibody recognizing the O-antigen of the lipopolysaccharide moiety. Cross-protection among *S. flexneri* serotypes and subtypes seems to occur, but there is no evidence to date that immunity is shared among *Shigella* species. Mucosal immunity is also important, as illustrated by the protective effect of breast-feeding on the severity of shigellosis in infants from endemic areas[385] and of passively transferred oral immunoglobulin in preventing experimental shigellosis in subjects.[386] Infection also induces cell-mediated immune responses, but their contribution to clinical protection has not been elucidated.

CLINICAL FEATURES

Shigellosis typically evolves through several phases. The incubation period is 1–4 days, but may be as long as 8 days with *S. dysenteriae*. First there is fever and other constitutional symptoms such as headache, malaise, anorexia and occasionally vomiting, followed in several hours by watery diarrhea. In a minority of cases, there is progression within hours to days to frank dysentery with frequent small stools containing blood and mucus, accompanied by lower abdominal cramps and rectal tenesmus. A variety of unusual but important extraintestinal manifestations may occur, including seizures (usually fever-associated), encephalopathy and metastatic infections such as meningitis, arthritis, and splenic abscess, infection of the vagina with bloody discharge, corneal infection and urinary tract infection. Hematologic complications include leukemoid reaction and HUS (following *S. dysenteriae* 1).

Most episodes of shigellosis in otherwise healthy persons are self-limited and resolve within 5–7 days without sequelae. Acute life-threatening complications are largely confined to infants and children from resource limited countries, particularly those with underlying malnutrition. Dehydration, electrolyte imbalance and hypoglycemia are the most common metabolic derangements and are associated with a poor outcome. Intestinal complications include toxic megacolon, rectal prolapse from tenesmus, and intestinal perforation. Sepsis is rare and seen mostly when there is malnutrition or immunodeficiency. Persistent diarrhea and malnutrition are the major long term sequelae resulting, at least in part, from a protein-losing enteropathy that follows *Shigella*-induced intestinal

damage. An uncommon late sequel seen primarily in adults is reactive inflammatory arthritis, alone or as part of a constellation of arthritis, conjunctivitis and urethritis known as Reiter syndrome. Persons with HLA-B27 haplotype are predisposed, accounting for about half of the cases.

DIAGNOSIS

The diagnosis should be suspected in patients with dysentery, febrile diarrhea or close contacts of patients with such symptoms. These symptoms in a child 1–4 years old should trigger the highest suspicion. If the patient presents with fever and diarrhea without macroscopic blood in the stools, the diagnosis of *Shigella* infection may be suggested by the presence of large numbers of leukocytes in the stool. Stool microscopy is also useful for distinguishing enteroinvasive bacterial infection from amebic dysentery or enterohemorrhagic *Escherichia coli* (EHEC). Moreover, EHEC and amebic dysentery are less likely to cause fever, and EHEC typically produces voluminous bloody stools rather than dysentery. On the other hand, bacterial pathogens such as nontyphoidal *Salmonella*, *Campylobacter jejuni*, *Yersinia enterocolitica* and enteroinvasive *E. coli* can cause bloody stools or dysentery accompanied by fecal leukocytes, as can a heavy *Trichuris trichiura* or *Schistosoma mansoni* infection.

Definitive diagnosis of *Shigella* infection is made by culturing the organism from a fresh stool specimen or rectal swab. Areas of fecal mucus are optimal for sampling. *Shigella* survives poorly in stool samples that are left in ambient temperature; therefore, if the sample cannot be promptly plated onto solid media, it should be inoculated into appropriate transport media and refrigerated. Culture of two or more stool specimens before initiation of antibiotic therapy increases the yield. Blood culture should be undertaken in toxic patients, young infants and those who are immunocompromised.

MANAGEMENT

Careful attention to the patient's fluid and electrolyte balance with correction of deficits and replacement of ongoing losses is a central feature of management. Agents that suppress intestinal motility, such as diphenoxylate, loperamide and opium-containing preparations, should not be given to children, debilitated or immunocompromised patients with known or suspected shigellosis, or to patients infected with antibiotic-resistant strains or with *S. dysenteriae* as they may increase the severity of dysentery by delaying clearance of the organism.

Many controlled clinical trials of patients with shigellosis have demonstrated that appropriate antibiotics significantly decrease the duration of fever, diarrhea, intestinal protein loss, and excretion of the pathogen. Most patients in these studies were infected with either *S. flexneri* or *S. dysenteriae*. The advantages of treating *S. sonnei*, which is usually self-limited, are less clear. Treatment is recommended for patients with severe disease, dysentery or underlying immunosuppression and should be administered empirically while awaiting culture and antibiotic susceptibility results. The major indication for treatment in mild disease is to decrease excretion and eliminate the potential for transmission. For susceptible strains, ampicillin, trimethoprim–sulfamethoxazole, nalidixic acid and pivmecillinam are good choices. Amoxicillin is less effective, presumably because of its rapid absorption and low fecal concentrations. For cases in which susceptibility is unknown or there is resistance to first line agents, a fluoroquinolone (such as ciprofloxacin), azithromycin or parenteral ceftriaxone can be used. The efficacy of ceftriaxone has been attributed to excretion of its active form in the bile; despite in vitro susceptibility, other cephalosporins such as oral cefixime and parenteral cefamandole are inconsistently effective, perhaps due to their lack of intracellular activity. Treatment can be administered orally except in seriously ill patients and is generally given for 5 days.

PREVENTION

Interruption of transmission by individual hygienic behavior such as hand washing is effective in interrupting outbreaks. Segregation of ill persons is useful in settings where hygienic practices are difficult to enforce, such as outbreaks occurring in institutions for the mentally handicapped. Antibiotics should not be used to prevent transmission.

Oral live attenuated vaccines and parenteral O-polysaccharide conjugate vaccines have been developed that show promise in early clinical trials, but as yet no effective vaccine is in use.[387] A polyvalent vaccine will be required to cover the *Shigella* serotypes of clinical and epidemiologic importance.

BACTERIAL INFECTIONS: *STAPHYLOCOCCUS*

Staphylococci are Gram positive cocci and include the coagulase positive *Staphylococcus aureus* which is responsible for most of the clinical problems. Coagulase negative staphylococci (CNS) include *Staphylococcus saprophyticus*, a cause of urinary tract infection, and *Staphylococcus epidermidis*, a skin commensal, which has become an increasing problem with the use of intravascular and other implantable devices.

STAPHYLOCOCCUS AUREUS

Staphylococci are relatively resistant to heat and drying, enabling them to survive for some months on a variety of surfaces or in dust. Their pathogenicity depends on various cell wall components, enzymes and toxins. Toxic shock syndrome toxin-1 (TSST-1), for example, is associated with toxic shock, exfoliative toxins A and B (ETA and B) with scalded skin syndrome,[388] and Panton–Valentine leukocidin (PVL) with abscesses and necrotizing pneumonia.[389] The production of beta-lactamases (penicillinases and cephalosporinases) is of particular clinical relevance, as these enzymes effectively inactivate beta-lactam antibiotics, and agents such as flucloxacillin or clavulanate-potentiated amoxicillin are required to overcome this.

Asymptomatic carriage of *S. aureus* is common, and the organisms can be found in the anterior nares and less often on the skin, particularly the perineum and axillae. This can be a problem in hospitals, where staff and patients can become carriers of resistant staphylococci, and can have serious consequences in obstetric units, burns units and surgical wards. Immunocompromised patients on broad spectrum antibiotics are particularly at risk. Since the 1960s, the prevalence of methicillin resistant strains of *S. aureus* (MRSA) and epidemic MRSA (EMRSA) has increased both in hospital and in the community. Local hospital infection control strategies vary in terms of patient isolation, barrier nursing and 'decontamination programs' with detergent baths and topical use of mupirocin (pseudomonic acid) to the anterior nares. Serious infection can occur with MRSA, and although strains are generally sensitive to vancomycin and teicoplanin, there are now occasional reports of vancomycin-resistant *S. aureus* (VRSA)[390] and vancomycin-intermediate *S. aureus* (VISA).

Bacteremia and septicemia

Septicemia and bacteremia with *S. aureus* is generally associated with a focus of infection such as osteitis, pneumonia or a severe skin infection and can be associated with intravascular devices such as intravenous cannulae, central lines and prosthetic heart valves. Severe systemic upset with fever is common, and weight loss and anemia can occur with prolonged illness. Staphylococcal bacteremia can progress to endocarditis with risk of damage to previously normal heart valves.

Toxic shock syndrome can be associated with tampon use or with other foci of infection, particularly where the skin integrity is compromised by trauma, surgical wounds, burns, chickenpox, eczema, etc. Symptoms include fever, headache, diarrhea, myalgia and confusion. Clinical features include pyrexia, hypotension, a widespread erythematous rash, particularly on the hands and soles (which later desquamate) and mucosal involvement with conjunctivitis and red, inflamed lips. It is a multisystem disease with frequent renal impairment, hepatitis or thrombocytopenia.

Successful treatment depends on rapid institution of antistaphylococcal therapy and general supportive measures, including surgical drainage or removal of tampon, as indicated (Table 28.29). Eradication of staphylococci from indwelling devices such as central lines is unlikely with antibiotic therapy alone and removal of the infected device is usually required. Staphylococci are generally penicillin resistant and suitable antimicrobial agents include flucloxacillin, second generation cephalosporins, rifampicin and fusidic acid. Clindamycin or erythromycin may be useful in combination with fusidic acid, particularly if there is a history of penicillin allergy or to treat suspected or proven community acquired MRSA infection. Aminoglycosides, such as gentamicin, have antistaphylococcal action and can be used in combination with other antistaphylococcal agents. Vancomycin or teicoplanin is prescribed for more resistant organisms. Usually 2 weeks of therapy is sufficient for uncomplicated bacteremia.

Skin infection

Intact skin is a powerful barrier against staphylococcal infection and most skin infection is fairly minor resulting in boils, pustules, furunculosis, carbuncles, styes, paronychia and impetigo. Topical therapy with mupirocin or fusidic acid ointment should suffice for the treatment of impetigo. Large abscess formation may require surgical drainage. Children who are prone to recurrent minor staphylococcal skin infections should be investigated for possible nasal carriage as they may benefit from a course of mupirocin applied to the anterior nares, and if necessary other family members may also be treated. In children with recurrent staphylococcal skin infection, consideration should be given to screening for neutrophil abnormalities, although the vast majority of these children are immunologically normal.

Table 28.29 Antimicrobial therapy for *Staphylococcus aureus* infection

Parenteral				
Flucloxacillin or cloxacillin	i.v. or i.m.	1 month to > 12 years	12.5 mg/kg	6-hourly
Fusidic acid	i.v. only	1 month–12 years	6–7 mg/kg	8-hourly
		12 years	500 mg	Diethanolamine fusidate
Vancomycin (infusion over 60 min, monitor levels)	i.v. only	> 1 month	15 mg/kg/d	
Oral				
Flucloxacillin		1 month–1 year	62.5 mg	6-hourly
		1–4 years	125 mg	6-hourly
		5–12 years	250 mg	6-hourly
		> 12 years	500 mg	6-hourly
Fusidic acid		1 month–1 year	12.5 mg/kg	8-hourly
		1–4 years	250 mg	8-hourly
		5–12 years	250–500 mg*	8-hourly
		> 12 years	500 mg*	8-hourly

*As sodium salt.

Cellulitis, a more deep-seated, spreading infection of the skin is an indication for systemic antimicrobial therapy. Orbital cellulitis carries risks of cavernous sinus infection and should be treated promptly with high dose intravenous antibiotics.

The scalded skin syndrome is discussed in Chapter 30.

Gastrointestinal infection
Food poisoning
Foodstuffs such as cooked meat products, cream, custard and pastry can be a source of staphylococcal food poisoning. The organism may be isolated from the food handlers involved, and often the food is found to have been undercooked and then refrigerated. Symptoms caused by the enterotoxin (which is heat stable) occur 2–5 h after consumption and result in an acute onset of sweating, abdominal pain, diarrhea and vomiting. The symptoms rarely last longer than a few hours but occasionally supportive therapy with intravenous fluids is required. Antibiotics are not helpful.

Pneumonia, osteitis, meningitis
These staphylococcal infections are discussed in Chapter 12.

STAPHYLOCOCCUS EPIDERMIDIS
With the increasing use of invasive procedures, this skin commensal has become an important pathogen, particularly in the neonate and in the presence of indwelling catheters and shunts. Children with ventriculoatrial shunts may have bacteremia, and ventriculoperitoneal shunts can lead to peritonitis. In this situation, eradication of infection with antimicrobial therapy may not be possible and relapse is common. Replacement of the infected device or catheter is, therefore, usually required.

Particularly in hospital acquired infection, resistance to many antimicrobial agents is common. Resistance to vancomycin is rare, though, despite its widespread use in this setting.

BACTERIAL INFECTIONS: *STREPTOCOCCUS* AND *ENTEROCOCCUS*

The large family of streptococci can be responsible for a variety of diseases and sequelae. Streptococci are Gram positive cocci, which tend to form chains. There are several classification systems based on serological or molecular biological techniques. A more traditional classification is based on the degree of hemolysis surrounding a colony on blood agar. Hemolysis can be complete (beta hemolysis), partial (alpha hemolysis) or absent (gamma hemolysis).

The beta hemolytic streptococci are responsible for most of the streptococcal disease in humans and are among the most common bacterial infections of childhood. Streptococci belonging to the other two groups are mainly commensals of the pharynx or gastrointestinal tract and tend to be less virulent pathogens.

THE BETA HEMOLYTIC STREPTOCOCCI
Beta hemolytic streptococci can be further classified into Lancefield groups depending on the serological characterization of the polysaccharide layer of the cell wall. Most human disease is caused by Lancefield group A streptococci (GAS), which include *Streptococcus pyogenes*. GAS can be further categorized into subtypes.

Beta hemolytic streptococci can produce disease by direct tissue invasion or by toxin production. Some strains have a hyaluronic acid capsule which is non-antigenic and has an inhibitory effect on phagocytosis. The cell wall is a complex structure built upon a peptidoglycan matrix. There are a variety of antigenic determinants, including the protein M antigen, which confer further resistance to phagocytosis and may act as a superantigen. Streptococci lacking this antigen are generally avirulent. The T antigens are useful for epidemiological tracing. The polysaccharide layer determines the Lancefield group. Lipoteichoic acid

is a further cell wall component, which influences membrane affinity and adherence to epithelial cells. Virulence also depends on the production of toxins. Several strains can produce the streptococcal pyrogenic exotoxins (SPE) A, B and C, previously known as erythrogenic toxins, which act as a superantigen triggering the rash of scarlet fever and the syndrome of streptococcal toxic shock syndrome. The two streptolysins O and S are responsible for the hemolytic action of streptococci and the estimation of the antistreptolysin O (or ASO) titer can be useful in diagnosing streptococcal infection. Persisting high ASO titers are seen, for example, in rheumatic fever. Other extracellular products, which are possibly involved in spread of infection and the pyogenic process, include DNases, hyaluronidases and streptokinase.

Epidemiology
GAS are principally carried in the pharynx and asymptomatic carriage occurs in 15–20% of children. Infection is spread by direct contact or droplet spread and outbreaks may occur particularly in dormitory-type accommodation in winter months. Food- or water-borne outbreaks have been reported. There have been changing patterns in streptococcal disease worldwide. Scarlet fever, for example, is less of a clinical concern than previously, although over the last few decades[391] there has been an increase in more severe invasive forms of disease such as necrotizing fasciitis.

Immunity
In view of the antigenic variety of the streptococcal strains, repeated streptococcal infection is possible. A child who has suffered from scarlet fever and developed immunity to the SPEs should be protected against further attacks of the syndrome.

Clinical features
The usual focus for GAS infection is the throat, and infection generally presents with symptoms and signs of acute tonsillitis. In children up to the age of 5 years the illness may be less specific. The incubation period is 2–4 days and the child usually complains of a sore throat and headache, is febrile and may have cervical lymphadenopathy. The pharynx may appear mildly inflamed or a more severe form of exudative pharyngitis may be present. Clinical discrimination from viral infection is not usually possible and uncomplicated carriage is always a possibility when streptococci are isolated from the throat swab. Classically, after 10 days of illness, a rise in the ASO titer will be apparent. Tonsillitis, otitis media, mastoiditis, sinusitis and the much rarer GAS pneumonia, impetigo or pyoderma, empyema, meningitis and septicemia are described elsewhere. Scarlet fever and erysipelas are unique to streptococcal infection.

Scarlet fever
Scarlet fever is caused by infection with an SPE producing strain of GAS. The usual portal of entry is via the pharynx and the syndrome classically follows acute streptococcal tonsillitis. However, the streptococci may gain access via broken skin following pyoderma, minor cuts, burns, surgical wounds or chickenpox infection.

Clinical features
The incubation period is usually 2–4 days and the illness may be of variable severity with sudden onset fever, headache, vomiting, sore throat and refusal to eat. In the past, severe illness was more common and delirium a frequent feature. The erythematous rash appears some 2 or 3 days after the onset of illness and classically is first seen in the axillae and groins with blanching on pressure (Figs 28.26 and 28.27). Within 24 h the rash spreads to the trunk and limbs. The face may be flushed and circumoral pallor is a common feature. Pastia's sign – linear petechiae in the flexures – may be helpful diagnostically. After a week or so, desquamation usually occurs starting on the face, then the trunk and limbs. Initially the tongue appears swollen with a yellowish white coating and prominent papillae. This is known as the 'white strawberry' tongue, which later becomes the 'red strawberry' tongue as the coating disappears.

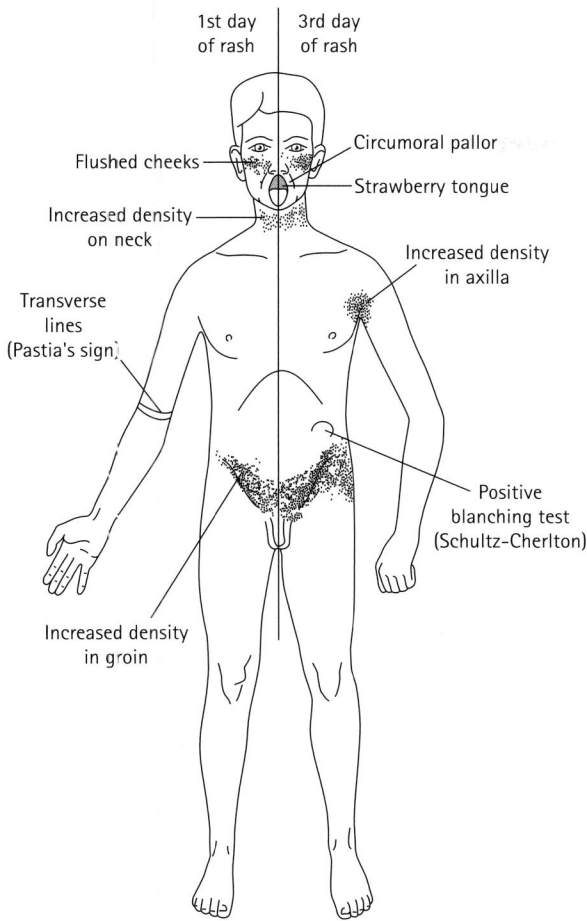

Fig. 28.26 The distribution and the development of rash in scarlet fever.

Untreated, the illness runs its course within 10 days or less. A high fever and tachycardia are common.

Albuminuria is a common finding and a polymorphonuclear leukocytosis is usual.

Since the availability of antibiotic therapy, serious complications are rare. Immediate complications include cervical lymphadenitis with more rarely abscess formation necessitating surgical drainage. Acute otitis media may develop and without treatment further complications including mastoiditis, meningitis or cerebral abscess may ensue. Involvement of the paranasal sinuses can lead to suppurative sinusitis. Other recognized local complications include peritonsillar cellulitis or abscess formation, laryngitis and retropharyngeal abscess.

Rarely, bacteremic spread can lead to metastatic foci of infection, and bronchopneumonia is a further complication, which may lead to empyema or suppurative pericarditis.

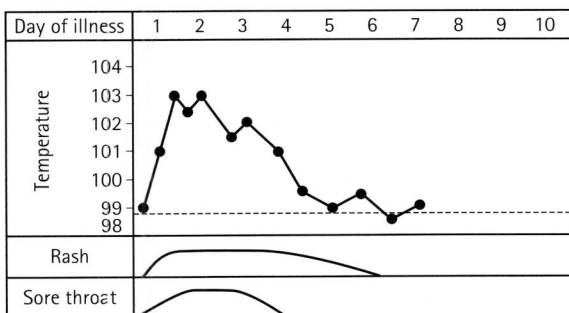

Fig. 28.27 The development of scarlet fever.

The later complications, occurring about 2–3 weeks after the onset of illness, include rheumatic fever, acute glomerulonephritis and erythema nodosum. Early antibiotic therapy should prevent such complications.

Differential diagnosis

Where acute tonsillitis is present the diagnosis is usually straightforward. With milder or subclinical pharyngitis the diagnosis may be less apparent and confused with other exanthemata. Measles is recognized by the prodromal catarrhal symptoms, diarrhea, conjunctivitis, the presence of Koplik spots and the different character and distribution of the rash. In rubella, the diffuse rash contrasting with the mild illness and the presence of predominantly occipital cervical lymphadenopathy are distinguishing features. Generalized lymphadenopathy with splenomegaly is often present in infectious mononucleosis; the blood film examination may reveal atypical mononuclear cells and Epstein–Barr virus (EBV) serology is positive. Other viral exanthemata run a shorter course and usually have leukopenia rather than polymorphonuclear leukocytosis.

Kawasaki syndrome may be difficult to differentiate. The rash, oral and peripheral changes are similar. The cervical lymphadenopathy of Kawasaki syndrome may be characteristically unilateral and matted, and the episcleritis with limbal sparing of Kawasaki syndrome is not usually seen in scarlet fever. In clinical practice, failure of a child with suspected scarlet fever to respond to antibiotics should arouse suspicion of Kawasaki syndrome.

A very similar rash may be seen with staphylococcal toxic shock syndrome but there is often an obvious focus of staphylococcal infection and the rash tends to be more severe on the palms and soles.

Drug rashes, particularly following antibiotic usage, can be scarlatiniform (scarlet fever-like). The other features of disease are not usually present, however, and the rash fades with the cessation of therapy.

Prevention and treatment

The main aim of antimicrobial therapy is to eradicate the infection and thereby prevent the sequelae of local suppurative disease or later rheumatic fever and post-streptococcal glomerulonephritis (Table 28.30). Penicillin is the drug of choice for the treatment of GAS. In severe cases intravenous or intramuscular administration of benzylpenicillin may be required initially. In milder cases, oral phenoxymethylpenicillin for 10 days is usually sufficient. Erythromycin is a suitable alternative in cases of penicillin allergy. Ampicillin and amoxicillin should be avoided, as if mistakenly given in infectious mononucleosis they can cause a severe rash and constitutional upset.

It is unusual to get multiple cases of scarlet fever in a family, although uncomplicated streptococcal throat infection may develop in other children.

Erysipelas

Erysipelas is a skin infection caused by any of the GAS, which can enter the skin through trivial wounds or abrasions. Children of all ages are susceptible and recurrent attacks often involving the same site can occur. Children with congenital lymphedema appear to be more at risk.

Clinical features

The illness may present with fever, malaise, vomiting and anorexia or the symptoms may be confined to the affected skin or occasionally the mucous membranes. A small erythematous patch may develop into a much larger area of affected skin, which becomes red, hot, painful, indurated and well demarcated by a raised edge. In infants, the periumbilical region is a common site, whereas in older children the extremities or the face are sites of predilection and both cheeks may be involved in a butterfly type of distribution. Facial erysipelas must be differentiated from the violaceous cellulitis caused by Haemophilus influenzae type b infection or the slapped cheek appearance of parvovirus B19 infection. Resolution of erysipelas starts centrally and may be followed by desquamation.

Table 28.30 Antimicrobial therapy for *Streptococcus pyogenes* infection

Parenteral				
Benzylpenicillin	i.m.	1–12 months	15 mg/kg	6-hourly
		1–4 years	150 mg	6-hourly
		5–12 years	300–600 mg	6-hourly
		> 12 years	600 mg–1.2 g	6-hourly
	i.v.	All ages	25–50 mg/kg	4–6-hourly
Erythromycin	i.v. only	1 month–12 years	8–12 mg/kg	6-hourly
Oral				
Phenoxymethylpenicillin		< 1 year	62.5 mg	6-hourly
		1–4 years	125 mg	6-hourly
		5–12 years	250 mg	6-hourly
		> 12 years	500 mg	6-hourly
Erythromycin		1 month–1 year	125 mg	6-hourly
		2–8 years	250 mg	6-hourly
		>8 years	500 mg	6-hourly

Blood cultures are frequently negative but after 10 days of illness there may be a rise in the ASO titer.

Erysipelas responds quickly to penicillin or erythromycin. It may be difficult to differentiate erysipelas from other soft tissue infection such as cellulitis, the more deep-seated infection caused mainly by staphylococcal infection, and in cases where doubt exists, antistaphylococcal antimicrobial therapy should also be prescribed, e.g. flucloxacillin.

Streptococcal pyoderma

Although most impetiginous lesions are caused by staphylococcal infection, localized purulent streptococcal infection of the skin (streptococcal impetigo or pyoderma) may result from secondary infection of wounds or burns. In children, particularly in the age range 2–5 years and living in tropical or subtropical climates, it mainly involves the lower limbs and may follow intradermal inoculation of streptococci by minor trauma or insect bites. Multiple lesions are common and begin as small papules, becoming vesicular with surrounding erythema. Pustule formation occurs and the lesions then enlarge and break down with formation of thick crusts. Systemic upset is not common but regional lymphadenitis is usually present. Ten days of penicillin therapy is advised although there appears much less risk of rheumatic fever with this type of infection.

Lymphangitis, characterized by red, linear streaks leading to the enlarged regional lymph nodes, may follow very minor skin infection or inoculation with streptococci. It may accompany cellulitis.

Streptococcus agalactiae (group B streptococcus)

Streptococcus agalactiae, or group B streptococcus (GBS), is a beta hemolytic streptococcus belonging to Lancefield group B, and is a major cause of neonatal infections, both early and late.

VIRIDANS GROUP STREPTOCOCCI

Viridans streptococci are usually alpha hemolytic but can be nonhemolytic. They are generally oropharyngeal commensals, and include *Streptococcus mutans*, *S. salivarius*, *S. sanguis* and *S. mitis* groups and three streptococci formerly known as the *Streptococcus milleri* group (*S. anginosus*, *S. constellatus* and *S. intermedius*). Even minor dental procedures can be complicated by a transient bacteremia, which is of no clinical consequence except for children with cardiac disease, either congenital heart disease, such as patent ductus arteriosus or bicuspid aortic valves, or acquired, such as rheumatic heart disease. Infective endocarditis is a risk in such cases. Regular dental care with additional antibiotic prophylaxis for dental procedures is advised for children who have a history of rheumatic fever or congenital heart disease.

ENTEROCOCCI

Enterococci are commensals of the intestinal tract. They can cause urinary tract infection, particularly in cases of structural urinary tract abnormality or neurological dysfunction of the bladder such as in children with lumbar or sacral myelomeningocele. *Enterococcus faecalis* and *E. faecium* are the major pathogens of the 18 types of enterococci seen in humans. *E. faecalis* can cause infective endocarditis and has emerged as a major cause of bacteremia in hospitalized patients. Enterococci are often penicillin resistant, and determination of the antibiotic sensitivity is important. In endocarditis, combinations of antimicrobial chemotherapy are advised, such as the synergistic combination of amoxicillin and an aminoglycoside such as gentamicin. Vancomycin is an alternative, but this treatment is threatened by the emergence of vancomycin resistant enterococci (VRE). Fortunately, few of these isolates appear clinically relevant and the organisms are often no longer evident after cessation of vancomycin or removal of infected lines and devices. There are concerns that VRE may cause more clinical problems in the future and drugs with activity against vancomycin resistant *Enterococcus faecium* include linezolid and quinupristin/dalfopristin.[352]

BACTERIAL INFECTIONS: TETANUS

Despite the availability of an effective active vaccination since 1923, tetanus remains a major health problem in resource limited countries and is still encountered in resource rich countries. At least 1 million cases require hospital treatment worldwide each year and there are approximately 400 000 deaths.[393] There are approximately 800 000 tetanus deaths each year, of which approximately 400 000 are due to neonatal tetanus.[393] Approximately 12–15 cases are reported per year in the UK and between 40 and 60 cases per year in the USA.[393]

ETIOLOGY

Tetanus is caused by a toxin released following infection with *Clostridium tetani*, a Gram positive, spore forming, obligate anaerobic bacillus. Tetanus typically follows deep penetrating wounds where anaerobic bacterial growth is facilitated. The most common portals of infection are wounds on the lower limbs, postpartum or postabortion infections of the uterus, nonsterile intramuscular injections and compound fractures. Minor trauma can lead to disease and in up to 30% of cases no portal of entry is apparent.[393]

EPIDEMIOLOGY AND PATHOGENESIS

Clostridium tetani is a ubiquitous inhabitant of the intestinal tract of many animals and commonly found in soil. The toxin binds to gangliosides on peripheral nerves, and the toxin is internalized. It is then moved by retrograde axonal transport to the central nervous system. The toxin prevents release of the inhibitory neurotransmitter (GABA) into the synaptic cleft. The alpha motor neurones are therefore under no inhibitory control and undergo sustained excitatory discharge causing the characteristic motor spasms of tetanus.

PREVENTION

Tetanus toxoid is produced by formaldehyde treatment of the toxin, its immunogenicity improved by absorption with aluminum hydroxide.[394] In the UK and USA it is administered to children between 2 and 6 months old (3 doses at 4–8 week intervals) with boosters at 15 months in the USA and at 4 years. A further dose is recommended in both the USA and UK within 5–10 years. In order to maintain adequate levels of protection, five additional booster doses should be administered to ensure life-long protection.[394] Minor reactions to the tetanus toxoid are estimated to be 1 in 50 000 injections. Severe reactions such as the Guillain–Barré syndrome and acute relapsing polyneuropathy are rare. Neonatal tetanus can be prevented by immunization of women during pregnancy.[395] Two or three doses of absorbed toxin should be given with the last dose at least one month prior to delivery. There is no evidence of congenital anomalies associated with tetanus toxin administered during pregnancy.[395] Maternal HIV and also malaria infection may limit the transfer of protective maternal antibodies. Passive immunization with human or equine tetanus immunoglobulin shortens the course and may reduce the severity of tetanus. The equine form, widely available throughout resource limited countries, has a higher incidence of anaphylactic reactions. In established cases, patients should receive 500–1000 IU/kg of equine antitoxin or 5000–8000 IU of human antitetanus immunoglobulin intravenously or intramuscularly. For prophylaxis 1500–3000 IU equine or 250–500 IU human antitetanus immunoglobulin should be given. Passive immunization should be administered as soon as possible after the injury; once the toxin is bound and internalized it will have no effect. In addition to passive immunization, active vaccination needs to be administered to all patients.

CLINICAL FEATURES

The incubation period (the time from inoculation to the first symptom) can be as short as 48 h or as long as many months after inoculation with *Clostridium tetani*. The period of onset is the time between the first symptom and the start of spasms. These periods are important in determining the prognosis: the shorter the incubation period or period of onset, the more severe the disease. Trismus (lockjaw), the inability to open the mouth fully owing to rigidity of the masseters, is often the first symptom. Generalized tetanus is the most common form of the disease, and presents with pain, headache, stiffness, rigidity, opisthotonus and spasms which can lead to laryngeal obstruction. These may be induced by minor stimuli such as noise or touch, or by simple medical and nursing procedures such as intravenous and intramuscular injections, suction or catheterization. The spasms are excruciatingly painful and may be uncontrollable leading to respiratory arrest and death. Spasms are most prominent in the first 2 weeks; autonomic disturbance usually starts some days after spasms and reaches a peak during the second week of the disease. Rigidity may last beyond the duration of both spasms and autonomic disturbance. Severe rigidity and muscle spasm necessitates paralysis for prolonged periods in severe tetanus.

DIAGNOSIS AND DIFFERENTIAL DIAGNOSIS

The diagnosis is a clinical one, relatively easy to make in areas where tetanus is seen frequently, but often delayed in resource rich countries where cases are less common. The differential includes tetany, strychnine poisoning, drug induced dystonic reactions, rabies and orofacial infection. In neonates the differential diagnosis includes hypocalcemia, hypoglycemia, meningitis and meningoencephalitis, and seizures.

TREATMENT

In patients with a deep wound, thorough debridement and toilet are critical to reduce the anaerobic conditions that the bacteria thrive in. Common complications in tetanus are those of prolonged periods in intensive care. Secondary infections are a frequent complication, most commonly associated with the lower respiratory tract, urinary catheterization and wound sepsis. Gram negative organisms, particularly *Klebsiella* and *Pseudomonas*, are common. Meticulous mouth care, chest physiotherapy and regular tracheal suction are essential to prevent atelectasis, lobar collapse and pneumonia, particularly as salivation and bronchial secretions are greatly increased in severe tetanus. Adequate sedation is mandatory before such interventions in patients at risk of uncontrolled spasms or autonomic disturbance and the balance between physiotherapy and sedation may be difficult to achieve. Energy demands in tetanus may be very high due to muscular contractions, excessive sweating and sepsis.

SPECIFIC TREATMENT

Penicillin is the standard antibiotic therapy for tetanus. The dose is 100 000–200 000 IU/kg/d intramuscularly or intravenously for 7–10 days. Metronidazole is a safe and effective alternative. Autonomic disturbance with sustained labile hypertension, tachycardia, vasoconstriction and sweating is common in severe cases. Profound bradycardia and hypotension may occur and may be recurrent or preterminal events. Diazepam has a wide margin of safety and a rapid onset of action, and is a sedative, an anticonvulsant and a muscle relaxant. However, it has a long cumulative half-life. Invariably, in the doses required to achieve adequate control of spasms, respiratory depression, coma and medullary depression are common. Magnesium sulfate has been used to reduce autonomic disturbance and help to control spasms.[396] There is very little information on follow-up of patients after tetanus; enuresis, mental retardation and growth delay have all been reported after neonatal tetanus.

PROGNOSIS

The prognosis in tetanus remains serious despite the best available treatment. Globally the mortality rate in neonatal infection is approximately 60%.[397] Older children and adults have a mortality rate of 10–30% depending on the availability of basic intensive care facilities.[393]

BACTERIAL INFECTIONS: TULAREMIA

ETIOLOGY

This disease derives its name from Tulare, a county in California, where it was first discovered amongst ground squirrels by McCoy in 1911. It is caused by a small, intracellular, nonmotile Gram negative coccobacillus, *Francisella tularensis*, that commonly causes disease in wild animals such as rabbits, hares, squirrels, foxes, rats and deer. There are four subspecies of the organism that are serologically identical but differ in biochemical properties and virulence.[398] *F. tularensis* subsp. *tularensis* represents over 90% of the isolates from North America and is highly virulent in man and rabbits.[399] It is usually recovered from rodents and arthropods. *F. tularensis* subsp. *holartica*, the type most commonly found in Europe and Asia, is less virulent in man and rabbits.[400] It is usually isolated from aquatic animals. The other two subspecies have only rarely been associated with disease in humans.

EPIDEMIOLOGY

The organism can be isolated from a wide variety of wild mammals, from domestic animals such as sheep, cattle and cats, and from the arthropods that bite these animals such as ticks, fleas and deer flies. Human infection occurs after a bite from an infected arthropod, by contact with an infected animal, by ingestion of a diseased animal or contaminated water, or by inhalation of infected secretions. Humans are highly susceptible to the organism, with fewer than 50 organisms required for infection. Tularemia occurs throughout the northern hemisphere, with large outbreaks reported in North America, the southern part of the former Soviet Republic, and northern Scandinavia. In the eastern part of the continental USA it occurs mostly in winter, related to the rabbit hunting season, whereas in the states west of the Mississippi River it occurs in summer when there is a preponderance of ticks. Human case-to-case contact has not been documented, though care must be taken in dressing discharging wounds. Tularemia is extremely infectious for laboratory workers, who must take exceptional care in the handling of infected material or cultures. Its high attack rate and virulence after inhalation has caused its frequent citation as a possible agent for bioterrorism.[401]

PATHOLOGY

There is a local lesion at the portal of entry and, at times, disseminated lesions throughout the body. Entry is usually through the skin, but may be via the conjunctiva, the respiratory tract or rarely the gastrointestinal tract. Dissemination occurs via the lymphatics or blood, and lesions may be found in the regional lymph nodes and in many other parts of the body. The local lesion is a painful, erythematous papule often with central ulceration and regional lymph node enlargement. The lesions are granulomatous, much like the lesions of miliary tuberculosis, but the center of the lesions is often necrotic and consists of polymorphonuclear leukocytes.

CLINICAL FEATURES

The incubation period ranges from 1 to 21 days but most cases occur 3–5 days after exposure. The severity of the disease depends on the route of entry, the subspecies involved, and the host's immune response. Children usually show more constitutional upset and less respiratory involvement than adults. Most frequently there is an abrupt onset of high fever, headache and malaise with or without regional adenopathy, chest X-ray changes, vomiting, and a cutaneous lesion at the site of entry. Sterile pyuria is also common. Rarely there may be pericarditis, osteomyelitis, meningitis, splenic abscesses or thrombophlebitis. Before antibiotics, reported mortality ranged from 7 to 30%. Six clinical syndromes have been described which occur according to the portal of entry. Most common is the *ulceroglandular syndrome* characterized by a primary painful maculopapular lesion at the point of skin entry with subsequent ulceration and slow healing. This is associated with painful, acutely inflamed regional lymph nodes that may ulcerate and proceed to abscess formation. Other forms of the disease include *typhoidal* tularemia, with high fever and hepatosplenomegaly, *pulmonary* tularemia, with pneumonia, pleuritis and hilar adenopathy, *ocular* tularemia, in which the eyelids become edematous and painful, *oropharyngeal* tularemia, in which the tonsils are covered by a pseudomembrane, and a *glandular* form in which no portal of entry can be identified.[402]

DIAGNOSIS

The circumstances of the disease onset, especially a history of bite or scratch or exposure to wild animals, should readily suggest the diagnosis in endemic areas. There is a significant risk to laboratory personnel when handling specimens so the laboratory should be informed if tularemia is suspected. Serology is the usual means of establishing the diagnosis: a four-fold or greater rise in serum agglutination titer to *F. tularensis* is evident after the second week of illness. Nonspecific, low titer cross-reactions may occur to *Brucella*, *Proteus* and *Yersinia* species. The organism can be cultured from infected sites on special media or by rodent inoculation, but this should be attempted only by personnel vaccinated against the organism.

PCR-based methods may be used to distinguish subspecies,[398] but are not routinely available.

The differential diagnosis depends on the presentation, but includes causes of skin lesions with regional adenopathy such as cat-scratch disease, causes of prolonged fever including brucellosis and salmonellosis (especially typhoid), and causes of atypical pneumonia.

TREATMENT

Streptomycin is the historical drug of choice for treatment of severe tularemia. However, as it is not widely available, gentamicin is an effective alternative although treatment failures have been reported.[403] Chloramphenicol should be added for tularemic meningitis. Options for outpatient therapy of older children include tetracyclines or the quinolones, although relapses have been reported after completion of therapy with both drugs.[404] Treatment is usually for 6–10 days, the duration depending on the severity of the illness.

PREVENTION

In endemic areas, opportunities for arthropod bites should be minimized by wearing protective clothing and regular tick inspections. Prevention also involves avoidance of contact with infected or potentially infected animals and insect vectors, adequate cooking of potentially infected meat and the boiling of water from springs and streams.

In the USA, a live attenuated vaccine is available for those repeatedly exposed to the organism such as laboratory technicians.[405]

BACTERIAL INFECTIONS: YERSINIOSIS AND PLAGUE

YERSINIOSIS[406,407]

Yersiniosis is caused by two species of enteric bacteria, *Yersinia enterocolitica* and *Yersinia pseudotuberculosis*. A wide spectrum of clinical manifestations occurs, including acute watery diarrhea, mesenteric adenitis, extraintestinal infection and bacteremia. Postinfectious sequelae such as arthritis or erythema nodosum are also common.

Microbiology and pathogenesis

Yersinia spp. are facultative anaerobic Gram negative coccobacilli which grow well on bile containing media. There are three human pathogens within the genus, *Y. pseudotuberculosis*, *Y. enterocolitica* and *Y. pestis*. Over 50 serogroups of *Y. enterocolitica* have been described. *Yersinia* infections occur through invasion of the gastrointestinal tract via a membrane protein, invasin, which binds to a cell surface ligand. Multiplication may occur within intestinal epithelial cells and Peyer's patches, with the potential for systemic spread.

Epidemiology

Yersinia enterocolitica infection occurs globally but is most common in temperate regions. Yersiniosis is a zoonotic infection but usually causes food-borne illnesses. The organism can be found in the gastrointestinal tract of a number of domestic and livestock animals. Infection of humans usually occurs after eating or drinking contaminated food or water; incompletely cooked pork is a major risk factor.[408] Infection may also occur by person-to-person or direct animal-to-person contact. Most infections are sporadic but a number of specific outbreaks due to contaminated food or water have occurred. Infants and young children are more susceptible to infection with *Y. enterocolitica* than adults.

Infection with *Y. pseudotuberculosis* is less common, apart from in Japan. Infection results from contact with both sylvatic and domestic animals and a number of birds. It usually affects patients aged between 5 and 20 years.

CLINICAL FEATURES[409]

The incubation period for acute yersiniosis is 3–7 days. *Y. enterocolitica* infection most commonly presents as acute gastroenteritis in young children with diarrhea, fever and abdominal pain, clinically indistinguishable from *Salmonella* or *Campylobacter* infection. Stools contain mucus, leukocytes and red blood cells. Patients may be symptomatic for up to 3 weeks and remain infectious over this period, due to shedding of organisms in the feces. Rare complications include diffuse ulceration of the small intestine and colon, perforation, intussusception and toxic megacolon.

Y. enterocolitica infection in older children most commonly causes mesenteric adenitis and terminal ileitis; this is also the most common manifestation of *Y. pseudotuberculosis* infection. The presentation mimics appendicitis. Diarrhea is unusual and the infection is usually self-limiting. Ultrasound and/or CT may help by demonstrating a normal appendix and enlarged mesenteric nodes. The differential diagnosis includes acute appendicitis or terminal ileal disease such as Crohn's or tuberculosis.

Y. enterocolitica bacteremia is rare and usually occurs in patients with other chronic medical conditions or immunosuppression. There is also a strong association with iron overload syndromes. Case fatality rates for *Y. enterocolitica* bacteremia range from 7.5 to 25%, but may reach 50% in patients with iron overload. Focal *Y. enterocolitica* infection can occur as a complication of bacteremia or occasionally in the absence of detectable bacteremia. *Y. pseudotuberculosis* bacteremia is much less common, but is also associated with chronic illness. Case fatality rates are extremely high in the immunocompromised population. In Japan, *Y. pseudotuberculosis* infection has been associated with renal failure in young children.

Secondary, immunologically mediated, postinfective complications may occur in up to 30% of patients following *Yersinia* infection. A reactive asymmetrical large joint polyarthropathy or erythema nodosum are the most common manifestations, occurring 1–2 weeks after the acute presentation. There is a strong association with the possession of HLA B27. Reiter syndrome, glomerulonephritis and myocarditis have also been described. Synovial fluid culture is normally sterile. Joint symptoms of reactive polyarthritis may last for several months.

Diagnosis

Definitive diagnosis of yersiniosis is by culture of the organism from stool, lymph nodes or blood. Isolation from stool may be optimized by using cold enrichment or cefsulodin–Irgasan–novobiocin (CIN) agar. High titers of *Yersinia* antibodies in a previously healthy individual are suggestive of infection but four-fold rises in titer are rarely found. Interpretation of serology is also complicated by low titers following yersiniosis in infants or immunocompromised patients, a high background prevalence of positive serology in some populations and cross-reactivity with *Brucella*, *Rickettsia* and *Salmonella* spp. Cultures are often negative by the time of appearance of postinfective symptoms.

Y. pseudotuberculosis may be found in sterile site samples, but is rarely isolated from stool. Serology is often the only mode of diagnosis available; antigens cross-react with those of *Y. enterocolitica*.

Treatment

Antimicrobial treatment does not shorten the course or severity of enterocolitis and is not indicated in uncomplicated cases. Localized infection, systemic disease or enterocolitis in an immunocompromised patient should be treated. *Y. enterocolitica* is resistant to most penicillins and first generation cephalosporins: amoxicillin–clavulanate combinations are also unsuitable due to variable minimum inhibitory concentrations. Aminoglycosides, chloramphenicol, tetracycline, co-trimoxazole and fluoroquinolones have been most effective in clinical practice: third generation cephalosporins may also be effective.[410] *Y. pseudotuberculosis* is sensitive to ampicillin and cephalosporins in addition to the drugs already discussed.

PLAGUE[411,412]

Epidemiology and pathogenesis

Plague is a zoonosis caused by *Yersinia pestis*. It occurs globally; approximately 2000 cases of plague are reported annually. Over 90% of cases occur in Africa, with current epidemics in the Democratic Republic of Congo and Madagascar; major active foci also exist in other parts of Africa, the Western USA, China and south-east Asia. Mammals, particularly rodents, act as host reservoirs. Fleas feed upon diseased hosts and organisms multiply within the midgut of the flea before being transmitted to humans or other mammals when the flea bites and regurgitates a blood meal. Human infection can also be acquired from direct contact with wild rodents or their predators (including cats), and person-to-person spread can occasionally occur in epidemics. Most human plague cases currently occur in rural settings with transmission from wild animals; epidemics in human settlements occur when domestic rat species become infected. Plague is a potential bioterrorism agent and this has led to an increased interest in the disease.

Clinical features

There are three main clinical forms of plague. *Bubonic* plague is most common. Bacteria multiply in regional lymph nodes following a flea bite, culminating 2–8 days later in systemic symptoms, fever, headache and malaise. Regional lymph nodes enlarge and become extremely tender with swelling and inflammation around the nodes: the bubo. Occasionally, pustules, eschars or papules occur at the site of flea bites. Most individuals develop a transient secondary bacteremia: in some this leads to septicemic or pneumonic plague.

Patients with *septicemic* plague present with Gram negative septicemic shock and may develop complications such as renal failure or DIC. Septicemic plague occasionally occurs in the absence of buboes; this presentation is more common in children.

Pneumonic plague is usually a complication of bacteremia and presents with cough, fever and hemoptysis: the chest X-ray may show bronchopneumonia, consolidation or cavitation. Large numbers of bacteria may be exhaled with the potential for respiratory spread to cause primary pneumonic plague.

Diagnosis

The patient's symptoms and an appropriate exposure history may lead to a clinical diagnosis of plague. Leukocytosis is common and liver function tests may be abnormal. *Yersinia pestis* may be demonstrated on smears from blood, bubo fluid or CSF: fluorescent antibody techniques increase the sensitivity. Definitive diagnosis depends upon culture of the organism, which grows readily on standard media. A rapid diagnostic test that detects plague antigens in blood has been developed and has helped considerably in field conditions, allowing confirmation of diagnosis within 15 minutes.[412] Serological tests are useful in retrospective diagnosis of plague.

Treatment

Case fatality rates may reach 30–50% in untreated plague. Streptomycin is the traditional drug of choice; gentamicin or doxycycline has been shown to be equally effective, with response rates of around 95%.[413] Seven days' therapy is required to prevent relapse: clinical improvement normally occurs within 3 days. Fluoroquinolones may also be effective, particularly for the rare strains with high level multidrug resistance, although clinical experience is limited. Ciprofloxacin is also indicated as prophylaxis for contacts of pneumonic plague.

Prevention

Plague vaccines are only usually administered to individuals at high risk in laboratories or field control teams: their efficacy against pneumonic plague is limited and frequent boosting is necessary. A number of new vaccines are being developed. Public education, reducing flea bites and rodent exposure, and avoidance of sick or dead animals are all measures that can help avoid infection.

INFECTIONS DUE TO VIRUSES AND ALLIED ORGANISMS

USE OF THE VIROLOGY LABORATORY BY THE CLINICIAN

VIROLOGY SPECIMEN COLLECTION AND TRANSPORT

When virus infection is suspected, it is important for the pediatrician to take a careful medical history and perform a thorough medical examination of the patient to decide the most likely viral pathogens causing an infection. The possible diagnoses should be discussed with the clinical virologist, so that appropriate specimens are collected and laboratory tests ordered. It is important to collect specimens for viruses as early as possible in the illness after the onset of symptom. Swabs and tissue specimens for viral culture should be placed in viral transport media, i.e. buffered media containing protein and antibiotics. The presence of antibiotics in viral transport media makes these specimens unsuitable for bacterial or fungal cultures. Separate swabs and specimens need to be collected if bacterial or fungal cultures are also required. Liquid samples such as CSF, bronchoalveolar lavage fluid or urine can be sent in clean sterile containers without transport media. Blood for virological tests should be sent in a tube containing an anticoagulant. Both heparin and EDTA are suitable for specimens for viral culture or antigen detection, but citrate should not be used. Heparin should not be used if polymerase chain reaction (PCR) testing of blood is to be performed, as it inhibits the reaction. All specimens for virological testing should be kept cold on ice after collection and during transport. Transport to the laboratory should be prompt and if there is a delay in transport the specimen should be frozen, preferably at $-70\,^{\circ}C$ rather than $-20\,^{\circ}C$, as this temperature often reduces virus viability. Most swabs are suitable for collection of specimens, e.g. cotton, Dacron, polyester and rayon, but calcium alginate may inactivate some viruses and inhibit PCR reactions. Swabs should have a metal or plastic shaft, as wood shafts can be toxic to cell cultures.

METHODS OF VIRUS DETECTION

There are five approaches to virus identification:
1. Sending patient material for direct examination by electron microscope.
2. Culturing body fluid or tissue for viruses.
3. Detecting viral antigen in clinical specimens.
4. Using PCR and nucleic acid probes to detect genomic material.
5. Identifying postinfection antiviral antibody by serological methods.

LABORATORY DIAGNOSIS OF VIRAL INFECTION

Respiratory viruses

Historically, cell culture techniques have allowed the detection of a wide range of viral pathogens which cause respiratory infections and also detect dual or mixed infections. However, traditional cell culture techniques are usually slow and often do not provide a diagnosis until the patient is recovering or has been discharged from hospital.

To enhance the clinical utility of viral diagnosis in respiratory infections, most laboratories now use virus specific fluorescent antibodies for direct identification of viruses in cells collected from the respiratory tract via nasopharyngeal aspirates, swabbing or bronchoalveolar lavages. There are now commercially available tools with monoclonal antibodies which are run simultaneously and can detect respiratory syncytial virus (RSV), influenza A, influenza B, parainfluenza viruses 1–3 and the adenovirus group. In addition these antibodies can be used to detect viruses in culture and decrease the culture time from 10–14 days to 3–5 days, thus improving the clinical utility of this test.[414] More recently molecular diagnosis using polymerase reverse transcription and polymerase chain reaction (RT-PCR) has increased the sensitivity of detection, but at a significantly increased cost.[415]

Rapid identification of respiratory viruses is important in health care, because it permits timely and appropriate cohorting (isolation) of patients to prevent nosocomial spread of disease and allows for prompt and appropriate clinical management, i.e. stopping unnecessary antibiotic therapy and commencing specific antiviral therapy for influenza or RSV if indicated.

Childhood exanthems

It is unusual to require laboratory diagnosis of common childhood exanthems such as measles, mumps and rubella and chickenpox, unless there is very severe or atypical disease.[416] Viral culture may be performed in these situations, but serological testing is used more commonly, with detection of IgM being most commonly performed by enzyme linked immunosorbent assay (ELISA) or immunofluorescence (IF) assay.

Enterovirus infection

Enteroviruses, now with more than 101 recognized members, are a common cause of many clinical syndromes including mild febrile illness, upper respiratory tract infections, viral pneumonia, exanthems, enanthems, myocarditis, pericarditis, aseptic meningitis, encephalitis and acute flaccid paralysis. Enterovirus infections are more prevalent in summer and early autumn in temperate climates, but can occur all year round. Enteroviruses are transmitted by the fecal–oral route; they replicate in the gastrointestinal tract, where they rarely cause gastrointestinal symptoms, but can cause diseases in other tissues or organs throughout the body.[417] During the acute illness, enteroviruses are excreted from the oropharynx for several days and continue to be excreted in the feces for several weeks. Most enteroviruses can be grown in tissue culture and usually take 4–8 days to detect. However, more recently PCR detection of enteroviruses has enabled more rapid diagnosis of enterovirus meningitis and encephalitis.

Gastrointestinal infection

Most viruses which cause diarrheal illnesses are not detectable by cell culture. Historically, viral gastrointestinal pathogens have been detected using electron microscopy, which is still used today. More commonly rotavirus, adenovirus or norovirus antigens are detected by immunological methods using ELISA, membrane enzyme immunoassay or latex agglutination. Potentially, PCR technology could be used to detect these viruses, but is not routinely available at present.

Arboviruses

Arboviruses (arthropod-borne viruses) include the alphaviruses and flaviviruses. These viruses are all transmitted by the bite of a hematophagous arthropod which transmits the virus to humans. As these viruses are transmitted by arthropods they occur seasonally, i.e. in the warm weather when arthropods are much more active and also are limited to specific geographic regions consistent with the distribution of the transmitting arthropod. Arboviruses are responsible for a significant amount of viral disease globally, e.g. dengue, yellow fever, Japanese encephalitis and West Nile virus.[418] Arbovirus infections may be asymptomatic. Clinical illnesses include mild febrile illness, acute hepatitis, viral arthritis, rash, hemorrhagic shock and encephalitis. Diagnosis of arbovirus infection is commonly performed by serology, commonly using ELISA technology to detect IgG and IgM antibodies.

Herpesviruses

The herpesviruses are a very large and diverse group of DNA viruses, of which eight have been recognized as the cause of infections in humans. Herpes simplex virus (HSV) types 1 and 2, cytomegalovirus (CMV), and varicella zoster virus (VZV) can be cultured from most sites by conventional cell culture or culture fluorescence. However, human herpes virus 6 (HHV-6), and HHV-7, HHV-8[419] and Epstein–Barr virus (EBV) cannot be cultivated. Diagnosis of central nervous system infections by HSV, CMV or VZV is now commonly done using PCR. Viral culture, while slower, can be performed. HSV and VZV can be detected in scrapings from vesicular skin lesions, using immunofluorescent antibody staining or PCR detection of a cell smear taken from the base of the vesicle. These assays are quite sensitive and specific.

Diagnosis of CMV infection in organ donors or recipients, neonates and pregnant women is usually performed using serology. Detection of IgM antibodies in the absence of IgG antibodies indicates acute infection in neonates and pregnant women while the presence of IgG antibodies indicates past infection in organ donors and recipients. The isolation of CMV from the urine and saliva of neonates in the first week of life is diagnostic of congenital CMV infection.

CMV infection and reactivation can cause significant disease in immunosuppressed patients, such as solid organ recipients, bone marrow transplant recipients, patients receiving chemotherapy and HIV positive patients. Culture for CMV alone is not adequate in these situations, as CMV shedding is quite frequent in immunosuppressed patients without the development of disease. The diagnosis of CMV disease in immunosuppressed patients is achieved by the detection of CMV in a biopsy of the affected organ. Detection of CMV in biopsy tissues can be achieved using histological evidence of CMV inclusions, evidence of CMV antigen, usually detected by immunoperoxidase antibody staining of tissue sections, or detection of CMV by culture or PCR. As tissue biopsies are very invasive, the detection of CMV viral load in blood as a surrogate marker for CMV disease or as an indicator for risk of development of CMV disease has become the standard of care. The usual method for detecting CMV in blood is a CMV antigenemia assay in infected leukocytes, using monoclonal antibody to the CMV late protein, pp65. By using a fluorescent label, CMV-infected cells can be counted using a microscope and the number per high power field determined, giving a relatively quantitative result. These assays can also be used to monitor the efficacy of CMV antiviral therapy in the prevention and treatment of CMV disease. More recently, detection of CMV DNA in blood using a quantitative PCR assay has been used.[420] Qualitative CMV PCR detection is adequate for the diagnosis of CMV retinitis by detection of CMV in aqueous or vitreous humor.

Serological methods are used for the diagnosis of primary EBV infection, whereas molecular methods are used to diagnose EBV-associated lymphoma of the brain and post-transplant lymphoproliferative disease. Diagnosis of acute EBV infection is performed with an EBV viral capsid antigen (VCA) IgM ELISA assay. Past infection of EBV can be determined by detecting IgG antibodies to VCA or Epstein–Barr virus nuclear antigen (EBNA). VCA IgG appears within one week of acute infection while EBNA IgG appears 1–2 months after acute infection. Quantitation of EBV DNA in serum can be used to monitor patients at risk for EBV associated lymphoproliferation; however, currently there are no established threshold levels of EBV DNA which indicate risk of disease.[421] These assays are most useful when run as serial assays to determine increases or decreases in EBV viral load in response to alterations in immunosuppression.

Hepatitis viruses

The hepatitis viruses are a group of unrelated DNA and RNA viruses that cause liver disease as the major clinical manifestation. Diagnosis of these infections is usually with serological techniques. More recently, quantitation of hepatitis B virus DNA and hepatitis C virus RNA has been developed to aid in monitoring antiviral therapeutic responses.

Human immunodeficiency virus infection

Human immunodeficiency virus (HIV) infection in infants greater than 18 months of age is confirmed with a positive HIV antibody test. The diagnosis of vertical HIV infection in an infant less than 18 months is achieved by culture of HIV or detection of HIV DNA in blood. Both these assays have a sensitivity of approximately 80% and are the current 'gold standard'. More recently, detection of HIV RNA (viral load assays) has been used. If using this assay, one has to be careful of the possibility of false positive results. Using these methods, greater than 90% of vertically infected HIV infants will be identified by 6 months of age.

Polyomaviruses

The human polyomaviruses, BK virus and JC virus, infect the majority of the population but remain latent in the kidneys after primary infection. Reactivation can occur when there is T cell immunodeficiency. BK viruria in bone marrow transplant patients is associated with hemorrhagic cystitis. JC virus causes progressive multifocal leukoencephalopathy (PML), seen primarily in AIDS patients.

Detection of BK virus can be achieved by cytologic examination of exfoliated urinary epithelial cells or by PCR detection of BK virus DNA in the urine or blood. JC virus is detected by PCR detection of DNA in CSF.[422] Alternatively, a brain biopsy of a patient suspected of PML may indicate histopathological changes consistent with the diagnosis of PML.

New viruses

More recently, newly discovered respiratory viruses have caused significant illness globally. In 2001, human metapneumovirus was discovered as a cause of bronchiolitis in infants and young children, clinically indistinguishable from that caused by RSV.[423] In 2003, the agent of severe acute respiratory syndrome (SARS), a coronavirus, was associated with a global outbreak of respiratory illness associated with high mortality.[424] There are ongoing concerns regarding pandemic avian influenza virus (H5) which has been spreading around the world both in avian populations and to a much lesser extent in humans since it was first recognized in Hong Kong in 1977. All three of these agents can be identified using molecular technology and PCR assays.

ANTIVIRAL SUSCEPTIBILITY TESTING

Antiviral therapy is now available for the management of many viral infections, including HIV, HSV-1 and 2, CMV, VZV, influenza A and B, RSV, hepatitis B virus and hepatitis C virus. It is anticipated that resistant viruses will invariably occur and increase in prevalence with increased use of antiviral agents. Antiviral resistance is defined as a decrease in susceptibility to an antiviral agent established by in vitro testing and confirmed by genetic analysis of the viral genome and biochemical analysis of the altered enzyme. Clinical failure of antiviral therapy may not always be due to antiviral resistance and consideration must be given to the patient's immunological status, the pharmacokinetic properties of the drug in a given patient, and patient compliance. Antiviral resistance is more likely to occur with long term or recurrent administration of intermittent or suboptimal therapy.

Laboratory assays to detect the viral susceptibility to an agent can be either phenotypic or genotypic assays. Phenotypic assays require growth of the virus in vitro in the presence of the drug and establishment of the concentration of antiviral agent resulting in 50% and 90% inhibition of growth. These assays have not been standardized or correlated with therapeutic success, as they have for antibacterial susceptibility testing, and are not routinely available.

On the other hand, genotypic assays which detect genetic mutations known to confer antiviral resistance are more widely available, especially in the management of HIV infected patients and the selection of anti-HIV therapeutic agents. The major limitation of genotypic assays is that they can only detect resistance caused by known mutations and will not detect new resistance mechanisms.

HIV INFECTION

EPIDEMIOLOGY

The first cases of pediatric acquired immune deficiency syndrome (AIDS) were described in 1982 and the causative agent, HIV, was first isolated in 1983. Since then, a large amount has been learnt about the disease and for resource-rich countries and even increasingly in resource-limited settings, antiretroviral therapies (ART) have had a major impact in reducing morbidity and mortality in HIV infected adults[425] and children,[426] as well as dramatically reducing transmission from mother to child.[427,428] However, the global HIV epidemic has continued, with an estimated 40 million people living with HIV worldwide in 2006 (Fig. 28.28). Whilst the global prevalence (proportion of the population living with HIV) appears to have plateaued, the total number of people

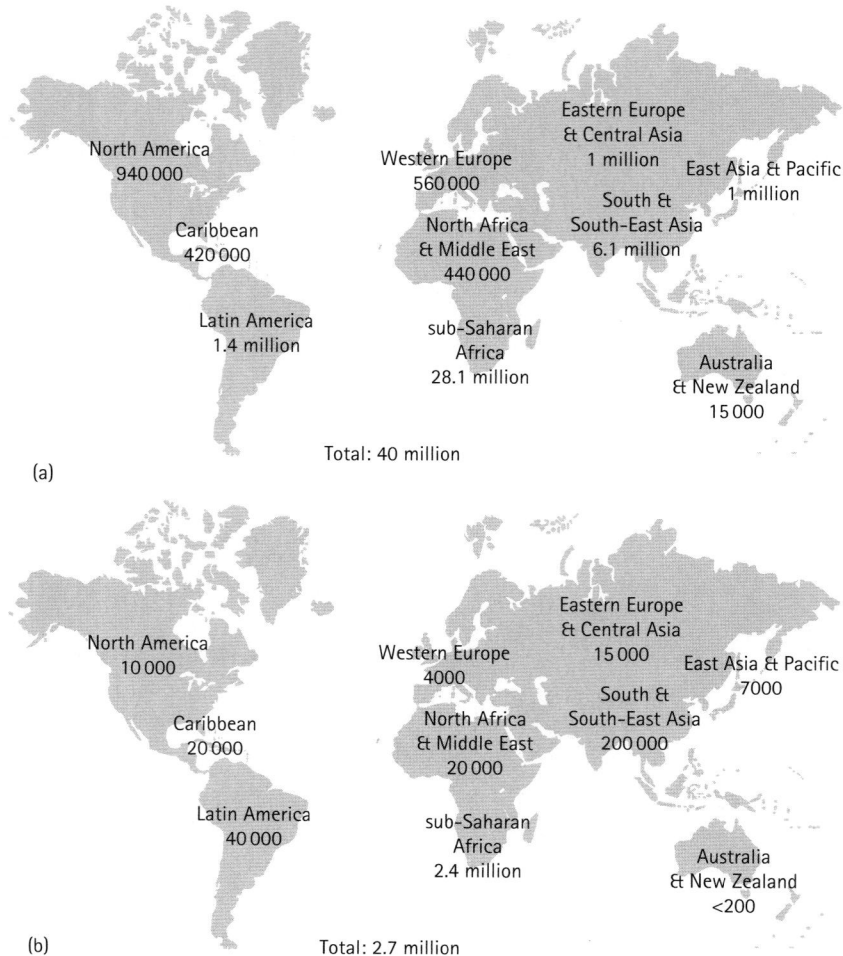

Fig. 28.28 (a) Adults and children estimated to be living with HIV/AIDS as of end 2001. (b) Children (< 15 years) estimated to be living with HIV/AIDS as of end 2001.

infected continues to rise with population growth and prolonged life expectancy from ART. About 95% of people infected with HIV live in resource-limited settings, with Africa continuing to bear the brunt of the epidemic (approximately 65% of global HIV infections), although incidence rates appear to have peaked in several African countries, and may even be falling in some countries (e.g. Kenya). Women are disproportionately affected by HIV, and HIV seroprevalence is over 20% among pregnant women in many sub-Saharan African countries. Because over 95% of pediatric infections are acquired from mother to child, this has major implications for HIV infection in children. In Africa, where almost 90% of the world's infected children live, HIV has reversed gains in child survival and has lowered life expectancy. In addition, large numbers of children have been orphaned. By the end of 2006, UNAIDS estimated that there were over 12 million children under 18 years of age in Africa who had lost their mother or both parents to AIDS,[429] placing enormous strains on communities already devastated by the social and economic impact of so many young adults prematurely dying.

The global HIV epidemic continues to grow outside Africa. Over half of the world's population lives in the Asia/Pacific region and in 2006 an estimated 8.3 million people were infected with HIV. Two thirds live in India, which now has the largest number of HIV infected persons of any single country.[429] Seroprevalence rates in pregnant women are over 1% in many states. The epidemic in Eastern Europe and Central Asia has seen a twenty-fold increase in the number of people living with HIV in under a decade; estimated at 1.5 million in 2006, the majority live in the Russian Federation and the Ukraine, where adult prevalence rates are

above 1%. While intravenous drug use is a major risk factor, increasing reports of new sexually transmitted infections suggest HIV is spreading into the general population.[429] Increasing availability of surveillance data from China provides estimates that at least 650 000 people are living with HIV, with highest prevalence rates seen in injecting drug users and sex workers.

Even in Western countries, prevention efforts appear to be stalling. Available information indicates that the number of newly infected people is no lower in 2006 compared with previous years, with 720 000 adults and children estimated to have acquired HIV in Western and Central Europe and 1.2 million in North America.[429] Overall HIV prevalence has risen in both regions, because ART is resulting in HIV infected individuals living longer, and also likely as a result of more people coming forward for testing (including in particular pregnant women). Thousands of infections are still occurring through unsafe sex between men, where complacency may be attributed to the fact that in the age of ART, HIV is seen as a treatable if not curable disease. However, it is also true that transmission rates of HIV are likely to be lower from persons on highly active ART (HAART) who will have lower plasma concentrations of the virus.[430] In the USA, there remain an estimated 25% of persons with HIV who have not been diagnosed, this proportion being higher in black African populations where HIV is now the leading cause of death in African American women aged between 25 and 34 years.[429] The proportion of persons with undiagnosed HIV is higher (around one third) in the UK. These persons are more likely to transmit HIV to their sexual partners as they are less likely to use barrier contraception and are not on HAART and therefore have higher levels of plasma viremia.

It is estimated that around 43% of transmission occurs around the time of seroconversion and thus generally before the infected person knows he or she has HIV infection.

By the end of 2006 there were an estimated 2.3 million children < 15 years old living with HIV infection worldwide, of whom 540 000 were newly infected and 360 000 died during 2006 alone; 87% live in sub-Saharan Africa.[429] Although contributing less than 1% of children infected with HIV worldwide, there are currently around 11 000 children living with HIV in North America and about 4000 in Western and central Europe, of whom over 1100 live in the UK and Ireland (www.chipscohort.org).[429] With dramatic decreases in transmission rates from mother to child in resource rich countries, new pediatric infections amongst babies usually occur only in countries where antenatal screening is not comprehensive and/or interventions to reduce mother-to-child transmission (MTCT) are not widely offered. Recent cases of MTCT in UK have been reported in infants of women with a negative HIV antibody test in early pregnancy who subsequently seroconvert during pregnancy or breast-feeding.[431] It is not surprising that pediatric infections in many countries of the north are increasingly in migrants from countries with a high prevalence of HIV infection. In the UK, over 75% of seropositive newborns are delivered to mothers born in sub-Saharan Africa, and whereas prior to 2000 approximately one third of HIV infected children were themselves born overseas, this proportion increased to around two thirds after 2003.[432] Similar patterns are being observed in many countries in Europe.[433]

Romania has the largest number of HIV infected children in Europe.[429] The majority belong to a cohort of children who were uniquely infected with HIV through contaminated blood products and needles in the late 1980s. Although many have died, there remain a considerable number of these children who are now teenagers in Romania. Maternal seroprevalence in Romania is about 0.3% in cities such as Costansa, on the Black Sea.

Surveillance for pediatric HIV infection

Unlinked anonymous monitoring of HIV through testing dried blood spots (Guthrie cards) collected on all newborns in many countries for metabolic screening, or antenatal bloods, can provide an unbiased estimate of the prevalence of HIV infection among women having live babies. This is a useful method of providing information about the extent of heterosexually acquired HIV infection in a population, particularly if monitoring is undertaken longitudinally. This might be done continuously or, if resources are scarce, it can be done intermittently (e.g. for 3 months each year). It is possible, while preserving full anonymity, to retain demographic information (e.g. mother's country of birth) which can then determine HIV seroprevalence among particular groups within a community as was done in North London, showing low HIV prevalence among women coming from Asian communities in

1998.[434] Data from anonymous serosurveys have also been combined with non-named confidential register data on HIV in pregnancy in order to provide an indication of the proportion of pregnancies being identified before or during pregnancy.[435] This can be a useful way to audit antenatal testing policy and provide local feedback to care providers (see below).

HIV antibody testing of Guthrie cards is being undertaken in the UK and covers approximately 70% of live births. In 2004, the HIV antenatal seroprevalence was 0.44% in Greater London and 0.11% in the rest of England, but women of sub-Saharan origin had a rate of 2.2%, over 30 times the rate of 0.07% in women born in the UK[436] (Fig. 28.29). Maternal seroprevalence rates in England and Scotland have risen from 0.16% in 2000 to 0.27% in 2004,[436] and this rise may in part reflect an increasing desire for HIV infected women on HAART and clinically well to have children, in the knowledge that the risk of MTCT with appropriate intervention is very low. In London in 2004, three quarters of seropositive newborns were delivered to mothers born in sub-Saharan Africa, and similar patterns are being observed in European countries such as France and Belgium. In Scotland, Ireland and southern Europe a higher proportion of seropositive children are still born to women with injecting drug use (IDU) as a risk factor, but here too the proportion of women acquiring HIV from heterosexual transmission is increasing.

Of 1441 children reported to the National Study of HIV in Pregnancy and Childhood (NSHPC) by June 2006, over 1300 are currently known to be living with HIV in the UK and Ireland. Over two thirds reside in London and were born to women who acquired HIV in sub-Saharan Africa. With dispersal of refugees to other cities in the UK, this is changing. Similarly, whereas the majority of HIV infected children in Scotland and Ireland are still white children born to mothers with IDU as a risk factor for acquiring HIV, this is changing and increasing numbers of mothers of more recently diagnosed HIV infected children acquired the disease through heterosexual contact, often abroad. Follow-up of infected children is being coordinated, along with follow-up of children in Europe participating in clinical trials [Paediatric European Network for Treatment of AIDS (PENTA)], through the Collaborative HIV in Paediatric Study (CHIPS) cohort which has over 1100 children in follow-up from over 40 centers and is coordinated through the MRC Clinical Trials Unit in London in collaboration with the Institute of Child Health (ICH) (www.chipscohort.ac.uk, www.pentatrials.org).[432]

With the advent of HAART, children with HIV are living longer and the average age of the cohort of infected children in the UK and Ireland is now around 8.5 years, with 12% being 15 years of age or older, and over 100 having transferred to adult clinics.[432] As children with HIV survive into adolescence they face many similar issues to other young people with chronic disease such as delayed growth, development and puberty and adherence to and the long term side-effects of drug therapy. However, these young people have the additional issues

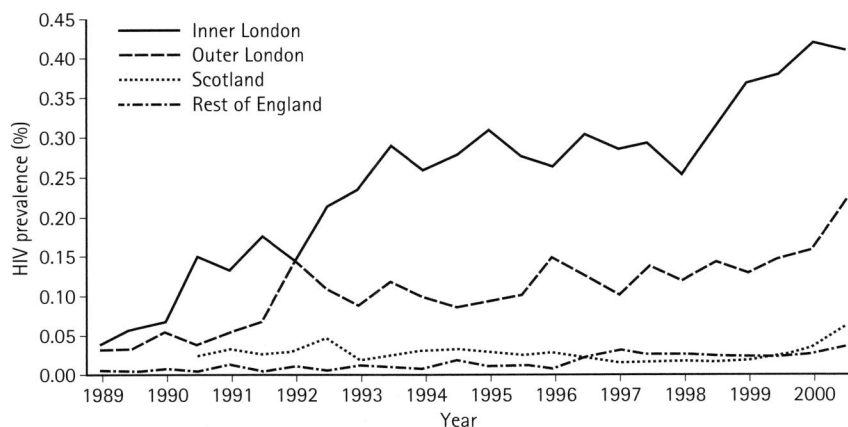

Fig. 28.29 Trends in prevalence of HIV infection in pregnant women by area of residence: 1989–2000.

of negotiating adolescence with a stigmatizing sexually transmissible disease. Many will also have lost a parent or will have to care for a sick family member. The complex medical, psychological and social needs of these young people require multidisciplinary team involvement with close liaison with adult colleagues when transitioning young people to adult services.[437]

MOTHER-TO-CHILD TRANSMISSION OF HIV

Mother-to-child transmission (MTCT) of HIV can occur during pregnancy, labor or breast-feeding.[438] In the absence of breast-feeding, approximately two thirds of transmission occurs around the time of delivery. In Europe and the USA, the rate of MTCT in the absence of breast-feeding prior to the advent of interventions was around 15–20%, compared with around 30–40% in Africa. Most of this difference is due to breast-feeding, which accounts for about one third of transmission in Africa.[439] Factors independently affecting the rate of transmission include the mother's clinical status, HIV viral load and CD4 cell count, particularly at the time of delivery, prematurity, factors around delivery such as duration of rupture of membranes and mode of delivery[438,440] (Table 28.31).

In the last 10 years, rates of MTCT in resource rich countries have fallen dramatically to 2% or less with strategies including use of anti-retroviral therapy, elective Cesarean section (CS) and refraining from breast-feeding.[427,441] Unfortunately in most resource limited settings, despite increased availability of at least some interventions to reduce MTCT, only about 10% of women are diagnosed in pregnancy and therefore have access to such interventions.[429]

Antiretroviral therapy to reduce MTCT

In 1995, the first placebo-controlled trial (the ACTG 076 trial) of zidovudine (ZDV) monotherapy, given to the mother antenatally from a median of 26 weeks by continuous intravenous infusion during labor, and then orally to the infant from birth for 6 weeks, resulted in a 67% reduction in MTCT in non-breast-feeding US and French HIV infected women compared with placebo.[442] This trial was followed by non-randomized studies to document the effect of ZDV monotherapy on MTCT in the clinical setting[427,441,443] and of non-randomized studies of double[444] and triple antiretroviral therapy. The results showed that ZDV was highly effective in reducing MTCT and, compared with historical controls, the use of double therapy was superior to monotherapy.[444] With triple therapy, MTCT rates below 1% are achievable among women with undetectable HIV viral load at delivery.[445] Cohort studies have documented reductions in MTCT over calendar time with increasing use of triple HAART in pregnancy (Fig. 28.30).[428]

The importance of low maternal plasma HIV viral load around the time of delivery in reducing the risk of MTCT has been demonstrated in subsequent trials.[446] However, it is not the only important factor and it is clear that ART reduces MTCT both by decreasing maternal viral load and by providing pre- and post-exposure prophylaxis to the infant. In an individual patient meta-analysis of women with low HIV RNA of < 10 000 copies/ml, the transmission rate was reduced from 10% to

Table 28.31 Factors associated with mother-to-child transmission (MTCT) of HIV

- Without interventions, the rate of MTCT was 15–20% in Europe, and 25–40% in Africa
- Most MTCT occurs around the time of delivery
- Increased risk is associated with:
  – late stage maternal disease
  – high maternal plasma viremia
  – prolonged rupture of membranes
  – invasive obstetric procedures
  – prematurity
  – breast-feeding

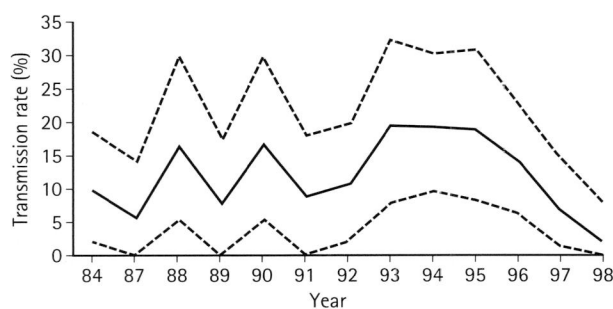

Fig. 28.30 Estimated vertical transmission rate (95% CI) in UK over time in non-breast-feeding women.
(From Duong et al 1999[428])

only 1% by the use of ZDV alone, which has only a minimal effect on maternal viral load (reduction by only about 0.3 log copies/ml).[447] This suggests that post-exposure prophylaxis to the fetus is also important, a factor borne out by the large impact on transmission of giving long acting nevirapine (NVP) to women during labor and to the baby.[448] Even if a woman has not received ART during pregnancy or delivery, ART given to the baby as soon as possible after birth is likely to have an effect on transmission. Guidelines for giving ART to pregnant women to reduce MTCT are available and are regularly updated.[449,450]

Trials have been conducted comparing different components of the ACTG 076 regimen and also evaluating other antiretroviral drugs. Most have taken place in resource-limited settings where an important goal was also to refine, simplify and reduce the costs of the initial ZDV regimen used in the ACTG 076 trial. A trial of ZDV monotherapy in non-breast-feeding women in Thailand showed that a 50% reduction of MTCT was possible by giving ZDV from 36 weeks' gestation, oral ZDV during labor and for 2 weeks to the baby.[451] However, another trial from Thailand emphasized that starting ART at 28 weeks added benefit compared with starting at 36 weeks,[452] suggesting that some in utero transmission may be prevented by ART. It is also true that if starting ART is left until 36 weeks, some women will go into premature labor having received minimal or no pre-labor ART.

Intrapartum ART alone does not appear to be useful[453] if given without postpartum prophylaxis to the baby. In HIVNET 012 undertaken in Uganda, a single 200 mg oral dose of NVP, given to the mother in labor, followed by a single oral dose of 2 mg/kg to the infant at 48 h (total cost US$4), led to a 40% reduction in MTCT at 16 weeks compared with intrapartum and neonatal (for 1 week) oral ZDV.[448] Follow-up to 18 months has shown continued efficacy of around 40% despite breast-feeding for an average of 9 months. However, probably due to its long plasma half-life,[454] nevirapine resistance rates of up to 75% in mothers and 46% in infants after single dose exposure have been reported.[455,456] As ART becomes increasingly available worldwide the therapeutic implications of NVP resistance for mothers and infants infected despite NVP are of increasing concern.[457,458] Methods to reduce rates of nevirapine resistance include the use of short course combination therapy to protect the nevirapine 'tail'. In the Treatment Option Study (TOPS) significantly reduced rates of NVP resistance were seen in women who received either 4 or 7 days of Combivir with single dose nevirapine (SD-NVP) when compared to women who received SD-NVP alone.[459,460] In a study from Malawi, infants who received SD-NVP plus AZT had lower rates of NVP resistance at 6–8 weeks of age than infants who received SD-NVP or mothers who had peripartum SD-NVP alone. Similar rates of MTCT were seen in all groups.[461] For those women who develop NVP resistance there are some data suggesting that these mutations fade over time. Women who had received peripartum SD-NVP had higher rates of virological failure when commencing subsequent NVP-based HAART than women who had received a placebo but only if they started HAART within 6 months of delivery.[462] Whether archived NVP mutations will continue to impact on the longer term response to subsequent

NNRTI-based regimens requires further follow-up. The balance between preventing transmission of HIV to infants whilst minimizing impact on maternal health and future HAART options is a complex issue requiring continuing research, during which time NVP continues to have a role in the prevention of MTCT in resource poor settings.

Reducing MTCT in well resourced settings

Whilst randomized controlled trials of HAART are lacking, in a European cohort HAART was associated with a fall in transmission from 11.5% to 1.2%, with a greater reduction (0.25% versus 1.92% respectively) if started prior to pregnancy compared to during pregnancy.[463] Prior to 2004, women commencing HAART in pregnancy would typically receive NVP with two nucleoside reverse transcriptase inhibitors (NRTIs), often ZDV and 3TC. Following reports of fatal fulminant hepatitis in pregnant women with good CD4 counts receiving NVP-based HAART, nevirapine is no longer recommended for pregnant women with good CD4 counts (>250 cell/uL) who are taking ART for the prevention of MTCT. Alternate regimens based on a protease inhibitor are used. NVP monotherapy is not recommended because of concerns about the development of resistance to all non-nucleoside reverse transcriptase inhibitor (NNRTI) drugs.

Problems with ART to reduce MTCT
Maternal pre-eclampsia and premature labor

Advances in the development of pharmaceutical interventions to reduce HIV MTCT are not without complications. Analysis of a Spanish cohort of HIV positive women delivering between 1985 and 2003 showed a marked reduction in MTCT but an increased risk of fetal death or pre-eclampsia with any form of HAART taken pre-pregnancy.[464] A European study found an increased risk of prematurity associated with combination therapy commenced before the pregnancy (OR 2.6, 95% CI 1.43–4.75),[465] but a US cohort reported similar rates of prematurity of 17% but no significant difference between mothers who had received ART and those who had not.[466] It is speculated that immune reconstitution due to ART may play a part in adverse pregnancy outcome.

Neonatal toxicity

In a French study of ZDV + 3TC, concerns were first raised about a possible link between mitochondrial dysfunction in HIV uninfected children and perinatal exposure to NRTIs.[467] This complication is also known to occur rarely in HIV infected individuals taking NRTIs. Retrospective analysis of other large cohort data failed to reveal other definitive cases.[468] Neonatal anemia, and neutropenia have been reported in uninfected infants perinatally exposed to NRTIs, but they rarely require transfusion and respond to discontinuing the NRTIs, although a small negative effect on hematopoiesis has been seen up to 18 months of age.[469] Although concerns about the potential carcinogenicity and reproductive effects of ART as well as mitochondrial toxicity remain, current evidence suggests that the benefit of ART in dramatically reducing MTCT far outweighs potential harm. Many countries are now setting up long term surveillance to follow all children born to HIV infected mothers, whether exposed or not to ARTs in utero. In the UK, the CHART study, the National Study of HIV in Pregnancy conducted at the ICH, assesses the long term health and development of ART-exposed children.

Effect of mode of delivery on MTCT

Several cohort studies have shown that factors around delivery contribute importantly to MTCT. In a meta-analysis of 15 large studies, including more than 5000 mother–child pairs from the USA and Europe, it was estimated that each hour longer in labor with ruptured membranes was associated with a 2% increase in the risk of MTCT.[470] A meta-analysis of these studies, a randomized European trial, and a European controlled trial, showed that among more than 8000 women the risk of transmission was 50% lower for babies delivered by elective CS prior to membrane rupture, compared with vaginal or emergency CS delivery.[471,472] Subsequent cohorts have shown that reduction of MTCT to around 2% is possible with ZDV, elective CS delivery and with not breast-feeding.[428,442] The question of how much additional reduction to transmission may occur if elective CS delivery is undertaken in women on HAART with undetectable HIV RNA viral load around the time of delivery is unclear[473] and is unlikely to be answered from controlled trials. However, as the risk is very low, most guidelines suggest that the women can undergo a normal vaginal delivery in this situation, but that membranes should not be ruptured prematurely, and invasive interventions during labor or delivery (e.g. use of scalp electrodes and instrumental delivery) should be avoided.[449,450] Increasingly, women on HAART with undetectable plasma viral loads are choosing vaginal delivery. This may be of particular importance for women returning to areas of the world where elective CS is not readily available for subsequent pregnancies.

Breast-feeding

HIV can be transmitted through breast milk.[474,475] Most transmission appears to occur early, and factors including HIV viral content in colostrum, immaturity of the infant gastrointestinal tract in the neonatal period, and the contribution of breast and nipple complications (e.g. mastitis and bleeding nipples which may increase the amount of virus in breast milk) all play a role. Breast milk transmission continues, however, throughout the duration of breast-feeding, posing extremely difficult dilemmas for policy in parts of the world where alternatives to breast-feeding are expensive, unsafe and culturally unacceptable, but where HIV prevalence is high.[476]

The current recommendation is that infants should continue to be breast-fed where infectious diseases and malnutrition are the main cause of infant mortality, because artificial feeding substantially increases the risk of illness and death.[476] Evidence suggests that mixed feeding is associated with a higher risk of transmission and therefore it has been recommended that women in these areas exclusively breast-feed for 4–6 months (which is anyway advocated for all women) and then wean as quickly as possible. After this time, the benefits of breast-feeding may be outweighed by the risk of HIV infection.[477] This strategy is likely to be more feasible than exclusive formula feeding, which in many settings is likely to increase infant mortality from other infections, to be socially unacceptable and unaffordable and risk a 'spill-over effect' on non-HIV infected mothers. Where infants of HIV infected mothers can be ensured uninterrupted access to nutritionally adequate, safely prepared breast milk substitutes, they are at less risk of illness and death from non-HIV related illness and their mothers should be encouraged not to breast-feed. Hopefully, larger prospective studies will help clarify the effects of exclusive breast-feeding followed by early weaning after short course anti-retroviral therapy on HIV transmission rates, and the morbidity and mortality of HIV infected and uninfected babies. The risk of transmission through breast-feeding in mothers with an undetectable plasma viral load on suppressive HAART is being assessed in studies in Africa.[478]

Other interventions to reduce MTCT

Other interventions that have been explored to reduce MTCT include trials of cleansing the birth canal and vitamin A supplementation during pregnancy. The rationale for the former is that the maximum risk of exposure appears to be around the time of delivery and, therefore, cleaning with chlorhexidine might reduce vertical transmission. However, clinical trials have failed to show significant reduction of MTCT with this approach.[479]

Observational studies suggested that low vitamin A levels were associated with increased MTCT.[480] Randomized trials have, however, failed to show a significant impact of supplementation with vitamin A on prevention of MTCT.[481]

ANTENATAL TESTING
In resource rich countries

The case for offering antenatal HIV testing is overwhelming. A recommendation that HIV testing should be offered to all women in pregnancy has been successfully implemented in most well resourced countries. In the UK, the universal offer of HIV testing during the antenatal period was endorsed in 1999 after an economic analysis showed that a universal offer policy was cost effective throughout the UK provided that a high uptake of testing was achieved.[482]

Statistical analysis of unlinked anonymous seroprevalence data with reported infections suggests that in 2004, 90% of infected women living in the UK were diagnosed prior to delivery and were therefore able to take up interventions to reduce MTCT. In most European countries and in the USA, a marked decrease in infected babies reflects the high proportion of pregnant women receiving appropriate care to reduce MTCT. However, a few infants continue to present with severe *Pneumocystis jiroveci*, previously called *P. carinii* pneumonia (PCP), and cytomegalovirus (CMV) infection[483] as a result of perinatal transmission of HIV from mothers who are unaware of their own HIV infection or from mothers who have seroconverted in pregnancy or during breast-feeding.[431] Discussions are underway in the UK to determine whether a second HIV antibody test in the later stages of pregnancy would be feasible and cost effective in further reducing the risk of MTCT.

In resource limited countries

In low income countries, ART to prevent MTCT is only one strand of a much more complex mesh of issues surrounding the prevention of vertical transmission.[484] With the available tools and knowledge that we have already, there is a strong argument for putting resources into providing antenatal diagnosis and the appropriate perinatal interventions. This undoubtedly requires a huge input of resources into the development of sustainable infrastructures in situations where antenatal care may currently be rudimentary.

Understandably, concerns have been raised that, rather than putting scarce resources into a 'magic bullet' of ART to pregnant women, efforts should be concentrated on the more difficult issue of preventing women getting infected in the first place. In sub-Saharan Africa pilot projects offering antenatal screening and intervention have been established since 2001, but the scaling up of these services has been disappointing, with less than 10% of infected pregnant women in sub-Saharan Africa offered intervention to prevent MTCT in 2006.[429] Preventing HIV infection in women will require both behavioral and biomedical interventions such as microbicides, several of which are currently being evaluated in phase III trials.

ETIOLOGY AND PATHOGENESIS

HIV is a retrovirus. Transmission occurs through sexual intercourse, via infected blood and blood products and by transmission from mother to child. Many of the clinical features of HIV can be ascribed to profound immune suppression, because HIV infects cells of the immune system and ultimately destroys them. An understanding of the way it does this is helpful in interpreting tests used in monitoring the disease and helps explain the difficulties in developing a vaccine for HIV.

The virus predominantly infects a subset of the thymus-derived lymphocytes carrying the surface molecule CD4, which binds the glycoprotein on the envelope of HIV called gp120. CD4 is also present on many monocytes and macrophages and on Langerhans' cells of the skin and dendritic cells of many other tissues. HIV also requires co-receptors to enter cells. Two of these, termed CCR5 and CXCR4, are of particular importance. These co-receptors are members of a family of receptors, expressed on the cells of lymphocytes, dendritic cells and cells of the rectal, vaginal and cervical mucosa, that function as receptors for chemokines that orchestrate the migration and differentiation of leukocytes during immune responses. Virus strains able to infect primary macrophages (R5 tropic viruses) use CCR5 as a co-receptor and these are detected early in infection, suggesting they are important for transmission. Further evidence for this comes from studies showing that individuals homozygous for a 32 pair deletion of CCR5 show increased resistance to being infected by HIV.[485,486] Both R5 and strains infecting T cells use CXCR4 as a co-receptor (T or X4 viruses) and they arise during the course of infection.

CD8 cytotoxic lymphocytes (CTL) capable of killing HIV infected targets develop early in primary HIV infection and are very important in the initial control of viremia.[487,488] Among CD8 cells, rapid expansion of strong T cell responses to multiple viral epitopes has been shown to be associated with better control of viremia following primary infection in adults. CD8 T cells kill infected cells and produce CD8 T cell antiviral factor (CAF) which inhibits viral replication. The breadth and strength of the CTL responses are determined by the degree of CD4 specific helper response, which may be determined by the level of HIV viremia and by genetic host factors. In adults who fail to control viral load, CTL responses are narrower and less marked. Because HIV replication is very rapid and errors occur in reverse transcription, these mutants can evade CTL response (escape mutants), i.e. the viral epitope mutates to 'escape' control by the CTL. Children surviving with perinatally acquired HIV have been shown to have more robust HIV-1-specific CD8 responses than was previously thought, comparable in magnitude and breadth to those of adults[489] and, as in adult studies, infants and children with unsuppressed viral loads had poorer CTL responses.[490]

In infants in whom the immune system is immature, the viral load rises over the first weeks after primary infection around the time of birth, and stays high throughout infancy. It then falls in the absence of therapy over the next 3–5 years (Fig. 28.31)[491,492] to reach a 'set point' which is much later after primary infection than in adults (set point at about 6 months). Unlike adults, infants have a highly active thymus which may 'work' to replenish CD4 cells destroyed by the virus. While this may appear to be advantageous, recent work has suggested these new thymic cells may quickly become infected with HIV and possibly delay reduction in HIV viremia in children on ART.[493]

As viremia starts to decline in adults, HIV antibody production increases. Detection of HIV antibodies is the principal way of making the diagnosis in adults and older children, as antibodies persist usually until death.

Polyclonal activation of B cells also occurs, resulting in high immunoglobulin levels in most children commencing during infancy, although infants with rapid disease progression may rarely be hypogammaglobulinemic. This polyclonal increase in immunoglobulin is in many cases nonfunctional, while antigen-specific antibody production is reduced, resulting in increased susceptibility to bacterial infections.

There are reports of both adults and children being exposed to HIV and remaining uninfected; these individuals have detectable HIV-specific CTL. In addition, individuals with strong CTL responses may have delayed disease progression (long term nonprogressors); the latter has also been associated with certain HLA type 1 alleles.[454]

The CD4 cell plays a central role in orchestrating the immune system, and their destruction by HIV accounts for much of the immunosuppressive

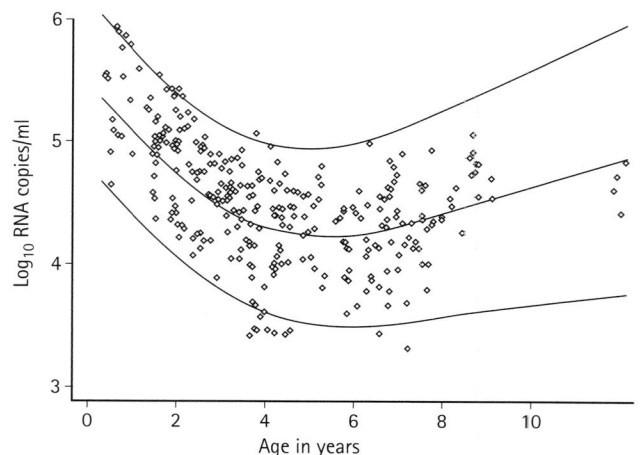

Fig. 28.31 Log$_{10}$ HIV-1 RNA plotted against age in untreated HIV infected children (fitted line and 95% CI). (From Gibb et al 1993[492])

effect of the virus. Following fusion into CD4 and other cells, viral core material enters the host cell and the genetic material encoded in RNA is converted to DNA by reverse transcriptase. This DNA 'provirus' is then integrated into the host genome. HIV replicates at an enormous rate with > 10⁶ particles being produced daily.[495] In addition, turnover of infected replicating CD4 cells is high, occurring approximately every 1.5 days. CD4 damage occurs both directly and through mechanisms resulting in apoptosis of infected cells. The exact role of both mechanisms is still debated. HIV in resting memory and long-lived cells both in the immune system and in other tissues remains latent for long periods of time and is largely responsible for persistence of the virus despite the ability of HAART to decrease virus to undetectable levels in plasma. In 1996, with the advent of HAART, there was great hope that the half-life of long-lived cells might be in the order of only a few years and that HIV eradication might be possible. Sadly this is not the case, and modeling exercises estimate the half-life of these long-lived infected cells to be around 70 years.[496] If HAART is stopped, even after plasma viral load has been undetectable for several years, HIV viral load rises again within 1–2 weeks, typically returning to the 'set point' seen prior to initiation of HAART. The virus also has a remarkable ability to mutate and develop resistance to antiretroviral drugs, as seen following single dose nevirapine exposure (see above). Mutant virus may remain in latent cells for many years but re-emerge if that drug is re-started in an individual.

Monitoring with CD4 and HIV RNA viral load

The most widely used markers for predicting disease progression in children, as in adults, are the CD4 cell count (or percentage) and viral load as measured by HIV-1 RNA in plasma.

Absolute CD4 counts are higher in young children than in adults and there is great within- and between-individual variability. CD4 percentages vary less with age, although they are still higher at very young ages as can be seen from percentile charts constructed from uninfected children born to HIV positive mothers (Fig. 28.32).[497] By around 4–5 years of age, the CD4 cell count number and range has fallen to nearer adult values. In children with HIV infection, as in adults, absolute lymphocyte counts and CD4 cell counts decrease with progression of the disease. Analyses of combined individual longitudinal data in untreated children prior to the advent of ART (HIV Paediatric Prognostic Markers Collaborative Study) have provided guidance for thresholds of CD4%, CD4 count and total lymphocyte counts (TLC) associated with a marked increase in disease progression at different ages.[498–500] These have formed the basis for new WHO guidelines[501]; clinicians can use a risk calculator (available on http://www.hppmcs.org/) to estimate risk of progression in an untreated child according to age and CD4% count or TLC level. Most pediatricians use CD4% up until the age of around 5 years when increasing account should be taken of the total CD4 count. Of particular note, in very young children, no marker is very good at predicting

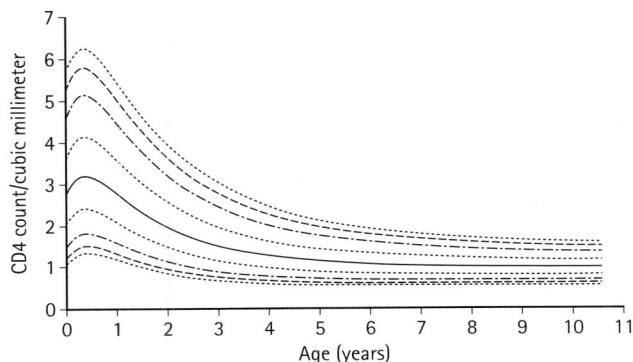

Fig. 28.32 CD4 lymphocyte counts in uninfected children by age: 3rd, 5th, 10th, 25th, 50th, 75th, 90th, 95th and 97th centiles. Created from data collected by the European Collaborative Study using the methods of Wade & Ades (1994).[497]

disease progression. Whereas, in adults, a CD4 cell count below 200 cells/mm³ is a useful predictor of risk of developing *Pneumocystis carinii* (*P. jiroveci*) pneumonia (PCP) and is therefore used to determine the time to start prophylaxis against this disease, during infancy even CD4 percentage is of limited predictive value.[502] After infancy, a CD4% greater than 25% is considered evidence of minimal immunosuppression, 15–25% moderate, and < 15% severe immunosuppression and these form the basis of the Centers for Disease Control (CDC) immunological classification of HIV in children.[503,504] The Revised WHO Clinical Staging and Immunological Classification of HIV/AIDS (2006) incorporates age-related immune classification from infancy through to adulthood.[501] Importantly, for the individual child the rate of fall of CD4% and at older ages of CD4 cell counts are of importance and should be taken into account when making decisions about when to start antiretroviral therapy. Further analyses of HPPMCS data are ongoing to try to define this more accurately.

Viral load as measured by plasma HIV RNA is an independent predictor of HIV progression in adults after the 'set point' has been reached. Several different assays are available in kit form with quality control (Roche, Chiron and NASBA). The Roche PCR version 1.5 and Chiron assays are widely used and include additional primers to ensure accuracy when measuring viral load in persons with different subtypes of HIV (e.g. subtype B is the most common virus subtype in white North Americans and Europeans but subtypes A, C and D are common in Africans). It is important to be aware that assay variability may be as high as 0.7 log and that results need to be interpreted on a log scale. Repeating results is advisable if treatment decisions are being taken based on viral load results; in general viral load is less predictive of disease progression than CD4% or count and used less to make decisions about starting therapy.[498] All assays are less precise at values above 750 000 copies/ml but all assays are more robust at low levels down to a cut-off of 50 copies/ml. In infants, HIV RNA is very high after infection around the time of birth and remains much higher (often 1 million copies/ml or more) than observed in adults for the first 2 years of life, gradually reducing by an average of about one log over the first 5 years of life in the absence of antiretroviral therapy (Fig. 28.33).[492,495]

LABORATORY DIAGNOSIS OF HIV

Enzyme linked immunosorbent assays (ELISA) for measuring HIV antibody are highly sensitive and specific for diagnosing HIV in adults and in children over 18 months of age. However, because of transplacental transfer of maternal antibody, all babies born to HIV infected women will have antibodies at birth which take a median of 10 months and a maximum of 18 months to clear. Other techniques, directed at viral components rather than the host immune response, are therefore required to diagnose HIV in young infants.

In Western countries, early diagnosis of HIV in infants has been improved significantly by polymerase chain reaction (PCR) techniques for detecting proviral DNA and RNA. Using these techniques, HIV infection can be definitively diagnosed in about 90% of infected infants by age 1 month and in virtually all by 3 months. HIV proviral DNA PCR is the preferred method for initial diagnosis. In a meta-analysis, 38% (90% CI = 29–46%) of infected children had positive PCR DNA tests by age 48 h, rapidly increasing in the second week with 93% of infected children (90% CI = 76–97%) testing positive by 2 weeks of age.[505]

HIV RNA tests may be more sensitive than DNA PCR for diagnosis, but limited data suggest lower specificity, immediately after birth. However, they may be alternatives if proviral DNA tests are not available and give additional information about the degree of viremia. Culture of HIV is time consuming and expensive and is no longer routinely undertaken. The detection of p24 antigen, both standard and immune-complex dissociated, although highly specific, is not as sensitive as DNA PCR. Nevertheless, detection of acid or heat dissociated p24 antigen by ELISA is considerably cheaper than PCR tests and is also technically less demanding, making it more promising as a diagnostic tool for resource limited settings; it is highly specific but less sensitive than proviral DNA.

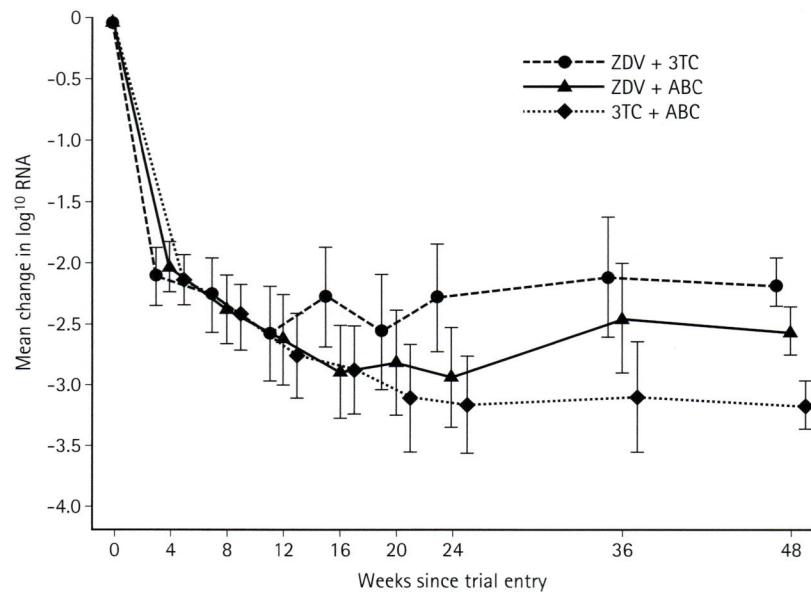

Fig. 28.33   Change in log[10] RNA after starting ART in the PENTA 5 trial. (From PENTA 2002[535])

Another laboratory clue that a child may have HIV infection is the presence of polyclonal hypergammaglobulinemia, which in the presence of CD4 lymphopenia should lead to a high suspicion of HIV infection.

In the last 5 years, there has been increased focus on developing cheaper ways of detecting early infection in infants. Although still outside the reach of most countries' budgets, early diagnosis using DNA PCR techniques is now available in many parts of South Africa and is being introduced into countries such as Uganda. Updated WHO guidelines recommend that treatment of symptomatic infants can start in the absence of a definitive diagnosis.[501] Early detection of infection among babies born to mothers who have received PMTCT is more problematic because, with reduced transmission rates, many babies have to be tested to detect a single infected baby. The issues of testing during breast-feeding also require attention; the WHO recommends that testing might be focused around timing of immunizations, and in women who wean at 6 months according to guidelines, after cessation of breast-feeding.[501] Debate continues about the best time to test if only one test per infant is available. However, unless it is undertaken early, it is clear that infected babies will die before there is time for diagnosis to occur.

CLINICAL ASPECTS IN WELL RESOURCED SETTINGS

HIV infected babies generally appear normal at birth, with birth weight in the normal range. Clinically one cannot usually detect any signs that a baby has HIV in the first days of life. Signs and symptoms develop over the first few weeks and most children have evidence of infection before 12 months of age. Anecdotally, axillary lymphadenopathy may be an early sign that a baby is infected. However, there is a wide spectrum and some infected children may not present to medical attention for several years, with a smaller number remaining asymptomatic into adolescence.

HIV can present with a spectrum of signs and symptoms in children. This is reflected in both the four-stage CDC classification[504] and more recently in the revised four-stage WHO classification system for children[501] (Table 28.32), and important differences between adults and children are summarized in Table 28.33. In the absence of antiretroviral

therapy or prophylaxis against PCP (see below), disease progression is faster than in adults, even in well resourced settings. Cohort studies reported in the early 1990s that 15–20% of children progressed to an AIDS-defining illness by 12 months of age.[506–508] Over half of this subset of perinatally infected children presented with PCP at around 3–6 months of age in the absence of using prophylactic co-trimoxazole. Data from prospective cohorts in Europe in the early 1990s reported overall survival rates in children on either no ART or only ZDV monotherapy of around 70% by 6 years and 50% by 9 years of age.[506–508]

Children with HIV infection frequently present with nonspecific signs and symptoms that are common in general pediatrics. The most usual clinical features associated with HIV infection include persistent generalized lymphadenopathy (particularly axillary), hepatosplenomegaly, chronic or recurrent diarrhea, prolonged or recurrent oral or diaper candidiasis, fever, recurrent otitis or sinusitis and chest infections. Children may also present with a picture of idiopathic thrombocytopenic purpura with no other signs and may be more prone to developing eczema, extensive molluscum, and recurrent allergic iritis and rhinitis. A typical and quite specific presentation is non-tender bilateral parotid enlargement, which may be associated with generalized cervical lymphadenopathy and X-ray appearances of lymphocytic interstitial pneumonitis (LIP) with hilar lymphadenopathy (see below). Such children often also have allergic rhinitis, tonsillar and/or adenoid enlargement and may present with sleep apnea. Herpes zoster (shingles) in childhood is uncommon and suggests a defect in cellular immunity justifying an HIV test in the absence of other explanations.

Persistent or recurrent oral candidiasis after the neonatal period, abnormal neurological signs, failure to thrive and poor growth in association with HIV are all indications of increasing immune deficiency and a poorer outcome. Conversely, thrombocytopenia does not indicate a poor prognosis and bilateral parotitis, lymphadenopathy and LIP (see below) are often associated with a relatively good prognosis. Details of the main AIDS (CDC stage C) presenting conditions are described below. Although the development of these conditions, along with immunological stage 3 disease, has been shown to be predictive of a poor outcome, the prognosis varies. For example, conditions such as recurrent

Table 28.32 Revised WHO clinical and immunological staging in adults and children with established HIV infection

HIV-associated symptoms	WHO clinical stage
Asymptomatic	1
Mild symptoms	2
Advanced symptoms	3
Severe symptoms	4

WHO-Proposed Immunological Classification for Established HIV Infection

HIV-associated immunodeficiency	Age-related CD4 values			
	< 11 months (%CD4+)	12–35 months (%CD4+)	36–59 months (%CD4+)	> 5 years (absolute number per mm³ or %CD4+)
None or not significant	> 35	> 30	> 25	> 500
Mild	30–35	25–30	20–25	350–499
Advanced	25–29	20–24	15–19	200–349
Severe	< 25	< 20	< 15	< 200 or < 15%

WHO Case Definitions of HIV For Surveillance and Revised Clinical Staging and Immunological Classification of HIV-Related Disease in Children:
WHO clinical staging of HIV/AIDS for children with confirmed HIV infection

Clinical stage 1
Asymptomatic
Persistent generalized lymphadenopathy
Clinical stage 2
Unexplained persistent hepatosplenomegaly
Papular pruritic eruptions
Extensive wart virus infection
Extensive molluscum contagiosum
Fungal nail infections
Recurrent oral ulcerations
Unexplained persistent parotid enlargement
Lineal gingival erythema
Herpes zoster
Recurrent or chronic upper respiratory tract infections (otitis media, otorrhea, sinusitis or tonsillitis)

Clinical stage 3
Unexplained moderate malnutrition not adequately responding to standard therapy
Unexplained persistent diarrhea (14 days or longer)
Unexplained persistent fever (above 37.5 °C intermittent or constant, for longer than one month)
Persistent oral candidiasis (after first 6–8 weeks of life)
Oral hairy leukoplakia
Acute necrotizing ulcerative gingivitis or periodontitis
Lymph node tuberculosis
Pulmonary tuberculosis
Severe recurrent bacterial pneumonia
Symptomatic lymphoid interstitial pneumonitis
Chronic HIV-associated lung disease including bronchiectasis
Unexplained anemia (< 8 g/dl), neutropenia (< 0.5 × 10⁹/L) and/or chronic thrombocytopenia (< 50 × 10⁹/L)
Unexplained refers to where the condition is not explained by other causes

Clinical stage 4
Unexplained severe wasting, stunting or severe malnutrition not responding to standard therapy
Pneumocystis carinii pneumonia (PCP)
Recurrent severe bacterial infections (such as empyema, pyomyositis, bone or joint infection or meningitis but excluding pneumonia)
Chronic herpes simplex infection (orolabial, genital or anorectal of more than one month's duration or visceral at any site
Esophageal candidiasis (or candidiasis of trachea, bronchi or lungs)
Extrapulmonary tuberculosis
Kaposi sarcoma
Cytomegalovirus infection (retinitis or infection of other organs with onset at age older than one month)
Central nervous system toxoplasmosis
HIV encephalopathy
Extrapulmonary cryptococcosis including meningitis
Disseminated nontuberculous mycobacterial infection
Progressive multifocal leukoencephalopathy
Chronic cryptosporidiosis
Chronic isosporiasis
Disseminated endemic mycosis (extrapulmonary histoplasmosis or coccidioidomycosis)
Cerebral or B cell non-Hodgkin lymphoma
Symptomatic HIV-associated nephropathy
Symptomatic HIV-associated cardiomyopathy

Table 28.33 Differences compared with adults

- Faster rate of disease progression, especially in infants (PCP and CMV)
- Lymphoid interstitial pneumonitis and parotitis common
- More bacterial infections
- Encephalopathy presents differently
- Growth failure occurs as well as wasting
- Kaposi sarcoma rare outside endemic areas
- Different immunology – developing immune system in uninfected children
- Higher numbers and more variation of CD4 cells
- Decline to adult values in mid-childhood
- CD4% is less variable and so is used in children under 5 years
- Different pattern of HIV RNA – decline of HIV viral load up to 5 years

CMV, cytomegalovirus; PCP, *Pneumocystis carinii* pneumonia.

bacterial infections were generally associated with a better prognosis in resource rich settings than HIV encephalopathy. According to the CDC disease classification, stage B disease includes a wide range of conditions with different predictive values.[504]

Infections

The T and B cell abnormalities resulting from HIV infection result in increased susceptibility to a wide range of organisms including fungi, mycobacteria, bacteria, protozoa and viruses. All infections occur at much higher rates than among HIV negative children, although rates of infection and hospital admissions for children on HAART are significantly lower than those reported in the pre-HAART era.[426] A recent analysis of children participating in clinical trials in the USA compared the incidence of infections in the era pre (n = 3331) and post HAART (n = 2767). The incidence rates of associated infections fell significantly following the introduction of HAART: bacterial pneumonia from 11/100 to 2.15/100 child years, herpes zoster from 2.9/100 to 1.11/100 child years and *Mycobacterium avium intracellulare* complex (MAIC) from 1.8 to less than 0.5/100 child years. Incidence rates of PCP, common in infants not on prophylaxis, fell from 1.3 to less than 0.5/100 child years.[509]

Opportunistic infections

Opportunistic infections, apart from PCP and primary disseminated CMV disease to which infants with rapidly progressive disease are particularly susceptible during the first 6 months of life, are usually a late complication of HIV infection and result from severe immunosuppression. The most common are esophageal candidiasis, multidermatomal varicella zoster, disseminated *Mycobacterium avium* complex (MAC), CMV infections, cryptosporidiosis, and more rarely, toxoplasmosis.[510] MAC should be considered in any child with advanced disease and unexplained fevers, weight loss and abdominal discomfort.

PCP infection (also termed Pneumocystis jiroveci pneumonia) and CMV

These infections are mentioned in greater detail as they present early, particularly in previously undiagnosed HIV infected babies, have a high mortality even in the era of HAART, and present differently in infants compared with older children and adults.

Among HIV infected babies who have not received PCP prophylaxis, PCP is a common first AIDS indicator disease, occurring most frequently in the first 6 months of life, with reported survival rates of only 38–62%.[483,511,512] CMV is often isolated at the time of PCP diagnosis from HIV infected adults and infants.[483,512] Between 1989 and 1999, PCP was the commonest AIDS defining diagnosis, occurring in 68% of reported infected infants born in the UK and Ireland.[512] In almost all, the mother was unaware of her HIV diagnosis before the child developed PCP.

PCP in infants with HIV infection should be treated with high dose co-trimoxazole (trimethoprim–sulfamethoxazole). An increased rate of reactions to co-trimoxazole has been reported with HIV infection in children, although interestingly this appears to be less common in black Africans.[483,513] Alternative therapies include pentamidine or atovaquone, both of which may also be used for prophylaxis against PCP (see below). As well as supportive treatment including ventilation, high dose steroids are recommended for PCP and in a few reports have been shown to improve outcome in children as well as adults with PCP.[483] However, concerns have been expressed about the use of steroids in infants dually infected with PCP and CMV.[483,512] In infants, CMV is a primary infection and corticosteroids could adversely affect the course of CMV disease. Infants with PCP should be investigated for CMV viremia and retinitis. Anti-CMV therapy should be strongly considered in infants with PCP who receive adjuvant corticosteroids until CMV co-infection has been excluded.

Babies presenting with multisite CMV disease may have retinitis, which should be actively sought. An association between CMV infection and HIV disease severity and progression has been hypothesized in children.[514]

Bacterial infections

Recurrent bacterial infections occur frequently in children with HIV infection, and include pneumonia, septicemia, meningitis, cellulitis, osteomyelitis, septic arthritis and skin and lymph node abscesses. The common causative organisms are similar to those seen in children with hypogammaglobulinemia and include pneumococci, non-typhi salmonellae, staphylococci, streptococci and *Haemophilus influenzae*, reflecting the B cell defect that accompanies destruction of the CD4 cells.

As noted above, despite the presence of hypergammaglobulinemia due to dysregulated polyclonal B cell activation, specific antibody responses are frequently absent either following infections or following immunizations, particularly in children with low CD4 counts. Studies of antibody levels following immunization with *H. influenzae* type b vaccine showed reduced levels in children with HIV infection compared with uninfected children, particularly in children with more progressive disease; in addition, antibody levels were not sustained.[515] Abnormal antibody function and avidity probably also play a role in the increased susceptibility to bacterial infections.

Lymphoid interstitial pneumonitis

Lymphoid interstitial pneumonitis (LIP) is characterized by multiple foci of proliferating lymphocytes in the lung interstitium and occurs in about 20–30% of vertically infected children, but is rare in adults or in children infected with HIV later in childhood. The cause of LIP is not clear. It may be an abnormal response to primary Epstein–Barr virus (EBV) infection or to HIV infection. Parotitis, prominent lymphadenopathy and very high immunoglobulin levels are frequently associated. It usually develops during the second year of life (and therefore should not be confused with PCP which is more commonly seen in infants under 6 months of age) and the child may have no clinical signs but persistent bilateral reticulonodular shadowing on chest X-ray. Alternatively in older children, clinical features may include chronic hypoxia and recurrent respiratory bacterial and viral infections with or without features of bronchospasm.[516]

The differential diagnosis includes other causes of interstitial pneumonitis including infection with *Mycobacterium tuberculosis*, which can be difficult to distinguish radiologically from LIP. Clinically, a child with bilateral infiltrates due to TB would be highly symptomatic, as opposed to LIP which may be clinically silent. A presumptive diagnosis of LIP is often made on clinical and radiological grounds, because definitive diagnosis requires lung biopsy. The symptoms and signs of LIP respond to antiretroviral therapy, although steroids were used in severe cases before the advent of HAART. Chest infections should be treated promptly and, where present, bronchospasm responds to bronchodilators. Without therapy clinical and radiological features may progress over time with increasing immunodeficiency. Older children diagnosed late may already have chronic lung disease such as bronchiectasis and present with a picture similar to cystic fibrosis (CF). Even with HAART, these children will continue to require treatment, similar to those with CF, for recurrent chest infections, including antibiotic prophylaxis, regular physiotherapy and nutritional support.

HIV encephalopathy

Encephalopathy due to effects of HIV infection on the central nervous system is seen most frequently in the subgroup of infants with rapid disease progression. The most common neurological manifestations are hypertonic diplegia, developmental delay (particularly affecting motor skills and expressive language) or acquired microcephaly. Cranial imaging studies may show basal ganglia calcification and cerebral atrophy and MRI scans may show evidence of white matter damage. Seizures are not usually a feature of HIV encephalopathy, which does not tend to affect the gray matter. In older children, presentation is more similar to that observed in HIV dementia in adults and may include behavioral change and memory loss.

HAART has reduced the incidence and prevalence of HIV encephalopathy and may arrest the progression of HIV encephalopathy in affected infants.[517] However, despite effective immune reconstitution on HAART, a proportion will have persistent motor and neurocognitive impairment requiring timely referral to child development services.[518,519]

Failure to thrive

Failure to thrive is a hallmark of HIV infection and is multifactorial in origin. In children, there is growth failure in addition to wasting. Failure to gain weight in adults has been related most closely to decreased intake and the same is probably true for children.

Malignancy

HIV infection greatly increases the risk of non-Hodgkin lymphoma (NHL) and Kaposi sarcoma (KS) in children and adults and is associated with more modest increases for other non-AIDS-defining malignancies.[520] The incidence of lymphoma has been estimated to be about 1000-fold higher in HIV infected children compared with the normal population.[521] In HIV infected adults, HAART has been shown to substantially reduce the risk of NHL and KS but not other non-AIDS-defining cancers.[522] Recently a similar response to HAART has been reported in pediatric cohorts.[523] Success of treatment for lymphoma often depends on the state of immunosuppression; response to standard chemotherapy may be good and has improved in the era of HAART. Decisions such as whether to stop HAART therapy during chemotherapy need to be made on an individual basis taking account of the stage of HIV disease, ability of the patient to tolerate both ART and chemotherapy, as well as consideration of possible drug interactions. Patients with refractory or relapsed disease with good immunology may now be considered for autologous bone marrow transplantation.[524]

Kaposi sarcoma (KS) is associated with human herpes virus 8 (HHV8) and is uncommon in children except for those from endemic areas for the disease in Africa. As in adults, cutaneous KS may regress with HAART alone but systemic disease may require additional treatment with liposomal daunorubicin. Cases have been reported of KS in both mother and child, suggesting MTCT of HHV8 may be responsible.[525]

CLINICAL ASPECTS IN RESOURCE LIMITED SETTINGS

The clinical aspects of HIV are similar in resource limited settings but several aspects differ. First, disease progression is much faster; about half of all infected children die in the first 2–3 years of life.[506,526] Second, background malnutrition and infections (including tuberculosis and bacterial infections) are common and may make it more difficult to distinguish HIV infected from uninfected children clinically. The revised four-stage WHO classification has been shown to have predictive value.[501,513]

MANAGEMENT

Testing for HIV

Recognizing HIV infection requires considering the diagnosis in children presenting with a wide range of pediatric conditions. All health professionals need to be able to hold a sensitive pre-test discussion with caregivers explaining the benefit of early diagnosis and the implications of a positive result for the family, including the fact that it will almost always indicate that the mother is HIV infected. To do this, there needs to

be communication and collaboration with adult colleagues, and where HIV infection is rare in children, involvement of adult counselors and health advisors as and when appropriate (see below), in line with the English Sexual Health and HIV Strategy published in July 2001.[527]

If a child is being adopted or entering long term foster care, consideration should be given to testing for HIV, hepatitis B and C; ideally maternal consent should be sought, to enable the mother to seek appropriate help for herself if any blood-borne viruses are detected, but if this is not possible, then the wishes of the adopting parents and welfare of the child should be of prime consideration.

Antiretroviral therapy

A detailed description of the many aspects of ART is beyond the scope of this chapter. This is a rapidly moving field with new drugs continually becoming available, and specialist input is required to manage children on ART. Guidelines for ART have been produced for adults[528,529] and children[530,531] and are regularly updated.

There are 20 drugs belonging to four different classes now available for treatment of HIV infection in adults; 15 have approval for pediatric use (Table 28.34). Two new drug classes, the integrase inhibitors and the CCR5 inhibitors, are currently entering phase 2/3 clinical trials in adults. In children, there is some lag in availability of drugs, particularly in the youngest children because of difficulties with development of appropriate formulations and undertaking of sufficient pharmacokinetic studies to assure correct dosing. The issue of formulations for older children who can take and prefer solid formulations but for whom only adult dosages exist means that in general simplification of HAART is more difficult for children. Fixed dose combination therapies for children with appropriate ratios and doses of drugs for children of different ages are urgently needed in resource limited settings where liquid formulations are particularly impractical because of logistics and cost.[532] However, with respect to licensing antiretroviral drugs for children, increasingly research is being undertaken in parallel in children, to ensure that pharmacokinetic and tolerability data are available in a timely manner. In addition to pharmaceutical company studies, there are two networks coordinating independent clinical trials in HIV infected children – the PACTG (now being replaced by IMPAACT) in the USA and the Paediatric European Network for Treatment of AIDS (PENTA, http://www.ctu.mrc.ac.uk/penta/trials.htm) in Europe. Both networks undertake trials addressing questions about management of ART in children (e.g. what to start with, when to switch, the value of

Table 28.34 Antiretroviral therapies

NRTIs	Protease inhibitors
– Zidovudine (ZDV)*	– Ritonavir *[†]
– Didanosine (ddI)*	– Nelfinavir *[†]
– (Dideoxycytidine*)	– Amprenavir ♦[†]
– Lamivudine (3TC)*	– Lopinavir ♦[†]
– Stavudine (d4T)*	– Indinavir ♦[†]
– Abacavir (ABC)*	– Saquinavir ♦
– Emcitarabine (FTC)♦	– Atazanavir
	– Fosamprenavir
	– Tipranavir
	– TMC114†
Nucleotide TRIs	**Entry inhibitors**
– Tenofovir ♦[†]	– T-20 ♦[†] (by injection)
NNRTIs	
– Nevirapine (NVP)*	
– Delavirdine ♦[†]	
– Efavirenz (EFV) [†]	
– TMC125 [†]	

*Pediatric formulation.
†Inadequate pharmacokinetic studies in infants.
♦Unlicensed in Europe.

resistance testing, whether HAART can be interrupted, etc.) as well as trials of specific drugs and drug combinations.

Combination ART has turned HIV into a treatable chronic disease of childhood. Until the mid-1990s, only one drug was available – zidovudine [ZDV, azidothymidine (AZT)]. Dual therapy was introduced in 1996/1997, followed by triple (HAART) therapy in 1997/1998 which has led to marked and sustained reductions in disease progression and mortality in HIV infected children in Europe, North America and Africa.[426,432,533,534] Eradication of HIV is not possible with current drugs, and even after virus has been suppressed below the level of detectability in plasma (< 5 copies/mm³ using highly sensitive HIV-1 RNA PCR) for several years in newly infected adults, HIV-1 RNA viral load rises promptly within 1–2 weeks after stopping therapy. Most children on HAART remain clinically very well, thriving normally, and are asymptomatic. However, the complexity of lifetime administration of ART should not be underestimated. With increasing numbers of drugs available, yet limited options for sequencing drugs within classes because of development of cross-resistance, it is important that expert consideration is given to when to start treatment, how best to sequence HAART regimens, and how the whole family (other family members will often be on HAART as well) receives cohesive medical (generally outpatient) management, which is facilitated by attendance at a 'family-based' clinic (see below).

Monitoring HAART

As discussed above, CD4 cell count or percentage and HIV-1 RNA viral load in plasma are useful predictors of disease progression, although much less so in infants than in older children and adults. In addition, they are used as surrogate markers for evaluating response to HAART, both as endpoints in clinical trials and for individual management of patients in clinical practice. In well resourced settings the usual aim of HAART is to suppress the plasma HIV-1 viral load rapidly below the lower limit of detection, typically < 50 copies/ml, and maintain it there for as long as possible with restoration of immune function. Within one month of commencing HAART in children, the plasma HIV-1 RNA viral load decreases substantially (Fig. 28.33)[535] and the CD4 lymphocyte count starts to increase. There are differences between adults and children of differing ages in both RNA and CD4 cell response to therapy.[536] Infants with very high HIV-1 RNA viral load may take a longer time to reach an undetectable viral load,[537] possibly because children are starting from a higher viral load than adults. This higher baseline viral load seen in children may be one of the reasons that children have been reported to achieve an undetectable HIV RNA viral load less commonly. However, it is also the case that attaining this goal has improved over time.[432]

Children's immune systems may also respond differently to HAART, due mainly to the fact that children have a much more active thymus than adults. Whereas in adults expansion of the CD45RO (memory cells) predominates, in children expansion is mainly of the CD45RA+ naive T cells which appear to be derived newly from the thymus.[538] Thus immune restoration in children may be more achievable than in adults, and studies are ongoing to evaluate further the quality of immune responses in children treated with HAART.

Most guidelines suggest that after starting HAART, children should have HIV-1 RNA viral load measured after one month and then both CD4 and viral load should be measured at 3 months to ensure that viral load is decreasing further and the CD4 cell count is starting to rise. Further measurements should be undertaken 3-monthly. Some centers perform tests more frequently, although the benefits of more intense monitoring have not been evaluated in clinical trials. Weight gain and growth are also important[539]; growth has been shown to be a sensitive marker of response to ART in HIV infected children, with significant differences reported in trials comparing different regimens, and reflecting HIV RNA response.[535] In resource limited countries with the advent of generic ART and cheaper drugs, and where the value of monitoring is being questioned because of cost, growth monitoring in children starting HAART may be a useful marker of response.

The goal of ART may vary according to the setting. Ideally, it is to achieve full virological suppression of HIV-1, restoration of both numbers and function of the immune system, and restoration of full growth and development for HIV infected children. This has to be balanced against the potential short and long term toxicity of ART and the effect of taking long term therapy on quality of life for the child and family. Frequently, and particularly in children, immunological and clinical responses to ART are good, but adherence issues and attention to maintaining adequate doses as a child grows[540] are vital to increase the proportion of children attaining undetectable viral load towards the near 100% figure observed in some adult cohorts. Where viral load is not fully suppressed, there is an increased likelihood of selection of resistant viral populations limiting future treatment options. A small number of heavily pretreated children and adolescents with multidrug resistant HIV (MDR HIV) have triple class HIV-1 associated resistance mutations and are awaiting drugs in development for future treatment options.[541]

When to start HAART

The PENTA 1 trial is the only trial addressing the issue of when to start ART in children, and, as in adults, showed no benefit from early therapy with ZDV monotherapy beyond about 6 months, due to the emergence of resistance.[542] There are no trials in children addressing the question of when to start triple combination therapy. When HAART initially became available, guidelines based on a 'hit hard, hit early' approach recommended starting early in the disease course. Subsequently, the development of cumulative adverse effects of long term HAART, as well as evidence of reasonable restoration of the immune system even when CD4 cell counts are low in adults and children, has resulted in adult guidelines being amended to start ART later in the disease course.[528,529] Guidelines for adults in the USA previously recommended starting therapy at a CD4 count < 500 cells/mm³ but subsequently became more conservative and in line with UK guidelines recommend starting all patients at CD4 cell count < 200 cells/mm³ and considering HAART for those between 200 and 350 cells/mm³.[528,529] In the last year, the pendulum has again started to swing towards earlier treatment, after the large SMART trial was stopped when it showed small but significant reduced incidence of disease progression in adults on ART even with high CD4 cell counts.[543] The question of conducting a large long term 'when to start HAART' trial which might also include older children is again being discussed.

In children, US guidelines have recommended starting HAART during infancy in all infected infants. In Europe, opinions are more divided but increasingly HAART is started either based on CD4% of < 35% or presence of any symptoms. Any infected infant not started on ART requires very close monitoring.[544] Highly encouraging results have been reported with three or more drug combinations in selected, infected infants, which demonstrate that complete viral suppression and maintenance of normal immune development can be achieved and sustained for at least 3 years.[545] However, there are concerns about the lack of HIV specific immune responses seen,[545] and the problems of resistance and toxicity in those whose regimens fail.[546] Nonetheless, these successes in infants treated early with HAART, as well as studies of adults treated during primary infection, have provided a rationale for early aggressive therapy of infants supported by recent studies suggesting an improved immune response to ART commenced in infancy.[546,547]

In infancy, viral load and CD4 cell counts are less predictive of outcome, and the anxiety this engenders tends to push towards starting HAART early as it can be difficult to distinguish the infant who will progress rapidly from the infant who remains asymptomatic for several years. However, the problem of inadequately defined pharmacokinetics for many drugs in infancy (and in particular, the PI class of drugs, such as nelfinavir in infants[548]) and the likely adverse consequences of early prolonged therapy, particularly the long term adverse metabolic effects of lipid abnormalities (PI class of drugs) and mitochondrial effects (nucleoside analogue class) are deterrents to such an approach. Despite these uncertainties many pediatricians continue to start all infants diagnosed under 6 months of age on HAART.

A number of factors need to be taken into account when starting ART in children (Table 28.35). Education of families, taking account of drugs other family members may be taking, as well as due care in choosing a regimen which the family can adhere to are important considerations. Considerable support is required to enable families to sustain high levels of adherence long term. Frequency of dosing has been a major development and once daily regimens are now feasible for children with well established once daily pharmacokinetics for drugs such as lamivudine and abacavir that were previously given twice daily.[550-552]

There is some evidence that adherence may be poorer among asymptomatic children who have never been ill. This disadvantage needs to be weighed against avoiding children becoming seriously ill before starting ART. Educating parents and carers about following CD4 and viral load as predictors of progression at monitoring visits is important to ensure that a consensus between health professionals and the family is achieved about the right time to start therapy. Viral load and CD4% can fluctuate, and at least two or three values should be obtained. Time spent on preparing and educating the family before commencing ART is always important. For children under 12 years the 'PENTA Calculator' (http://www.ctu.mrc.ac.uk/penta/) can be a useful tool in decision making and help parents and carers to further understand the risk of disease progression.

Older children presenting for the first time are a selected group who do not have rapid disease progression. For these children it is reasonable to monitor CD4 counts and only offer treatment if counts are declining steadily below 20% or counts are between 200 and 350 as in adults (Table 28.35).[5C1] There is no consensus level of viral load above which treatment should be started in children.

Which ART to start

When starting HAART, most prescribers would initiate triple therapy with two NRTI drugs and one PI or one NNRTI. Intensive induction with quadruple combination therapy, sparing at least one class of drugs, reducing to a maintenance regimen of three drugs when the plasma viral load is well maintained at undetectable levels is another possible option and has been used in infants with extremely high levels of plasma viremia in some centers. The PI drugs are difficult to formulate into palatable suspensions for children compared with the NRTIs and NNRTIs. No large randomized clinical trials in children or adults provide evidence to conclude that PI-containing or PI-sparing regimens have greater long term clinical efficacy. This question and when to switch therapy is being addressed in a randomized controlled trial of children in Europe and the US starting therapy randomized to either PI- or NNRTI-based HAART (PENPACT 1 trial; www.pentatrials.org).

Data from the UK and Ireland CHIPS cohort show that most children start HAART with a triple regimen and over time there has been a shift from a PI- to an NNRTI-based regimen.[426] NVP is the main NNRTI in young children, but efavirenz is increasingly being used in children over 3 years. The main PI was nelfinavir, but increasingly this is being replaced by ritonavir boosted lopinavir (Kaletra). NRTI fixed drug combination tablets are increasing being made available in adult doses to reduce pill burden and ease adherence, thereby potentially improving response to therapy. Combivir (ZDV+3TC), Trizivir (ZDV+3TC+ABC), Kivexa (3TC+ABC) and Truvada (TDF+FTC) are available, the latter two formulations administered once daily. However, no combination liquid formulations are available. Use of crushed whole or half tablets requires care as some pills (e.g. Combivir) have these drugs unevenly distributed through the tablet. Fixed drug combinations containing an NNRTI with

Table 28.35   WHO recommendations for initiating ART in HIV-infected infants and children according to clinical stage and availability of immunological markers[549]

WHO pediatric stage	Availability of CD4 cell measurements	Age-specific treatment recommendation	
		≤11 months	≥12 months
4	CD4	Treat all	
	No CD4		
3	CD4	Treat all	Treat all, CD4-guided in those children with TB, LIP, OHL, thrombocytopenia
	No CD4		Treat all[c]
2	CD4		CD4-guided
	No CD4		TLC-guided
1	CD4		CD4-guided
	No CD4		Do not treat

WHO age-specific recommendations for starting ART on immunological markers

Immunological marker	Age-specific recommendation to initiate ART			
	< 11 months	12–35 months	36–59 months	>5 years
%CD4	<25%	<20%	<15%	<15%
CD4 count	<1500 cells/mm³	<750 cells/mm³	<350 cells/mm³	<200 cells/mm³

WHO TLC criteria for severe HIV immunodeficiency requiring initiation of ART; suggested for use in infants and children with clinical stage 2 and where CD4 measurement is not available

Immunological marker	Age-specific recommendation to initiate ART			
	< 11 months	12–35 months	36–59 months	>5 years
TLC	<4000cells/mm³	<3000cells/mm³	<2500cells/mm³	<2000cells/mm³

What HAART to start?
Either: 2 NRTI + 1 PI (PI: NFV or lopinavir/r)
plus NRTI combinations: ZDV + ddl; ZDV + 3TC; ddl + d4T, d4T + 3TC; 3TC + ABC
Or: EFV + 2 NRTI (if over 3 years)
NVP + 2 NRTI (all ages)
Or: 3 NRTI: ZDV + 3TC + abacavir

two NRTIs are already available as generic formulations in resource limited countries, and a combined once daily pill of efavirenz, emtricitabine and tenofovir is available for adults and can be used for older adolescents in well resourced settings.

There is considerable inter- and intra-patient variation in drug levels achieved even when using standard ART doses for size. The role of therapeutic drug monitoring (TDM) has not been clearly defined in pediatrics but is frequently used in many centers. A randomized controlled trial assessing the impact of differing levels of TDM compared to no TDM (PENTA 14) was recently halted due to low levels of recruitment. TDM is definitely indicated where there is the possibility of drug interactions and can provide additional information regarding individual pharmacokinetics, absorption and adherence.

Adherence

It has become very clear from adult and pediatric studies that adherence is one of the principal determinants of both the degree and duration of virological suppression.[553] In one study, children whose caregivers reported no missed doses in the previous week were more likely to have an undetectable viral load (50% versus 24%).[554] The reasons for non-adherence are complex and multifactorial. Adherence is difficult to assess in the clinic. No pediatric intervention studies aimed at improving adherence have been conducted. Outpatient attendance and adherence are poorer in adolescents and young adults, increasing their risk of virological failure and the evolution of resistance.[555]

Changing therapy

Virological failure requires investigation into the potency of the regimen, including checking that the child is on the correct dose (which may be higher than the recommended dose in drug packet inserts)[548,550] and that the child has not outgrown their dose, checking for possible pharmacokinetic interactions with other drugs or food, and checking on adherence. These should all be done before switching therapy. A recent study demonstrated that children were frequently underdosed with antiretrovirals, a continuing issue for growing infants and children whose dosing is calculated on weight or surface area.[540] The level of viremia in children that should prompt a switch in therapy is the subject of an ongoing trial discussed above. Adult guidelines recommend switch consideration for sustained viral rebound, defined as two plasma viral loads at least one month apart > 400 copies/mm³, for patients whose viral loads have previously been undetectable.[528,529] Occasionally, despite virological failure, families and doctors may wish to continue the current regimen when the child is clinically and immunologically stable, and there is not an obvious easy palatable regimen to switch to. However this may lead to accumulation of resistance mutations and therefore fewer options for subsequent therapy. The choice of the new regimen will depend on the prior ART history, drug toxicity, availability of new drugs/formulations and adherence, and may be guided by resistance testing.

Resistance

Resistance testing is recommended for treatment of naive adults prior to initiation of HAART as transmitted resistance is well recognized and has also been reported in infants following mother-to-child transmission.[556] As the availability of ART increases worldwide, baseline resistance testing may be considered for children if there is any uncertainty regarding ART exposure either for the child directly or the mother prior to or during pregnancy or breast-feeding.[530] Resistance testing is increasingly routinely performed in children on HAART with virological failure, although virological or immunological benefit was not demonstrated in a recently published pediatric trial with long term follow-up[557] and results from short term adult studies are conflicting. Further validation of resistance testing is difficult as, like TDM, it has increasingly become part of standard care.

Toxicity

Children on HAART are now surviving into adult life, but as the length of exposure to HAART grows, the long term side-effects are becoming increasingly apparent. Lipodystrophy (LD) is defined as abnormality in lipid metabolism resulting in dyslipidemia (high lipids) and body changes characterized by truncal obesity alongside disfiguring loss of fat on the face and in the periphery. A European cross-sectional study reported fat redistribution in a quarter of children. Increased risk was associated with more advanced disease, female gender, use of protease inhibitors and of stavudine, which are similar risk factors to adults.[558,559] However, studies are hampered by the lack of a standard definition of LD in the growing child, and many reports are clearly subjective although efforts are being made to standardize assessments.[560] Hyperlipidemia is being increasingly reported but there is uncertainty as to the level of hyperlipidemia that should precipitate a treatment switch or addition of lipid lowering drugs. Insulin resistance resulting in hyperglycemia and occasionally exogenous insulin dependence is seen in adults and occasionally in pediatric cohorts and has been associated with length of time on PI-based HAART.[561] Adult cohorts have reported an increase in cardiovascular events when compared to the general population. HIV itself has a pro-inflammatory effect on the endothelium but coupled with the metabolic complications described above. concern is growing about the cardiovascular risk in adult life for children with perinatally acquired HIV infection.[562]

A high prevalence of bone demineralization has been reported in children in association with HIV infection and HAART, raising concerns of risk of progression to osteopenia and osteoporosis in early adult life. The optimum management strategy is currently unclear and requires further consideration.[563,564] Mitochondrial toxicity, at least in part due to the inhibition of DNA polymerase by nucleoside analogues, has rarely been associated with severe, even fatal, lactic acidosis in children on HAART.[565] Asymptomatic hyperlactatemia occurs more frequently but may be temporary and current evidence does not support routine lactate measurements for children on HAART.[566] Unexplained nausea, vomiting, fatigue and/or neurological deterioration in a child on HAART should prompt assessment of lactic acid status and consideration of mitochondrial toxicity.

As toxicity associated with long term continuous ART becomes more apparent, strategies to reduce ART exposure, including structured treatment interruptions (STI) and immune therapies, are being evaluated in children and adults. Recent trials of STIs in adults have been halted early due to an excess of clinical adverse events in patients off treatment, although overall absolute risk of events in the SMART trial was small.[543] Interim analysis of a pilot European pediatric trial (PENTA 11) was satisfactory. The argument prevailed that STI in children has a compelling rationale and may be safer because of a more active immune system; the trial is continuing, with a parallel trial also continuing in Botswana. The cost/benefit for children may be different to adults as they potentially face a lifetime of ART with its cumulative toxicities.

Prophylaxis against opportunistic infections
Co-trimoxazole prophylaxis for prevention of PCP

There is good evidence from randomized trials in adults with HIV that co-trimoxazole is very effective at preventing PCP and this is the drug of choice. Dapsone or inhaled pentamidine can be used in the event of hypersensitivity to co-trimoxazole but they are less efficacious. The evidence for efficacy of co-trimoxazole in preventing PCP in infants with HIV is indirect, and comes from studies showing decreased PCP after the introduction of guidelines recommending starting all babies on co-trimoxazole.[567,568]

The MTCT rates are now so low in Europe and the USA that, coupled with the ability to exclude HIV infection by 3 months of age, the need for PCP prophylaxis has decreased and can be restricted to babies born to mothers who do not take interventions in pregnancy to reduce MTCT, or have a high risk of MTCT (e.g. because of detectable HIV RNA viral load at delivery) or babies where the mother is reluctant for the baby to be tested early in life.[449] Prophylaxis can be stopped once it has been established that the baby is uninfected. Infected infants should continue prophylaxis throughout the first year of life, as CD4 counts are unreliable indicators of PCP risk. Thereafter, it is not unreasonable to stop prophylaxis unless the CD4 count is under 15%.

Guidelines for PCP prophylaxis in adults permit discontinuation of both primary and secondary PCP prophylaxis when the CD4 cell count is above 200 cells/µL for greater than 3 months in response to HAART. Although evidence is more limited in pediatric populations, most practitioners consider discontinuation of primary and secondary prophylaxis when the CD4 count has increased above 200 cells/µL or 15% on HAART,[568] and the majority of children on HAART in the UK are not on PCP prophylaxis. A prospective study in children over 2 years in the US supported the safe withdrawal of OI and PCP prophylaxis following immune reconstitution in response to HAART.[569] In all children, whether or not they are on HAART, guidelines recommend restarting co-trimoxazole when the CD4% falls below 15% or 200 cells/µL.

Prophylaxis against other infections
Co-trimoxazole has also been shown, in a large placebo controlled trial of Zambian HIV infected children aged 1–14 years (mean age 4.5 years), to reduce mortality by 43%.[513] The efficacy was maintained over a period of 18 months and occurred despite high background prevalence of *S. pneumoniae* and non-typhi *Salmonella* species with resistance to co-trimoxazole. The trial also showed a reduction in hospital admissions and use of antibiotics in the arm treated with active drug. Although most causes of death and hospital admissions were presumptive diagnoses, it appeared that reduction in bacterial lung infections was the most likely mode of action and PCP was not observed in nasopharyngeal aspirates.[534] Updated WHO guidelines recommend that all HIV infected children in resource limited settings continue to receive co-trimoxazole prophylaxis while awaiting HAART.[501] The question about continued benefit of co-trimoxazole prophylaxis in the presence of HAART requires further evaluation.

In well resourced countries, as a result of advances in antiretroviral therapy, there has been a shift in focus from diagnosing and managing opportunistic infections to restoring and maintaining cellular immunity with HAART and thereby preventing opportunistic infections.

HIV infected children who are contacts of individuals with open pulmonary TB should be carefully assessed, bearing in mind skin testing is frequently unhelpful because of anergy. If there is no evidence of infection, prophylactic isoniazid for 6 months, or isoniazid plus rifampicin for 3 months is recommended. Prophylaxis against *Mycobacterium avium-intracellulare* in children is not recommended because of adverse reactions and the potential for resistance and breakthrough on single agents such as rifabutin.

Primary prophylaxis against CMV is not recommended. With respect to secondary prophylaxis following CMV infection, infants who have had CMV usually reconstitute their immune systems very well, obviating the need for secondary prophylaxis.

For most other established opportunistic infections, such as cryptosporidiosis for which there were few useful therapeutic options, the best treatment is HAART, which should be started as soon as possible if a child presents initially with HIV infection and an acute opportunistic infection. Immune reconstitution disease, which may occur particularly in severely immunocompromised children, may make opportunistic infection symptoms worse initially. Some individuals with immune reconstitution disease may require steroids in addition to HAART and specific therapy for opportunistic infections.

Immunizations
Children with HIV infection should be immunized according to normal schedules with both live and killed vaccines. The exception is that BCG is not advised for children with HIV infection in low prevalence areas because of the risk of dissemination. However, it should be given in areas of high TB prevalence and this, in the author's view, should include babies born to African women in the UK who have a high rate of TB and may also return to Africa either to live or to visit. In line with current UK vaccination schedules, inactivated polio vaccine (IPV) is to be preferred to live oral polio vaccine because of theoretical concerns about paralytic poliomyelitis in contacts of children excreting live virus. Pneumococcal polysaccharide vaccine has been recommended for HIV infected children over 2 years of age, but a trial of its use in adults with HIV in Africa showed no benefit. Conjugate pneumococcal vaccine should be given to children under 2, in line with national UK guidelines. Annual influenza vaccination is also recommended. All children with HIV should be screened for hepatitis A, B and C co-infection; hepatitis A and B vaccination should be offered to those who are susceptible to infection.

The efficacy of all vaccines is improved among children who have immune reconstitution following ART. Children immunized before starting ART in whom responses are inadequate should be revaccinated.

Passive immunization of symptomatic children with CD4% < 15% is recommended if they are in contact with varicella zoster virus (VZV) and are either VZV naive or have no detectable specific antibodies to VZV. Varicella zoster immunoglobulin (VZIG) ideally should be given within 72 h of contact. VZIG may prolong the incubation period to 28 days, so clinicians need to consider isolating these patients at clinic visits. Similarly, normal human immunoglobulin should be given for susceptible symptomatic children in contact with measles. The role of oral aciclovir in preventing VZV infection following contact has not yet been ascertained but it is used by some pediatricians.

Regular intravenous immunoglobulin infusions (400 mg/kg every 28 days) should only be given to children with recurrent bacterial infections despite good compliance with HAART and co-trimoxazole prophylaxis, or those with proven hypogammaglobulinemia. Higher doses may be useful in the management of thrombocytopenia (0.5–1.0 g/dose every day, for 3–5 days). However, in the era of HAART, the number of children requiring such therapy should be minimal.

Supportive care
Unlike most other severe chronic diseases of children, HIV simultaneously affects family members including the parents and other siblings. The parents' own health, their social isolation and feelings of guilt compound the difficulties of caring for a sick child. An effective well coordinated multidisciplinary team is required to address the changing needs of infected children and their caregivers. Continuity of care needs to be developed between inpatient and outpatient services, local referring hospitals and the community. Ideally adults and children should be treated in family based units.[570] All too often parents will ignore their own health needs because they put their children first.

The work of the multidisciplinary team has increasingly shifted towards ways of helping families achieve long term adherence to HAART. As children survive longer, meeting the needs of adolescents and planning transition to adult clinics is placing new demands on services. The decision as to who should be informed should be tailored individually. Families may need help in explaining the diagnosis to older children. This needs to be undertaken at the child's pace, and is frequently most effectively achieved in gradual steps. It is not mandatory to tell staff at schools, as universal precautions should be employed for all children with injuries. The risk of transmission from casual contacts in school or daycare settings is virtually zero. Ensuring that adolescents are well informed and responsible before they become sexually active is a priority and pediatric family clinics in London are setting up specific adolescent clinics with their adult colleagues. Peer support for adolescents is important to help young people with HIV come to terms and live with their disease.

The multidisciplinary team should include a dietician, as nutritional problems and growth faltering are not uncommon even in the era of HAART and particularly in children with chronic lung disease. Balanced supplements are sometimes required and enteral feeding through gastrostomy tubes may be necessary. Gastrostomy tubes have been used with success to allow unpalatable medicines to be given, particularly in children on multiple therapies such as in TB co-infection, those with neurological impairment, or in children who have failed first/second line therapy due to poor adherence. In addition, dietary and exercise advice is increasingly needed to prevent and treat obesity in HIV infected children on HAART.

Pain management is important in late stage disease. Complementary therapies frequently used in adults with late disease, such as aromatherapy, may be useful and require evaluation. With the continuing success of HAART, there are currently very few children in industrialized countries needing palliative or terminal care. However a small number of children and adolescents in Europe and more in the USA have multidrug resistant virus and urgently require novel therapies.

Prevention remains the top priority in managing HIV infection in children. Reducing national perinatal transmission rates to below 2% is an achievable target that can only be realized if HIV infected mothers can be identified prenatally and offered appropriate interventions. Antenatal detection rates in most European countries and the USA have reached high levels for several years and continued effort by health professionals, public health planners and community organizations is essential.

EXANTHEMATA

MEASLES (MORBILLI AND RUBEOLA)

Measles is a viral disease of high infectivity, which presents with an acute catarrhal illness, fever, and characteristic Koplik spots on the buccal mucous membranes followed by a distinctive maculopapular rash. There is a high incidence of serious complications of the respiratory and nervous systems. In large cities and towns, measles is most likely to occur in infants and preschool children, but in rural and less crowded urban areas the principal incidence is between the ages of 5 and 10 years. Measles is extremely rare under 3–4 months of age, because of protective maternal antibody, but authenticated cases have occurred.

In some countries measles outbreaks have shown a characteristic biennial periodicity but such a pattern is by no means universal and the introduction of active immunization has altered the natural epidemiology of the disease.

Mortality

In resource limited countries, where malnutrition is common, measles may have a mortality as high as 25% and produce serious complications.[571] Children are at increased risk of dying for a year after their measles due to impaired cellular immunity. Inhibition of macrophage production of interleukin-12, a cytokine important for driving cell mediated immunity, by binding of measles virus to CD46, a cellular protein that regulates complement, is thought to be partly responsible for this immunosuppression.[572] Measles can cause devastating outbreaks when the virus is introduced into naive populations such as on remote islands. Although the morbidity and mortality are lower in highly immunized, industrialized countries, outbreaks can still occur if a population of unimmunized children, usually preschool, is allowed to develop. In more exposed communities, measles is now comparatively mild and its morbidity and mortality lower, although occasional deaths still occur in the UK. Children who contract measles when in remission from acute leukemia or who have other conditions in which immunity is compromised are at particular risk.

Etiology

Measles virus is an RNA virus of the paramyxovirus family, genus *Morbillivirus*, and morphologically resembles the parainfluenza viruses. It is usually transmitted by droplet infection from the respiratory tract of a case before, or close to, the onset of the rash. Entry mainly occurs through the respiratory tract, but infection through the intact conjunctiva has been postulated. Clinically significant antigenic variation has not been described. An attack is usually followed by life-long immunity and there is little or no authenticated evidence of second attacks of measles except in individuals with severe immunological defects. Subclinical infection can probably occur but is rare.

Clinical features

Measles has an incubation period of 8–14 days. A mild illness may occur at the time of infection but most cases develop a prodromal illness some 3–5 days before the eruptive stage. The main features of this illness are pronounced catarrh, characterized by a constantly running nose, conjunctivitis and a harsh dry cough. Fever and irritability are usually present and there may be a fleeting scarlatiniform or morbilliform rash. Koplik spots, the most pathognomonic sign of measles, appear during this stage and are seen as small, grayish white lesions on the buccal mucosa close to the posterior molar teeth; they are usually quite numerous but may be scanty or occasionally cover the entire lining of the cheek. They can be difficult to demonstrate and the angle of the inspecting light is critical; having faded, they are replaced by a dry, matte appearance on the mucosa, which has a ground-glass-like surface.

The true rash of measles (Fig. 28.34)[573] starts behind the ears and along the hairline. Fever, which will have lessened at the end of the prodromal period, may now rise again to 39–40 °C (Fig. 28.35),[573] and the eruption spreads rapidly to involve the face. The lesions are maculopapular in character and of a dusky hue. Over the next two days the eruption spreads downwards and becomes generalized; marked confluence of the spots develops and this gives a blotchy appearance.

The extent and severity of the rash shows wide variation. In some, especially the younger cases, the eruption may be unusually sparse and modification by maternal antibody has been suggested. There is frequently some degree of hemorrhage or diapedesis into the rash giving it a purpuric quality and subsequent skin staining. This should not be confused with the rare, and usually fatal, hemorrhagic measles in which extensive bleeding occurs into the skin and from the mucous membranes. In the immunocompromised child, the rash occasionally does not develop.

Fading of the rash can be surprisingly rapid but it usually disappears quite slowly, beginning to fade on the third day in the order of

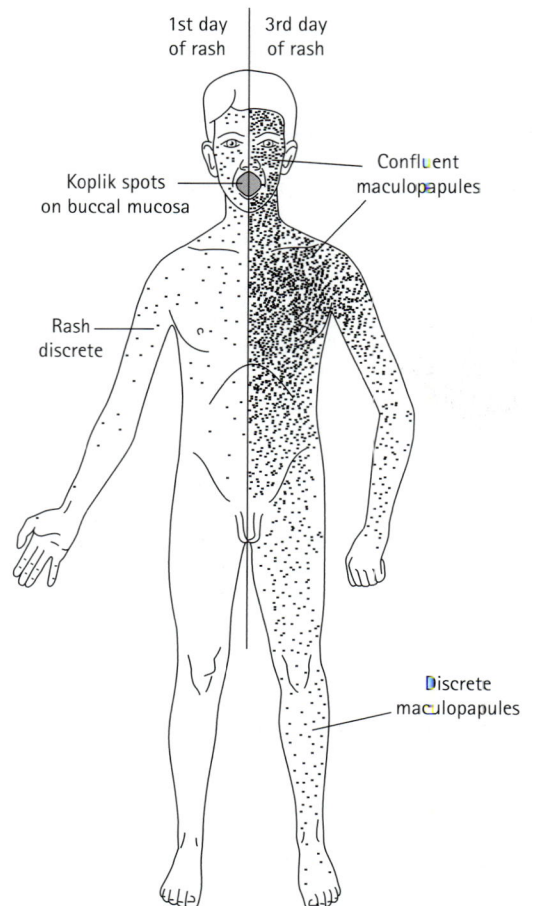

Fig. 28.34 The distribution and the development of rash in measles. **(From Krugman & Ward 1968[573])**

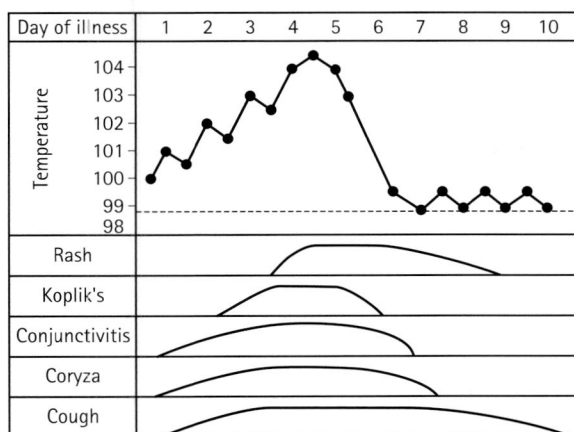

Fig. 28.35   The development of measles. (From Krugman & Ward 1968[573])

appearance; the rash may be largely gone from the face and upper trunk by the fourth day though persisting on the lower extremities. After a further 3–4 days a brownish staining appears, probably due to capillary hemorrhage and, on occasions, this staining can be very intense. In severe cases, a fine desquamation may occur at the site of the rash, but this does not usually involve the hands and feet like scarlet fever.

Complications

Respiratory

Measles virus always attacks the respiratory tract causing some degree of laryngotracheobronchitis. An element of bronchitis is universal and can be severe, extending even to bronchiolitis; the latter can be complicated by acute mediastinal emphysema. Croup may be prominent. Viral damage may denude the respiratory tract of its protective lining and allow the aspiration of bacteria. Bronchopneumonia may result and the severity will depend on the nature of the aspirated material. Staphylococcal pneumonia can be life threatening.

In a few instances measles virus involvement of the respiratory tract may spread to the lung parenchyma, giving rise to the condition known as giant cell pneumonia. This complication may be prolonged and is often fatal, and the illness may be accompanied by little or no rash. It is usually found in association with underlying disease such as HIV infection, leukemia, or other immune deficiency with impaired T cell function. In view of its atypical nature, this illness is often undiagnosed during life and the true diagnosis is made as a result of autopsy findings.

Ophthalmic

Some degree of conjunctivitis and keratitis occurs in every case of measles. It is typically exudative, nonpurulent and nonfollicular and can be characterized by Koplik spots. When pseudomembranes or corneal ulcers occur they are the result of secondary bacterial infection. Optic neuritis and retinitis are associated with measles encephalitis.

Ear

Involvement of the middle ear used to be commonplace and could result in suppurative otitis media, chronic perforation or mastoiditis. The lessening severity of measles and prompt antibiotic treatment has reduced the incidence of these complications to a low level.

Gastrointestinal tract

Severe oral inflammation due to secondary infection by bacteria, *Treponema vincentii*, or thrush can occur but cancrum oris is only likely to be seen where malnutrition is rife. Cancrum oris (noma) is a gangrenous form of stomatitis that commences with a dusky red spot on the inside and outside of the cheek. This rapidly spreads to form a sloughing gangrene of the gums and jaws and in extreme cases teeth

may be shed. The breath develops a peculiarly foul odor and death can supervene.

Gastroenteritis is common in measles in non-industrialized countries and can be prolonged; it probably results from direct viral involvement of the gut with or without superinfection with organisms such as *Cryptosporidium*. Appendicitis can occur in measles though abdominal pain is more commonly due to associated mesenteric adenitis.

Enlargement of the spleen is more frequently encountered in measles than is generally realized.

CNS

Measles, with its pronounced constitutional upset and high fever, is often complicated by febrile convulsions. These are most commonly encountered at the start of the eruptive stage and either settle spontaneously or in response to simple sedation; they should not be assumed to be indicative of encephalitis.

True postinfectious encephalomyelitis occurs in from 1 in 1000 to 1 in 5000 cases of measles and has a mortality of about 10% and leaves about 15% with neurological residua. It normally presents after 7–14 days, when the rash is subsiding, but can commence earlier in the disease and rarely even before the rash. Drowsiness, fits, a recrudescence of fever, focal neurological signs and progressive coma suggest that severe cerebral involvement is occurring. In some cases the process may arrest at this juncture and be followed by rapid improvement; in others there is a steady deterioration and death. Between these extremes there are patients in whom recovery is slow and permanent cerebral damage likely.

Rarely subacute sclerosing panencephalitis (SSPE) may complicate measles infection, though not apparently measles immunization. In SSPE, measles virus becomes latent in the cerebrum following primary infection and is then reactivated, usually 5–10 years later, by some unknown stimulus. An alternate hypothesis suggests that a partially immune individual is reinfected by measles which then provokes this unique form of encephalitis. It is more common in children in whom primary measles occurs before 1 year of age.

Others

Uncomplicated measles tends to produce leukopenia, and significant thrombocytopenia is occasionally encountered. Epistaxis is a common and occasionally troublesome feature.

There is a traditional but unconfirmed belief that measles may activate or predispose to tuberculosis. Diagnostic difficulty is provided by the fact that measles may suppress the Mantoux reaction for several weeks.

Diagnosis

Provided the medical attendant is consulted at its inception, measles can be diagnosed on clinical grounds with a fair degree of accuracy. Immunofluorescence can be used to detect measles virus antigen in respiratory secretions if rapid diagnosis is needed. Difficulties can arise when an opinion is required later in the disease.

Neutralizing, complement-fixing and hemagglutination-inhibiting antibodies to measles develop during the illness and appropriate serological tests can confirm their presence. Detection of measles IgM on a single specimen is the simplest method for diagnosis. Measles IgM can be detected from 3 days after the onset of the rash for about a month. Sensitivity rates, however, vary according to the type of assay used and the time after the onset of the rash, with the hemagglutination-inhibiting antibodies assay being the most sensitive and complement fixation the least (87% and 37% of cases, respectively, 3 days after the onset of the eruptive phase).[574] The demonstration of a significant rise (four-fold or greater) in antibody titer to measles virus confirms the clinical diagnosis. The hemagglutination-inhibition and complement fixation tests are usually employed, on account of the ease and rapidity with which they can be performed.

Measles virus can be isolated in primary tissue cultures of human kidney, human amnion or monkey kidney, and several other tissue culture systems have been used. The growth rate of measles virus in tissue culture is relatively slow and serological tests will often yield a positive result before the virus has been isolated and identified. During the late prodromal stage of the illness virus can be recovered from the nasopharynx, urine, conjunctival secretions and blood. By the second day of the rash, virus isolation becomes more difficult, though the urine may continue to contain virus for a further 2 days. In the immunocompromised child, there may be prolonged shedding of measles from the sites after the initial infection.[575]

In SSPE, measles antibody in high titer is demonstrable in the serum many years after a typical attack of measles. Antibody may also be detected in the CSF and the ratio of this antibody to that in the serum may be of diagnostic significance. Brain biopsy can confirm the diagnosis of SSPE where facilities for electron microscopy and immunofluorescence are available.

Differential diagnosis

Kawasaki disease can cause a morbilliform rash with fever, conjunctivitis and lymphadenopathy and can be quite difficult to distinguish clinically from measles. The milder illness of rubella with its pinker rash and selective involvement of the suboccipital glands is usually distinguishable. The rash of infectious mononucleosis can cause confusion but its other clinical and laboratory features usually lead to the correct interpretation. Enteroviral infections associated with a rash are usually more transient and lack the catarrhal involvement. Influenza virus infections, both A and B, can occasionally cause a morbilliform rash with respiratory symptoms and fever. In roseola infantum, the rash is very like measles, but as it appears the fever falls and the child is well, in contrast to measles. Scarlet fever and drug eruptions have readily distinguishing features.

Treatment

There are currently no antiviral agents available with demonstrated efficacy in vivo against measles virus. Ribavirin has been shown to inhibit measles virus replication in vitro, and there are anecdotal reports of its use either intravenously or by aerosol to treat severe pneumonitis or encephalitis in the immunocompromised child.[576] However, this treatment remains experimental in the absence of data from a randomized controlled trial.

Amongst the earliest complications that may require treatment are croup and febrile convulsions. These are managed symptomatically (see Chs 20 and 22).

Secondary bacterial infection, superimposed on viral damage to the respiratory tract, will require treatment. Staphylococcal pneumonia is the most feared complication, and if bacterial pneumonia is suspected antistaphylococcal antibiotics should be used. Prophylactic antibiotics are unnecessary, as confirmed by a recent systematic review on the subject.[577]

Mastoiditis should not occur if adequate treatment of otitis media is given early, but if it does occur surgical drainage is required. Any sign of secondary infection of the conjunctiva should be treated with appropriate antibiotics, and chloramphenicol eye ointment smeared on to the lids often proves efficacious.

It is rare for gastroenteritis to be so severe as to cause fluid and electrolyte depletion but where this occurs appropriate measures require to be taken. True appendicitis can present in the course of measles.

Postinfectious encephalitis requires intensive supportive treatment, including anticonvulsants for seizures. The use of corticosteroids remains controversial, but many clinicians feel such therapy warrants trial in severe cases whose progress is unsatisfactory.

Preventive measures
Quarantine

Because this disease is highly infectious and the maximum infectivity is before the rash appears, quarantine measures are frequently ineffective. However, any child who is suffering from a severe, debilitating disease should be protected from exposure whenever possible. In the hospital setting, appropriate quarantine measures should be in place for up to

4 days after the onset of the rash while the child is infectious via the respiratory route. The immunocompromised child with measles should be placed on respiratory isolation for the duration of the illness.

Passive immunization

Passive immunization has been used as post-exposure prophylaxis against measles for many years, although the evidence for it is sparse. Normal human immunoglobulin (gamma globulin) is used (0.2 ml/kg intramuscularly for normal children, 0.5 ml/kg for immunocompromised children, maximum dose 15 ml). The use of passive immunization is particularly important when immunocompromised children, for whom active immunization is contraindicated, are exposed to measles.

Active immunization

In the early years of measles vaccines, an inactivated measles vaccine was used which not only failed to protect against infection but resulted in the children developing severe, atypical illness with giant cell pneumonitis when exposed to wild-type virus.

Live, attenuated measles vaccines are highly protective and have very few side-effects. Where they have been used to immunize whole populations, acute measles, encephalitis and subacute sclerosing panencephalitis have virtually disappeared. In countries where immunization rates are relatively low, there are many cases of acute encephalitis, with several children each year dying or handicapped as a result.[578] Measles vaccine is readily inhibited by maternal antibody and may be ineffective if given before 1 year of age. If it is wished to protect a child exposed to measles who has no contraindications to immunization and is over 1 year old, then measles vaccine is preferable to passive immunization. Many countries now give measles vaccine in conjunction with mumps and rubella vaccines (MMR) in the second year of life, and a second dose may be given at school entry or at 12–14 years old. The only contraindication to measles vaccine is immune deficiency (including high dose but not low dose steroids). Anaphylactic egg allergy is no longer considered to be a contraindication.[579] HIV infection is not a contraindication unless the patient is severely immunocompromised; on the contrary, as they are at high risk from wild-type measles virus, every attempt should be made to immunize HIV positive children against measles. Measles continues to be a significant public health concern despite an effective vaccine. Recent outbreaks in countries such as the USA[580] and UK[581] where endemic infection was considered to be virtually eliminated have highlighted the need for sustained high vaccination coverage in areas where wild-type virus no longer circulates. There is also concern that infants, who are at greater risk of severe disease, are becoming susceptible to measles earlier in their first year due to declining levels of maternal antibody.[580]

RUBELLA (GERMAN MEASLES)

Postnatal rubella is characterized by its mild nature and relative freedom from complications. Some of the original accounts of the disease emanated from Germany and because of this and a certain similarity to measles, the name of German measles became a popular, if ill-conceived, descriptive title.

Etiology

Rubella virus is an RNA virus of the Togaviridae family. It was first cultured and identified as recently as 1962. Since then it has proved possible to grow it quite readily on suitable tissue cultures, a factor that has considerably enhanced our knowledge of the disease. Transmission is primarily through droplet spread of infected nasopharyngeal secretions from a few days before to up to 14 days after the onset of the rash.

Incidence

The true incidence of rubella is difficult to assess as infection is subclinical in a sizable proportion of cases. Even the clinical illness itself has no pathognomonic features, a point that is substantiated in surveys where rubella antibody levels correlate poorly with the history of previously suspected infection. By early adult life as many as 90% of city dwellers may show serological evidence of previous rubella but the figure can be much lower in rural communities. Rubella is less common in preschool children than, for example, measles and in one survey less than 10% of children under 2 years showed evidence of previous infection, though this figure had risen to 25% between the ages of 2 and 5 years. By 12 years of age, 80% had antibody, suggesting the bulk of infection occurs between 6 and 12 years of age.

Clinical features

Rubella has an incubation period of 14–21 days, with an average of 17 days. In children it is rare to have a significant prodromal illness and the first indication of rubella infection is the appearance of a rash over the face (Fig. 28.36).[573] This soon spreads to cover the trunk and later the limbs. The basic lesions are fine, pink macules which, originally discrete, can soon coalesce over the face and trunk. The rash usually disappears within 2–3 days but may persist for as long as 5 days. Occasionally it has a duration measured in hours and in this instance can be readily missed. A biphasic type of rash, with complete regression in between, has been described and a small area of the eruption may persist on the medial aspect of the thighs after the main rash has subsided. Small purpuric spots sometimes appear on the soft palate but have no diagnostic significance, as other infections are associated with a similar enanthem.

Lymph node enlargement is an important feature of the disease. It may appear as much as a week before the rash, though usually just before, and may persist for some time after the eruption has faded. The cervical, postauricular and suboccipital glands are most commonly involved, can be tender and are sometimes unassociated with any rash.

In adolescents and adults, especially female, prodromal symptoms are more likely and include malaise, headache, stickiness of the eyes,

conjunctivitis and fever. In children the temperature rarely rises above 37.1–37.4 °C but in adults it can attain 39.5–40.0 °C (Fig. 28.37).[573]

The clinical stigmata of congenital rubella are described in Chapter 12.

Complications

In general, complications are unusual though a higher incidence is encountered in certain epidemics and some seem age or gender dependent.

Polyarthritis may be a sequel of rubella. It usually commences when the rash has subsided, is more common after florid eruptions and occurs in adults, especially women, rather than in children. The small joints of the hands and the wrist joints are most often involved but the large joints can also be attacked. The condition usually resolves within 2 weeks.

Postinfectious encephalitis, myelitis and polyradiculitis may follow an attack of rubella and have a similar pathology to these syndromes when they occur after other infections. However, in rubella they appear to have a better prognosis.

Thrombocytopenia is quite common in the course of the illness and may become clinically manifest as purpura. Epistaxis, hematuria and melena can also develop. Some cases of so-called 'idiopathic thrombocytopenic purpura' can be shown by laboratory tests to have resulted from subclinical rubella infection. Leukopenia is frequently found at the height of the illness and there may be an increase in plasma or Turk cells.

Diagnosis

Owing to the lack of pathognomonic features, one cannot rely on a clinical diagnosis of rubella and, whenever confirmation is important, laboratory tests (in the form of appropriate serological studies) should be used.

A serological diagnosis depends on the demonstration of a significant rise in antibody titer (four-fold or greater) when a sample of serum collected at the onset of the illness and a further sample taken 2–3 weeks later are compared.

Antibodies to rubella virus may be detected by hemagglutination-inhibition, neutralization, complement-fixation or radial hemolysis test. Nowadays, the hemagglutination test is generally preferred, owing to its reliability and the ease with which it can be performed.

Following infection both neutralizing and hemagglutination-inhibition antibodies persist, at a variable titer, for a long time whereas complement-fixation antibodies disappear more rapidly.

Virus may be recovered with relative ease from the nasopharynx during the last week of the incubation period and for up to 2 weeks thereafter. It is less readily isolated from the urine and blood. However, many laboratories do not offer viral culture for rubella.

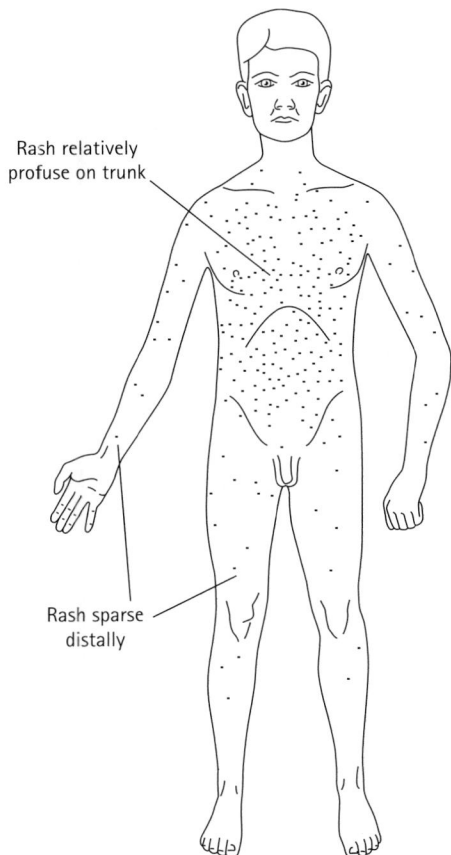

Fig. 28.36 The distribution and development of rash in rubella. (From Krugman & Ward 1968[573])

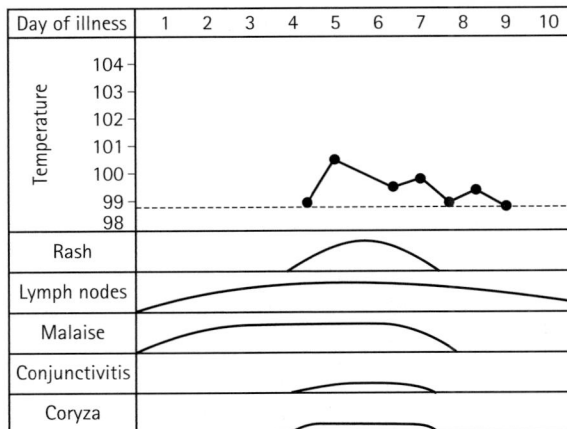

Fig. 28.37 The development of rubella. (From Krugman & Ward 1968[573])

Differential diagnosis

Rubella may be confused with many common exanthemata and other skin eruptions. Differentiation from measles, glandular fever and drug eruptions does not present great difficulty but scarlet fever can cause confusion. Enteroviral infections accompanied by a rash, especially those associated with ECHO virus infection, provide the greatest diagnostic challenge. The presence of the herald patch, the distribution over the trunk and the complete well-being of the patient help to distinguish pityriasis rosea.

Resort to laboratory tests is always desirable when doubt exists in regard to a suspicious rash in a pregnant woman or her contacts.

Treatment

There is no specific treatment for rubella. A rapid recovery is to be expected. Prodromal symptoms rarely cause trouble but analgesics may be needed when polyarthritis occurs. Neurological complications are managed along the usual lines for such conditions.

Prevention

As a general rule, preventive measures are unnecessary in view of the mild nature of the disease. However, the situation is quite different in the case of women in early pregnancy, and attempts to prevent rubella were traditionally made using intramuscular normal human immunoglobulin. Evaluation of this procedure proved difficult, but laboratory-confirmed cases of rubella occurred despite immunoglobulin. Attenuated live rubella vaccines are now widely used and in general stimulate reasonable antibody levels. Opinions differ as to how they are best employed. Some recommend they are given to girls around puberty and non-immune pregnant women postpartum (selective immunization) while others believe children of both sexes should be given the vaccine in early childhood, usually in conjunction with measles and mumps vaccine as MMR, in an attempt to reduce the pool of infection in the community (universal immunization). Although terminations of pregnancy are frequently performed on pregnant women who have been inadvertently immunized there have been no cases of congenital rubella syndrome caused by the vaccine.

ERYTHEMA INFECTIOSUM (FIFTH DISEASE, SLAPPED CHEEK DISEASE)

This disease may occur at any time of year, but outbreaks in primary school children are classically in the winter and spring. Joint involvement may occur. Children with shortened red cell survival can develop profound anemia (aplastic crises), including children with endemic malaria,[582] and sickle cell disease.[583] Infection during pregnancy can lead to hydrops fetalis.

Etiology

Erythema infectiosum is caused by parvovirus B19 (human parvovirus), a small, single-stranded DNA virus. Spread is by droplet infection, although as the virus can be seen in plasma during infections, it could be transmitted by blood products. Erythrocyte precursors are particularly susceptible to the virus, causing a mild fall in hemoglobin (of about 1 g/dl) in normal individuals but profound anemia in those whose red cell survival is already shortened.

Clinical features

B19 infection may be asymptomatic or may cause a mild febrile illness with rash. In children the first sign of infection is usually marked erythema of the cheeks or slapped cheek appearance often with relative circumoral pallor (Fig. 28.38). In volunteer studies, however, there is an initial febrile episode with headache, chills, myalgia and malaise associated with viremia and the rash appears about 7 days later (Fig. 28.39). Then 1–4 days after the slapped cheeks an itchy, erythematous, maculopapular rash develops on the trunk and limbs. As the rash on the limbs clears it leaves a lacy, reticular pattern. The rash may fluctuate over the next 1–3 weeks and a hot bath, for example, may lead to recrudescence of an evanescent rash.

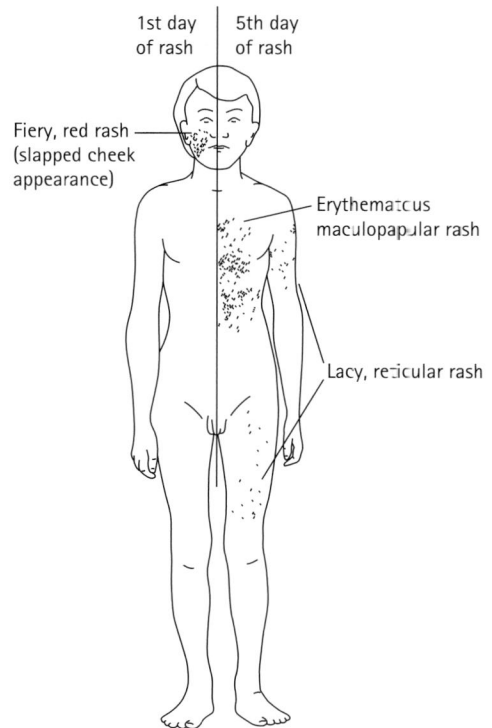

Fig. 28.38 The distribution and development of rash in erythema infectiosum (fifth disease).

Complications

Arthritis or arthralgia is more common in adults, but certainly can occur in children. It usually appears 1–6 days after the rash but there may be no history of rash at all. Arthritis is characteristically transient and asymmetrical, affecting wrists, knees, ankles, elbows and fingers, though it may persist for weeks or even months.

Children with a shortened red cell survival, such as those with sickle cell anemia, thalassemia major, hereditary spherocytosis or other hemolytic anemias, may have severe aplastic crises with hemoglobin levels falling as low as 1–2 g/dl and no reticulocytes.

Children with malignancy, particularly acute leukemia, or with HIV infection may develop prolonged anemia from chronic parvovirus B19 infection.

Infection during pregnancy can result in hydrops fetalis due to fetal anemia, which may be fatal, but no congenital syndrome has been described in babies of infected mothers who delivered at term.[584]

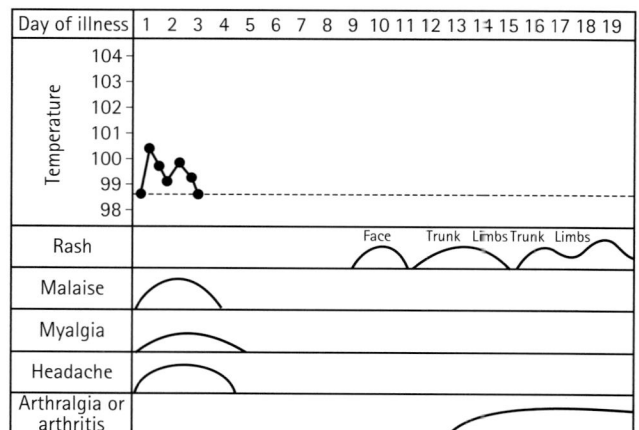

Fig. 28.39 The development of erythema infectiosum (fifth disease).

Encephalitis with or without neurological sequelae has rarely been reported after clinical erythema infectiosum, but it is not certain that this is a true complication of B19 infection.

Diagnosis

Erythema infectiosum may closely mimic rubella, and the two diseases can circulate concurrently. The slapped cheek appearance with circum-oral pallor can be mistaken for scarlet fever.

The diagnosis can be made serologically by demonstrating parvovirus B19-specific IgM on an acute serum sample, although it is always better to get a paired sample in case there is a late rise in antibody. The virus can be detected by electron microscopy or PCR of plasma of patients with aplastic crises. This is particularly important in patients with sickle cell disease in whom severe anemia might be due to sequestration or pneumococcal sepsis. DNA probes and PCR have been used to detect the viral genome in stillbirths with hydrops fetalis and to demonstrate persisting antigen in children with leukemia and chronic anemia.

Treatment

There is no specific treatment. Isolation of patients is unnecessary since they are no longer infectious when the rash appears.

Arthritis may require salicylates or nonsteroidal anti-inflammatory agents. Children with aplastic crises may require blood transfusion until the red cell aplasia resolves spontaneously after 1–2 weeks.

ROSEOLA INFANTUM (SIXTH DISEASE, EXANTHEM SUBITUM, THREE DAY FEVER)

Roseola infantum is a common disease of infancy, characterized by fever and the appearance of an erythematous maculopapular rash as the fever defervesces. It may be confused with measles clinically. It is generally benign.

Etiology

Human herpesvirus 6 (HHV-6) is the main causative agent of roseola.[585,586] HHV-7 is responsible for most clinical cases of roseola infantum which are HHV-6 negative.[587] These double-stranded DNA viruses are members of the herpesvirus family, and as such, persist for the life of the host with frequent asymptomatic reactivation. There are two variant strains of HHV-6: type A and type B. Most of the primary infections in childhood are due to type B infection, and nearly 80% of children acquire HHV-6 by 2 years of age.[588] Primary HHV-6 infection is usually symptomatic and often results in presentation for medical evaluation.[588]

Clinical features

The illness starts abruptly with fever and some anorexia and irritability although in general the child appears relatively well. Mild cough, coryza, diarrhea and vomiting rarely occur. The pyrexia of 38.9–40.6 °C persists for 3–5 days, then falls precipitously as the rash appears (Fig. 28.40).[573] The rash is erythematous, with discrete macular or maculopapular

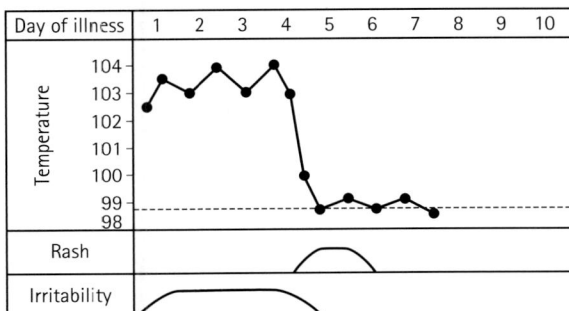

Fig. 28.40 The development of exanthem subitum. (From Krugman & Ward 1968[573])

lesions, and starts on the trunk and neck, sometimes spreading to the face and limbs. It lasts 1–2 days. Cervical lymphadenopathy is common and may sometimes be prominent: the suboccipital, posterior cervical and posterior auricular nodes are most commonly involved. There is no characteristic enanthem, although there may be pharyngitis, small exudative follicular tonsillar lesions, or small ulcers on the soft palate, tonsils and uvula.

For the first day or two of fever the white count is often elevated with a neutrophil leukocytosis, but then may fall as low as 3000/uL (3×10^9/L) predominantly lymphocytes with an absolute neutropenia.

A number of clinical syndromes (bone marrow suppression, pneumonia, hepatitis, encephalitis) have been associated with reactivation of HHV-6 in the immunocompromised, although a causal link has been difficult to prove.[586]

Complications

Convulsions may occur in association with roseola.[589] These are usually febrile convulsions but encephalitis has rarely been described, sometimes with severe residua such as hemiparesis or mental retardation. Rarely thrombocytopenic purpura may occur following roseola.[586]

Diagnosis

The diagnosis of roseola infantum is primarily clinical, although it can now be confirmed serologically. PCR assays to detect HHV-6 DNA are available, but cannot distinguish an acute infection from reactivation. The characteristic fever chart and discrete rash that does not become confluent distinguish roseola from other childhood exanthemata including measles. The rash may be confused with a drug rash if antibiotics have been given and a vaccine reaction may cause confusion if the illness comes on soon after immunization.

Treatment

There is no specific treatment. There are anecdotal reports of treatment of HHV-6 infection in immunocompromised children with ganciclovir, but there is no evidence to support efficacy from clinical trials. Antipyretics may lessen the risk of convulsions, but if these occur, encephalitis should be considered and the child treated appropriately.

HERPESVIRUSES

CHICKENPOX (VARICELLA)

Chickenpox is a common and highly infectious disease caused by varicella zoster virus (VZV). In general, chickenpox is relatively benign and has a virtually worldwide distribution. However, chickenpox is not endemic in some isolated areas and if introduced to such a community a more serious disease may occur. It can also prove severe and even fatal in neonates, when contracted by a patient on immunosuppressive drugs and rarely in previously healthy children and adults.[590]

Immunity following chickenpox is usually life-long and second primary attacks are rare. Like all herpesviruses, however, the virus can remain latent and recur years later, in the case of VZV, in the form of zoster (shingles).

Etiology

Chickenpox is transmitted from person to person by direct contact, droplet or airborne spread; infection can also arise through articles recently contaminated by an infected person. Viral entry is through the upper respiratory tract mucosa or via the conjunctiva. Infectivity is maximal during the prodromal period 1–2 days before the eruption of the rash and has completely waned by the time the eruption becomes crusted. In the immunocompromised, infectivity may continue after crusting has occurred if new lesions continue to develop.

The causative agent, VZV, is a large DNA herpesvirus. The virus is highly specific for humans and is very difficult to grow in culture in the laboratory.

Clinical features

Chickenpox is predominantly a disease of childhood and usually occurs between 2 and 8 years of age. Cases may occur in infancy. Peripartum intrauterine infection can lead to varicella neonatorum (see below) which, untreated, has a mortality up to 20%. Postnatal infection can cause classical chickenpox of a lesser severity occurring only in babies whose mothers have not had chickenpox.

Following an incubation period of 10–28 days, usually around 16 days, the disease starts with mild malaise and fever (Fig. 28.41).[573] In children prodromal symptoms may be absent and the illness begins with a rash. Older children and adults have more definite prodromata and symptoms include malaise, fever, headache, sore throat and backache.

The rash (Fig. 28.42)[573] commences as a crop of macules, which within hours pass through a papular stage to become vesicular; the vesicles persist for 3–4 days, becoming pustular and finally forming a crust. The spots are superficial and the vesicles may be round, oval, elliptical or irregular in shape; they are often surrounded by a red areola. The rash is usually mild in children vaccinated against varicella with the Oka vaccine and may be atypical (maculopapular with few or no vesicles).[591]

Evolution of the rash occurs by a series of crops, and lesions at different stages may be seen. The trunk is principally involved but spots also appear over the face, scalp and the proximal parts of the limbs. Lesions tend to be more abundant on covered rather than exposed parts of the body.

In mild cases the entire eruption may consist of a few spots; less often, the rash is almost generalized, extending to the distal parts of the limbs including the soles and palms. By the time of vesiculation there is often an intense pruritus. In some patients crusts can be very tenacious and 2–3 weeks may elapse before their separation is complete.

An enanthem is usually found and presents as vesiculation over the palate, tongue or buccal mucous membranes; the conjunctivae and vagina may be similarly affected.

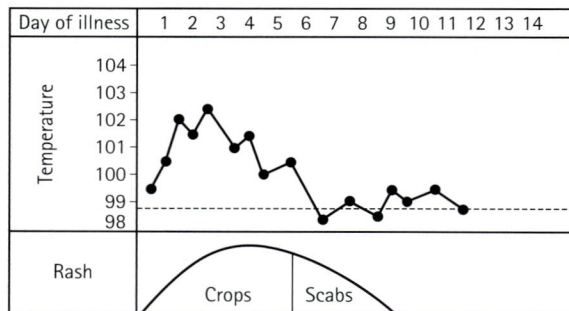

Fig. 28.41   The development of chickenpox. (From Krugman & Ward 1968[573])

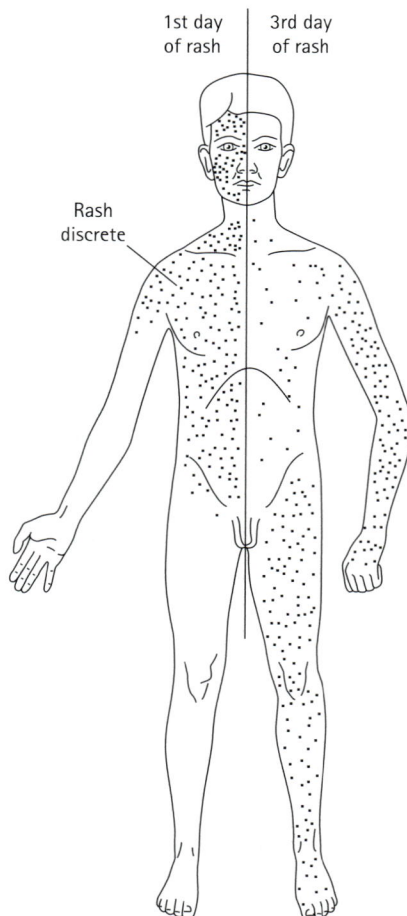

Fig. 28.42   The distribution of rash in chickenpox. (From Krugman & Ward 1968[573])

Hemorrhagic chickenpox

In this there is usually a marked constitutional disturbance and high fever. Extensive bleeding into the vesicles develops and the lesions become black; areas of ecchymosis can appear on otherwise uninvolved skin. Bleeding may occur from mucous membranes and present as hematuria or melena. Both children and adults may contract this form of chickenpox and it has been particularly reported in patients receiving corticosteroids or cytotoxic drugs suggesting the importance of cell mediated immunity as well as antibody in recovery from infection. It can be associated with profound thrombocytopenia (purpura fulminans) and is often fatal.

Varicella gangrenosa

This form of the disease usually results from severe secondary bacterial infection (usually due to group A streptococci) of the vesicles which may extend down to muscle. These lesions are slow to heal and can leave considerable scarring. Occasionally this form of varicella appears to start ab initio before any apparent secondary infection.

Varicella neonatorum

If the maternal rash appears less than 7 days before delivery or up to 2 days after delivery there is a risk that the baby will receive a large inoculum of virus without maternal antibody. Such babies are at very high risk of disseminated disease with death from pneumonitis, and should be protected at birth by giving zoster immune globulin (ZIG) (reviewed in Heuchan & Isaacs 2001[592]). Since this does not always protect them,[593] families of these infants should be informed of the risk of severe disease and early treatment with acycloguanosine (aciclovir) commenced promptly if symptoms develop. Babies whose mother's rash develops 7 days or more before or 3 days or more after delivery are at low risk. Postnatally acquired chickenpox is nearly always mild although if the mother has not had chickenpox the use of ZIG should be considered for a neonate exposed to the virus.

Varicella bullosa

Bullous varicella may occur in children, the lesions developing into large bullae with a positive Nikolsky sign. It is due to superinfection with a toxin-producing Staphylococcus aureus, and the prognosis for full recovery without scarring is excellent. Treatment is with antistaphylococcal antibiotics.

Complications
Sepsis

Secondary skin infection is the commonest complication. Abscesses may form locally or in regional lymph nodes. Cellulitis, erysipelas and scarlet fever can also develop. Bacteremic spread may give rise to pneumonia, osteomyelitis and septic arthritis. Common infecting organisms include group A streptococci and S. aureus.

Neurological

Postinfectious encephalitis can occur and usually starts as the rash reaches maturity. The most common manifestation is a pure cerebellar ataxia with an excellent prognosis. Complete recovery is virtually invariable, usually rapidly, though it may rarely take some weeks. Acute disseminated encephalomyelitis (ADEM) is a more sinister but rarer form of post varicella encephalitis with cerebral demyelination giving rise to long tract signs, cranial nerve lesions, convulsions, etc. Examination of the CSF may show a mild lymphocytic pleocytosis and slight elevation of the protein content. About 10% of cases of Reye syndrome occur secondary to chickenpox. Transverse myelitis, acute infantile hemiplegia and Guillain–Barré syndrome have been described complicating varicella.

Pneumonitis

Pneumonitis is usually seen in adults and immunocompromised children (and varicella neonatorum) and may present with acute respiratory distress or hemoptysis; diffuse nodular infiltration is seen on X-ray of the chest. The diagnosis is often obscure until the typical exanthem develops. Some cases die and, in those who recover, miliary calcification may be seen in the lung fields some years later.

In normal children, pneumonia complicating chickenpox is most likely to be bacterial, due to *S. pneumoniae*, group A streptococcus or occasionally *S. aureus*.

Others

Myocarditis, pericarditis, endocarditis, hepatitis and glomerulonephritis have rarely been reported. Appendicitis may also occur and can present before the eruptive phase; this sometimes leads to cross infection in pediatric surgical wards. Keratitis and conjunctivitis are rare and usually benign. Arthritis may mimic septic arthritis but the latter should always be excluded by examination of the joint fluid because septic arthritis can complicate chickenpox. If ampicillin is prescribed a drug eruption may occur as with EBV infection, probably as a result of drug–hapten interaction.

Congenital varicella

If the mother contracts chickenpox up to 20 weeks' gestation, there is about a 2% risk of the baby developing congenital varicella syndrome with cicatricial scarring of the limbs, cortical atrophy, hypoplasia of limbs, digital defects, retinitis or cataracts. Maternal chickenpox in the second 20 weeks of gestation may result in an inapparent primary infection in the fetus, and causes shingles in the first years of life in about 1% of exposed children.

Diagnosis

The clinical course of varicella and the nature of the rash are usually typical and a firm clinical diagnosis can be made. Rapid diagnosis can be by direct immunofluorescence (DFA) of cells scraped from the base of a vesicle and placed directly on a slide. DFA can also be performed on respiratory secretions obtained by nasopharyngeal aspirate or bronchoalveolar lavage for the diagnosis of infection in the immunocompromised.

VZV can be isolated from vesicle fluid collected during the first 3 or 4 days of the rash, but rarely from other sites. Tissue culture for varicella is not widely available. Detection of VZV DNA in body fluids or tissues by PCR is a sensitive technique that may be helpful in the diagnosis of VZV infection in the immunocompromised child.

A number of serological assays are available for diagnosis of past VZV infection that vary in their sensitivity. These have application in deciding if an exposed individual needs passive immunoprophylaxis. They can also be used to make a retrospective diagnosis of VZV infection if a significant rise in varicella IgG has occurred during the illness. In this setting, it is necessary to test two sera – an acute sample collected within a day or two of the onset of the illness and a convalescent sample collected 2 or 3 weeks later.

Differential diagnosis

Chickenpox can be confused with impetigo, scabies, dermatitis herpetiformis, eczema herpeticum or vaccinatum and erythema multiforme. In most of these the absence of the typical, centripetal distribution and cropping of varicella helps in the differentiation.

Treatment
General

No treatment is usually required and bed rest is probably unnecessary except in ill patients. Simple analgesics will control prodromal symptoms where these are troublesome. Aspirin should not be given because of the risk of Reye syndrome. Calamine lotion will normally soothe pruritus; if not, an antihistamine should be tried. If the enanthem is unusually severe careful oral toilet is needed and lesions on the conjunctiva should be protected from secondary infection. Treatment with aciclovir is indicated if infection develops in immunosuppressed cases, and in any patient with severe disease.

Sepsis

In convalescence, simple antiseptics should control superficial skin infection. More severe sepsis will require appropriate antibacterial chemotherapy, which should be guided by swabbing of the affected lesions and by cultures of the blood and of any pus. Flucloxacillin will adequately treat hemolytic streptococcal infection or staphylococcal infection until culture results are available.

Encephalitis

No specific treatment is available for the neurological complications and the usual supportive measures will be employed. Some clinicians favor the use of corticosteroids in severe cases despite the unhappy association of chickenpox with these drugs. It is argued that the encephalitis is of allergic origin and that by this stage of the illness there is sufficient antibody response to prevent further dissemination of the virus. In practice no serious untoward effects have been reported where steroids have been used in this condition although it is difficult to assess how much this therapy contributes to any recovery. Similarly the role of aciclovir in treating varicella encephalitis is unclear.

Others

Cases of severe varicella pneumonitis and profound thrombocytopenia have also been treated with aciclovir and corticosteroid drugs but an accurate evaluation of their benefit is impossible. Appendicitis should be treated surgically.

Prevention

The live attenuated Oka strain varicella vaccine is available in some countries for use in healthy children over 12 months of age or adults who have not had varicella. It has been shown to be highly effective (approximately 85% of children) in preventing clinical disease post exposure.[594] However, clinical disease in vaccinated persons is contagious and can sustain transmission, prompting the question of whether a two-dose regimen is required to prevent transmission during outbreaks. The Oka vaccine has been shown to be safe in solid organ transplant recipients post transplantation,[595] and in HIV infected children with CD4+ T cell counts ≥ 200 cells/μl (or 15%).[596]

The infectivity of chickenpox is such that the strictest isolation measures may fail to prevent its spread. In the community, it is usual practice to isolate a child from school or day care until the rash has become crusted. In the hospital setting, a child with active chickenpox should be quarantined in respiratory isolation while the rash remains vesicular.

Postexposure prophylaxis

In the case of patients who are receiving corticosteroid drugs or cytotoxic drugs, every effort should be made to prevent exposure to chickenpox and herpes zoster for reasons already described. If such exposure should occur then hyperimmune chickenpox gamma globulin (ZIG) has been shown to modify severity even if it does not always prevent the disease, and should be given. The use of ZIG in neonates has already been discussed. Chemoprophylaxis with aciclovir after exposure to VZV reduced the likelihood of clinical disease in a few small case control studies,[597–599] but has not been assessed in a properly evaluated randomized controlled trial and is not routinely advocated.[600] Postexposure immunization with the Oka VZV vaccine has been shown to protect against or modify chickenpox in nonrandomized cohort studies.[601] It is thought to be most effective if given within 5 days of exposure.

HERPES ZOSTER (ZOSTER: SHINGLES)

The clinical relationship between chickenpox and herpes zoster has long been recognized. The virus causing the two syndromes is identical, and is referred to as the varicella zoster virus (VZV). Non-immune persons may develop chickenpox when exposed to herpes zoster but the converse rarely occurs. The inoculation of children with virus obtained from zoster patients has resulted in clinical chickenpox which has then spread to other children as chickenpox.

Following an attack of varicella, the virus survives in a latent form in the sensory root ganglia of the cord and brain, a situation with similarities to latent infection by HSV. After an interval of many years, but sometimes earlier, the virus becomes activated by local precipitating factors or by some depression of protective immunological mechanisms. Virus then spreads along the sensory root in question; adjacent motor areas of the cord, or other parts of the cerebrum, may become involved. A degree of systemic spread can also occur which provokes a modified form of chickenpox. Such modification may result from the antigenic stimulus provided by the reactivated virus, and the very high antibody levels found early in the course of herpes zoster support this impression.

Patients who develop zoster are usually elderly, but the disease does occur in children and younger adults. In young children, pain is much less marked than in adults, and zoster is not suggestive of immune deficiency or malignancy. There is often a history of maternal varicella during pregnancy or early neonatal varicella: it is thought that varicella at a time of relatively poor immunity is more likely to result in childhood zoster. In a few instances, primary infection by VZV appears to provoke zoster rather than chickenpox; the explanation is not known. On occasion zoster may also occur simultaneously with a primary attack of chickenpox.

For reasons alluded to above, zoster is seen quite frequently in persons suffering from leukemia or other malignant disease and can follow radiotherapy.

Clinical features

Zoster may start with constitutional disturbance or progressive pain over a particular dermatome, although in children zoster may be pain free. Clusters of macules and papules appear on the skin overlying the dermatome, rarely crossing the midline. These soon vesiculate and the vesicles formed may be larger than in chickenpox and tend to coalesce. Extensive crusting follows, which slowly separates to expose a raw, ulcerated area. This will bleed readily and is susceptible to secondary infection. Healing is slow, vitiligo may develop after months or years and the involved skin is often anesthetic. Enlargement of the regional lymph nodes is very common.

Acute pain tends to subside as crusting sets in, but extreme irritation and neuralgia may persist for months and even years (post-herpetic neuralgia). In children the illness tends to be much milder, pain is mild or absent and recovery is considerably quicker.

Thoracic segments are most commonly involved in the community, but zoster of the trigeminal nerve, and usually of the ophthalmic division, is the commonest variety seen in hospital.

Geniculate herpes is of special interest and is frequently misdiagnosed; in this form of zoster, vesicles appear on the meatus and pinna of the ear. Pain may be experienced in the throat, in or behind the ear, and taste may be lost over the anterior two thirds of the tongue. Facial paralysis, sometimes permanent, may result. This condition is sometimes referred to as the *Ramsay Hunt* syndrome. A modified generalized rash over the trunk and face is seen in many cases provided examination is sufficiently diligent. Other features include involvement of the adjacent motor root with resultant paralysis, which can be permanent, and meningitis, encephalitis or myelitis can be encountered.

Occasionally zoster occurs without any accompanying rash, the so-called 'zoster sine herpete'.

Diagnosis

Prior to the appearance of the skin eruption diagnosis is difficult in children, in whom zoster is rather unexpected. Diagnoses such as pleurisy or fibrositis may be made but the difficulties are quickly resolved when the classical rash, along the line of a nerve, makes its appearance. If it is in a distribution that looks dermatomal, HSV infection may sometimes be mistaken for zoster. Laboratory tests are referred to in the section on chickenpox.

Treatment

The illness is usually mild in children and simple analgesics such as paracetamol will usually control pain. Relief may follow the application of a dusting powder of zinc oxide or the use of cold sprays.

Ophthalmic zoster requires special care because of the danger to the eyes. Topical or systemic antivirals may be needed for ophthalmic VZV. Consultation with an ophthalmologist is advisable.

In some instances, particularly severe zoster may show a dramatic response to treatment by corticosteroid drugs. However, their general use is not advised and they are best avoided in zoster affecting the eye and wherever any underlying immunological defect may be present. Aciclovir may be needed for immunocompromised children or those with severe zoster.

High doses of the live attenuated Oka vaccine (known as the 'zoster vaccine') have been shown to reduce disease incidence and severity in the elderly,[602] but the vaccine has not been evaluated for use in children or young adults.

Prognosis

This is usually good. Post-herpetic neuralgia is uncommon in children. Certain paralyses can prove permanent and impairment of vision has followed ophthalmic zoster. Such complications are more commonly found in adult cases.

HERPES SIMPLEX VIRUS

Primary infection by *Herpesvirus hominis* (HSV) usually occurs in early childhood and is generally subclinical. However, in a small percentage of children it may produce a variable clinical illness, the main features of which include localized vesiculation on some part of the body and a sharp constitutional reaction. Some children avoid infection altogether and may reach adolescence or adult life with no immunity to this virus. This is more likely to occur when they have been brought up in rural, as opposed to urban, areas and, as with many other viral infections, an attack in adult life can often be more severe.

An interesting feature of this virus is its ability to persist in a latent form once the primary infection, whether clinical or subclinical, has subsided. In some people, the virus becomes reactivated by certain non-specific stimuli at various times in their lives and the resultant clinical manifestations tend to differ from those seen with a primary infection. Reactivation of HSV with asymptomatic shedding or, less commonly, clinical disease is a common event after the initial infection.[603]

Etiology

HSV is a DNA virus surrounded by a membrane and is approximately 150–180 nm in diameter. There are two strains, HSV types 1 and 2. HSV type 2 primarily infects the genital tracts of adults, and infection in the pregnant woman near term can result in serious infection in the newborn infant. HSV type 1 is primarily oral, although type 2 can cause oral disease and type 1 can infect the genitalia.

Clinical features

A variety of different syndromes may result from primary infection by HSV beyond the neonatal period. Neonatal HSV disease is discussed in Chapter 12.

Acute herpetic gingivostomatitis (ulcerative stomatitis)

This, the commonest manifestation, commences with a sharp constitutional reaction with high fever, malaise, anorexia and irritability. The patient, usually a young child, has difficulty feeding due to pain in the mouth. Inspection, often hampered by severe discomfort, reveals marked swelling and inflammation of the gums which may bleed at the merest touch. Deeper inspection will reveal the typical shallow ulcers, white in color, on such sites as the tongue, palate, gums, buccal mucosa and tonsils. In mild cases, the ulcers are few; in more severe examples there may be a contiguous sheet of ulcers involving all the sites mentioned. Saliva tends to flow from the mouth and satellite lesions form down the chin or cheek where the child dribbles. Considerable swelling of the face and neck may accompany or even precede the appearance of lesions and cause diagnostic confusion. Mild cases subside rapidly but the worst may take up to 2 weeks before the local lesions disappear. Younger children may implant the virus onto other sites such as the sucked finger or perineal region, where vesiculation will develop. The isolation of HSV2 from an oropharyngeal lesion in a child prior to puberty should raise the question of sexual abuse.

Perineal herpes (acute herpetic vulvovaginitis)

This is a less common primary manifestation, though it may be underdiagnosed in view of confusion with severe napkin and other eruptions in the same area. It is diagnosed far more often in girls, though primary perineal herpes sometimes occurs in boys. Some degree of constitutional upset will again herald the infection, to be followed by painful vesiculation over the perineum, which may extend into the vagina in girls. Lesions close to the external urethral orifice may cause difficulties with micturition and regional adenitis may develop. The lesions usually subside without scarring despite the likelihood of secondary infection. Reactivation occurs over the buttocks, thighs or perineum.

Traumatic herpetic infection

The intact skin appears relatively resistant to this virus but primary infection may arise over the site of abrasions and burns. An interesting variety is the herpetic whitlow of the finger which is sometimes seen in nurses who contract the infection by virus entering such lesions as needle puncture wounds or the abrasions that can result from opening glass phials – lesions that are common on the nurse's hand. Here again there may be a marked constitutional upset and regional lymphadenitis.

Acute herpetic keratoconjunctivitis

Primary herpetic infection of the eye is a serious presentation of this infection though relatively rare. The majority of cases are due to HSV1, although HSV2 eye disease may occur as a consequence of neonatal infection. Normally only one eye is involved and cases present with constitutional upset and pain. Marked reddening and edema appear on the affected conjunctiva, the cornea becomes hazy and the eye will usually close. Vesicles appear around the lids and a purulent discharge often occurs. So long as the infection remains superficial the condition will usually subside without complications in 10–14 days. Deeper involvement may give rise to keratitis disciformis, hypopyon keratitis or iridocyclitis, all of which may be followed by scarring; however, these are more commonly encountered in recurrent herpetic infection. Recurrent herpetic keratitis has been shown to be an immune-mediated phenomenon.[604]

Kaposi varicelliform eruption (KVE) or eczema herpeticum

Children with eczema are prone to superinfection of the involved skin by a number of organisms including HSV. The disease starts with a particularly sharp constitutional upset and vesicles then appear on the skin and are most intense at the eczematous areas. An experienced observer may readily recognize the condition; more often the true diagnosis is unappreciated and extensive secondary infection accompanied by a marked serosanguinous discharge will develop. Further crops of vesicles may appear and the child's condition may deteriorate further. The most severe cases may be fatal without aciclovir therapy. In the remainder there is a slow recovery over a period of 3–4 weeks.

Primary herpetic meningoencephalitis

Previously considered an infrequent infection, modern virological techniques have shown that herpetic meningoencephalitis is more common than was believed. The signs of CNS involvement may appear shortly after a primary lesion at some other site but there is usually no clinical evidence to indicate the basic etiological agent. Cases may present as mild forms of aseptic meningitis or as a rapidly fatal form of encephalitis principally involving the temporal lobes. Recently, a genetic etiology for HSV encephalitis was demonstrated in two children with autosomal recessive deficiency in the intracellular protein UNC-93B, resulting in impaired cellular type I interferon responses.[605]

Clinical features: recurrent herpes

Exacerbations of latent HSV infection may be provoked by a variety of nonspecific stimuli which include upper respiratory infections, any febrile illness, gastrointestinal upsets, overexposure to sunlight and emotional upsets. Drugs and certain foods have also been incriminated.

Whatever the excitant, recurrent herpes presents as a crop of tiny vesicles which are sometimes painful and after a few days will dry up to form a scab. They may erupt on almost any part of the skin or on the mucous membranes of the mouth, conjunctivae or genitalia. The most usual site is on the skin around the nose and mouth (cold sores). Exacerbations tend to recur at the same site in any particular individual. Recurrent herpes gives rise to little or no constitutional upset or fever but the excitant, such as lobar pneumonia, may do so.

Diagnosis

The clinical features are often diagnostic in themselves but resort to laboratory aid is of help in certain instances. The procedures most commonly employed are:

1. growth of the virus in tissue culture;
2. demonstration of viral antigens in the material by a fluorescent antibody technique;
3. detection of HSV DNA in CSF or other bodily secretion or tissue by PCR.

Other procedures that may be employed are:

4. demonstration under the electron microscope of herpesvirus particles in material taken from a lesion;
5. antibody estimations on acute and convalescent serum samples to show specific IgM or a significant rise in IgG during a suspected primary infection;
6. histological evidence of intranuclear inclusions and giant cells.

Primary herpes

The oral lesions of primary herpetic gingivostomatitis may be confused with a variety of conditions such as thrush, tonsillitis, Vincent's stomatitis, agranulocytosis and leukemia. Careful clinical and laboratory studies readily differentiate most of these but herpangina, due to infection by coxsackie viruses group A, can cause genuine confusion; however, gingivitis does not normally accompany herpangina, but is common in herpetic infections. Virus studies may be needed in doubtful cases. Herpetic vulvovaginitis is readily confused with ammoniacal dermatitis which has been secondarily infected. Impetigo of the vulva is usually accompanied by involvement elsewhere. Kaposi varicelliform eruption (eczema herpeticum) may be confused with bacterial superinfection of eczema, with eczema vaccinatum and occasionally with varicella. Herpetic meningoencephalitis is difficult to diagnose on clinical grounds; usually virological studies are required to make a conclusive diagnosis.

Recurrent herpes

Recurrent herpes produces a fairly precise diagnostic picture, but on occasion can resemble herpes zoster. The absence of pain, lack of a definable neurological distribution and differing nature of the vesicles should differentiate these conditions.

Treatment

As a rule, primary oral herpetic infections do not require other than supportive treatment. Children with severe gingivostomatitis may have feeding difficulties due to pain, and careful coaxing will be needed to ensure adequate hydration; cleansing of the mouth is also difficult on account of this pain. Irritating acidic fluids should be avoided and diet restricted to cold, bland drinks during the most acute phase. Superinfection by *Candida* may occur but this usually responds to treatment by the local application of nystatin suspension; secondary bacterial infection rarely warrants any antibiotic therapy though this may be required in herpetic vulvovaginitis. Intravenous aciclovir should be reserved for children requiring hospital admission for intravenous rehydration.

Eye involvement is best managed by an experienced ophthalmologist. Herpetic infections are amongst the few viral diseases in which highly successful treatment by antiviral agents has been reported; topical 5-iodo-2-deoxyuridine (IDU) or aciclovir are effective in herpetic eye infections.[606] Intravenous aciclovir is the treatment of choice for herpes simplex encephalitis, for KVE and for any manifestations of HSV disease in a neonate.

CYTOMEGALOVIRUS INFECTIONS

Cytomegalovirus (CMV) is a DNA virus of the herpesvirus group and as such, after the primary infection, causes latent infection with frequent subclinical reactivations for the life of the host. It is ubiquitous in the community, and in the immunocompetent host usually results in asymptomatic infection. CMV infection of the fetus and newborn (congenital and perinatal CMV infection) is discussed in Chapter 12. CMV can cause life-threatening disease in immunocompromised patients with HIV infection, or post solid organ or bone marrow transplantation, either after a primary infection or when a latent infection becomes reactivated.

Clinical features

In immunocompetent older children and adults, CMV infection is usually asymptomatic. On occasion, it may present with fever, cough, headaches and pains in the back and limbs. The clinical picture is one of infectious mononucleosis, with lymphadenopathy, hepatosplenomegaly and sometimes jaundice. Examination of the peripheral blood reveals the presence of atypical lymphocytes, and there is a varying degree of derangement in liver function tests. Hemolytic anemia can occur, and cold agglutinins, cryoglobulins and antinuclear factor may be present. Ampicillin may cause a rash as in EBV infection. CMV may produce a pneumonitis but this is usually seen in premature neonates with postnatally acquired infection or in children suffering from underlying diseases such as chronic hepatic disorders, leukemia and other malignancies.

A febrile illness with features suggesting infectious mononucleosis may also be encountered in patients who have recently undergone open heart surgery or organ transplantation and investigation of obscure postoperative illness in such cases should include tests for CMV infection. In patients with immune deficiency, particularly AIDS patients, CMV may cause pneumonitis, hepatitis, encephalitis or myelitis, severe retinitis and colitis. HIV infected children who acquire CMV during the first 4 years of life have been shown to have a more rapid progression to AIDS than those who remain CMV negative.[607] CMV is a frequent cause of hepatitis, pneumonitis or graft rejection in solid organ transplant recipients and is associated with increased rates of co-infection with other opportunistic pathogens in these individuals. The virus is usually acquired from the donor organ or blood products, although reactivation of latent host CMV may also occur.

Laboratory diagnosis

Histological lesions due to CMV infection are characterized by large cells containing intranuclear and cytoplasmic inclusion bodies. The inclusion-containing cells may be widely disseminated.

Rapid viral diagnosis using DNA probes or by early immunofluorescence testing of tissue cultures (so-called 'shell vial cultures') or detection of the CMV pp65 antigen in blood is particularly useful in the management of suspected CMV infection in immunocompromised patients.

A clinical diagnosis may be confirmed by:
1. isolation of the virus from urine, peripheral blood mononuclear cells, or other secretions;
2. demonstration of a significant rise in antibody titer during the illness;
3. the presence of typical histological lesions in a biopsy specimen, e.g. liver;
4. typical inclusion bodies in cell deposits of fresh urine.

With improved virological techniques, efforts should always be made to grow CMV when infection is suspected. Suitable specimens are fresh urine samples and saliva swabs but these specimens must be delivered to the laboratory with minimum delay as the virus easily loses its infectivity. Isolation of the agent is usually carried out in tissue cultures of human fibroblasts.

Quantification of the amount of CMV DNA or antigen in blood or other secretions to monitor recurrence and allow early pre-emptive therapy in the immunocompromised child is currently being evaluated.[608]

Differential diagnosis

CMV infections acquired in later life may mimic a variety of febrile states but infectious mononucleosis is the most likely condition to cause confusion. Where jaundice occurs, infectious hepatitis, serum hepatitis and leptospirosis require exclusion.

Prevention

Blood products from CMV antibody negative donors should always be given to preterm neonates and immunocompromised patients, particularly post-transplant or HIV infected patients. Alternatively, as the virus is cell associated, filtration or freezing of the donor blood to remove white cells also reduces the risk of acquired CMV infection.

Passive immunoprophylaxis of transplant patients with immunoglobulin is partially successful in reducing the risk of CMV infection. Seropositive CMV patients may reactivate when immunosuppressed, and interferon but not aciclovir reduces this risk.

Treatment

Ganciclovir, a derivative of aciclovir, has been successfully used to treat immunocompromised patients with CMV retinitis, enteritis and pneumonitis.[609] In adult patients, 70–80% cease excretion of CMV within a week, with the exception of marrow transplant patients with CMV pneumonitis, of whom somewhat fewer respond. However, relapse occurs in about half when ganciclovir is stopped, it causes significant marrow suppression, and the drug is incorporated into the host genome. Milder CMV disease can be treated with oral valganciclovir.

Foscarnet causes less marrow suppression, although transient renal impairment may occur. There are few controlled data on its use in CMV infections in childhood. Cidofovir is another antiviral agent with activity against CMV. Its main use is in CMV retinitis or prophylaxis in the organ transplant population.

Prophylaxis with oral antiviral agents in solid organ transplant recipients to prevent CMV disease has been recently demonstrated to be successful in a meta-analysis.[610]

Prognosis

Congenital CMV infection has a variable outcome. Normal individuals who contract CMV infection rarely suffer any sequelae, but in immunocompromised patients, blindness due to retinitis, graft rejection and death from pneumonitis, hepatitis and disseminated CMV infection or opportunistic infection may occur.

EPSTEIN–BARR VIRUS

EBV is the cause of infectious mononucleosis or glandular fever, a disease primarily of older children, adolescents and young adults. An almost identical syndrome can be caused by CMV and *Toxoplasma gondii* as well as EBV. An anginose form of glandular fever primarily affecting the tonsils is seen in younger children under 5 years of age. EBV is a DNA virus and like the other herpesviruses can persist in a latent state and reactivate. It has a worldwide distribution, is potentially oncogenic and has been linked with nasopharyngeal carcinoma, Burkitt lymphoma and other lymphomas, particularly in immunocompromised patients. It can also cause lymphoproliferative syndromes post transplant or in the HIV infected individual.

Etiology and epidemiology

Primary infection of the lymphoid tissue of the nasopharynx may be asymptomatic or may lead to symptomatic infection of lymph nodes. Humans are the only source of EBV, transmission is by the respiratory route and the virus is of low infectivity, usually requiring intimate oral contact. The 'kissing disease' refers to its spread among adolescents and young adults by this route. Epidemics are unusual. The virus persists in the nasopharynx and the uterine cervix. The virus primarily infects B lymphocytes but the atypical mononuclear cells seen in the blood film are activated T lymphocytes.

Clinical features

The anginose form of glandular fever is characterized by fever and sore throat with moderate or marked cervical lymphadenopathy. The tonsils are red and inflamed and there is often exudative folliculitis with white exudate. Other lymph nodes and spleen are rarely enlarged and the clinical picture is not readily distinguishable from acute streptococcal tonsillitis, except that EBV is more likely to cause palatal petechiae.

Glandular fever often starts insidiously with malaise, anorexia and fever, and sore throat is usually a prominent symptom. Occasionally the patient merely has malaise and fever for 1–3 weeks with chills and sweats (febrile form of infectious mononucleosis) and presents with pyrexia of unknown origin. Generally, however, there is marked enlargement of posterior and anterior cervical lymph nodes, and the suboccipital, postauricular, axillary, epitrochlear and inguinal nodes may also be enlarged (glandular form). The tonsils may be inflamed with exudate and rarely this can be sufficient to impair swallowing and even breathing. Splenomegaly is usual and hepatomegaly may also be present, sometimes with jaundice.

Skin eruptions occur in about 10–15% of cases. Most common is a widespread maculopapular rash but morbilliform, scarlatiniform, purpuric and urticarial rashes may occur. Ampicillin (or amoxicillin) causes a particularly florid, confluent maculopapular rash in EBV infection, and the ampicillin rash may be seen less commonly in conjunction with other herpesvirus infections, such as CMV and chickenpox.

In Duncan syndrome, or X-linked lymphoproliferative disease, affected males are unable to control EBV infection and develop generalized lymphadenopathy and hepatosplenomegaly which persists and is rapidly fatal. These patients usually have persistently high levels of IgG antibodies to the viral capsid antigen (VCA).

EBV may be responsible for the lymphoid interstitial pneumonitis that can occur in children with HIV infection, since the EBV genome has been demonstrated in lung biopsy specimens from these patients. It can also cause CNS and other lymphomas in patients with HIV infection.

Complications

Threatened obstruction of the airway may occur in the severe anginose variety, especially when there is secondary edema in the neck. Neurological complications include aseptic meningitis, cranial nerve palsies (including Bell's palsy), encephalomyelitis, transverse myelitis and Guillain–Barré syndrome. Cardiac involvement may present as myocarditis or as transient arrhythmias. Other complications include pneumonitis, orchitis, rupture of the spleen, hemolytic anemia, thrombocytopenic purpura and various ocular manifestations; hepatic involvement has been referred to previously. A prolonged illness with fatigue and relapses over many months has occasionally been described in children, in association with raised EBV antibodies. Chronic EBV infection is not a common cause of the 'chronic fatigue syndrome' or myalgic encephalopathy (ME).

EBV is thought to be the cause of Burkitt lymphoma and of nasopharyngeal carcinoma, in both of which tumors the EBV genome can consistently be demonstrated.

Diagnosis

Five main points arise in the diagnosis of glandular fever: a suggestive clinical picture, typical changes in the peripheral blood, a positive heterophile antibody test, IgM antibody to EBV, and certain nonspecific changes in other laboratory tests.

Blood changes

Most important is the presence of large, atypical mononuclear cells which have an irregular nucleus, whose cytoplasm contains vacuoles, and which have characteristic pale staining of the cellular cytoplasm. Often there is a leukocytosis of $10–20 \times 10^9$ cells/L and sometimes the predominant cells are initially polymorphonuclear. However, atypical monocytes and lymphocytes soon appear, or may be present from the outset, and these can represent from 5 to 50% of the total leukocyte count. Other changes in the blood include occasional leukopenia and rare instances of profound thrombocytopenia and transient autoimmune hemolytic anemia.

Heterophile antibody test (Paul–Bunnell reaction)

There is massive B cell activation in acute EBV infection resulting in an outpouring of nonspecific antibodies. Sheep red cell agglutinins (heterophile antibodies) develop frequently by the second week of infectious mononucleosis, but occasionally not for 2 or 3 weeks, so an early negative test should be repeated.

Sheep red cell agglutinins are not specific for infectious mononucleosis and may occur in other conditions. However, by means of absorption tests using guinea pig kidney and ox erythrocytes the specificity of the test may be increased. The following are the salient features:
1. Antibodies present in infectious mononucleosis are not absorbed by guinea pig kidney but are absorbed by ox erythrocytes.
2. Antibodies found in normal serum are not absorbed by ox erythrocytes but they are absorbed by guinea pig kidney.
3. Antibodies found in serum sickness are absorbed by both guinea pig kidney and ox erythrocytes.

Agglutinins to horse erythrocytes may also be present in the serum of a patient suffering from infectious mononucleosis and in many laboratories a test based on the agglutination of horse erythrocytes is in use. This is the basis of the rapid slide test, the 'Monospot' test. This test may sometimes be negative early in the disease and if EBV is suspected should be repeated. The test is unreliable under 5 years of age, owing to false negative results.

EBV antibody tests

The presence of specific EBV anti-VCA IgM antibody indicates a recent or current infection, whereas the presence of IgG antibodies to the VCA or nuclear antigen (EBNA) merely indicates an infection with EBV some time in the past. Only a small proportion of affected patients show a rise in IgG to VCA, so the IgM test is preferred to show acute infection.

Nonspecific laboratory tests

In well over half the cases some derangement of liver function tests will be found. Most often there is a mild or moderate rise in the serum alanine aminotransferase (AAT) or glutamic pyruvate transaminase (SGPT) level but the alkaline phosphatase and serum bilirubin levels may also rise. Usually these changes are transient but in cases with clinical evidence of hepatic involvement the derangement in liver function tests is more marked.

On occasion, a false positive Wassermann reaction occurs in infectious mononucleosis. High antistreptolysin 'O' titers may be found, probably due to an anamnestic reaction.

The detection of EBV DNA by PCR or in situ hybridization in saliva or tissue of an immunocompromised child may indicate a lymphoproliferative syndrome.

Differential diagnosis

Infectious mononucleosis may be diagnosed too readily. Young children with mild fever and lymph node enlargement in the neck are more likely to have a respiratory viral infection.

Cases that present with fever and little else may be confused with influenza, brucellosis or typhoid; those with a sore throat need to be differentiated from streptococcal or other viral tonsillitis, diphtheria, agranulocytosis and leukemia. Glandular enlargement may be mistaken for toxoplasmosis, CMV infection or reticulosis, and the icteric form of the disease has to be distinguished from infectious hepatitis, leptospirosis and, occasionally, from obstructive liver disease.

The skin eruption of glandular fever has produced confusion with measles, rubella, secondary syphilis, Kawasaki disease and drug rashes.

Treatment

There is no specific treatment. Aciclovir has virtually no in vivo activity against EBV. The disease tends to be mild in children, but simple analgesics may be required to ease pain and gargles to soothe the sore throat. There is increasing evidence that antibiotics can do more harm than good, as toxic skin eruptions appear to follow their use, and ampicillin is especially incriminated in this direction. However, in cases where significant secondary infection is fully substantiated, antibiotics may need to be employed. Corticosteroids can have a dramatic, symptomatic effect but should be reserved for cases where edema of the airway is severe or where life-threatening complications such as thrombocytopenic purpura or severe neurological involvement are encountered. Reduction of immunosuppression or bone marrow transplantation may be of value in the management of EBV lymphoproliferative diseases.[611]

Prognosis

The prognosis is good and children recover more quickly than adults, though some cases run a protracted course and patients may take months to recover their full health. Death is rare and usually results from rupture of the spleen or severe neurological involvement. Recurrences in the immediate convalescent phase can occur but are usually short-lived.

VIRAL AND ALLIED INFECTIONS OF THE RESPIRATORY TRACT

Infections of the respiratory tract are frequent and ubiquitous. They are the most common cause of illness in almost any age group and have a predilection for the extremes of life. Agents that are capable of attacking one part or another of the respiratory tract include viruses, rickettsiae, mycoplasmas and fungi.

Respiratory infection frequently results from a combination of different organisms because, once the initial assault has damaged the defensive mechanisms within the air passages, secondary infection is readily superimposed. This often renders it difficult to prove the primary cause. Nevertheless, detailed studies on the etiology of acute respiratory tract infection indicate that up to 85% of such disease may be initiated by a virus.

In the ensuing account a description is given of the various viruses and allied organisms which play a significant role in the production of infective respiratory disease.

INFLUENZA

Influenza is an acute infectious disease of variable severity with an emphasis on general illness rather than on symptoms arising from the respiratory tract. It tends to occur in pandemic form every few years. In most instances the disease is a benign condition, but it may have a devastating effect in some normal children. Disease is often more severe with an increased mortality in immunosuppressed patients or those with chronic cardiorespiratory disease.

Etiology

Influenza viruses are RNA viruses of the orthomyxovirus family. There are three antigenic types: A, B and C. Infection by type C is relatively uncommon, results in mild or inapparent illness and does not produce epidemics. Type B virus produces significant illness, followed by reasonably effective immunity. Outbreaks or small epidemics may occur, especially in schoolchildren, but are often of a localized nature. Some variation in antigenicity of type B virus occurs and outbreaks appear sporadically at intervals of 3–6 years.

Most clinical, virological and epidemiological interest is focused upon type A viruses, as these produce the most noteworthy outbreaks or epidemics and, when major new variants emerge, pandemics. Pandemics have usually been identified by titles that reflect the suspected geographical origin, as in 'Asian flu' or 'Hong Kong flu'. The World Health Organization has devised a more definitive classification of influenza viruses which reflects the nature of mutation more precisely.[612] Influenza strains that cross the species barrier pose an increasing pandemic threat as shown by the recently identified avian influenza A strain (H5N1).[613]

Structurally, influenza viruses comprise a central core of ribonucleoprotein with a covering envelope. From this envelope spikes containing hemagglutinins project and between these spikes are mushroom-shaped protrusions composed of neuraminidase.

Each basic type of influenza (A, B or C) has its own distinctive ribonucleoprotein consisting of the S or soluble antigen. Protein antigens on the viral surface are related to hemagglutinins (the H antigens) and to neuraminidases (the N antigens). In the case of type A viruses minor changes may occur year by year, producing what is known as antigenic drift. However, at intervals usually exceeding a decade, major changes take place producing antigenic shift. The virtually new type A virus that emerges as a result of antigenic shift has thus acquired the potential to produce a pandemic.

Strain designation of influenza viruses is, therefore, based on the following points:

1. identification of the S antigen – that is, whether the virus is type A, B or C;
2. the host origin – when isolated initially from man, no specific identification is recorded but, if from an animal source, a suitable suffix is appended;
3. the geographical origin;
4. the strain number and the subtype of the hemagglutinin and neuraminidase identified;
5. the year of isolation.

Without an appreciation of the relatively complex antigenic structure and its variation, an understanding of the epidemiology of influenza is difficult.[614] Furthermore, effective vaccination requires using vaccines whose antigenic components accurately reflect the strain of influenza virus prevalent at the time of use.

Epidemiology

Man is the principal reservoir of infection and the disease is transmitted by direct contact, through droplet infection and by articles that have been freshly soiled with discharges from the nose or throat of infected persons. Infectivity appears to persist for 4–5 days after the clinical onset of the disease. Occasional cases originate from animals, e.g. pigs or chickens. In view of the high infectivity of influenza and the rapidity of modern travel, an epidemic can soon develop pandemic proportions. Human infection with avian influenza A strain (H5N1) was initially described in Vietnam, but the virus has now been isolated from individuals in most parts of the world.[613] It infects humans in contact with diseased birds and is associated with high mortality rates due to respiratory failure. At the current time, only low levels of human to human transmission of H5N1 have been shown to occur, but an increase in transmission efficiency via this route could result in a major world pandemic.

Pathogenesis

Influenza infection causes necrosis of ciliated respiratory epithelium and this commences in the nose and spreads downwards to the trachea and bronchi. Edema and leukocyte infiltration follow causing pharyngitis, tracheitis and bronchitis; in severe cases considerable exudation of blood and edema fluid may occur and enter the alveoli with resultant pneumonia.

Primary respiratory damage from influenza virus may in itself produce a severe illness, but secondary bacterial infection is more often the cause of fatal pneumonia; organisms such as *Staphylococcus aureus* and *Klebsiella pneumoniae* are particularly dangerous in this context.

Clinical features

The incubation period of influenza is short and ranges from 1 to 3 days. In children over 5 years of age there is a sudden onset of fever, headache and shivering, with pains in the limbs and back. Anorexia, listlessness and malaise may also be experienced and in some instances, particularly in children, nausea and vomiting may be unduly pronounced. Abdominal pain ('gastric flu') can be a prominent symptom. A dry, painful cough, discomfort in the throat, hoarseness and nasal discharge are usual.

The temperature may reach 39–40 °C, but apart from signs of pharyngitis, objective physical findings are few and in uncomplicated cases clinical and radiographic examination of the chest is usually clear. Leukopenia will be found in uncomplicated cases and the ESR becomes moderately elevated.

The illness usually runs a short course and is followed by rapid improvement. Some patients experience a period of mental and physical lethargy in convalescence but seriously complicated cases are rarely seen outside epidemics.

In younger children and infants influenza A typically causes high fever (over 39 °C) and upper respiratory tract infection with coryza, cough, irritability and pharyngitis. Otitis media, laryngotracheitis, bronchitis, bronchiolitis indistinguishable from that due to RSV, and pneumonia may all occur. Vomiting and diarrhea are frequent in infants. Febrile convulsions are frequent, as are fleeting erythematous rashes, which can be morbilliform. Despite these manifestations, a recent large scale epidemiological study in the USA confirmed that a significant burden of influenza disease in infants and young children goes unrecognized.[615] The risk of severe lower respiratory tract involvement is greater in immunocompromised children, and in children with neurological and neuromuscular disease.[616]

In neonates the picture is nonspecific, with apneic episodes, lethargy, poor feeding and impaired circulation. Outbreaks may occur in neonatal units.

Diagnosis

At epidemic times, a clinical diagnosis of influenza has a high likelihood of being correct, but such a diagnosis in a sporadic case can often be incorrect. Other respiratory viral infections and some quite unconnected diseases may present with a similar clinical picture and a specific diagnosis depends on definitive laboratory tests.

Virological confirmation of influenza can be established by serological studies or by demonstrating the presence of influenza virus. The latter can be isolated from pharyngeal swabs, nasal swabs or throat washing during the acute stage of the illness and can be grown in the amniotic cavity of chick embryos or in tissue cultures. Influenza may be isolated in monkey kidney tissue cultures. During epidemics, immunofluorescence using an antiserum to the epidemic strain to test nasopharyngeal secretions can be used for rapid diagnosis. Complement-fixation, neutralization and hemagglutination-inhibition tests are available for the serological study of antibody responses to infection with influenza. In all these tests it is desirable to show a significant (four-fold or greater) rise in antibody titer during the illness.

Complications

Viral complications such as myocarditis, polyneuritis, encephalitis and psychosis are rarely seen in childhood cases. Secondary bacterial infection of the respiratory tract is more likely and pneumonia, otitis media and purulent sinusitis may occur. Death can result from severe overwhelming infection by influenza virus itself, though a fatal outcome is more likely to result from secondary bacterial infection. Acute myositis may be severe, particularly affecting the calves, with a raised serum creatine phosphokinase (CPK). Reye syndrome has sometimes followed influenza infection.

Treatment

In mild cases this is essentially symptomatic. Bed rest is advisable and pain will be eased by simple analgesics such as paracetamol (acetaminophen). Troublesome cough may respond to codeine or similar preparations. Bacterial complications may require antibiotic treatment, whenever possible guided by appropriate laboratory studies. Amantadine and rimantadine have been successfully used to treat severe infection in immunocompromised children or those with underlying chronic illnesses. The neuraminidase inhibitors are a new class of antiviral agents that have been shown to be effective in the treatment of severe influenza in high risk patients.[617,618] Zanamivir is an inhaled preparation, and oseltamivir is an oral preparation. Their use in childhood disease is still under evaluation.

Prophylaxis

The extreme infectivity of influenza renders such measures as isolation and quarantine virtually ineffective. There is evidence that killed virus vaccine can significantly reduce the incidence of influenza, although the sudden emergence of a fresh influenza A mutant may render it impossible to produce the specific vaccine in time to influence an outbreak. Annual influenza vaccination should be considered for the child over 6 months with chronic pulmonary, circulatory or neuromuscular disorders, or with chronic renal disease or diabetes mellitus, or with immunosuppression (including HIV infection). Postexposure prophylaxis with amantadine or the neuraminidase inhibitors has been shown to be effective in preventing illness in adults and children.

In the USA, annual influenza vaccination is now recommended for all children aged 6–59 months, using either a trivalent inactivated influenza vaccine or a live attenuated vaccine.[619] Previously unvaccinated children under 9 years should receive two doses the first year.[619] In other countries, including the UK and Australia, annual influenza vaccination is recommended for children at high risk of severe influenza.

PARAINFLUENZA VIRUS INFECTIONS

The parainfluenza viruses are RNA viruses of the *Paramyxovirus* group. They are more closely related to mumps and Newcastle disease viruses than to influenza.

Four antigenic varieties, called 1, 2, 3 and 4, are recognized, although type 4 has no known role in causing disease in humans. Types 1, 2 and 3 have frequently been isolated from cases of acute laryngotracheobronchitis (croup), bronchitis, bronchiolitis and pneumonia in infants and children, and less often from rhinitis and pharyngitis. They are undoubtedly the commonest cause of acute laryngotracheobronchitis, in which other viruses such as influenza A, RSV and ECHO viruses play a lesser role.

Serological studies indicate that infection, especially with type 3, is common in preschool children. Type 3 infection is endemic and occurs at any time of the year. Type 1 infection tends to occur in summer or autumn outbreaks every second year while type 2 outbreaks are less predictable.

Laboratory diagnosis

Parainfluenza viruses can be isolated from nasal and pharyngeal swabs. The viruses are relatively labile so these swabs should be placed in virus transport medium and delivered to the laboratory with minimum delay. Antigen detection by immunofluorescence or ELISA is increasingly available. Serological diagnosis is rarely helpful, other than in epidemiological studies, because of heterotypic antibody rises among the three types and related viruses, particularly mumps.

Treatment

There is no specific treatment available. Symptomatic treatment of laryngotracheobronchitis with steroids or adrenaline (epinephrine) for severe airways obstruction may be indicated. Ribavirin has been used to suppress infection in immunocompromised hosts.

A live attenuated parainfluenza type 3 vaccine is currently in clinical trial in young infants.[620]

RESPIRATORY SYNCYTIAL VIRUS INFECTIONS

Respiratory syncytial virus (RSV), first identified in 1956, is now recognized to be amongst the most important agents causing respiratory infection in infants and young children worldwide. RSV is an RNA paramyxovirus. The virus grows well in many tissue cultures. In contrast to members of the myxovirus group, to which it shows some resemblance, RSV has no hemagglutinins so does not cause hemagglutination, but produces a fusion protein which causes in vitro and in vivo fusion of cells to form syncytia. Only two antigenic strains of RSV have been described.

Clinical features

RSV has been found in association with several clinical syndromes including mild upper respiratory tract infection, croup, bronchitis, bronchiolitis and pneumonia. Its principal association is with acute bronchiolitis in infants below 1 year of age. Epidemics of RSV infection occur annually in late autumn and winter in temperate climates. Outbreaks are mainly found in urban communities. In tropical climates there is not such a clear-cut annual epidemic. Nosocomial infections can be a major problem in hospitals.

Bronchiolitis is described elsewhere and although infection by influenza viruses, parainfluenza viruses, human metapneumovirus, mycoplasmas, adenoviruses and rhinoviruses may produce a similar picture, few clinical respiratory syndromes have so close an etiological association as bronchiolitis and RSV infection.

Neither maternal nor acquired antibody protects absolutely against RSV, so RSV can infect neonates. Reinfections throughout childhood are common, but successively milder. Preterm infants with symptomatic RSV bronchiolitis appear to have worse lung function at follow-up.[621] High RSV viral load is associated with more severe disease.[622] Toddler-age children may develop bronchitis or pneumonia, school-age children more commonly develop otitis media, while adults get a severe cold with sore throat. Infants with mutations in the Toll-like receptor 4 (TLR4) gene complex involved in the innate immune response to RSV are especially prone to severe disease.[623]

Laboratory diagnosis

The ideal specimen is a nasopharyngeal aspirate of mucus. Rapid viral diagnosis by immunofluorescence (or ELISA) has greatly aided the management of infants with bronchiolitis. The virus can be isolated successfully in various tissue culture systems, but as it is relatively unstable it is recommended that the specimen should be inoculated directly into the cultures without previous freezing. If the specimen has to be stored for a few hours it should be kept in virus transport medium at 4 °C.

Serology can be used in children over 6 months of age, usually by complement-fixation test on paired sera. Under this age there is often no IgG response.

Treatment

Treatment is primarily supportive with supplemental oxygen and/or fluids. Nebulized ribavirin may be indicated in proven severe RSV infection in infants at high risk, particularly those with pre-existing cardiopulmonary disease or immune deficiency.[624–626]

Prevention

Two agents have recently become available for the prevention of RSV in high risk infants (those born prematurely < 35 weeks' gestation, or those with underlying chronic lung disease, cardiac disease or immunosuppression). RSV intravenous immunoglobulin (RSV IVIG) from pooled donors is administered intravenously, and palizumab is a mouse monoclonal antibody to the RSV protein that is given intramuscularly. Both are given monthly during the RSV season and have been shown to significantly reduce the number of cases of hospitalized RSV bronchiolitis in at-risk groups,[627–629] but are expensive. The cost effectiveness of these agents in the UK has been questioned based on local data.[630]

HUMAN METAPNEUMOVIRUS

Human metapneumovirus (MPV) is an RNA virus that was discovered in 2001 in the respiratory isolates of young children.[681] It has been found to be a cause of respiratory illness in all age groups.[631–634] It is a member of the *Paramyxoviridae* family and has four major genotypes that fall into two antigenic subgroups (A and B). Humans are the only source of infection and transmission is thought to occur through contact with infected secretions. Infection occurs in yearly epidemics, peaking in late winter to spring.[632–634] Co-infection with other viral pathogens is common. Seroprevalence studies suggest that virtually all children have been exposed to MPV by the age of 5.[631]

Clinical features

The clinical features of MPV are similar to those of RSV.[630,631,633] It causes respiratory illnesses of both upper and lower respiratory tract, including bronchiolitis in infants and croup. Disease in normal hosts is usually mild, although MPV can occasionally cause severe pneumonitis. Preterm infants and children with underlying pulmonary or cardiac disorders or with immunodeficiency are at risk of severe disease from MPV, although RSV is a more common pathogen in this group.[635] Immunocompromised children may have persistent shedding of MPV.[635] Severe disease in children with HIV infection is usually associated with pneumococcal superinfection.[637] Like RSV, recurrent infections occur throughout life.

Laboratory diagnosis

There are currently no commercially available tests for the diagnosis of MPV. MPV can be isolated by culture of respiratory secretions, and MPV viral nucleic acid can be detected by RT-PCR in reference or research laboratories.[632,634]

Treatment

Treatment is supportive with supplemental oxygen and attention to hydration as required.

Prevention

Control of nosocomial MPV infection requires contact precautions, with particular attention to hand washing after contact with infected respiratory secretions.

ADENOVIRUSES

The first isolation of an adenovirus took place in 1953 from fragmented human adenoids grown in tissue culture, hence the name. Subsequently a number of different strains, chiefly types 1, 2, 5 and 6, were isolated from cultures of tonsils and adenoids. Outbreaks due to these agents have been encountered in children at boarding schools, at summer camps and amongst those attending communal swimming pools. Outbreaks in adults mainly involve military recruits. The nature of the clinical illness produced shows considerable variation and overlap but some relatively specific syndromes are included.

Adenoviruses are DNA viruses. They are relatively stable to changes in temperature and pH. They are widespread in nature and have been isolated from monkeys, pigs, dogs, birds and cattle, as well as from man. They may persist for weeks or even months in the upper respiratory tract.

Clinical features

Adenovirus infections are principally diseases of childhood, occurring mostly in children under 5 years old. Certain adenovirus types show a pronounced age association. Immunocompromised hosts are at risk of severe disease from adenovirus.[638]

Amongst syndromes recognized to be associated with adenoviral infection are the following:

Acute febrile pharyngitis

This syndrome has a high endemic rate in infants and young children and mainly results from infection by types 1, 2 and 5. It can also occur in epidemic form when type 3 is usually involved.

Pharyngoconjunctival fever (PCF)

Most commonly associated with infection by type 3, and less frequently with types 7A and 14, this syndrome can also follow infection by types 1, 2, 5 and 6. Epidemics occur in children, some associated with swimming pools. Symptoms include sore throat, headache, myalgia, eye discomfort, abdominal pain and back stiffness. Examination often reveals pharyngitis and unilateral or bilateral follicular conjunctivitis.

Acute respiratory disease (ARD)

Uncommon in children, ARD is usually found in military recruits. It is most commonly due to infection by types 4 and 7, less often by types 3 and 14. The main clinical features include pharyngitis, cough, hoarseness and chest pain.

Viral pneumonia in infants

Adenoviruses may cause severe pneumonia, and outbreaks have been reported in hospital nurseries. Types 3, 7 and 21 have caused the most severe, sometimes fatal, cases. Infection may disseminate (see below) or may result in bronchiolitis obliterans, bronchiectasis or unilateral hyperlucent lung. In immunocompetent infants hospitalized with severe adenovirus infection, disease severity correlates with serum LDH and oxygen saturation at admission.[639]

Ocular syndromes

Two specific ocular syndromes are associated with adenovirus infection. The first is called *epidemic keratoconjunctivitis* and is associated with type 8 infection; the second, *follicular conjunctivitis*, usually results from infection by type 3 and may expand into the fuller syndrome of pharyngoconjunctival fever.

Disseminated disease

Adenovirus types 7 and 21 are particularly prone to cause pneumonia and disseminate to involve the liver (hepatitis), heart (myocarditis or pericarditis) and CNS (meningitis or encephalitis). This is more likely in immunocompromised patients.

Gastroenteritis

Noncultivable enteric adenoviruses (types 40 and 41), seen on electron microscopy of feces, have been associated with gastroenteritis.[640]

Laboratory diagnosis

Adenoviruses can be grown in a wide range of tissue cultures. These viruses are relatively stable and can readily be isolated from throat swabs and feces. In respiratory disease, a pharyngeal swab should be sent to the laboratory in virus transport media. Growth may be slow, so cultures should be incubated for at least 3 weeks before being regarded as negative.

Serological evidence of infection is by detecting complement-fixing antibodies to adenoviruses in acute and convalescent serum samples. Antigen detection by immunoassays and detection of viral DNA by PCR in body fluids may aid in diagnosis of adenovirus infection in the immunocompromised.

Treatment

Treatment is largely supportive. The new antiviral agent, cidofovir, has been used with some success in the treatment of severe adenoviral infections in children post bone marrow transplantation.[641]

MUMPS (EPIDEMIC PAROTITIS)

To mump is an old English word meaning to mope. Mumps is an acute infectious disease characterized by nonsuppurative enlargement of the salivary glands, particularly the parotids. It results from infection by mumps virus, one of the myxoviruses, and is associated with an unusually diverse range of complications. Infection may be inapparent in as many as 30% of cases and the illness may present with a complication and no history of preceding salivary gland involvement.

Epidemiology and etiology

Mumps is an endemic disease of urban communities which occasionally occurs in epidemic proportions, especially in certain closed communities. Spread is by droplet infection or from recently contaminated articles and close contact is required. The relatively high incidence in adults bears witness to the comparatively low infectivity of the disease, though when mumps is introduced into a naive community, a serious and widespread outbreak may follow. There have been recent outbreaks of mumps in young adults in the UK.[642]

The responsible agent is an RNA virus. Man appears to be the only reservoir and the portal of entry is through the mouth or nose. Infectivity may extend from several days before the illness to several days after the first sign of salivary gland involvement. Virus has been isolated from the blood in the prodromal stage and from the urine up to 14 days after the commencement of clinical illness. It is not clear whether spread to the salivary glands occurs locally or through the bloodstream.

Clinical features

The main incidence occurs between 5 and 15 years of age; mumps is relatively uncommon in younger children and in adults over 30 years.

The incubation period is between 14 and 21 days and the illness may commence with malaise, fever, headache and anorexia; these prodromal symptoms may be absent. Salivary gland involvement commences 1–2 days later and the parotid glands are the most frequently affected. Pain develops around the ear and a swelling appears which extends forwards from the lobe of the ear, downwards over the angle of the jaw and backwards behind the pinna, which is usually pushed outwards. The swelling may be so trivial as to escape casual inspection or be very marked and exquisitely tender. Often only one parotid is involved initially, followed, in 75% of cases, by swelling of the other parotid 1–5 days later. Less often simultaneous and synchronous swelling of both parotids occurs.

Submandibular salivary gland involvement can easily be overlooked as the soft tissues under the jaw readily absorb such swelling, unless it is particularly marked, and it is often the concomitant swelling of the parotids that directs attention to it. Sublingual involvement is much less common but is extremely painful and can be seen readily beneath the upturned tongue.

In addition to salivary gland involvement, the orifice of Stensen's duct may be swollen and the mouth rather dry. Fever is present in the majority of cases, may reach 40 °C and persist for up to a week; in fact, cases without salivary gland involvement may present as examples of unexplained fever and recover without the true diagnosis being appreciated, though in others the later development of a typical pattern of complications may indicate mumps to be the cause.

There may be some degree of leukopenia in mumps though certain complications, such as meningitis and pancreatitis, may provoke a leukocytosis.

Complications

Complications are common and varied.

CNS

Aseptic meningitis is the commonest complication and may present before, coincidentally with, or after, the illness. The CSF will show a lymphocytic pleocytosis and the count may exceed 1000 cells/μl. The protein content may be moderately raised and the glucose level is usually normal. However, the latter is occasionally decreased in mumps meningitis and where no salivary gland enlargement occurs to indicate the diagnosis, confusion with tuberculous meningitis has occurred. Other less common complications include postinfectious encephalitis, myelitis and polyradiculitis. Although usually unilateral, bilateral nerve deafness, often complete, can also occur, as may transient facial paralysis. The virus is easily isolated from the CSF of patients with mumps meningitis, which is generally benign. The postinfectious encephalitis is, however, more severe; although complete recovery is usual, neurological sequelae and even death may occur. Virus can be grown from the CSF, but an immune-mediated mechanism is more likely to contribute to pathogenesis.

Orchitis

Orchitis may occur in 20% of postpubertal males and in younger children can occasionally occur in an undescended testicle. The involvement is usually unilateral but even after severe orchitis, sterility is rare, and males with orchitis should be firmly reassured of the good prognosis.

Pancreatitis

A significant degree of pancreatitis is rare and this complication is over-diagnosed. Salivary gland enlargement by itself raises the serum amylase level but when the pancreas is significantly involved intense pain will occur with rigidity of the abdominal wall and there is often a marked leukocytosis.

Other complications

These include oophoritis, mastitis, bartholinitis, myocarditis, hepatitis, thyroiditis and thrombocytopenic purpura. An occasional case of diabetes mellitus has also been reported following mumps.

Laboratory diagnosis

Viral confirmation of mumps depends on isolation of the virus or the demonstration of a significant rise in antibody titer during the illness.

Mumps virus can be cultured from saliva swabs and urine during the acute illness and from the CSF in cases complicated by meningitis.

Serological tests are readily available to demonstrate a significant rise in antibody titer during the illness and the complement-fixation test is most commonly employed. In this test, two specific antigens, soluble (S) and viral (V), are often used. In general, antibody to S antigen rises earlier in the illness than antibody to V antigen, but whereas S antibody may only persist for a few months, the V antibody is present for a very long period. Hemagglutination-inhibition and virus neutralization tests are also of help where available.

Differential diagnosis

In children, the differential diagnosis is more limited than in adults as in the latter one may encounter more diseases that involve the salivary glands. Conditions that cause lymph node enlargement produce most confusion but careful clinical examination should resolve the difficulty. Pyogenic submandibular abscesses and glandular fever can prove more perplexing and in these instances the blood picture and serum amylase estimations can be helpful. Suppurative parotitis may be considered where there is overlying inflammation and where pus can be expressed from the appropriate salivary duct. Recurrent parotitis is quite common in children. It is not due to repeated attacks of mumps. Sometimes an underlying allergic disorder, sialectasis or duct calculi may be found. Other conditions which may require exclusion are tumors, Mikulicz syndrome, uveoparotid fever in sarcoidosis, HIV infection, tuberculosis and dental conditions.

Treatment

There is no specific treatment. Pain may be relieved by simple analgesics and the application of heat to the glands can prove soothing. The mouth should be kept clean and a fluid diet is needed until swelling subsides. Neurological complications are managed along customary lines though the diagnostic lumbar puncture in mumps meningitis often produces dramatic relief of headache. In orchitis the testes should be supported and ice bags may ease the discomfort; there is no evidence that corticosteroid drugs, stilbestrol or incision of the tunica albuginea significantly alter the course of this complication.

Prognosis

This is generally good and a fatal outcome exceedingly rare, although permanent brain damage and deafness have been described. Sterility

is most unlikely. One attack of mumps appears to provide life-long immunity.

Prevention

Injections of human anti-mumps immunoglobulin have been used prophylactically and appear beneficial if given sufficiently early in the incubation period. Live vaccines are safe and produce a good antibody response with long immunity though the duration has not been fully substantiated. They can be used to immunize contacts, and are incorporated into the MMR vaccine for routine immunization in many countries.

COXSACKIE AND ECHO VIRUS INFECTIONS

Respiratory illness in association with these enteroviruses is usually mild.

Certain coxsackie viruses produce specific respiratory syndromes. Some group A serotypes can cause herpangina and certain group B viruses are the agents responsible for causing pleurodynia (Bornholm disease). Agents from both groups of coxsackie viruses have been found in association with mild febrile respiratory disease and one strain, coxsackie A21 (Coe virus), has been recovered with particular frequency from outbreaks in young servicemen.

ECHO viruses are not usually regarded as respiratory pathogens, but they have been found in the throat or feces during upper respiratory disease. Amongst serotypes isolated in these circumstances are ECHO viruses types 6, 11, 19 and 20.

The laboratory diagnosis of infections due to coxsackie and ECHO viruses is described in the section specifically devoted to these agents.

RHINOVIRUS INFECTIONS

Rhinoviruses are the main cause of the common cold. There are many serologically distinct types. They belong to the large group of picornaviruses, meaning small RNA viruses, but unlike coxsackie and ECHO viruses they are acid labile at pH 3.

The common cold is probably the most ubiquitous infection in man and the illness tends to be more severe in children than in adults, with an acute catarrhal inflammation involving the nose, nasopharynx and accessory sinuses. The onset is usually abrupt and is accompanied by a copious watery discharge, which may later turn mucopurulent even in the absence of bacterial superinfection. Little or no fever occurs and constitutional symptoms are mild.

Apart from their ability to produce the common cold, rhinoviruses have been found in association with acute wheezing episodes in children and with pneumonia.[643]

Laboratory diagnosis

Nasopharyngeal aspirates in virus transport medium, nose swab or throat swab collected during the acute stage of the respiratory illness should be sent to the laboratory for the isolation of rhinoviruses. Serology is generally unhelpful. ELISA and PCR for rhinovirus have been developed but are not widely available.

CORONAVIRUSES AND SARS

Human coronaviruses (HCV) are probably almost as frequent a cause of colds and acute upper respiratory tract infections as rhinovirus infections.[644] Coronaviruses have also been associated with wheeze and pneumonia.[645] The exact frequency of HCV infections has been difficult to ascertain because coronaviruses are difficult to grow and can often only be isolated in tracheal organ cultures. The diagnosis can be made by ELISA on respiratory secretions or serologically by detecting antibody to one of the two main serotypes, 229E and OC-43. PCR is not widely available.

During 2002–2003, there was an acute outbreak of a severe atypical pneumonia, originally in China and Hong Kong, that did not respond to routine antimicrobial therapies.[646,647] The disease was labeled severe acute respiratory distress syndrome (or SARS). Commonly known viruses and bacteria were not isolated and eventually a novel coronavirus, SARS-CoV, was confirmed to be the causal agent.[648,649] The syndrome was characterized by fever of 38 °C or more, respiratory symptoms (cough, dyspnea), myalgia and marked infiltrates on chest X-ray which were often out of proportion to the degree of symptoms. Most patients did not experience upper respiratory tract symptoms. Gastrointestinal symptoms were present in 10% of patients. Severe disease was associated with deranged liver function enzymes, thrombocytopenia and leukopenia, and respiratory failure, and was associated with high mortality. Infected children < 12 years of age experienced only mild disease and rarely progressed to respiratory failure or death.[648,649]

Transmission of SARS-CoV is by contact with respiratory secretions, although urine, stool and blood can also be a source of infection. Infected individuals are most contagious during the second week of the illness. In the 2003 outbreak, high rates of human to human transmission were reported in exposed health care workers.[648,649] Routine diagnostic tests are not available for SARS-CoV, and the diagnosis is usually made by the combination of known exposure, clinical features and failure to isolate other pathogens. The virus is difficult to isolate in cell culture. Research laboratories have confirmed the infection by molecular techniques, serology or by immuno-electron microscopy. Although severe SARS has been treated with steroids, ribavirin and interferon alfa, there is no antiviral agent with proven efficacy against this virus.[648,649]

REOVIRUS INFECTIONS

In 1954, a new group of respiratory-entero or reovirus agents was recognized. It had originally been thought to belong to the ECHO virus group. Since then three distinct types (1, 2 and 3) have been serologically differentiated though they share a common complement-fixing antigen.

Following these preliminary investigations reoviruses have been isolated from many different animal hosts in widely separated areas. These viruses have also been recovered from rectal and throat swabs taken from children suffering from mild respiratory disease, diarrhea, and occasionally fatal pneumonia.

A recent seroprevalence study in the USA suggests that reovirus infections are common during early childhood.[650] However, the exact role of reoviruses in producing human disease is largely undetermined. The family Reoviridae also includes the rotaviruses, which are associated with gastroenteritis.

Laboratory diagnosis

Reoviruses can be isolated from pharyngeal swabs and nasal secretions, but are more commonly recovered from feces.

Acute and convalescent samples of serum are required for hemagglutination-inhibiting antibody titer estimations; a four-fold, or greater, rise in titer during the illness is evidence of infection with a reovirus.

Rotaviruses are difficult to culture and diagnosis depends on electron microscopic examination or ELISA tests on feces.

CHLAMYDOPHILA PSITTACI (PSITTACOSIS)

Psittacosis is a zoonosis contracted from birds or objects they have contaminated. It was originally considered that infection could only result from birds of the psittacine group (psittacosis) but it is now appreciated that infection may arise from many other birds, both wild and domesticated (ornithosis), and animals such as sheep and goats.

Chlamydophila (formerly *Chlamydia*) *psittaci*, the causative organism, is antigenically and genetically distinct from the genus *Chlamydia* in which it was previously grouped.[651] This obligate intracellular organism appears to occupy an intermediate position between viruses and rickettsiae and shows sensitivity only to certain antibiotics.

Clinical features

The presentation is usually with high fever, chills, headache, myalgia, chest pain, anorexia and fatigue. A dry cough may become productive

and fine crackles may be heard. The pulse may be relatively slow. Contact with a sick bird is suggestive, but there may be no history of bird or animal contact. Chest radiography may show perihilar infiltrates, atelectasis or even consolidation. Children and adolescents seem less susceptible to psittacosis than adults. However, this may merely reflect the fact that less specific illness is produced in the young and the diagnosis may therefore be overlooked.

Laboratory diagnosis

A clinical diagnosis of psittacosis can be confirmed by serological tests. Treatment can suppress antibody responses. The estimation of complement-fixing antibodies in acute and convalescent samples of serum is a reliable and popular test which avoids the hazards involved in the isolation of a highly infectious agent but does not distinguish between other species of *Chlamydia* or *Chlamydophila*. The acute serum sample should be collected as early in the illness as possible and a convalescent sample taken about 2 weeks after the onset of the illness. It is often worthwhile examining a third sample of serum obtained after a further 2 weeks. A four-fold, or greater, rise in antibody titer during the illness is indicative of infection with a member of the psittacosis–lymphogranuloma venereum group of agents.

The psittacosis agent can be isolated from blood in the early stages of the illness and later from pleural fluid and infected tissues by reference laboratories where appropriate controls are enforced to prevent infection in personnel.

Sensitive immunoassays for *C. psittaci* are available in some reference laboratories.[652]

Prognosis

Spontaneous recovery is to be expected, but where the diagnosis is confirmed during the clinical illness, tetracycline (except in children less than 8 years old) or erythromycin may reduce symptoms and hasten convalescence.

CHLAMYDOPHILA PNEUMONIAE

C. pneumoniae is closely related to *C. psittaci*, and cross-reacts with it in complement-fixation serological tests. Infection can be subclinical or result in mild to moderate respiratory illnesses. The prodrome may include a sore throat, and there is often a protracted cough persisting up to 6 weeks with a biphasic course.[653] Serological surveys suggest it is a not uncommon cause of pneumonia in children, particularly in resource limited countries. Treatment is as for psittacosis.

CHLAMYDIA TRACHOMATIS

C. trachomatis, acquired by passage through an infected birth canal, can cause a pneumonitis usually at 3–11 weeks of age. There may be a history of maternal vaginal discharge and the infant may have had conjunctivitis. The infant is afebrile with a characteristic staccato cough. There are often crackles and wheezes on auscultation. About half the infants have otitis media with a pearly white tympanic membrane. The radiographic appearance is of diffuse pulmonary infiltrates with peribronchial thickening and focal consolidation. Definitive diagnosis is by culturing *C. trachomatis* or detecting antigen in a nasopharyngeal aspirate or conjunctival swab, or by detecting specific IgM by immunofluorescence. PCR and other nucleic amplification techniques can be used to detect *C. trachomatis* DNA in genital swabs or urine from the mother. They can also be used on conjunctival swabs from the infant, but the test has not proved sensitive when performed on infants' pharyngeal specimens. Presumptive evidence can be obtained by demonstrating characteristic inclusions on conjunctival scrapings if there is active conjunctivitis. Treatment of conjunctivitis is with erythromycin 40 mg/kg/d 6-hourly for 14 days. Parents should be alerted of the signs of infantile hypertrophic pyloric stenosis, which is associated with erythromycin use in infants < 6 weeks of age, although the link has not been proven to be causal.[653]

Chlamydia pneumonia can be treated with erythromycin as before or with azithromycin 20 mg/kg orally once daily for 3 days. The parents should also be treated.

MYCOPLASMA PNEUMONIAE

Mycoplasma pneumoniae is a common cause of atypical pneumonia in childhood but can also cause a variety of clinical syndromes. It is not a virus but a pleuropneumonia-like organism (PPLO) that lacks a cell wall and belongs to the distinctive genus of mycoplasmas.

Clinical features

M. pneumoniae may give rise to inapparent infection, mild upper respiratory tract infection, bronchitis, bronchiolitis, bronchopneumonia and bullous myringitis both in adults and children. Epidemics occur every 3–4 years. *M. pneumoniae* may have an etiological role in some cases of Stevens–Johnson syndrome and can also cause myocarditis, pericarditis, arthritis and encephalitis. When it causes pneumonia, the radiological appearance may be of bilateral, diffuse reticular infiltrates or of consolidation, including lobar consolidation. Small pleural effusions can occur.

Laboratory diagnosis

Isolation of *M. pneumoniae* from sputum, throat washings or pharyngeal swabs is possible, but the agent grows slowly.

For serological studies, acute and convalescent samples of serum should be collected. Various serological tests are available, but the complement-fixation test appears popular and reliable. A single high titer of IgG antibodies to *M. pneumoniae* on an acute serum sample may be helpful, since there is often a fairly long history of illness. Detection of *M. pneumoniae* IgM by immunofluorescence does not distinguish an acute infection from one in the recent past, as the antibody may persist for many months.

Cold agglutinins are present in the serum in many cases and may be useful in acute management, although their detection is not specific for *Mycoplasma* infection.

Treatment

Mild respiratory illnesses caused by *Mycoplasma* are usually self limiting and do not require treatment. Pneumonia caused by *M. pneumoniae*, where a diagnosis is made during the active stage of illness, can be treated with tetracycline (25–50 mg/kg/day) or doxycycline (2.5 mg/kg up to 100 mg twice daily) in children over 8 years old, or with erythromycin (30–50 mg/kg/day) or with one of the newer macrolides such as clarithromycin or azithromycin in younger children. There is no evidence that antimicrobial treatment alters the course of nonrespiratory forms of *Mycoplasma* disease.

VIRAL INFECTIONS OF THE CNS (INCLUDING MENINGITIS, ENCEPHALITIS, MYELITIS AND POLYNEURITIS)

See Chapter 22 (Infectious and inflammatory disorders of the CNS).

LYMPHOCYTIC CHORIOMENINGITIS

Lymphocytic choriomeningitis (LCM) virus was first recognized in 1934, and is classified as a member of the Arenavirus group. It occurs in mice.

Sporadic cases and small outbreaks of LCM aseptic meningitis in man have been reported in Europe and the USA, in circumscribed areas where infected mouse colonies have been shown to exist.[654] Although originally suspected to be a common cause of aseptic meningitis, it is now known to have a very small role except in these endemic areas.

Clinical features

The incubation period of LCM lies between 7 and 14 days. Any age group may contract the disease, if in contact with the relevant infected mouse colonies. The clinical picture and the abnormalities in the CSF are identical with those found in other types of viral meningitis and etiological diagnosis can only be made by laboratory studies. LCM can also cause mild respiratory illness and occasionally pneumonia. Orchitis, myopericarditis, arthritis or alopecia may rarely occur. The prognosis is usually excellent, although an occasional fatality has been reported in infants. No specific treatment is indicated. Control of infected mouse colonies should be undertaken by expert rodent exterminators.

Laboratory diagnosis

LCM virus can be isolated from blood in the initial febrile phase of the illness, and from CSF after the onset of meningitis. The virus can be propagated in young mice and in various tissue cultures.

Complement-fixing and neutralizing antibodies appear in the patient's serum following infection and a serological diagnosis can be made by demonstrating a significant rise in antibody titer during the illness. The antibodies tend to be produced rather late in the illness, so the convalescent serum sample for complement-fixing antibodies should be collected about the third week of the illness and that for neutralizing antibodies about 6 weeks after the onset of the disease.

RABIES (HYDROPHOBIA)

Rabies, the most feared of all zoonoses, has been a recognized disease of man since early times.[655] Spread to man may occur from a wide variety of warm-blooded animals which demonstrate variable susceptibility. Although this susceptibility is extremely high in such animals as foxes, jackals and wolves, it is only moderate in others including the dog. However, as man has a closer association with domestic animals, such as the dog, they provide a greater risk to him. In any particular geographical area, enzootic or epizootic infection may predominate in only one or two species of wild animal. In Central and South America the dominant animal is the vampire bat, in Russia the wolf, in North America the bat and skunk, and in Europe the fox.

Certain areas of the world are currently free of rabies including New Zealand, certain Pacific islands, parts of Scandinavia and the UK. In an attempt to retain this position, the movement of animals is governed by strict regulations including compulsory quarantine of animals, but such measures can be severely stretched. Enzootic rabies was eradicated from the UK in 1922, but fears exist that the current epizootic form amongst foxes in Europe, which has spread rapidly westwards over recent years, may result in the reintroduction of rabies.

Infection can follow the licking of abraded skin or mucosa by an infected animal as well as by a bite. Airborne infection from bats to man can also occur in caves where they are roosting. In most instances suspicion will arise that the animal concerned is rabid, especially where the furious form of the disease occurs. Should the less dramatic, dumb form occur, however, the true nature of the illness is not so readily suspected.

Clinical features

The incubation period may be as short as 10 days or as long as 7 years, but is usually between 1 and 3 months. Wounds on the hands, forearm and neck are especially dangerous and in them or where there is extensive biting at any site, the incubation period may be shortened. Age may also be a factor, and cases in young children tend to have a shorter incubation period.

The onset of clinical illness is heralded by a prodromal period of 2–7 days. Indefinite sensory changes may be experienced at the site of the bite, together with such nonspecific features as slight fever, headache, malaise, nausea and sore throat. Paresis and paralysis then develop and the muscles of deglutition go into spasm at any attempt to swallow (hence the term hydrophobia). Increasing depression and anxiety become apparent and the patient may become very withdrawn.

The disease may now enter a stage of excitement (furious rabies) with alternating manic activity and calm. The patient will remain lucid but fearful and the spasms in the throat become more violent. Cranial nerve palsies may develop and generalized convulsions become frequent. Death follows in virtually every case, from either cardiac or respiratory arrest. Less often the picture is not so florid and a progressive ascending paralysis occurs, giving rise to the so-called 'dumb' form of the disease.

Clinical diagnosis
A classical case, following a significant bite, provides a clearly recognizable clinical picture. Otherwise, forms of viral encephalitis, bulbar poliomyelitis, hysteria and tetanus may produce similar features and cause diagnostic confusion. Encephalitis can occur following antirabies vaccination with the old vaccines and produce a similar picture to that of rabies itself, but this has not been recorded following the human diploid cell vaccine.

Laboratory diagnosis
Rabies virus is probably not a single antigenic species and four rabies-related viruses are recognized. These agents have a marked predilection for nervous tissue but multiply in other organs such as the salivary glands. Within the nervous system the main pathological process is an encephalomyelitis leading to the development of inclusion bodies, particularly within the hippocampus. These inclusions are known as Negri bodies.

During life, the laboratory diagnosis of rabies depends on testing such specimens as saliva, CSF and conjunctival secretions by animal inoculation and immunofluorescent techniques. Viral antigens may be detected in skin biopsies. The rapidly fatal outcome, and the confusion which serum or vaccine can introduce, may render serological tests unhelpful.

If the suspected animal is available, it should be sacrificed and the brain examined for rabies virus antigens by hybridization techniques.

After death, specimens of brain tissue should be inoculated intracerebrally into mice. The specimens should also be subjected to rabies immunofluorescent tests and examined for Negri bodies. These tests should yield results within 1–2 days. However, if they are inconclusive, the results of mouse inoculation must be awaited, and it may take up to 3 weeks to declare this test negative.

Treatment
The treatment of clinical rabies is largely symptomatic, but intensive supportive therapy including artificial ventilation has been employed and at least two cases of proven rabies have survived following such measures. Appropriate steps must be taken to avoid possible spread to the attendants and to the immediate environment.

Postexposure prophylaxis
Local treatment of the wound. This can prove highly beneficial and should not be overlooked or delayed. Ideally wounds should be thoroughly cleansed using a 20% soap solution and after washing any residual soap away with water, a 0.1% quaternary ammonium compound such as cetrimide should be applied. Alternatives include 40–70% alcohol or tincture and aqueous solutions of iodine. Should none of these agents be immediately available, extensive cleansing with clean water should be used as early as possible and the chemical agents employed when practicable. Primary suturing of the wounds should be avoided and human rabies immunoglobulin (HRIG) should be infiltrated into the tissue beneath the wound. If there is any suspicion of exposure to tetanus, tetanus prophylaxis should be instituted.
Special systemic treatment. The aim of prophylaxis by vaccination is to induce a rapid antibody response which may prevent clinical disease developing. The human diploid vaccines are safe and highly effective. The site and frequency of injections for postexposure prophylaxis will depend on the vaccine used. If the human diploid cell vaccine is used, vaccination should commence as soon as possible after the incident and injections should be given by deep subcutaneous or intramuscular injection on days 0, 3, 7, 14 and 28. As antibodies do not develop for some days, immunoprophylaxis with HRIG should be given intramuscularly as well as infiltrating the wound[656] of those not previously immunized,

ideally within 24 hours. Treatment may be discontinued if the suspect dog or cat remains healthy after observation for 5 days. Other animals may require longer observation.

Pre-exposure prophylaxis
Prophylaxis by the human diploid cell rabies vaccine may be used for those at high risk of contracting rabies, e.g. laboratory staff or veterinary staff in endemic areas. Immunization is not routinely recommended for those visiting endemic areas.

NEURODEGENERATIVE VIRUS DISEASES
Subacute sclerosing panencephalitis (SSPE)
See Chapter 22 (Infectious and inflammatory disorders of the CNS).

Rubella panencephalitis
See Chapter 22 (Infectious and inflammatory disorders of the CNS).

Progressive multifocal leukoencephalopathy
This disease is a demyelinating disease caused by infection of astrocytes and oligodendrocytes with one of two papovaviruses, JC virus or simian virus 40 (SV40). The more common of the two to cause disease, JC, is named after the initials of the first affected patient, a 38-year-old man with Hodgkin disease who developed progressive multifocal leukoencephalopathy.

All cases have been in patients who are immunosuppressed, e.g. post renal transplant, have a malignant lymphoproliferative disorder or have a chronic disease such as tuberculosis or sarcoidosis. All areas of the brain and spinal cord may be affected. The usual presentation is early dementia with confusion, impaired cerebration and labile affect. Focal weakness often progresses to hemiparesis and later to bilateral long tract signs. Blindness, aphasia and ataxia are usual, with death occurring in less than 6 months. Detection of JC viral nucleic acid in the CSF by PCR analysis may be helpful in making the diagnosis of progressive multifocal leukoencephalopathy, but the sensitivity of the assay varies widely between laboratories.

PRION DISEASES: TRANSMISSIBLE SPONGIFORM ENCEPHALOPATHIES
The transmissible spongiform encephalopathies (TSE) of man are a rare, neurodegenerative, fatal group of disorders in which there is progressive degeneration of neurones with demyelination and gliosis of gray matter, causing a spongiform appearance of the brain, and the accumulation of a rare protein or prion (proteinaceous infectious agent). Their existence was first postulated by Pruisner in his analysis of the pathogenesis of scrapie in sheep.[657] Prions are thought to cause neuronal dysfunction and pathology when an alpha helical protease-sensitive form of the prion converts to a protease-resistant protein form associated with a structural predominance of beta sheet. Human TSE disorders include Creutzfeldt–Jakob disease (CJD), variant-Creutzfeldt–Jakob disease (v-CJD), Gerstmann–Straussler–Scheinker disease, kuru and fatal familial insomnia.[658] They closely resemble two animal diseases, scrapie and transmissible mink encephalopathy.

Kuru was the first TSE to be identified over 40 years ago. It was initially thought to be caused by a slow virus. In kuru, the cerebellum is most affected, and the disease is characterized by a progressive ataxia with a shivering tremor (the word 'kuru' means shivering). The incubation period is up to 20 years. It was acquired by the women and children of the Fore tribe in New Guinea who ate the brains of dead kinsfolk.

CJD is a progressive dementia with varying neurological features. Myoclonus, ataxic tremor, spasticity and parkinsonian features have all been described. CJD is sometimes familial. Cases have occurred in children who received human growth hormone from human pituitary extracts unwittingly infected with the agent and through brain and eye surgery.

The TSE of most relevance to pediatricians is v-CJD. It was first identified in the UK in 1996,[659] and there is evidence to suggest it is linked to exposure to tissues from cattle infected with bovine spongiform encephalopathy (BSE),[660,661] although the route of infection and indeed much about the natural history of this disease remains unclear despite analysis of the dietary history of people with v-CJD.[662] There appears to be a genetic component to the disease, as all patients identified to date are homozygous for methionine at codon 129 of the 'PRNP' gene.[658] v-CJD is distinguished from CJD by a younger age at onset and some distinguishing clinical features such as a psychiatric presentation, altered pain sensation and the absence of the periodic electroencephalographic complexes seen in CJD. Neurological signs such as ataxia and myoclonus occur later in the illness than in CJD. Amyloid plaques and bilateral, increased thalamic densities may be seen on MRI.

Treatment

No specific treatment for prion diseases is available. Supportive therapy is indicated for the sequelae of the neurodegeneration.

INFECTIONS DUE TO ENTEROVIRUSES

Poliomyelitis (infantile paralysis, acute anterior poliomyelitis)

Poliomyelitis has been a disease of man for many centuries, but has become more virulent since the late nineteenth century.

In the great majority of infected people, poliomyelitis is a harmless subclinical event; nevertheless, severe epidemics can arise with remarkable rapidity and the mortality and morbidity that result demonstrate that the fear in which the disease is held is well founded.

Epidemiology

Man appears to be the main reservoir of polioviruses in nature, although the great apes can also develop poliomyelitis. In temperate climates, epidemics occur in summer months. The large epidemics of the early 1950s were associated with a higher attack rate and greater severity in older children and young adults in countries with a high standard of living. A possible explanation was that improved hygiene standards led to a diminished rate of subclinical infection in infancy. In countries where vaccination rates are low, poliomyelitis is still primarily a disease of infants and young children.

The Expanded Program of Immunization of the World Health Organization, having as one of its goals global eradication of polio, has led to a steady decline in the world incidence of poliomyelitis since 1973, and a 95% decline in cases worldwide.[663] Intense wild-type poliovirus activity is now limited to the Indian subcontinent and sub-Saharan Africa.[663] In the rest of the world there are rare cases of vaccine-associated paralytic poliomyelitis attributable to the oral poliovirus vaccine.

Etiology

There are three strains, polioviruses types 1, 2 and 3, which show little antigenic overlap. They are particularly small RNA viruses. Poliovirus type 1 has been associated with most of the major epidemics and shows the greatest propensity to cause paralytic forms of the disease, whereas type 2 causes sporadic cases or small outbreaks with a low incidence of paralysis; type 3 occupies an intermediate position. Clinical severity is increased by age and pregnancy. Excessive muscular activity in a recently infected person makes a paralytic form of the disease more probable as do intramuscular injections into the limbs and other minor, traumatic procedures. Recent tonsillectomy predisposes to bulbar poliomyelitis and corticosteroid drugs can have an adverse effect. Antibody is clearly important as there is a higher incidence in patients with antibody deficiency.

The disease is spread by direct contact with infected persons through pharyngeal secretions and feces. Infectivity is probably maximal early, and oral–oral spread may be more common than fecal–oral spread.

Rarely paralytic poliomyelitis may result from oral vaccine strains which revert to virulence.

Pathogenesis and pathology

Polioviruses enter the body via the oral route and multiply in the tonsillopharyngeal tissues and intestinal wall. The virus passes to regional lymph nodes. Infectivity of the pharyngeal secretions disappears rapidly, but there is continued excretion into the bowel and polioviruses can be isolated from the feces for weeks and sometimes months.

The viruses probably pass to the bloodstream from the infected lymph nodes and can be isolated from the blood on occasion. The mode of passage thereafter to the nervous system is not fully understood.

In man, the pathological lesions in the CNS are mainly found in the anterior horns of the spinal cord but the posterior horns and intermediate columns may be involved. The essential lesion is neuronal damage, and though some neurones will die, others may recover. Meningitis occurs, and in some cases there is an extensive encephalitis involving motor cells in the medulla and pons, the vestibular nuclei and the motor and premotor areas of the cerebral cortex. Sometimes the lesions are concentrated in the medulla with little damage at lower levels in the cord.

Clinical features

Poliomyelitis is highly infectious and has an incubation period of 1–3 weeks. Most people infected will have an inapparent illness, which can only be demonstrated by retrospective serological surveys or by examination of contacts in the course of an actual epidemic. Paralytic disease virtually only occurs in unimmunized children or adults, as the virus still circulates in the community.

The minor illness. People infected by polioviruses may respond with a mild, insignificant illness whose features may include fever, anorexia, headache, lassitude and gastroenteritic symptoms. The title of 'abortive poliomyelitis' was sometimes used to describe this condition, now more commonly referred to as the minor illness.

The major illness (nonparalytic or preparalytic poliomyelitis). The major illness may immediately follow the minor or there may be a short gap of apparent recovery. Occasionally the minor illness does not occur.

In the preparalytic stage of the major illness, the symptoms simulate those of aseptic meningitis with neck stiffness and a positive Kernig sign. The patient has headache, vomiting, malaise, fever, and may develop pain and stiffness in the neck and back. Patients may also complain of an aching pain and spasm in the limbs.

Lumbar puncture normally shows a mild CSF pleocytosis (either polymorphonuclear or lymphocytic) and slight to moderate elevation of the protein content.

A variable percentage of cases presenting with this picture will gradually improve over the ensuing 7–10 days and thereafter make an uninterrupted recovery (nonparalytic poliomyelitis). Others, unfortunately, proceed to paralysis, starting some 2–3 days later. Occasionally, paralysis comes on earlier or the preparalytic stage is absent.

Paralytic poliomyelitis. *Spinal paralysis.* The cervical and lumbar segments of the cord are most frequently involved and patchy, asymmetric paralysis in the limbs results. This may be trivial and can be confined to part of one muscle group when it is easily overlooked. Unilateral involvement of the dorsiflexors of the feet, of the quadriceps or of the deltoids is a common finding. The paralysis is of lower motor neurone type.

Spinal respiratory paralysis. This form is usually associated with rapid, severe limb paralysis, and neuronal damage may then extend through the central part of the cord. Paralysis of the abdominal muscles may show itself by a weak cough. Lower intercostal involvement may be symptomless to the patient at rest and only evident to the examiner. Eventually such signs as tachypnea, tachycardia, cyanosis, a rising blood pressure and mental confusion will become apparent. In some instances, the signs of increasing ventilatory failure are difficult to distinguish from those of bulbar involvement or encephalitis, which can be present simultaneously.

Bulbar poliomyelitis. This form may be seen with unusual frequency in some epidemics and can be associated with recent tonsillectomy. Difficulty in swallowing is the cardinal sign and the subject is unable to clear mucus and saliva from the throat. There is a reluctance on the part of the patient to breathe deeply, in case secretions become aspirated into the lung. Such symptoms arise from pharyngeal involvement and further spread may cause weakness of the flexors of the neck, facial paralysis, external ocular palsies and, occasionally, true laryngeal paralysis. Extension to the respiratory center, with totally irregular breathing and periods of apnea, has a grave prognosis and involvement of the circulatory center will result in circulatory collapse and an irregular, rapid pulse. Involvement of these vital centers is usually fatal.

Vaccine associated paralytic poliomyelitis (VAPP). The World Health Organization defines VAPP as 'acute flaccid paralysis in a vaccine recipient 7 to 30 days after receiving oral polio vaccine, with no sensory or cognitive loss and with paralysis still present 60 days after the onset of symptoms'.[664] It occurs in about one case in every 750 000 first doses distributed,[665] and has led to reintroduction of the inactivated Salk vaccine into the routine immunization schedule in many industrialized countries including the USA, the UK and Australia.

Laboratory diagnosis

Isolation of poliovirus from the patient is the method of choice. Polioviruses grow well in a variety of tissue cultures, and if specimens are collected early in the illness, successful virus isolation is not difficult. Virus may be recovered from throat swabs early and from the feces for several weeks after the onset. CSF should be cultured for polioviruses but, unlike coxsackie and ECHO viruses, these are found infrequently.

Acute and convalescent samples of serum should be obtained and tested for a significant rise in antibody titer during the illness; tests for both complement-fixing and neutralizing antibodies are available.

Differential diagnosis

Paralytic poliomyelitis may be confused with a variety of disorders including Guillain–Barré syndrome, botulism, localized paralysis following specific infections such as mumps or infectious mononucleosis, paralytic episodes in sickle cell disease, myasthenia gravis and familial periodic paralysis.

Particular forms of poliomyelitis can be specially confusing, such as isolated facial paralysis which may mimic Bell's palsy, and bulbar paralysis which can be mistaken for tetanus. Pseudoparalysis may be found in acute rheumatism, osteomyelitis, fractures, scurvy, congenital syphilis and hysteria.

A true poliomyelitis-like illness can follow infection by other enteroviruses such as coxsackie, ECHO viruses and enterovirus type 71. Wherever possible, the diagnosis of any case of clinical poliomyelitis should be supported by virus isolation and positive serological tests.

Complications, course and prognosis

Nonparalytic poliomyelitis. There are no complications of nonparalytic forms of poliomyelitis. However, unsuspected paralysis may be detected in cases of this type once they become mobilized and this is particularly seen in the back muscles, the strength of which is difficult to assess whilst the patient remains in bed.

Spinal paralytic poliomyelitis. Some recovery may occur in the first 4 weeks following paralysis. Improvement thereafter is much slower. In muscles where the neuronal supply has been severely affected, permanent paralysis with extremely rapid wasting will result.

Spinal respiratory paralysis. At the height of the illness in this group, various cardiac irregularities and even cardiac failure may occur, secondary to the respiratory complications or as a direct effect of the virus on the myocardium.

Major complications include pneumonia, hypertension, urinary retention and constipation. Renal calculi are not uncommon.

Bulbar poliomyelitis. This form of poliomyelitis is of great seriousness if it spreads to the vital centers in the medulla. However, in those cases without involvement of these centers there is remarkably full and quite

rapid recovery of the cranial nerves. Involvement of the diaphragm may be permanent.

Late effects (post-polio syndrome). People with paralytic polio may develop new symptoms many years later, characterized by pain in muscles, weakness, fasciculation, breathlessness and problems with speech and swallowing. The mechanism is unknown.

Treatment

Spinal paralysis. The mainstay of therapy is physiotherapy, emphasizing passive movement, and hydrotherapy if available. Paralytic limbs should be supported and splinting may prevent contractures.

Patients may remain fecal excretors of poliovirus for several weeks and infection control precautions must be used.

In children, lack of growth in severely paralyzed limbs may lead to significant shortening, and skilled orthopedic advice is needed in such instances.

Spinal respiratory paralysis. Ventilatory support may be required and a constant watch for the incipient onset of respiratory insufficiency must be maintained. Late diagnosis may cause hypoxia and increased neuronal damage. Where respiratory paralysis is marked, ventilation is best achieved by the use of intermittent positive pressure ventilation combined with tracheostomy.

Bulbar poliomyelitis. Mild cases whose major defect is inability to swallow can often be managed conservatively with nasogastric tube feeding and suction of secretions. These patients often do well and undergo spontaneous recovery in 2–3 weeks. More severe cases require tracheostomy. Even in severe cases the prognosis is good and the tracheostomy can often be closed within a few weeks.

Prevention

Virtually all cases of paralytic poliomyelitis occur in children who have not been immunized. Poliomyelitis outbreaks are unlikely to occur in a community where a high level of protection by immunization is maintained. Active immunization can be produced by either killed virus vaccines (Salk type) or live attenuated virus vaccines (Sabin type). The former require to be given by injection and the latter by the oral route. A full primary course of either type involves three doses with a booster. In general, Sabin type vaccines result in higher humoral antibody levels, are easy and painless to administer and also produce local immunity in the gut. Children with immune deficiency are at increased risk of paralytic polio and should be immunized with the killed vaccine. Children with HIV infection can receive either live or killed vaccines, but if there is a relative at home with AIDS who might be infected by the vaccine virus, Salk (killed) vaccine should be given.

Non-polio enterovirus infections

The coxsackie and ECHO viruses, nonclassified enteroviruses and polioviruses are called enteroviruses and are classified with rhinoviruses into a larger group known as the picornaviruses (pico = small, RNA viruses). The agents in this group have a similarity in size, a similar nucleic acid core (RNA) and other common physical and chemical properties. Clinical and epidemiological studies show that the coxsackie and ECHO viruses are widely distributed in man and can cause a considerable variety of clinical syndromes. However, they have not demonstrated the same propensity to produce such large and serious epidemics as polioviruses.

Coxsackie virus infections

The existence of this group of viruses became apparent in 1948 when unidentifiable, filterable agents were isolated from the feces of two children in whom a clinical diagnosis of paralytic poliomyelitis had been suspected. These children resided in Coxsackie in New York State and the large group of similar viruses subsequently identified has been named after this town. At the present time there are approximately 30 different varieties of coxsackie viruses and these have been classified into two groups, known as A and B; 24 of the strains have been allocated to group A and the remaining 6 to group B.

Some, but not all, viruses of the coxsackie groups may be grown on suitable tissue cultures but all produce a characteristic histopathological effect when injected into suckling mice.

Coxsackie group A virus diseases

Relationship of group A viruses to disease. Viruses of this group may be isolated from a variable percentage of healthy individuals; as a result their isolation from a sick patient must not necessarily be construed as a diagnostic event.

Herpangina. This is one of the most clearly defined clinical syndromes caused by infection with coxsackie A viruses. It is most commonly seen in infants and children, though it can occur in adults. The onset is characterized by fever, anorexia and pain in the throat; other features include headache, abdominal pain and myalgia. Infection will normally derive from another human and the agent may be transmitted from nasal secretions as well as from the feces. The incubation period lies between 3 and 5 days and fecal infectivity may last for several weeks.

Local examination of the mouth will usually reveal hyperemia of the pharynx and characteristic papulovesicular lesions, approximately 1–2 mm in diameter and surrounded by an erythematous ring. Most commonly the lesions are present over the tonsillar pillars, soft palate and uvula, although the tongue may be involved. It is rare to find more than five to six lesions and these soon enlarge and form shallow ulcers. The illness will usually subside within a week and few complications are found in children. Second attacks may result from infection by different antigenic strains. The clinical picture is highly suggestive, but laboratory studies are required for full confirmation, and at least nine different group A viruses are known to produce this syndrome.

CNS involvement. Aseptic meningitis is the most common clinical manifestation and may result from infection by several different coxsackie A virus strains. As with other types of viral meningitis, young children are most likely to be involved and the incidence is rather higher in boys. There is no characteristic clinical picture that differentiates this from other causes of viral meningitis, although in a few instances one of the more specific syndromes associated with group A infection may be present simultaneously. On occasion non-polio enterovirus infection may be associated with paralytic disease that is clinically indistinguishable from poliomyelitis. Coxsackie virus A7 is the most frequently implicated, but other strains such as A9 have also been involved. Severe and fatal encephalitis has been described in a small number of cases of coxsackie A virus infection.

Hand, foot and mouth disease. Most cases of hand, foot and mouth disease are due to infection with coxsackie virus A16, but other coxsackie viruses (usually A5 and A10), ECHO viruses and enterovirus 71 have all caused cases or outbreaks.

Hand, foot and mouth disease usually presents with little or no constitutional upset. Reluctance to feed may be an early sign in babies. Examination of the mouth often shows mild ulceration of the tongue and pearly white vesicles, sometimes surrounded by a red halo, and further examination shows lesions on the palms and soles. The lesions are mainly found over the ventral surface of the fingers and toes and have a characteristic distribution along the sides of the feet. Some children also have a maculopapular rash over the buttocks which may extend on to the thighs and mimic Henoch–Schönlein purpura. Fever is rarely marked and there is little associated lymphadenopathy.

A fully developed case is extraordinarily characteristic and once seen is readily recognized thereafter. The mouth lesions can be confused with herpetic gingivostomatitis and herpangina as the peripheral lesions are painless and may be overlooked. An occasional case has been confused with scabies.

Outbreaks of this syndrome are usually small and tend to occur in the summer months. Subclinical infection of family contacts can be demonstrated by the isolation of viruses and the prognosis is excellent.

The association between HFM disease caused by enterovirus type 71 and brainstem encephalitis is described below.

Miscellaneous coxsackie A virus infections. Coxsackie A viruses have been isolated from children suffering from a febrile illness with a rash, from cases of pharyngitis and from cases of benign pericarditis. They have also been associated with mild undifferentiated respiratory tract infection, especially coxsackie A21 virus (previously known as Coe virus), with acute febrile lymphadenitis, gastroenteritis, tracheobronchitis and pleurodynia.

Laboratory diagnosis. The isolation of most coxsackie group A viruses is not difficult provided suitable specimens are sent to the laboratory. Suitable specimens include vesicle fluid, throat swabs, feces and CSF, depending on the clinical syndrome under investigation. Serological tests on acute and convalescent serum samples can be carried out, but owing to the large number of serotypes this is not a practical procedure unless an agent has been isolated. The coxsackie virus complement-fixation test frequently employed cross-reacts with all enteroviruses and is not very sensitive. Detection of viral RNA by PCR is now generally available and more sensitive than culture.

Coxsackie group B virus diseases

Bornholm disease or epidemic pleurodynia. This disease, first recognized clinically over a century ago, results from infection with certain group B coxsackie viruses. Children and young adults are usually involved and more severe cases occur in the latter.

After an incubation period of 2–4 days, the illness commences in a nonspecific manner with fever, malaise and headache. However, the characteristic pain will soon follow. This is principally experienced over the lower chest and may be associated with acute dyspnea. A clinical diagnosis of pleurisy can be made, even if no friction rub is audible and X-ray of the chest is clear. Pain may also be felt lower down the trunk and this may spread over the abdomen and simulate an acute surgical condition. Palpation over the affected muscles may reveal exquisite tenderness and this can have a band-like distribution suggestive of a neurological disorder or shingles.

In many instances the illness subsides within a few days but it may run a relapsing course and last for as long as 3–4 weeks. Several members of a family may be attacked in quick succession and show a wide variation in the severity.

Bornholm disease requires to be differentiated from pleurisy and pneumonia. Acute appendicitis and cholecystitis have been mimicked by an abdominal presentation but milder varieties, without significant pain, can be confused with influenza. In general, there is no significant leukocytosis and this may be helpful in the differentiation of pyogenic infection.

Outbreaks are small and often confined to family units. However, an epidemic can be more widespread and in these instances the correct clinical diagnosis may be made with reasonable accuracy. Nevertheless, full confirmation requires detailed virological assessment.

CNS involvement. All six group B coxsackie viruses can cause *aseptic meningitis*. The age incidence is similar to that encountered in aseptic meningitis due to other viruses. Clinical differentiation from other possible causes is impossible, although pleurodynia is an occasional accompaniment. Severe and fatal encephalitis has been described in only a small number of cases, as has mild paralytic disease.

Neonatal or infant coxsackie B virus myocarditis. Coxsackie viruses B1–5 can all cause myocarditis, but types B3 and B4 most frequently. The illness usually commences within the first 2 weeks of life though older babies have been involved. Most neonatal cases are probably caused by vertical spread from an infected mother, and a maternal history of respiratory or gastrointestinal illness is common. Nursery outbreaks can also occur.

Clinical features (see Ch. 21). The presentation can be abrupt or more insidious. Presenting symptoms include feeding difficulties, lethargy, fever, cyanosis, respiratory distress and shock. Cardiomegaly, tachycardia, hepatomegaly and electrocardiographic changes soon appear. Involvement may not be confined to the cardiovascular system. In up to one third of cases, there are central nervous signs such as convulsions, neck stiffness, and coma with CSF changes.

The prognosis is poor, and up to 75% of cases die in spite of intensive therapy. At autopsy an intense inflammatory infiltration and necrosis is found in the myocardium and changes may also be found in the liver, pancreas, suprarenal glands, bone marrow and CNS.

Differential diagnosis. Myocarditis is difficult to diagnose in a neonate. Most cases are initially considered to be some form of acute respiratory disorder (e.g. respiratory distress syndrome), other overwhelming infections or congenital heart disease.

Treatment. Infants with this condition require intensive nursing in hospital. Oxygen, diuretics and inotropes may be required. The heart is often very sensitive to digoxin and low doses may be needed if used.

Pericarditis and myocarditis due to coxsackie B viruses in older children. Acute pericarditis in older children and adults is a syndrome where the causative role of coxsackie B viruses (types B1–5) is well established. Less often, myocarditis may also occur in these age groups but, unlike infection in neonates, the prognosis is generally good. Clinical recovery is quite rapid and although the electrocardiographic changes can take some months to resolve, recovery seems complete and there is little evidence of any permanent cardiac damage. Rare cases of myocarditis are fulminant and fatal.

Miscellaneous coxsackie B virus infections. Group B coxsackie viruses can be associated with mild respiratory tract illness, febrile illness with an exanthem and orchitis. They are also reputed to cause endocardial fibroelastosis, the infection of the fetus occurring in utero.

Laboratory diagnosis. The six types of coxsackie group B viruses can be readily isolated in the laboratory either in tissue cultures or suckling mice. Virus can be grown from throat swabs, feces, CSF and in some cases from other organs, e.g. myocardium and testis. Acute and convalescent samples of serum should be sent to the laboratory so that, if present, a significant rise in antibody titer during the illness can be shown. Serological tests may be of special value if a coxsackie group B virus has been isolated as in this instance the sera need only be tested for an antibody rise against this specific isolate. In all cases it is advisable to try to isolate a virus from the patient as early in the illness as possible. Detection of viral RNA by PCR is available in many laboratories.

ECHO virus infections

Agents of this group are named after the initial letters of their original name, enteric cytopathogenic human orphan viruses. There are some 30 distinctive serotypes and their association with aseptic meningitis, encephalitis and paralytic diseases is well documented. They may also cause respiratory tract infections, gastroenteritis, myocarditis and exanthemata of a rather nonspecific character. Subclinical infection with this group is common. Infections may be sporadic or occur in moderate sized epidemics.

A number of different types of ECHO viruses have been associated with each of the various clinical syndromes that this group may cause and most types have been found in association with more than one syndrome. A few of the identified types have not, as yet, been found in association with obvious disease. In general, infection by this group of agents is relatively benign and, except in neonates, few fatalities have been described. They spread in a fashion similar to polioviruses and coxsackie viruses.

Clinical syndromes

A considerable number of different ECHO virus types can cause *aseptic meningitis*, which may be sporadic or in epidemics. In general, the prognosis is good and in many instances the cases are clinically indistinguishable from those produced by other viral infections. However, in some there is a rash and where this is seen in a reasonable proportion of cases in any outbreak of aseptic meningitis, it often indicates that an ECHO virus is responsible.

Sporadic cases of *poliomyelitis-like illness* with paralysis have been reported in association with confirmed ECHO virus infection. The paralysis is usually mild and reversible, but permanent residual paralysis can occur. Cases of *encephalitis* due to ECHO viruses have also been reported,

occasionally fatal. Children with antibody deficiency can get chronic ECHO virus encephalitis and/or myositis.

Mild upper respiratory illness has been found in association with a few ECHO viruses, particularly types 11, 19 and 20. ECHO viruses 5, 11, 14, 18, 19 and 20 have been associated with gastroenteritis in infants and young children.

ECHO viruses have been isolated in association with sporadic cases of pleurodynia, pericarditis and myocarditis. However, as these agents may be cultured from many otherwise healthy people their etiological relationship should not necessarily be assumed.

Where rashes do occur as a result of ECHO virus infection they tend to be of a fine, maculopapular character, have a widespread distribution and fade rapidly. Generally there is no classical distribution or typical enanthem, although lesions may be papular, arranged in lines and located peripherally, the so-called 'papular acro-located syndrome' (PALS).

Neonatal ECHO virus infection can disseminate and cause massive hepatic necrosis, disseminated intravascular coagulation, bleeding and usually death. Such severe cases are acquired vertically (from the mother) and a maternal history of peripartum illness with diarrhea or abdominal pain is common. Although nursery outbreaks may occur, most horizontally acquired or nosocomial cases are relatively mild, although occasionally complicated by meningitis and myocarditis.

Laboratory diagnosis

The ECHO viruses can be readily isolated in tissue culture, or enteroviral RNA can be detected by reverse-transcriptase PCR. Specimens usually required by the laboratory are CSF, throat swabs and feces depending on the clinical manifestations of the illness. Serology is not sufficiently sensitive to be useful clinically.

Enteroviruses types 68–71

In addition to the spectrum of symptoms outlined above, this group of enteroviruses is also associated with specific syndromes. Enterovirus type 70 has been isolated from patients with acute hemorrhagic conjunctivitis. Enterovirus type 71 (EV71) is associated with hand, foot and mouth syndrome. In Australia, Malaysia, Taiwan and Japan, outbreaks of EV71-associated hand, foot and mouth disease in children have been followed by severe neurological symptoms such as brainstem encephalitis often with neurogenic pulmonary edema, and by Guillain–Barré syndrome, acute transverse myelitis, cerebellar ataxia, opsomyoclonus, benign intracranial hypertension and febrile convulsions.

Treatment

No specific therapy is available. In a small, uncontrolled case series, the antiviral agent pleconaril was used in severe enteroviral infection in infants and immunocompromised children.[666] However, efficacy data from randomized controlled trials are as yet unavailable. Intravenous immunoglobulin and interferon have been used to treat chronic enteroviral infection in immunodeficient children. None of these agents is reportedly effective against EV71-associated disease.

VIRUSES AND THE GASTROINTESTINAL TRACT

Many viral agents may inhabit the intestinal tract without producing obvious clinical illness. As a result, when such agents are cultured in the presence of gastrointestinal symptoms, their etiological role is difficult to establish. Nevertheless epidemiological studies in the recent past seemed to indicate that some agents, such as certain ECHO viruses, may be involved in outbreaks of diarrhea in infants. The picture has, however, changed in the last few years as a wide variety of new viral agents has been discovered by electron microscopy of feces. Notable amongst these are *rotaviruses* and *noroviruses*, including *Norwalk virus*.

GASTROENTERITIS

Viruses associated with gastroenteritis include rotaviruses, noroviruses including Norwalk, caliciviruses, coronaviruses, astroviruses, adenoviruses, stool parvoviruses and enteroviruses. The role of rotaviruses and Norwalk virus is most clearly established, but other viruses can cause limited cases or outbreaks of infantile diarrhea.

Rotaviruses were initially found on electron microscopy of duodenal biopsies taken from children with diarrhea in Australia in 1973. Since then these agents have been found to be common worldwide and their presence may be detected by a variety of methods. Several different human types have been identified as well as many animal varieties. Species specificity appears incomplete.

Between 1 and 7 days after infection, but usually within 2 days, the affected child starts to vomit and develops a low grade fever. Watery diarrhea soon follows and, although mucus may be seen in the stools, blood is rarely present. The vomiting stops after 1–2 days, but diarrhea persists even if intravenous fluids are started with no oral intake. Nonspecific respiratory symptoms may occur and, although the illness terminates in about 5–7 days, virus may be found in the stool for up to 10 days.

The peak age of attack is between 6 and 24 months of age, mainly from 9 to 12 months. There is a slight male preponderance. Asymptomatic cases may be found in older members of the household. Neonatal infection occurs and has been associated with a clinical picture resembling necrotizing enterocolitis. However, neonatal infection is often subclinical, perhaps due to the presence of maternal antibody. It is suggested that breast-feeding can be protective.

Up to 50% of hospitalized cases of infantile gastroenteritis and a lower proportion of community cases are caused by rotaviruses.[667] Transmission is by the fecal–oral route. In temperate climates it is mainly a winter disease, although cases can occur throughout the year. Serological surveys show that up to 90% of children aged 3 years or over possess antibody to rotaviruses, and surveys in the adult population show figures of up to 70%.

Treatment of gastroenteritis due to rotavirus infection is along standard lines. Fatalities are rare in industrialized countries and usually in otherwise debilitated children. A variety of complications have been found but the role of rotaviruses in their production is not firmly established.

A tetravalent rotavirus vaccine was licensed in the USA in 1998 and introduced into the routine schedule. It was then voluntarily withdrawn from the market in 1999, due to a possible rare association with intussusception that was detected in post-licensing surveillance.[668] New rotavirus vaccines are safe and effective and have not been associated with intussusception.

The *Norwalk virus*, which was first discovered in 1972, and other caliciviruses are also known to produce gastroenteritis. Outbreaks have usually occurred in older children with secondary cases in adults, some involving schoolchildren and their teachers. These agents, first discovered in the USA and certain Far Eastern countries, are now found on a worldwide basis. After an incubation period of some 2 days the illness starts with nausea and vomiting. Diarrhea, abdominal cramps and fever follow in about half of those involved but symptoms usually abate within a day or so. Treatment is purely symptomatic.

Enteric adenoviruses are the second most important cause of viral diarrhea of infancy, in terms of hospitalization, and often cause prolonged diarrhea with or without vomiting. Astroviruses rarely result in hospital admission but can cause winter vomiting and may cause rare outbreaks in hospitals.

INTUSSUSCEPTION

Intussusception involves the invagination of a portion of the intestine into an adjacent portion. A study found *adenovirus infection* in 34% of Vietnamese and 40% of Australian children with intussusception, but no association with rotavirus, other enteric pathogens or oral polio vaccine.[669] It is thought that adenovirus infection causes inflammation of the Peyer's patches that acts as a focus for the intussusception. Adenoviruses have also been isolated from regional lymph glands in children with mesenteric adenitis and, as this condition is considered to be associated with the development of intussusception, the possible etiological role seems strengthened.

The association between intussusception and a live attenuated rotavirus vaccine, although not with wild-type rotavirus infection, is further evidence that intussusception may follow virus infections of the gastrointestinal tract.

OTHER CONDITIONS

Attempts to establish an association between viral infection and appendicitis have not proved very rewarding. Pancreatitis is a recognized complication of mumps and has occasionally been found in association with infection by coxsackie viruses.

LABORATORY DIAGNOSIS

In general, the main pathogens responsible for viral gastroenteritis, rotavirus, enteric adenoviruses, caliciviruses and astroviruses cannot be readily isolated by culture.[670] Although these agents may be demonstrated in stools by negative staining electron microscopy this has largely been replaced by enzyme immunoassays or PCR for rotavirus and enteric adenoviruses.

OCULAR DISEASES CAUSED BY VIRUSES AND ALLIED ORGANISMS

It is now recognized that viral and chlamydial infections of the eye constitute a larger proportion of ocular disease than was formerly appreciated. In part this stems from the enormous advances in viral technology but many ocular diseases are now recognized to have a viral basis because chemotherapy has cleared secondary bacterial infection and revealed the true, underlying viral pathogenesis.

In most instances viral infection of the eye presents as part of a systemic infection which may manifest itself by direct tissue invasion or indirectly through neural involvement, as in the viral encephalitides. Examples of viruses that may act this way are CMV and HSV in the congenitally infected or immunocompromised. However, some viral infections seem to involve the eye selectively, including certain adenoviral infections, trachoma, inclusion conjunctivitis and acute hemorrhagic conjunctivitis.

ADENOVIRUS INFECTIONS OF THE EYE

Two main ocular syndromes are associated with adenovirus infection – *pharyngoconjunctival fever* and *epidemic keratoconjunctivitis*.

Pharyngoconjunctival fever

Pharyngoconjunctival fever may result from infection by several types of adenoviruses, most commonly type 3. Clinically it may present as unilateral or bilateral follicular conjunctivitis, often with fever, pharyngitis and mild preauricular lymphadenopathy. The conjunctivitis shows follicular hypertrophy and a mild transient keratitis is sometimes develops.

Children are most often affected and cases may occur sporadically or in epidemics, sometimes associated with swimming pools.

Epidemic keratoconjunctivitis

This disease presents as an acute keratoconjunctivitis with follicular hypertrophy of the conjunctiva and marked preauricular lymphadenopathy. A distinctive keratitis then develops and about a third of the cases have pseudomembranes.

Large epidemics may occur and adults are involved rather than children. Infection is usually due to adenovirus type 8 and spread may occur through ocular instruments, infected eye-droppers and contaminated solutions used in hospitals, first aid stations and surgeries. Complete recovery usually occurs but permanent impairment of vision can occasionally result.

Laboratory diagnosis

Ocular infection with an adenovirus can be confirmed by culture or PCR. Swabs or scrapings in virus transport medium should be sent to the laboratory for virus isolation. The adenoviruses are not difficult to grow.

TRACHOMA AND INCLUSION CONJUNCTIVITIS (see Ch. 12)

Chlamydia have properties intermediate between viruses and bacteria, and show sensitivity to certain antibiotics. *Chlamydia trachomatis* is the cause of trachoma, inclusion conjunctivitis, afebrile pneumonitis and lymphogranuloma venereum.

Trachoma

Trachoma is a specific form of keratoconjunctivitis that first involves the upper tarsal follicles. Later upper limbal changes appear followed by pannus formation and the development of Herbert's peripheral pits. The disease is mainly encountered in tropical areas where water is scarce. In such areas there is often a very high incidence. Permanent scarring and blindness may occur, especially where adequate facilities for treatment are not available.

All ages are affected, but the disease is especially common in children and is often associated with secondary infection. Theories to explain the spread have included person-to-person contact, infection through fomites and dissemination by flies.

Treatment

Among drugs which may be used are sulfonamides, tetracycline and less often erythromycin. Opinions differ as to the efficacy and mode of treatment. However, where topical therapy is conscientiously applied over a period of several weeks or even months, a good response can be anticipated. Some advocate supplementation by oral therapy.

Inclusion conjunctivitis

This condition is caused by certain strains of *Chlamydia trachomatis* that may reside in the genital tract and produce cervicitis or urethritis. There is a danger of spread to infants during their passage through the birth canal, resulting in inclusion blennorrhea. Older children and adults may contract inclusion conjunctivitis from swimming pools contaminated by urine or genital tract discharge.

Treatment of inclusion conjunctivitis is also by sulfonamides or topical broad spectrum antibiotics. However, the response is quicker than in trachoma and treatment need not be so prolonged. The prognosis is also better and permanent scarring does not occur. Neonates with inclusion conjunctivitis should be treated with oral erythromycin 10 mg/kg/dose 6-hourly for 14 days because of the risk of progression to afebrile pneumonitis.

Laboratory diagnosis

The agents are situated in the epithelial cells of the conjunctiva, and for successful culture epithelial scrapings or eye swabs in special transport medium should be sent to the laboratory. Cultural methods consist of inoculation of suitable tissue cultures and then, after incubation, examination under the microscope for typical inclusion bodies. Direct microscopy on Giemsa-stained smears may reveal typical inclusions. ELISA antigen detection tests and PCR that avoid the need for culture and give a rapid diagnosis are increasingly being used.

ENTEROVIRUS 70 (ACUTE HEMORRHAGIC CONJUNCTIVITIS)

This condition is caused by enterovirus type 70, which has been isolated from the conjunctiva of affected patients. Extensive outbreaks have been reported from Africa, Pakistan, India and South America. The disease appears to have an incubation period of about 24 hours and to be highly contagious in unhygienic and crowded conditions. The infection is of sudden onset with swelling, congestion, watering and pain in the eye. The most characteristic sign is subconjunctival hemorrhage of varying intensity, which may sometimes be accompanied by corneal keratitis. The disease is not influenced by antibiotics and symptoms usually subside within 1–2 weeks.

Laboratory diagnosis

Conjunctival scrapings or swabs should be sent to the laboratory where suitable tissue cultures can be used to isolate the causative agent.

VIRAL INFECTION OF THE LIVER

Acute inflammation of the liver may be caused by a number of viruses including hepatitis viruses A to E, CMV, adenoviruses, picornaviruses, HSV, EBV and the viruses of diseases such as yellow fever and rubella.

HEPATITIS A VIRUS INFECTION OR INFECTIOUS HEPATITIS (EPIDEMIC HEPATITIS, EPIDEMIC JAUNDICE OR CATARRHAL JAUNDICE)

This disease has an incubation period of 15–50 days (average 30 days) and is mainly found in young children. It is also quite common in older children and young adults but the attack rate declines with increasing age though a higher proportion of severe and complicated cases may be found in these older age groups. Pregnant women may contract a particularly severe form.

Infectious hepatitis occurs worldwide and epidemic periodicity varies greatly in different communities. The responsible agent, hepatitis A virus, is present in both blood and feces at the peak of the illness and persists in the feces for a relatively short time. Susceptible human volunteers have been fed filtered fecal extracts and virus could be found in the feces of those who developed jaundice from 14 to 26 days before the onset of icterus and for over a week thereafter. Furthermore, although at least two thirds of the recipients displayed no clinical evidence of hepatitis, subclinical evidence of infection was found on serial examination by appropriate liver function tests. This indicates a ratio of 1:2 for clinical, as opposed to subclinical, infection and this impression is further substantiated by epidemiological studies in naturally occurring epidemics.

Although infectious hepatitis is mainly transmitted by the fecal–oral route through contamination of food and water, transmission may also occur from blood, urine, nasopharyngeal secretions and saliva. Large epidemics usually occur in institutions and closed communities and, in some of these, infection of a communal water supply has been responsible. Prevention of waterborne outbreaks of this type is difficult, although carefully controlled super-chlorination may be effective. Outbreaks have also followed the ingestion of raw oysters and raw clams infected by sewage. Infection may also result from the use of imperfectly sterilized instruments, syringes and needles that have been contaminated by infected blood or blood products.

The diagnosis, differential diagnosis and detailed treatment of infectious hepatitis are referred to elsewhere (Ch. 19). Complement-fixation tests, immune-adherence hemagglutination, ELISA and radioimmunoassay can be used to detect specific IgM and IgG antibody to hepatitis A virus. The presence of specific IgM antibody indicates a recent infection with hepatitis A virus. In the majority of childhood cases the illness is mild and treatment need not extend beyond simple bed rest and a moderate period of convalescence.

Mortality amongst otherwise healthy, well-nourished individuals is as low as 0.1–0.2% but can rise to 2 or 3% in the poorly nourished. Death may either be early from fulminating hepatitis leading to acute hepatocellular failure or occur considerably later from chronic liver damage.

Prevention

Killed vaccines are safe and effective,[671] and indicated for older children and adults at long term risk. Human normal immunoglobulin is effective prophylaxis and should be given to adult and child contacts of index cases and to people traveling for short periods to areas with poor sanitation.

HEPATITIS B (SERUM HEPATITIS, AUSTRALIA ANTIGEN-POSITIVE HEPATITIS)

Hepatitis B is enormously important. Worldwide, there are about 200 million chronic carriers of hepatitis B virus (HBV), which is one of the most important causes of liver cirrhosis and hepatoma. HBV can be transmitted either vertically (mother to child) or horizontally (from an infectious contact). Infection is endemic in some parts of the world, notably South East Asia where carriage rates may exceed 15%. About half of all carriers will die liver-related deaths.

The incubation period is 60–160 days, much longer than hepatitis A. Virus antigen can be detected in the blood up to 3 months before jaundice occurs and often for many years after clinical recovery. The virus is mainly transmitted via infected blood and is highly infectious, far more so than HIV. Infected blood transfusions, needle sharing by intravenous drug abusers, tattooing and ritual scarification are all well-documented means of spread. The virus can be sexually transmitted and the incidence is high in many homosexual communities. Vertical spread is common and is thought to be mainly peripartum rather than transplacental, thus being largely preventable by intervention immediately after birth. Most vertically infected babies become chronic carriers. About a quarter to a third of asymptomatic HBV carriers remain infectious and go on to develop liver fibrosis[672] or carcinoma (hepatoma).[673,674] The virus is also found in breast milk, although breast-feeding has not been shown to be a clear risk factor for transmission. Clinical features of hepatitis B infection are discussed elsewhere.

Etiology

In 1965, geneticists investigating inherited variations in human plasma proteins discovered an unusual protein antigen in the serum of an Australian aborigine. This antigen, originally called Australia antigen (Au), and now hepatitis B surface antigen (HBs), was found to be associated with hepatitis of long incubation. On electron microscopy of serum three particles are identifiable. Dane particles, 42 nm in diameter, are complete virus comprising an inner core containing double-stranded HBV DNA within a core antigen (HBc) and surrounded by an outer coat of surface antigen (HBs). A further antigen, the e antigen, a component of the inner core, may also be seen (Fig. 28.43). The detection of e antigen in the absence of e antibody correlates with high infectivity. Subjects may be:

1. HBs antigen positive, with no e antigen or e antibody detected – these will be mainly chronic carriers;
2. HBe antigen positive, but e antibody negative – usually also HBs positive – are highly infectious: usually suggests recent, active infection, but can be chronic HBe Ag positive carriers;
3. HBe antibody positive – recovery phase, much less infectious.

Tests commonly used to detect the presence of HBV antigens and antibodies include hemagglutination tests and ELISA tests, which are often used to screen sera for surface antigen (HBs), and radioimmunoassays which are more sensitive.

Detection of HBs antibody indicates either recovery from acute HBV infection or a response to immunization. Presence of HBc IgM antibody indicates acute HBV infection, while HBc IgG antibody is detected following infection but not immunization (which uses only surface antigen).

Prevention

In many countries, blood or blood product donations are routinely screened for surface antigen (HBs) and antenatal screening of all pregnant women or those from high risk groups allows intervention to prevent vertical transmission. Great care should be taken when handling blood and excreta from HBV positive patients because of the high infectivity, although any person doing so should have been immunized.

Passive immunization with specific immunoglobulin is given for accidental contamination with infected blood, e.g. in the laboratory or from a syringe and needle from a drug abuser. It reduces vertical transmission if given to infected mothers in the first 72 h (ideally < 12 h) after birth.[675] There appears to be no additional benefit by giving further doses of HBV immunoglobulin beyond the newborn period.[675]

Recombinant DNA hepatitis B vaccines are now widely available. All health care personnel likely to come into contact with HBV positive patients (e.g. doctors, dentists, nurses, midwives, students, laboratory staff) should receive a course of three doses of the vaccine.

Babies of mothers who are in the above risk groups 1 (HBs positive) and 2 (HBe antigen positive) are at high risk of becoming chronic carriers without intervention. Indeed this will be the case in up to 90% of babies of HBe antigen positive mothers. Such babies should receive both passive HBV specific immunoglobulin and be actively immunized with hepatitis B vaccine, which provides additional protection against vertical transmission over HBV immunoglobulin alone.[675] Babies of mothers in group 3 (HBe antibody positive) are at lower risk but may rarely develop acute hepatitis, and there is a risk of later horizontal transmission from the mother or an infected sibling. They should therefore be immunized and many would feel they should also receive specific immunoglobulin.

Many countries are now advocating universal neonatal hepatitis B immunization.

Treatment

Pegylated interferon alpha and lamivudine have been used in the treatment of chronic hepatitis B disease in adults, and shown to be effective at reducing HBV viral load and inducing HbeAg seroconversion in some patients.[676,677] Lamivudine has been given to HBV infected women in the last weeks of pregnancy to reduce the risk of vertical transmission with variable success.[678] The use of these agents for the treatment of chronic HBV infection in children has also been reported in small case series,[679] but the efficacy of these therapies has not been fully evaluated.

HEPATITIS C (TRANSFUSION-ASSOCIATED NON-A, NON-B HEPATITIS)

Hepatitis C virus is a small single-stranded RNA virus that is a member of the flavivirus family. It is the cause of the great majority of transfusion-associated hepatitis.

The structure of hepatitis C virus (HCV) was determined by molecular biology techniques in 1988. There are multiple HCV genotypes and subtypes, each of which carries a different long term prognosis. Serological tests have been developed to screen blood products, and PCR testing for the presence of viral nucleic acid is widely available. The virus is extremely difficult to grow.

HCV has an incubation period of around 30–60 days. Transmission is mainly via blood transfusion or by needle sharing between intravenous drug abusers. Screening of donated blood for the presence of hepatitis C antibodies has greatly reduced the risk from blood transfusion. HCV

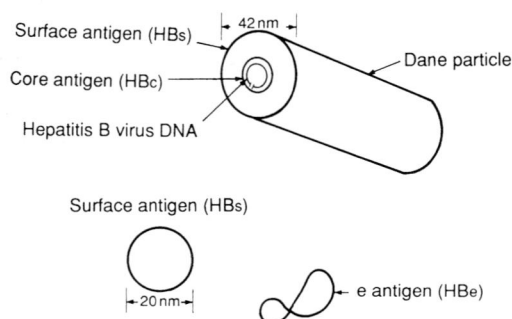

Surface antigen (HBs)
Core antigen (HBc)
Hepatitis B virus DNA
42 nm
Dane particle

Surface antigen (HBs)
20 nm
e antigen (HBe)

Fig. 28.43 Diagrammatic representation of electron microscopic appearance of hepatitis B virus.

is more resistant to inactivation than HBV or HIV, and blood products such as intravenous immunoglobulin have occasionally transmitted HCV despite viral inactivation steps.

Vertical transmission from mother to fetus occurs in about 5% of pregnancies, and is thought to occur antenatally or perinatally almost exclusively in the setting of high maternal viral load in the serum. Maternal co-infection with HIV is associated with a higher risk of transmission.[680] Other risk factors have been poorly defined. As yet unconfirmed associations include prolonged rupture of membranes, and invasive fetal monitoring[681] and female sex of the infant.[682] Elective Cesarean section does not confer protection from vertical transmission.[682] HCV RNA and antibody have been detected in breast milk,[683] although breast-feeding has not been shown to be associated with transmission to the infant by hepatitis C positive women.[684] Nevertheless, a theoretical risk remains and the decision of a hepatitis C positive woman whether to breast-feed should be made on an individual basis. The diagnosis of perinatally acquired HCV is usually based on the detection of HCV antibody and/or HCV RNA by PCR. The presence of maternal antibody makes interpretation of serological assays difficult in children less than 18 months. At 12 months, up to 10% of uninfected children remain HCV seropositive, but this figure has dropped to 0.1% by 18 months.[685] PCR for HCV RNA is sensitive over 1 month of age and is specific, but the test is expensive. Any positive PCR test should be repeated to exclude false positive results, and because of the possibility of viral clearance.[685]

Childhood HCV infection is largely asymptomatic,[686] but a high proportion of those infected with HCV become chronic carriers and may progress to cirrhosis. A large cohort study from Italy of HCV infected children has shown a shift in the dominant HCV genotype from genotypes 1 and 2, associated with poorer response to therapy and reduced viral clearance, to genotypes 3 and 4, with genotype 3 associated with a better prognosis.[687] Nevertheless, it is estimated that childhood HCV disease will have an important economic impact on direct medical costs in the next decade, as the burden of pediatric HCV infection increases.[688] Interferon alfa therapy alone or with ribavirin is effective in reducing viral replication in around 40% of adult chronic carriers, although half of these responders will relapse when interferon is stopped. Experience with the use of these agents in HCV infected children is increasing. Treatment may be considered for the child with severe hepatitis C induced liver disease, which should be managed by a pediatric hepatologist.[689]

Children with hepatitis C infection should be immunized against hepatitis A and hepatitis B to protect against further insults to the liver.

DELTA AGENT (HEPATITIS D)

The delta agent is a defective RNA virus which requires HBV for its own synthesis. This is one of the most important examples of viral co-infection described. The delta agent was detected by immunofluorescence studies of liver cell nuclei of chronic HBV carriers. Delta antigen and antibody are detected by radioimmunoassay or ELISA and have never been demonstrated other than in association with HBV. The delta agent is most prevalent in intravenous drug abusers in Italy and the Mediterranean but has been detected worldwide. It appears to be a risk factor for acute hepatitis in drug abusers. About half of HBs positive hemophiliacs in the USA and Italy have anti-delta antibodies.

HEPATITIS E (ENTERIC NON-A, NON-B HEPATITIS)

Hepatitis E is the enterically transmitted form of non-A, non-B hepatitis and is transmitted by the fecal–oral route. It is of major importance in resource limited countries as a cause of hepatitis due to waterborne epidemics, which mainly affect young adults, but rarely children. The mortality can be as high as 40% in pregnant women. The viral genome has been cloned and sequenced, and serological tests and PCR assays are available.

HEPATITIS G

This single-stranded RNA virus of the flavivirus family usually results in an asymptomatic infection. It can cause chronic infection, but rarely hepatitis. It has been documented in adults and children, especially those whose mothers are co-infected with HCV or HIV.[690] It can be diagnosed by detection of viral RNA by PCR.

HEPATITIS – THE ROLE OF OTHER VIRUSES

Other viral infections may involve the liver.

CMV is known to attack the liver in 85% of newborn infants suffering from cytomegalic inclusion disease; the same virus may also cause hepatitis when older children or adults contract the acquired form of the infection. *Infectious mononucleosis*, due to EBV, is frequently accompanied by some degree of liver involvement; most often this will reveal itself as a mild derangement of liver function tests though some cases will manifest obvious jaundice. Infection by *arboviruses* may cause a similar picture; yellow fever produces a more specific and severe form of hepatitis.

HSV infection of the newborn can manifest as severe and often fatal hepatitis.

Lastly, there are instances where transient liver involvement has been found in a variety of viral infections including ECHO viruses types 4 and 9, coxsackie viruses, adenoviruses and lymphocytic choriomeningitis virus. In most the involvement has been extremely mild with full recovery, although severe hepatitis may occur.

MISCELLANEOUS VIRAL INFECTIONS

ORF (CONTAGIOUS PUSTULAR DERMATITIS OF SHEEP, CONTAGIOUS ECTHYMA OF SHEEP)

This is a common and widespread viral infection of sheep and to a lesser extent of goats. In general infection is from animal to animal but virus can persist in the soil of affected pastures for several months. Lambs are most commonly involved and they develop a papulovesicular eruption on the mouth, lips and non-hair-bearing areas of the skin. Transmission to man is relatively rare and the main incidence is in springtime. The infection is most commonly encountered in shepherds, farm and abattoir workers. However, children can be infected owing to their liking for handling young lambs.

Orf virus is included amongst the poxviruses and has certain similarities to the virus of molluscum contagiosum. It can be grown with difficulty on tissue culture but is usually identified by electron microscopy. Scrapings from the base of the bullae are preferred to vesicle fluid in these studies.

Clinical features

Lesions, which are usually but not exclusively single, most commonly appear on the hand or forearm. Initially there is an area of infiltration presenting as brawny edema but this soon develops into a flaccid bulla. However, on puncture a rather clear serosanguinous fluid is obtained. There is little or no constitutional upset but the progression of the lesion is slow and may take 6–8 weeks before it finally heals. No specific treatment is available or required in view of the benign nature of the condition but it is wise to protect the lesion with dressings to counteract the possibility of secondary infection.

MOLLUSCUM CONTAGIOSUM

This viral disease (see also Ch. 30) is seen in children more often than in adults. The responsible agent is a DNA virus belonging to the pox group but serologically unrelated to vaccinia or variola; it is readily identified by electron microscopy of the curettings from a lesion or on the histological appearances of a biopsy. Transmission is by close contact but infectivity is low.

Clinical features

Molluscum contagiosum is unassociated with any constitutional upset and presents as a chronic viral infection of the epidermis. Lesions, which may be multiple, take the form of pinkish white or flesh-colored, dome-shaped nodules between 2 and 8 mm in diameter and most show a central depression or umbilication. They may appear on the face, arms, legs, buttocks, scalp or genitalia but sparing of the palms of the hands and the soles of the feet is a characteristic feature. Occasionally the margins of the eyelids are involved and chronic follicular conjunctivitis can supervene (Fig. 28.44). HIV infection may be associated with disseminated molluscum.

Treatment

The disease is benign and self-limiting. Treatment is advised only to prevent spread by autoinoculation or to others. Treatment is simple and consists of the removal of the lesions with a sharp curette. Other methods include electro- or cryocautery. The lesions will usually heal without scarring and recurrence is rare.

TRANSFUSION TRANSMITTED (TT) VIRUS

TT virus is a DNA virus that was first identified in 1997 in the serum of a patient with post-transfusion hepatitis of unknown etiology.[691] To date, there has been no disease association with this virus. It can be detected in the serum of 2% of healthy blood donors in the UK, and can be transmitted by transfusion, by fecal–oral spread and vertically.[692]

ARENA VIRUSES CAUSING HEMORRHAGIC FEVER

Lassa fever

Lassa fever was first reported from Lassa in Nigeria in 1969. The Lassa virus shows some morphological and antigenic similarities to lymphocytic choriomeningitis virus. It is one of the arenaviruses and it is widely distributed throughout West Africa. It is one of five African viruses (yellow fever, Lassa, Ebola, Marburg and Congo-Crimean) that cause hemorrhagic fever. The natural host is the rat *Mastomys natalensis*.

The virus is transmitted from person to person by close contact. It causes a diffuse serositis, hemorrhage and shock and is often fatal. Intravenous ribavirin reduces mortality from Lassa fever and is the treatment of choice. Additional treatment involves the use of plasma from a convalesced patient. For the adult 250–500 ml are used. Stocks of this are held in Nigeria, Sierra Leone, the London School of Hygiene and Tropical Medicine and the Communicable Disease Center, Atlanta, Georgia, USA. Strict isolation of patients is mandatory.

Marburg virus disease (green monkey disease, vervet monkey disease, Jo'burg virus disease)

Marburg virus disease was first recognized in Germany in 1967 in personnel who had handled a consignment of African green monkeys

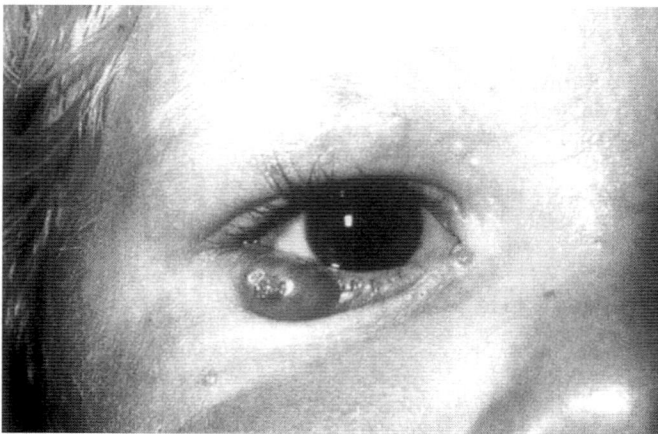

Fig. 28.44 Molluscum contagiosum.

(*Cercopithecus aethiops*) from Uganda. Outbreaks have occurred in Sudan and Zaire. The Marburg virus is long, rod shaped (rhabdovirus-like) and does not appear to possess antigenic affinity with other known viruses. Although the Marburg outbreak appeared to follow contact with African green monkeys, no similar infections have been recognized as a result of other contacts with these monkeys and such monkeys suffer 100% mortality if experimentally infected. Thus the natural host and possible vectors are unknown.

The disease is highly infectious and carries a high mortality: 7 of the 31 Marburg cases died. Secondary cases appear to have a better prognosis than primary cases. There is as yet no protective vaccine. Strict isolation and barrier nursing of patients is necessary.

Ebola virus disease

This disease is clinically indistinct from Marburg virus disease. The virus is morphologically identical to the Marburg virus, but antigenically distinct. The disease has been found in the Sudan and Zaire.

INFECTIONS DUE TO ARBOVIRUSES (TOGAVIRUSES)

The principal feature linking the viruses of this group is the fact that all are arthropod borne (hence the name) and well over 200 such agents have been recognized. Most viruses in this group are natural parasites of animals or birds and multiply in arthropod vectors, which are unharmed by the process. Infection in the human may take several forms; most commonly encephalitis of varying severity results. Other diseases produced include yellow fever, dengue and sandfly fever. Arboviruses may also result in mild influenza-like illness. Children are particularly susceptible to this group of diseases. The arboviruses are subdivided into a number of families: Bunyaviridae (sandfly fever virus, Hantaviruses), Togaviridae (western equine encephalitis virus, eastern equine encephalitis virus), Flaviviridae (yellow fever virus, dengue viruses, West Nile virus), Reoviridae and Rhabdoviridae. They may also be classified according to the clinical syndromes they produce.

Arboviruses group A

Some 20 arboviruses are included in this group, the best known being the viruses of eastern and western equine encephalitis, and more recently West Nile virus.[693] These present in humans as aseptic meningitis or meningoencephalitis of varying severity. Children tend to be more seriously affected and death may result. Those who survive the illness may have permanent mental retardation, deafness, epilepsy and paralysis. Mortality may vary with age and the responsible virus. On average, 5% of patients may die, but this figure is often considerably higher following infection by certain viruses, reaching 74% in eastern equine encephalitis.

Other viruses of this group produce a mild dengue-like illness and most have their animal reservoir in wild or domestic birds. Their arthropod vectors are culicine and anopheline mosquitoes.

Arboviruses group B

This, a larger group, can be divided into (1) *mosquito-borne* and (2) *tick-borne* sections. The best-known disease associated with the former is yellow fever. The latter are mainly associated with a variety of encephalitic illnesses.

Yellow fever (yellow jack)

Yellow fever has been a recognized clinical entity for over 300 years, and in 1881 Carlos Finlay suggested that *Aedes aegypti* spread the infection. This theory was substantiated by the classical studies of Walter Reed and his colleagues working on mosquitoes and yellow fever in Cuba.[694] Yellow fever occurs in parts of Africa, South America and central America, but not Asia. The last cases of infection acquired in the UK occurred in the latter part of the nineteenth century, when ships arrived carrying infected *A. aegypti*.

Disease may vary from a mild fever to a fulminant hepatitis with jaundice, hepatic necrosis, hemorrhage and shock. In the jungle it is predominantly an adult disease. Where infection occurs in an urban community, all ages and both sexes are equally affected.

There is no specific treatment.

Elimination of the responsible vector is of prime importance and infection has been eradicated from certain areas where this has been diligently performed. Vaccination with the 17 D attenuated strain of virus is compulsory for travel to endemic areas and immunity will usually last for up to 6 years. Complications of immunization are confined to an occasional case of benign encephalitis, usually encountered in young infants, and the vaccine is not recommended under 9 months of age if exposure to mosquitoes can be avoided.

Dengue fever

Dengue fever is mosquito-borne like yellow fever, is also caused by a virus from group B, and the same vector, *A. aegypti*, is involved. The disease is widespread and is mainly found in warm areas, including Australia, Greece, Japan, India, Malaysia and Hawaii. So far, four antigenic varieties, known as types 1, 2, 3 and 4 have been described.

Clinical features. There is an incubation period of 5–9 days. The illness starts with high fever, malaise, headache, pain in the eyes, backache and excruciatingly painful limbs (it is sometimes called breakbone fever). Between the third and fifth days, a maculopapular, scarlatiniform or petechial rash appears and lasts up to 4 days. Following this there is usually a rapid recovery. Occasionally, however, particularly in children, the disease progresses to a severe hemorrhagic form, dengue hemorrhagic shock syndrome (DHSS), which may be fatal (see Hemorrhagic fevers below). It is thought that DHSS follows prior sensitization with a different strain of dengue virus, and is an example of antibody-mediated enhancement of disease.

Control. Eradication of the vector is desirable. Dengue viruses are poor antigens, which has frustrated efforts to produce effective vaccines.

Hemorrhagic fevers

A number of virus infections may occur in a hemorrhagic form, e.g. Lassa fever, yellow fever and measles. The arboviruses, particularly the Chikungunya (group A) and dengue (group B) viruses, are also prone to cause hemorrhagic disease. Hemorrhagic fever due to the mosquito-borne Chikungunya virus has been reported in Africa, India and Thailand. In South East Asia, hemorrhagic fever due to dengue virus is transmitted by the bite of the *A. aegypti* mosquito which is common in urban areas.

The hemorrhagic fevers affect mainly children. Patients develop fever, erythematous or petechial rashes, hepatosplenomegaly and bleeding that may be mild or severe. The majority of patients recover, but some develop shock and die. Thrombocytopenia is common. In fatal cases there are gross effusions into the serous cavities, petechial hemorrhages on the surface of organs and bronchopneumonia. Treatment is symptomatic. In shocked cases, intravenous plasma should be administered, together with the usual measures for collapsed patients.

Hemorrhagic fever with renal syndrome

This name is used for several similar conditions including Korean hemorrhagic fever and nephropathica epidemica occurring in Scandinavia, central Europe, Russia, China, Japan and Korea.[695] At least two viruses, Hantaan (Hantavirus) and Puumala, transmitted by arboviruses from rodents, are implicated. The clinical manifestations are fever, shock, massive proteinuria followed by acute renal failure, and thrombocytopenia and bleeding with bruising, hematuria, hematemesis and melena. With supportive treatment, the mortality is low.

Tick-borne arbovirus infections

These including louping ill (a disease of sheep in Scotland and northern England; rarely aseptic meningitis can occur if man is infected by an infected tick), Russian spring–summer encephalitis (western and eastern forms), Omsk hemorrhagic fever and Kyasanur Forest fever. Illness associated with this group may range from aseptic meningitis to severe and even fatal encephalitis, although the prognosis is better than with

infection by group A strains. On occasion paralytic disease simulating poliomyelitis can occur and Omsk fever is usually characterized by bronchopneumonia and hemorrhage from various orifices.

Arboviruses group C and unclassified arboviruses

Group C, comprising seven viruses, is responsible for influenza-like illness in parts of South America. Amongst the unclassified infections, sandfly fever is perhaps the best documented illness.

Sandfly fever (phlebotomus fever, papataci fever)

This illness results from infection by one of the unclassified arboviruses. It is relatively common in countries bordering the Mediterranean and occurs in parts of Africa, Russia, India and China. The responsible vector *Phlebotomus papatasii*, often called sandfly, is extremely small and may pass through mosquito nets. Infection in these sandflies may be permanent, due to trans-ovarian infection, and no definite animal reservoir is known. Several different strains of virus have been isolated with established immunological variation.

Clinical features. The incubation period is 3–7 days. Onset is sudden and rigors may occur. Headache, pain behind the eyes, muscular aching and fever are typical features. Occasionally photophobia, neck and back stiffness occur and mimic meningitis. After 3 or 4 days there is an abrupt termination by crisis. Severe apprehension often accompanies this illness and acute depression may follow an attack for a short time. Leukopenia is common. A clinical diagnosis is readily made in endemic areas or during an outbreak.

There is no specific treatment and the prognosis is good. Control is confined to attempts at eradication of the vector in its breeding grounds.

RICKETTSIAL INFECTIONS

Rickettsial infection in man produces a number of different diseases, spread over a wide geographical area. The resultant illnesses have certain basic similarities and all but one are characterized by some form of skin eruption. Definitive clinical diagnosis can be difficult and confirmatory laboratory tests are desirable. A simple classification of rickettsial infection is shown in Table 28.36.

Rickettsiae have biophysical properties that place them in an intermediate position between viruses and bacteria and are small coccobacilli, usually less than half a micrometer in diameter, with rigid cell walls. They contain both RNA and DNA, but are obligate intracellular parasites and are sensitive to certain antibiotics.

LABORATORY TESTS

Procedures to isolate the causative organisms exist, but should only be undertaken by a laboratory well equipped to deal with the risks involved. In view of the hazards involved in isolation, serological methods of diagnosis are usually employed.

The Weil–Felix agglutination reaction, used for several years, depends on the fact that patients with certain rickettsial infections develop agglutinins in their serum during the illness which agglutinate some strains of Proteus organisms, namely OX 19, OX 2 and OXK. There are now a number of other serological assays available in specialist reference laboratories. If possible, paired sera should be examined in the Weil–Felix test, but agglutinins may appear as early as the fifth or sixth day after the onset of the fever and usually reach a peak during the second or third week. Detection of rickettsial DNA in the blood or tissue by PCR may allow the diagnosis to be made earlier in the illness.

TYPHUS FEVER (EPIDEMIC LOUSE-BORNE TYPHUS FEVER)

Historical writings suggest that typhus fever (classical or historic typhus) has been a scourge of humanity for many centuries. Typhus fever and war are inextricably linked. Although the responsible agent may be endemic in many parts of Europe, serious epidemics only arise

Table 28.36 Rickettsial diseases: causal agents, vectors, reservoirs and differential Weil–Felix reactions

	Disease	Causal rickettsiae	Principal vectors	Animal reservoir	Geographic occurrence
Typhus	Epidemic (louse-borne typhus)	R. prowazekii	Lice	Man	Worldwide
	Brill–Zinsser disease	R. prowazekii	–	Man	Worldwide
	Endemic murine (flea-borne) typhus	R. mooseri	Fleas	Rats	Worldwide
	Scrub typhus (mite-borne) (Tsutsugamushi fever)	R. tsutsugamushi	Mites	Small rodents	Japan, South East Asia, Pacific
Spotted fevers	Rocky Mountain spotted fever	R. rickettsii	Ticks	Small rodents	East and west USA
	Mediterranean fever (fièvre boutonneuse)	R. conorii	Ticks	Small rodents and dogs	Mediterranean, Caspian and Black Sea, Africa, South East Asia
Rickettsialpox		R. akari	Mites	House mice	USA, Russia, Korea
Q fever	Query fever	R. burnetii	Occasionally ticks	Cattle Sheep Goats Bandicoots	Worldwide

during times of war or in their aftermath, due entirely to the increased infestation by lice that occurs in these periods. Epidemics occur chiefly in winter when people are crowded together for warmth and shelter, enhancing chances of spread of the louse. Following the 1914–1918 war, it was estimated that 30 million cases of typhus occurred in Russia alone, and some 10% of these probably died. In the 1970s, large epidemics occurred in central Africa (Ruanda–Burundi).

The responsible organism is *Rickettsia prowazekii* and transmission is by the body louse *Pediculus corporis* or the head louse *Pediculus capitis*. The lice become infected by biting a human who is carrying the specific rickettsiae in the blood. Subsequent spread of the infection results from the infected feces of the lice rather than by an actual bite, and the irritation set up on the human body by the infestation results in the organisms being scratched into the skin. Infection may also result from the inhalation of louse feces in dust. At times fleas may act as a vector and also convey the infection through their feces.

Clinical features

The incubation period is 6–15 days. There are three main clinical phases – prodromal, invasive and eruptive.

Prodromal symptoms, not always present, include mild headache, lassitude, weakness and pyrexia. The invasive stage is characterized by a sharp rise in temperature, severe headache and generalized aching. Rigors may occur and the fever may reach 40–41 °C. The pulse is rapid, the blood pressure reduced and a variable degree of prostration develops. A wide variety of additional symptoms and signs may be encountered including suffusion of the conjunctivae, facial flushing, photophobia, deafness, tinnitus, vertigo and cough.

The characteristic rash arises about the fifth day of illness and the initial lesions, comprising pinkish red macules, appear on the trunk and soon spread to the limbs. Most cases show sparing of the face, palms and soles. In mild cases the rash may develop no further, but in the more severely ill the eruption becomes hemorrhagic or even purpuric. During this eruptive phase the mental state becomes dulled. Stupor, delirium and coma may follow. Hypotension also becomes more intense and oliguria with azotemia is common. Severe cases will die between the 9th and 18th day of illness. Those who recover slowly improve after 2 weeks, the mental recovery being more rapid than the physical. Typhus is usually accompanied by leukopenia and normochromic anemia.

Complications

Bronchopneumonia, otitis media, skin sepsis, arterial thrombosis and gangrene are all encountered. Less often there may be areas of skin necrosis and secondary infection of the salivary glands. Prolonged hypotension has a grave prognosis.

Differential diagnosis

Typhus may be readily considered and diagnosed at epidemic times, but sporadic cases can cause considerable confusion. Amongst diseases that may require differentiation are other rickettsial infections, typhoid fever, measles, malaria and meningococcal septicemia.

Treatment

In children, doxycycline 5 mg/kg/d 12 hourly (max 200 mg) or chloramphenicol 75–100 mg/kg/d (max 2 g) or tetracycline 50 mg/kg/d is used and should be continued until the temperature has settled for 48 h. Antibiotics should be re-instituted if there is clinical relapse.

Careful nursing and general supportive measures are required. A high protein diet is desirable and transfusion of blood or plasma may be needed. Electrolyte imbalance can readily occur and requires appropriate correction. Oxygen may be given for pulmonary complications and digoxin for cardiac failure.

Prognosis

The disease is rarely fatal in children, but about 10% of young adults and 60–70% of people over 50 may die.

Control

Killed vaccines prevent deaths, although not necessarily infection. Scrupulous hygiene is desirable and insecticides should be used to eliminate lice: DDT, lindane and malathion have proved effective.

BRILL–ZINSSER DISEASE (RECRUDESCENT TYPHUS)

This condition represents a recrudescence of epidemic louse-borne typhus that occurs years after the primary attack. It is usually mild and the illness is drastically modified. Skin rashes are usually absent and the prognosis is good. In view of its atypical clinical nature and the fact that a case may arise when no other typhus infection is occurring, diagnosis is difficult. Less markedly abnormal laboratory tests can also be misleading. However, if a diagnosis is made, treatment is along the lines employed for epidemic typhus. The real danger of Brill–Zinsser disease is to the community. If epidemiological factors are favorable, especially if the environment is heavily louse infested, an epidemic could arise from such a case.

MURINE TYPHUS (ENDEMIC FLEA-BORNE TYPHUS FEVER)

This disease is clinically similar to classical epidemic typhus but is milder and has a much lower fatality rate (2%); the management and treatment are also similar. The responsible agent is named *Rickettsia mooseri* and it is usually spread to man from its animal host by the rat flea (*Xenopsylla cheopis*).

Widely distributed throughout the world, the disease appears to be on the decline, probably owing to stricter control of rats. It is more common in summer when rats are more numerous and has a higher infection rate amongst persons in the food trade where rats may abound. Unlike lice, which die from *R. prowazekii*, the rat flea is not killed by the multiplication of *Rickettsia mooseri* in its tissue. Control depends on flea eradication and extermination of rats.

SCRUB TYPHUS (TSUTSUGAMUSHI FEVER)

This disease, known by many different names according to the locality where it occurs, is transmitted to man by the bite of the larvae of different species of chigger-like mites; best known of these are *Trombicula akamushi* and *Trombicula deliniensis*. The responsible agent is known as *Rickettsia tsutsugamushi* and the cycle of infection involves chiggermite and various wild rodents. Clinical features are again like those of other rickettsial infections though fairly mild. A diagnostic finding in some is a small necrotic ulcer or eschar where the responsible mite has attached itself to the skin and introduced the infection. The disease occurs in the south west Pacific and South East Asia between Japan, the Solomon Islands and Pakistan.

Treatment is with doxycycline 5 mg/kg/d 12 hourly (max 200 mg) or chloramphenicol 75–100 mg/kg/d (max 2 g) and the mortality is under 5%. Elimination of the disease is difficult and mite-infested areas are best avoided. Alternatively protective clothing, treated with a mite repellent, should be used. Vaccines have not proved effective in this condition.

ROCKY MOUNTAIN SPOTTED FEVER

This disease results from infection by *Rickettsia rickettsii* which is transmitted to man through a variety of ticks which are both the vector and the common reservoir for the responsible agent. Some rodents, dogs and sheep also act as additional but less prolific reservoirs. The clinical course has many similarities to classical typhus but the incubation period is often shorter (2–5 days in severe cases). Furthermore, the rash is usually more pronounced and frankly petechial. It can also be more widespread and may take some time to subside.

Complications, differential diagnosis, laboratory findings, treatment and management are all similar to epidemic typhus. Reported mortality rates have varied between 3 and 90% with an average, for all ages, of 20%. Despite its name, this disease is now much more common in the eastern than the western USA. In the western USA, adult males are most frequently attacked, whereas in the east children are most commonly affected.

Control is difficult owing to the disseminated nature of the vector in the wild, and where possible it is best to avoid tick-infested areas or to ensure that adequate protective clothing is worn.

TICK TYPHUS FEVERS (FIÈVRE BOUTONNEUSE)

There are three tick-borne spotted fevers caused by rickettsiae which share the same group-specific antigen as *Rickettsia rickettsii*, the cause of Rocky Mountain spotted fever, but have distinct type-specific antigens.

Rickettsia conorii causes fièvre boutonneuse, which is also called Mediterranean fever along the Mediterranean, Black and Caspian sea littorals; called Kenyan tick typhus and South African tickbite fever; and called Indian tick typhus in South East Asia. *Rickettsia australis* causes Queensland tick typhus in eastern Australia. *Rickettsia sibirica* causes Siberian tick typhus which occurs throughout central Asia.

The main animal reservoir is dogs. These tick typhus fevers are clinically similar. A small, indurated lesion, the tache noire, develops at the site of the tick bite, and central necrosis gives way to eschar formation. There is regional lymphadenopathy. The tick typhus fevers are much milder than Rocky Mountain spotted fever, with a mortality under 1%. Antibiotic treatment is as for the latter disease.

RICKETTSIALPOX

Due to *Rickettsia akari*, this disease is usually transmitted to man by a mite and the house mouse is the main animal reservoir. Epidemics tend to occur where mice and mites are found together, primarily in urban populations worldwide.

The illness is comparatively mild. The incubation period is 10–21 days. Fever is usual and a mild rash develops, most closely resembling adult chickenpox. Death is extremely rare. Doxycycline is the drug of choice.

Q FEVER (QUERY FEVER)

This disease results from infection by *Coxiella burnetii* and usually presents as an influenza-like illness with fever and headache, often followed by an atypical pneumonic illness. Unlike other rickettsial infections, Q fever is unaccompanied by a rash.

C. burnetii is an obligate intracellular parasite which is highly pleomorphic and contains both RNA and DNA. It is more resistant to chemical and physical agents than other pathogenic rickettsiae and is relatively sensitive to certain antibiotics.

The natural reservoir of *C. burnetii* is animals such as cattle, sheep and goats, as well as certain ticks, and the latter are probably involved in animal-to-animal spread. Infection in humans may arise from the handling of infected meat and placentae, the inhalation of infected dust in farmyards and the consumption of infected raw milk. Cases are most likely to be found in farm workers, slaughtermen and shepherds. Where milk is the vehicle of transmission, the disease may occur without any apparent occupational link and involve children.

Clinical features

Q fever is less commonly diagnosed in children than in adults because the illness produced in younger age groups is less severe and less intensively studied.

There is usually an incubation period of 2–3 weeks and the illness starts abruptly with fever, rigors, headache, malaise and weakness. In some instances the illness may terminate in approximately 1 week without any further progression, but in most diagnosed cases the patient goes on to develop a cough and chest pain. Physical signs may be absent or minimal, although the chest X-ray may show pneumonitis.

Severe cases may have symptoms for up to 3 weeks and radiological abnormalities can take a similar period to resolve. Inapparent infection can also occur. Occasionally Q fever presents with meningoencephalitis and diagnosis can be difficult.

Complications

Q fever, or rickettsial, endocarditis has only been seen in people with pre-existing valvular disease of the heart and the clinical presentation is with culture negative subacute bacterial endocarditis. Granulomatous hepatitis and bone granulomas have been described.

Laboratory diagnosis

C. burnetii can be isolated in laboratory animals or fertile hen's eggs. However, as it is a significant biohazard to laboratory workers, serological tests are preferred to confirm a clinical diagnosis, and a complement-fixation test or immunofluorescence is used on acute and convalescent sera. Detection of nucleic acid by PCR or hybridization techniques is also available.

Treatment

Prodromal symptoms require symptomatic treatment. Once the diagnosis is made, doxycycline (5 mg/kg/d up to 200 mg) or tetracycline (25 mg/kg/d) or chloramphenicol should be given in standard dosage for 2 weeks.. Therapy should not be withheld where the diagnosis is retrospective and the patient has recovered, because it is important to eradicate the infection and avoid the possibility of chronicity. Endocarditis has a grave prognosis.

PROTOZOAL INFECTIONS

AMEBIC INFECTIONS

Amebae are characterized by two forms – the motile, feeding trophozoite and the cyst. The cyst has a rigid wall, resistant to environmental conditions, which allows it to survive for variable periods without feeding. The major ameba of importance to man is *Entamoeba histolytica*, which is anaerobic and an obligate parasite of the gut. It has to be differentiated from other nonpathogenic gut amebae, e.g. *E. dispar*, *E. coli* and *E. hartmanni*. There are a number of free-living aerobic amebae which are found in the soil and feed on bacteria in muddy water. In dry conditions the cysts may be dispersed by wind. Species that are pathogenic to man and may cause meningoencephalitis are *Naegleria fowleri* and the opportunist *Acanthamoeba culbertsoni* and *Balamuthia mandrillaris*.

AMEBIASIS

Amebiasis is caused by *E. histolytica* and is transmitted by the fecal–oral route. Sources of infection include sewage contamination of water supplies, infection by food handlers and direct fecal contact from person to person, as may occur in mental institutions. Transmission by sexual contact, including oral and anal sex, also occurs. Rarely, amebic colitis or liver abscess may present within the neonatal period.

Infection occurs worldwide, with a high prevalence in resource limited countries where hygiene is poor.

E. histolytica cannot be differentiated by microscopy from the morphologically identical but nonpathogenic *E. dispar*. Methods required include stool antigen tests, culture characteristics, zymodeme analysis and molecular techniques, such as PCR.[696–698] *E. histolytica* trophozoites characteristically demonstrate active erythrophagocytosis. *E. dispar* is 9 times more prevalent than *E. histolytica* and is the most likely species when 'amebic cysts' are detected in stools of asymptomatic subjects in any part of the world. Up to 10% of asymptomatic carriers of *E. histolytica* develop invasive disease; the remainder clear the infection within a year.[696,698]

Why *E. histolytica* is activated to invade is not known. Malnutrition, pregnancy, ulcerative colitis, immunosuppression, corticosteroids and intercurrent infection by bacteria or parasites may be precipitating factors. Inflammatory bowel disease should not be treated with corticosteroids until amebiasis has been excluded.

The incidence of disease does not necessarily correlate with prevalence of infection. Invasive disease is reported particularly from South East Asia, Natal (South Africa), the west coast of Africa, Mexico and parts of South America. In the USA, infection is associated especially with children of Hispanic origin.

Pathogenesis and pathology

Infection occurs from ingestion of cysts, which, on digestion, release trophozoites in the intestine. The trophozoites feed on bacteria and fecal matter in the cecum and further down the colon. When they reach areas where the feces are more solid, they encyst and the cysts are passed in the stool. Trophozoites may be detected in the stool even if there is no intestinal hurry. The presence of either trophozoites or cysts in stool is not necessarily indicative of invasive disease. However, the presence of hematophagous trophozoites (containing ingested red blood cells) is usually suggestive of invasion. Invasion is accomplished by lytic enzymes secreted by the trophozoites which result in tissue necrosis and erosion of blood vessels, but with a surprising lack of inflammatory response. Initial lesions are small superficial erosions. With progression, they penetrate the muscularis mucosa and may expand to produce flask-shaped ulcers. Further extension may result in intestinal perforation, but more commonly the parasite is carried to the liver in the portal vein, and rarely to other organs such as the lung, heart or brain. The colonic lesions may vary from small pinhead erosions confined to the cecum and rectosigmoid to extensive, deep, confluent ulcers extending throughout the colon. It is probable that the majority of amebae

reaching the liver do not cause detectable disease. Possibly, an area of tissue necrosis is necessary for the disease to be established. As in the bowel, liver abscess is characterized by localized necrosis without much inflammatory response, unless there is secondary infection.

Clinical features

The major organs affected in invasive amebic disease are the colon, the liver and adjacent organs, such as the right lung, pericardium and rarely the skin or eye.

Intestinal amebiasis

Intestinal amebiasis has a wide spectrum of severity. It may occur within a few weeks of infection or be delayed several months. There may be mild, intermittent diarrhea with blood and mucus, usually with no systemic upset or fever. Severe, fulminating dysentery is associated with watery, blood-stained, mucoid stools resulting in dehydration, electrolyte disturbance and toxemia. Abdominal pain, tenesmus and tenderness may be present. Perforation, which is often multiple with slow leakage, and peritonitis may occur. Other complications include hemorrhage, ameboma, stricture, intussusception and rectal prolapse. Chronic or relapsing dysentery may occur unless the initial attack has been managed by adequate chemotherapy and nutritional support. Ameboma is a complication of previous amebic dysentery and presents as a tender mass in the cecum or colon.

Enlargement of the liver may occur without evidence of an abscess, presumably the result of toxic products transported in the portal vein from the diseased bowel.

Amebic liver abscess and related disorders

Amebic liver abscesses may be single or multiple and more often involve the right lobe. Multiple abscesses are common in young children (Fig. 28.45). The liver is tender and, if the abscess is situated anteriorly, a mass is commonly visible (Fig. 28.46). There is nearly always fever and usually anemia, leukocytosis and raised erythrocyte sedimentation rate

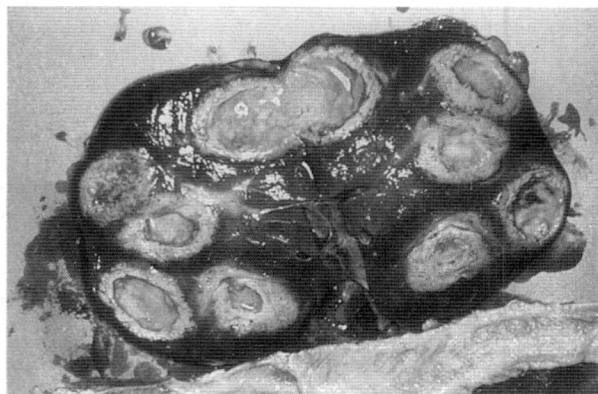

Fig. 28.45   Typical multiple amebic abscesses in the liver of an infant aged 8 months.

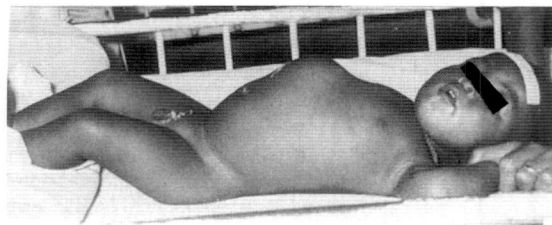

Fig. 28.46   An African infant of 10 months with a large amebic liver abscess presenting as a fluctuant mass in the epigastrium.

(ESR) and often also alkaline phosphatase. Jaundice is infrequent and serum transaminases are usually not raised. There is dysentery or a history of previous dysentery in only half the cases. In over two thirds of cases, elevation and immobility of the right diaphragm produces corresponding signs in the right lung.

Complications of amebic liver abscess include secondary bacterial infection, extension, or rupture into the peritoneal cavity, the pleural cavity and/or the lung. Involvement of the left lobe of the liver may result in a pericardial effusion or rupture into the pericardium. Rarely, there may be extension to abdominal organs including the stomach, gut or kidneys. Blood-borne spread may result in a brain or lung abscess.

Skin

Cutaneous amebiasis may be associated with rupture of a liver abscess, colostomy stoma or a laparotomy incision. In infants, amebic abscess of the perineum may result from direct contact with infected feces (Fig. 28.47).

Diagnosis

The diagnosis of amebic dysentery is based on the finding of motile, hematophagous E. histolytica trophozoites in feces. Red cells and bacteria but few leukocytes are usually present. Examination of a freshly passed warm stool (within 30 min of being passed) is important because, when the stool cools, the amebae stop moving and release the contained red cells in their vacuoles. Three or more stool examinations may be necessary and both direct and concentrated methods should be used. E. histolytica stool antigen test is more sensitive than microscopy and can differentiate E. histolytica from E. dispar. Endoscopy may demonstrate amebic ulcers, which are usually shallow, covered with a yellowish-gray exudate and contain numerous hematophagous trophozoites. Biopsy should be taken from the edge of the ulcer. The intervening mucosa is often relatively normal in appearance. Serum antibody titers to E. histolytica may be raised in two thirds of cases early in disease and in over 90% during convalescence.[697] In endemic areas, positive serology in young children suggests infection, but in older children does not distinguish between past and current infection.

The definitive diagnosis of amebic liver abscess is made by aspiration of bacteriologically sterile pus. The pus is usually gray-yellow at the first aspiration and only at subsequent aspirations takes on the pink or red-brown 'anchovy-paste' color. Amebae are seldom detected in necrotic material from the center of the abscess, but are more common in the walls of the cavity and thus are more likely to be detected in the last portions of the aspirate.

In most cases an ultrasound scan can localize and delineate the size of the abscess cavity. Ultrasound, CT and MRI have equal sensitivity in detecting amebic abscesses. Differential diagnosis includes pyogenic liver abscess, subphrenic abscess and hydatid disease. X-ray and screening may demonstrate a raised diaphragm with reduced movement and there may be an effusion or other signs of inflammation at the lung

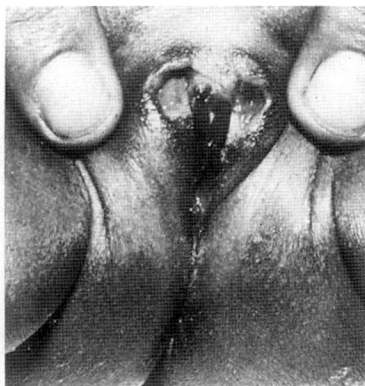

Fig. 28.47 Cutaneous amebiasis involving the vulva in an infant aged 5 months.

base. Usually there is a leukocytosis and a raised ESR. Antibody titers are usually high and may be detected in serum in over 95% of cases later on in disease.[697] ELISA has high sensitivity and specificity and usually becomes negative 6–12 months after response to treatment, whereas indirect hemagglutination titers may remain raised for many years. For unknown reasons, infection is only detected in the stool in about one third of cases, and usually only cysts are present.

Management

Chemotherapy of invasive amebiasis must include drugs which can eliminate amebae both from the tissues and the lumen of the bowel. Metronidazole and tinidazole (longer half-life) achieve both but are less effective as luminal amebicides.

For asymptomatic patients, and following invasive disease, the luminal amebicide diloxanide furoate is given, using 20 mg/kg/d in three divided doses for 10 days. Paromomycin 25–35 mg/kg/d in three divided doses for 7 days is an alternative. In endemic areas, older asymptomatic children are usually not treated, as reinfection is so common.

In symptomatic intestinal disease, metronidazole or tinidazole is recommended. Metronidazole 35–50 mg/kg/d in three divided doses orally is given for 7–10 days depending on the severity of the infection. Side-effects such as nausea and a metallic taste in the mouth may make compliance difficult. Alternatively, oral tinidazole 60 mg/kg is given as a single daily dose for 5 days. Both drugs may also be given intravenously. In severe colitis, correction of fluid and electrolyte imbalance is important, and gastric suction is necessary when there is ileus. Blood transfusion may be required. Broad spectrum antibiotics may be necessary if septicemia or other infection is suspected. Perforation of the bowel with leakage into the peritoneum may require surgery.

For liver abscess, metronidazole or tinidazole is usually effective and is given in doses similar to intestinal disease. Diloxanide furoate or paromomycin should be given to eradicate the bowel infection.

Indications for aspiration of the abscess include: suspected pyogenic abscess (particularly when there are multiple lesions), a palpable mass, a markedly raised diaphragm, failure of symptoms to remit after 72 h of drug therapy, and abscess in the left lobe. Aspiration, by relieving the pressure within the liver tissues, allows better drug penetration of the abscess. Surgical evacuation may be necessary for multiple or inaccessible abscesses, or when secondary infection has occurred. For needle aspiration, a wide-bore needle with a three-way tap should be used and the abscess cavity evacuated fully. Aspiration is usually through the right chest wall at the point of maximum tenderness, or through the abdomen if the abscess is superficial. Aspiration should be guided by ultrasound scan. If repeat aspiration is required, or in the case of drug resistance, percutaneous catheter drainage for 24–48 h may be undertaken.[699]

Resolution of the abscess cavity may take many months. Follow-up should be arranged to ensure complete eradication of infection, otherwise relapse may occur.

Intrathoracic and intraperitoneal rupture of amebic liver abscesses usually responds to standard anti-amebic chemotherapy.

As humans and primates are the only reservoirs of E. histolytica, eradication of disease is possible and vaccines are being developed with this aim.

NAEGLERIA AND ACANTHAMOEBA

Two distinct types of meningoencephalitis are caused by free-living amebae: primary amebic meningoencephalitis by Naegleria fowleri, and granulomatous amebic encephalitis usually by Acanthamoeba culbertsoni or Balamuthia mandrillaris.[700]

Primary amebic meningoencephalitis

This is an acute necrotizing meningoencephalitis caused by N. fowleri which gains access to the nasal cavities and results in direct invasion of the nervous system through the olfactory apparatus. There is usually a history of swimming under water or diving in warm fresh water or hot springs. Cysts transmitted in dust may colonize the nasal cavities of children. The cerebrospinal fluid (CSF) has changes similar to bacterial meningitis, viz. a predominant neutrophil count, often accompanied by red cells, a raised protein (usually > 1 g/L) and low glucose concentration. Careful search for trophozoites should be undertaken on fresh CSF. Nasal secretions or washings should also be examined for amebae.

The course of the disease is usually rapidly fulminating within 3–6 days. Intravenous and, if necessary, intraventricular (through a reservoir) amphotericin is the main treatment. In addition, parenteral fluconazole is usually given by the intravenous (and intrathecal) route and rifampicin orally. Duration of therapy is 8–10 days.

Granulomatous amebic encephalitis

This is a slowly progressive disease, occurring usually in immunocompromised individuals, although sometimes no immune defect can be demonstrated.[701] Infection by acanthamoeba may result from swallowing or inhaling cysts, or by direct skin or corneal contact. The CSF shows a lymphocytosis, a raised protein and low or normal glucose. Acanthamoeba may be detected in histological specimens. Sometimes the trophozoites may be detected by wet mount of CSF and subsequently cultured. Serology may also be of value.

Severe brain damage may have occurred by the time the diagnosis is made. Suggested drugs for treatment include polymyxin B, pentamidine isetionate, co-trimoxazole, ketoconazole and flucytosine.

Successful outcome is more likely in immunocompetent children.

Acanthamoeba keratitis

Most cases of acanthamoeba keratitis are associated with use of contact lenses, owing to a combination of abrasions of the cornea and contamination of the lens from washing in homemade solutions, especially fresh or tap water.[702]

Treatment is difficult and often requires keratoplasty. Local application of a combination of biocides, e.g. 0.02% polyhexamethylene biguanide plus 0.1% propamide isetionate and neomycin, is used. Local chlorhexidine may also be of value.[702] Corticosteroids are required to control inflammation. Only fresh, sterile, commercial solutions should be used to clean contact lenses.

Research on vaccines to prevent acanthamoeba keratitis is in progress.

BALANTIDIASIS

Balantidium coli is a parasite of pigs which may colonize the colon of man producing a disease similar to *E. histolytica*, but extracolonic disease does not occur. Treatment is with metronidazole or tetracycline for 8–10 days.

CRYPTOSPORIDIOSIS

Cryptosporidium spp. are second only to the enteric viruses in importance as causes of diarrheal disease in children. There are a number of different species of *Cryptosporidium*, some of which infect humans (Table 28.37). *C. muris* was first described by Tyzzer in 1907 as an asymptomatic infection of the gastric glands of mice. *C. parvum* was first described also by Tyzzer in 1912 in the intestines of mice. *C. meleagridis* was described as a cause of diarrhea in turkeys by Slavin in 1955 and since then the number of different *Cryptosporidium* species has expanded, contracted and then expanded again. It was first described as a human pathogen in 1976[703,704] and thought to be zoonotic. Interest in cryptosporidiosis increased, first because it was possible to diagnose infection by microscopic examination of stained fecal smears and second because of its association with AIDS.[705,706] It was originally thought of as a zoonotic infection, but person-to-person transmission was described in 1983[707] and it is clear that both anthroponotic and zoonotic transmission occur.

Originally *Cryptosporidium* was classified as a member of the subclass *Coccidosina* in the phylum *Apicomplexa*. However, recent molecular

Table 28.37 *Cryptosporidium* species

	Major hosts	Minor hosts
C. hominis	Humans	Cattle, dugong, sheep
C. parvum	Cattle, sheep, goats, humans	Deer, mice, pigs
C. meleagridis	Turkeys, humans	Parrots
C. felis	Cats	Humans, cattle
C. canis	Dogs	Humans
C. wrairi	Guinea pigs	Humans
C. baileyi	Chickens, turkeys	Other birds, humans
C. muris	Rodents, Bactrian camels	Humans, rock hyrax, chamoix
C. andersoni	Cattle, Bactrian camels	Sheep
C. bovis	Cattle	
C. galli	Finches, chickens	
C. serpentis	Snakes, lizards	
C. saurophilum	Lizards	Snakes
C. molnari	Fish	

phylogenetic studies and the detection of extracellular stages have placed it closer to the Gregarines than Coccidia.[708]

Cryptosporidium spp. have a complex life cycle (Fig. 28.48) which can be simplified to (a) replication within the host and (b) the excreted infective form. The infective form is the oocyst, which is excreted in large numbers during acute infection (Fig. 28.49). It is highly resistant to disinfectants and is sufficiently small (c. 6 μm) to be able to pass through some water filtration units. The oocysts are infective as soon as they are excreted. Under the influence of gastric pH and duodenal enzymes, the oocyst excysts to release four sporozoites. These attach to and penetrate the enterocytes. Their location is just beneath the enterocyte membrane (Fig. 28.50) sometimes termed 'intracellular but extracytoplasmic'. It then undergoes cycles of asexual and sexual reproduction culminating in the production and excretion of the thick-walled oocysts. *C. hominis*

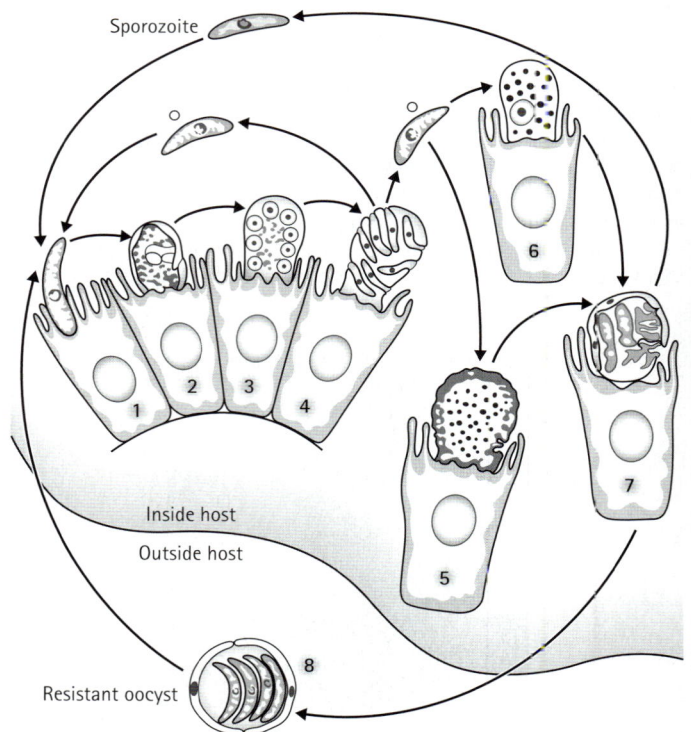

Fig. 28.48 The life cycle of *Cryptosporidium*.

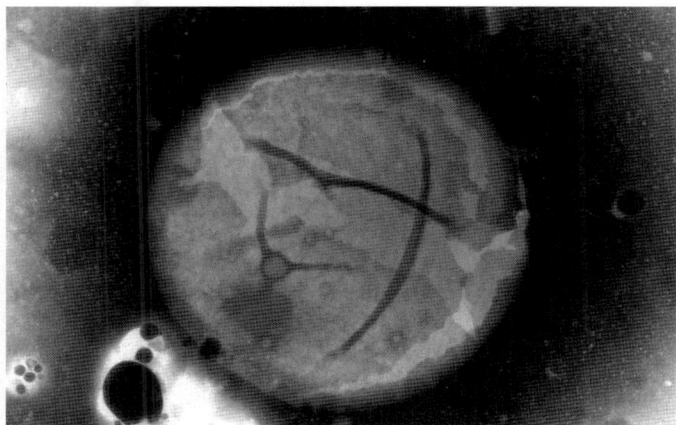

Fig. 28.49   An oocyst of *Cryptosporidium hominis*.

has a 9.2 megabase genome encoded on 8 chromosomes, the full sequence of which has recently become available.[709]

EPIDEMIOLOGY

Cryptosporidiosis has a worldwide distribution, being detected in every country where it has been sought. There are an estimated 250–500 million cases each year in Africa, Asia and Latin America.[710] It is an important cause of traveler's diarrhea and outbreaks can occur in crèches and day care centers. School visits to farms where children handle farm animals and then eat without washing their hands are another risk activity. In addition, *Cryptosporidium* can be acquired by the waterborne route. The largest such outbreak occurred in Milwaukee, USA, and affected 403 000 people.[711] It was related to a water treatment failure, although the fecal coliform count (the standard measure of water quality) was within normal limits.

Large numbers of oocysts are excreted during acute infection and the infective dose is low (30–300 oocysts), varying by *Cryptosporidium* species.[706] In some volunteer experiments one oocyst was able to initiate infection. Transmission of *C. hominis* is usually considered to occur by person-to-person transmission, directly or indirectly, and the other species by zoonotic transmission. However, *C. hominis* has been detected in cattle and *C. parvum* can be transmitted person to person. Most of the cases of cryptosporidiosis are due to *C. hominis* and *C. parvum* followed by *C. meleagridis*, *C. canis* and *C. felis*.[712–714] *C. muris* is rarely a cause of human disease.[712,715] In the UK and other temperate countries there is a distinct seasonality with peaks in spring and to a lesser extent in autumn.[705,710,716]

The impact of cryptosporidiosis is greatest in children, and prevalence rates are much higher in children in resource limited countries (5–19%) compared to industrialized (<4%) countries.[705] The highest prevalence (19%) was recorded among children in Gaza.[717] Although children have the highest prevalence of infection, cryptosporidiosis can occur at any age. The youngest recorded case was 3 days and the oldest 95 years old.[716] Patients immunocompromised by AIDS, immunosuppression, congenital immune deficiency or cytotoxic therapy are at risk of severe and prolonged cryptosporidiosis (see ref. 705).

PATHOLOGY AND PATHOGENESIS

Cryptosporidiosis is usually acquired by ingestion but there have been instances where it was acquired by the airborne route.[718] The shortest incubation period is presumed to be 3 days in a neonate who acquired infection intrapartum.[719] In a large study of Finnish travelers visiting Leningrad the mean incubation period was 7.2 ± 2.4 days with a median of 8 days.[720] Infection affects the small and large intestine in immunocompetent hosts but can spread along mucosal planes to the biliary tree, pancreas, liver, sinuses and lung in immunocompromised patients.

The mechanisms by which *Cryptosporidium* causes diarrhea are not entirely clear. Possible mechanisms include malabsorption and a local intestinal inflammatory response with increased production of prostaglandins and several cytokines.[721] In addition, *Cryptosporidium* delays apoptosis in infected cells but promotes it in adjacent enterocytes.[721] The histopathologic appearance of the intestine in cryptosporidiosis shows minimal inflammatory infiltrates with blunting of villi (Fig. 28.51). Electron microscopic examination of infected mucosa shows minimal damage to the brush border (Fig. 28.49).

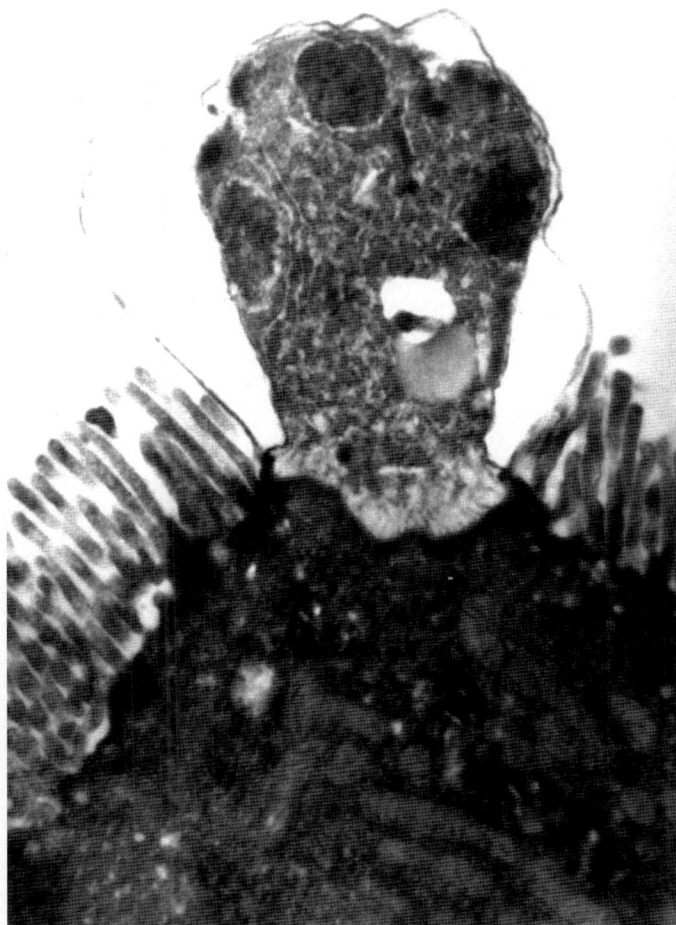

Fig. 28.50   A trophozoite of *Cryptosporidium hominis* just beneath the enterocyte membrane.

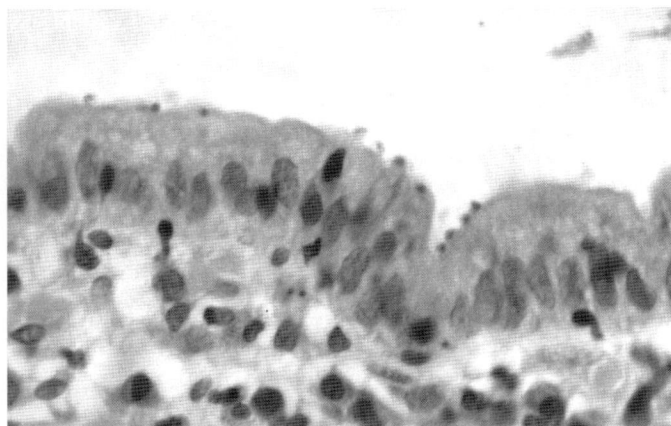

Fig. 28.51   Duodenal mucosal biopsy stained by hematoxylin and eosin showing villous blunting and cryptosporidia on the luminal surface.

CLINICAL FEATURES

The clinical features vary according to whether the patient is immunocompromised or has an intact immune system.[705,710,716]

Immunocompetent children

The severity of disease varies across a spectrum from a short mild illness to one of prolonged watery diarrhea lasting over 6 months which has been mistakenly diagnosed as celiac disease. Anorexia (60–70% of cases), vomiting (50–75%), fever > 38 °C (25–50%) and abdominal pain (50–90%) are commonly described. The stool is watery (60–100% of cases), green (60–70%) and has a particularly offensive odor (80–100%). The stool frequently varies from 3 to 20 per day with 60–70% of children producing > 5 stools per day. The average duration of diarrhea is 12–14 days but with a wide range (5–60 days).[722,723] On average, patients excrete oocysts for 10–14 days after cessation of diarrhea.[724] In approximately one third of children the diarrhea is intermittent with bouts lasting for 2–3 days with 1–2 days quiescence until the next bout. Up to a third of children have respiratory tract symptoms,[723] which might be related to the presence of *Cryptosporidium* in a case of laryngotracheitis in a child in Papua New Guinea.[725]

Cryptosporidiosis is not a major cause of severe dehydration in well-nourished children,[705] but is in children from resource limited countries.[725] A major feature is loss of weight and failure to thrive, which occurred in 25% of children admitted to a Liverpool children's hospital.[723]

Immunocompromised patients

Although there is a spectrum of severity, cryptosporidiosis in immunocompromised patients is much more likely to be severe and also less likely to be self-limiting. The diarrhea is often described as profuse, voluminous and cholera-like. A stool frequency of up to 71 per day and a volume of 17 liters per day have been recorded in adults.[716] Another feature of cryptosporidiosis in immunocompromised patients is the occurrence of extraintestinal infection, which can involve the lung, sinuses, biliary tree or liver.

The immune deficits associated with severe cryptosporidiosis include B cell deficiency (hypo- or agammaglobulinemia, IgA deficiency), B and T cell deficiency (severe combined immunodeficiency, HIV/AIDS), immunosuppressive therapy (cytotoxic drugs, steroids, transplants), malnutrition, diabetes and measles.

DIAGNOSIS AND DIFFERENTIAL DIAGNOSIS

The first human cases of cryptosporidiosis were diagnosed by examination of duodenal biopsies.[703,704] However, it was soon realized that patients with cryptosporidiosis excrete sufficiently large numbers of oocysts for them to be detected by microscopic examination of stained fecal smears. Stains now include modified Ziehl–Neelsen, Kinyoun and Safranin methylene blue.[705] An auramine phenol method has greater sensitivity as on UV illumination the oocysts fluoresce apple-green against a dark background. Such tests are labor intensive, and detection of copro-antigens by commercially available enzyme immunoassay kits allows large numbers of samples to be processed rapidly.[726] However, their efficiency depends upon the quality of the antibody used, they may not detect all species of *Cryptosporidium*, and recently one test was recalled because of problems with false positives.

Genome detection by PCR amplification of the 18S rRNA gene is a sensitive diagnostic tool and coupled with restriction fragment length polymorphism (RFLP) analysis will provide assignment to species. However, it is not commercially available.

Finally serological diagnosis by detection of antibody is possible, which although valuable for population-based surveys of exposure is not useful for acute diagnosis.

TREATMENT

In most cases of infection in immunocompetent children only supportive therapy is needed. The infection is self-limiting. This is not the case in immunocompromised patients and a large number of drugs (> 150) have been tried in the treatment of cryptosporidiosis. Paromomycin and spiramycin produce symptomatic improvement but no alterations in oocyst excretion. A new agent, nitazoxanide, has been licensed for treatment of cryptosporidiosis and in double-blind placebo-controlled trials shows great promise.[727] The only other intervention possible is to decrease the immune suppression by giving antiretroviral drugs in AIDS or stopping chemotherapy for malignancies.

CONTROL MEASURES

Great emphasis on personal hygiene is needed to limit person-to-person spread. In particular hand washing after toileting and nappy changing are very important. It is the mechanical effect of hand washing that is important as the thick-walled oocysts of *Cryptosporidium* are very resistant to most disinfectants and detergents. Prevention of waterborne disease is very difficult as evidenced by the Milwaukee experience.[711] The providers of potable water in the UK continuously screen the water to try to prevent infection. Boiling or freezing water should kill the oocysts. There is no vaccine to prevent cryptosporidiosis and as yet we still do not have a sound understanding of immunity to cryptosporidiosis.

PROGNOSIS

Except in immunocompromised or malnourished children, the prognosis is very good providing there is adequate nutrition during the recovery phase. However, one study from Guinea-Bissau indicated that cryptosporidiosis in infancy was associated with a higher subsequent childhood mortality rate.[728]

GIARDIASIS

The enteric protozoan *Giardia* is a major cause of diarrheal disease of humans and other animals including dogs and cats. Although frequently referred to as *Giardia lamblia* in the medical literature, this has no taxonomic validity. *Giardia duodenalis* is the species affecting most mammals including humans, companion animals and food animals.[729] Other recognized species are *G. agilis* in amphibians, *G. muris* in rodents, and *G. psittaci* and *G. ardae* in birds. The vegetative form of *G. duodenalis* or trophozoite is a pear-shaped flagellate protozoan 12–15 μm long and 5–9 μm wide (Fig. 28.52). It has two nuclei and four symmetrically arranged flagella originating from basal bodies at the anterior poles of the nuclei. The concave

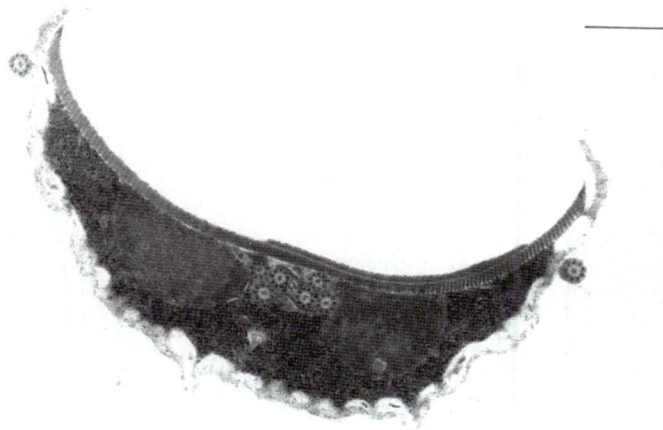

Fig. 28.52   Thin section electron micrograph of *Giardia duodenalis* showing the ventral disc and flagella in cross-sections.

ventral surface has a ventral disc composed of microtubules, which are used by the protozoan for attachment to intestinal cells. The trophozoites are unusual among eukaryotes in having only a few rudimentary intracellular organelles.[730] The infective form is the cyst which is excreted in feces. It can survive water chlorination and for months in cold fresh water. The cysts are quadric-nucleate, ovoid and 7–10 μm in length. The genome is small and consists of approximately 12 million base pairs on five chromosomes encoding an estimated 5000 genes.

EPIDEMIOLOGY

Giardiasis has a worldwide distribution and it is estimated that some 200 million people in Africa, Asia and Latin America have symptomatic infection and there are approximately 500 000 new cases each year.[731] It is an important cause of traveler's diarrhea and there is an increasing incidence of outbreaks in day care centers and crèches. Spread is fecal–oral, especially when hygiene is poor. Waterborne spread is increasingly important and, since a number of animal species can harbor *G. duodenalis*, a proportion of cases could be zoonotic.[732] Cyst concentrations excreted in feces are 150–20 000/g, but in contrast the infective dose is 10–100 cysts.

The impact of giardiasis is greatest in children. Prevalence rates are significantly higher in resource limited (20–30%) compared to resource rich (2–5%) countries. Recurrent and prolonged infections are not uncommon and some children may excrete cysts for long periods asymptomatically. Patients with hypo- or agammaglobulinemia are at particular risk of chronic giardiasis, but HIV and AIDS do not apparently increase the risk greatly.

Recently it has been shown that strains infecting humans can be subdivided on the basis of 18S rRNA gene sequences into two major groups. These are called assemblages A and B and there are clusters of genotypes within the two assemblages.[729] Not only are these subdivisions useful for epidemiologic purposes, but it also appears that assemblage A isolates tend to be associated with intermittent diarrhea and assemblage B with more severe, persistent diarrhea.[733]

PATHOLOGY AND PATHOGENESIS

Histologic changes in duodenal biopsies from cases of symptomatic giardiasis vary from entirely normal through partial, subtotal and total villous atrophy. Approximately 20–25% of patients will have normal villous architecture and <10% subtotal villous atrophy.[734] On electron microscopic examination there can be shortening and disruption of microvilli even in biopsies appearing normal on light microscopy.

Following ingestion, cysts are excysted by the sequential exposure to low pH in the stomach and higher pH in the duodenum, which activates giardial proteases.[735] Interestingly, the newly excysted protozoa express different surface antigens (variant surface proteins, VSP) to those expressed by the trophozoite before it was encysted. The trophozoites then can be found free in the small intestinal lumen (here motility by flagella is important to prevent flushing out) and closely apposed to the enterocyte surface, often embedded in mucin. Most often their ventral surface is towards the enterocyte surface and it is thought that attachment is by the ventral disc; however, they also have a mannose-binding lectin on their surface. The trophozoites reproduce by binary fission and it is thought that bile salts stimulate growth. Trophozoites encyst in the small intestine when they are at high cell densities and this is stimulated by high bile salt concentrations, lipid metabolites and neutral pH. How diarrhea is induced is not entirely clear. Suggestions include the trophozoites acting as a mechanical barrier to prevent nutrient absorption (which is unlikely), structural and ultrastructural damage to enterocytes, and malabsorption. Recently it has been demonstrated that giardiasis is accompanied by disruption of inter-enterocytic tight junctions perhaps mediated by anexin-like alpha giardins.[736]

CLINICAL FEATURES

There are three clinical forms of giardiasis:
1. asymptomatic excretion of cysts;
2. acute diarrheal disease which is usually short and self-limited;
3. chronic diarrhea with malabsorption, weight loss and failure to thrive.

The asymptomatic carrier state can occur in children or adults but whether carriage follows symptomatic infection or carriage occurs with no prior disease is unclear. There is no information on whether the asymptomatic carrier has subclinical enteropathy. However, it is clear that carriers can act as a reservoir of infection for others.

Acute giardiasis follows an incubation period of 3–20 days (mean 7 days) and the illness usually lasts 2–4 weeks, but may last as long as 7 weeks. Diarrhea (in over 90%) is the major feature and weight loss occurs in 60–70%. Other features are abdominal discomfort, flatulence, nausea and vomiting (in 30%). Approximately half the patients will have signs of steatorrhea. In patients with cystic fibrosis, giardiasis may worsen the malabsorption of fat and fat soluble vitamins.

A proportion of those with acute giardiasis (estimated to be about 30%) go on to develop chronic diarrhea, most often with steatorrhea. Weight loss can be great, with fat malabsorption in about 50%. In infants and young children this can cause failure to thrive. In some cases malabsorption of vitamins such as B_{12} or folate can lead to macrocytic anemia. Secondary lactase deficiency may occur and does not necessarily resolve with successful therapy.

DIAGNOSIS AND DIFFERENTIAL DIAGNOSIS

Giardiasis should be considered in cases of acute or chronic diarrhea. Specific diagnosis is by detection of the protozoon, its antigens or genome either in stool or duodenal fluid obtained by endoscopy, a nasoduodenal tube or a weighted nylon thread ('string-test'). Stool is the most appropriate specimen, but more invasive specimen collection is indicated when there is a high index of clinical suspicion yet stool samples are repeatedly negative. Although trophozoites are shed in the initial phase of acute diarrhea, giardiasis is most often confirmed by detection of cysts on microscopy of wet-mount or formalin–ethyl acetate concentrated stool samples. A single stool sample will detect giardiasis in 70% of cases and examination of three samples on separate days will detect it in 85%. The sensitivity of microscopy can be increased by using anti-*Giardia* fluorescent labeled antibody (direct immunofluorescence). In general, antigen detection by ELISA is more efficient and cost effective.[737] A number of commercial kits are available, including one that can simultaneously detect *G. duodenalis*, *Entamoeba histolytica* and *Cryptosporidium parvum*.[738] Diagnosis by genome detection, for example by PCR, is at present experimental.

TREATMENT

There is no evidence of benefit in treating asymptomatic infection. At least five classes of drugs – nitroimidazoles (metronidazole, tinidazole), benzimidazoles (albendazole), acridine dyes (mepacrine), nitrofurans (furazolidone) and nitazoxanide – are used for treating symptomatic giardiasis. A recent systematic review has concluded that drug treatment was associated with an improved cure rate (odds ratio 11.5; 98% confidence interval 2.3–58). Of the longer course regimens, metronidazole was the most effective (OR 2.4; 95% CI 1.2–4.4) with a smaller relapse rate. Tinidazole, which has a longer serum half-life than metronidazole, was best of the single dose regimens.[739] Unfortunately, there are few trials in children. The generally accepted regimen in children is metronidazole 15 mg/kg/d in three doses for 7–10 days. Mepacrine may be used as second line therapy (50 mg twice daily for children 1–5 years and 100 mg twice daily for children 5–10 years). Its use is limited by its bitter taste and induction of vomiting. In the USA, either metronidazole or furazolidone is preferred (tinidazole is not licensed for giardiasis). Furazolidone comes as a suspension, is given four times daily (6 mg/kg/d) for 7–10 days, and is less effective than metronidazole.

CONTROL MEASURES

In nurseries, crèches and child care centers, personal hygiene should be emphasized. Hand washing by staff and children should be stressed, especially after toileting and nappy changing. In outbreaks, attempts should be made to identify and treat all of those with symptomatic giardiasis. Those with symptomatic giardiasis should be excluded from work or nurseries until the diarrhea ceases. Although such infection control measures will decrease transmission, it must be remembered that routes other than direct person to person (e.g. waterborne, zoonotic) are possible. Recently, a vaccine has been licensed for the prevention of giardiasis in dogs and cats.[740] The vaccine, which is made from killed whole trophozoite preparations, proved highly effective. This could be of benefit to humans, firstly in decreasing an animal reservoir for zoonotic transfer and secondly by paving the way for a human vaccine.

PROGNOSIS

The prognosis is excellent, except in immunocompromised children, when relapse is common and treatment may need to be continued for prolonged periods. At the same time, attention must be paid to adequate nutrition and the treatment of concurrent infections.

LEISHMANIASIS

Leishmaniasis is caused by infection with a number of species of protozoan parasites of the genus *Leishmania*. It occurs in many parts of the world, including southern Europe, and is particularly problematic in Central and South America, the Middle East, South Asia, China and East Africa. An estimated 1–2 million new cases occur annually. Most forms of leishmaniasis are zoonoses with rodent or canine reservoirs of infection; man and other vertebrate hosts become infected by the bite of sandflies (genera *Phlebotomus* and *Lutzomyia*). Clinical syndromes are determined by the infecting species and range from self-limiting cutaneous lesions to potentially fatal visceral leishmaniasis.

LIFE CYCLE AND PARASITE BIOLOGY

Leishmania are transmitted by sandflies of the genus *Phlebotomus* in the Old World and *Lutzomyia* in the New World. Sandflies take in blood containing the aflagellate stage (amastigotes) from a hemorrhage made in the skin by their mouthparts. The amastigotes divide at least once before changing into the motile flagellate stage (promastigotes). These develop within the gut over 4–14 days and migrate forward to become inoculated when the sandfly attempts to take its next blood meal.[741] The intracellular stage in the vertebrate host (including man) is a small uninucleate ovoid body (2–5 μm long and 1–2 μm wide) containing a kinetoplast with a flagellar remnant and known as the amastigote (also referred to as the Leishman–Donovan body). The amastigote predominantly infects cells of the reticuloendothelial system and multiplies repeatedly by binary fission, eventually destroying the host cell.

Parasite biology

Two major subgenera of importance in human leishmaniasis can be distinguished by the site of development within the sandfly vector: *Leishmania* subgenus *Leishmania* (*L. donovani*, *L. mexicana*, *L. tropica* and *L. major*) and *Leishmania* subgenus *Viannia* (*L. braziliensis* complex).[742] Leishmania that infect man are morphologically similar apart from minor variations in size of amastigotes. However, isoenzyme profiles, DNA characterization, PCR, monoclonal antibody techniques and serotyping can all be used to distinguish species.[743] Culture of leishmania can be performed using specialized media. Some *Leishmania* species grow poorly in culture, and culture characteristics have been used to differentiate *L. braziliensis* which is slow growing from *L. mexicana*.

The important leishmania affecting man and the clinical syndromes that they cause are summarized in Table 28.38.

VISCERAL LEISHMANIASIS (KALA AZAR)

Visceral leishmaniasis (VL) is caused by leishmania of the *L. donovani* complex (*L. donovani*, *L. infantum* and *L. chagasi*).

Table 28.38　Summary of human leishmaniasis

Parasite	Geographical distribution	Animal reservoir	Disease
Visceral leishmaniasis (*Leishmania donovani* **complex**)			
L. donovani	India, Bangladesh, China	None	VL PKDL
	Kenya	(Dog)	VL PKDL
	Sudan and Ethiopia	Rodents	VL (CL) (MCL)
L. infantum	Mediterranean littoral, Central Asia, China	Canine sp.	VL (CL) VL CL
L. chagasi	Central and South America	Canine sp.	VL
Old World cutaneous leishmaniasis			
L. tropica	Middle East to India	(Dog)	CL (dry), LR
L. aethiopica	Ethiopia and Kenya	Rock hyrax	CL DCL
L. major	Africa, Middle East and Asia	Rodents	CL (wet)
American cutaneous leishmaniasis (*Leishmania mexicana* **complex**)			
L. mexicana	Mexico, Belize, Guatemala	Forest rodents	CL (DCL) Chiclero's ulcer
L. amazonensis	Brazil–Amazon basin	Forest rodents	CL DCL
American mucocutaneous leishmaniasis (*Leishmania braziliensis* **complex**)			
L. braziliensis	Brazil, Amazon forest, Peru, Ecuador, Bolivia, Venezuela, Colombia, Paraguay	Uncertain, forest animals	CL and MCL
L. guyanensis	North Amazon, Guyana	Sloth, lesser anteater	CL MCL
L. panamensis	Panama, Costa Rica	Sloth	CL (MCL)
L. peruviana	Western Andes	(Dog)	CL (Uta)

CL, cutaneous leishmaniasis; DCL, diffuse cutaneous leishmaniasis; LR, leishmania recidivans; MCL, mucocutaneous leishmaniasis; PKDL, post kala azar dermal leishmaniasis; VL, visceral leishmaniasis.

Epidemiology

L. donovani is endemic and epidemic in north-eastern India and Bangladesh, predominantly affecting young adults and children. Infection is confined to man and no animal reservoirs have been identified. The vector, *P. argentipes*, is peridomestic and readily feeds on man. The parasite is similar in East Africa, where the disease is widespread with endemic foci and occasional epidemics, particularly in association with population movements and land development. Children are predominantly affected. Rodents are reservoirs of disease in Sudan, but no animal reservoir has been identified in Kenya. Transmission is often seasonal due to fluctuations in sandfly populations.

L. infantum is widely distributed through the Mediterranean littoral, southern Europe, the Middle East, southern regions of the former USSR and China. In endemic areas, children under 5 are predominantly affected although infection may occur at any age in visitors or the immunosuppressed. The domestic dog is an important reservoir host; wild canines and foxes also act as reservoirs.

L. chagasi in South and Central America resembles *L. infantum* clinically and epidemiologically. Infection occurs in Amazonian Brazil, Bolivia, Paraguay, Argentina, Colombia and Venezuela. Children are predominantly affected and both domestic and wild canines and foxes are reservoir hosts.

Pathogenesis

After inoculation into the skin, the promastigotes convert to amastigotes in skin macrophages. These disseminate throughout the reticuloendothelial system and amastigote-laden macrophages are found in liver, spleen, bone marrow, lymphatic tissue and occasionally the skin. Progressive splenomegaly, hepatomegaly, anemia and thrombocytopenia result.

Clinical features

Subclinical or asymptomatic infection is common and protects against subsequent infection; clinical disease only occurs in 10–20% of infections. The clinical features of visceral leishmaniasis are similar throughout the world. A small cutaneous lesion may occur at the site of inoculation, but is usually not observed. After a variable incubation period (usually 4–6 months), symptoms develop. Classical clinical features are a triad of fever, splenomegaly and anemia. However, the spectrum of VL ranges from an acute febrile infection with anemia, pancytopenia and splenomegaly to a protracted illness slowly progressing over 2 or more years with severe anemia and massive splenomegaly. *L. infantum* infections are usually more acute than infection with *L. donovani* but acute forms of *L. donovani* occur, especially in children. *L. infantum* may also cause simple cutaneous leishmaniasis in adults in Southern Europe.

Fever is frequent, commonly remittent or intermittent, and may have a characteristic double diurnal periodicity. In very acute forms, fever is high, with prostration, toxemia and minimal splenomegaly. However, many patients remain active despite high fever and some patients with chronic infection may be afebrile for prolonged periods. Most patients develop progressive splenomegaly and hepatomegaly; in chronic infections, the spleen may be grossly enlarged, smooth and hard. Generalized or localized (often cervical) lymphadenopathy occurs in some geographical areas and may be present in the absence of hepatosplenomegaly or other features of visceral leishmaniasis.

Patients with chronic disease are pale and, especially in India, develop an earthy grey color with areas of hyperpigmentation (kala azar). In Africa a diminution in skin pigmentation is more typical. Chronic VL leads to progressive wasting, nutritional skin changes and hair changes similar to those observed in kwashiorkor. Pancytopenia with associated immunosuppression leads to secondary infections such as pneumonia, bronchitis, meningitis and tuberculosis. Episodes of diarrhea are common and may be due either to secondary infection or submucosal infiltration with leishmania-laden macrophages. Patients are rarely jaundiced but dependent edema and ascites occurs. Hemorrhagic features, especially recurrent epistaxis, are common; major or fatal hemorrhagic episodes may occur.

Visceral leishmaniasis and HIV

Visceral leishmaniasis is an important opportunistic infection in HIV, particularly in Southern Europe. Most cases occur in young adults but pediatric cases of co-infection have been reported. Both classical and atypical presentations with pulmonary, skin and gastrointestinal infection occur; fulminant infection without splenomegaly is also recognized. Leishmania serology is frequently negative, but parasites are usually easy to find in appropriate samples.

Laboratory findings

The hematological features of visceral leishmaniasis are classically moderate to severe normocytic, normochromic anemia with hemoglobin levels of 6–8 g/dl, accompanied by neutropenia and thrombocytopenia, commonly $80–100 \times 10^9$/L. Lymphocytes are usually in the normal range and circulating eosinophils reduced or absent from the peripheral blood. The serum albumin is reduced and there is a substantial elevation of immunoglobulins, predominantly IgG.

Diagnosis[744,745]

A parasitic diagnosis may be made by microscopy or culture of bone marrow or splenic aspirates. Splenic aspiration is more sensitive and reasonably safe in the absence of disturbed hemostasis or thrombocytopenia. Marrow aspiration is preferable in acute illness or in the presence of thrombocytopenia or disturbed hemostasis. Leishmania may also be identified by examination of the buffy coat and in lymph node and liver biopsy specimens. Smears are fixed in methanol and stained with Giemsa or Leishman that stain the cytoplasm of the amastigote blue, the nucleus pink or violet and the kinetoplast bright red. Culture is generally less sensitive than direct smear examination, but will detect some smear negative cases.

Anti-leishmania antibodies may be detected by a number of techniques, including IFAT, ELISA, and direct agglutination tests (DAT). ELISA and DAT techniques are highly sensitive and specific. High titers are associated with active disease and fall slowly after treatment. Rapid field diagnosis may be made by use of immuno-chromatographic strips which use recombinant antigens. PCR techniques can be used to detect leishmania DNA in peripheral blood and marrow with high sensitivity and specificity.

Differential diagnosis

Visceral leishmaniasis should be considered in the differential diagnosis of acute or chronic fever accompanied by hepatosplenomegaly and anemia, especially when there is a history of residence in an endemic area. Many other infections including malaria, especially *P. malariae* infection, typhoid, brucellosis, relapsing fever and tuberculosis (which may coexist with visceral leishmaniasis) should be considered. Splenomegaly must be differentiated from schistosomiasis, tropical splenomegaly syndrome and lymphoma or leukemia.

Treatment[744,745]

Pentavalent antimonial compounds remain the treatment of choice for most cases of visceral leishmaniasis. Two preparations are in common use: sodium stibogluconate containing 100 mg antimony (Sb) per ml (Pentostam) and methylglutamine antimonate containing 85 mg Sb per ml (Glucantime). Response rates are usually around 90%, but antimonial resistance, particularly in Bihar, India, is an increasing problem, and some regions report failure rates of up to 60%.

Sodium stibogluconate is administered by daily intravenous or intramuscular injection. The dose is 10–20 mg/kg Sb per day for 20–30 days. Children normally receive 20 mg/kg/d. Rapid extensive renal clearance occurs and dose adjustments should be made if renal function is poor. Common side-effects in adults include arthralgia, myalgia, biochemical and clinical pancreatitis, mild increase in liver enzymes and marrow suppression. The drug appears to be better tolerated by children.[746,747] Minor ECG changes are common; prolonged Q-T interval and dysrhythmias may occur in high dose regimens used for the treatment of antimony-resistant infections. Anaphylactic shock is a rare complication following administration. Sodium stibogluconate has been used in pregnancy without untoward effects on the fetus.

Amphotericin B. Both conventional and lipid formulations have been proven to be effective in various regimens lasting for between 10 and 40 days depending upon geographical location and the immune status of the patient. Standard amphotericin B is now the first line of therapy in some areas of India. Lipid formulations are better tolerated, have the theoretical advantage of being preferentially being taken up by macrophages and can be used in shorter courses of 10 days. They are currently the treatment of choice if expense does not preclude their use. Reported efficacy in children in Mediterranean VL is over 95%.[748]

Pentamidine. This may be effective, but resistance appears to develop rapidly and relapse is not uncommon. The main concern is toxicity, particularly the development of diabetes mellitus. The drug is now rarely used, except in areas of high resistance to antimonials or in patients who relapse.

Aminosidine (paromycin) is an aminoglycoside that has high efficacy and is well tolerated. It is administered intravenously or by intramuscular injection at a dose of 12–20 mg/kg/d for 3–4 weeks. Phase three trials with new formulations are currently underway.

Miltefosine is a new oral drug that is emerging as a very effective treatment option. It is given in a 4-week regimen at 2.5 mg/kg daily and is effective against antimony resistant strains. Cure rates are over 90% in children.[749,750]

Supportive and symptomatic treatment is important in addition to chemotherapy. Intercurrent bacterial infections are common and should be appropriately treated and attention paid to correcting nutritional status and vitamin deficiencies. Patients with hemorrhage should receive vitamin K. Blood transfusions are often required for the treatment of anemia in children.

Response to treatment

Fever normally subsides and patients start to feel better in the first week of treatment. Hemoglobin and white cell counts improve over 2–4 weeks while the splenomegaly reduces more gradually over subsequent weeks or months. Patients should be followed up for at least one year to detect relapse.

Relapse and nonresponsiveness

Relapse normally occurs within 6 months and relapse rates vary considerably depending upon the geographical location and the initial treatment regimen. Treatment of relapse is usually with prolonged courses of sodium stibogluconate, but depends upon geographical patterns of resistance. Pentamidine, aminosidine, amphotericin B and liposomal amphotericin have all been used successfully to treat relapse. Systemic interferon-gamma may be useful as an adjunctive therapy in resistant infections. HIV infected individuals are more likely to relapse and may need maintenance therapy.

Post kala azar dermal leishmaniasis

Post kala azar dermal leishmaniasis (PKDL) is most commonly seen in Indian visceral leishmaniasis (20%) and less often in African infections (1–5%). Following treatment of visceral disease, cutaneous lesions develop with symmetrical depigmented lesions especially on exposed surfaces. Lesions progress to become papular or nodular and mucosal surfaces may be involved with abundant leishmania (*L. donovani*) in lesions. Treatment with pentavalent antimonial compounds is effective although lesions also heal spontaneously.

CUTANEOUS LEISHMANIASIS
Epidemiology

L. tropica and *L. major* cause cutaneous leishmaniasis in the Middle East, Afghanistan, the southern Mediterranean, Sudan and sub-Saharan Africa. Clinical infection in endemic areas occurs mainly in children.

L. tropica has a human reservoir and transmission is mainly urban whereas *L. major* occurs in rural areas with rodent reservoirs.

L. mexicana and *L. braziliensis* cause cutaneous leishmaniasis in Central and South America. *L. mexicana* has a reservoir in forest rodents in Central and South America and particularly affects the pinna of the ear in forest workers, notably chicleros (chewing gum collectors). *L. braziliensis* has a reservoir in domestic animals and forest rodents. Cutaneous lesions may progress to mucocutaneous leishmaniasis (espundia).

Clinical features

Clinical features of cutaneous leishmaniasis are similar throughout the world with some slight differences between species. Typically, after an incubation period of several weeks, a localized, small, raised cutaneous nodule occurs, surrounded by a zone of erythema. The lesion grows slowly and central shallow ulceration may occur. Lesions remain raised above the level of normal skin; ulcers are shallow and do not have undermined edges. Lesions continue to progress for 6–24 months followed by spontaneous healing eventually leaving a slightly depressed papery scar. Satellite lesions may develop and regional lymphadenopathy is found in some forms. Lesions may be single or multiple and are more common on the face, hands, feet or limbs. *L. tropica* tends to cause single lesions lasting for 1–2 years with little tissue reaction and sometimes non-ulcerating lesions, whereas lesions in *L. major* are often multiple with a greater degree of ulceration and tissue reaction. Spontaneous healing occurs in 50% of lesions by 3 months in *L. major* or *L. mexicana*, 10 months in *L. tropica* and much longer in *L. braziliensis*.

Diffuse cutaneous leishmaniasis

In the Ethiopian highlands and western Kenya, *L. aethiopica* causes initial skin lesions similar to *L. tropica*. In very rare cases, leishmania disseminate throughout the skin to cause widespread, often symmetrical, lesions that resemble lepromatous leprosy. Similar syndromes occur in Central and South America due to infections with *L. mexicana* and *L. amazonensis*. A cell-mediated immune response to leishmania antigens is absent.

Leishmania recidivans

This is an unusual form of cutaneous leishmaniasis found in the Middle East and caused by *L. tropica*. The initial chronic skin lesion heals but then groups of lesions resembling lupus vulgaris occur around the healed scar. Leishmania amastigotes are difficult to find but the leishmanin skin test is strongly positive.

Mucocutaneous leishmaniasis

L. braziliensis complex infections cause single, often self-healing, primary lesions of the skin. However, in less than 10% of cases, subsequent metastatic spread to the oro-nasopharynx may occur (espundia). The time interval between initial infection and mucosal infection varies from a month to many years. The nasal septum is often involved initially causing symptoms of nasal stuffiness and epistaxis. Granulomatous lesions cause necrosis and destruction of cartilage and soft tissue and extend to involve the nose, mouth, tongue and soft palate. Lesions may ultimately involve the pharynx and larynx. Secondary infection is common and contributes to tissue destruction. Aspiration pneumonia occurs in the late stages and may be fatal.

Diagnosis of cutaneous leishmaniasis

The likelihood of finding parasites depends upon the infecting species and the stage of the lesion. Parasites are more numerous in early lesions and in *L. tropica* and diffuse cutaneous leishmaniasis. Aspirates and slit smear preparation from the raised margins of a lesion, dermal scrapings and biopsies are all useful. Care should be taken to reduce the chance of bacterial contamination of samples. Multiple sampling and a combination of techniques increase the chances of a successful diagnosis. Samples should be examined microscopically and cultured on appropriate media. Impression smears should be made from biopsy samples. Although histology is less sensitive in detecting parasites, it is useful in excluding other causes of the lesion. Mucocutaneous disease is often difficult to diagnose due to the limited number of parasites. PCR may be helpful on lesion aspirates or biopsies and may distinguish between different species complexes. Species diagnosis may also be made on cultured parasites by isoenzyme analysis or other DNA diagnostic techniques.

The leishmanin skin test (a test of delayed hypersensitivity using leishmanial antigen) may become positive during the course of infection, but is now rarely used for diagnosis. Serodiagnostic tests are of limited value for the diagnosis of cutaneous disease but may be helpful for the diagnosis and follow-up of mucocutaneous disease.

Important differential diagnoses for cutaneous leishmaniasis include superficial mycoses such as sporotrichosis, cutaneous mycobacterial infections, yaws, syphilis, sarcoidosis and neoplasms. In mucosal disease, histoplasmosis, paracoccidioidomycosis and midline granuloma must also be considered.

Treatment[751]

Many cutaneous leishmaniasis lesions heal spontaneously without specific treatment. Local treatment should include cleansing and antibiotics to control secondary infection and covering to prevent secondary contact lesions. Local infiltration with antimonials is used in some areas for treatment of early non-inflamed lesions to accelerate healing.[752] This can be painful. Topical paromomycin may be effective in *L. major* infection; success rates in other species are variable.[744,745]

Oral agents such as allopurinol and imidazoles (ketoconazole, itraconazole) have been used for cutaneous leishmaniasis with variable and generally disappointing results. Miltefosine may be effective orally for American cutaneous leishmaniasis.[753]

In *L. braziliensis* areas where mucocutaneous leishmaniasis occurs, all leishmanial lesions must be treated with prolonged systemic pentavalent antimonials (20 mg/kg stibogluconate for 20 days) to prevent metastatic spread. The clinical response may be poorer in children under 5.[754] Systemic therapy is also indicated for multiple or potentially disfiguring lesions of any species; shorter, lower dose courses may be adequate for *L. major* or *L. tropica*. Established mucocutaneous disease is difficult to treat and may require prolonged courses of systemic antimony or amphotericin. Diffuse cutaneous leishmaniasis is resistant to pentavalent antimonials but may respond either to combinations of aminosidine and antimonials or to prolonged courses of pentamidine.

CONTROL OF LEISHMANIASIS

Control centers upon vector control and reduction in the reservoir host. In central Asia, the simultaneous use of rodenticide and insecticide in gerbil burrows has reduced markedly the incidence of *L. major* infection. Similarly, control of stray dog populations and residual insecticide spraying have reduced *L. infantum* infection in many areas. Effective control can be achieved by medical surveillance of the population at risk when man is the major host reservoir. Insecticide spraying of houses is useful for peridomestic vectors such as in Indian visceral leishmaniasis. Control remains problematic in the vast forested areas of the Americas; the use of insecticides in tropical rain forests is impractical and control of the extensive reservoir of infected wild animals equally impossible. A number of candidate vaccines have been developed but clinical trials have been disappointing in both cutaneous and visceral leishmaniasis. A number of studies suggest that treated or untreated bednets reduce the risk of visceral leishmaniasis.[755]

MALARIA

Malaria is a disease of humans caused by infection with one or more of four species of protozoa of the genus *Plasmodium* (*Plasmodium falciparum*, *Plasmodium vivax*, *Plasmodium malariae* and *Plasmodium ovale*). It is usually acquired through the bite of an infected female *Anopheles* mosquito, although it may also follow the transfer of infected blood as in blood transfusion, or transplacentally or by the use of contaminated syringes. Worldwide some 45 *Anopheles* species effectively transmit malaria, although the identity, behavior and importance of local vectors vary widely with geographic location. The most effective vector is probably *Anopheles gambiae* – a mosquito that is widely distributed in tropical Africa. *P. falciparum* is the most pathogenic of the malaria parasites and infections with it must always be regarded as serious and potentially life threatening. The other three species tend to cause less serious illness, although on occasion a lethal nephrosis may complicate *P. malariae* infections.

THE PARASITE LIFE CYCLE

Malaria parasites undergo a complex stage of asexual development in the human host and a stage of sexual development (sporogony) which occurs partly in man and partly in the mosquito vector.[756]

Asexual development in man

This begins with the introduction of infective forms (sporozoites) in mosquito saliva during the biting act. Sporozoites circulate for less than 60 min, eventually gaining access to parenchymal liver cells either directly or after passage through Kupffer cells. The invasion process may entail specific ligand–receptor interaction. Once within the hepatocyte, the sporozoite initiates the exoerythrocytic (EE) phase of asexual development during which it grows and undergoes repeated nuclear fission (schizogony), eventually producing a cyst-like schizont filled with daughter parasites (merozoites). This phase usually proceeds without interruption and both the time taken to schizont maturity and the number of merozoites produced vary with the identity of the plasmodial species involved. *P. falciparum* completes its EE development fastest (about 5 days) and produces most merozoites per schizont (about 30000). The other species are slower and less prolific, the respective values for *P. malariae*, for example, being about 15 days and about 15000 merozoites. In two parasite species, *P. vivax* and *P. ovale*, some sporozoites initiate this uninterrupted EE stage of development but some do not. These latter, on entering hepatocytes produce small unicellular forms (hypnozoites) which persist without development for periods varying from several weeks to many months. Eventually the hypnozoites, activated by mechanisms as yet not known, resume growth and proceed to schizont maturation and merozoite liberation. Hypnozoites are currently widely believed to give rise to the relapsing parasitemias which characterize *P. ovale* and, particularly, *P. vivax* infections and which can occur even after drug treatment has effectively eliminated erythrocytic parasites. Hypnozoites do not develop in infections with *P. falciparum* and *P. malariae* and in these species recrudescence of parasitemia is generally considered to be due to persistent erythrocytic infection.

Merozoites liberated from EE schizonts are short lived and must find and enter a red blood cell within a few minutes. Within the erythrocyte each grows rapidly through ring form and uninucleate trophozoite stages eventually to form a schizont containing merozoites. On schizont rupture, the merozoites enter the bloodstream, attach to and penetrate fresh erythrocytes and again begin the cycle of erythrocytic asexual development. Attachment and penetration by merozoites are complex operations, which require specific ligand–receptor interactions. Erythrocyte invasion by *P. vivax* appears to require a ligand that is associated with Duffy blood group antigens, while attachment of *P. falciparum* merozoites to red cells requires one associated with sialic acid on the erythrocyte membrane. Age of the red cell also influences invasion by merozoites: *P. vivax* preferentially invades reticulocytes – a feature which tends to limit the density of parasitemia attained by this species – while *P. falciparum* can invade red cells of all ages.

The duration of the erythrocytic phase of asexual development and the merozoite yield per schizont vary with the plasmodial species. *P. malariae* has the longest cycle (72 h, i.e. quartan periodicity); the remaining species have cycles of about 48 h duration (i.e. tertian periodicity). *P. falciparum* has the greatest capacity to replicate and the merozoite yield of its schizonts is in the range 8–32. For the others the yields are 8–24 for *P. vivax*, 4–16 for *P. ovale* and 8 for *P. malariae*. The ability of *P. falciparum* to replicate rapidly in both the hepatic and erythrocytic phases of development partly accounts for the severity of the illness this species causes.

The time taken for parasites to become detectable in the peripheral blood following sporozoite inoculation is termed the prepatent period, while the time from infection to the onset of symptoms is termed the incubation period. While the two periods may be of equal duration, more usually the incubation period is about 2 days longer.

Late in its asexual erythrocytic cycle *P. falciparum* withdraws from the peripheral circulation and sequesters in deep vasculature. The phenomenon, which probably contributes importantly to the serious pathological effects that this *Plasmodium* causes, is effected by the binding of receptors on the surface of red cells infected with nearly mature parasites to ligands exposed on the surface of the endothelial cells lining deep blood vessels. Sequestration does not occur in the course of infections with the other plasmodial species that infect man.

Sexual development

In the course of blood stage schizogony in the human host some merozoites differentiate, by mechanisms which are not yet understood, to give rise to male and female sexual forms (gametocytes). In the case of *P. vivax*, gametocytes are formed early after the release of merozoites from the liver (before clinical symptoms), while *P. falciparum* gametocytes are generated after a number of erythrocytic cycles. Early treatment of fever with antimalarial drugs may therefore prevent gametocyte formation in *P. falciparum* but not in *P. vivax* infections. When mature, gametocytes circulate in the blood but do not undergo further development unless they are ingested by an anopheline mosquito during feeding. Once in the midgut of the mosquito, the female (macrogametocyte) escapes from the enclosing erythrocytic membrane and becomes a macrogamete. The male (microgametocyte) undergoes a process of exflagellation during which eight slender, uninucleate filaments (microgametes) are extruded and break free. Each microgamete seeks a macrogamete and, if successful, penetrates and fertilizes it. The two nuclei fuse and a zygote is formed. This is probably the only point in the life history of the parasite that genetic recombination occurs. The diploid zygote then undergoes meiosis and, as an ookinete, migrates to penetrate the epithelium of the mosquito midgut wall where it comes to rest on the external surface. There it rounds up, becomes an oocyst and begins a series of nuclear divisions. Oocyst maturity is reached after a period which is dependent on the identity of the plasmodial species and the ambient temperature to which the mosquito is exposed. It may be 1–4 weeks, or longer. At maturity the oocyst is filled with as many as 10 000 daughter parasites (sporozoites), each some 10–15 µm in length and feebly motile. The sporozoites escape at oocyst rupture and travel in the hemocelomic fluid to the salivary glands where they accumulate in the acinal cells to be discharged with saliva when the mosquito next feeds.

Infected humans constitute the only known source of mosquito infection for *P. falciparum*, *P. vivax* and *P. ovale*. For *P. malariae* some apes and monkeys may constitute reservoirs of infection in addition to humans.

EPIDEMIOLOGY

Despite widespread operations promoted by the World Health Organization between 1955 and 1975 with the aim of achieving global eradication, malaria remains probably the most prevalent, important, communicable disease throughout much of the tropical and subtropical world, the greatest burden of disease being in sub-Saharan Africa. Estimates of the world annual incidence of malarial illness have ranged from 200–450 million episodes[757] to over half a billion.[758] The much-quoted estimate of around 1 million malaria deaths annually in Africa, >75% of them in children, is supported by available evidence.[759] Over the past 25 years *P. falciparum* parasites have become increasingly resistant to chloroquine and other currently available antimalarial drugs.

This development appears to have been accompanied by an increase in malaria-attributed mortality in some endemic areas[760] and has required the development of new drug policies for malaria control and new regimens for chemoprophylaxis for travelers and other at-risk groups.

Many factors influence the epidemiology of malaria. Atmospheric temperature is important. For successful development in the mosquito vector, *P. vivax* requires a sustained temperature of at least 16 °C, while *P. falciparum* requires one of 20 °C. The geographical limits of *P. vivax* transmission are thus more widely set than those of *P. falciparum*. Other factors relate to the identity and biology of the *Plasmodium*, the identity and behavior of the vector, the social and economic customs of human populations and the topography and climate of the region. It follows, therefore, that the epidemiological pattern of the infection is not uniform but varies considerably between and within countries.

Where transmission occurs the measurement of endemicity has, in the past, relied on establishment of spleen rates and parasite positivity rates in ambulant children aged 2–9 years. Thus categories classified as hypo-, meso-, hyper- and holoendemic were characterized by both spleen and parasite rates of <10%, 11–50%, constantly >50% and constantly >75% respectively. In hyperendemic areas spleens in adults were frequently enlarged; in holoendemic areas they were not (this observation was attributed to the greater acquisition of immunity in holoendemic areas).

However, the widespread use of antimalarial drugs in areas where malaria is endemic has adversely affected these classical indices of endemicity and they are less useful today than formerly. This change has prompted the use of seroepidemiological techniques in the identification of malaria transmission and the measurement of its intensity. These techniques detect and quantify specific malaria antibody in serum and establish age-specific profiles for prevalence and titer. Briefly, profiles which show little change with age denote low transmission while profiles showing values which rise rapidly with age denote high transmission.[761]

Epidemiologically malaria presents in two extremes, one of which is stable and shows little change from one year to another, and the other which is unstable and may fluctuate violently in intensity at regular or irregular intervals. Stable malaria is most in evidence in areas where transmission rates are high; it is characterized by rates of mortality and morbidity which are high in infants and young children and which fall to low, even negligible, levels as age advances and effective immunity is acquired. Unstable malaria occurs where transmission rates remain low for periods of several years then suddenly increase greatly for climatic or other reasons; it is characterized by the occurrence of epidemics in which morbidity and mortality are conspicuous at all ages. Acquired immunity is not a feature of unstable malaria, save possibly at the end of a protracted epidemic period. Between the extremes of stability and instability, a range of intermediate epidemiological presentation occurs.

IMMUNITY

Malarial immunity may be innate, i.e. genetically determined, or acquired. Innate immunity may be due to a lack of ligands on the erythrocyte surface which bind to specific receptors on the merozoite surface at an essential stage in the invasion process, or to the presence of abnormal intramembranous erythrocytic components, which inhibit, but do not totally prevent, growth of the parasite within the red cell. An example of the former is the freedom from *P. vivax* infection that is apparent in people whose erythrocytes lack Duffy blood group antigens, while an example of the latter is the partial protection and survival advantage towards *P. falciparum* infections that heterozygosity for the sickle cell gene confers.[762]

Acquired immunity may be passive or active. Passive immunity due to the transplacental transfer of specific IgG malarial antibodies from mother to fetus probably accounts, at least in part, for the relative resistance to malaria that infants born in highly endemic areas show over the first few months of life. Acquired active immunity develops slowly in response to infection with malaria.[763] The first evidence is an ability to restrict the clinical effects of infection despite the persistence of high density parasitemia. This 'clinical' immunity is usually discernible in young children in highly endemic areas around the third to fourth year of life. Later, an ability to restrict parasite density develops and slowly strengthens throughout later childhood and adolescence to reach maximum expression in adult life. When fully developed, malarial immunity is species, strain and stage specific.

Acquired active immunity entails the collaboration of different cell populations, notably T cells, B cells and macrophages, during which specific and nonspecific humoral factors are elaborated which restrict parasite growth and replication.[764] Knowledge of how this complex response is assembled and controlled remains incomplete. T cells play a central role and their recognition of, and response to, defined malarial antigens are probably controlled by immune response (Ir) genes. Sensitized T cells respond to antigen by replication and the secretion of lymphokines which promote further T cell replication and diversification, induce replication of B cells with antibody production and activate macrophages.

Specific malarial antibodies belong to the immunoglobulin classes G, M and A. They function by agglutinating parasites and parasitized cells, inhibiting interactions between host cell surface ligands and parasite receptors, mediating cellular cytotoxicity and phagocytosis and inhibiting sequestration of mature asexual erythrocytic forms of P. falciparum in deep vasculature. Antibodies do not kill parasites directly through the activation of complement. Natural malaria infection induces synthesis of a wide range of antibodies directed against specific parasite antigens. Thus antibodies with specificity for the antigens of sporozoites, EE forms, asexual blood stages and sexual stages can be detected and titrated in the sera of residents of endemic areas.

The killing of parasites, which is probably carried out mainly by activated macrophages and cytotoxic T cells, involves release from the host cells of toxic oxygen derivatives and occurs principally in spleen and liver. However, other killing mechanisms exist. Interferon-gamma released by sensitized T cells has been observed to kill EE stages in hepatic cells, while tumor necrosis factor (TNF) liberated from macrophages stimulated with endotoxin has been reported to inhibit replication of both EE and erythrocytic stages of the parasite.

PATHOLOGY

The pathogenic sequences that develop in malaria are attributable to events that arise during the asexual erythrocytic stage of development of the parasite in man.

Anemia is common and is due partly to the rhythmic invasion and destruction of erythrocytes by parasites and partly to additional mechanisms, such as dyserythropoiesis and immune hemolysis following sensitization of nonparasitized red cells.[765] Bone marrow changes in dyserythropoiesis include erythroblast multinuclearity, karyorrhexis, incomplete and unequal nuclear division and cytoplasmic bridging. The marrow may contain large amounts of stainable iron and show evidence of phagocytosis of defective red cell precursors by macrophages. Whether these changes are initiated by toxic substances liberated by the parasite, or represent the nonspecific effects of macrophages rendered hyperactive by parasite antigens remains to be ascertained. The sensitization of uninfected red cells occurs commonly in malaria, often involves C3 and/or IgG and can be detected by the direct antiglobulin test (DAT) using specific antisera. DAT positivity of red cells, which is frequent in patients with falciparum malaria, has been found to be associated with enhanced blood destruction, but the association appears to be relatively uncommon.[765]

A characteristic feature of P. falciparum infections is the collection ('sequestration') of large numbers of late-stage parasites in the venules and capillaries of a variety of organs.[766] This results from the ability of this parasite, in the later stages of its development in the red cell, to display a number of proteins – known as P. falciparum erythrocyte membrane protein-1 (PfEMP-1) – on the red cell surface, by which the parasitized red cell attaches to host receptors on the microvascular endothelium.[767]

PfEMP-1 is a family of proteins encoded by recently identified highly variable var genes.[768] It is possible that sequestration is augmented by adhesion between parasitized erythrocytes, a phenomenon that can be demonstrated in vitro.[769] Sequestration is believed to be the mechanism underlying some of the clinical complications of P. falciparum infection, including the coma and convulsions of cerebral malaria. It is not known how sequestration may lead to tissue dysfunction: one possibility is that the huge number of actively metabolizing parasites consume oxygen and glucose at the expense of neighboring tissue, or produce toxic metabolites, including lactate, that may affect cellular function. Another possibility is that sequestration stimulates the release of host transmitters, such as nitric oxide, that may have a local effect on blood flow or on the conduction of nerve impulses. Host cytokines, too, are released and these may make endothelial cells more adhesive for the surface of parasitized red cells, thus augmenting sequestration.[770]

In some children with fatal cerebral malaria, histological changes include accumulations of platelets and microthrombi in cerebral and other microvessels.[771] CT scans of children surviving cerebral malaria with neurological sequelae show areas of brain infarction that may result from such vascular occlusions. Fortunately the majority of children and adults treated for cerebral malaria recover without neurological sequelae,[772] suggesting that microvascular occlusions from microthrombi are not a usual or major component of the pathology.

In children dying of encephalopathy with P. falciparum parasitemia, autopsies indicate that in a considerable proportion (about a quarter in one series[773]) the diagnosis may be a condition other than malaria, the parasitemia in these cases being incidental. This underlines the fact that, when a high proportion of a population is parasitemic, the diagnosis of severe malaria requires careful judgment and will sometimes be mistaken. This can result in failure to treat severe bacterial infection, often with fatal consequences.

Enlargement of the spleen and liver is common in acute and chronic infections and, on section, both organs are dark from the accumulation of malarial pigment (hemozoin). Evidence of phagocytosis of parasites, parasitized cells and hemozoin is usually present in the splenic pulp and in the sinusoidal macrophages and Kupffer cells of the liver.

In P. falciparum infections an acute diffuse glomerulonephritis may occur in which deposits of immunoglobulins, complement and malarial antigens are detectable in the mesangium and capillary loops. This is usually transient, but in non-immune adults with P. falciparum malaria it may lead to acute renal failure, usually characterized pathologically by acute tubular necrosis, from which recovery is usual if the patient can be sustained by supportive care and dialysis until renal function is restored. In P. malariae infections, however, a much more progressive and frequently lethal nephropathy may develop, again with evidence of antigen/antibody deposition. In children these lesions may progress despite antimalarial treatment to total glomerular sclerosis with secondary tubular atrophy. Clinically, the manifestations of a nephrotic syndrome develop with severe generalized edema and ascites accompanied by heavy proteinuria and hypoalbuminemia.

During pregnancy, P. falciparum may attain very high densities in the maternal placental blood and cause damage to the syncytiotrophoblast. Placental infection is associated with reduced infant birth weight and, in endemic areas, the association is most marked in first pregnancies. Occasionally, parasites cross the placenta, giving rise to congenital infection in the infant at or soon after birth. In endemic areas such infections seldom persist or cause disease in the neonate, but if the mother is a 'non-immune' individual, the baby may develop an illness with fever, anemia and jaundice.

Thrombocytopenia commonly occurs in P. falciparum infections for reasons that remain poorly understood. It usually occurs independently of changes in other measures of coagulation (prothrombin time, partial thromboplastin time) or to plasma fibrinogen concentrations and is usually unaccompanied by bleeding. Spontaneous bleeding may occur associated with disseminated intravascular coagulation (DIC), but this is an uncommon clinical feature of severe malaria in adults and is rare in children.

CHEMOPROPHYLAXIS

Large scale continuous chemoprophylaxis for children is not recommended in endemic areas, the main reason being that it is economically and logistically almost impossible to achieve over the long term on a national scale. It may be a useful measure, however, in focal high risk communities, such as refugees who have moved from a nonmalarious to an endemic area. Theoretical but unproven disadvantages of community-wide chemoprophylaxis include interference with the development of acquired immunity, enhancement of the development and spread of drug resistance and risk of toxicity from long term drug usage.

For individuals traveling from nonmalarious to malarious areas, however, chemoprophylaxis remains an important means of protection.

Drug prophylaxis should be seen as only one component of prevention. At least as important is sleeping under a permethrin-impregnated net (malaria-transmitting mosquitoes bite mainly in the middle of the night). Other measures can help: application of insect repellents [dimethylphthalate (DMP) or dimethyl-m-toluamide (DEET)] to exposed skin areas over periods of mosquito activity, the screening of houses and the use of knock-down insecticides in bedrooms before retiring.

Most prophylactic drugs should be taken for at least a week before travel (mainly in order to ensure acceptability) and for a month after exposure ends (to eliminate parasites that have developed in the liver in the intervening time).

Expatriates from a non-endemic country who intend to reside with their children for many years in a country with P. falciparum transmission must decide whether to take drug prophylaxis over the long term. The decision must be based on the extent of local risk, its seasonality, the local pattern of parasite resistance to various antimalarial drugs, and the availability of prompt health care. With screening and indoor residual spraying of the home and consistent use of insecticide-impregnated bednets, the risk may be low enough to avoid prophylaxis, provided that any fever is promptly diagnosed and treated. Expatriates may consider using chemoprophylaxis only during seasons of increased transmission or when visiting parts of the country where transmission is known to be high.

No prophylactic regimen, even if adhered to fully, guarantees protection against malaria absolutely. If a febrile illness develops during or up to 6 months after the period of exposure, malaria remains a possibility and should be investigated accordingly. Parents should be advised to ensure that physicians attending illness in children after return from endemic areas are aware of the need to exclude a diagnosis of malaria. Similarly, parents who live in endemic areas and are visited from time to time by children being educated in non-endemic areas should ensure that guardians and school authorities are alerted to the need to exclude malaria as a diagnosis in any illness developing in the repatriated child.

When contemplating the need for chemoprophylaxis in particular instances, the physician should ascertain the risk to which the child is or will be exposed, the duration of exposure, the pattern of drug resistance of malaria in the area to be visited, and possible drug toxicity. Useful information on disease incidence and drug resistance in the malarious countries of the world is to be found in the periodic reviews published by the World Health Organization in its Weekly Epidemiological Record.

Suggested chemoprophylactic regimens[774] (see also www.prodigy.nhs.uk/malaria_prophylaxis) are as follows:

1. Where only P. vivax malaria exists, prophylaxis should be by chloroquine proportional to an adult dose of 300 mg (two tablets) once weekly or by proguanil (Paludrine) proportional to an adult dose of 200 mg (two tablets) daily (see Table 28.39).
2. Where P. falciparum transmission occurs, options include:
   - Atovaquone–proguanil (Malarone), daily. This has the advantage of very little known toxicity and of attacking liver stage as well as blood stage parasites, so that it need be taken for only a week after exposure ends. Malarone is expensive.
   - Mefloquine (Lariam) once weekly. The weekly dosage is an advantage, but is easier to forget. Various side-effects are

Table 28.39 Age-related dosage of antimalarial drugs for chemoprophylaxis in children

Age	Fraction of adult dose
< 6 weeks	1/8
6 weeks–1 year	1/4
1–5 years	1/2
5–12 years	3/4
> 12 years	Adult dose

commonly reported, including insomnia and vivid dreams. Mefloquine should not be given to children who have a history of epilepsy or psychiatric disease.

Various prophylactic regimens used in the past are no longer recommended as prophylactics, although some of the component drugs remain important for treatment. Amodiaquine as a weekly prophylactic has been associated with occasional hepatic necrosis or neutropenia; weekly pyrimethamine–dapsone (Maloprim) with occasional agranulocytosis; and weekly sulfadoxine–pyrimethamine (SP, Fansidar) with Stevens–Johnson syndrome. Doxycycline, a useful prophylactic in adults, is contraindicated in children.

Continuous chemoprophylaxis is indicated for indigenous children in malarious areas who are homozygous for the sickle cell gene, because malaria may precipitate a crisis. Malaria increases viral load in adults with HIV infection,[775] but it is not yet known whether chemoprophylaxis against malaria will improve life expectancy in children with HIV infection or AIDS. Co-trimoxazole prophylaxis is beneficial in HIV infected children[776] and co-trimoxazole is an efficacious antimalarial drug, but it is not known whether or to what extent the benefit of co-trimoxazole is dependent on its antimalarial activity.

VACCINATION

A safe and effective vaccine for malaria is not yet available. Several candidate vaccines, making use of antigens from various combinations of sporozoite, erythrocytic and sexual stages of P. falciparum, are undergoing development or clinical trials. Promising results have been obtained among children in Mozambique in trials of the candidate vaccine RTS,S, a product consisting of sequences of the circumsporozoite protein of the P. falciparum merozoite linked to hepatitis B surface antigen and combined with the adjuvant ASO2.[777] In a double-blind randomized trial in children aged 1–5 years, the vaccine demonstrated 30% (95% CI 11%, 45%) protection against clinical malaria, 58% (16%, 81%) against severe malaria disease and 45% (31%, 56%) protection against P. falciparum infection, a benefit that was shown to persist over a subsequent year of observation.[778] Trials of this vaccine continue, with the aim of assessing its benefit when administered to young infants within existing standard EPI schedules.

CLINICAL FEATURES

The manifestations of malaria in an individual are determined by the infecting species of Plasmodium and the resistance or immunity of the host.

Each of the four species of parasite causing human malaria may produce a febrile illness with nonspecific symptoms including anorexia, malaise, headache, chills, rigors, sweating, irritability and failure to eat and drink. Symptoms begin about 10 days after the infective mosquito bite, but longer incubation periods are common, especially with the nonfalciparum malarias, and sometimes the first symptoms are not experienced until months or years after exposure. Diarrhea, vomiting and cough are common, but not severe, early symptoms. Febrile convulsions commonly complicate sudden rises of temperature in young children. The pattern of fever is irregular at first; the classical periodicity appears only if the illness is protracted and untreated, when P. malariae may cause quartan fever (72 h between spikes), P. vivax and

P. ovale tertian fever (48 h intervals) and *P. falciparum* subtertian fever (less than 48 h intervals). The liver and spleen may become palpable during the first few days of fever; the spleen may become enlarged during the course of a single episode, and may become very large after repeated or untreated infections.

Anemia develops, its degree being greatest in those with the heaviest or most protracted infections. Minor abnormalities of hepatic enzymes may be found, but jaundice is unusual even in severe falciparum malaria.

The most important distinction between species in their clinical effects is in the capacity of *P. falciparum* to cause, in susceptible individuals, a rapidly progressive severe ('complicated') disease, which may be fatal. Most of the many deaths from malaria every year are due to *P. falciparum* infections in young children living in endemic areas, the majority in sub-Saharan Africa.

In endemic areas the patient's first encounter with *P. falciparum* may be in utero. Parasitemia is common in pregnant women, and both placenta and cord blood may contain parasites at the time of delivery. Babies born to infected primigravid mothers may have a low birth weight but are otherwise unaffected. Parasitemia usually clears rapidly in the newborn, who remains relatively resistant to falciparum malaria for the first few months of life, probably because of a combination of maternal antimalarial antibodies and the fact that parasites grow less successfully in fetal than in adult hemoglobin. Occasionally (rarely in endemic areas) the newborn goes on to develop congenital malaria, features of which may include fever, failure to feed, anemia, jaundice and hepatosplenomegaly. Severe disease begins to affect children in endemic areas after the first few months of life, and for the next few years. During this time the majority of children are increasingly able to tolerate parasitemia with few or no symptoms, and malaria-related mortality decreases later in childhood.

In areas where there is little or no malaria transmission, children are susceptible to infection and severe disease at any age, and congenital malaria is sometimes seen.[779]

Acute *P. falciparum* infections

P. falciparum malaria usually presents as a febrile illness similar to that caused by other species of malaria. In a proportion of patients, however, complications develop which may threaten life. The most important manifestations of severe malaria in children are altered consciousness, labored breathing (due to acidosis) and severe anemia. These features may occur singly or in any combination.[780] A variety of metabolic complications may develop, resembling those that may complicate any severe systemic infection (reviewed in ref 781). Hypoglycemia may accompany any of the above syndromes and is associated with increased mortality, especially when the hypoglycemia is profound.[782] Some of the organ complications of falciparum malaria which are common in non-immune adults are uncommon in children. Renal failure, pulmonary edema and disseminated intravascular coagulation are less likely to develop in children, and are not present in most of those who die of falciparum malaria.

Cerebral malaria (CM)

When impaired consciousness in a child with falciparum malaria cannot be explained by the presence of hypoglycemia, seizures or a transient postictal state, and no other causative disease is present, the term 'cerebral malaria' is used.

Clinical measurements of the depth of coma are helpful in defining severity.[772]

CM develops rapidly. In the majority of children febrile symptoms precede coma by 2 days or less; in some the interval is only a few hours. Most patients have been feverish, irritable, listless and unable to eat or drink prior to losing consciousness. Convulsions are common and sometimes herald the onset of coma. In CM there is no postictal recovery of consciousness as occurs after a febrile convulsion. Other symptoms that may precede coma include vomiting and cough; minor looseness of stool may occur, but severe diarrhea is unusual.

The rectal temperature may exceed 40 °C, and is usually sustained during the first day or two of treatment. Occasionally a patient with CM may be afebrile when first examined, and rarely may remain so throughout the illness. Tachycardia is appropriate to the degree of fever, and the systolic blood pressure is normal in most patients. Dehydration is not clinically obvious, but vigorous fluid therapy in some patients leads to correction of acidosis and to improved tissue perfusion, suggesting that hypovolemia is commonly important. Respiration is rapid; in some patients breathing is stertorous, in others deep suggesting acidosis. About 5% of children with CM are jaundiced. The heart and lungs are normal on examination. The abdomen is soft; the liver may be moderately enlarged and the spleen may be palpable. In a minority of children with CM a shock-like state, with hypotension, cold peripheries and a wide core-to-skin temperature difference, may develop. Anemia is clinically apparent in some patients, and may develop during the course of illness in others.

The most striking clinical features are neurological. By definition the patient is unconscious and cannot be roused. Coma may be profound, the child being unable to withdraw from or localize a painful stimulus, and unable to moan or cry in response to pain. With less severe neurological impairment, motor and vocal responses to pain are retained but the patient is unable to watch or recognize familiar people. Corneal and pupillary reflexes are usually intact, but brainstem reflexes may be lost in the most severely ill. Retinal hemorrhages are common. Some of the most severely ill patients have papilledema.[783] Recently two further features have been identified that constitute a characteristic 'malarial retinopathy' not seen in other infections: these are areas of discrete retinal whitening, and a silver, orange or white appearance of some of the smaller vessels, usually in a patchy distribution.[784,785]

In some patients the motor picture suggests decerebration or decortication, with symmetrical rigidity or posturing of limbs, which may be sustained or repetitive. These may represent underlying seizure activity. It is not uncommon for patients to be opisthotonic. Focal asymmetrical twitching movements of the face or of a limb may be witnessed, sometimes (not invariably) proceeding to a generalized convulsion. If available, electroencephalography may reveal cerebral seizure activity in some cases in whom there is minimal or absent convulsive movement. Both overt and subtle seizures may occur in the absence of extremes of fever, and they cannot be regarded as febrile convulsions. The plantar reflexes may be abnormal. Abdominal reflexes are almost invariably absent.

The peripheral blood film reveals ring stages of *P. falciparum*. Occasionally parasites may be scanty, and rarely absent, in the blood film of a child with CM, perhaps as a result of the synchronous sequestration of mature parasites, and especially in a non-immune child; parasitemia is usually revealed with repeated examination at intervals of a few hours. In an endemic area, in a child with suspected CM who has scanty or moderate peripheral parasitemia, alternative diagnoses must be considered with particular care, as peripheral parasitemia may be an incidental finding in a child whose encephalopathy is due to something else. The likelihood that *P. falciparum* is the cause of a cerebral disease increases with the density of the parasitemia; it is not uncommon for up to 20% of red cells to be parasitized, and in some patients the figure exceeds 50%.

The packed cell volume may be normal or may be reduced; it usually falls further as the illness progresses. Life-threatening anemia may develop rapidly in patients with hyperparasitemia. Commonly the fall in hematocrit exceeds what would be predicted from the level of parasitemia. The peripheral white cell count is normal in the majority of patients but may be elevated in the very ill. The most severely affected patients are acidotic. There are minor abnormalities of hepatic enzymes, and the plasma creatinine may be mildly elevated. Plasma sodium, potassium, chloride, phosphate and calcium concentrations may show mild abnormalities but are commonly normal. Plasma and cerebrospinal fluid (CSF) lactate levels are abnormally raised in some patients, commonly in association with hypoglycemia. CSF opening pressure is raised in most patients, and fluctuates over time.[786] The mean and distribution of opening pressures were similar in a series of patients with fatal and nonfatal CM, and the pathogenetic importance of raised intracranial pressure remains uncertain.[787] The CSF is clear with normal cell counts and protein concentration.

A significant proportion of patients with CM are hypoglycemic when first admitted to hospital.[782,788] These patients do not differ from others in their duration of preceding illness, fasting or coma, or by any distinctive physical signs, but they tend to be younger and are more likely to be profoundly unconscious, to exhibit motor abnormalities and to have elevated levels of lactate and alanine in the plasma.

Even with optimal treatment, the mortality among children admitted to hospital with CM is 10–20%. The cause of death is not known, and in most cases cannot be attributed to renal, cardiac, pulmonary or hematological complications of malaria. Presenting features associated with an increased risk of death in children with CM include profound coma, age under 3 years, hypoglycemia, witnessed convulsions, motor abnormalities (hypertonicity, posturing), extreme hyperparasitemia (> 20% of red cells parasitized), acidosis, lactic acidemia and leukocytosis (> 15×10^9 white blood cells/L).[772]

In patients who survive CM, the duration of coma after the start of treatment ranges from a few hours to several days, the average duration being about 30 h. The change from deep coma to full consciousness may be dramatically rapid, and usually occurs before the temperature has fallen to normal and before parasitemia has cleared. The great majority of children who survive CM make a full neurological recovery; 5–10% of patients, however, suffer neurological sequelae, including hemiparesis, spasticity and cerebellar defects, from which a gradual recovery is made in some patients over the subsequent months. Risk factors for the development of sequelae are the same as those associated with mortality. Areas of intracerebral infarction have been demonstrated by computerized tomography in some children with neurological sequelae after CM.[789] Long term follow-up studies suggest that children recovering from CM are at increased risk of epilepsy in subsequent years, and that some may have cognitive and learning defects.[790]

Anemia

Anemia is a component of most episodes of malarial illness. In areas endemic for P. falciparum severe anemia (hemoglobin concentration < 5 g/dl) is an important clinical consequence of acute or recurrent malaria.[791]

The history of fever and associated symptoms may be similar to that of any malarial illness, but it is common for a child to present without such symptoms, or for anemia to be identified when a child is examined for an unrelated complaint. Some children with severe malarial anemia develop respiratory distress, which is usually due to acidosis resulting from impaired tissue perfusion and oxygenation.[792] Less commonly, breathlessness is due to cardiac failure, with enlarging liver, and a gallop rhythm on auscultation of the heart.

Peripheral blood films reveal parasitemia and a normochromic normocytic or, in chronic infections, hypochromic anemia. The reticulocyte count is inappropriately low. Unconjugated bilirubin may be increased in the plasma, free hemoglobin may be present in plasma and urine, and the plasma haptoglobin concentration is usually decreased or absent in the acute stage of the illness. The bone marrow shows normoblastic erythropoiesis with minimal dyserythropoiesis and increased myeloid precursors.[765] Unless other diseases are present, serum and red cell folate values are normal. Serum iron may be normal or moderately reduced, but there is usually normal or increased stainable iron in the bone marrow.

After the start of treatment for acute malaria, the hemoglobin level falls further in proportion to, or in excess of, the degree of parasitemia. In endemic areas, many children have a positive direct antiglobulin test. Reticulocytosis begins within a few days, and the hemoglobin level rises rapidly in convalescence.

Severe anemia recurs within a few weeks or months in an important proportion of children admitted to hospital for treatment of severe anemia. The role of malaria in this recurrence, and the potential for its prevention by antimalarial drugs, is under investigation.

Hyper-reactive malarial splenomegaly

Some children with protracted or frequent P. falciparum infection develop hyper-reactive malarial splenomegaly, a condition in which massive enlargement of the spleen is accompanied by raised serum IgM, high titers of antimalarial antibody, and hepatic sinusoidal lymphocytosis.[793] Splenomegaly resolves slowly with prolonged antimalarial treatment.

DIAGNOSIS AND DIFFERENTIAL DIAGNOSIS

Delayed diagnosis of P. falciparum malaria can have tragic consequences. In endemic areas it is a justifiable policy for all fevers without another obvious cause to be regarded as malarial and treated accordingly. In non-endemic areas a history of travel should alert the physician to the possibility of malaria, even if travel was many months or years ago. Malaria should be considered in puzzling clinical situations, even in individuals who have not traveled to an endemic area, as mosquitoes may transmit plasmodia after 'commuting' on an aeroplane ('airport malaria'), and parasites may be transmitted transplacentally or by needle-stick injury. Malaria should be considered in the differential diagnosis of all fevers accompanied by cerebral complications, acidosis or anemia, and in patients with fever who develop hypoglycemia, acute renal failure, disseminated intravascular coagulation or pulmonary edema.

The diagnosis of malaria depends on finding the parasite in the peripheral blood. Thick smears stained with Field's or Giemsa stain, and thin films stained with Leishman's, Giemsa or a modified Field's stain, allow identification of the species and density of malaria parasitemia. There have been occasional well-authenticated reports of fatal falciparum malaria in which blood films were repeatedly negative during life. Treatment should therefore not be withheld from a patient with an illness suggestive of malaria even if films are negative. In such patients blood films should be repeated at intervals during treatment, when parasitemia may be revealed. Serological methods of identifying malarial infection are valueless for individuals in endemic areas, and of limited use to the clinician seeing patients elsewhere. Serology identifies past or current infection, and may help towards diagnosis in a patient with recurrent fever in a non-endemic area in whom parasitemia cannot be found on repeated testing. Antigen-detecting test strips and DNA probes can identify parasitemia; these methods are valuable in clinical and epidemiological research, but have not become standard methods for use in clinical practice.

In high transmission areas where more than half of the child population may be parasitemic but apparently well at any given time, diagnosis of malaria as the cause of an illness must be speculative and will sometimes be wrong. In the comatose child, finding the distinctive ophthalmoscopic changes of malarial retinopathy (Fig. 28.53) strengthens the confidence with which the illness can be attributed to malaria. Other possible causes of the patient's clinical disease must also be considered.

A proportion of children with malaria have bacteremia, which may be either the principal or an additional cause of the child's illness.[794] Nontyphi bacteremia is particularly associated with malaria and severe anemia in infants and young children.

TREATMENT OF UNCOMPLICATED MALARIA

Most countries in endemic areas now have a national malaria control program with a stated policy of first line therapy for the treatment of presumed or proven malaria. In many areas it is a (necessary) part of national policy to base treatment on a presumptive diagnosis of malaria in the child with no obvious alternative explanation for fever. The correct drug, dosage and route are important. In general, antimalarial drugs should be given by mouth unless the patient is too ill to swallow. It is usual to prescribe additional symptomatic treatment, e.g. paracetamol, to reduce high fever, myalgia and headache.

In response to strong recommendations from WHO and funding bodies, countries are moving to adopt combination therapies as first line

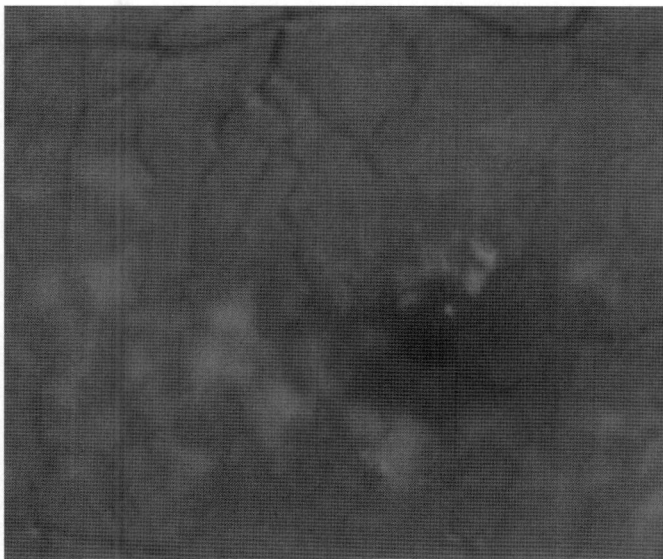
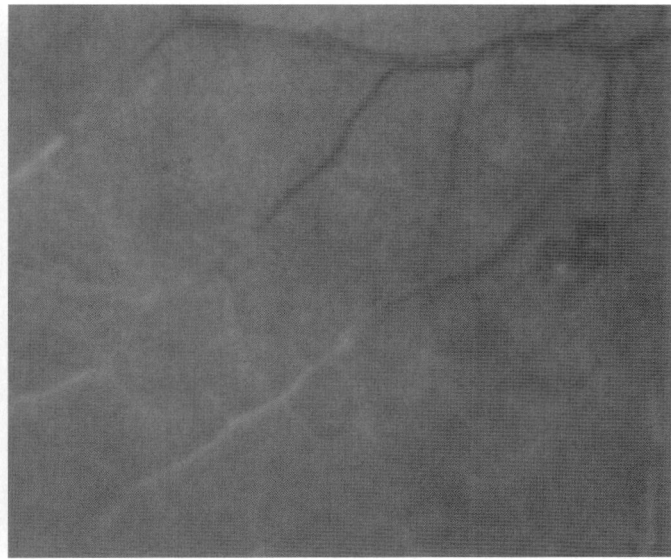

(a)   (b)

Fig. 28.53 Ophthalmoscopy in a child with cerebral malaria, showing (a) patchy retinal macular whitening, close to the fovea, (b) whitening of vessels, and two white-centered hemorrhages.

antiparasitic treatment in areas with a predominance of *P. falciparum* (i.e. most of sub-Saharan Africa). Artemisinin-containing combination therapies (ACTs) are preferred because of the rapid antiparasitic action of artemisinin drugs, their lack of toxicity, and the expectation that combination with another drug will prevent or delay the evolution of drug resistance to each component drug.[795]

Combination therapies that are being increasingly introduced include: artemether–lumefantrine (Coartem) – the only combination yet available (2006) for which the different components are co-formulated in the same tablet; amodiaquine plus artesunate; and amodiaquine plus sulfadoxine–pyrimethamine. The first of these must be given twice daily for three days, the others once daily for three days. Chlorproguanil–dapsone–artesunate (CDA) is a further option for which large scale field evaluations remain to be completed.

Policies usually include a second line therapy if the first line fails or is contraindicated in an individual. If a child vomits more than one attempted dosing by mouth, parenteral or rectal therapy with quinine or an artemisinin drug may be given.

Treatment of nonfalciparum malaria
Chloroquine is the treatment of choice for acute nonfalciparum malaria. Some *P. vivax* infections are chloroquine resistant, but since *P. vivax* does not progress to life-threatening disease, a trial of chloroquine is justified.

P. vivax and *P. ovale* malaria (unless acquired congenitally or by blood transfusion) may relapse if treatment does not include a drug to eliminate hepatic hypnozoites. Primaquine (0.25 mg/kg daily for 2 weeks) will achieve this, but is not worth giving in areas where reinfection is inevitable, and it should not be given to children under the age of 5 years. Primaquine causes severe hemolysis in patients with glucose-6-phosphate dehydrogenase deficiency; the red cell concentration of this enzyme should therefore be measured before the drug is given; if low, an alternative method of radical cure is weekly chloroquine for 6 months in prophylactic doses. Primaquine need not be given after malaria due to *P. falciparum* or *P. malariae*. Primaquine has the additional action of killing gametocytes of all species of malaria parasites; it therefore has the potential to reduce transmission and has occasionally been used for this purpose in areas of moderate endemicity, a function now more safely achieved using artemisinin drugs.

MANAGEMENT OF SEVERE (COMPLICATED) FALCIPARUM MALARIA
Malaria due to *P. falciparum* differs from disease due to other plasmodial species in that *P. falciparum* infections may progress to severe and complicated disease. In the patient with falciparum malaria treatment must therefore be undertaken urgently; complications must be foreseen, recognized and treated; and the antimalarial drugs must be carefully chosen and correctly and promptly administered. Most of the deaths in children admitted to hospital with severe malaria occur before specific antiparasitic drugs can be expected to affect the disease: supportive care during the early phase of management is therefore critically important.

Supportive measures
Hypoglycemia
This complication should be suspected in any child with impaired consciousness, convulsions or acidosis, whether at the time of admission or during the course of treatment. Glucose should be administered as 10% or 20% solution by slow intravenous injection (0.5 g/kg). (If only 50% glucose is available, it should be diluted two- to three-fold with normal saline before being infused over a few minutes.) The blood glucose concentration must be measured again at hourly intervals until the patient's condition improves.

Convulsions
Hypoglycemia and hyperpyrexia should be corrected. Prolonged seizures should be treated with the optimal available drug regimen: drugs which may be used include lorazepam, diazepam, paraldehyde, phenytoin or phenobarbital, using drugs in sequence if convulsions prove refractory.

Acidosis
Deep or labored breathing due to acidosis is a common presentation of severe malaria in children. Possible contributory (and often additive) causes are dehydration, severe anemia, shock, repeated convulsions and hypoglycemia, all of which should be looked for and corrected in the acidotic child (see below under Severe anemia).

Hyperpyrexia
Hyperpyrexia (rectal temperature > 39 °C) should be corrected by administration of oral or rectal paracetamol (15 mg/kg 4–6-hourly). Although important to reduce the risk of seizures in infants and for

symptomatic relief in the conscious child, antipyretic measures have not been demonstrated to affect the prognosis in severe malaria.[796]

Severe anemia

Because of the increasing risk of transmission of HIV by blood in parts of the world where malaria is endemic, blood transfusion should only be given if life-threatening anemia is present or can be predicted on the basis of the hematocrit and level of parasitemia on admission. Blood transfusion is particularly important for the child with severe anemia and respiratory distress.[797] Most children with severe malarial anemia who are breathless have acidosis rather than heart failure, and may be in urgent need of fluid volume replacement.[792]

Exchange transfusion has been advocated and successfully used for patients with hyperparasitemia, but no controlled trials have been done to prove the superiority of this measure. In countries with limited resources for blood transfusion and with high prevalence rates of HIV infection, exchange transfusion is not justifiable as a method for treating severe malaria.

Fluid therapy

This must be sufficient to correct hypovolemia, acidosis and oliguria. When a child has both volume depletion and encephalopathy, there is a therapeutic dilemma: infusion of isotonic electrolyte solution may correct hypovolemia but increase the risk of cerebral edema.[798] In this situation an infusion of albumin, plasma or other plasma expander may be safer (in the anemic child, whole blood will serve all of the needed functions). Current studies are in progress to provide appropriate guidelines. The usual precautions are important to avoid overhydration and the risk of pulmonary edema. Acute tubular necrosis is uncommon as a complication of P. falciparum malaria in children, but if it occurs peritoneal or hemodialysis may be required.

Antibiotics

Some children with severe malaria are bacteremic, the proportion differing between studies and sites. In a series in Kenya the overall rate of bacteremia among 421 children with malarial coma or severe anemia was 8.6% and mortality was three-fold higher in these patients than others, prompting the authors to recommend routine antibiotic treatment for patients with severe malaria.[794] Other studies have indicated a more specific association between severe malarial anemia (SMA) and nontyphoidal salmonella bacteremia, especially in infants and toddlers, suggesting that antibiotics should be considered in the management of SMA in very sick children and in those not responding to antimalarial and hematinic

therapy. Policies for antibiotic use in various severe malaria syndromes may best be decided on the basis of local experience.

In a child with malarial coma, it may be impossible on physical examination to exclude a diagnosis of bacterial meningitis. Since asymptomatic parasitemia is common in endemic areas, parasitemia in the febrile unconscious child cannot be assumed to be the cause of the disease. Some clinicians prefer to perform a lumbar puncture in these circumstances, to clarify the diagnosis. If lumbar puncture is deferred because of the child's clinical condition, antibiotics should be given to cover the possibility of bacterial meningitis.

There is no place for heparin, dexamethasone or dextran in the treatment of CM.[799]

Antimalarial drugs for severe malaria

For severe or complicated P. falciparum malaria, the antiparasitic treatment of choice depends on the context. Recent multicenter studies in South East Asia[800] have shown that intravenous artesunate is superior to quinine in the treatment of adults with severe malaria, but there were insufficient children in these studies to detect a comparable difference among children. Africa differs from South East Asia in two important respects relating to the treatment of severe malaria: (1) in Africa most patients are children, while in South East Asia most patients are adults; and (2) in Africa quinine resistance is unknown among P. falciparum isolates, while partial quinine resistance is well described in South East Asia. Studies are therefore under way to compare parenteral quinine with intravenous artesunate in African children with severe malaria.

Meanwhile, for children in Africa, parenteral quinine remains the drug therapy of choice for severe malaria. If quinine is unavailable, quinidine is an equally effective alternative. Appropriate schedules for treatment are given in Table 28.40.

Quinine may cause severe hypotension if given by rapid intravenous injection, so a dilute solution (1–2 mg/ml) must therefore be infused slowly (over 3 or more hours). If the intravenous route is problematic or impossible, quinine may be given by intramuscular injection in the same doses, the solution (diluted to contain 60 mg/ml) being divided and administered in two sites simultaneously. Parenteral quinine is known to stimulate the secretion of insulin from the pancreatic beta cells, but hypoglycemia in children being treated for malaria is usually due to the disease rather than to drug therapy.[782] If intramuscular quinine is used in the treatment of a comatose child, supplementary glucose must be given or the blood glucose level checked frequently.

Oral drugs should replace parenteral as soon as a patient can take them. If given as the only drug treatment, quinine must be continued

Table 28.40 Drug treatment of acute malaria. In this table the first regimen listed in each section is the treatment of choice

Diagnosis	If patient can take oral drugs	If patient unable to take oral drugs
Malaria due to P. vivax, ovale, malariae, and uncomplicated CQ-sensitive falciparum malaria	Oral CQ: 10 mg/kg first dose then 5 mg/kg after 6, 24 and 48 h Or: AQ, same doses	CQ: 10 mg/kg over 8 h in saline or 5% dextrose; then 5 mg/kg by similar infusions ×3 (total 25 mg/kg in 32 h) Or: CQ i.m. or s.c. 2.5 mg/kg 4-hourly to 10 doses. Substitute oral CQ when possible
Uncomplicated falciparum malaria of doubtful CQ sensitivity	S/P single dose (S: 25 mg/kg, P: 1.25 mg/kg) Or: oral AQ as above Or: oral MQ 15 mg/kg first dose, then 10 mg/kg after 8 h	As for complicated falciparum malaria
Severe or complicated falciparum malaria	QN: i.v., first dose* 16.7 mg/kg over 4 h in 5% dextrose, then 8.3 mg/kg over 2–4 h each, 8-hourly, until oral drug can be taken (viz. quinine 8.3 mg/kg 8-hourly) to complete 7-day course Or: QN i.m. 8.3 mg/kg 8-hourly as solution containing 60 mg/ml. Give supplementary glucose. Substitute oral quinine as soon as possible, 8.3 mg/kg 8-hourly to complete 7-day course Or: quinidine i.v. 7.5 mg/kg 8-hourly, each dose over 4 h in 5% dextrose, until oral treatment can be taken; this may be QN 8.3 mg/kg 8-hourly or quinidine 7.5 mg/kg 8-hourly. Total course 7 days	

*The first dose of i.v. quinine should be reduced to 8.3 mg/kg if the patient has received any quinine or mefloquine in the two preceding days.
CQ, chloroquine; AQ, amodiaquine; QN, quinine; MQ, mefloquine; S/P, sulfonamide–pyrimethamine combination, e.g. Fansidar. All doses of CQ, QN and quinidine refer to base, not salt (8.3 mg quinine base = 10 mg quinine dihydrochloride).

for at least 7 days. Alternatively, once oral treatment is resumed, quinine may be replaced by a locally efficacious oral combination therapy (as used for uncomplicated *P. falciparum* malaria).

MALARIA CONTROL

Since the epidemiology of malaria varies greatly between and even within countries, control measures which are effective in one area may prove ineffective in another. It is important, therefore, that national control programs be designed having regard to local epidemiological, social and economic circumstances.

There are currently four principal methods of malaria control relevant to the well-being of children in areas of intense transmission:

1. *Prompt recognition and treatment of both mild and severe disease* at all levels of the health service, with referral to a larger health facility when necessary. This requires appropriate diagnostic policies (often including presumptive diagnosis of fever as malarial), effective, safe and affordable treatment schedules, competent health staff, and health facilities that are accessible to the majority of people. Because health services are inevitably distant from the homes of many rural people, complementary strategies are needed, and several are being assessed. These include administration of antimalarial drugs for treatment or prevention by village health workers,[801] the training of shopkeepers in appropriate prescribing and dosages (most first line treatment for malaria in village communities is obtained from local grocery stores),[802] schemes to involve traditional healers in treatment or referral of patients with malaria, and making rectal artesunate available at village level for the early treatment of the convulsing or unconscious child.[803]

2. *The use of insecticide-treated nets (ITNs) or curtains.* Several controlled trials and a meta-analysis have demonstrated that sleeping under ITNs can reduce all-cause child mortality in communities.[804] Inevitably there is concern that such results depend on the presence of a scientific team, providing materials and encouraging their use. A study in Tanzania showed a 27% increase in child survival among ITN users in the context of a bednet program promoted by social marketing, i.e. without the involvement of an investigative team.[805] Impregnated nets and curtains therefore have a potentially important place in malaria control, which may depend on local culture and malaria transmission patterns. The need for annual re-impregnation of nets poses a challenge to sustainability; new methods (the 'permanet') may make re-impregnation unnecessary.

3. *Intermittent presumptive treatment (IPT).* Pregnant women, especially primigravidae, are at increased risk of malaria, and placental malaria is associated with low birth weight and increased infant mortality. Provision of two, three or more therapeutic doses of an antimalarial drug such as pyrimethamine–sulfadoxine (Fansidar) between the fourth and eighth months of pregnancy, irrespective of symptoms or parasitemia – intermittent presumptive treatment in pregnancy, or IPTp – reduces placental malaria and improves birth weights.[806] IPTp is now an instrument for control of malaria-induced morbidity in many endemic countries. *Intermittent presumptive therapy for infants (IPTi)* proved promising in an East African study, in which infants given a therapeutic dose of sulfadoxine–pyrimethamine at 2, 3 and 9 months of age, irrespective of fever or parasitemia, had fewer episodes of malaria and of severe anemia during the first year of life than controls.[807] Some (not all) subsequent studies have shown similar benefits, and multicenter trials of IPTi are in progress. Similar studies in older age groups of children (IPTc) are being considered.

4. *Indoor residual spraying (IRS)* – the spraying of the inside walls of dwellings with residual insecticide – was a mainstay of the malaria eradication campaigns in 1950–70, parts of which were spectacularly successful. But IRS encountered both political and vector resistance, was poorly sustained, and was never adequately achieved in Africa. IRS is now receiving renewed attention as novel methods and capacities are acquired, and it is being increasingly explored as a promising component of malaria control programs.

There is growing optimism that vaccination will, within the next few years, become a further weapon in the armamentarium available to fight malaria.

The success of any method or combination of methods of control is likely to be materially influenced by the degree to which the causes and consequences of malaria are appreciated by populations and by the willingness of communities to participate in, and even finance, specific operations.[799]

Meanwhile the international community is becoming more aware of the fact that tools for malaria control exist, and that their deployment needs expenditure on materials, infrastructure, health systems and staff development. Commitments of funding from major donors have increased in recent years and will need to be sustained if real progress is to be made.

TOXOPLASMOSIS

Toxoplasmosis is mainly of importance to pediatrics as a congenital infection (see p. 1202). Infection acquired after birth can cause choroidoretinitis or infectious mononucleosis and can cause significant disease in persons with underlying T cell immunodeficiencies. Occasionally, signs of congenital infection may not manifest until late in childhood or early adulthood.

The birth prevalence of congenital toxoplasmosis infection across Europe ranges from 1 to 10 per 10 000 newborns.[808] In the UK, only 10% of women show evidence of past infection with toxoplasmosis, whereas in France up to 55% of pregnant women show antibodies to toxoplasmosis on antenatal screening.

ETIOLOGY

The causative organism, *Toxoplasma gondii*, is, in its free active state, a small, crescentic protozoan, which is a strict intracellular parasite multiplying only within the cytoplasm of the nucleated host by binary fission or, probably more frequently, by internal budding (endodyogeny). The active form, responsible for acute infection, stimulates an immunological response by the host. At the same time, cyst forms of the parasite develop in any tissue, but chiefly in nervous tissue or striated muscle, and may persist for the life of the host.

PATHOGENESIS

T. gondii infects virtually all species of mammals and several species of birds. The cat family is the definitive host. Cats usually acquire the infection after eating infected rodents, birds or uncooked meat. After primary infection, they shed millions of oocysts in their feces for up to 14 days. Oocysts may remain viable in soil for many months, and are not found on the cat fur, thus explaining the failure to link cat exposure with the risk of human toxoplasmosis infection.[809]

Humans are most commonly infected after ingestion of tissue cysts in raw or poorly cooked meat, or by ingestion of soil, food or water contaminated with oocysts. Infection from meat has been shown to be responsible for up to two thirds of all new infections in pregnant women.[810] Traditionally pork, lamb, goat or game meats hold the highest risk for human infection, although undercooked beef has been shown to be a risk factor for toxoplasmosis seroconversion,[810] possibly due to combination with cheaper meats.[809] Congenital toxoplasmosis infection usually occurs as a result of placental infection after a primary infection in a pregnant woman. The risk of transmission and the clinical outcome after maternal toxoplasmosis infection vary with the trimester of pregnancy, with the first trimester having the lowest risk of transmission to the fetus but the highest risk of damage.

Transmission has also been rarely documented in children after blood or blood product transfusion, heart or bone marrow transplantation[811,812] and through infected breast milk.[813]

CLINICAL FEATURES

Acquired infection with *T. gondii* is uncommon in the UK in children under 5 years. Serological surveys suggest a peak acquisition of infection in early and mid teens. The disease is nearly always asymptomatic. The commonest manifestation, if clinical signs do occur, is lymphadenopathy, particularly of cervical nodes, which may be accompanied by no ill health, or may be accompanied by fever and prostration and resemble severe infectious mononucleosis. Muscle pain may also occur due, it is believed and occasionally confirmed, to infection of voluntary muscle. Acquired toxoplasmosis may also result in hepatosplenomegaly, lymphocytosis, and, rarely, pneumonitis, acute hepatitis, arthritis or cardiac arrhythmias (due to lesions in the region of the conducting system). The occurrence of cardiac failure due to toxoplasma infection of the myocardium is conjectural. Isolated visual disturbance due to toxoplasmosis retinitis in childhood used to be thought to be due to reactivation of an undiagnosed congenital infection, but is equally commonly due to acquired infection.[814]

Acquired toxoplasmosis infection has been documented in immunodeficient children with HIV infection, or post bone marrow or solid organ transplantation, but it occurs much less commonly than in adults. Toxoplasmosis in the immunocompromised child may manifest as encephalitis, pneumonitis or even a multiorgan systemic disease.

DIAGNOSIS AND DIFFERENTIAL DIAGNOSIS

Acquired toxoplasmosis should be considered in any case of unexplained lymphadenopathy, particularly when maximal in, or confined to, the cervical region, whether or not it is accompanied by pyrexia. Lymph node enlargement in acquired toxoplasmosis may persist for several months, leading to the consideration of lymphoma and tuberculous lymphadenopathy in the differential diagnosis.

In the immunocompromised child, it enters the differential diagnosis for neurological disease (encephalitis, meningoencephalitis, brain abscess), for interstitial pneumonitis, and for myocarditis.

Laboratory diagnosis

The most common laboratory aids to the diagnosis include serology, isolation of the organism, histology and the direct detection of *T. gondii* DNA in infected tissues or fluids by polymerase chain reaction (PCR). Other diagnostic methods used less commonly today include skin testing and the Sabin–Feldman dye test, which depends upon the inhibition by antibody-containing serum of methylene blue staining of laboratory cultures of *T. gondii*. The diagnosis of a congenital infection postnatally is discussed in Chapter 12.

Serological methods remain the most commonly used method for diagnosis. Acute infection in the older child or adult may be diagnosed by a four-fold rise in toxoplasma-specific IgG by indirect immunofluorescence, or enzyme immunoassay. Toxoplasma-specific IgM can be detected by 2 weeks post infection, and usually declines by 6 months, but at times may persist for months (and occasionally over a year) after the initial infection. Thus the detection of toxoplasma IgM may indicate either an acute or a recent past infection. Positive results should be confirmed by multiple tests in different laboratories, given a false positive rate of up to 2%. If timing of the infection is critical, as in the case of a pregnant woman, the presence of IgA and IgE antibodies to toxoplasmosis which decline more readily than IgM, and IgG avidity (high avidity suggests an infection > 12 months prior) may be helpful in differentiating an acute infection from a past infection. However, some suggest that even current serological assays cannot predict the time of infection within the first year after infection (reviewed in Petersen et al[815]).

The detection of *T. gondii* DNA by PCR in amniotic fluid is now commonly used for the prenatal diagnosis of congenital toxoplasmosis.

Sensitivity rates of up to 90% have been reported, but there is a wide range in the quality of assays available, with false positive rates ranging from 0 to 10% reported in some laboratories (reviewed in Petersen et al[815]). Other applications of the assay are on cerebrospinal fluid, or peripheral white blood cells in the immunocompromised or congenitally infected infant.

Culture of *T. gondii* from lymph node biopsy material, amniotic fluid, placenta or, less often, other tissue fluids is possible, although generally less widely used than serological methods. The organism can be cultured in suitable laboratory animals, particularly mice, embryonated eggs and tissue cultures. The most reliable of these procedures is that of intraperitoneal inoculation of mice. Histological examination of biopsy material is also of value, limited chiefly by the availability of suitable material. Cysts can be identified readily, but vegetative forms are recognized with difficulty.

In the immunocompromised child, such as those with HIV infection, the ability to document seroconversion to toxoplasmosis is impaired. A diagnosis must be made by demonstrating the organism by PCR, culture or histology in infected tissues, or presumptively by characteristic findings on imaging that respond to an empirical trial of antiparasitic therapy.

Dermal hypersensitivity to injection of a suspension of killed toxoplasma is indicated by a delayed tuberculin type response. There is good correlation between a positive skin test and a positive dye test titer of 1:8 or more. The test may be negative in very recent infections and is used chiefly in epidemiological surveys in man.

TREATMENT AND PROGNOSIS

Treatment of acquired toxoplasmosis infection in childhood is usually only indicated for active ocular infection or severe disease in other organs.

Treatment of congenitally infected infants is discussed in Chapter 12. Antibiotics, other than spiramycin, have proved to be of little value in the treatment of acute toxoplasmosis. Sulfonamides have proved disappointing and sulfones too toxic in the doses required. The most effective form of chemotherapy is a combination of pyrimethamine and sulfadiazine for a total duration of 3–4 weeks. The hematological toxic effects of pyrimethamine, due to its antifolic acid action, can be prevented or reversed by folinic acid. Spiramycin, though less toxic than the pyrimethamine and sulfadiazine combination, is clearly less effective. An alternative is the use of a combination of trimethoprim and a sulfonamide, e.g. co-trimoxazole. Life-long suppressive therapy with these agents is indicated for HIV infected children after toxoplasmosis encephalitis.

In the pregnant woman, spiramycin may be given in early pregnancy for suspected primary toxoplasmosis to prevent transmission to the fetus, and after 17 weeks' gestation, pyrimethamine and sulfadiazine may be used for confirmed fetal infection to reduce the risk of transmission or complications in the child. However, a recent systematic review of randomized trials of antiparasitic treatment of toxoplasmosis in pregnancy concluded that there was still insufficient evidence available to determine whether such treatment has a positive effect on clinical outcomes or risk of transmission.[816]

Chemoprophylaxis to prevent reactivation of toxoplasmosis should be considered in the significantly immunosuppressed child with HIV infection or prior to heart transplantation.

TRYPANOSOMIASIS

AFRICAN TRYPANOSOMIASIS: SLEEPING SICKNESS

Human African trypanosomiasis (HAT) is caused by two 'subspecies' of *Trypanosoma brucei* which are transmitted by the bite of the tsetse fly. Sleeping sickness is widely distributed in 36 countries in sub-Saharan Africa. Approximately 18 000 cases are reported annually to the WHO, with an estimated total burden of 50–70 000.

T. b. gambiense occurs in west and central Africa and causes a disease which is slow in onset and progression (Gambian sleeping sickness). Infected humans provide long term sources of infection for the tsetse and the *T. b. gambiense* disease is largely an anthroponosis. Infection with *T. b. rhodesiense* occurs in east and south east Africa and causes an acute illness that is often lethal within a few months (Rhodesian sleeping sickness). It is a true zoonosis: infection is maintained within wild ungulate reservoirs. Both forms most commonly infect adults but any age may be affected; infection is 2–3 times more common in adults than children in *T. b. gambiense* endemic areas.[817]

Life cycle

In the tsetse fly, stumpy trypomastigotes ingested with the blood meal transform into slender midgut forms. These eventually reach the salivary gland and transform via epimastigotes to the infective metacyclic trypomastigote. After inoculation, the metacyclic trypomastigotes are converted into long slender forms in the subcutaneous tissue of the host. Blood forms are polymorphic with both slender and stumpy forms. The continual movement of the trypomastigote is activated by a flagellum and a fold of membrane which is lifted up by the motion of the flagellum – the 'undulating membrane'. Three 'subspecies' of *T. brucei* group exist; *T. b. brucei*, which is not infective to humans, cannot be distinguished morphologically from *T. b. rhodesiense* and *T. b. gambiense*. However, biochemical techniques, DNA analysis and isoenzyme characterization can distinguish different *T. brucei* populations. *T. b. rhodesiense* comprises two distinct zymodemes; the 'Zambezi' group in southern Africa and the 'Busoga' group in east Africa associated with more acute severe disease. *T. b. gambiense* is less variable.

Epidemiology

The reported number of infections has declined considerably over the last 6–7 years, because of improved surveillance and control measures in some regions. However, recent epidemics have occurred in areas such as DRC, Angola and Sudan, partly because of breakdown of control measures and population movement due to civil unrest. *T. b. gambiense* accounts for the vast majority of cases of trypanosomiasis.

T. b. gambiense is restricted to west and central Africa and is transmitted by 'palpalis group' tsetse (*Glossina palpalis*, *G. tachinoides* and *G. fuscipes*), which inhabit dense vegetation along rivers and in forests. Vectors feed on man at water collecting points and river crossings. The man–fly–man cycle of transmission may maintain the disease in the absence of an animal reservoir; infected individuals may be asymptomatically parasitemic for years. Although human parasites infect both wild and domestic animals, their epidemiological significance remains uncertain.

T. b. rhodesiense is usually transmitted by 'morsitans group' tsetse (*G. morsitans*, *G. pallidipes* and *G. swynnertoni*) in East African woodland savannah and lake shores. Most infection is sporadic such as in Tanzania when game hunters or honey gatherers are bitten by *G. morsitans* which transmit disease from the bushbuck host, or in south east Uganda and western Kenya where fishermen are bitten by *G. pallidipes* on lake shores. However, epidemics have occurred in western Kenya and in south eastern Uganda with infections occurring in both sexes and all age groups. The vector is *G. f. fuscipes*, a 'palpalis group' tsetse which invades *Lantana camora* thickets close to human habitation; domestic cows may play an important part in maintaining infection in such situations. Imported trypanosomiasis is also relatively rare, but an increased number of cases have been reported over the last 5 years in Europe and the USA as a result of exposure in game parks. Congenital infection with *T. b. rhodesiense* and *T. b. gambiense* does occur, but appears to be very rare.

Pathogenesis and pathology

Pathological processes are similar but vary in intensity between *T. b. gambiense* and *T. b. rhodesiense*. Parasites inoculated into the subcutaneous tissue multiply locally, forming a trypanosomal chancre, with edema and an infiltrate of polymorphonuclear leukocytes, lymphocytes and plasma cells. Parasites travel to regional lymph nodes where they continue to multiply and cause parasitemia 5–12 days after infection. Waves of parasitemia occur, each differing in its surface antigens (particularly variant surface glycoprotein) as the parasite attempts to avoid the host immune response.

Hyperplasia of the reticuloendothelial system, with lymph node and spleen enlargement, occurs as a response to infection; lymph nodes may subsequently become atrophic and fibrotic. Morular cells (Mott cells) are found; these are plasmacytes that may have an important role in the production of IgM. Blood parasites invade the central nervous system via the choroid plexus leading to the second stage of infection, a meningoencephalitis. A lymphocytic meningoencephalitis and focal vasculitis with perivascular infiltrates occurs particularly in the frontal lobes, pons and medulla. Parasites in the CNS are accompanied by changes in the cerebrospinal fluid with a raised protein concentration and the presence of mononuclear cells, particularly lymphocytes. Parasites can also be identified in the CSF.

The succession of variable antigens induces a profuse production of IgM antibody in the serum and it is also locally produced in the central nervous system by plasma cells and the morular cells. Immune complex damage (type III hypersensitivity) may cause less common lesions of the kidney, lungs, liver and heart. Expression of cell-mediated immunity, induction of cell-mediated immunity and expression of humoral immunity have been shown to be impaired in *T. b. gambiense* infections in man.

Clinical features
The trypanosomal chancre
The primary lesion (trypanosomal chancre) is a painful, erythematous and edematous swelling at the site of the bite that appears within 2 or 3 days. Skin vesicles and ulceration may develop and the chancre heals with residual scarring over 2–3 weeks. Chancres commonly occur in *T. b. rhodesiense* infection but are less common in *T. b. gambiense*. As the chancre develops, the regional lymph glands become enlarged and tender.

The hemolymphatic (first) stage
Waves of irregular remittent fever, in association with the waves of parasitemia, occur 5–12 days after the bite. This is most marked in *T. b. rhodesiense* infections; in *T. b. gambiense* the hemolymphatic stage may be mild, subclinical or asymptomatic. Febrile episodes, sometimes with rigors, are accompanied by malaise, headache, muscular tenderness, joint aches and weight loss. An annular erythematous rash (circinate erythema) may be visible, particularly on the trunk in the fair skinned. Generalized lymphadenopathy may develop, especially in *T. b. gambiense*. Winterbottom's sign, posterior cervical triangle lymphadenopathy, occurs in *T. b. gambiense* due to the predilection for *G. palpalis* to bite on the head. Edema may affect the ankles or feet or face, producing a dull expressionless facies. Irritability, insomnia and confusion may occur even in the early stage. The spleen and liver may enlarge. In the acute stage of *T. b. rhodesiense* infection, tachycardia is common; pleural or pericardial effusions may occur and myocarditis with arrhythmias or cardiac failure may lead to death.

Meningoencephalitic (second) stage
Meningoencephalitis is an inevitable consequence of untreated human African trypanosomiasis. In *T. b. gambiense*, it tends to occur after months or years while in *T. b. rhodesiense* it occurs early, often during the febrile illness, and progresses rapidly to a fatal outcome. Children develop meningoencephalitis more rapidly than adults. A wide variety of neurological signs occur. Behavioral changes and sleep disturbances are often the first signs; inappropriate diurnal somnolence with insomnia and agitation at night are common. Patients become apathetic, lacking in attention and may exhibit trance-like states. Behavior becomes inappropriate, aggressive or overtly paranoid. Nutritional deficiencies, intercurrent infections and progressive emaciation result. Generalized weakness, unsteadiness of gait, expressionless facies, slurred speech, tremors of the limbs, hyper-reflexia and delayed deep hyperalgesia all occur. In advanced disease, focal epileptic attacks, profound ataxia, choreoathetosis and psychotic changes may be followed by coma and death. There is little variation in symptoms or signs between adults and

children, apart from the incidence of malnutrition, which may be as high as 50–60% in children with second stage disease.[818]

Diagnosis[819]

Clinical diagnosis of African trypanosomiasis may be difficult. Although the presence of a chancre is pathognomonic, the hemolymphatic stage must be differentiated from a wide range of febrile illnesses including malaria. Differential diagnosis of second stage disease includes other causes of meningoencephalitis, particularly cryptococcal and tuberculous meningitis in the HIV infected, and psychiatric illness. Routine laboratory tests show a normal total white cell count, raised ESR, anemia, thrombocytopenia, low serum albumin and elevated serum IgM. Bilirubin and transaminases may be raised. Hematological abnormalities, including coagulopathy, are particularly prominent in acute *T. b. rhodesiense*. A parasitic diagnosis must be attempted in all suspected cases.

Parasitological diagnosis

In the early stages of *T. b. rhodesiense* infection, parasitological diagnosis is usually simple, as the concentration of trypanosomes in the blood or aspirates of trypanosomal chancres is high. Organisms can be seen by single or repeated microscopic examination of wet films or thick blood or aspirate fluid films stained with Field's stain or Giemsa. Blood film microscopy is less reliable in *T. b. gambiense*; repeated examination of blood films and concentration techniques are more often required. However, organisms are readily seen in fresh lymph node aspirates. Trypanosomes may also be identified in CSF, various effusions and marrow smears.

Concentration methods increase the sensitivity of microscopy; microhematocrit centrifugation and microscopic examination of the area above the buffy coat are commonly used. The quantitative buffy coat technique (QBC), where motile trypanosomes are stained with fluorescent acridine orange, tubes centrifuged and examined by fluorescent microscopy, is rapid and sensitive.[820] The miniature anion exchange centrifugation technique (MAEC[821]) involves passing a sample of blood through a DEAE-cellulose anion exchange column, which allows trypanosomes to pass into a collecting tube which is centrifuged and examined. This technique is sensitive but difficult in field conditions.

Once trypanosomiasis is diagnosed or suspected, the CSF must be examined, preferably within 15 min of lumbar puncture. Increase in cell count (more than 5 cells/mm³), protein elevation, CSF IgM or trypomastigotes in the centrifuged deposit indicate CNS involvement.

Immunodiagnosis

Immunodiagnostic tests include IFAT, ELISA, CFT and IgM estimation. IFAT is valuable in epidemiological investigation and screening of populations and suspects but provides only presumptive evidence of infection. A card agglutination test for trypanosomiasis (CATT) has been developed for the diagnosis of *T. b. gambiense*. The test provides a rapid field test for preliminary screening of populations in endemic areas. Positive serological tests require confirmatory parasitic diagnosis prior to treatment.[822] Antigen detection techniques (CIATT) have also been developed and appear to be sensitive and specific; they have potential for following the response to therapy.[823]

Treatment[824]

Treatment should be started as soon as possible after making a parasitological diagnosis although nutritional disturbances or intercurrent infection should first be treated in view of the toxicity of treatment. Routine use of antihelminth and antimalarial drugs is common. Examination of the CSF is mandatory to distinguish early stage from late stage disease as CNS involvement requires different, more toxic therapy. Lumbar puncture should not be performed until at least one dose of suramin (or pentamidine) has been given to clear parasites from the blood and prevent inoculation into the CSF at the time of LP.

Treatment of hemolymphatic trypanosomiasis

Suramin is effective in treatment of the hemolymphatic stage of both *T. b. rhodesiense* and *T. b. gambiense* disease and will rapidly clear the parasitemia in both early and late sleeping sickness. Pentamidine is the first line therapy for *T. b. gambiense* but is not effective in *T. b. rhodesiense*. Neither suramin nor pentamidine is effective in meningoencephalitis.

Suramin. Suramin is given intravenously with a test dose of 5 mg/kg on day 1 followed by 20 mg/kg on days 3, 7, 14 and 21. Fever nausea, vomiting and urticaria are common side-effects: renal toxicity may occur.

Pentamidine. Pentamidine is usually given intramuscularly at doses of 4 mg/kg base daily or on alternate days for 7 days. Intravenous administration avoids local side-effects that include sterile abscesses, but requires close supervision. Side-effects include syncope and hypotension, vomiting and abdominal pain, especially in the first half hour after administration. Peripheral neuritis is a rare complication and severe hypoglycemic reactions may occur during the course of treatment. Adrenaline and glucose should be available when treatment with pentamidine is given.

Meningoencephalitic (late stage) trypanosomiasis

Melarsoprol. Melarsoprol (Mel B) is an arsenical compound which enters the CNS. Use is limited to late stage trypanosomiasis because of its toxicity. A variety of different treatment schedules have been used. In *T. b. rhodesiense* infection, melarsoprol is usually given in three or four courses, each course lasting three days and separated by a week, giving a total dose of 35–37.5 ml melarsoprol. Regimens which use lower doses initially and increase through four courses of treatment may be less toxic.

Many regimens have been advocated for treatment of *T. b. gambiense*. Recently, shortened 10-day regimens (2.2 mg/kg daily) have been used for *T. b. gambiense* with no loss of efficacy, and no increased relapse.[825,826]

Thrombophlebitis is a frequent complication of melarsoprol treatment; extravasation causes severe local reactions. The major side-effect is a *reactive arsenical encephalopathy* (RAE), which occurs in up to 5% of patients, usually after the third or fourth dose. The onset is usually sudden with neurological deterioration, confusion, convulsions and coma. It occurs more commonly in severe meningoencephalitis and is fatal in 10–50% of cases. In *T. b. gambiense* (but not *T. b. rhodesiense*) prophylactic prednisolone significantly reduces the incidence of RAE.[827] Other toxicity common with melarsoprol includes agranulocytosis, aplastic anemia, thrombocytopenia and peripheral neuropathy. Melarsoprol should not be given as initial therapy to parasitemic patients; it may cause a Jarisch–Herxheimer-like febrile reaction after the first injection. Treatment normally leads to a striking improvement in the mental and physical condition of patients with sleeping sickness, but there is increasing concern about rising relapse rates.

Eflornithine (difluoromethyl-ornithine, DFMO). This drug has been used for the treatment of both early and late stage *T. b. gambiense* with good results but is poorly effective in *T. b. rhodesiense*. The drug is given intravenously in a dose of 100 mg/kg 6-hourly for 14 days (4 g/m² for young children); oral preparations are being evaluated. Major side-effects are diarrhea and reversible marrow depression. Response rates vary from 73 to 97% with some geographical variability; shorter courses are less effective. Recent studies suggest that eflornithine may be more effective and safer than melarsoprol in some settings,[828,829] although efficacy may be reduced in those who are HIV positive.

Nifurtimox. (an oral agent) has occasionally been used in the treatment of *T. b. gambiense*. As a single agent it has high relapse rates, but when used in combination with a low dose 10-day course of melarsoprol, the combination regimen was superior to a standard melarsoprol regimen.[830]

Follow-up and relapse

Patients should be seen 3 months after treatment and followed up for 2 years to identify relapse which occurs in 5–20% of those treated, usually presenting as a chronic meningoencephalitis without a peripheral parasitemia. Follow-up should include routine lumbar puncture to identify a rising cell count or protein. Relapse in *T. b. gambiense* following treatment with suramin or pentamidine should be with melarsoprol; eflornithine can also be used in the treatment of relapse after melarsoprol therapy. Relapse in *T. b. rhodesiense* is usually treated with a second course of melarsoprol; nifurtimox may be effective, but more data are needed.

Control of sleeping sickness

There are two major components of control activities: detecting and treating human cases and vector control. Sleeping sickness caused by *T. b. rhodesiense* is usually detected at fixed medical units in rural areas when patients present with the symptoms of early parasitemia (passive surveillance). In *T. b. gambiense*, limited clinical symptoms in the early stage mean that active surveillance for infected individuals is necessary. Active surveillance may also be useful in *T. b. rhodesiense* epidemics. Blood film examination is used to screen for *T. b. rhodesiense*, but in *T. b. gambiense* CATT tests or gland aspiration are frequently used for initial population screening. Diagnoses should be confirmed parasitologically; serologically positive but parasite negative individuals should be followed at regular intervals. Community education may play a large part in encouraging early diagnosis and reducing the number of parasitemic individuals. There is no role for mass community prophylaxis: it may mask second stage infections and lead to resistance.[824]

Vector control measures used include destruction of tsetse habitats and insecticide spraying. Insecticide-impregnated (and/or odor-baited) traps have been very effective in reducing fly populations without the environmental problems associated with widespread application of insecticides.

AMERICAN TRYPANOSOMIASIS: CHAGAS' DISEASE

Chagas' disease is endemic throughout most countries of South and Central America. It is caused by *Trypanosoma cruzi*, which is transmitted to humans by triatomine bugs. Acute *T. cruzi* infection is usually benign; the major public health and socioeconomic significance of the disease arises from the chronic stages of the disease. Improved control has led to a reduction in disease: approximately 10 million are infected with an estimated 14 000 deaths annually.

Life cycle of *Trypanosoma cruzi*

The organism occurs in three distinct forms: amastigotes found in tissues of mammalian hosts, epimastigotes found in the digestive tract of the triatomine bug, and trypomastigotes found in mammalian blood. After ingestion by the vector, trypomastigotes change and multiply as epimastigotes and in the succeeding 2–4 weeks develop into metacyclic trypomastigotes in the gut of the bug. Infective forms, excreted with the feces, enter through an abrasion in the skin or through intact mucous membranes such as the conjunctiva. Within 1–2 weeks trypomastigotes circulate in the bloodstream. After an undetermined period, the trypomastigote invades tissue cells and is transformed into the amastigote.

Epidemiology

T. cruzi infect over 100 mammalian species; the commonest wild hosts are rodents and small marsupials. Many triatomine bugs are sylvatic and maintain infection among reservoir hosts. Three species have adapted to human dwellings: *Rhodnius prolixus*, *Triatoma infestans* and *Panstrongylus megistus*. Human infection usually occurs from transmission between man and domestic animals. There may be hundreds or thousands of bugs in a household due to factors such as poor housing, thatched roofs and lack of wall resurfacing. Up to 40–50% of bugs may be infected in some locations. Most transmission occurs rurally but peri-urban transmission is increasing as a result of the rapid urbanization occurring throughout much of South America.

Chagas' disease may also be acquired by blood transfusion, although widespread serological screening has decreased transmission considerably. Congenital disease is an important public health problem in rural areas of endemic transmission, occurring in up to 10% of seropositive women.

Pathogenesis

Parasites multiply at the site of entry which may lead to a chagoma, consisting of interstitial edema and focal inflammation. Parasites reach the blood but soon disseminate to enter cells, particularly histiocytes, neuroglia, smooth muscle, cardiac muscle and skeletal muscle cells. Amastigotes develop within cells to form pseudocysts. Pseudocyst rupture may lead to the development of acute inflammatory foci with tissue damage, such as the destruction of conducting tissue in the heart. A small proportion of individuals have acute complications, but in the vast majority the inflammatory reaction subsides and parasitemia and multiplication of parasites in the tissues is reduced by the immune response. Mechanisms of the chronic complications of Chagas' disease remain uncertain; tissue damage, neuronal loss and an autoimmune response are all likely to be important.[831]

Clinical features

Acute Chagas' disease

Acute Chagas' disease is usually an illness of children but can occur at any age. The acute phase of Chagas' disease is asymptomatic in over two thirds of affected infants and children. If symptomatic, the acute phase lasts for 1–3 months and resolves spontaneously. A chagoma may occur at the portal of entry. The skin over the chagoma becomes hard and may desquamate. Romaña's sign, unilateral eyelid edema and chemosis, is one of the classical syndromes associated with acute Chagas' disease, occurring when bug feces contaminate the conjunctiva.

One to two weeks later, a febrile reaction develops, often associated with headache and myalgia. Vomiting, diarrhea, lymphadenopathy, moderate hepatosplenomegaly and meningoencephalitis may all occur. Myocardial involvement, causing varying dysrhythmias to myocarditis and cardiac failure, may occur; these complications may occasionally be fatal. Meningoencephalitis in the very young has a bad prognosis. Leukocytosis and lymphocytosis accompany the parasitemia.

Following the acute phase, if untreated, low level infection may persist asymptomatically for many years (sometimes termed indeterminate phase). Between 15 and 40% of these patients will develop chronic Chagas' disease.

Chronic Chagas' disease

Chronic symptomatic disease is rarely a pediatric problem, usually occurring between the ages of 15 and 50 years. It is characterized by the reappearance of clinical disease 10–20 years after infection. In adults, classical manifestations are the development of a biventricular congestive cardiomyopathy or cardiac rhythm disturbances. Complete right bundle branch block with left bundle hemi-block is the most common abnormality; AV block, extrasystoles and Stokes–Adams attacks also frequently occur. Inflammatory changes and destruction of parasympathetic ganglion cells in muscle may also eventually lead to mega-esophagus and megacolon.

Congenital Chagas' disease

Congenital infection with *T. cruzi* occurs in between 2 and 10% of maternal infections. Infection is associated with abortion, stillbirth and severe illness or death in early infancy in a high proportion. Clinical features include cardiac problems, mega-esophagus, pneumonitis and meningo-encephalitis. Transmission is also thought to occur through breast milk.

Chagas' disease in the immunocompromised

Chagas' disease in immunocompromised individuals is an increasing problem in South America due to HIV infection and the use of immunosuppressive drugs in transplant patients. Reactivation of latent *T. cruzi* infection or transplantation of an infected organ can cause the recurrence of parasitemia and the development of an intense myocarditis or severe neurological problems if careful monitoring and pre-emptive therapy is not used.[832]

Diagnosis

Parasitic diagnosis

A specific diagnosis, demonstrating *Trypanosoma cruzi* in the peripheral blood, is usually easy in the early acute illness. The parasite appears as a C- or S-shaped trypomastigote with a prominent kinetoplast in Romanowsky-stained thick or thin films. Centrifugation steps on separated red cells or lysed blood increase the sensitivity of microscopic examination. Culture requires specialized media and is difficult to perform outside a laboratory. Xenodiagnosis is a method for detecting sub-patent parasitemia in chronic infections (and occasionally in acute infection) by allowing triatomine bugs to feed on the individual patient: it is preferable to animal inoculation which is unreliable. Bugs are then dissected to look for gut infection after 20–40 days. PCR methods have published sensitivities of 60–100% when compared with serology; the technique may be more sensitive in children than in adults. It may also be particularly useful in the early detection of congenital infection.[833]

Serological diagnosis

An initial IgM response and life-long IgG response may be detected by a number of serological tests, including complement-fixation tests, indirect fluorescent antibody tests and enzyme-linked immunosorbent assays. Approximately 50% of individuals with positive serology will also be positive using xenodiagnosis, but there is a poor specificity with false positive tests from other parasitic infections, particularly leishmaniasis, and autoimmune disorders.

Following the response to therapy is difficult; xenodiagnosis may be negative in those with low parasite burdens and serological tests often remain positive after parasitological cure. PCR may be particularly useful in this situation.[834]

Treatment

Chemotherapy in Chagas' disease is problematic. Two drugs have been widely used: nifurtimox (8 mg/kg body weight daily for 60–90 days) and benznidazole (6–10 mg/kg body weight daily for 30 or 60 days). The latter is now more commonly used as it is better tolerated. Benznidazole side-effects are more common in adults than in children and occur in 4–30% of cases; hypersensitivity reactions cause rashes and fever, vomiting and peripheral neuropathy. Treatment in acute disease suppresses parasitemia, shortens the course of the acute illness and helps to prevent complications and deaths from acute myocarditis or meningoencephalitis. However, elimination of parasites and prevention of chronic illness only occurs in 50–70% of patients.

The value of treatment in the indeterminate and chronic phase is less certain; results of clinical trials vary both geographically and according to the stage of the infection. Standard recommendations have been that chemotherapy is of no benefit. However, increasing evidence and a Cochrane review suggests that treatment of patients with benznidazole in the indeterminate phase (chronic asymptomatic) leads to parasite clearance in around 60% of patients (measured by negative serology or xenodiagnosis) and reduces the proportion developing ECG changes or progressing to heart disease.[835,836]

Both allopurinol and itraconazole have been used for treatment of chronic disease with parasitological cure in 40–50% and normalization of ECG abnormalities in 36–48% of individuals; itraconazole appears to be superior in preventing the development of new ECG changes.[835,837,838] Further work is needed to evaluate the true value of chemotherapy in chronic disease. Heart failure is usually treated with vasodilators such as ACE inhibitors; digitalis may aggravate arrhythmias. Pacemakers are commonly implanted for heart block. A number of surgical procedures are used for mega-esophagus and megacolon. Treatment of symptomatic congenital infection is often unsatisfactory. Recent evidence suggests that routine screening of babies of seropositive mothers with treatment of positive infants is a safe and effective approach.[833,839]

Control

No vaccine exists for Chagas' disease. Major preventative efforts center upon control of transmission. Chagas' disease is predominantly a disease of poverty, which leads to poor quality housing and the inability to control domestic triatomine bugs. In recent years, control programs have been effective in countries in the southern cone of South America (Argentina, Brazil, Bolivia, Chile, Paraguay and Uruguay) with a reduction in incidence of between 60 and 99% from 1983–1997.[840]

Seroprevalence surveys are used to indicate areas and dwellings at risk, and pyrethroid insecticides are used for the spraying of housing and peri-domestic buildings; the use of fumigant canisters may also be useful. Community surveillance is then used to detect residual or new infections and further spraying performed. Housing improvements and health education help to promote sustainability. Programs to control blood transfusion transmission are based on routine serological testing and usually combine serological tests for HIV and hepatitis B as well as T. cruzi. If seropositive blood has to be used, the addition of gentian violet 24 h before is effective and safe in preventing transmission.

FUNGAL INFECTIONS

Fungi form a large and very diverse kingdom but only a small number are pathogenic for humans. Fungi are eukaryotes, that is, unlike bacteria, they have a nucleus and intracellular organelles. They also possess a cell wall composed of chitin. Infections are conveniently divided into superficial, subcutaneous and systemic or deep mycoses. In addition, an increasing number of opportunist fungi cause infection in immunocompromised children (Table 28.41).

Fungi can grow in a unicellular mode (yeasts) or a multicellular mode, when cells elongate and multiply to form long filaments called hyphae and collectively form a mycelium. Some fungi are dimorphic, existing as a yeast at one temperature but forming multicellular hyphae at another. Rather confusingly, some are given different names when in the different forms. Thus *Cryptococcus neoformans* is the name as a yeast and *Filobasidiella neoformans* is its hyphal form. *Actinomyces* and *Nocardia* spp. are not fungi but branching bacteria, but are more conveniently included in discussions of fungal disease (Table 28.42). Treatment of subcutaneous and systemic mycoses is most often by antifungals such as polyenes (e.g. amphotericin B) or imidazoles (e.g. ketoconazole) (Table 28.42). To prevent repetition, information on dosage, mode of administration and side-effects and toxicity is included at the end of the chapter.

ACTINOMYCOSIS

ETIOLOGY

Actinomycosis is an infection with a worldwide distribution that affects humans and other animals such as cattle and canines. *Actinomyces* spp. are Gram positive, non-spore-bearing, short or filamentous bacilli, which may exhibit true branching. Although *Actinomyces israelii* is the major pathogen, other species including *A. gerencserai, A. meyeri, A. naeslundii, A. odontolyticus, A. pyogenes, A. radicidentis* and *A. viscosus* do cause human infection. *Actinomyces* spp. can be found as commensals in the oral cavity, gastrointestinal tract and female genital tract.

PATHOGENESIS

Actinomyces spp. are incapable of invading normal tissues and thus require trauma to the mucous surface to initiate disease. This can result from mechanical (accidental or surgical) trauma, primary bacterial or viral infection or malignancy. In addition, this damage will produce injury that renders the tissue anaerobic which facilitates growth of the bacterium. Little is known of virulence determinants of *Actinomyces* spp. and, for example, toxins have not been detected. The commonest sites of actinomycosis are the cervicofacial region (60% of cases), abdomen (25%) and lungs (15%). In addition, *A. naeslundii* and *A. viscosus* are associated with periodontal disease and *A. radicidentis* with dental radiculitis. In actinomycosis there is a dense cellular infiltrate with abscess and sinus formation. The small yellow particles (sulfur granules) characteristic of actinomycosis occur especially with infection due to *A. israelii*.

CLINICAL FEATURES

Actinomycosis is uncommon in children but a case series has been reported.[841] Cervicofacial actinomycosis presents as an indurated swelling in the mandibular region. Subsequently one or more sinuses develop. Less commonly, the tongue, pharynx, lacrimal glands or bone can be affected. Regional lymph nodes tend not to be affected. Local spread to

Table 28.41 Medically important fungi

Superficial mycoses		
	Dermatophytes (tinea capitis, tinea cruris, tinea pedis, tinea unguium, endothrix, ringworm)	Epidermophyton floccosum Microsporum audouinii (M. gryseum, M. canis) Trichophyton rubrum (T. mentagrophytes, T. verrucosum, T. terrestre, T. violaceum, T. schoenleinii, T. tonsurans)
	Pityriasis versicolor	Malassezia (Pityrosporum) furfur
	Black piedra	Piedraia hortae
	Tinea nigra	Cladosporium werneckii
	Candidiasis (mucous membrane)	Candida albicans (C. tropicalis, C. parapsilosis)
Subcutaneous mycoses		
	Sporotrichosis	Sporothrix schenckii
	Chromomycosis	Phialophora verrucosa, Phialophora (Fonsecaea) pedrosoi, Cladosporium carrionii
	Mycetoma	Actinomadura madurae, Nocardia asteroides, N. brasiliensis, Streptomyces somaliensis
	Rhinosporidiosis	Rhinosporidium seeberi
	Zygomycosis	Basidiobolus haptosporus Conidiobolus coronatus
Systemic mycoses		
	Histoplasmosis	Histoplasma capsulatum
	Cryptococcosis	Cryptococcus neoformans
	Blastomycosis	Blastomyces dermatitidis
	Coccidioidomycosis	Coccidioides immitis
	Paracoccidioidomycosis	Paracoccidioides brasiliensis
	Penicilliosis	Penicillium marneffei
Opportunist pathogens		
	Aspergillosis	Aspergillus fumigatus
	Candidiasis	Candida albicans and other species
	Mucormycosis	Mucor spp.
	Pneumocystosis	Pneumocystis carinii

cause brain or spinal cord abscesses has been reported. In these cases there is usually a mixed bacterial population.

Thoracic actinomycosis can occur by aspiration of oral bacteria, hematogenous spread, or local spread from cervical or abdominal lesions. Thus the initial focus can be in the bronchial tree or lung parenchyma. Subsequently, multiple abscesses develop which form sinuses that traverse the chest wall. The main clinical features are chest pain, fever, productive cough and weight loss. Abdominal actinomycosis presents with fever, neutrophilia, chronic abdominal pain and an inflammatory mass. Sinus formation is uncommon. Most often abdominal actinomycosis follows a perforated appendix.[842] Pelvic actinomycosis occurs most often in association with intrauterine contraceptive devices (the coil) and is thus very uncommon in children. Disseminated actinomycosis is uncommon in pediatric practice but has been reported.[843]

DIAGNOSIS AND DIFFERENTIAL DIAGNOSIS

Cervicofacial actinomycosis is part of the differential diagnosis of an indurated swelling of the mandibular region, especially if there is sinus formation. Specific diagnosis is by bacteriological culture of aspirated pus, sinus discharge, biopsy tissue or fine needle aspirations, but care must be taken to avoid contamination by commensal bacteria. Cultures should be kept anaerobically at 35–37 °C for up to 14 days. More rapid diagnosis can be obtained by examination of crushed sulfur granules stained by Gram stain where filamentous, branching or beaded Gram positive bacteria will be seen. It must be distinguished from other chronic suppurative lesions of the cervical region including chronic pyogenic osteomyelitis and tuberculosis. Thoracic actinomycosis may be confused with other chronic lung infection, including bronchiectasis and pulmonary tuberculosis.[844] Culture of sputum, bronchial aspirates or biopsy material will confirm the diagnosis.

The mass of abdominal actinomycosis can mimic an appendix abscess, abdominal tuberculosis or intra-abdominal carcinoma.[843] Laparotomy with culture of pus or biopsy material is necessary to establish the diagnosis. Serologic diagnosis is unreliable.

TREATMENT AND PROGNOSIS

Benzyl penicillin is the treatment of choice. It is given in high doses, intravenously for 2 weeks at least, then orally for 6–8 months. This may be accompanied wherever possible with surgical drainage. For penicillin-allergic patients, tetracycline and perhaps ciprofloxacin can be tried. The prognosis is generally good, although thoracic actinomycosis may require even more prolonged and energetic treatment.

ASPERGILLOSIS

ETIOLOGY

Aspergillosis is a fungal infection with a worldwide distribution. There are over 90 Aspergillus species described and 19 have been associated with human disease. However, most infections are due to Aspergillus fumigatus, A. flavus and to a lesser extent A. niger. Aspergillus spp. are widely distributed in the environment and some cause infection in other animals. Aspergillus is a member of the Eumycetes (true fungi) and produces a mycelium with a fruiting body, the conidium, from which spores are released into the atmosphere. The spores can be found in air sampled anywhere on earth.

EPIDEMIOLOGY AND PATHOGENESIS

Most disease manifestations involve the lung. In general, community acquired disease tends to be non-invasive aspergillosis and hospital acquired disease either non-invasive or invasive aspergillosis. In addition,

Table 28.42 Subcutaneous and systemic mycoses

Disease	Causative organism	Geographical distribution	Predominant clinical features	Treatment
Actinomycosis	*Actinomyces israelii*	Worldwide	Abscesses and sinuses in face and neck, lungs, abdomen	Benzyl penicillin
Aspergillosis	*Aspergillus* spp.	Worldwide	Granulomata of lungs, skin or generalized, aspergilloma	Nystatin aerosol, i.v. amphotericin B or oral itraconazole or ketoconazole
North American blastomycosis	*Blastomyces dermatitidis*	North America	Granulomata of lungs or generalized	i.v. amphotericin B or oral itraconazole or ketoconazole
South American blastomycosis	*Paracoccidioides brasiliensis*	South America	Ulcerating granulomata of oropharynx, lungs or generalized	i.v. amphotericin B or oral itraconazole or ketoconazole
Candidiasis	*Candida* spp. usually *C. albicans*	Worldwide	Usually superficial infection. Systemic resembles septicemic illness	i.v. amphotericin B with or without 5-flucytosine or oral fluconazole i.v. caspofungin
Chromoblastomycosis	*Cladosporium werneckii Fonsecaea compacta F. pedrosoi Phialophora verrucosa Rhinocladiella aquaspersa*	Tropics	Nodular, verrucose, tumors, plaque or cicatricial lesions of skin and deeper tissues	Surgery and i.v. amphotericin B, with 5-flucytosine, itraconazole or ketoconazole but mixed results
Coccidioidomycosis (San Joaquin Valley fever)	*Coccidioides immitis*	North and South America	Influenza-like illness. Progressive pulmonary or central nervous system infection in minority	i.v. amphotericin B or 5-flucytosine or i.v. miconazole or oral itraconazole
Cryptococcosis (torulosis)	*Cryptococcus neoformans*	Worldwide	Chiefly central nervous system infection, meningoencephalitis, or focal lesion but can cause pneumonia	i.v. amphotericin B or oral fluconazole
Histoplasmosis	*Histoplasma capsulatum*	Central USA	Granulomata in lungs, or in miliary distribution	i.v. amphotericin B or oral itraconazole or fluconazole
Mycetoma (Madura foot, maduromycosis)	Actinomycetoma *Actinomadura madurae A. pellotieri Nocardia brasiliensis N. madurae Streptomyces somaliensis* Eumycetoma *Madurella grisea M. mycetomatis Pseudallescheria boydii*	Tropics	Localized chronic infection involving skin, subcutaneous tissue and bone (nodule, sinuses and discharge)	Surgery (removal of lesions, amputation). Actinomycetoma: dapsone plus streptomycin. Eumycetoma: griseofulvin or imidazoles plus penicillin (but poor results)
Mucormycosis	*Mincor* spp. *Absidia corymbifera Rhizomusco* spp. *Rhizopus* spp.	Worldwide	Rhinocerebral, rhino-orbital, cardiac involvement, pulmonary, gastrointestinal, skin and soft tissue, bone involvement	i.v. amphotericin
Nocardiosis	*Nocardia asteroides* or *N. brasiliensis*	Worldwide	Pulmonary suppuration, occasionally central nervous system infection	Sulfonamides
Penicilliosis	*Penicillium marneffei*	South East Asia	Generalized infection especially in immune compromised patients with skin, bone, liver, spleen and lung involvement	i.v. amphotericin and oral itraconazole
Pneumocystosis	*Pneumocystis carinii*	Worldwide	Acute or subacute pneumonia in children immunocompromised by HIV, malnutrition or cytotoxic drugs	Oral co-trimoxazole, nebulized pentamidine
Rhinosporidiosis	*Rhinosporidium seeberi*	India and Ceylon	Polypoid tumors of mucous membrane – nose, nasopharynx, conjunctival sac. Gelatinous lesions, bleeding easily. Diagnosis by microscopic examination of crushed fragments of polyp. Pulmonary and nasopalatal types with tissue destruction may occur in the patients subject to severe metabolic disturbance	Surgical removal
Sporotrichosis	*Sporothrix schenckii*	Worldwide	Subcutaneous nodule (usually on hands or feet) which enlarges and adheres to skin and breaks down to form chronic ulcer. Satellite nodules develop by lymphatic spread. Usually localized but may be widely disseminated. Diagnosis by culture of exudates or scrapings or antibody tests. Extracutaneous forms involving muscles, lungs eyes, CNS, urinary tract and wide dissemination may occur	For lymphangitic form, potassium iodide 30 mg/kg/d up to maximum tolerance. For disseminated form i.v. amphotericin B or oral itraconazole

mycotoxins such as aflatoxin may contaminate cereals, groundnuts and other foods. Aflatoxin is a potent carcinogen but its role in human disease remains to be clarified. The non-invasive manifestations of aspergillosis are extrinsic allergic alveolitis (EAA), allergic bronchopulmonary aspergillosis (ABPA) and aspergilloma. In the former two, disease results from an allergic response to *Aspergillus* spp., a type III hypersensitivity response in EAA and type I in ABPA. An aspergilloma is a fungal mycelial ball that develops in a pre-existing lung cavity. In each case, the fungus is acquired by inhalation. Invasive pulmonary aspergillosis occurs in those immunocompromised by radiation, steroids or chemotherapy, especially if there is neutropenia. An increase in numbers of cases is often preceded by building work in or near the hospital, which increases atmospheric contamination by aspergillus spores. Dissemination from invasive pulmonary aspergillosis can result in metastatic foci in most organs of the body.

CLINICAL FEATURES AND DIAGNOSIS

ABPA in pediatric practice is particularly associated with cystic fibrosis, but may also occur in asthma. It presents insidiously with worsening bronchospasm and less commonly low grade fever. Up to two thirds of patients expectorate brownish sputum, which contains aspergilli. Eight diagnostic criteria (aspergillus precipitins, aspergillus specific IgE, chest radiographic infiltrates, blood eosinophilia > 500/mm³, *A. fumigatus* skin test, total serum IgE > 1000 ng/ml, bronchiectasis, cough and wheeze) are widely used,[845] but must be applied regularly to be of benefit.[846]

Invasive pulmonary aspergillosis occurs most often in the setting of relapse of the underlying condition or post bone marrow transplant[847] and presents with unremitting fever, new pulmonary infiltrates, dyspnea and unproductive cough. These, together with hemoptysis and tachycardia, can mimic pulmonary embolus. Massive hemoptysis is rare. Radiographic changes are variable, but most often, patchy bronchopneumonic infiltrates or nodular densities are seen. After 2–3 weeks, cavitation may occur. Dissemination is clinically indistinguishable from bacterial septicemia in immunocompromised patients. The presentation of metastatic disease, which can occur almost anywhere, will depend on the site of infection. Specific diagnosis depends upon culture of aspergilli from the infective site but blood cultures are very rarely, if ever, positive. Since aspergilli are so frequently present in the environment it is also necessary to demonstrate tissue invasion by histologic examination.

TREATMENT, PROGNOSIS AND PREVENTION

Allergic bronchopulmonary aspergillosis requires early therapy with oral corticosteroids and addition of high dose inhaled steroids may be of benefit. Recurrence is common. The natural history of aspergillosis is variable but only a minority of children resolve spontaneously. If there is evidence of some pulmonary invasion from the aspergilloma, antifungal therapy with amphotericin B or oral itraconazole may be beneficial. Surgical removal is necessary, for example, if there is life-threatening hemoptysis; however, this does carry a risk of inoculating fungi into the field of surgery.

For invasive pulmonary or other aspergillosis, surgical drainage, debridement or resection is most important with antifungal therapy acting as an adjunct. Amphotericin B is the gold standard for therapy, and addition of 5-flucytosine might be of benefit. Itraconazole given orally is licensed for therapy but long term administration will be needed. The prognosis is generally poor but it is difficult to distinguish the relative contributions of the aspergillosis and the underlying condition.

BLASTOMYCOSIS

ETIOLOGY

Blastomyces dermatitidis is a dimorphic fungus. It exists as a yeast in human infection and when cultured at 37 °C, but in a mycelial form at room temperature or in the environment. Two serotypes and several genotypes have been described. *Paracoccidioides brasiliensis* is also dimorphic. In human lesions, it is found as a double-walled ovoid or round yeast 4–40 μm in diameter. In culture at 19–28 °C or in the environment it has a mycelial form. Isolates of *P. brasiliensis* vary greatly in their ability to cause disease.

EPIDEMIOLOGY AND PATHOGENESIS

Although sometimes referred to as North American blastomycosis, *B. dermatitidis* infection has been reported in North and South America, Europe, Africa and Asia. Within North America it has been reported from the mid-west and south east USA and parts of Canada. It appears that the environment along waterways is an important reservoir and infection is probably acquired by inhalation. Humans and other animals can be infected but person-to-person transmission does not occur and children are rarely infected. *P. brasiliensis* infection was originally called hyphoblastomycosis but is now known as South American blastomycosis, or, more correctly, paracoccidioidomycosis. It is limited to Central and South America from Mexico to Argentina but most cases (80%) are reported from Brazil. It is found in soil and is thought to be acquired by inhalation. It is rare in women, adolescents and children. Person-to-person transmission does not occur.

CLINICAL FEATURES

It is likely that most infections with *B. dermatitidis* are asymptomatic, but when clinically apparent can range from acute self-limiting pneumonia to disseminated infection. Occasionally, the acute pneumonia does not resolve and chronic pulmonary blastomycosis occurs, which is clinically indistinguishable from pulmonary tuberculosis or histoplasmosis. Cutaneous lesions are the most frequent manifestations of disseminated infection. These begin as subcutaneous nodules or papules. They then become ulcerated with raised irregular borders and a crusted center. Histologically these are granulomas.

P. brasiliensis causes a spectrum of disease ranging from acute pulmonary infection with or without mucocutaneous involvement to a progressive disseminated form with involvement of the mucocutaneous tissue, reticuloendothelial system and adrenals. It may also give a miliary appearance in the lung.

DIAGNOSIS AND DIFFERENTIAL DIAGNOSIS

Blastomycosis, although uncommon in children, should be suspected in patients from endemic areas with granulomatous and ulcerating lesions of the skin or mucous membranes, especially if it is of long duration or there is involvement of other organs. Acute pulmonary blastomycosis is difficult to diagnose clinically, as it presents as an influenza-like illness or with pleuritic pain. The chronic form is indistinguishable from tuberculosis, histoplasmosis or coccidioidomycosis. Specific diagnosis is by demonstrating the presence of *B. dermatitidis*, by culture of lesions or sputum, and for superficial lesions, biopsy stained by methenamine silver (the yeasts may not stain by hematoxylin and eosin).

Paracoccidioidomycosis has similar differential diagnoses to blastomycosis. Since children may present with an acute or subacute form with large numbers of yeast in the reticuloendothelial system and fungemia, specific diagnosis can also be aided by blood culture.

Treatment and Prognosis

Without treatment the mortality rate of blastomycosis is over 60%. Amphotericin B is the mainstay of therapy but higher doses are needed. Treatment should continue until symptoms resolve and continue for 3–4 months thereafter. Even with this, relapses occur in 10–20% of patients (up to 5 years later). Oral ketoconazole or, better still, itraconazole appears as effective as amphotericin B but there are no trials directly comparing the regimens. Treatment should continue for at least 6 months. Ketoconazole is effective in 85% of cases of paracoccidioidomycosis and relapse rates are low (0–11%) if therapy is continued for at least 6 months. Itraconazole appears superior to ketoconazole.

CANDIDIASIS

ETIOLOGY AND EPIDEMIOLOGY

There are almost 200 *Candida* species and they have a worldwide distribution. They exist in budding yeast, hyphal or pseudohyphal forms (Fig. 28.54). *Candida albicans* is the commonest species found both as a commensal, particularly in the mouth, rectum, vagina or on skin, and as a pathogen. The others are found less commonly as commensals but *C. glabrata* can be found in the mouth, rectum or vagina and *C. parapsilosis* and *C. tropicalis* on skin. Infections occur particularly in neonates and immunocompromised children, especially those with T cell defects.

PATHOGENESIS AND CLINICAL FEATURES

Different *Candida* spp. have differing virulence but *C. albicans* is the most competent pathogen. Virulence factors include adhesins, ability to switch from yeast to hyphal (invasive) forms, production of proteolytic enzymes, antigenic variability and host mimicry. In addition to these, however, there need to be breaches in the skin or mucosa, alterations in the normal flora (usually due to antibacterial therapy), or underlying conditions such as immune deficiency (congenital or acquired), diabetes mellitus or implanted devices.

Superficial candidiasis (thrush)

Oral thrush typically occurs in neonates. Adherent gray-white plaques on removal reveal a raw, red base. They are usually found on the tongue, gums or gingival mucosa but may extend into the esophagus or trachea, especially in HIV/AIDS. There may also be scaly, macular or vesicular, erythematous perianal lesions. In skin areas that are moist, occluded or irradiated, candidiasis can occur as intensely erythematous intertriginous lesions. These can be papular, plaque-like or confluent with surrounding satellite lesions. Commonly involved sites include the axillae, inguinal regions, perineum and digital web spaces. *Candida* spp. can also cause onychomycosis which, unlike that due to dermatophytes, is painful.

Chronic mucocutaneous candidiasis

This includes a heterogeneous group of patients with T cell deficits, some of which are highly specific to *Candida* spp. Most cases present in infancy or early childhood with oral thrush or perineal candidiasis which may become more widespread or just persist with localized lesions.

Deeper candidiasis

Candidal infection of deeper tissues and organs occurs rarely in otherwise healthy patients. Oral or esophageal candidiasis may be complicated by extension of infection to the intestine, typically with symptoms of diarrhea, abdominal pain and pruritus ani. The child may present with a celiac-like syndrome. In pulmonary candidiasis, the symptoms of fever and productive cough, sometimes with hemoptysis, are nonspecific. On radiological examination, patchy consolidation is seen, and cavitation may occur with infections of sufficient duration. Pulmonary candidiasis

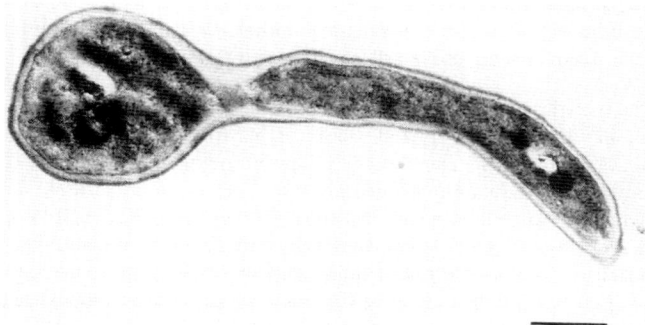

Fig. 28.54 A thin section electron micrograph of *Candida albicans* showing a pseudohypha (bar = 1 µm).

should be not diagnosed too readily on the evidence of culture of *Candida* from sputum, since the organism may be isolated in a proportion of healthy individuals, and particularly from hospital patients.

Disseminated *Candida* infection, although very uncommon in infancy and childhood, is thought to be increasing in frequency and has been reported in neonates, debilitated infants and children, particularly those treated with antibiotics or corticosteroids, or with diseases of the reticuloendothelial system, and in patients requiring prolonged intravenous therapy. Several *Candida* species have been isolated from such patients, whose clinical features are those of septicemia. Disseminated candidiasis, which may be confirmed by blood culture should be suspected when a septicemic illness supervenes in premature neonates, debilitated infants, or children in the course of antibiotic therapy, especially in the presence of a portal of entry for the organism such as an indwelling intravenous cannula.

The isolation of *Candida* from a specimen of urine obtained by suprapubic aspiration is highly suggestive of disseminated infection but must be interpreted in the light of other clinical data. Urinary tract infections with *C. albicans* do occur, especially in neonates or in association with indwelling urinary catheters. In neonates infection can ascend to produce fungal balls in the renal pelvis. The appearance of papular lesions on the skin containing *Candida* has been noted in preterm infants under such circumstances.

Candida endocarditis, though rare, has been reported in childhood. Previously damaged heart valves are the site of localization of infection in a patient with disseminated *Candida* infection.

DIAGNOSIS AND DIFFERENTIAL DIAGNOSIS

Oral thrush can usually be diagnosed on observation of the typical lesion, which may be confused with deposits of milk. The latter can be scraped off without effort, revealing a normal mucosal surface. Candidal napkin rash may be confused with ammoniacal dermatitis and, although it is common for the two lesions to coexist, the sharply demarcated edges of the former and its association with oral thrush should suggest the diagnosis. Confirmation of superficial candidiasis is readily made by the finding of typical pseudohyphae on microscopic examination and by culture of the organism from swabs from superficial lesions. Yeast cells are not significant in feces as they occur in 15% of normal children but hyphal forms occur only with invasion of mucous membranes and their presence can therefore be taken as an indication of enteric candidiasis.

The clinical and radiological features of pulmonary candidiasis can be confused with a number of subacute and chronic bacterial infections of the lungs. The presence of characteristic predisposing circumstances should suggest the diagnosis, especially if pulmonary cavitation is present. Laboratory confirmation is best made by repeated sputum culture, or preferably, by culture of tracheal or bronchial aspirates.

In disseminated candidiasis the organism can be isolated by blood or urine culture.

TREATMENT AND PROGNOSIS

Oral candidiasis is best treated by local application of antifungal agents. Preparations in common use are suspensions of nystatin (100 000 units/ml) and miconazole (2% in a gel). Gentian violet (1% aqueous solution) is by far the cheapest but it is messy, may produce excoriation of buccal mucosa, and generally fails to eradicate the fungus from the lower alimentary tract; it is now little used in Western countries. Nystatin and miconazole are probably equally effective. Nystatin is given in a dose of 1.0–2.0 ml dropped in the oral cavity 4 to 6 hourly for 7–10 days while miconazole gel is applied as 5.0 ml, two to four times each day. Apparent failure of such treatments is seldom, if ever, due to the presence of antibiotic-resistant species of *C. albicans*. While resistance to nystatin and amphotericin B by *Candida* species other than *C. albicans* can readily be induced in vitro, only a minor degree of diminished antibiotic sensitivity can be induced in *C. albicans*. A dose of 1 ml of nystatin by oral instillation 6 hourly may be inadequate; higher and more frequent doses should be employed if the infection appears to be unresponsive. In perianal forms or candidiasis of skin or nails, topical nystatin (100 000 units/g of ointment) or miconazole is effective. Oral therapy with either antibiotic is effective in candidal enteritis.

In the treatment of candidiasis of deeper structures and organs, oral nystatin therapy is not recommended, since absorption from the gastrointestinal tract is poor. Oral ketoconazole may be effective. In pulmonary candidiasis, nystatin may be administered by aerosol, e.g. 500 000 units in 15 ml distilled water. In systemic candidiasis and candidal endocarditis and probably in pulmonary candidiasis, the most effective treatment is the intravenous administration of amphotericin B. Recent reports have indicated that the liposomal amphotericin B (AmBisome) treatment is less toxic and at least equally effective.[848] Flucytosine has the advantages over amphotericin B of oral administration and lower toxicity. Many strains of *C. albicans* are resistant, however, and the drug cannot be administered parenterally to those patients too ill to take it by mouth. It should be reserved for those patients in whom amphotericin B has proved to be too toxic. Echinocandins such as caspofungin are also useful in treating such infections.

The prognosis of superficial candidiasis is excellent; that of candidal enteritis has to be guarded. Disseminated candidiasis carries a poor prognosis, largely related to the nature of the predisposing conditions. Meningeal candidiasis, however, may run a surprisingly mild course.

CHROMOBLASTOMYCOSIS

ETIOLOGY, EPIDEMIOLOGY AND PATHOGENESIS

This is the commonest infection by the dematiaceous or black pigmented fungi. A number of fungi including *Fonsecaea pedrosoi*, *F. compacta*, *Phialophora verrucosa*, *Cladosporium carrionii*, *Rhinocladiella aquaspersa* and, less commonly, *Exophiala jeanselmei* cause chromoblastomycosis. Although most common in the tropics, cases have been reported from more temperate regions such as Europe and the USA. The habitat of each of the fungi is soil, decomposing vegetation and woodland. Humans most often become infected by traumatic implantation of such material for example when walking barefoot. Person-to-person transmission has not been described.

CLINICAL FEATURES, DIAGNOSIS AND TREATMENT

Chromoblastomycosis usually begins as a small pink papule which enlarges to a nodule. Over time it evolves to a scaly, fissured pink brownish plaque which eventually becomes verrucose. Eventually thick, crusted, hyperkeratotic masses occur which are prone to secondary infection, leading eventually, after many years, to lymphatic blockage and elephantiasis. The differential diagnosis includes blastomycosis, lupus vulgaris, leishmaniasis and tertiary syphilis. Specific diagnosis is by histologic examination and isolation of the fungi, which requires up to 6 weeks incubation at both 25 and 37 °C. Treatment is difficult. For small lesions, wide surgical excision is possible. Itraconazole for 6–24 months is effective in above 60% of cases. Amputation may be required.

COCCIDIOIDOMYCOSIS

ETIOLOGY AND EPIDEMIOLOGY

Coccidioides immitis is a dimorphic fungus which exists as a mycelial saprophyte in soil but as an endosporulating spherule in the human lung. Infection is acquired by inhalation of arthroconidia from soil and is particularly prevalent in the San Joaquin Valley in California. Although most cases occur in and around this area, cases have been described in Central (Guatemala, Honduras) and South America (Venezuela, Colombia, Paraguay, Bolivia, Argentina). It may also occur when dust storms blow the arthroconidia into other areas.

PATHOGENESIS

Inhalation of arthroconidia results in a disease attack rate of about 40%. Once in the lungs the arthroconidia convert to the spherule-endospore phase within 3 days. This causes an initial influx of neutrophils and an inflammatory response which changes to a mononuclear cell infiltrate with granulomata once the spherule-endospore phase is well established. The spherules are too large (20–150 µm) to be ingested by neutrophils or even macrophages but they are important in defense presumably because they can engulf the released endospores (c. 2–5 µm). A brisk T_H1 (T helper type 1) response is needed for recovery from infection.

CLINICAL FEATURES

Most often coccidioidomycosis is a somewhat prolonged influenza-like illness, often with pneumonia, which follows an incubation period of 1–3 weeks. In 90%, recovery is complete; the remainder are left with pulmonary cavities and nodules.[849] Nonpulmonary features include fever, malaise, headache, arthralgia, myalgia and skin rashes. Approximately 25% of patients develop erythema nodosum 6–16 days after onset of symptoms. In about 1% of patients, there is dissemination with skin (subcutaneous abscesses), bone, meningeal and even miliary manifestations. Dissemination is particularly found in immune compromised patients including cardiac allograft recipients (5% of those in Arizona) and those with HIV/AIDS.

DIAGNOSIS AND DIFFERENTIAL DIAGNOSIS

Coccidioidomycosis should be suspected in children in or from endemic areas, especially if non-white, who develop an acute febrile illness. Primary pulmonary coccidioidomycosis especially with erythema nodosum can be confused with primary tuberculosis, and the postprimary nodular or cavitating disease with secondary tuberculosis. Diagnosis can be confirmed by culture of sputum, pus or blood (if disseminated), but the laboratory should be warned since this is a significant pathogen that will need special containment. The coccidioidin skin test (similar to tuberculosis) will become positive within 21 days of infection. Serologic tests such as complement-fixing titers are available and useful for confirmation of diagnosis.

TREATMENT AND PROGNOSIS

Primary coccidioidomycosis seldom requires more than symptomatic treatment. Amphotericin B, the most effective drug, should, in view of its toxicity, be reserved for severe primary or postprimary pulmonary disease. Intravenous amphotericin B therapy is, however, essential in disseminated coccidioidomycosis and, where there is infection of the central nervous system, may be given by intrathecal infection. Until recently, the only alternative form of therapy was intravenous miconazole but oral itraconazole has been shown to be of value and of relatively low toxicity.

The prognosis of primary coccidioidomycosis is excellent, while that of postprimary pulmonary disease is good. Disseminated coccidioidomycosis carries a poor prognosis, especially with meningeal infection, unless treated vigorously and at an early stage.

CRYPTOCOCCOSIS

ETIOLOGY AND EPIDEMIOLOGY

Cryptococcus neoformans exists as a yeast in mammalian infections and on artificial culture but in a mycelial form in the environment. *C. neoformans* has a worldwide distribution and there are two variants: *C. neoformans* var. *neoformans* and *C. neoformans* var. *gattii*. *C. neoformans* is subdivided into four serotypes (A–D). *C. neoformans* var. *neoformans* falls into serotypes A and D, and var. *gattii*, serotypes B and C. The former is associated with soil, especially that contaminated by pigeon droppings and causes infection in patients immunocompromised by HIV/AIDS, chemotherapy or steroid administration. The latter is associated with the tropics and has been isolated from debris around *Eucalyptus camaldulensis*, the Australian red river gum tree. It causes infection in immunocompetent individuals. Although infection occurs in all age groups, children are less often infected.

PATHOGENESIS AND CLINICAL FEATURES

Infection is acquired, it is thought, by inhalation of the fungus. Person-to-person transmission does not occur. Virulent strains of *C. neoformans* have a thick polysaccharide capsule (Fig. 28.55) that protects them from phagocytic killing by macrophages and neutrophils. In the lungs, they can cause pneumonia but this occurs in less than 15% of patients with cryptococcosis. Most often the organism passes through the lungs silently to infect at secondary sites. The major manifestation is chronic meningitis with headache, personality changes, dementia and focal neurologic signs. It can be entirely asymptomatic early in the infection and, especially in HIV/AIDS patients, neck stiffness and fever are not major presenting features (< 50% of cases). In approximately 15% of cases of cryptococcosis there is skin or bone involvement. The cutaneous manifestations can be acneiform, abscesses, ulcers, granulomas or plaques.

DIAGNOSIS AND DIFFERENTIAL DIAGNOSIS

Specific diagnosis depends on demonstrating the fungus or its capsular antigen in CSF, blood or other infective sites. However, it must be remembered that *C. neoformans* can be present in sputum in the absence of disease. In CSF the cellular response varies. In AIDS patients, the cell count is low (< 5/mm³) whereas in non-AIDS patients it ranges from 10 to 300/mm³, but in each case there is a prevalence of lymphocytes (> 80%). *C. neoformans* will stain violet on Gram stain (Gram positive), but the India ink stain is best for demonstration of the yeasts. This is a negative stain because the stain does not penetrate the yeast but shows it with its thick polysaccharide capsule against a black background. There are commercially available latex agglutination kits for detection of capsular antigen in CSF or serum. These can also be used to measure response to therapy. Finally *C. neoformans* can be cultured on suitable fungal culture medium. The differential diagnoses include other bacterial and viral causes of acute or chronic meningitis or meningoencephalitis, in particular tuberculous meningitis, and for the skin lesions molluscum contagiosum, penicilliosis and histoplasmosis, especially in AIDS patients.

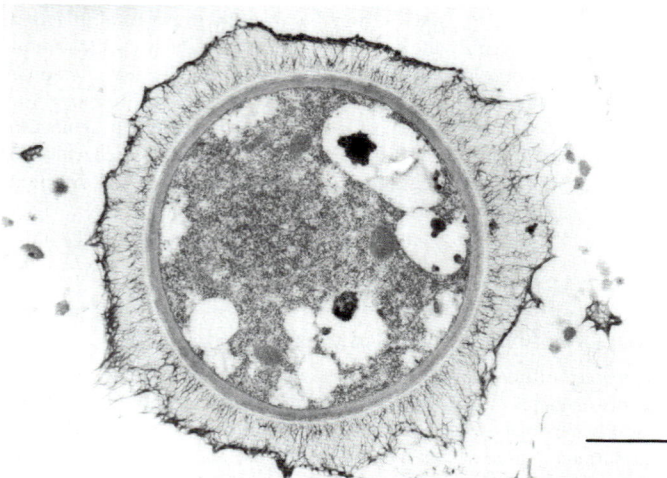

Fig. 28.55 A thin section electron micrograph of *Cryptococcus neoformans* showing its thick polysaccharide capsule (bar = 1 μm).

TREATMENT AND PROGNOSIS

For non-AIDS patients a combination of amphotericin B and 5-flucytosine for 6 weeks is curative in 75% of patients. In AIDS patients a number of regimens have been tried, principally because relapse is common after stopping therapy. Amphotericin B with or without 5-flucytosine for 2 weeks followed by 8 weeks of therapy with either fluconazole or itraconazole appears optimal in these cases. This is then followed by long term oral suppressive therapy with fluconazole. However, with the advent of combination antiretroviral therapy for HIV/AIDS the outlook is much better.[850] In addition to frequent relapse, obstructive hydrocephalus is a major complication of cryptococcal meningitis.

HISTOPLASMOSIS

ETIOLOGY AND EPIDEMIOLOGY

Histoplasma capsulatum is another dimorphic fungus which undergoes reversible morphologic variation according to the environment in which it is placed. Its normal habitat is soil, especially below where birds and bats have roosted. Here it exists in a mycelial form with hyphae bearing macroconidia (8–14 μm diameter) and microconidia (2–5 μm), which are the infective forms. At temperatures above 35 °C *H. capsulatum* grows as a yeast (2–3 × 3–4 μm) and this is the form found in human infections. Histoplasmosis is endemic in North America (especially the Ohio and Mississippi valleys) and Latin America, but cases have been reported from Europe and Asia. The taxonomy of *H. capsulatum* is currently under discussion. Three varieties are recognized: *H. capsulatum* var. *capsulatum*, *H. capsulatum* var. *duboisii* (which causes African histoplasmosis) and *H. capsulatum* var. *farciminosum* (which causes skin ulcers in horses and mules) but genetic analysis suggests *H. capsulatum* might harbor six species.[851] It is estimated that there are 200 000–500 000 cases each year worldwide. In endemic areas of the USA, it is estimated that 90% of the population have been exposed with frequent re-exposure.[852]

PATHOGENESIS AND CLINICAL FEATURES

Infection occurs when microconidia are inhaled. Most often this occurs when individuals disturb soil or dust containing microconidia, but they can travel for miles in the wind. In the lungs, the spores germinate to the yeast form, which elicits an influx of neutrophils, macrophages and lymphocytes and formation of granulomas. The yeasts are able to survive within macrophages,[853] and may persist for years within the reticuloendothelial system. Infection is more likely to progress, persist or disseminate if there is abnormal T cell function. Infection is also likely to disseminate in infants under 2 years,[854] but there is often an associated T cell defect. With exposure to a low infective dose, only 1% of patients develop clinical disease, but the rest have serologic evidence of infection. With a higher inoculum only 10–50% are asymptomatic. Most clinically expressed infections are self-limited and include acute pulmonary histoplasmosis, mediastinal lymph node enlargement, pericarditis and rheumatologic manifestations.

Approximately 80% of the symptomatic cases are of acute pulmonary histoplasmosis, which presents as a 'flu-like' illness with fever, chills, headache, myalgia and a nonproductive cough. This usually resolves within a few weeks. More diffuse pulmonary disease leading to respiratory insufficiency can occur with a higher infecting dose. The rheumatologic manifestations include erythema nodosum with arthralgia or frank arthritis, which can persist for months. Pericarditis occurs as an inflammatory complication of pulmonary disease. Chronic pulmonary histoplasmosis is very rare in children. It occurs mostly in middle-aged men with chronic obstructive airways disease. Disseminated histoplasmosis is a progressive illness with extrapulmonary spread of the fungus. It can occur following acute infection or years later. In infants it presents as fever, splenomegaly and/or hepatomegaly.[854] Subsequently, shock, liver or renal failure and central nervous system involvement can occur. Cutaneous or mucosal granulomas in children in endemic areas should also be considered as possible histoplasmosis.

DIAGNOSIS AND DIFFERENTIAL DIAGNOSIS

Diagnosis requires a high index of clinical suspicion in a child living in, or coming from, an endemic region. Specific diagnosis requires a battery of tests including histology, antigen and antibody detection and fungal culture of bone marrow, spleen, lymph node, liver or bronchoalveolar lavage samples.[854] The histoplasmin skin test is not useful, especially in those with T cell impairment and disseminated disease. The differential diagnosis includes pulmonary or miliary tuberculosis.

MYCETOMA[855]

Mycetoma is a chronic, subcutaneous granulomatous disease caused by either fungi (eumycetoma) or branching bacteria (actinomycetoma). It has a worldwide distribution and is endemic in a belt between latitudes 15°S and 30°N, which encompasses Senegal, Sudan, Somalia, Mexico, India and parts of Central and South America. In Sudan it is estimated that there are 300–400 new cases each year, mostly in males aged 20–40 years, but children may rarely be affected. The clinical triad of subcutaneous nodules, sinuses and discharge is suggestive. The differential diagnosis includes Kaposi's sarcoma, neurofibroma, malignant melanoma, syphilitic osteitis and bone tuberculosis, but specific diagnosis can be made by histologic examination. Culture is difficult and takes a long time. Surgical treatment is to remove all affected tissue, which can involve amputation of affected feet or hands. Actinomycetoma can be treated with dapsone and streptomycin for 1 month. Medical treatment of eumycetoma is much more difficult. Griseofulvin, ketoconazole or itraconazole have had mixed success but treatment must be continued for 1–10 years.

NOCARDIOSIS

ETIOLOGY AND EPIDEMIOLOGY

Nocardia spp. are Gram positive, acid alcohol fast, nonmotile, branching bacteria in the suborder *Corynebacterineae* that are closely related to the actinomycetes. There are 20 *Nocardia* spp. but most human infections are by *Nocardia asteroides* and less commonly by *N. farcinica* and *N. nova*. In tropical countries infection can also be by *N. brasiliensis* and *N. africana*.[856] *Nocardia* are environmental organisms living in soil and decaying vegetation. Person-to-person spread does not occur, and although *Nocardia* spp. can cause infections in animals they are not zoonotic. Primary infections do occur but most infections occur in immunocompromised individuals.

PATHOGENESIS AND CLINICAL FEATURES

Infection is acquired either by inhalation or direct inoculation into the skin. Characteristically *Nocardia* spp. produce abscesses and granulomas. Virulent strains of *N. asteroides* can evade phagocytic killing by inhibiting phagolysosome fusion or acidification of phagosomes.[857,858] Dissemination is much more likely to occur if there is some form of immune compromise and has been reported in HIV/ AIDS when it may involve the skin, kidneys and adrenals. In 5% of patients it involves the central nervous system either as diffuse meningitis or abscesses.

Pulmonary infection is found in 75% of patients with nocardiosis, alone or in association with disseminated infection, and may produce no symptoms. In other patients malaise, cough, fever and dyspnea may develop. Hemoptysis is an uncommon symptom. Involvement of the central nervous system may result in the clinical features of meningoencephalitis, or, if the lesion is a single abscess, of a localized intracranial or intraspinous tumor. Primary cutaneous nocardiosis can present as cellulitis or as an abscess with or without lymphadenitis and can be mistaken for *Streptococcus pyogenes* or *Staphylococcus aureus* infections.[859] *Nocardia* spp. are also pathogens in mycetoma.

DIAGNOSIS AND DIFFERENTIAL DIAGNOSIS

There are no typical symptoms and signs, and the pulmonary form may readily be confused with other suppurative lung conditions. Radiological examination of the chest similarly provides no characteristic features, the most common being patchy infiltration perhaps with cavitation. Specific diagnosis depends upon laboratory help but unfortunately *Nocardia* spp. are difficult to recognize and identify in the routine diagnostic laboratory, compounded by the fact that they are slow growing.

TREATMENT AND PROGNOSIS

Prior to the advent of the sulfonamides, nocardial infection was usually fatal, and at present the outlook is poor, partly because of the nature of the predisposing conditions and partly because of delay in diagnosis.

The treatment of choice is prolonged administration of sulfonamides or co-trimoxazole. Treatment may be necessary for several months, and may be combined with surgery. It is recommended that sulfonamides be given in a dose adequate to maintain a blood level of not less than 10 mg/100 ml.

Treatment with antibiotics, including benzyl penicillin and chloramphenicol, has been reported to be successful on occasions and, as indicated by sensitivity of the organism in vitro, may be given in addition to sulfonamides.

PENICILLIOSIS

This is an emerging infection which is the third commonest opportunist infection in HIV infected patients in South East Asia.[860] Most cases are due to *Penicillium marneffei* but occasional cases of *P. chrysogenum* occur.[861]

Approximately 80% of patients with penicilliosis are immunocompromised. Penicilliosis can present as cutaneous or disseminated infection or both. The skin lesions are usually umbilicated papules resembling molluscum contagiosum. Disseminated disease usually presents as fever, weight loss and anemia. Specific diagnosis is by isolation of the fungus from skin, bone marrow or blood. Mild to moderate disease can be treated with itraconazole or ketoconazole but severe disease will require amphotericin B. There are no controlled trials of therapy.

SPOROTRICHOSIS[862]

Sporotrichosis is caused by the dimorphic fungus *Sporothrix schenckii*. It grows as a saprophyte in decaying vegetation and infection occurs following traumatic inoculation into the skin. Some cases have been transmitted by domestic cat scratch.[863] It has a worldwide distribution but, for example, is the commonest subcutaneous mycosis in Latin America. Infection is often related to occupation (e.g. farmers, florists, gardeners) and occurs most often in adults, although infections do occur in children.[864] The initial nodule at the inoculation site enlarges becoming red, pustular and ulcerating in turn. Extension occurs up the lymphatics to draining lymph nodes which themselves enlarge and drain to the skin. Spontaneous healing can occur but most often the lesions persist with gradual extension and scarring. Diagnosis depends upon demonstrating *S. schenckii* in lesions by immunohistochemistry or immunofluorescence. Fungal culture, however, provides the definitive diagnosis. There are no controlled trials of therapy, but oral itraconazole for 3–12 months has cure rates of 89–100%. Saturated potassium iodide (10 drops diluted in fruit juice three times daily) can be used in a resource poor setting but it is poorly tolerated. If disease is unresponsive to itraconazole, it might be necessary to use amphotericin B.

ANTIFUNGAL CHEMOTHERAPY[865]

Only a small number of antifungal drugs are available for treatment of systemic mycoses and there are very few controlled trials to demonstrate efficacy, none in children. Most of the antifungals act on the fungal cell membrane by either chelating ergosterol (polyenes) or inhibiting its synthesis (imidazoles, triazoles). 5-Flucytosine is a nucleoside analog that inhibits fungal transcription.

POLYENES

Nystatin is a microcrystalline suspension so should not be given parenterally. It is very effective in treating superficial infections due to sensitive fungi and resistance has developed very slowly if at all. Amphotericin B is active against a wide range of fungi in vitro including *Candida* spp., *C. neoformans*, *H. capsulatum* and *Aspergillus* spp. However, up to 40% of *P. marneffei* are resistant and the agents of chromoblastomycoses are usually resistant as are those causing eumycetoma.

For systemic mycoses, amphotericin B must be given intravenously by slow infusion but can also be given intrathecally, intraventricularly or intraperitoneally. The lyophilized powder must be reconstituted in 5% dextrose solution (not saline, which may cause it to precipitate) and is given as a slow infusion over 4–6 h at a concentration of 100 µg/ml. Usually treatment begins with a dose of 0.25 mg/kg/d with a gradual increase up to about 1 mg/kg/d as can be tolerated. A daily dose of 1.5 mg/kg/d should not be exceeded. For intrathecal use, doses of 0.1–0.5 mg or even 1 mg have been given to children according to weight and tolerance of the drug. Only 2–5% of the daily dose of amphotericin B is excreted in urine in the active form, and in experimental animals 20% is excreted in bile. The fate of the major part of the administered dose is unknown, but there are reports of detection of the drug in liver, spleen and kidney one year after cessation of therapy. There are no trials delineating duration of therapy, but treatment is usually given for 1–3 months depending upon the rate of clinical and laboratory improvement. Amphotericin B has a high toxicity profile. During a 4–6 h infusion, 50–90% of patients experience fever, chills, malaise, muscle and joint pains, nausea and vomiting. The major side-effect is nephrotoxicity: glomerular filtration rates fall by 40% in most patients and stabilize to 20–60% after multiple doses. Toxicity is manifest by increased blood urea and creatinine levels and the appearance of red cells, white cells and casts in the urine. If blood urea rises above 16.7 mmol/L or creatinine above 170 µmol/L treatment should be stopped until levels return to normal. Hematological side-effects occur in 75% of patients, most frequently a normochromic, normocytic anemia, and cardiac arrest, hepatotoxicity, neurotoxicity and allergic reactions do occur but are rare.

Encapsulating amphotericin B in liposomes (AmBisome, Abelcet) or in a colloidal dispersion (Amphocil) gives better tolerance and fewer side-effects in doses up to 3–5 mg/kg/d.

FLUCYTOSINE

5-Flucytosine is a fluorinated pyrimidine that was originally developed as an antineoplastic drug. Its mechanisms of action are, on conversion to 5-fluorouracil in the fungus, to act as an analog of uracil, inhibiting protein synthesis and to inhibit thymidylate synthetase and thus DNA synthesis. It has a narrow spectrum of activity but is usually active against *C. albicans* and *C. neoformans*. However, resistance even in these fungi can develop, so it is most often used in combination with amphotericin B. It is well absorbed orally and is usually given at 50–100 mg/kg/d in four divided doses in neonates and children. Although less toxic than amphotericin B, it can cause bone marrow suppression, cutaneous reactions (particularly in AIDS patients) and diarrhea. The risk of bone marrow suppression is greater with concomitant amphotericin B therapy and appears more likely in children. For these reasons, it is advisable to measure peak (2 h post oral or 30 min post intravenously) and trough (just prior to dose) serum levels twice weekly during therapy. Peak levels should not exceed 100 mg/L and the trough is around 25 mg/L.

IMIDAZOLES

Of the licensed imidazoles, clotrimazole is solely a topical agent, while ketoconazole can be given topically or orally and miconazole topically or intravenously. Miconazole has a broad range of antifungal activity in vitro but is less active against *Aspergillus* spp., *Hansenula* (now *Pichia*) *anomala* and *Mucor* spp. It is particularly useful for topical application in dermatophyte infections and in oral and cutaneous candidiasis. Intravenous miconazole should be considered in patients unable to tolerate amphotericin B and as an alternative to the latter drug in systemic infections with *Candida* resistant to flucytosine.

Recommended dosage for oral candidiasis is 5 ml of miconazole gel (20%) two to four times per day. For systemic infections, an ampoule containing 200 mg of miconazole should be diluted with 5% dextrose or physiological saline solution and administered by slow intravenous infusion three times daily. In children, the total daily dose is of the order of 40 mg/kg body weight.

Toxic effects are in general less frequent and less severe than those encountered with amphotericin B therapy. They include gastrointestinal, mental and liver enzyme disturbances. The poor water solubility of miconazole necessitates the use of a lipophilic solvent causing major problems with venous irritation and occlusion.

Ketoconazole has an even better antifungal spectrum of activity. It is a less toxic alternative to amphotericin B but does cause gastrointestinal problems (in 3–40%) and hepatocellular damage (most often in females over 40 years). Its use has been reported in systemic candidiasis, coccidioidomycosis and histoplasmosis. An appropriate dose is 3 mg/kg daily orally for a child and 200–400 mg once daily for an adult. Treatment should be maintained for 10 days, in the case of oral thrush, and for at least 1 month in the case of systemic infections. Less than 10% of either drug is excreted in urine, so they are of little use in urinary tract infections.

TRIAZOLES

The two major antifungals in this recently introduced class of drugs are fluconazole and itraconazole. Fluconazole has high bioavailability, and peak serum concentrations are similar by either the oral or intravenous routes. It is active against most *C. albicans* and *C. neoformans* but some other *Candida* spp. (e.g. *C. krusei*) are resistant. Its main clinical use is in treating cryptococcosis and candidiasis. In children over 4 weeks, recommended doses are 3 mg/kg/d for mucosal candidiasis, 6–12 mg/kg/d for systemic candidiasis or cryptococcosis and 3–12 mg/kg/d for prophylaxis in neutropenic children. Neonates aged 2–4 weeks should be given similar doses but every 2 days, and those aged 2 weeks and under every 3 days. Fluconazole is generally well tolerated with nausea, vomiting, abdominal pain and diarrhea in less than 5%. Asymptomatic elevation of hepatic aminotransferase enzymes occurred in 12% of children after 4 days of intravenous therapy.[866] About 80% of the drug is excreted by the renal route. Itraconazole has an even broader spectrum of activity being active against most *Candida* spp., *H. capsulatum*, *B. dermatitidis*, *C. immitis*, *P. braziliensis*, *P. marneffei*, *A. flavus* and *A. fumigatus*. It has an equally broad clinical use for infections by the above and in sporotrichosis, chromoblastomycosis and phaeochromomycosis. For the latter two, response depends on the infecting fungus. The dose is 2.5–5 mg/kg daily by the oral route. The duration of therapy depends upon the infection being treated. Itraconazole has a good safety profile but very little of the drug is excreted in urine.

ECHINOCANDINS

This novel class of antifungals includes caspofungin, micafungin and anidulafungin. They inhibit $\beta(1,3)$-D-glucan synthesis in the fungal cell wall. They are clinically effective in invasive candidiasis and candidemia but less effective in aspergillosis.[867] They have little or no activity against the rest of the fungi described here.

HELMINTH INFECTION

Helminth or worm infections occur worldwide, although in warmer, moister areas, especially where standards of hygiene are low, the range of species and prevalence tends to be greater and multiple infections are common. Because children tend to live more closely with nature and with their pets, many helminth infections are more common in children than in adults. Reviews listing the estimated prevalence of the variety of worm infections in humans worldwide indicate that a vast health problem exists. New and emerging helminth zoonoses continue to be identified.[868]

Many tentative prevalence figures are undoubtedly underestimates. One review[869] concluded that there are more trematodes infecting humans than any other group of animal parasites, over 75 species, mostly acquired from poorly prepared or cooked food.[870]

Helminth infections are by no means confined to tropical or resource limited countries and the increase in travel and of refugee movements in recent years has led to an increasing awareness in resource rich countries of the dangers of imported diseases.[871]

Helminth infections differ in most cases from those caused by viruses, bacteria or protozoa, in that the clinical effects exhibited by the host are mostly related to the worm load carried, and the latter in turn is usually related to the infective dose. The controversy regarding the possible adverse effects of helminth infections and the value of anthelmintic treatment on cognitive function and learning or educational ability remains unresolved, but the concept may well be valid.[872,873]

The common parasitic helminths infecting humans include the Nematoda (roundworms) and Platyhelminthes (flatworms) which comprises the Trematoda (flukes) and Cestoda (tapeworms). Less commonly humans may be infected with such worms as the Acanthocephala (thorny headed worms).[874]

The control of human helminth infections usually depends on a detailed knowledge of the epidemiology and life cycles of the species concerned – the aim being to break the cycle. The following principles are utilized, either alone or in combination, depending upon the species:

1. treatment of infected individuals, including mass treatment;
2. control of animal reservoirs where such exist;
3. hygiene, which includes education and provision of adequate and acceptable toilet facilities;
4. vector control where applicable;
5. the wearing of shoes where infection occurs from the soil through the skin;
6. instruction in food preparation and cooking;
7. immunization – a field which continues to be of great interest.

Of all the above, the most important method for the control of human helminthiases remains education combined with improved sanitation and personal hygiene. However, mass de-worming may play an important role in the control of some helminthiases and, in relation to immunization, Maizels et al[875] expressed the view that 'vaccines are the one major goal of the helminthological community'.

NEMATODES (ROUNDWORMS)

Nematodes are nonsegmented worms, round in transverse section with separate sexes. They possess both gut and body cavity (pseudocele). Species particularly important to humans include amongst others: *Ascaris lumbricoides, Toxocara canis, Enterobius vermicularis, Ancylostoma duodenale, Necator americanus, Trichuris trichiura, Strongyloides stercoralis, Trichinella spiralis, Onchocerca volvulus, Loa loa, Wuchereria bancrofti, Mansonella perstans, Mansonella ozzardi* and *Brugia malayi*.

ASCARIASIS

The intestinal roundworm *Ascaris lumbricoides* is cosmopolitan but variable in distribution, thriving in a moist climate, temperate or tropical, and especially under conditions of overcrowding. Ascariasis (like trichuriasis) tends to have a lower prevalence and worm load at higher altitudes.[876] The adult ascarids, male and female, live in the lumen of the small intestine, maintaining only an intermittent attachment to the mucosa. The gravid female lays an average of 200 000 eggs each day. Newly excreted eggs may remain dormant for a long period. If conditions are suitable they develop into an infective egg in about 2 weeks, in which condition they can remain viable for months or years until ingested.[877] The only hosts of these worms are humans, although cases of human infection with *A. suum*, the pig ascarid, have also been recorded. The life cycle of *A. lumbricoides* is depicted in Figure 28.56.

Clinical features

In 80% of cases the only manifestation of ascariasis is the asymptomatic passage of eggs and adult worms in the stool. Symptoms are related to three phases of the ascarid's life cycle:

1. invasion and migration of larvae;
2. presence of a large adult worm load;
3. migration of adult worms from their normal habitat.

To this one may add symptoms associated with the development of true allergy to the ascarid.[878]

Ascariasis is potentially serious and can contribute to a significant proportion of abdominal emergencies in children.[879]

Larval pneumonitis

The initial migration of larvae through the intestinal wall and via the portal circulation to the lungs may, in the case of heavy infection, or with repeated reinfections, cause a characteristic and often seasonal clinical picture.[880] The patient develops a dry spasmodic cough with intermittent wheezing and breathlessness, transient rhonchi and crackles in the lung fields; rarely, hemoptysis occurs. There may be malaise, with fever as high as 40°C, discomfort over the liver, and urticarial rashes. Radiological examination of the chest reveals diffuse, mottled opacities, peribronchial infiltration or areas of pneumonitis. Marked eosinophilia is present. Symptoms and signs subside after 2 or 3 weeks and the eosinophilia generally diminishes to 3–5% of the total white cell count. Chronic lung disease occasionally results from repeated larval onslaughts. Severe pulmonary infiltration with asthma, eosinophilia and raised IgE levels can occur in children infected with *A. suum*.

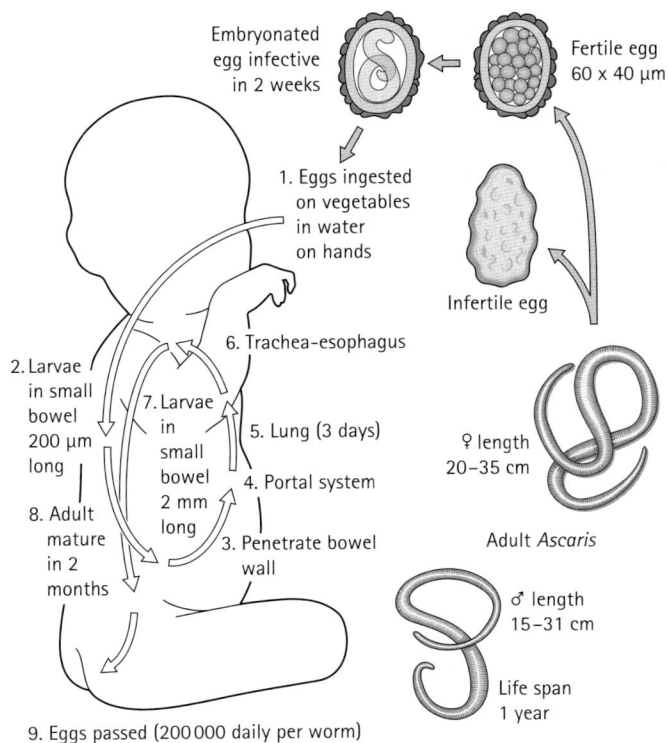

Fig. 28.56 Character and life cycle of *Ascaris lumbricoides*.

Worm load

Although some features of intestinal ascariasis are of an allergic nature, in the healthy child on a normal diet it is unlikely that the presence of a few ascarids will cause any significant disturbance.[880] A large worm load will, however, drain off a considerable proportion of a child's nutritional intake and in children can be associated with impaired lactose digestion and absorption.[879] Heavy infections are usually seen in underprivileged communities where nutrition is already inadequate. The combination of malnutrition, vitamin and iron deficiency, and the almost invariable presence of intestinal parasites of other types, makes the part played by ascarids difficult to assess. However, studies in Colombia have shown that steatorrhea and D-xylose malabsorption associated with heavy loads of *Ascaris* improved after de-worming. These children are ill, stunted and marasmic, with abdominal distention. Colicky abdominal pain is frequent. There may be low grade fever and a mass of worms can often be palpated abdominally. Toxins from ascarids may play a part in producing the chronic illness.

Intestinal complications associated with a heavy worm burden are frequently seen in hyperendemic areas.[881] A bolus of worms (usually both dead and living) may impact, particularly near the ileo-cecal junction (Fig. 28.57). A mass of ascarids may also precipitate temporary obstruction from spasm, cause inflammatory reactions and adhesions, or lead to volvulus or intussusception.

Migration of adult worms

Under certain circumstances, particularly with high fever, gastrointestinal upset or ineffectual anthelmintic therapy (e.g. the use of tetrachlorethylene for a concomitant hookworm infection), an ascarid may migrate from its normal habitat in the bowel and be vomited, or wriggle up the esophagus and emerge through the nose. Lodgment in the appendix or Meckel's diverticulum can result in obstruction and perforation. The common bile duct may be blocked by a roundworm, leading to severe upper abdominal pain, vomiting, tenderness and enlargement of the liver, a palpable gallbladder, and jaundice. Pancreatitis is a further complication. Other manifestations of the migrating ascarid include intestinal perforation with peritonitis, chronic peritonitis due to the presence of eggs, soft tissue or liver abscess, laryngeal impaction and even the passage of a worm per urethram. Ascarids can also penetrate perforations, suture lines and into drainage or suction tubes.

Roundworm sensitivity can produce a variety of allergic manifestations: nasal, pulmonary, dermal, or gastrointestinal.[880]

Diagnosis

Larval pneumonitis (Löffler syndrome) is generally suggested by the presence of eosinophilia, but other parasites can produce this syndrome (Table 28.43), and proof of diagnosis can only be obtained if a larva is identified in the sputum. Adult worms may later be passed in the stool or seen on radiological examination (Fig. 28.58) of the abdomen using barium. Diagnosis, however, rests almost wholly on finding eggs in the stools (Fig. 28.59), except in the event of early infection or a population of purely male worms. Serological and intracutaneous tests are available but as yet are of little practical value although they have been used in epidemiological surveys.[882]

Treatment

No treatment is known to remove migrating larvae, although some have claimed success using piperazine or pyrantel. The pneumonitis responds dramatically to prednisone.[880] Albendazole is a very valuable, broad spectrum anthelmintic with a wide activity against intestinal nematode species. It is generally well tolerated at doses recommended for these helminths and has, in fact, been designated as a 'WHO essential agent'. It is given at a dose of 400 mg as a single dose (200 mg for children < 10 kg).[877,880,883,884]

Two anthelmintics highly effective in ascariasis and with minimal side-effects are pyrantel embonate/pamoate (10–20 mg/kg, max. 750 mg) and mebendazole (100 mg 12-hourly for 3 days; children < 10 kg 50 mg 12-hourly for 3 days). Levamisole is also effective and

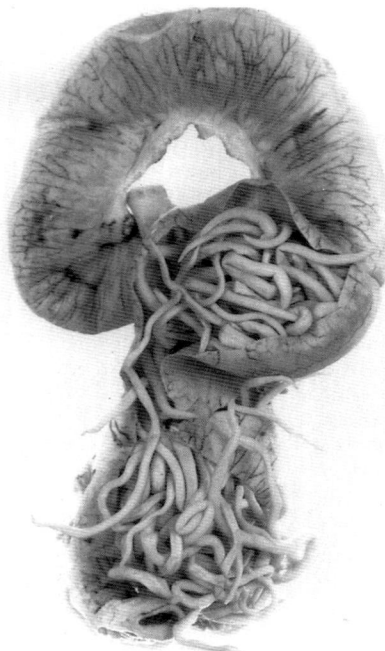

Fig. 28.57 Intestinal obstruction by *Ascaris lumbricoides* in a 14-year-old boy.

Table 28.43 Worms and fly larvae giving rise to pulmonary infiltrations, visceral larva migrans and cutaneous larva migrans

	Pulmonary infiltration with eosinophilia	Visceral larva migrans	Cutaneous larva migrans
Ancylostoma braziliense			×
Ancylostoma caninum			×
Ancylostoma duodenale	Rare		
Angiostrongylus cantonensis		×	
Anisakis species		×	
Ascaris lumbricoides	×	Rare	
Ascaris suum	×	×	
Capillaria hepatica		×	
Dirofilaria species	×	×	
Fly larvae			
Dermatobia species		×	
Gasterophilus species			×
Hypoderma species			×
Gnathostoma species		×	×
Necator americanus	Rare		'Ground itch'
Schistosoma species			'Swimmer's itch'
Strongyloides stercoralis	×	Rare	'Ground itch'
Toxocara canis	×	×	
Toxocara cati	Uncertain	Uncertain	
Uncinaria stenocephala			×

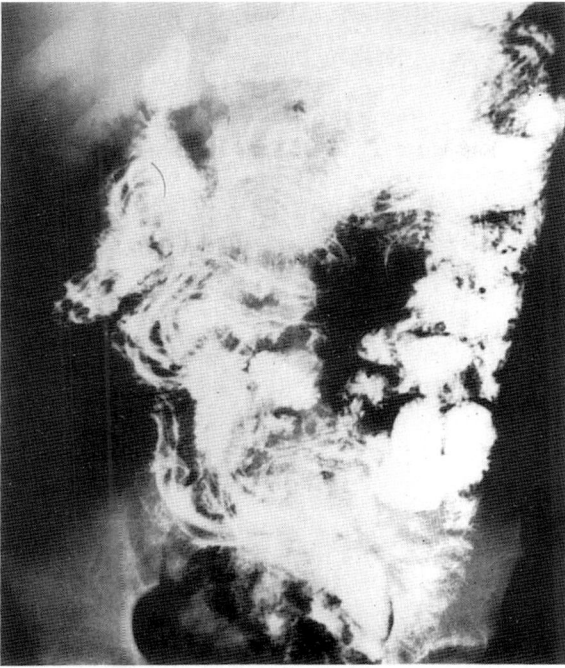

Fig. 28.58 *Ascaris lumbricoides.* Barium follow-through showing infestation in small bowel with worms coated with barium.

piperazine has been used with success in the past. Tiabendazole, although effective, is best avoided owing to its side-effects.[885,886]

Overall, albendazole seems to be the drug of choice for ascariasis but, while results can be achieved quickly with chemotherapy, they are only temporary in the absence of other control measures. Prevention of ascariasis depends on improving living conditions and the sanitary disposal of feces, on preventing contamination of drinking water and raw vegetables, and on education in hygiene. There is evidence too, to indicate that the mass delivery of anthelmintic treatment to children may be an important option in the control of geohelminth infections, including ascariasis. The 1993 World Development Report of the World Bank[887] includes mass de-worming in its 'essential package of health interventions' and school-based mass delivery is singled out as one of the most cost-effective measures – a concept supported by studies such as that of Guyatt.[888]

TOXOCARA CANIS AND VISCERAL LARVA MIGRANS

Toxocara canis is a close relative of *Ascaris*. Its natural hosts are the young dog and the fox, in which it undergoes a cycle essentially similar to *Ascaris* in humans (Fig. 28.60). The cycle in dogs is complicated by the development of immunity with expulsion of adult worms by the animals at about 6 months of age. In pregnant bitches, however, this immunity is lost and dormant larvae in the tissues are reactivated or reinfection occurs, resulting in the puppies being infected in utero and being born with worms. Children ingest infective eggs from dirt contaminated with dog feces or directly from the animals themselves, especially young puppies or lactating bitches.[889] The larvae, after penetrating the intestinal wall, are incapable of completing their pulmonary migration in an unnatural host and wander aimlessly, never to find their intestinal habitat. They pass through, or become encysted in liver, lungs, kidneys, heart, muscle, brain or eye, causing an intense local response from the tissue.

Clinical features

The child (most commonly 1–5 years of age) with visceral larva migrans (VLM) shows failure to thrive associated with pica (90% of cases), anemia (Hb < 9 g/dl in 45%), fever (80%) and enlargement of liver (65%) and spleen (45%). There is cough (80%), bronchospasm and wheezing (63%).[889] A single organ may bear the brunt of the infection so that pulmonary symptoms or neurological abnormalities due to brain involvement (convulsions, disturbances of consciousness, hemiparesis) may predominate. Intense and persistent eosinophilia lasting months or years and reaching levels as high as 80×10^9/L is characteristic and may be the only abnormality found. Serum globulin levels are raised, particularly IgM, IgG and IgE, and elevated titers of anti-A and anti-B isoagglutinins have been described in 39% of cases. Transient chest shadows are recorded in about 50% of cases and the CSF may show an eosinophilia where the CNS is involved. The infection usually runs a chronic, benign course of 18 months or so and generally the prognosis is good, although deaths have been reported.

Ocular manifestations of toxocariasis (ocular larva migrans, OLM) may be the only evidence of the disease. The age of maximal ocular involvement is higher than that of systemic involvement, the average age being about 7–8 years. Loss of sight in the affected eye generally results, and usually only one eye is involved. A diagnosis of ocular toxocariasis should be considered when there is inflammatory detachment of the retina or retinitis of the posterior pole in a child, especially in one with geophagic habits, who has contact with young dogs. The diagnosis can be confused with retinoblastoma, which may lead to the unnecessary surgical removal of an eye in a child with ocular toxocariasis.

It appears, therefore, that there are two toxocaral syndromes in humans:
1. larvae in the eye, presenting as granulomatous pseudotumors of the retina (OLM);
2. generalized toxocariasis with numerous larvae in the liver and other organs and associated with fever and eosinophilia (VLM).
Because ocular lesions are seldom found in the generalized forms, and because ocular disease is almost entirely confined to children, it has been postulated that ocular toxocariasis could be the manifestation of congenital infection of the child from an infected mother, in a similar fashion to the transplacental infection of puppies. This

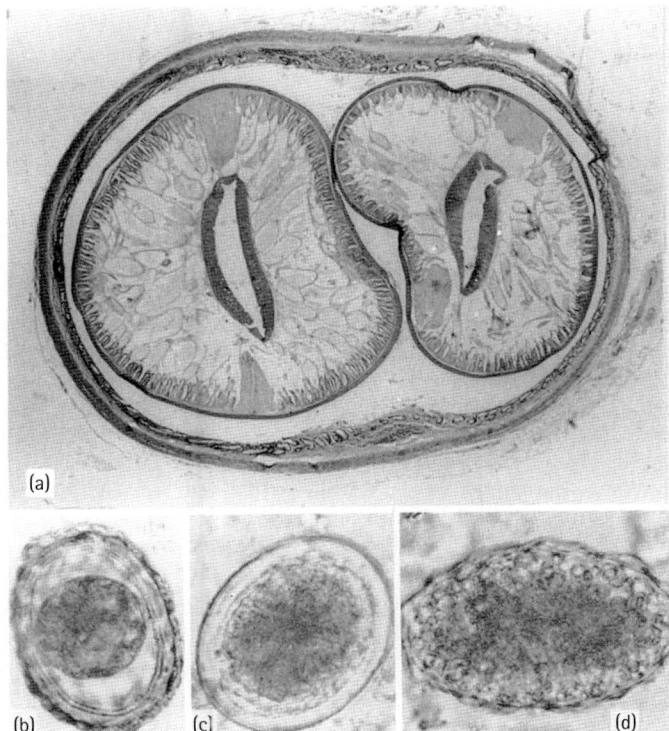

Fig. 28.59 (a) Pair of *Ascaris* in appendix (approx. × 10). (b) Fertilized egg of *Ascaris lumbricoides* (approx. × 600). (c) Decorticated fertilized egg of *A. lumbricoides* (approx. × 600). (d) Unfertilized egg of *A. lumbricoides* (approx. × 600).

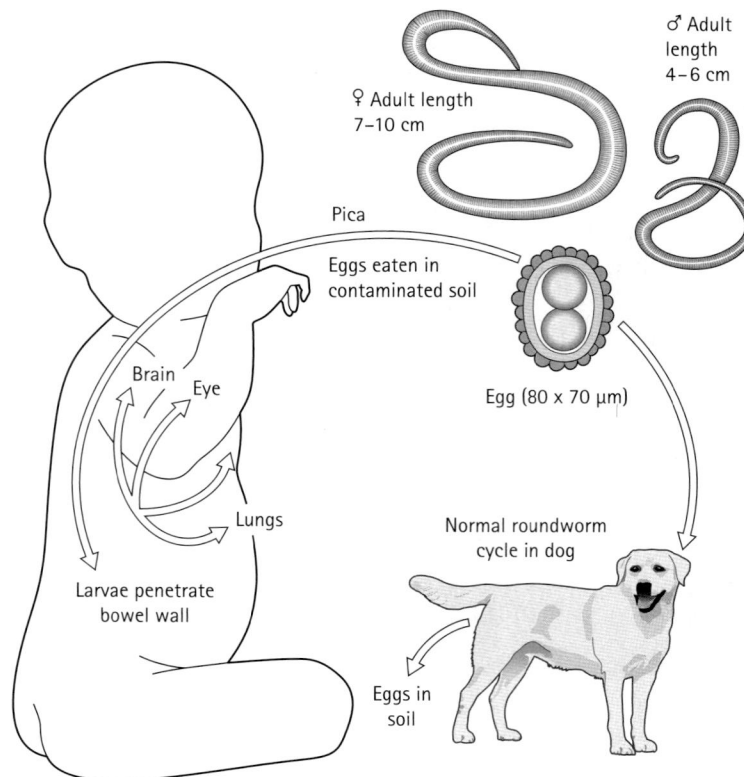

Fig. 28.60 Character and life cycle of *Toxocara canis*.

hypothesis, if true, would have important implications for expectant mothers. Similarly, contact with cats or cat litter might entail risk of fetus-damaging infection due to toxocariasis from *Toxocara cati* as well as toxoplasmosis.

It has been suggested that the eosinophilia so often seen in children suffering from lead poisoning resulting from pica may well be due to concurrent *Toxocara* infection. Physicians managing children with lead intoxication should be aware of this possibility and treat the toxocariasis concurrently.

A similar clinical syndrome can be caused in children by filarial parasites of animal origin and by larvae of other types[889] (Table 28.43). It still remains unclear whether *T. cati* (the cat roundworm) can be responsible for systemic larva migrans, and another dog ascarid, *Toxascaris leonina*, previously thought to be non-infective to humans, should be considered as a potential cause of visceral larva migrans.

Diagnosis
Acquisition of a puppy in the preceding year has proved to be a good suggestive indicator of *Toxocara* infection in symptomatic patients.[889] The diagnosis can only be established with certainty, however, by a biopsy (generally of the liver) or, undesirably and rather drastically, after enucleation of the eye. Skin tests and serological tests such as the indirect fluorescent antibody test and the *Toxocara* enzyme immunoassay (EIA) are available with the latter having a reported sensitivity of 78% and a specificity of 92%.[889,890] It is worth noting that 2–7% or more of symptomless adults and up to 23% of children with no symptoms may have detectable *Toxocara* antibodies.[889,891]

Fluorescein angiography, ultrasound and CT scans are also described as useful adjuncts to diagnosis.[890]

Treatment
Diethylcarbamazine (DEC) (2 mg/kg 8-hourly for 7–10 days) is reportedly effective.[883,890] An alternative regimen is up to 6 mg/kg in divided doses for 3 weeks.[889] Repeated courses may be necessary and if respiratory distress or myocardial involvement develops, corticosteroids may be life-saving.

Tiabendazole at a dose of 50 mg/kg per day for 3–5 days or 25 mg/kg for 1–4 weeks has also been recommended in the past and has been considered especially useful for early ocular cases where diethylcarbamazine should not be used, as the cellular response it elicits could aggravate visual problems. Corticosteroids are also important in controlling ocular lesions and should be given before the DEC is started.[890] Albendazole (400 mg 12-hourly for 3–5 days) has shown promise and flubendazole has also proved encouraging.[890,892]

Overall, however, the chemotherapy for toxocariasis remains unsatisfactory.

Prevention
While the dangers of infection from pets cannot be overstressed, this is a very emotive issue. Hungerford[893] stated: 'In our stress distorted society, pets...may be the critical factor in maintaining or restoring mental health or happiness to an only child, or to a psychotic, mentally distraught or lonely child or adult.'

The answer, therefore, is not destruction of pets, but regular and routine de-worming of dogs, especially puppies and pregnant bitches, with mebendazole, fenbendazole, piperazine or pyrantel pamoate. Also important is education to impress upon children and expectant mothers the need to wash their hands after handling pets and not to allow dogs to lick them on the face. Dogs and cats should also be prevented from defecating where children play (sandpits, etc.).

ENTEROBIUS VERMICULARIS (OXYURIASIS)
Enterobius vermicularis (threadworm, pinworm, seatworm) is common worldwide, but unlike most nematodes it is more prolific in temperate and cold climates. The incidence is highest in schoolchildren from 5 to 9 years with another peak at 30–49 years.[894] Boys and girls are equally affected. Enterobiasis is particularly common in highly populated

districts, institutional groups, and among members of the same family. Incidences as high as 40–50% have been reported and in institutions such as mental hospitals, prevalence may reach 90–100%. The absence of a prolonged developmental stage outside humans (Fig. 28.61) favors reinfection and transmission from child to child. Hands are contaminated by scratching the perianal area where eggs are deposited, and by contact with soiled underclothing, nightclothing or bedding. Infection is also acquired by inhalation of egg-containing dust, which may be disseminated from bedclothing by shaking, or movements of the sleeper. At room temperature eggs survive for 2–3 weeks. Furthermore, retroinfection may occur when the eggs hatch on the perianal area and larvae find their way back through the anus into the intestinal tract.

The usual habitat of the threadworm of both sexes is the caecum and adjacent appendix, lower ileum, and colon. The worms are free in the intestinal lumen or lie with their heads attached to the mucosa. Gravid females migrate to the lower colon and rectum and crawl through the anus to deposit thousands of sticky eggs on the anal verge and perineum at night, usually dying thereafter. It is worth emphasizing that dogs and cats play no part in the transmission of enterobiasis to humans.

Clinical features

Threadworm infection is generally asymptomatic. The most common manifestation is anal pruritus due to migration of the worms and the presence of eggs. Restless sleep, nightmares, teeth grinding, and perhaps bed-wetting may result. In up to 20% of girls, vulval irritation and vaginal discharge are caused by threadworms and can persist for years[877] and night crying may be due to a threadworm in the vaginal introitus. Excoriation and pyogenic infection can follow from constant scratching.

It is most unlikely that threadworms play any significant part in causing the variety of symptoms commonly attributed to them. For example, threadworms are no more common in children with recurrent abdominal pain than in those without pain. Similarly, threadworms are found as often in normal appendices as in appendices showing acute or chronic inflammation, so that they are not considered to play any material role in the production of appendicitis, although appendiceal blockage resulting in a simulated chronic appendicitis may occur at times.[894]

Nail biting, nose picking, masturbation, convulsions, hyperkinesis and other behavior disturbances are also often erroneously ascribed to these parasites.

Very heavy infections can, however, result in catarrhal inflammation of the bowel from the attachment and irritation of worms, resulting in gastrointestinal disturbance. Intestinal obstruction has even been reported. Rarely, heavy infections have led to invasion of the bowel and appendiceal walls, peritoneum or viscera by larvae and immature worms. In their external migration gravid threadworms may occasionally crawl up the vagina into the uterus and Fallopian tubes or into the urethra and bladder depositing eggs in these sites with resulting low grade salpingitis, cystitis or urethritis, and cases are on record of worms penetrating the intestinal wall, probably through a pre-existing mucosal breach, to reach the peritoneal cavity.

Enterobiasis may be associated with infection by the protozoan flagellate, *Dientamoeba fragilis*, which is believed to be transmitted within the egg of the threadworm and may be a cause of diarrhea.[895]

Eosinophilia is usually absent in enterobiasis but may occur in up to 12% of cases.

Diagnosis

Often the first evidence of infection is the discovery of the adult worms in the feces, particularly after enemas, or on the perineum. Worms may be clearly visible on proctoscopy. The most widely used and effective method of obtaining eggs from the perianal region is the adhesive cellulose tape method. The adhesive side of a piece of transparent tape is applied to the anus and surrounding skin – either directly or wrapped round a test tube – and the tape then transferred adhesive side down to a glass slide. The adhering eggs are clearly visible under a microscope (Fig. 28.62a). The test is best performed in the morning before bathing or defecation, and in view of the irregular migrations of gravid worms at least three examinations should be made on consecutive days. Eggs are found in the stools in only 5–10% of cases, but five perianal swabs reveal eggs in 97% of infections.

Treatment

Drugs of choice for enterobiasis include mebendazole, albendazole and pyrantel embonate/pamoate. Mebendazole given in a single dose of 100 mg (one tablet) stat. is recorded as giving a cure rate of about 95% with no or very few side-effects.[877] Although some authorities advise that mebendazole should not be used in children < 2 years of age, others accept that a dose of 50 mg can be used for a child < 10 kg.[884] Albendazole is also reported as effective, at a dose of 400 mg orally (200 mg in children 10 kg or less).[896] Neither mebendazole nor albendazole should be used during pregnancy.[884]

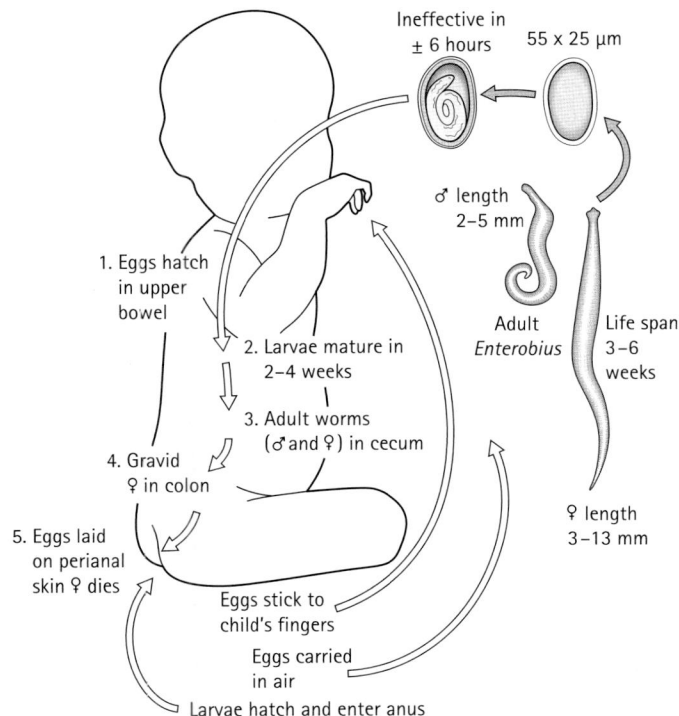

Fig. 28.61 Character and life cycle of *Enterobius vermicularis*.

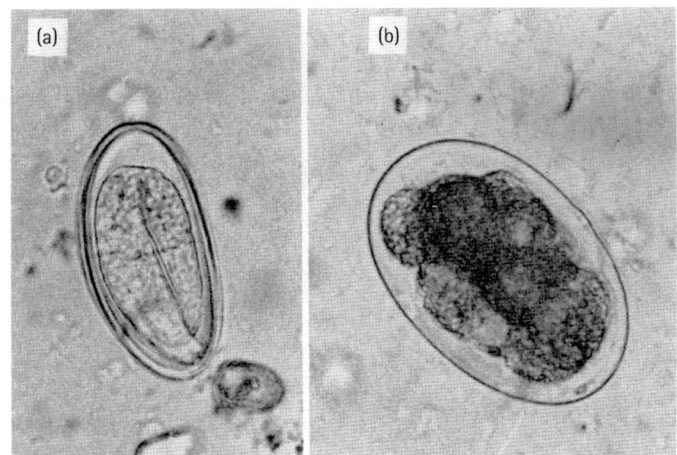

Fig. 28.62 (a) Fully developed egg of *Enterobius vermicularis* (approx. × 600). (b) Hookworm egg (approx. × 600).

Pyrantel 11 mg/kg is also very effective as a single dose treatment, giving cure rates greater than 90%. Side-effects are usually mild (e.g. nausea and vomiting), occurring in about 3% of cases.[877,886]

Piperazine citrate and pyrvinium pamoate are no longer in general use for enterobiasis, and tiabendazole, while efficacious, has unpleasant side-effects.

When a child is treated for enterobiasis, the whole family should be treated, and a second course should be given after 3 weeks. Unfortunately, reinfection is the rule rather than the exception. Intractable family infections can be controlled by the treatment of all family members with 100 mg (50 mg for children <10 kg) mebendazole a week for 12 weeks.

Prevention of recurrence is extremely difficult, particularly in crowded communities and in humid temperate climates, which facilitate prolonged survival of eggs. Personal cleanliness is essential and this includes cutting fingernails, regular hand washing before meals and after using the toilet, washing the anal area on rising, and regular changing of underclothing and bed linen.

HOOKWORM (ANCYLOSTOMIASIS)

Ancylostoma duodenale (Old World hookworm) and *Necator americanus* (tropical hookworm) are morphological variants, tropical hookworm being rather smaller with differences of fine morphology.

Hookworm occurs in most tropical and subtropical areas of the world, with *A. duodenale* distributed mainly around the Mediterranean littoral and *N. americanus* in south and central Africa and southern America. Both species are, however, widely distributed today in Asia as well as in most other tropical countries. In South East Asia and Brazil, *A. ceylanicum* infections of humans occur as well and *A. malayanum* is yet another species from humans.[877] Hookworm is one of the world's chief causes of anemia.

A. braziliense, one cause of cutaneous larva migrans (Table 28.43) and a natural parasite of dogs and cats, is widely distributed throughout tropical and subtropical areas, while the common dog hookworm *A. caninum* is also widely distributed, and *Uncinaria stenocephala* infects dogs in temperate regions. These latter two species can also cause cutaneous larva migrans in humans and it is claimed that in northern Queensland in Australia, *A. caninum* may be a cause of eosinophilic enteritis in humans as discussed by Smyth.[897]

The excreted egg, in favorable damp, shady conditions, hatches on the soil in about 2 days, releasing a rhabditiform larva which develops 8–10 days after hatching into the infective (filariform) larva. This larva penetrates the skin of the host, although *A. duodenale* is believed also to enter via the oral route with fecally contaminated food and water and may infect by the transmammary and transplacental routes from infected mother to child.[898] The life cycle in humans from larval penetration to oviposition lasts about 5 weeks (Fig. 28.63). The adult worm may survive within its host for 7 years or longer.

Adult worms are attached to the wall of the jejunum, or, less commonly, the duodenum, by their buccal capsules, sucking blood from their hosts. Each worm may suck up to 0.5 ml of blood per day; thus heavy worm loads may result in a loss of 100–150 ml/day. Significant damage is therefore produced by hookworms, but clinical manifestations depend on the host's general resistance, on the worm load, and on the child's dietary intake and iron reserves.

Clinical features
Larval invasion
Penetration of the skin, usually of the feet or buttocks, by the filariform larvae may produce, within minutes, a series of wheals, which soon develop into an itchy, papular and vesicular eruption ('ground/dew itch'). The rash may become ulcerative or pustular, but generally

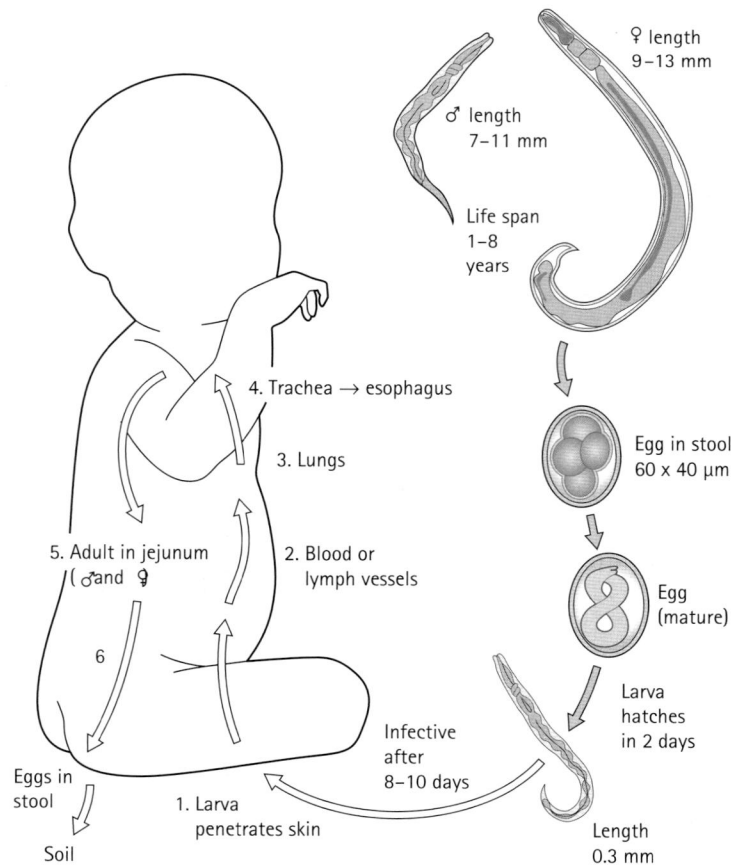

Fig. 28.63 Character and life cycle of hookworm.

subsides within 10 days and the larvae do not wander within the skin as in the case of cutaneous larva migrans (see below).

Migration through the lungs

After penetration of the skin, larvae reach the small intestine via the heart and lungs as in ascariasis.

Respiratory symptoms are unusual in children except in the case of heavy or repeated infections, particularly of *N. americanus*, when there may be cough, sore throat, bloody sputum and pulmonary changes on X-ray (Table 28.43).

Adult worms in the intestine

A distinction should be made between hookworm infection (where patients carry a subclinical worm load) and hookworm disease, which results from heavy worm loads and inadequate diet. Where heavy infections occur, symptoms develop 2–7 weeks after initial infection and consist of abdominal discomfort especially after meals, anorexia and sometimes nausea and vomiting. There may be intermittent diarrhea, general debility and undue tiredness. Once the adult worms are well established, there is little disturbance to the child, provided that the intake of iron, vitamins and protein keeps pace with the chronic blood loss produced by the parasites. When diet is inadequate and worm load heavy, severe hookworm disease results, characterized by profound iron deficiency anemia, hypoalbuminemic edema, cardiac failure and even death. It has been estimated that 100 worms will cause a daily loss of 4 mg of iron. A balanced diet easily compensates for this loss, but iron deficiency soon develops on a marginal dietary intake. Children with heavy hookworm infections are stunted, marasmic and anemic; their skin is dry and their face puffy. All aspects of development are retarded. An important concomitant which makes hookworm infection much more serious is sickle cell anemia.

A marked eosinophilia (40%) is characteristic of early hookworm infection. It reaches maximum intensity at about 3 months after initial infection and then diminishes gradually to levels of 5–20%. A partially effective protective immunity seems to develop in hookworm infection.[899,900]

Diagnosis

This depends on finding the eggs (Fig. 28.62b) in the feces, and an egg count should be performed if a causal relationship with a concomitant iron deficiency anemia is to be established. An egg count > 2000 eggs/g of feces is generally considered to be of clinical significance.

In old stool specimens rhabditiform larvae are occasionally found and can be distinguished from those of *Strongyloides* by the short buccal chamber and larger genital primordium of the latter.

Eggs similar to those of hookworms can be recovered from humans infected with *Trichostrongylus* spp., *Oesophagostomum* spp. and *Ternidens deminutus*. The eggs of the former species are more pointed than those of hookworm and the eggs of *T. deminutus* are significantly larger than those of the hookworm species. These infections can be treated as for hookworm.[901]

Treatment

Albendazole is reported to be effective against the migrating larval stages of the human hookworms, *A. duodenale* and *N. americanus*.[902] The avermectins (ivermectin) have shown promise against all stages of hookworm development including migrating larvae.[877] Children with severe anemia, malnutrition or a heavy worm load should receive preliminary supportive treatment in the form of blood transfusion, high calorie and protein diet, vitamins and iron therapy before definitive treatment of the worms. A highly effective anthelmintic for hookworm infection is albendazole and at a single dose of 400 mg (200 mg for children 10 kg or less) it has also proved highly effective against a wide range of other intestinal helminths.[877,884] Albendazole is additionally reported to have ovicidal activity against hookworm, ascariasis and trichuriasis, making it especially valuable in integrated control programs for these infections.[902] Mebendazole also gives excellent cure rates for both species

of hookworm at a dose of 100 mg twice a day for 3 days or 50 mg for children 10 kg or less – and with few or no side-effects.

Pyrantel embonate/pamoate (11 mg/kg, max. 750 mg) is effective for *A. duodenale* given in a single dose regimen,[903] but for *N. americanus* needs to be given as a multiple dose treatment.

Other treatments for hookworm include phenylene diisothiocyanate and bephenium hydroxynaphthoate.

The preventive aspects of hookworm are complex and include education of the public into the mode of spread of the disease, provision and proper usage of latrines, improvement of diet, and, where the incidence is high, mass population treatment. The wearing of shoes will also help to prevent infection. Studies from Papua New Guinea by Quinell et al[903] suggest that host susceptibility differences may explain why different individuals are predisposed to heavy or light burdens. Interest continues regarding the possibility of vaccination against hookworm infection.[898,900,904]

CUTANEOUS LARVA MIGRANS (CREEPING ERUPTION, SAND WORM)

Clinical features

The larvae of the dog hookworms, *A. braziliense*, *A. caninum* and *U. stenocephala*, together with certain other parasites (Table 28.43), can produce in humans a long-lasting skin eruption which differs from that caused by 'human' hookworms. The larva, after penetrating the epidermis, is unable to enter the bloodstream or lymphatics and instead burrows just below the corium, traveling up to an inch a day. Papules mark the site of entry and advancing end of the larva and the tunneling causes slightly elevated, erythematous and serpiginous lines which itch intensely (Fig. 28.64). Vesicles may form along the course of the tunnels and scaling develops as the lesions age. The most common sites in children are the buttocks and the dorsum of the feet, but any area can be affected. The eruption generally disappears after 1–2 months, but may persist for 6 months or longer. The diagnosis is clinical.

Treatment

Topical tiabendazole 15% cream is the treatment of choice and can easily be made from the oral preparation by dissolving 500 mg tablets in a water base, if not commercially available. Ivermectin (children > 5 years) 200 μg/kg orally as a single dose, or albendazole 400 mg (200 mg for a child < 10 kg) orally, once daily for 3 days, is also effective.[884] Cryotherapy is unpleasant, ineffective and no longer used.

TRICHURIS TRICHIURA (TRICHOCEPHALIASIS, WHIPWORM)

The whipworm, so called for its thin anterior lash-like end (Fig. 28.65), is widely distributed, being most common in hot, damp environs. The adult nematode frequents the cecum but can occur in the appendix, colon or

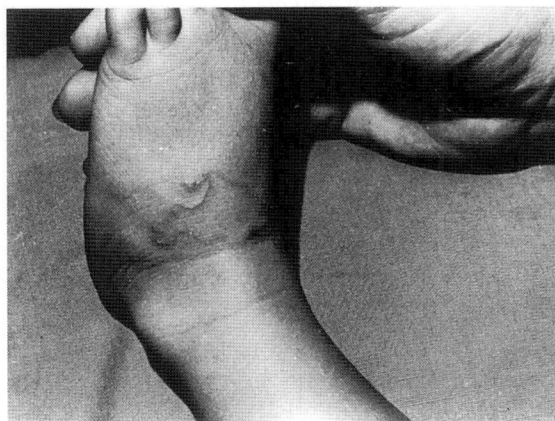

Fig. 28.64 Cutaneous larva migrans.

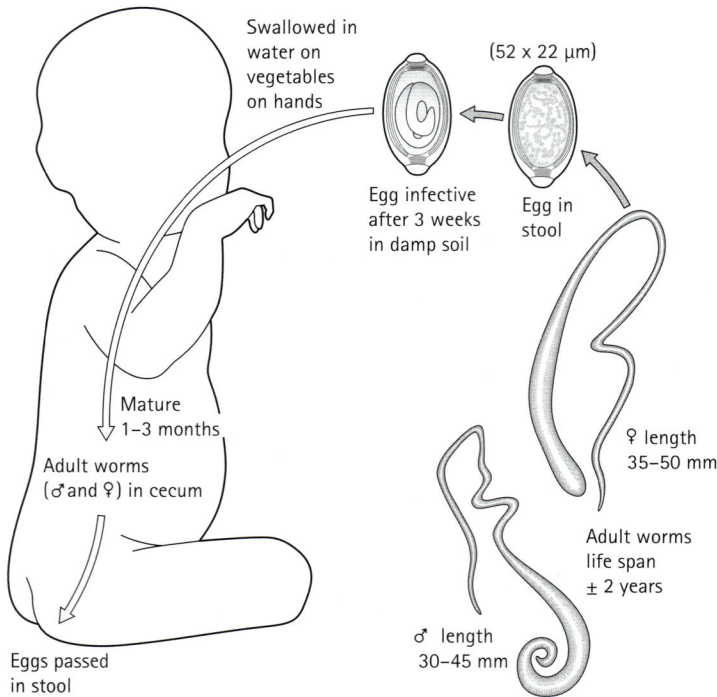

Fig. 28.65   Character and life cycle of *Trichuris trichiura*.

terminal ileum, its thin anterior extremity threaded or embedded in the mucosa. Eggs pass out with the feces and mature on the soil in about 2–3 weeks. Children usually acquire whipworm by sucking fingers or objects contaminated with fecal-polluted soil containing infective eggs, but contaminated vegetables and fly-borne contamination of food are also important means of spread. Trichuriasis is by no means confined to the tropics[905] and may prove troublesome in mental institutions.

Trichuris vulpis, the dog whipworm, may occasionally infect humans.[891]

Clinical features

Whipworm infection is often asymptomatic but should not be under-rated as a pathogen in humans.[905] Heavy worm loads may be responsible for intestinal symptoms including abdominal pain, which is most marked in the right iliac fossa simulating appendicitis, bloody diarrhea, tenesmus, and sometimes mild pyrexia. Heavy loads can lead to marked anemia, weight loss, and a picture closely resembling hookworm disease or amebic colitis. Clubbing of the fingers and toes is seen and is reversed with eradication of the infection. Rectal prolapse is a well-recognized complication. Trichuriasis often causes insidious disease and is frequently associated with growth retardation.[906]

Diagnosis

This is readily accomplished by finding the characteristic eggs (Fig. 28.66) in the stools. A barium enema may assist in diagnosis (Fig. 28.67).

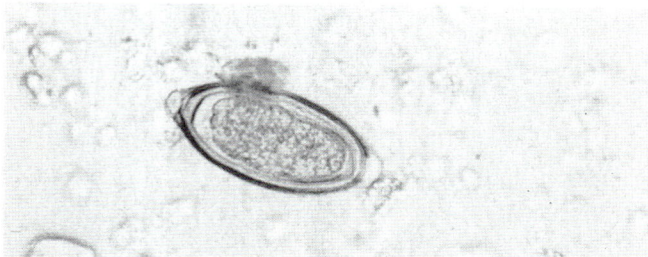

Fig. 28.66   Egg of *Trichuris trichiura* (approx. × 600).

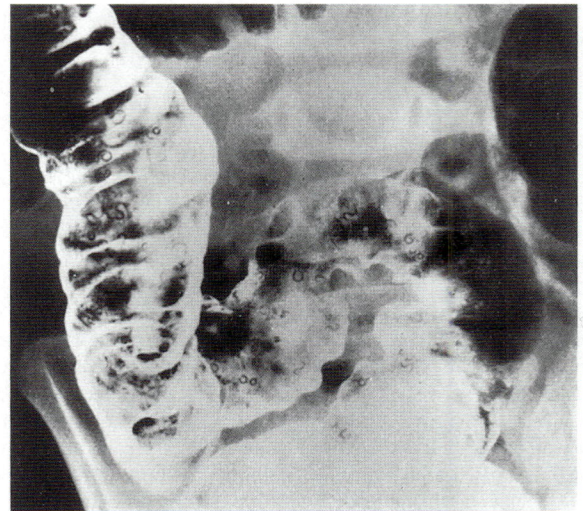

Fig. 28.67   *Trichuris trichiura*. Double contrast barium enema examination showing infestation and numerous small circular or sigmoid defects in barium coating of colon.

Treatment

Albendazole at a dose of 400 mg, or 200 mg for children 10 kg or less, given once, is the drug of choice,[884] but mebendazole can also be used at a dose of 100 mg (50 mg for a child 10 kg or less) 12-hourly for 3 days.[877] Difetarsone has been reported to be most useful in the treatment of whipworm, and oxantel pamoate is also reported to be effective.[877]

STRONGYLOIDES STERCORALIS (STRONGYLOIDIASIS)

Strongyloides stercoralis (sometimes termed 'threadworm' in the American literature) has a human cycle closely resembling hookworm, except that autoinfection is common and a free-living cycle can occur if external conditions are favorable (Fig. 28.68). Strongyloidiasis is most common in tropical or semitropical climates but may occur sporadically in temperate regions. The minute adult worms are to be found in the crypts of Lieberkuhn glands in the upper part of the small intestine, where they burrow into the mucosa.

In central Africa, *Strongyloides fülleborni* is often found in humans and a similar species is reported to cause 'swollen belly syndrome' in infants about 6 weeks of age in Papua New Guinea (PNG).[907] The species in PNG has been designated as *S. fülleborni Kellyi*, and infants as young as 18 days of age can become infected, possibly by transmammary infection, as may also occur with *S. fülleborni* in Africa.[908]

Clinical features

Skin penetration by filariform larvae may cause a transient prickling sensation, but following heavy infection there is a pruritic petechial rash with local edema. Internal and external autoinfection frequently occurs, especially in immunodeficient patients or patients on immunosuppressant drugs or corticosteroids, larvae in the feces entering through the rectal mucosa, anus or skin in the perianal region. This gives rise to an often recurring eruption resembling cutaneous larva migrans (termed larva currens) but of shorter duration. Generalized urticaria is sometimes seen as a result of hypersensitivity. Eosinophilia is common. Clinical manifestations of pulmonary migration of larvae are infrequent, but respiratory symptoms can occur and, rarely, chronic lung disease develops due to larvae maturing within the lung.

In chronic strongyloidiasis the presence of the adult worms in the intestine is often asymptomatic.[909] A heavy worm load causes epigastric pain, episodes of acute appendicitis,[896] bowel upset often with bloody diarrhea, iron deficiency anemia and debility. Infection can last 20 years or more, owing to constant internal and external autoinfection.[910]

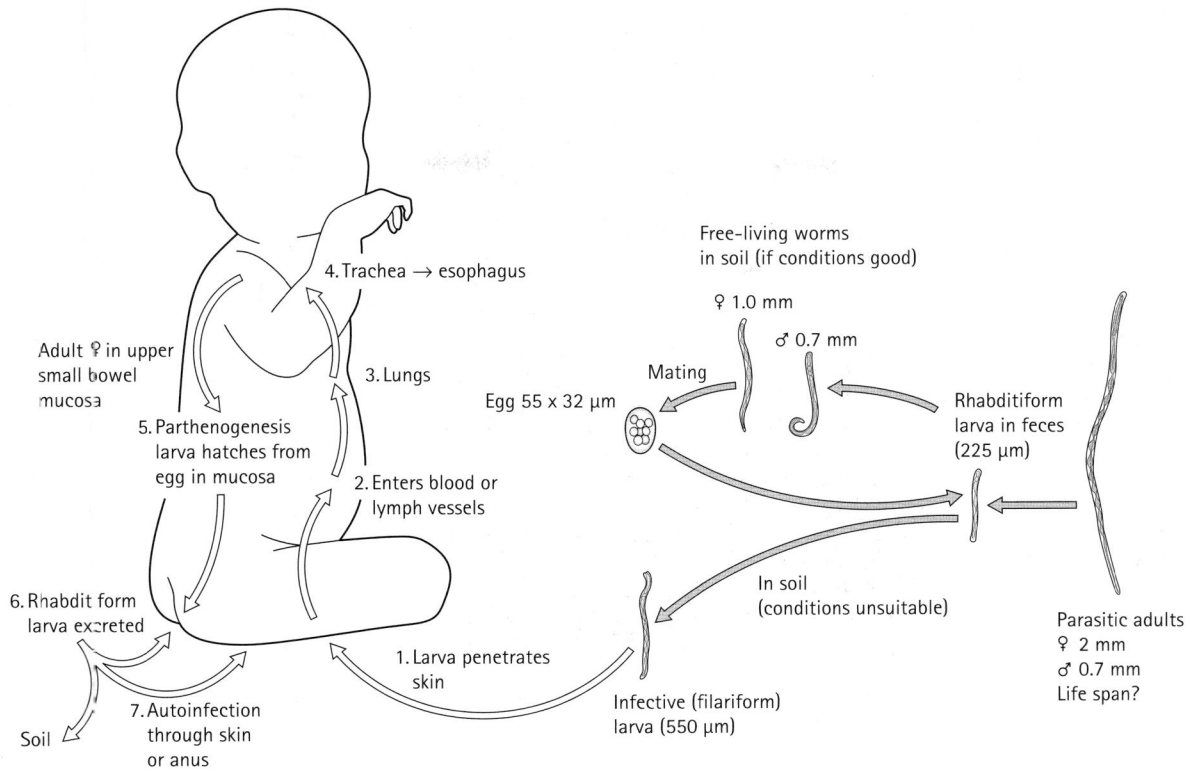

Fig. 28.68 Character and life cycle of *Strongyloides stercoralis*.

In immunocompromised patients, fatal infection can occur, but it is noteworthy that despite the HIV/AIDS pandemic in sub-Saharan Africa and elsewhere, *S. stercoralis* has not proved an important opportunistic pathogen, although an epidemiological association between strongyloidiasis and HTLV-1 has been reported.[901,909] *Strongyloides* hyperinfection syndrome may be complicated by Gram negative bacteremia in both immunocompromised and non-immunocompromised individuals and has a high mortality.[911,912]

Diagnosis

Considerable eosinophilia is usual and can be an important diagnostic indicator in some circumstances.[910] Diagnosis of *S. stercoralis* is established by demonstrating rhabditiform larvae (Fig. 28.69a) in fresh stools (repeat examinations may be necessary) or duodenal fluid. A useful method for diagnosing *S. stercoralis*, giardiasis, and other upper intestinal parasites is duodenal drainage or the use of the duodenal capsule (Enterotest), or 'string test'; a special pediatric size is available. The capsule, containing a length of thread and 3-ply nylon yarn, is swallowed while the protruding free end of thread is held at the mouth. The yarn within the capsule plays out, and within 3–4 h the line has almost invariably extended to the duodenum or jejunum. The gelatin capsule dissolves. The nylon yarn is then pulled back through the mouth and the adhering mucus examined for parasites.

Serological tests such as EIA are available in some countries, with sensitivities in the order of 80–90% and specificities of about 90%. These tests do not usually differentiate present from past infection and may cross-react with other nematode infections.[890]

In *S. fülleborni* infections, fully embryonated eggs (Fig. 28.69b) are passed in the feces. They are similar in appearance to hookworm eggs but much smaller, about 50 × 36 μm in size, are fully developed at time of passage[901] and hatch after about 2–3 h.

Treatment

Because of the dangers of autoinfection, especially in the immunocompromised, strongyloidiasis must always be treated when diagnosed.[913]

The treatment of choice for strongyloidiasis is now albendazole 400 mg 12-hourly, orally for 3 days (children 10 kg or less 200 mg), repeated after 7 days if the infection is disseminated.[884,902] Ivermectin 200 μg/kg orally each day as a single dose for 1–2 days can also be used

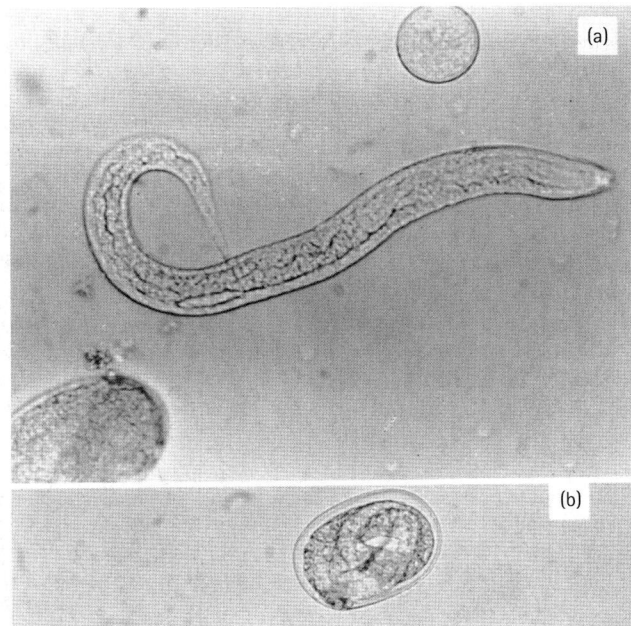

Fig. 28.69 (a) Rhabditiform larva of *Strongyloides stercoralis*. Note short buccal cavity and large genital primordium. Also in the field, an *Entamoeba* cyst and a hookworm egg (approx. ×600). (b) Egg of *Strongyloides fülleborni*. Note its small size. It contains a fully developed, motile larva when passed (approx. ×600).

for children > 5 years of age.[884,913,914] Tiabendazole, which is effective (25 mg/kg 12-hourly, orally, given morning and evening for 3 days up to a maximum total of 3 g daily), is an alternative, but can have unpleasant side-effects.[884,913]

ANGIOSTRONGYLIASIS

Angiostrongylus cantonensis is a natural parasite in the lungs of rats over much of the world, human infection being recorded from Indonesia, Papua New Guinea, Northern Australia, Africa, the Pacific, South East Asia, Cuba and Puerto Rico. The intermediate hosts are snails (such as the giant African land snail *Achatina fulica*) and slugs, which are eaten by the rodents. Humans become infected by eating certain edible snails or by accidental ingestion of small infected slugs on food plants or ingestion of paratenic (or 'carrier') hosts such as edible crustacea.[915]

In humans, larvae migrate to the brain causing eosinophilic meningitis, with neck stiffness, photophobia, pyrexia, decreased consciousness and vomiting.

The diagnosis can be suspected when large numbers of eosinophils are found in the CSF in patients with a history of eating snails or perhaps crustacea. Blood eosinophilia may also be present. Occasionally adults or larvae of *A. cantonensis* can also be detected. Surgical intervention may be necessary.[916] No effective specific treatment is presently available and may in any case be inadvisable as dead worms cause more clinical problems than live ones. However, mebendazole (100 mg 12-hourly for 5 days) together with corticosteroids (30–60 mg/day) is recommended for *A. cantonensis*.[890,913]

Other forms of angiostrongyliasis include an abdominal form caused by *A. costaricensis* in several Latin American countries. This species causes intestinal and liver lesions similar to those caused by *Toxocara*. It is usually diagnosed at surgery and has an epidemiology similar to *A. cantonensis*.[917] This species may require a higher dose of mebendazole than that recommended for *A. cantonensis*.[913]

HELMINTHOMA

Nodules in the bowel wall which contain the adult worms (helminthomas) can be caused by the nodular worms which belong to the genera *Oesophagostomum*, occurring naturally in simian and ruminant hosts, and the false hookworm, *Ternidens deminutus*, a natural parasite of non-human primates. These are known in Central Africa to cause human disease characterized, particularly in *Oesophagostomum*, by tumor-like granulomatous reactions in the wall of the colon.[918] *Ternidens* infections in humans have also been reported from Surinam and Thailand.[919,920] Eggs of these species are hookworm-like but those of *Ternidens* are larger in size.[901]

The drug treatment of choice for the expulsion of the adult worms is mebendazole (100 mg 12-hourly for 3 days). Albendazole is promising.[901,918]

ANISAKIASIS (ANISAKIDOSIS)

Anisakiasis in humans is caused by the larval stages of some 30 genera of anisakid nematodes, of which the most common are *Anisakis*, *Contracaecum*, *Terranova* and *Pseudoterranova*.[896,921] These helminths are intestinal parasites of a range of fish-eating vertebrates, including dolphins, and the larval stages of the worm are found in intermediate hosts such as small fish (e.g. mackerel, herring, salmon), squid or octopus.[922,923] Humans become infected when they eat raw or undercooked fish.

The ingested worms live in the human gastrointestinal tract or penetrate the tissues, giving rise to abscesses or eosinophilic granulomata.

Clinically the infection may be asymptomatic or mild with nausea, vomiting, epigastric pain and often an eosinophilia, which may exceed 40%. Rarely, death may result from peritonitis following perforation of the gut.[922]

While the infection has for many years been recognized in Japan, an increase has been noted in the USA owing to better diagnostic techniques.[923] Diagnosis is established at laparotomy, by X-ray or, most reliably, by endoscopy. Serological tests for diagnosis include the radioallergosorbent test (RAST) and counterimmunoelectrophoresis.

The most effective treatment, where possible, is removal of worms from the stomach by endoscopy. Prevention is best achieved by removing worms from fish prior to eating and by thorough cooking of fish. No effective anthelmintic treatment is presently available,[922] but Shorey et al[890] express the view that mebendazole might have some value, and albendazole at a dose of 400 mg 12-hourly for 21 days proved promising in one case.[921]

TRICHINOSIS

The genus *Trichinella* contains at least four species, the best known being *Trichinella spiralis*. This species has a cosmopolitan distribution, usually being transmitted to humans by eating inadequately cooked, infected pig meat, although outbreaks from other meat sources (e.g. horse meat) are recognized.[924,925] The disease may occur in outbreaks (Fig. 28.70). Trichinosis due to *T. spiralis* is rare in communities which shun pork and in those with vigilant agricultural control, but human disease, especially with other species (e.g. *T. pseudospiralis*, *T. nelsoni*, *T. britovi* or *T. nativa*), may follow eating the meat of other species of animal. Adult *T. spiralis* infect humans, pigs and rats, as well as other animals. Porcine infection usually results from the ingestion of either infected rats or garbage containing uncooked pork meat.

Clinical features
Human trichinosis is frequently mild or symptomless. Although symptoms may occur as early as 24 h following a pork meal, it is usually during the incubation period of 5–7 days or longer,[926] in which the ingested larvae mature into adults, that a clinical picture resembling food poisoning develops – nausea, vomiting, diarrhea and abdominal pain. This phase lasts about 5 days and is followed by signs and symptoms as the larvae enter the bloodstream and encyst in the muscle, a phase lasting a further 2–3 weeks. There is pyrexia, edema of the face and eyelids, splinter hemorrhages under the fingernails, tender lymphadenopathy and myalgia, often extreme. Cough may occur and in severe cases the illness may suggest encephalitis or myocarditis. Marked eosinophilia is usual. Final encystment of the larvae occurs only in voluntary muscles, particularly those of the diaphragm, throat, chest wall, extrinsic ocular apparatus and tongue, and patients may die of toxemia or myocarditis. The encysted larvae may live for many years.

Diagnosis
Diagnosis in the early stages can be made by finding worms in the feces, but in the later stages of the disease, diagnosis is established by muscle biopsy. Intracutaneous and fluorescent antibody tests, together with other serological procedures, are useful adjuncts.[890,926]

Treatment
Albendazole (400 mg for 3 days; 200 mg for children 10 kg or less) is the drug of choice. Mebendazole (200–400 mg daily for 3 days and then 400–500 mg for 10 days) is also recommended.[890,913]

There is evidence that tiabendazole (25 mg/kg per day 12-hourly for 5 days; max. 3 g daily) rapidly kills off migrating larvae and relieves the symptoms.[883] If taken early, the drug also kills larvae in the bowel but is not lethal to the adult worms. Corticosteroids, previously recommended for the treatment of trichinosis, should be restricted to critically ill cases,[916] and then only used in conjunction with anthelmintics.

PARACAPILLARIA PHILIPPINENSIS (CAPILLARIASIS)

It has long been known that the nematode *Capillaria hepatica* can cause a visceral larva migrans-like syndrome in people who have eaten meat (e.g. infected liver) or sand containing the eggs of the worm. Infected

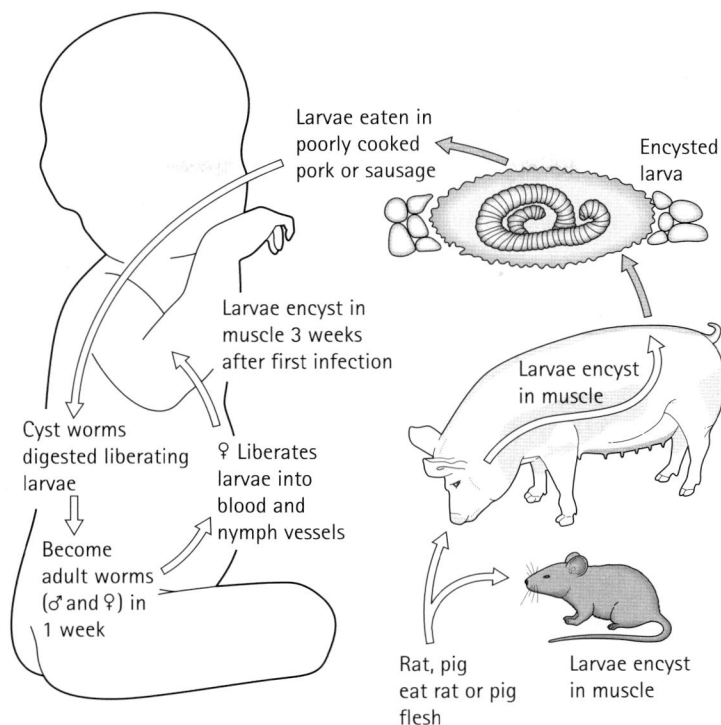

Fig. 28.70 Character and life cycle of *Trichinella spiralis*.

children exhibit such symptoms as fever, eosinophilia, abdominal pain and hepatomegaly, with large numbers of typical eggs being found in the liver on histological examination.

Another species of the genus, *Paracapillaria philippinensis*, has also been shown to be an important cause of epidemic diarrhea in humans in South East Asia and the Middle East. Clinical features in these cases include abdominal pain, malabsorption and diarrhea, which is often severe and not uncommonly fatal (35%) without medical care.[927]

P. philippinensis is a parasite of the small intestine, and is believed to be a zoonotic infection from birds and freshwater fish. Humans become infected by ingestion of eggs or infected raw fish, the usual intermediate host, and the host parasite load may increase as a result of autoinfection.[896]

Capillaria aerophila is found in the lungs of cats, and occasional human infections have been recorded.[890,896]

Diagnosis of capillariasis is based upon histology or finding eggs and larvae in feces. The eggs are like those of *Trichuris*, but the polar plugs are inset and the shells are striated or pitted. *C. hepatica* eggs can be found as spurious 'transit eggs' in feces of patients who have recently eaten infected liver.[928]

Tiabendazole has been used for treatment, but side-effects and relapses are common.[927] Mebendazole (200 mg 12-hourly for 20 days) and albendazole (400 mg daily for 10 days) are reported to be effective for the treatment of capillariasis.[896,913]

DRACUNCULOSIS (DRACONTIASIS)

Despite its bizarre mode of propagation, the guinea worm (*Dracunculus medinensis*) is widely distributed in equatorial Africa, the Middle East and India. However, with new international efforts to improve drinking water supplies, dracontiasis eradication may well be achievable.[929]

Clinical features

Children from the age of 2 years may be infected by drinking water containing *Cyclops*, a tiny crustacean which is infected with the larvae of *Dracunculus*. During the asymptomatic incubation period, lasting approximately 1 year, the guinea worm matures in retroperitoneal tissues. The male, having fertilized the female, apparently dies. The gravid female, often over 100 cm in length by 1.5 mm in width, then migrates

through the subcutaneous tissues to distal parts of the extremities, usually the lower limb, to form a large pruritic papule. This vesiculates, then bursts leaving a shallow ulcer. On immersion in water the worm's uterus prolapses through the ulcer releasing myriads of larvae. Occasionally adult worms may develop in ectopic sites.

Papule formation may be associated with a marked allergic reaction (vomiting, diarrhea, urticaria and bronchospasm).

Secondary infection of sinuses, subcutaneous cysts, sterile abscesses and periarticular fibrosis with joint deformity are recognized complications. Calcified worms may be discovered on radiological examination.

Treatment

The ancient technique of repeatedly stimulating the parturient worm with cold water, grasping the uterus which then protrudes, and then cautiously winding the worm round a stick an inch or two per day is still used. However, drug treatments recommended for dracontiasis include the use of niridazole (12.5 mg/kg 12-hourly for 7–10 days) and tiabendazole which has also been reported to be effective at a total dose of 25 mg/kg orally daily for 3 days.[883] Metronidazole is also claimed to be highly effective at an oral dose for children of 7.5 mg/kg (max. 250 mg) 8-hourly for 5–10 days.[883,885,913]

FILARIASIS

Filariasis is included among the diseases given priority by the United Nations Development Program/World Bank/WHO Special Program for Research and Training due to the huge number of people infected and the enormous burden of morbidity affecting whole communities in endemic regions.[930]

Humans are the primary hosts to several species of filariae, the adult worms living in the tissues. The adult female worms produce eggs which hatch to release pre-larval microfilariae. These are ingested by an appropriate blood-sucking arthropod vector, in which they undergo metamorphosis to form infective larvae. Important characteristics of the principal human filariae are shown in Table 28.44).

During the early stages of all filarial infections moderate to high eosinophilia is usual, but this gradually diminishes in those who have

Table 28.44   Types of filaria worms responsible for human disease

Type and distribution	Insect vector	Important features of microfilaria	Human adult worm location
Onchocerca volvulus, west, central and east Africa, Guatemala, Mexico, and Surinam	*Simulium* black flies	Do not occur in blood, but in skin as unsheathed intradermal microfilariae (microfilariae may penetrate eye)	Subcutaneous tissue
Mansonella perstans, tropical and subtropical areas mainly of Africa and South America	*Culicoides* midges	Occur in blood. Nonperiodic. Unsheathed. Nuclear column extends into tip of thick blunt tail	Mesenteric, perirenal and retroperitoneal tissues
Mansonella ozzardi, South America	*Culicoides* midges	Occur in blood. Nonperiodic. Nuclear column does NOT extend into tip of thin, pointed tail	Mesentery and serous body cavities
Wuchereria bancrofti, tropical and subtropical areas throughout the world	Many mosquitoes belonging to the genera *Culex, Aedes, Anopheles*, and *Mansonia*	Occur in blood. Nocturnal periodic. Sheathed. Nuclear column does NOT extend into tip of thin pointed tail	Lymphatic tissue
Brugia malayi, B. timori, East Indies and Southern Asia	Many mosquitoes belonging to the genera *Mansonia, Culex*, and *Anopheles*	Occur in blood. Nocturnal periodic. Sheathed. Nuclear column extends into tip of tail with single spaced nuclei in terminal bulb and subterminal swelling	Lymphatic tissue
Loa loa, west and central Africa	*Chrysops* flies	Occur in blood. Diurnal periodic. Sheathed. Nuclear column extends into tip of thick blunt tail	Subcutaneous tissue

been infected for long periods. Apart from *Onchocerca volvulus*, where microfilariae are found in skin snips, parasitological diagnosis is best achieved by using stained blood films or concentration techniques applied to peripheral blood. However, very promising and effective serological tests for the detection of circulating filarial antigen have been developed.

Onchocerca volvulus

Onchocerciasis is a filarial disease transmitted to humans by bites from black flies of the genus *Simulium*. It is characterized by subcutaneous nodules, containing adult worms of *O. volvulus*, by skin eruptions due to microfilariae, and by serious eye disease. The condition is only seen in Central Africa and in parts of South America (Table 28.44), especially along the banks of fast flowing rivers, in which the flies breed.

Clinical features

Adolescents are most commonly affected, but children down to 1 year of age may be afflicted. Signs of disease begin to appear after 4–18 months, and the commonest manifestation is the *Onchocerca* nodule. These subcutaneous fibrous nodules (onchocercomata), each containing one or more adult worms, vary from a few millimeters to about 3 cm in diameter and become fully developed within a year of exposure. In Africa, they tend to occur most commonly in the pelvic region, especially over the hips and on the buttocks, while in Latin America the head is more usually involved. Nodules do not generally give rise to much discomfort, but at times they may be painful, and secondary infection with abscess formation can occur. The number and size of nodules increases with intensity of infection.

Typical skin lesions (onchodermatitis) consist of an intensely itchy, papular dermatitis, with edema in the early stages, progressing to lichenification and atrophy ('lizard skin'). Large numbers of microfilariae are present in the skin, and involvement may be generalized or limited to one area of the body. Transient urticaria is often the only skin manifestation, and indeed the condition may be entirely asymptomatic despite the presence of microfilariae in the skin. General well-being is seldom disturbed.

Ocular lesions (river blindness), due to microfilariae penetrating the eyes, represent the most serious feature of onchocerciasis and are a frequent cause of blindness in endemic areas. They occur especially when the disease is present in the upper half of the body and are more common in South America. Children rarely show advanced ocular lesions, but hyperemia of the conjunctiva and nummular keratitis may be seen in older children. Any part of the eye can be involved.

Diagnosis

Diagnosis is best established by demonstrating microfilariae in skin snips and the adult worms on nodule biopsy. Serological tests, including tests for antigen, are also available in onchocerciasis but there may be some cross-reaction with other filarial species (e.g. *Mansonella ozzardi*) in areas where they coexist.[931] Microfilariae are not uncommonly found in urine.

Treatment

Microfilariae are killed by diethylcarbamazine, but the drug is no longer considered justified for the treatment of onchocerciasis due to the common and often severe adverse reactions that it causes. Ivermectin is now accepted as the treatment of choice for onchocerciasis at a single dose of 150–200 µg/kg for both adults and children.[913,932–934] As it kills only the microfilariae but not the adult worms, treatment is long term and may need to be repeated every 3–6 months for 2–3 years.[890,935,936] It has been found, however, that adding doxycycline (100 mg daily for 6 weeks) to the ivermectin regimen significantly enhances microfilarial suppression by sterilizing female worms through depletion of the symbiotic *Wolbachia* bacteria.[937,938] The use of ivermectin for mass treatment has given hope for the effective control of this disease. Suramin is lethal to the adult worms but it may cause severe adverse reactions. Excision of nodules, especially those near the eyes, is sometimes recommended prior to chemotherapy, because of the danger of ocular involvement. Regular urine tests should be made as the drug is nephrotoxic. Amocarzine and albendazole are also being evaluated for efficacy in the treatment of onchocerciasis.[896]

Vector control requires the simultaneous application of control measures (spraying with appropriate insecticides) over whole river systems.

Loa loa

Loa loa is transmitted by flies of the genus *Chrysops*, which are infected by sucking human blood containing microfilariae. These are present in blood during the daytime, thus corresponding with the diurnal biting habits of most *Chrysops*. The disease is endemic in western and central Africa. Adult worms are found migrating through subcutaneous tissues, the male being some 3 cm and the female 6 cm in length. They may remain viable for as long as 30 years.

Clinical features

Symptoms of loiasis are usually trivial. The most characteristic manifestation is a recurrent, painless, puffy, pink swelling, often referred to as a calabar, or fugitive, swelling. This lesion marks the journey of the adult worm in the subcutis. It develops over a period of 3–4 h and may acquire a diameter of 10 cm or more, before subsiding in a few days. The upper extremities and eyelids are most often involved and on occasions the thin worm may be seen rapidly traversing the bulbar conjunctiva and sometimes accompanied by periorbital edema. The appearance of the calabar swelling is frequently associated with fever and malaise. Eosinophilia is present.

Some patients remain afilaremic, no microfilariae being found in the peripheral blood despite intensive investigation.[939]

Treatment

Diethylcarbamazine is used in the treatment of loiasis but can cause severe adverse reactions in people with microfilarial counts > 2000 mf/ml blood.[940] It is usually recommended that the drug be given in slowly increasing doses.[913]

Day 1: 50 mg (child 1 mg/kg) after food;
Day 2: 50 mg (child 1 mg/kg) 8-hourly;
Day 3: 100 mg (child 1–2 mg/kg) 8-hourly;
Days 4–21: 3 mg/kg 8-hourly.

In afilaremic patients, side-effects can be controlled by steroids and/or antihistamines. In patients with large numbers of microfilariae in their blood, meningoencephalitis may result from lysis of dead microfilariae and thus in these patients benefits of treatment must be weighed against the danger of the side-effects. In these people, steroids and antihistamines may not be effective in preventing side-effects.

Ivermectin (200 µg/kg stat repeated every 6–12 months) has been recommended[890] while mebendazole and albendazole have also been tried.[939]

Wuchereria bancrofti and Brugia malayi

Infections by Wuchereria bancrofti, Brugia malayi and B. timori (termed 'lymphatic filariasis') occur in the tropics and in some semitropical areas, being transmitted by various species of mosquito. The adult female and male worms (some 85 mm and 40 mm in length respectively) attain maturity in the lymphatic system about 1 year following entry to the body, after which time the nocturnal periodic sheathed microfilariae are demonstrable in peripheral blood between 10 pm and 2 am. Some Pacific strains of W. bancrofti are nonperiodic.

Clinical features

First infection may occur in children but the full clinical picture may take many years to develop. As with other filarial diseases, the early phases may be entirely asymptomatic or associated with florid allergic manifestations. The commonest manifestations of the mature filariae are acute and recurring lymphangitis. The affected lymph node, together with its afferent vessel, usually in the groin, is painful and tender. The lymphatic vessel becomes palpable and cord-like and is associated with a linear red streak in the overlying skin. This stage is often accompanied by pyrexia, malaise, nausea and headache. Dreyer et al[941] believe that acute attacks of lymphatic filariasis can be divided into a number of clearly defined clinical syndromes. The acute attacks, which subside after several days, have a variable periodicity of weeks or months, gradually becoming less severe, often with persistence of residual subcutaneous swelling. Recurrent funiculitis may occur and involvement of intra-abdominal lymph nodes may give rise to the clinical picture of peritonitis. Chylous ascites, chyluria, varicose groin nodes, hydrocele and elephantiasis are classical end results but as they arise from chronicity over many years, emphasis on this aspect is out of place in a pediatric context. Nevertheless, early manifestations of chronic disease may sometimes appear in the late years of childhood.

Work by Hightower et al[942] has suggested that children born to mothers infected with W. bancrofti are more susceptible to this infection than those born to uninfected mothers.

Tropical eosinophilia syndrome. In some patients, an abnormal response to W. bancrofti infection results in a clinical picture which reflects a specific allergic sensitization to filarial antigens, a condition known as tropical pulmonary eosinophilia or tropical eosinophilia syndrome. These patients present with cough, asthma-like symptoms, respiratory distress and eosinophil counts of 3000/mm³ or greater. X-ray of the lungs usually shows extensive changes. These patients often do not develop filaremia, hence the term 'occult filariasis'.

A similar condition can be caused by infection with Brugia malayi and perhaps by infection with nonhuman filariae.

Diagnosis

The clinical diagnosis of lymphatic filariasis based on symptoms can now be greatly aided by ultrasonography and lymphoscintigraphy.

The recovery of typical sheathed microfilariae in midnight blood slides and occasionally in urine will establish the diagnosis. Concentration techniques may need to be used to recover microfilariae from the blood.

In the case of tropical pulmonary eosinophilia, diagnosis is made clinically and confirmed by serology or rapid response to diethylcarbamazine.[943]

It is worth noting that visitors to endemic areas who contract lymphatic filariasis often do not develop a microfilaremia, which can make parasitological confirmation of the infection impossible. Thus the development of an EIA test (TropBio, Australia) to detect circulating filarial antigen has provided a major breakthrough in the diagnosis of lymphatic filariasis, the test for W. bancrofti being highly specific and very sensitive. Antigen-detecting tests, including DNA detection from blood spots, have also been developed for B. malayi, show great promise and are very cost-effective.[944–946]

Treatment

Diethylcarbamazine rapidly removes circulating microfilariae but large doses are required to kill adult worms. The dosage regimen for children utilizes increasing doses as for loiasis.[883,885,913] There is often an acute exacerbation during therapy, for which antihistamines should be given. Ivermectin, which has significantly fewer side-effects than diethylcarbamazine, is also very effective in the treatment of lymphatic filariasis. It kills microfilariae but not adult worms and the single oral dose of 150–200 µg/kg should be repeated at yearly intervals. Albendazole and doxycycline are also mentioned as showing promise.[938]

A single oral dose of ivermectin has been recommended for controlling lymphatic filariasis al[934,947] and the use of yearly or 6-monthly doses of ivermectin or the regular use of salt fortified with diethylcarbamazine has proved invaluable in the control of this condition in endemic regions. The control of lymphatic filariasis is a public health problem which is neither easy nor straightforward.[948] Even small areas omitted from a general filariasis vector control program due to, for example, difficult terrain, have the potential to disperse the infection.[949] As Molyneaux[950] says: 'environment remains a key determinant in changing patterns of vector-borne infections. Changes are rapid and vectors have the capacity to change equally rapidly, a capacity not matched by health systems'. He believes less time will be spent in future on developing new pesticides for insect vector control, and that the emphasis will be on genetic approaches to make insects less effective vectors.

Mansonella perstans and Mansonella ozzardi

Mansonella perstans has had many recent changes in its name[951] and is widely distributed in those tropical and subtropical areas which favor the habitat of the vector. The unsheathed microfilariae are transmitted by Culicoides midges from person to person, and the adult worms develop in the mesentery, perinephric and retroperitoneal tissues where they may survive for many years (Table 28.44).

Clinical features

This form of filariasis is often held to be harmless, but symptoms can be associated with infection, particularly in people visiting from non-endemic regions. Infection with these helminths may result in lethargy, arthralgia, urticaria and headache. Less frequently calabar-like swellings around the eye ('bung eye'), and pericardial or pleural effusions occur. Among indigenous inhabitants of endemic areas *M. perstans* is often asymptomatic.

The period from exposure to the appearance of nonperiodic microfilariae in the blood is unknown.

Diethylcarbamazine is ineffective in treatment of mansonellosis,[890,940] but trichlorophone has been used with success. Albendazole (400 mg bd for 30 days), mebendazole (100 mg 12-hourly for 30 days)[913] or a combination of mebendazole and levamisole have all been reported as effective.[940] The judicious use of corticosteroids is valuable in severe cases. Ivermectin (150 μg/kg stat p.o.) is reported to be effective in the treatment of *M. ozzardi* but not *M. perstans*.[890,940]

In rain forest areas of Central Africa, a related species, *M. streptocerca*, infects humans. Microfilariae of this species are unsheathed and have a curled tail with nuclei extending to the tip. The adult and microfilariae of this species are found in skin, and diagnosis is by skin snips as for *Onchocerca*. Symptoms include dermatitis, with macules and papules. Infection is more common in older people than in children.

M. ozzardi in South America is a species with many clinical similarities to *M. perstans*. In the past it has been considered a commensal, but studies have suggested that this parasite may also not be as harmless as is often believed (Table 28.44).

Dirofilaria immitis

The dog heartworm is a common filarial nematode infecting dogs in most tropical regions of the world including parts of the USA and northern Australia. It is transmitted by mosquitoes.

Occasional human cases are diagnosed during serological surveys or on biopsy for investigations of pulmonary 'coin' lesions found on X-ray.[897] Cases of pleural effusion, intraocular infection and eosinophilic meningitis are also caused by *D. immitis* in humans. Most cases of dirofilariasis are recorded in adults, but clinical infections are seen at times in children and Hungerford[893] believes that dirofilariasis is much more common in Australia than is believed at present.

As *D. immitis* infection in humans does not usually exhibit a filaremia, diagnosis is usually made on biopsy of a lung lesion or on removal of a worm from the eye. Skin tests or serological tests are unhelpful.

Other species of *Dirofilaria* are also recorded from humans, usually from subcutaneous tissue or from the conjunctival sac.

CESTODES (TAPEWORMS)

The cestodes are platyhelminths, which are dorso-ventrally flattened, have no gut or body cavity and are hermaphroditic. Adult tapeworms have a characteristic morphology with a scolex armed with suckers and sometimes hooks, an unsegmented neck region and a long segmented strobila.

Life cycles are complex, with the adult tapeworms living in the gastrointestinal tract of the vertebrate definitive hosts and larval stages occurring in a range of vertebrate or invertebrate intermediate host species. Larval forms vary from the free-living, ciliated coracidium larva and worm-like procercoid and plerocercoid (sparganum) larvae of the pseudophyllidean tapeworms (e.g. *Diphyllobothrium latum*) to the cysticercoid, cysticercus (bladderworm) or hydatid larvae of the cyclophyllidean tapeworms.

Humans can become infected with a range of cestode species and mostly harbor the adult tapeworm although human infection with larval cestodes includes sparganosis (*Spirometra* sp.), cysticercosis (*Taenia solium*) and hydatidosis (*Echinococcus granulosus*).

The main cestodes relevant to humans are *Taenia saginata*, *Taenia solium*, *Hymenolepis nana*, *H. diminuta*, *Dipylidium caninum*, *Diphyllobothrium latum*, *Echinococcus granulosus*, *E. multilocularis* and *Inermicapsifer madagascariensis*.

TAENIASIS

Taeniasis is caused by infection with adult *T. saginata* or *T. solium* (Table 28.45). In both these infections, the adult tapeworm is found in the

Table 28.45 Characteristics of *Taenia saginata* and *Taenia solium*

	Taenia saginata	Taenia solium
Parasite		
Scolex	4 suckers only	Crown of hooklets and 4 suckers
Length	5–20 m	3–15 m
Lateral branches of uterus	15 or more	8–13
Intermediate host	Cattle	Pig, but occasionally man
Final host	Man	Man

intestinal tract of humans – the only definitive host. The intermediate hosts harboring the larval stage (cysticercus) of the tapeworm are cattle in *T. saginata* (the beef tapeworm) and usually pigs in *T. solium* (the pork tapeworm). However, in the case of *T. solium*, in addition to pigs, a wide range of mammals, including humans, can harbor the cysticerci.

It has been suggested that in the Asia-Pacific region, other, but as yet incompletely defined, species of *Taenia* may infect humans.[952,953] One such species found in Indonesia, Taiwan and Korea morphologically resembles *T. saginata* but is acquired from pork and has been named *T. asiatica*.[870,896]

Infection with adult *Taenia* results from ingestion of infected meat and, as such, is not common in very young children.

Taenia saginata (the beef tapeworm)

The beef tapeworm is cosmopolitan, occurring in almost all countries where beef is eaten. It is especially common where local eating habits favor the consumption of raw or undercooked beef. The cysticerci in the beef can even survive salting and a moderate degree of drying.

The adult worm is harbored in the human intestine, attached by its scolex to the mucosa of the small intestine. It may reach 20–25 m in length and gravid proglottids (or segments), their uteri packed with eggs, break from the strobila singly or in chains of 2–5 segments, and either migrate actively out of the anus or pass out passively with the feces.

These proglottids crawl about on the ground releasing eggs, which are also liberated when the proglottid dies and disintegrates on pasture land. Eggs lying on the grass are ingested by grazing cattle (Fig. 28.71). The oncosphere (hexacanth) larva is released in the intestine, penetrates the intestinal wall using its six hooklets and is carried via the bloodstream to the heart and voluntary muscles, especially the tongue, shoulder

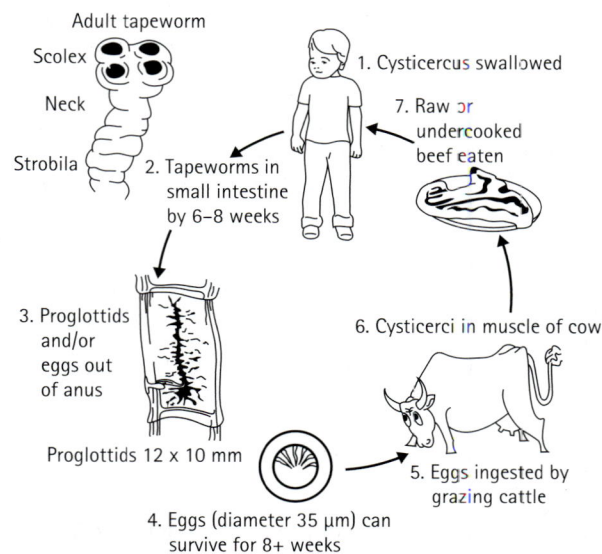

Fig. 28.71 Life cycle of *Taenia saginata*.

and masseter muscles. Here it loses its hooklets, develops an inverted scolex with suckers but no hooks and changes into a bladderworm (or cysticercus) larva, termed *Cysticercus bovis*, over about 3 months. These cysticerci are about 8 × 5 mm in size and meat infected with them is commonly termed 'measly' owing to its spotted appearance.

When ingested, the cysticercus evaginates the scolex and elongates into the adult stage. Humans eating such 'measly' beef raw or undercooked thus become infected with adult tapeworm. Gravid segments are shed about 3 months after infection.

Epidemics of 'measles' in cattle have not uncommonly resulted from cattle grazed on pastures fertilized with untreated effluent from sewage outlets. Such cattle become infectious about 3 months after ingestion of eggs.

Clinical features

In most cases infection with *T. saginata* is quite symptomless, the only feature being the intermittent passing of segments. In 5–50% of cases, eosinophilia may occur while abdominal pain, weight loss, malaise, an increase or decrease in appetite and such allergic features as urticaria and pruritus ani may be seen.

Adult tapeworms absorb digested food through their cuticles and thus they compete for food with the host and in this process food deprivation and digestive upset may occur.

Rarely, intestinal obstruction results and at times proglottids wander into the appendix and, impacting there, may cause obstructive appendicitis.

Diagnosis

Diagnosis is generally made when proglottids are seen in the stool. These can readily be identified by pressing them between two glass microslides and counting the number of uterine branches on each side of the central stem. In *T. saginata*, there are usually 15 or more primary uterine branches on each side.

In the cases where proglottids cannot be found, eggs (Fig. 28.72) may be detected in the feces or on anal tapes as used for *Enterobius*, a process which is more effective for recovery of *T. saginata* eggs than stool examination. Eggs of *T. saginata* and *T. solium* are identical.

Treatment

The treatment of choice for *T. saginata* infection is praziquantel as a single oral dose of 10–20 mg/kg.[883,884] Niclosamide is also effective, being usually given without purgation at a dose of 1 g (11–34 kg) or 1.5 g (34 kg and over), which should be chewed before swallowing.[883] The worm is passed in a partially digested state. Treatment can be followed, if desired, by a saline purge after 2 h.

Treated patients should be re-checked 3 months after treatment to assess cure. With modern anthelmintics it is not feasible to examine post-treatment stools for the scolex.

Prevention of *T. saginata* infection depends upon avoidance of consumption of raw or undercooked beef and hygienic disposal of human feces to prevent infection of cattle.[870] Freezing of meat (−10 °C for 10 days) is also reported to be effective in killing cysticerci.

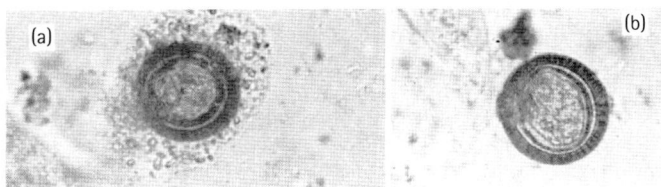

Taenia solium (the pork tapeworm)

T. solium is widely distributed, but less so than the beef tapeworm. It is common, however, in Africa, Asia, Latin America and parts of eastern Europe.

The life cycle of *T. solium* (Fig. 28.73) is similar to that of *T. saginata* but with some very important differences. In both species humans comprise the only definitive host and may harbor one or more tapeworms. In *T. solium* infections humans become infected with the adult tapeworm after eating raw or undercooked 'measly' pork containing cysticerci. The range of intermediate hosts of *T. solium* is wider than that of *T. saginata* and, besides pigs, can include the domestic dog. In fact, in areas where dogs form a significant part of human diet, they may serve as an important source of human *T. solium* infection. Humans too can become infected with cysticerci of *T. solium* (known as *Cysticercus cellulosae*) after ingestion of eggs, a condition termed cysticercosis.

The adult *T. solium* is, on average, a little shorter than *T. saginata*, reaching about 15 m in length. The scolex has both suckers and a double row of hooks. The cysticerci of both species are essentially similar, but again the invaginated scolex of *C. cellulosae* has hooks which are absent in *C. bovis*.

Clinical features

Taeniasis solium. Infection with the adult *T. solium* is much the same as with the adult *T. saginata* except that proglottids of the pork tapeworm are less mobile than those of the beef tapeworm and so such features as appendiceal blockage are more rare. Most cases are asymptomatic, but diarrhea and constipation have been recorded and a moderate eosinophilia may develop.

Cysticercosis. The greatest danger in infection with *T. solium* is the danger to others of infection with eggs via food or water (heteroinfection) and the danger to the patients themselves of autoinfection by external means (hand-to-mouth transfer of eggs) or internal means (vomiting up and re-swallowing of proglottids).

The clinical effects of cysticercosis are essentially dependent upon the number and sites of the cysticerci. Cysticerci can develop almost anywhere in the body: beneath the skin (subcutaneous cysticercosis); in the myocardium; in the muscles; within the eye or in the brain (cerebral cysticercosis or neurocysticercosis). If within the ventricles of the brain the cysticerci can become greatly enlarged resulting in a racemose cyst.

Usually cysticerci do not cause clinical symptoms until they die, swell and calcify – a process which occurs about 3 years or longer after infection. Whether or not they cause symptoms is also dependent upon their site. In the muscles, heart or beneath the skin they are relatively benign but within the eye they can cause retinal detachment, loss of vision and even blindness. If sited in the brain they may result

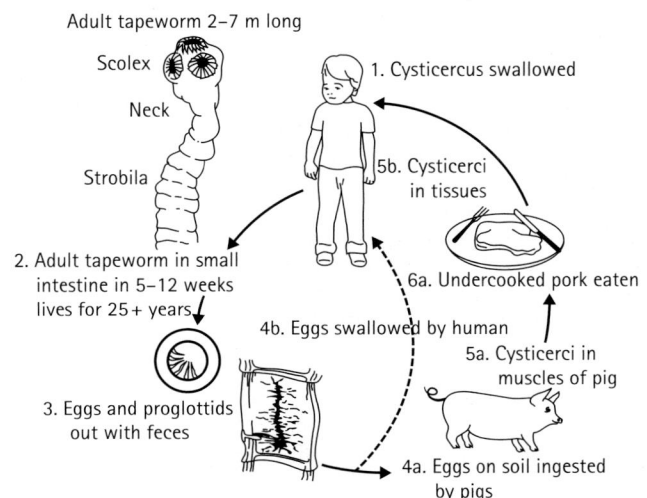

Fig. 28.72 Complete egg of *Taenia* sp., the embryophore being surrounded by the remains of the vitelline cell. (b) Other egg has lost all traces of the vitelline cell and consists only of the oncosphere larva surrounded by its thick, striated embryophore (approx. × 600).

Adult tapeworm 2–7 m long
Scolex
Neck
Strobila
1. Cysticercus swallowed
2. Adult tapeworm in small intestine in 5–12 weeks lives for 25+ years
3. Eggs and proglottids out with feces
4a. Eggs on soil ingested by pigs
4b. Eggs swallowed by human
5a. Cysticerci in muscles of pig
5b. Cysticerci in tissues
6a. Undercooked pork eaten

Fig. 28.73 Life cycle of *Taenia solium*.

in neurological disorders, personality changes or epileptic convulsions. Neurocysticercosis is a common cause of epilepsy among Africans in southern Africa and, although more common in adults, it has even been recorded in children as young as 3 years of age.[954] Death can follow hydrocephalus resulting from blockage of the ventricular spaces.

Diagnosis

Taeniasis solium. Diagnosis of infection with adult *T. solium* is established by the finding of eggs (indistinguishable from those of *T. saginata*) in feces (Fig. 28.72) or by the passing of typical gravid proglottids. The proglottids of *T. solium* have fewer than 13 lateral uterine branches on each side and so can be differentiated from those of *T. saginata* although some degree of overlap may occur. (Note: gloves must be worn when examining proglottids for counting of the uterine branches, as eggs of *T. solium* are infective to humans.)

Cysticercosis. Cysticercosis can be diagnosed by palpation and biopsy of cysticerci if accessible and their microscopic examination after squashing between two glass microslides or after histological sectioning.

In patients in whom cysticercosis is clinically suspected confirmation can sometimes be obtained by radiology, where calcified cysticerci are visible as millet seed-shaped shadows in the muscles or small spotted areas on skull X-ray (Fig. 28.74a,b). X-rays are also useful in differentiating cerebral cysticercosis from CNS infection due to *Angiostrongylus*, *Gnathostoma* and *Paragonimus*.[955]

Eosinophils can at times be found in the CSF of patients with cerebral cysticercosis. About 25% of patients with cerebral cysticercosis will be found to harbor adult *T. solium* in their intestines or have a history of such infection.

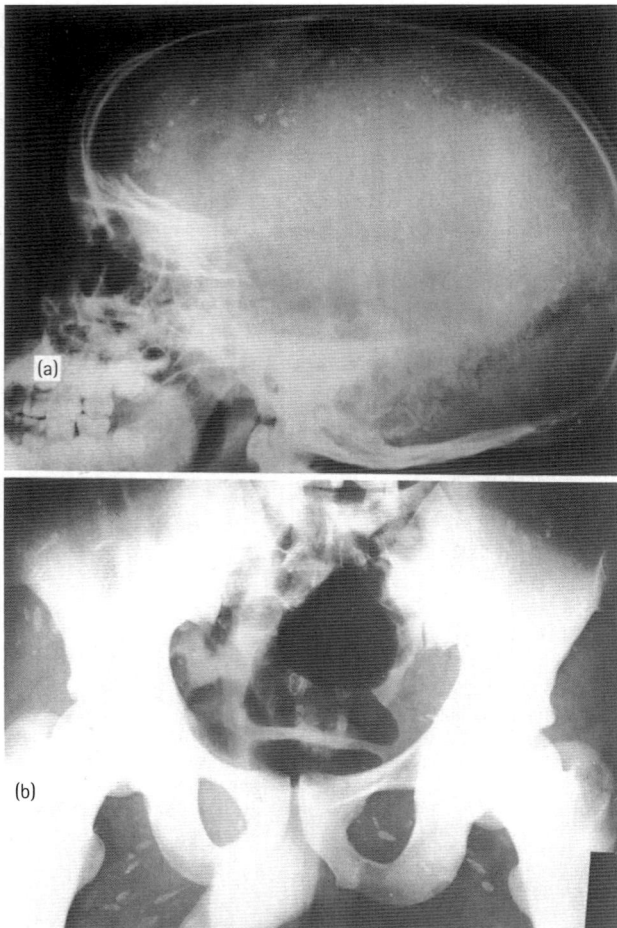

Fig. 28.74 (a) Cerebral cysticercosis. (b) Calcified cysticerci visible in the muscles in X-ray of pelvis.

Serological tests for blood or CSF are available for the diagnosis of cysticercosis.[955–957] In addition, tests have been developed to detect cysticercal antigen in CSF.

CT scans are of great value, not only for the diagnosis of cerebral cysticercosis, but also for an assessment of the length of infection and for post-treatment progress evaluation.[955,957,958]

Treatment

Treatment for *T. solium* is similar to that for *T. saginata*, with praziquantel or niclosamide being the drugs of choice.[913,959] Mepacrine, while effective, tends to cause nausea and vomiting and should thus be avoided because of the danger of regurgitation of proglottids into the stomach and re-swallowing them.

Cysticercosis. Albendazole (5 mg/kg 8-hourly for 8–15 days) is probably the treatment of choice for cysticercosis.[890] Although clinical studies have shown that praziquantel at a dose of 25–50 mg/kg/d in three divided doses for 14 days may be effective for the treatment of cysticercosis,[883,885,886,913,960] it is frequently associated with side-effects in neurocysticercosis and its use is not universally accepted in this situation.[883,961]

A number of authors have argued that the risks of cysticidal therapy in neurocysticercosis sometimes outweigh the benefits, and should be considered for each individual patient.[890,913,962] The simultaneous administration of steroids may help reduce inflammatory complications which can follow the death of the cysticerci after anthelmintic treatment.[896]

Surgical removal of cysticerci is seldom feasible, especially if the cysticerci are numerous and deep seated.

Anticonvulsants to control fits, steroids to control raised intracranial pressure and occasionally surgery to control hydrocephalus may be required for controlling the fits in neurocysticercosis.

Prevention of *T. solium* infection and cysticercosis is essentially the same as for *T. saginata*. Cysticerci can be destroyed during cooking by heating the meat to 50 °C.

Hymenolepis spp.

Two species of this genus of tapeworm infect humans, *Hymenolepis nana* (the dwarf tapeworm) and *H. diminuta* (the rat tapeworm). These are small tapeworms, reaching only 40 mm in length for *H. nana* and 40 cm in length for *H. diminuta*.

Hymenolepis nana

H. nana is harbored in the small intestine of the human (or sometimes rodent) host and the gravid proglottids disintegrate in the gut so that eggs pass out in the feces. When an egg is ingested by another person, it releases an oncosphere into the small intestine, and this burrows into a villus, forming a cysticercoid. It develops here before leaving the villus after about 14 days to grow into an adult tapeworm in the intestinal lumen (Fig. 28.75).

Because of its direct person-to-person mode of transmission, *H. nana* is a common tapeworm in resource limited countries and tends to be more common in children than in adults. In a survey in Zimbabwe, 18.7% of children were infected with *H. nana*, but only 3.8% of adults.[963]

Diagnosis is based on detecting characteristic *H. nana* eggs (Fig. 28.75). The treatment of choice is praziquantel or niclosamide as for taeniasis.[886,913] Praziquantel at a dose of 25 mg/kg has a cure rate of 98.5% and minimal side-effects.[964]

Hymenolepis diminuta

The rat tapeworm, *H. diminuta*, is common in many parts of the world in rats and mice. Its intermediate hosts are fleas and flour beetles. Children may become infected when they accidentally swallow the intermediate host – often with insect-infested meal or flour.

Diagnosis of *H. diminuta* infection is based on finding the eggs in feces. These eggs differ from those of *H. nana* in being larger, rounder, lemon yellow in color, and having a striated shell and no polar filaments.

Treatment is as for *H. nana*.

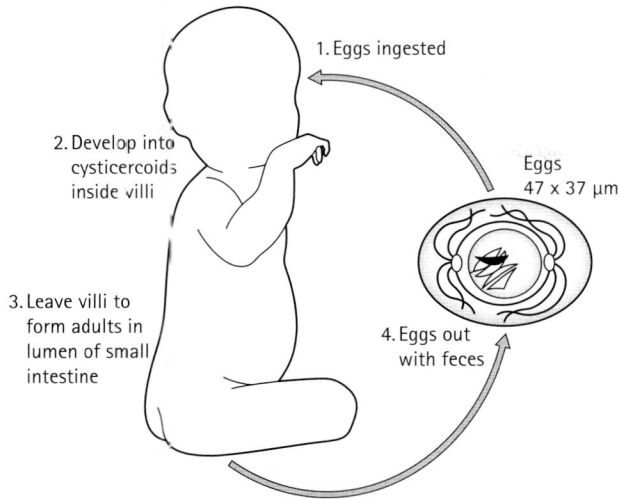

Fig. 28.75 Life cycle of *Hymenolepis nana*. Egg inset (approx. ×600).

Neither *H. nana* nor *H. diminuta* causes serious clinical effects, but abdominal pain, diarrhea, loss of appetite and eosinophilia may occur when loads are heavy. One problem with *H. nana* is a build-up of worm load as a result of external autoinfection by ingestion of eggs.

Dipylidium caninum

This tapeworm is worldwide, commonly infecting both dogs and cats. The intermediate hosts are fleas, such as the common dog and cat fleas (Fig. 28.76a), which contain the cysticercoids, and infection of the final host occurs when the flea is swallowed. Children can become infected when they accidentally swallow a flea or when they are licked on the mouth by a dog which has been 'fleaing' itself and has cysticercoids on the tongue.

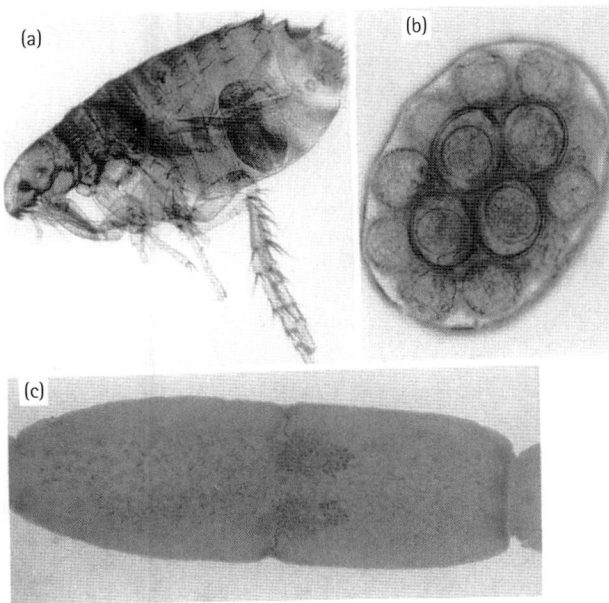

Fig. 28.76 (a) *Ctenocephalides* sp. – dog flea intermediate host of *Dipylidium caninum* (approx. ×50). (b) Egg capsule of *Dipylidium caninum* (approx ×600). (c) Stained gravid proglottid of *Dipylidium caninum*. Note characteristic double set of reproductive organs and twin genital pores (approx. ×20).

Dipylidium caninum is a relatively small tapeworm (20 cm long) and usually causes little discomfort, although at times diarrhea, fever, restlessness and even convulsions have been recorded.

Diagnosis is made when actively motile proglottids with two genital pores (Fig. 28.76c) are found by the mother on nappies or when typical egg capsules (Fig. 28.76b) are found in the feces on microscopic examination.

Niclosamide is reported to be effective in treatment although in some cases repeated treatments with this drug have failed.[965] The recommended drug of choice is praziquantel at a single dose of 5–10 mg/kg.[965]

Diphyllobothrium latum

The adult fish tapeworm can reach 20 m or more in length. It is a common tapeworm of a variety of fish-eating mammals, including dogs and cats, in Scandinavia, the Baltic, South America, the Great Lakes of North America, parts of the Middle and Far East and Indonesia, while occasional cases are encountered in other parts such as Labrador and Australia.[896,959]

The scolex of this species has sucking grooves, and eggs are shed from the gravid proglottids to pass out with the feces.

When the eggs fall into water, a ciliated coracidium larva develops and is released through the operculum into the water. This is ingested by the microscopic crustacean, *Cyclops*, in which a procercoid larva is formed. When the *Cyclops* is eaten by a fish, the procercoid changes into a plerocercoid (sparganum) larva in the muscles of the fish. Finally the life cycle is completed when the fish is eaten by the mammalian definitive host (Fig. 28.77), which may include humans.

Clinical effects of heavy worm loads include diarrhea, abdominal pain, generalized weakness[959] and occasionally intestinal obstruction. *D. latum* is also recorded as causing a megaloblastic (macrocytic) anemia in susceptible patients who have a genetic predisposition and who are on a diet deficient in vitamin B_{12}, by competition with the host for this vitamin – especially when the worm is attached high up in the small intestine. Eosinophilia is not usually a feature of infection.

Diagnosis is based on finding typical operculate eggs in the feces (Fig. 28.78). Proglottids in the feces can be recognized by their centrally situated uterus and genital pore.

The recommended treatment is praziquantel 2.5–10 mg/kg orally as a single dose for people >4 years old. Niclosamide 1 g orally as a single dose for children 11–3 kg is an alternative.[890,913] Whichever anthelmintic is used, concurrent vitamin B_{12} should also be given if the patient is anemic.

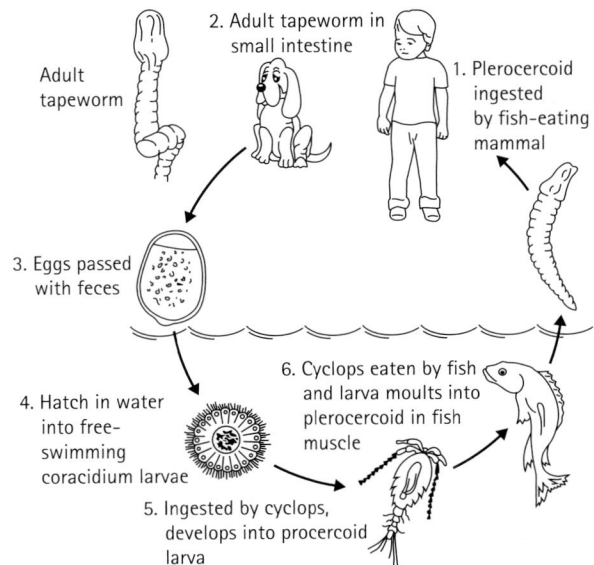

Fig. 28.77 Life cycle of *Diphyllobothrium latum*.

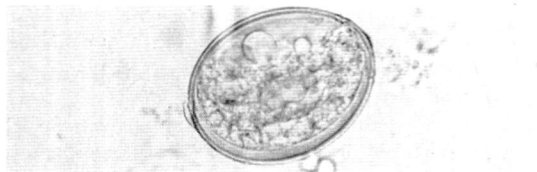

Fig. 28.78   Operculate egg of *Diphyllobothrium latum* (approx. × 600).

A common source of human infection is eating raw or smoked fish, so cooking fish is an important preventive measure.[870] Freezing fish (−10 °C for 15 min) is also effective in killing plerocercoids.

The plerocercoids of certain species belonging to the related genus, *Spirometra*, the adults of which inhabit the intestines of dogs, can infect humans and cause a condition called sparganosis. These elongated plerocercoid (sparganum) larvae can infect humans after ingestion of infected frogs or *Cyclops* with water (East Africa, North America) or by application of infected frog flesh to skin ulcers or eye wounds as poultices. Plerocercoids in the frog muscle migrate into the human flesh where they settle – a condition occurring in South East Asia.

These spargana can encyst in any tissues. Perhaps the commonest manifestations are nodules about 2 cm in size under the skin with painful surrounding edema. They can be detected radiologically as elongated shadows and can usually be removed surgically if accessible. One species of sparganum can bud and proliferate so spreading through the tissues.

ECHINOCOCCOSIS (HYDATID DISEASE)

Echinococcosis (hydatid disease) in humans is caused by the larval stage of *Echinococcus granulosus* and to a much lesser extent by *E. multilocularis*, *E. oligarthrus* or *E. vogeli*.

The life cycle of *E. granulosus* is shown in Figure 28.79. The small adult tapeworms (Fig. 28.80a) live in the intestine of the dog and related canids such as dingoes in Australia. After ingestion of the eggs by the intermediate hosts, which are usually sheep or sometimes cattle and in

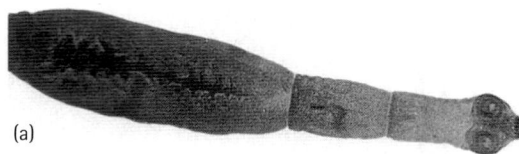

(a)

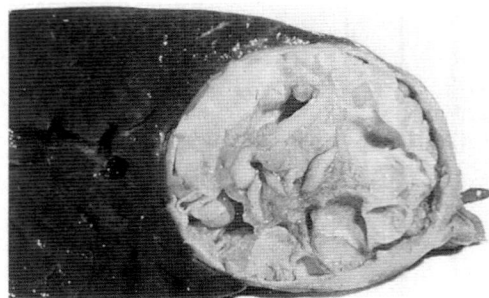

(b)

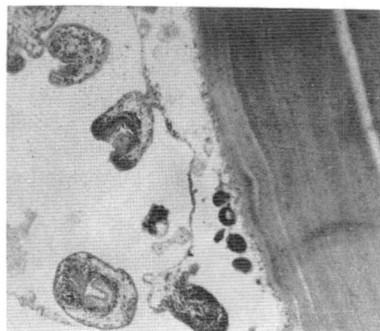

(c)

Fig. 28.80   (a) Adult *E. granulosus*. Note scolex and proglottids (approx. × 12). (b) Hydatid cyst in human liver. (c) Histological appearance of the wall of a pulmonary hydatid cyst.

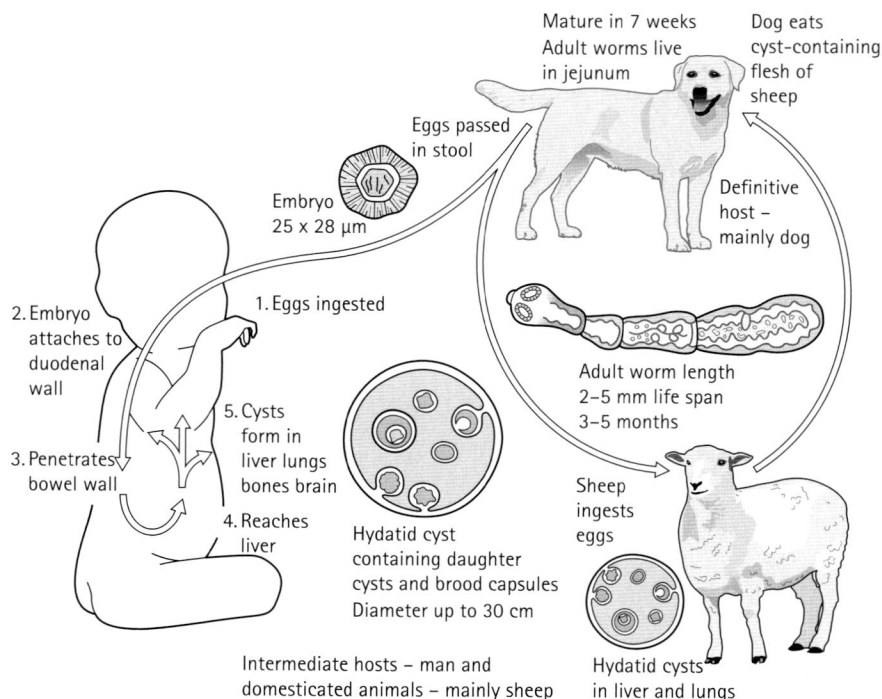

Fig. 28.79   Character and life cycle of *Echinococcus granulosus*.

Australia wallabies or other marsupials, the larval tapeworms develop into hydatid cysts in the viscera. Humans can also become infected when they ingest the tapeworm eggs, and children are particularly at risk because of their often intimate contact with dogs. They may pick up eggs contaminating the animal's coat or from the dog's tongue after being licked.

The infection is particularly common in rural sheep and cattle farming areas, especially where dogs are used for herding. It is widespread throughout Africa, Australasia, Asia, the Near East and South America and is also found in the Mediterranean, the USA and the UK.[871,966] *E. multilocularis* is widespread in the northern hemisphere, with human cases being common in parts of the former USSR, China, northern Japan, Alaska and central Europe, including possible spread into eastern Germany.[966-968] Cycles involving wild animals are also found in certain parts of the world.

In hydatidosis due to *E. multilocularis*, wolves, coyotes and foxes are the definitive hosts, and small field rodents serve as the natural intermediate hosts. Urban cycles involving the domestic cat and house mouse have been demonstrated.

The incidence of echinococcosis is decreasing in some areas owing to regular anthelmintic treatment of dogs and strict controls prohibiting the feeding of offal to dogs,[969] and global control has been mooted.[970]

Clinical features

Because development of cysts is slow, an infection acquired in childhood may only become clinically evident in adulthood, but manifestations of the disease in children are by no means uncommon.

The most frequent sites for cysts are the liver (Fig. 28.80b) and lungs (Fig. 28.80c). Spleen, peritoneum, kidneys, bone, orbital fossae, brain, heart and reproductive organs may also be invaded. In children, lung disease is reported to be the commonest form. Cysts sited in parenchymatous organs are large unilocular, well-circumscribed, fluid-filled structures in *E. granulosus* infections.

In bone, the parasite ramifies along bony canals, eroding bone and later involving the medullary cavity to form a large osseous cyst, which often results in spontaneous fracture. The much rarer *E. multilocularis* infection may produce complex, multilocular alveolar cysts with a gelatinous matrix and this alveolar hydatid disease has a 93% mortality within 10 years of diagnosis.[970]

Many cases of hydatid disease are silent. When symptoms occur they are usually those of a slow-growing tumor, with pressure on, or blockage to, the affected organ. Thus, recurrent pyrexia, paroxysmal cough, chest pain, hemoptysis and even expectoration of cyst fluid and membrane (should rupture occur into a bronchus) may occur as manifestations of pulmonary hydatidosis. Abdominal pain, vomiting, hepatomegaly and obstructive jaundice may indicate liver involvement. Intracranial localization can produce symptoms and signs indistinguishable from those of a tumor. Orbital cysts produce proptosis.

Sensitivity to cyst contents, resulting from slow leak of fluid, may develop with resulting allergic symptoms, notably urticaria. Severe anaphylaxis and even death can follow rupture of a cyst, while secondary metastatic cysts may develop in other parts of the body following such rupture.

Diagnosis

Diagnosis depends initially upon clinical awareness. A moderate eosinophilia is almost invariably present in childhood cases, except during febrile illnesses.

Often an X-ray provides the first indication of hydatid disease, especially in thoracic cases (Fig. 28.81). Ultrasound or CT scanning may be required to demonstrate the cystic nature of the lesion.[957] Serological tests may be helpful in confirming diagnosis. The historic Casoni skin test is no longer used because better serological tests are available, including the indirect hemagglutination test, a hydatid ELISA test and the improved immunoelectrophoresis, Arc 5 test and the double diffusion Arc 5 test.

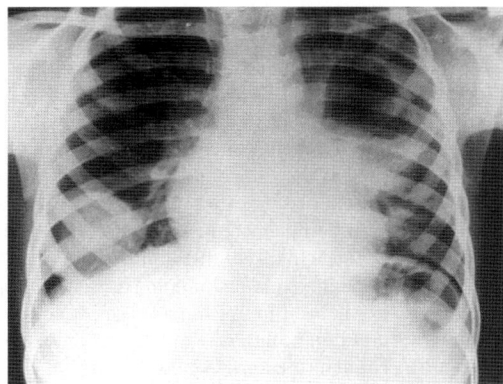

Fig. 28.81 Hydatid cysts in lung. Noncalcified cyst in right lung. Cyst in left lung has ruptured into a bronchus and contains fluid and air.

Pulmonary hydatids appear less serologically active than cysts in other parts of the body. After surgical removal of hydatid cysts, antibodies may be detectable in low titers for a while, but sooner or later disappear completely.

At times a cyst in the lung may rupture and diagnosis can then be made by finding hydatid sand or hooklets in the sputum. The latter are easily detected by using a standard Ziehl–Neelsen or auramine stain with UV microscopy, as they are intensely acid fast.

If hydatid cysts are suspected, diagnostic aspiration must *not* be attempted because of the danger of anaphylaxis and metastatic spread.

If children vomit what appear to be hydatid cysts, care should be taken to confirm their nature microscopically by the presence or absence of a germinal membrane (Fig. 28.80c), as gel cysts, closely resembling small hydatids, can easily mislead the unwary. These gel cysts may be vomited, by children up to 2 years, after ingestion of commercial fruit gels containing carrageenan.

Treatment

Treatment is surgical, if cysts are accessible, but due precautions must be observed to prevent release of hydatid fluid and to sterilize cysts prior to removal, using a scolicidal agent. Shorey et al[890] have summarized an approach to the treatment of uncomplicated hepatic hydatids using *p*uncture; *a*spiration of cyst contents; *i*ntroduction of a scolicidal agent such as alcohol or hypertonic saline; *r*e-aspiration of the solution – termed PAIR therapy.

Results of chemotherapy for hydatid cysts using mebendazole have been disappointing, but albendazole can be used as an adjunct to surgery or for the treatment of inoperable hydatids at a dose of 400 mg bd for 28 days, repeated as necessary or as 15 mg/kg/d in 2 doses (max 800 mg) for 28 days and repeated as necessary.[913,965] Albendazole can also be used in the treatment of infection with *E. multilocularis*, but treatment of multilocular hydatidosis remains largely surgical drainage.[958]

Prevention

While highly successful control programs have resulted in decreases in the prevalence of hydatid disease in Tasmania and New Zealand, elsewhere the disease remains common and may even be spreading.[871,966,970]

Dogs should not be allowed access to offal, to limit canine infection, and their regular treatment with an effective teniafuge such as praziquantel is indicated. In endemic areas this de-worming should be carried out every 2 months.

ANOPLOCEPHALID TAPEWORMS

This group of cestodes includes *I. madagascariensis*, *Raillietina* spp. (tapeworms of rodents with various arthropod intermediate hosts probably involved) and *Bertiella studeri* (a monkey cestode). Human infection with *I. madagascariensis* is particularly common in southern Africa but it has been sporadically reported also from a number of other tropical and sub-tropical areas. Outside Africa, the parasite seems to have dispensed with a need for a rodent reservoir.

These cestodes may reach 42 cm in length and their small, actively motile proglottids are shed in the stool and have the appearance of rice grains; they contain characteristic parenchymatous egg capsules.

I. madagascariensis most frequently involves children between the ages of 1 and 5 years, and while the infection is usually asymptomatic, anorexia, asthenia, anemia and abdominal pain have occasionally been attributed to it. It has been found to be the most common tapeworm affecting white children in Zimbabwe and more cases in African children are coming to light as awareness increases.[971,972]

Niclosamide is the treatment of choice for *I. madagascariensis*, one tablet (0.5 g) repeated in 1 h, while niclosamide or praziquantel is recommended for *Bertiella studeri*.[972]

TREMATODES (FLUKES)

Trematodes are parasitic helminths belonging to the class Platyhelminthes (flat worms). Trematodes are dorsoventrally flattened worms which have a gut, no body cavity and possess an oral and a ventral sucker. Most are hermaphrodite, except the schistosomes. The flukes have a complex life cycle involving various species of aquatic snail as intermediate hosts. Trematodes infecting humans include blood flukes (*Schistosoma*), liver flukes (*Fasciola, Clonorchis, Opisthorchis*), intestinal flukes (*Fasciolopsis, Heterophyes, Metagonimus*) and lung flukes (*Paragonimus*).

BLOOD FLUKE INFECTION (SCHISTOSOMIASIS OR BILHARZIASIS)

Schistosomiasis has been increasing as a hazard to humans through the construction of dams and the movement of human populations.

Adult blood flukes live in the veins of the final host. There are three main species which infect humans: *Schistosoma japonicum*, *S. mansoni* and *S. haematobium*[973] (Table 28.46). *S. japonicum* is a zoonotic species which frequents the superior mesenteric veins of humans and causes a more virulent and rapidly progressive illness than the other species, involving mainly the small and large intestine and liver. Adult *S. mansoni* worms live in the inferior mesenteric veins with resultant damage to the colon and liver while *S. haematobium* is found in the veins of the vesical plexus of humans, the disease thus predominantly affecting the urinary tract.

Other blood flukes less commonly recorded in humans include *S. intercalatum* (Central and West Africa), *S. mekongi* (Viet Nam), *S. malayensis* (Malaysia), *S. bovis* (in North Africa and Iraq) and *S. mattheei* (in southern Africa). The latter two are zoonotic species of cattle and sheep.

The life cycle of the human blood flukes is shown in Figure 28.82.

Pathogenesis and clinical features

Humans are usually infected by direct penetration of the cercariae through intact skin. The pathological changes in schistosomiasis are produced by cercariae, schistosomulae, adult worms and eggs – by their physical presence, by virtue of metabolic products or from the body's immune response to the infection. The severity of the disease depends primarily upon the number of parasites that can gain entry to the body and mature.

Despite the wealth of knowledge that has accumulated regarding the pathophysiology of schistosomiasis, the extent of ill health and mortality caused by this disease is still debatable.[974]

While large sections of a population may harbor the parasites, many individuals come to terms with the disease and suffer virtually no morbidity, owing to an interplay of factors such as immunological tolerance, worm load and rate of reinfection. The role of protective immunity in schistosomiasis continues to be a subject of debate.[975] Increased prevalence and intensity of infection in childhood lend credence at least to

Table 28.46 Geographical distribution of schistosomiasis (After Warren & Mahmoud 1975[973])

Species	Distribution				
	Africa	Middle East	Asia	South America	Caribbean
S. mansoni	Egypt Libya Sudan South of the Sahara Malagasy Republic	Yemen* Aden* Saudi Arabia*		Brazil Surinam Venezuela	Puerto Rico Dominican Republic* Guadeloupe Martinique St Lucia
S. japonicum			Malaysia* [1] China Japan Philippines Sulawesi* Thailand* Laos* [2] Kampuchea*[2] Vietnam[2] India[†]		
S. haematobium	Widespread including Malagasy Republic and Mauritius[†]	Lebanon Iran* Turkey Iraq Jordan Yemen Israel Saudi Arabia			

*Very small focal areas.
[†]Focal distribution.
[‡]Limited foci have been reported in Portugal in the past.
[1]Species known as *S. malayensis*.
[2]Species known as *S. mekongi*.

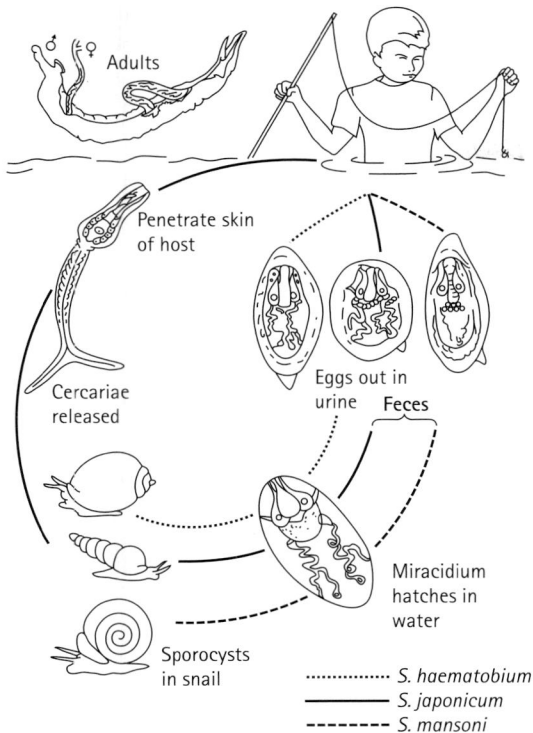

Fig. 28.82 Life cycle of schistosomes.

some protective immunity playing a part.[976] The immunity involved in schistosomiasis is complex,[975] being described as concomitant immunity, whereby the adult worms are not affected by the host's immune response to the infection, but newly invading cercariae are destroyed.[977–980]

The later stages of schistosomiasis generally take many years to develop so that the spectrum of clinical disease in children is narrowed. Nevertheless, such late manifestations as portal hypertension, calcification of the bladder and even vesical carcinoma are by no means rare in adolescents living in hyperendemic areas. A further difference in the disease as it affects children compared with adults is related to the caliber of blood vessels. Because of the smaller and more tenuous venous plexuses and collaterals, schistosomes are less able to migrate to sites far removed from their normal habitat in children than in older persons. The relative lack of immunity in young patients renders them more liable to severe systemic disturbance during the early stages of the disease. Determinants of infection in human communities are varied and involved.[981]

Clinical features can be related to the phase of parasitic invasion, and symptomatology is generally, but not always, proportionate to worm load. The pathogenesis of schistosomiasis is complex but it is essentially an immunological disease.[982–985]

Penetration of cercariae
At the time of penetration, within a few hours to a few days of exposure, a dermatitis termed swimmer's, or Kabure, itch may develop and last for 2–3 days. The condition is more common in non-indigenous inhabitants. It can also be caused by avian or mammalian schistosomes in countries where human schistosomiasis is unknown. For example it is quite common in Australia where it is sometimes termed 'pelican itch' and in the USA where it is known as 'seabather's eruption'. These latter cercariae, however, die while attempting to penetrate the skin. A prickly sensation is followed by intense itching and an urticarial, papular or occasionally vesicular rash appears, lasting from a few hours to several days.

Migratory/toxemic stage: the Katayama syndrome
Having passed through the skin, the cercariae lose their tails and the resulting schistosomulae enter the lymphatics, pass to the veins and travel to the heart and hence to the lungs to circulate freely in the systemic circulation. Many die, but those that gain access to the portal system reach the liver where they mature into adult male and female worms. Rarely, worms mature in other ectopic sites such as veins of the brain and spinal cord. Coupling takes place in the liver and the male transports the female against the flow of blood to their sites of predilection where egg laying begins. The prepatent period in schistosomiasis (i.e. from infection to egg laying) is normally about 5–9 weeks.

During the migratory stage of the life cycle with a crescendo just prior to egg laying, the patient may develop an illness known as the Katayama syndrome due to antigenic challenge by the parasitic metabolites in the non-immune host. Malaise, pyrexia, liver tenderness and splenomegaly occur. Eosinophilia is constant. Urticaria, joint and muscle pains, cough, abdominal discomfort and diarrhea may also occur. Encephalopathy, myocarditis and anaphylactoid purpura are reported complications.[896]

Katayama syndrome is most common in S. japonicum infections, but can also occur when a previously uninfected individual is exposed to a heavy invasion by S. mansoni cercariae.

Early egg laying stage
Many eggs laid by female worms in the submucosal venules of the intestine or bladder pass through the tissues and are discharged in the feces (S. japonicum and S. mansoni) or urine (S. haematobium). This early egg laying stage may be associated with dysenteric symptoms or with dysuria, frequency and terminal hematuria.

Late egg laying stage – pathology of chronic schistosomiasis
Initially eggs pass through the tissues relatively easily but as infection progresses, marked tissue reaction occurs, eggs can no longer pass through the tissues so readily, and many are swept back by the flow of blood to be deposited elsewhere.

The morbidity of chronic schistosomiasis is mainly related to the presence of eggs,[985] which initially stimulate a granulomatous reaction characterized by a pseudotubercle, rich in eosinophils. This is followed by degeneration and calcification of the eggs with much reactive fibrosis. The principal pathological effects are as follows.

Genitourinary system. S. haematobium is the principal cause. The early bladder lesions usually occur on the trigone where deposition of phosphates round the egg deposits imparts a velvety appearance termed 'sandy patches'. Subsequent mucosal proliferation may produce multiple papillomata before ulceration, calcification (Fig. 28.83) and fibrosis lead to diminished bladder capacity. A similar process may involve the ureters, especially at their lower ends, leading to ureteric stricture and consequent hydronephrosis. This complication can also occur from vesical reflux

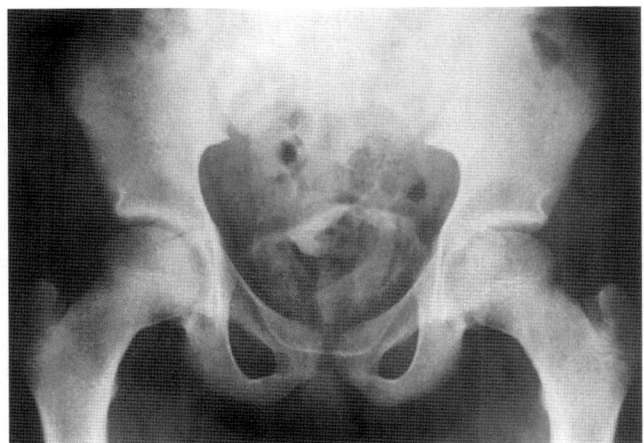

Fig. 28.83 X-ray showing bladder calcification due to schistosomiasis in a 10-year-old girl.

in the absence of overt ureteric involvement. Vesical or ureteric calculi may occur. An important long term complication is the predisposition of the bladder affected by schistosomiasis to develop carcinoma, usually of squamous cell type. The pathogenesis of bladder carcinoma in *S. haematobium* infection is complex and has still not been fully elucidated. While most common in adults, it is recognized to occur in adolescents. Genital lesions are usually diagnosed after puberty. These include epididymo-orchitis (often with associated secondary hydrocele), salpingo-oophoritis and chronic cervicitis. Large schistosomal granulomata (bilharziomas) consisting of masses of eggs enveloped in granulation tissue may involve the skin of the perineum and vulva. The lesions have a warty papillomatous appearance and when situated at the urethral meatus such a lesion is indistinguishable from a caruncle. Cutaneous schistosomiasis may rarely involve other parts of the body, and bilharzial granuloma of the conjunctiva has even been described in children.

An extended bacteremia with *Salmonella typhi* or *S. paratyphi* can occur, including a prolonged urinary carrier state, in concurrent *S. haematobium* infections.

Bacteriuria is generally considered to be more common in patients with *S. haematobium* than in uninfected controls.

Intestinal tract. Involvement of small bowel is usually only seen in *S. japonicum* infection but schistosomiasis of the colon may be due to both *S. japonicum* and *S. mansoni*. Eggs of *S. haematobium* may also be encountered in rectal snips taken from the lower part of the rectum. Mucosal involvement of the bowel gives rise to a similar appearance to that seen in the bladder with a velvety roughening of the mucosa. This may be associated with dysentery in the early egg laying phase of the disease, especially with *S. japonicum* infection. Gross lesions of the bowel are rare, but on occasions papillomata, granulomata, ulcers, stricture and fistulae occur. The appendix is frequently involved and signs of chronic appendicitis are common, although acute obstructive appendicitis consequent upon fibrosis is a rare complication.

Liver. Hepatic fibrosis may result from the presence of eggs of *S. mansoni* or *S. japonicum* with formation of granulomata and healing by fibrosis leading to thick tracts of periportal fibrous tissue traversing the liver in different directions. This 'pipe stem' fibrosis (Symmers' liver) gives the surface of the liver an irregular bosselated contour due to tethering of the capsule. In the later stage, eggs are scanty and may even be absent from biopsy material, in which the essential features are of preserved liver architecture associated with gross thickening of the portal tracts by collagenized bands of fibrous tissue. Kupffer cells usually contain schistosomal pigment. Liver involvement can lead to portal hypertension with ascites and splenomegaly, which is occasionally massive ('Egyptian splenomegaly'). Anemia is frequent and may be due to chronic hemorrhage from varices or to associated 'hypersplenism'. There is usually only mild impairment of liver function and thus the results of portal systemic shunting procedures usually give good results in selected cases. Splenectomy combined with lienorenal anastomosis is a helpful procedure if there is associated hypersplenism.

A relationship has been postulated between schistosome infection and carcinoma of the liver.

Cardiopulmonary systems. Lung involvement is usually the result of pulmonary embolization by eggs of *S. haematobium*. Though generally rare, it is reported with some frequency from Egypt. Two forms of lung disease occur:

1. a bronchopulmonary form, characterized by parenchymal egg granulomata: chronic bronchitis and bronchiectasis may result;
2. a cardiovascular form, due to occlusion of pulmonary arterioles by obliterative endarteritis, resulting in Ayerza's syndrome with cor pulmonale.

Nervous system. Eggs may lodge in any part of the CNS, generally seeded there by gravid females ectopically situated in nearby veins. Migrating schistosomulae may also be arrested in the nervous system if treatment is administered during the early migratory phase of the disease. However, neurological complications are unusual in schistosomiasis, cerebral involvement being best known with *S. japonicum* and spinal cord lesions with *S. mansoni* and *S. haematobium*.

Neuroschistosomiasis may well be more common than is currently recognized and is probably underdiagnosed according to Hughes and Biggs.[957]

It has been claimed that school performance can be adversely affected by chronic schistosomiasis.

In patients infected with *S. mansoni*, glomerulonephritis has been reported due to the deposition of immune complexes (IgM and IgG) in the kidney.

Laboratory diagnosis

Confirmation of the diagnosis of active schistosomiasis can only be obtained by finding typical viable eggs (Fig. 28.84a,b,c). Eggs can be recovered by examination of urinary deposit (*S. haematobium*) or from stool (all other species) by direct smear (including a Kato smear), sedimentation or water centrifugation.[986] Flotation techniques are not satisfactory and formol ether concentration kills the eggs with the result that no report can be made on egg viability as judged by miracidial activity or flame cell activity. Confirmation of viability of the egg is important to differentiate active disease from past infection.

Egg recovery is not easy and as many as 20% of infected persons may not pass eggs. Repeated examination of stool and urine specimens, the latter collected at midday, is essential. If urine or stools fail to reveal

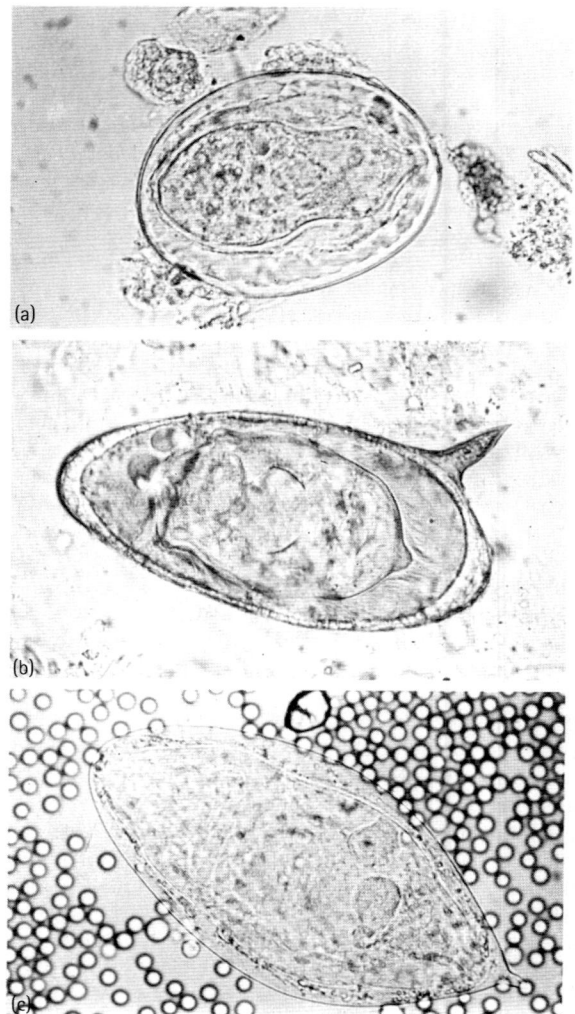

Fig. 28.84 (a) Egg of *Schistosoma japonicum* (approx. × 600). (b) Egg of *Schistosoma mansoni* (approx. × 600). (c) Egg of *Schistosoma haematobium* (approx. × 1000).

eggs, a rectal snip may prove rewarding in *S. japonicum*, *S. mansoni* and *S. haematobium* infections. In fact a single rectal snip gives more positives than three urines and stools. Cystoscopy may be indicated where urinary symptoms are present, the cystoscopic picture depending on the worm load.

A type I response skin test and various serological tests are available. These may be negative in early disease and positive results may indicate present or past infection, so a positive result is not, in itself, an indication for treatment. However, these tests often provide good negative screens to exclude a diagnosis of schistosomiasis and are particularly useful in screening returned travelers from endemic regions.

Treatment

The treatment of choice for all forms of schistosomiasis, and the only effective and safe treatment for *S. japonicum* infections, is praziquantel.[886,987-989] This drug is designated as a 'WHO essential agent', being extremely safe and highly effective when given as a single dose of 40 mg/kg (can be divided into two doses) for *S. haematobium* and *S. mansoni*[913,965,988,989] and at a dose of 60 mg/kg divided into three doses and given in a single day for *S. japonicum*.[884,885,965,990]

Of the other treatments available for schistosomiasis, metrifonate, an organophosphorus compound, appears to be less effective for treatment in cases of infection with *S. haematobium* than praziquantel.[989] It is not used for other species of schistosome. The dose used for children is 7.5 mg/kg per fortnight for a total of three doses.[885] Although side-effects are minimal, some have been recorded. The drug does depress cholinesterase levels and caution is needed in cases where patients may require some form of surgery necessitating the use of the muscle relaxant, suxamethonium. Oxamniquine is only effective against *S. mansoni* infections. The dose regimen is 10–20 mg/kg given as a single or divided doses over 1–2 days after food.[883,885,913,965,988,990] High cure rates and few side-effects are recorded.[886] This drug is useful for treating children orally at a rate of 20 mg/kg/d in 2 doses for 1 day.[913] Antischistosomal drugs such as the antimonials, niridazole and hycanthone have been superseded by the newer, more effective and safer compounds.

Prevention

As reinfection often follows successful treatment,[989] the control of schistosomiasis remains a priority. However, control is complex and generally employs a two-pronged attack on the life cycle of the fluke. The first is aimed at eliminating the snail population. Planned water systems for irrigation, which give a flow rate too high for survival of snails, are an ideal, but not always feasible method. Nontoxic molluscicides such as Frescon or Bayluscide have been found effective.

The experimental introduction of snail-eating predators and parasites has not had any lasting effect.

The second approach to control is aimed at preventing pollution of waterways by human excreta and involves public health education combined with provision of adequate and effective toilet facilities. In some control projects, mass treatment of infected humans has been used in conjunction with snail control. However, these aspects of prevention are ineffective in the case of *S. japonicum* which is extensively propagated by rodents. In *S. japonicum*, cercariae can be prevented from penetrating the skin by using topical applications of niclosamide or niclosamide-impregnated leggings.

Mass de-worming, repeated chemotherapy and the provision of safe water supplies through pump systems have all been proposed for the control of schistosomiasis.[991]

By 1988, schistosome vaccines were entering phase 1 trials[992] and research continues into the development of vaccines and chemoprophylaxis. The results to date appear to be encouraging, but there are concerns about the application of vaccine programs.[993-996]

OTHER TREMATODES

The life cycles of these flukes involve a variety of snail hosts with infective metacercariae settling on plants or aquatic invertebrates or vertebrates[870] (Table 28.47).

Liver fluke infection

The main trematode infections of the liver are fascioliasis, caused by the cattle and sheep liver flukes *Fasciola hepatica* (temperate regions) and *F. gigantica* (tropical Africa, Asia and Hawaii); clonorchiasis caused by *Clonorchis* (*Opisthorchis*) *sinensis* in the Far East; and opisthorchiasis, caused by *Opisthorchis felineus* in parts of Europe and Asia or *O. viverrini* in Thailand.

Clinical features

Infection with these flukes results when the metacercariae are ingested with aquatic plants (*Fasciola*) such as watercress to which the encysted metacercariae are attached, or in undercooked fish (*Clonorchis*, *Opisthorchis*).[870]

Symptoms of liver fluke infection depend largely upon the worm load and mild infections are often asymptomatic. Heavier infections tend to produce a triphasic response with an initial phase of invasion being accompanied by irregular fever and eosinophilia. Diarrhea and urticaria are common and there may be tender hepatomegaly. This phase lasts for about 4 weeks and is followed by an asymptomatic latent period

Table 28.47 Life cycles of intestinal and lung flukes

	Fascioliasis	Clonorchiasis	Opisthorchiasis	Fasciolopsiasis	Paragonimiasis
Adult fluke ↓	30 × 10 mm F. hepatica F. gigantica Liver	15 × 5 mm Cl. sinensis Liver	9 × 5 mm O. felineus O. viverrini Liver	50 × 15 mm F. buski Small intestine	12 × 6 mm Paragonimus spp. Lung
Egg ↓	Feces	Feces	Feces	Feces	Sputum/feces
Miracidium ↓	Free-swimming ↓	Ingested by snail ↓	Ingested by snail ↓	Free-swimming ↓	Free-swimming ↓
Snail ↓					
Cercariae ↓					
Metacercaria ↓	Water plants	Freshwater fish	Freshwater fish	Water plants (water chestnut)	Crabs and crayfish
Definitive host	Plant eater: sheep, cow human	Fish eater: dog, cat, pig, human	Fish eater: dog, human, seals	Water chestnut eater: pig, human	Crab/crayfish eater: dog, cat, human

usually lasting several months before the stage of obstructive jaundice occurs. Rarely the parasites of *F. hepatica* may settle in ectopic sites such as the pharynx after eating raw liver and mature there with resulting local reaction. Pharyngeal fascioliasis is known in the Middle East as *halzoun*. Individual worms may migrate into the liver parenchyma resulting in liver abscess formation. Eosinophilia is often present and the ESR is usually raised.

In Thailand, cholangiocarcinoma has been found to be associated with infection by *O. viverrini*.[997]

Local prevalences are often dependent upon social customs and dietary habits, and epidemic outbreaks of fascioliasis have been recorded.[997,998]

Diagnosis

The diagnosis is usually based upon the finding of typical operculate eggs in the feces (Fig. 28.85) although in some infected patients stools are consistently negative for eggs. The finding of eggs of *Fasciola* in the feces must be regarded with caution, as persons eating infected cattle or sheep liver can pass 'transit eggs' and this condition of spurious infection or false fascioliasis must be distinguished from true fascioliasis by the examination of repeat stool specimens.[928]

Treatment

On the whole, treatment of liver fluke infection remains unsatisfactory. For fascioliasis, treatment now consists of triclabendazole 12 mg/kg orally once daily for 1–2 days.[890,913,916] Bithionol 50 mg/kg orally in divided doses on alternate days for 2–3 weeks has been used,[965] and chloroquine, dehydroemetine and praziquantel have also been tried. Drug treatment of choice for clonorchiasis and opisthorchiasis is praziquantel 25–75 mg/kg/d in 3 doses for 1–2 days with albendazole (10 mg/kg for 7 d) as an alternative.[890,913,965]

Intestinal fluke infections

Many species of fluke infect the human intestinal tract[870,999] including the large intestinal fluke *Fasciolopsis buski* in parts of South East Asia, the small intestinal fluke *Heterophyes heterophyes*, in the Nile Delta and Far East, *Metagonimus yokogawai* in the Far East and eastern Europe and *Brachylaima* sp. in Australia.[1000]

Infection with these flukes results from ingesting metacercariae with aquatic vegetation (*F. buski*), with raw or undercooked fish (*H. heterophyes* and *M. yokogawai*) or by snail ingestion (*Brachylaima*). As in the case of liver fluke infection, a local high prevalence may be caused by local eating habits.[870,998]

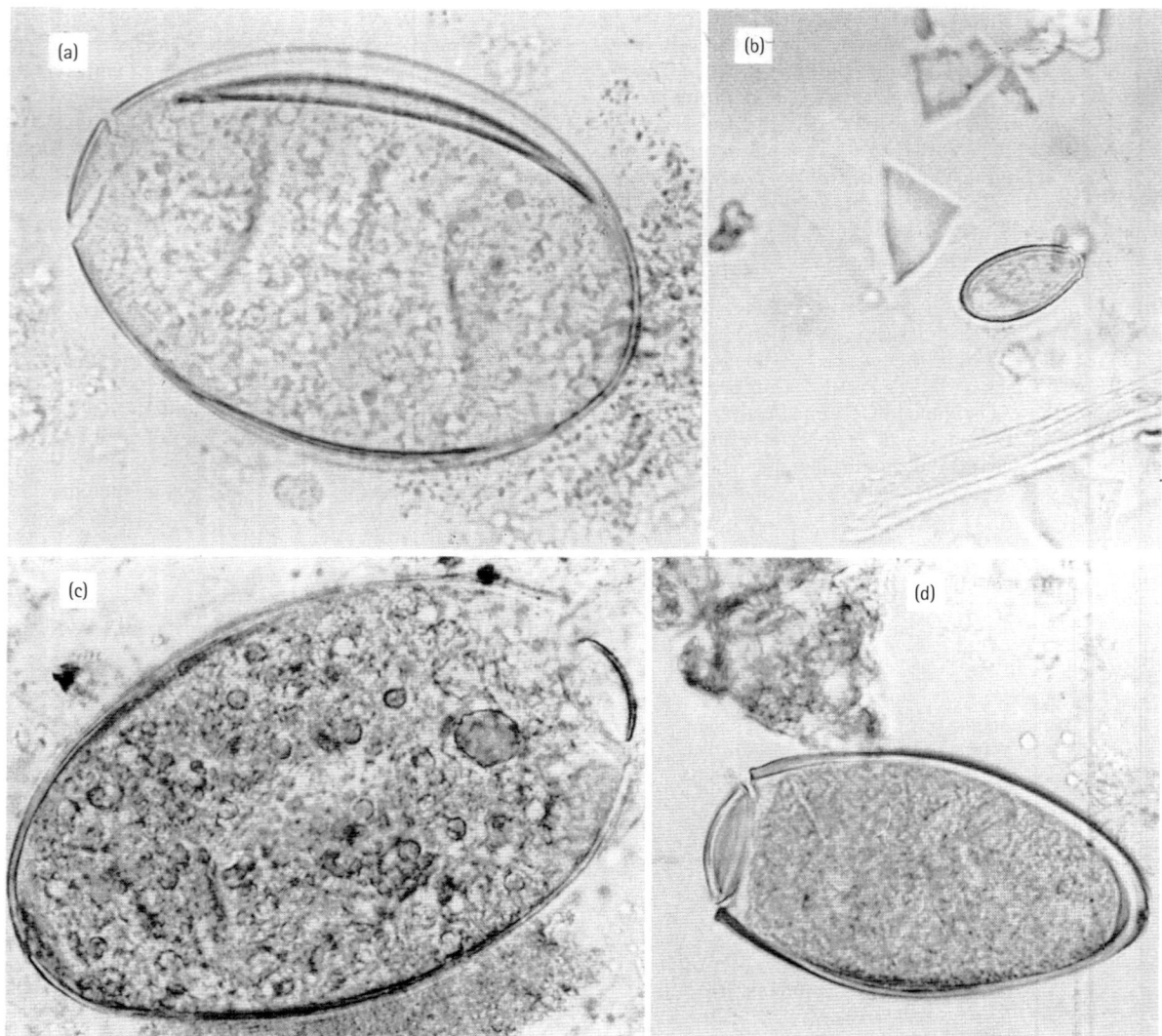

Fig. 28.85 Eggs of (a) *Fasciola hepatica* – ruptured to demonstrate operculum (approx. × 600); (b) *Opisthorchis sinensis* (approx. × 600); (c) *Fasciolopsis buski* – ruptured to demonstrate operculum (approx. × 600); (d) *Paragonimus westermani* (approx. × 600).

Symptoms of intestinal fluke infection may vary from a mild inflammatory reaction at the site of worm attachment in the small intestine to ulceration or abscess formation in the bowel wall, associated with severe bloody diarrhea.

Infections due to *F. buski* may result in vague abdominal symptoms, ascites and edema, probably as a result of protein-losing enteropathy and toxaemia.[999] An eosinophilia may be present, and iron deficiency anemia is common in fasciolopsiasis.

Diagnosis
As with liver fluke infection, diagnosis is made by finding typical operculate eggs in the feces of infected patients (Fig. 28.85).

Treatment
Intestinal fluke infections due to *F. buski*, *Heterophyes heterophyes* and *Metagonimus yokogawai* in children can be treated with praziquantel in a dose of 75 mg/kg in three doses for 1 day.[883,885,913,965] Niclosamide has also been used to treat intestinal fluke infections, while tetrachlorethylene has been described as an effective and cheap anthelmintic.[886,896]

Lung fluke infection
Human lung fluke infection is caused by 11 species of the genus *Paragonimus*. In the Far East, South East Asia and the Philippines, the species involved is *P. westermani* while in central and west Africa (and probably South Africa) the species is *P. africanus* or *P. uterobilateralis*. In the western hemisphere, *P. mexicanus* and *P. kellicotti* are the more common species.[896]

Infection occurs with the ingestion of the metacercariae in crabs and crayfish. Again local high prevalences are largely dependent upon dietary habits and culinary practices of preparing and cooking the crustacean intermediate hosts.[870,998] However, an interesting epidemic is on record which resulted from the use of crab juice as an antipyretic for children suffering from measles.

Symptoms of lung fluke infection are often suggestive of pulmonary tuberculosis, which may also often be present concurrently. The onset is insidious with cough and chest pain. Hemoptysis is usual, with copious blood-tinged sputum containing many eggs. Bronchiectasis and pulmonary fibrosis are late results, and finger clubbing is often present. An eosinophilia may occur and variable symptoms may result from flukes developing in ectopic sites, e.g. transverse myelitis and skin ulceration. In a small percentage of patients with paragonimiasis, the adult worms may settle in the CNS resulting in epilepsy, hemiplegia, visual impairment or an eosinophilic meningitis.[957]

Diagnosis
The diagnosis of paragonimiasis is established by finding the characteristic asymmetrical operculate eggs in sputum or feces (Fig. 28.85). X-rays, CT scans and serology may all prove useful.

Treatment
The drugs of choice are bithionol (or Bitin) at a dose of 30–40 mg/kg in divided doses given orally every other day for 10–15 days, or the newer derivative of bithionol, Bitin-S, given at a dosage regimen of 10–20 mg/kg every other day for 10–15 days. Praziquantel is very effective at a dose of 75 mg/kg/d in three doses for 2 days[883,885,886,913,965] and may be used in conjunction with corticosteroids if there is CNS involvement.[890]

Side-effects include diarrhea, nausea, vomiting and abdominal pain, but these are mild and soon subside.

ACANTHOCEPHALA
This group of helminths, the thorny-headed worms, are intestinal parasites of rats throughout the world. They are characterized by a proboscis covered with rows of recurved hooklets and have as their intermediate hosts insects such as cockroaches. The only species recorded from humans are *Moniliformis moniliformis* and *Macracanthorhynchus hirudinaceus*.

Humans, especially children, are occasionally infected after accidental ingestion of the intermediate host.[874] The worms live in the small intestine and diagnosis is made by passing adult worms or finding eggs in the feces. Spurious transit eggs can be passed by humans after eating of rodents as food.

Pyrantel pamoate and tiabendazole appear to be ineffectual, and mebendazole (Vermox) is the drug of choice, at a dose of 100 mg (one tablet) twice a day for 3 days.

FLIES, FLEAS, MITES AND LICE

MYIASIS

Myiasis is the infection by fly maggots of tissues of living animals, including humans. The larvae of a number of fly species may penetrate the skin of children or enter wound tissue.[1001] While the maggots of some myiasis-causing fly species only feed on dead and necrotic tissue (and even today are sometimes used in the medical treatment of wounds), the maggots of species such as the screw worm flies (*Callitroga americana* in the New World and *Chrysomyia bezziana* in the Old World) can be dangerous, as they extend their activities from necrotic to healthy tissue around the wounds.

Various clinical forms of myiasis are recognized: cutaneous (including wound infection), gastrointestinal, ocular, aural and urogenital. The clinical relevance varies according to the site and the species of fly involved, but infection of the sinuses and nasal cavities may be the most dangerous.[1002]

The tumbu, or putsi fly, *Cordylobia anthropophaga*, is found in tropical and subtropical Africa, and recently in Northern Europe.[1003] The large pale brown tumbu deposits her eggs on shady soil contaminated with urine, or damp clothing, where they hatch to release larvae in about 3 days. Laundry placed out to dry is an ideal site for oviposition, especially if laid out on grass or on the ground, so thorough ironing of clothes is desirable in endemic areas. The larvae penetrate intact skin where they grow rapidly, and unless removed, abandon the host and drop onto the ground in about 8 days to pupate.

Cutaneous lesions, which may be single or multiple, can occur on any part of the skin, particularly the waist, back (Fig. 28.86a) and feet. The characteristic lesion is a tender, large, furuncular swelling with a dark, central pore (Fig. 28.86b). Following application of petroleum jelly, the pore widens revealing movement of the posterior spiracles. The larva, about 0.5–1.0 cm in length, may then be squeezed out or grasped with forceps and extracted. Secondary infection of these lesions is rare.

In South America, the eggs and larvae of the tropical warble fly *Dermatobia hominis* may be transferred to the human skin by flies, mosquitoes or ticks and produce similar papular lesions.

Cutaneous myiasis is being increasingly recognized as an imported infection in many nontropical areas.[1003]

In areas of the world where sheep are farmed, the sheep nasal bot fly, *Oestrus ovis*, has been at times recorded as causing ophthalmomyiasis, a self-limiting but extremely painful condition.

Other larvae (e.g. those of *Gasterophilus*) may produce itching skin lesions related to the wanderings of the larvae, or tender short-lived subcutaneous cystic swellings. *G. intestinalis* can cause intestinal myiasis.

Maggots of some fly species tend to infest neglected wounds with excess necrotic tissue, even in hospital situations, and can be controlled by adequate wound toilet.

Myiasis may occur rarely in mucous membrane-lined orifices such as the mouth, anus and vagina, and in the eye. One species, *Auchmeromyia luteola*, lives in cracks and crevices of floors in Africa, coming out at night to suck blood from the sleeping human host.

TUNGIASIS

Tungiasis is infection with the jigger (or chigoe) flea, *Tunga penetrans*, originally endemic to South America, but now also endemic in central Africa and parts of India.

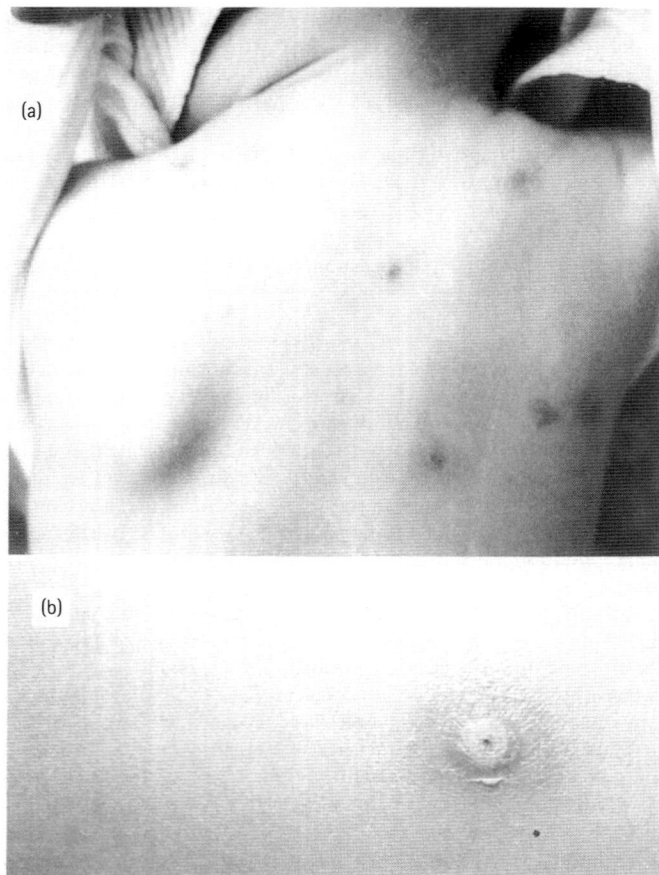

Fig. 28.86 (a) Child with multiple putsi lesions on back. (b) Lesion due to *Cordylobia anthropophaga* on leg to show characteristic appearance.

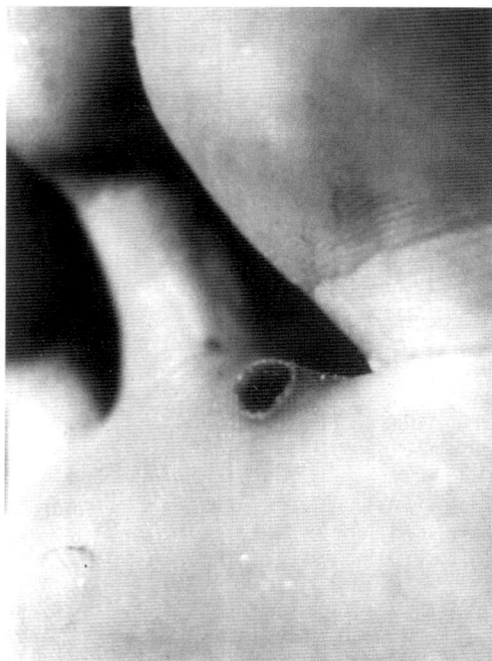

Fig. 28.87 Lesion due to jigger flea (*Tunga penetrans*). (Courtesy of Dr K. Ott)

The adult fleas live in soil or in the dust and cracks of earth floors of houses. After mating, the female flea penetrates the skin of the host (rodents, dogs, cats or humans) and develops in the epidermis under the stratum corneum, her abdomen swelling tremendously with developing eggs. The initial small lesion becomes inflamed and erythematous, developing into a pustule which may crust over or even form a suppurating ulcer if secondarily infected by bacteria. Lesions mostly occur on the feet, especially under the toenails or between the toes (Fig. 28.87). Itching, pain and even regional lymphadenopathy are common.

Eggs are expelled by the female flea, fall to the ground and form free-living larvae and pupae in the soil.

Diagnosis is made by finding the flea in the lesion and carefully removing it. In unsuspected cases, diagnosis may be made after biopsy of the lesion and finding the fragmented flea in the lesion.

Treatment consists of a careful removal of the flea, without rupturing it, using a sterile needle, followed by a cleaning of the wound with chloroform and a careful curetting of the affected area.

Jiggers are a potential source of tetanus in unimmunized children.

DEMODICIDOSIS

The hair follicle mite, *Demodex folliculorum* (Fig. 28.88), is one of the commonest parasites of the human skin, with infection rates of 25% or higher.

Human infection is probably acquired by direct person-to-person contact, often at a very young age (e.g. suckling babies infected from their mother). Human infection with other species of *Demodex* from animals has not been ruled out.

The mites live in the pilosebaceous glands and hair follicles especially of the face, scalp, external ear and breast. They are common in the eyelids and mites can often be found clinging to removed eyelashes.

Clinically the condition may be asymptomatic or infected hair follicles may result in the formation of 'blackheads' with crops of red papules appearing on the forehead. In heavy infestations, or in sensitized patients, dermatitis may follow, with scaling of the skin. Demodicidosis may be associated with HIV infection, causing an acute papulo-nodular rash, usually localized to the head and neck.[1004]

Diagnosis is established by finding the mites, often in sero-purulent fluid expressed from the lesions, or in biopsied specimens of skin in which mites can be found.

Treatment consists of good hygiene, soap and water together with sulfur ointment or gamma-benzene hexachloride if necessary.

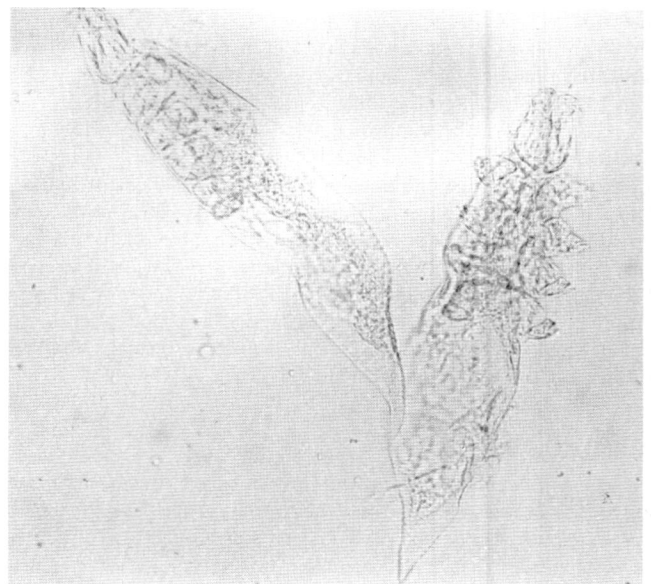

Fig. 28.88 *Demodex folliculorum* (approx. × 300).

SCABIES (see Ch. 30)

Scabies is a disease caused by the mite *Sarcoptes scabiei* (Fig. 28.89b). It occurs worldwide, especially in areas of crowding and in countries with a low standard of living. Scabies appears to sweep the world in cyclical pandemics.[1003,1005] It can afflict both rich and poor alike, and is more common in women and children.[1006] Most cases of human scabies are contracted from other infected humans, but occasionally animal strains of the scabies mite can infect humans.[1002]

The gravid female mites burrow into the horny layers of the skin, forming tunnels (Fig. 28.89c) in which the eggs are laid. The female mite lives for about one month, laying 2–3 eggs daily, which hatch in 3–4 days into six-legged larvae. These migrate to the surface and then burrow into the skin again and moult into eight-legged nymphs before becoming adults about 10 days after hatching. On average, each patient is infested with only 10–12 mites at any one time and much of the observed symptomatology is due to sensitization of the host to the mite and its products.[1007,1008]

CLINICAL FEATURES

Although the main sites infested can vary with the age of the patient, the commonest sites found to harbor mites include the hands (especially the sides of the fingers and the interdigital spaces), the finger webs, the wrists, the elbows, the feet, the penis and the scrotum, the buttocks and the axillae, with a lesser involvement of the body. The head and face is spared in most cases, except in infants.[1006,1009]

The feeding activities of the mites and host sensitization result in itching and the development of an extensive rash, which does not correlate with the predilection sites of the mites (Fig. 28.89a).

The characteristic lesions of scabies are the burrows in the skin, but there may also be pruritic papules, vesicles and pustules. Often there is eczematization and crusting of the lesions, especially when they are secondarily infected by bacteria. Scabies lesions can provide an entry site for infection with Group A beta hemolytic streptococci and thus glomerulonephritis may follow scabies.[1009]

Scabies may present in variable forms.[1006] In some healthy persons and in patients on corticosteroids, scabies may present with minimal signs and symptoms. In young children, vesicles rather than tunnels are often the rule, while in some patients the disease occurs in the nodular form. In mentally handicapped patients, debilitated patients and the immunosuppressed, extensive crusted or 'Norwegian scabies' is sometimes seen and in HIV infected individuals scabies can be particularly severe and persistent. In such cases the infestation is highly contagious and large numbers of mites can be found.

A common feature of scabies is the characteristic nocturnal itching, especially when the patient is warm in bed.

The infestation is transmitted by direct contact, including sexual contact. Fomites such as clothing and blankets generally play no part in the transmission of scabies.

DIAGNOSIS

Scabies is usually diagnosed clinically and should be considered in any patient presenting with an itchy rash covering the whole body but sparing the head and face.[1008,1010] In infants, scabies may present in an atypical form which can involve the face.[1006] Confirmation by the finding of mites is often difficult, even extensive lesions being associated with very few mites. Mites or their fecal pellets can sometimes be found in the tunnels after careful removal of the horny layers of skin. An improved method of obtaining mites is to scrape a suspect lesion and then float the mite out using mineral oil.

TREATMENT

The treatment of scabies involves the widespread application of topical preparations. Permethrin 5% cream or benzyl benzoate 25% emulsion are the treatments of choice.[1006,1008–1010] Full strength benzyl benzoate can cause an unpleasant stinging, so for children and sensitive adults it should be used diluted to half strength and in children under 2 years should be diluted with 3 parts water. Monosulfiram and crotamiton are possibly less effective, but the latter is said to have some antipruritic activity. Gamma-benzene hexachloride 1% has in the past proved to be cheap and effective,[1009] but is toxic if ingested. It should not be used in premature babies and should be used with care in pregnancy and in infants under 1 year of age.[1011] Children younger than 2 months can be treated with 5% sulfur cream daily for 2–3 days.[884,1006]

Resistance to both lindane and the pyrethroids (including permethrin) has been recorded and it may be difficult to distinguish resistance from incomplete treatment.[1009]

For adequate treatment and control, *all members of the family must be treated whether or not they exhibit symptoms*, or relapses and treatment failure will result.[1006] In conditions of overcrowding and poor hygiene, the regular use of monosulfiram soap prevents reinfection.

For mild scabies a single treatment should suffice but moderate or severe scabies might require re-treatment after 14 days. Symptoms may persist due to sensitization to treatment, and some patients have a 'parasitophobia' and see imaginary parasites; in these cases over-treatment must be avoided.

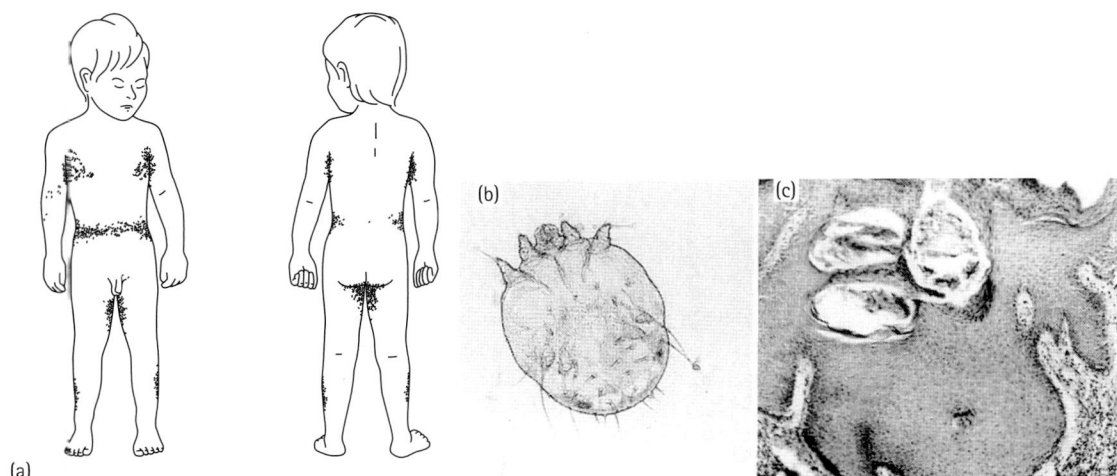

Fig. 28.89 (a) The distribution of the rash in scabies. (b) Adult *Sarcoptes scabiei* (approx. × 100). (c) Histological section of skin in scabies showing tunnels (approx. × 300).

Giving a child a hot bath before treatment for scabies commences is unnecessary.

Many animal parasitic mites (e.g. *Dermanyssus* and *Ornithonyssus* from rodents or birds and mange and cheyletid mites from dogs and cats) as well as many free-living and nonparasitic mites can attack humans and cause an extensive rash with a severe dermatitis and an itchy allergic reaction resulting in the formation of papules, vesicles and skin blotches. This condition can be very distressing and infestation usually derives from pets, animals nesting in roofs, straw and other packing materials.[1012]

The use of oral ivermectin (200 µg/kg orally as one dose for children > 5 years together with scabicides)[884,1006] may be required for the treatment of crusted scabies; toxicity can be a problem.[1008,1009] One review[1013] found no difference in clinical cure rates between crotamiton and lindane or benzyl benzoate and sulfur and concluded 'the evidence that permethrin is more effective than lindane is inconsistent. Lindane, permethrin and ivermectin appear to be associated with rare but serious drug reactions'. More research is needed on the safety and effectiveness of ivermectin and malathion compared to permethrin, on community management, and on different regimens and vehicles for topical treatment.

LOUSE INFESTATION

Humans can become infested with three types of lice: the head louse (*Pediculus humanus capitis*; Fig. 28.90); its morphologically identical, but behaviorally different variant, the body louse (*P. h. corporis*); and the crab or pubic louse, which forms a distinct species, *Pthirus pubis*. All three types are confined to humans worldwide and tend to be more prevalent in areas with poor living standards.[1014]

PEDICULUS HUMANUS CAPITIS (THE HEAD LOUSE)

P. h. capitis is worldwide in distribution. Its incidence is subject to unpredictable increases and decreases, with sporadic extensive pandemics. The prevalence varies from country to country and from year to year but may reach 60% or more of schoolchildren.[1007,1014]

Head lice tend to be confined to the scalp but are occasionally found on other hairy parts of the body. The insects live close to the scalp and feed on blood which they obtain with their sucking mouthparts. After mating, the female louse lays 6–8 eggs every 24 h. These eggs or 'nits' (Fig. 28.91) are glued tightly to the hairs close to the scalp and hatch in about 7 days into nymphs, which feed and pass through three instars before becoming adult in 10–11 days.[1014]

Head louse infestation is usually asymptomatic but heavy infestations may be manifested by scalp pruritus and, with secondary bacterial infection, by cervical gland enlargement.

Pediculosis capitis is found in people of all ages but is most common in children aged 3–13 years, and maximal at 6–9 years. Although not

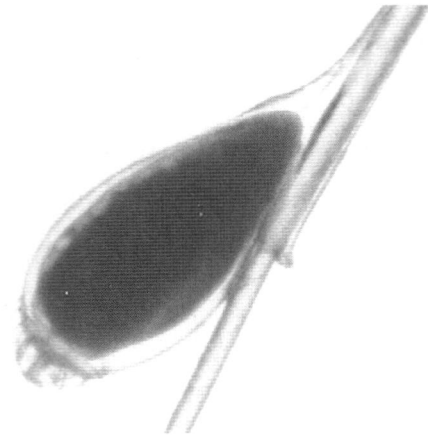

Fig. 28.91 Egg of crab louse (*Pthirus. pubis*) attached to hair (approx. × 60).

directly correlated to hair length, head lice are more common in girls than in boys. Both rich and poor alike are afflicted, but infestation is more frequent in low socioeconomic areas.

Diagnosis of pediculosis capitis is based on careful examination of the scalp for lice or their eggs. This is greatly facilitated using a hand lens. A more effective method for diagnosis involves treating dry hair with white conditioner, combing it with a fine tooth 'nit' comb, and examining the comb or, better still, the combings spread on a sheet of paper for nits.[1015,1016]

Head lice can only be controlled by regular inspection and treatment of infected cases *and all their family members*, whether or not lice or nits can be found in the latter. Dead nits remain tightly attached to the hairs and may have to be combed out with special fine toothed 'nit combs'.

In the past, DDT has been used for treatment, but its toxicity and resistance in the lice led to its replacement by gamma-benzene hexachloride (gamma BHC, gamma HCH; lindane). However, resistance is being recorded to HCH and this, plus its toxicity, has resulted in its being considered obsolete in many parts of the world.[1007,1017,1018] It is being replaced by safer preparations such as carbaryl, malathion and the synthetic pyrethroids such as permethrin. Of these, malathion (a 0.5% preparation in a spirit base) is the most widely used. It is twice as safe as HCH and has the added but variable advantage of possibly being residual for at least a month, through bonding to the hair. Additionally, malathion and carbaryl are reported to be ovicidal killing both lice and nits, a feature absent in HCH which is not ovicidal. However, the concept of an inherent ovicidal efficacy for malathion and carbaryl has been challenged.[1019] Repeat treatments after a week or so might be advisable, irrespective of the insecticide used. Pyrethrins, especially those in a mousse formulation, may also be effectively used to treat head lice,[1014] with the third generation synthetic pyrethroids such as permethrin proving the most promising.[1017,1018] Permethrin, synergized pyrethrum and malathion are all effective in head louse treatment and the choice between them really depends on local resistance patterns.[1020] All these preparations are toxic to some extent and care should thus be exercised in their use, with particular care being taken to avoid accidental ingestion or contact with eyes. Shampoos and lotions are both available, but lotions are far superior.[1014,1021,1022] Developing resistance to head louse preparations may prove a problem, albeit a sometimes controversial one.[1014,1020,1023] Ivermectin may be considered for the treatment of more difficult cases.[1024]

The use of levamisole for pediculosis, although considered to be safe and economical by some,[1025] does not really seem a practical alternative to the more conventional methods of head louse control.

An alternative, non-insecticidal approach to the treatment of head lice involves applying hair conditioner to wet hair, then combing the hair thoroughly using a fine toothed comb to remove the lice and their eggs, a technique known as 'bug-busting' in the UK.

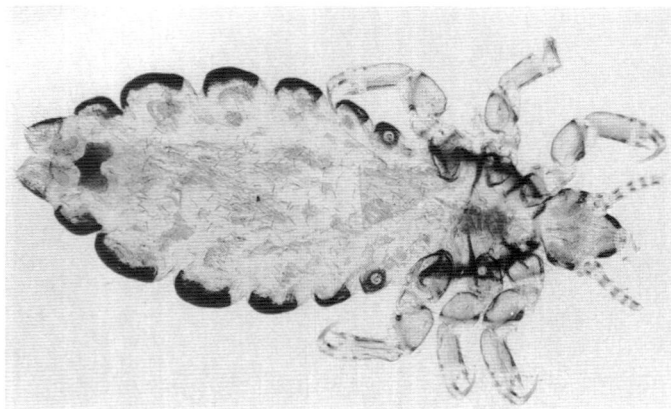

Fig. 28.90 Photomicrograph of adult *Pediculus humanus capitis* – the head louse (approx. × 50).

This does need dedication to ensure that the process is effectively carried out and results of its efficacy compared to insecticidal treatment vary.[1026-1028]

In the control of head lice, sterilization of clothing, bedding, combs, etc., is unnecessary, as insecticide treatment of the hair will provide sufficient protection from re-invasion by the short-lived lice that have strayed from the head.

In community control programs, education and involvement of all participants, parents, education and health professionals, as well as hairdressers, is necessary, and anti-louse preparations should be changed on a regular basis to prevent the emergence of resistance.

PEDICULUS HUMANUS CORPORIS (THE BODY LOUSE)

P. h. corporis is identical to the head louse in appearance, but differs in that it lives on the clothing and only visits the skin to suck blood. The eggs are glued to the clothing, especially the seams, and hatch in about one week to nymphs, which like those of the head louse, develop into adults in 7–10 days.

Pediculosis corporis may be characterized by the presence of feeding punctures appearing as small papules which, in sensitized patients, may become swollen, pigmented and hardened, a condition formerly known as vagabond's disease or *morbus errorum*.

Body lice are more limited to areas of overcrowding and poorer standards of living but may reach epidemic proportions during periods of social upheaval and unrest such as war, earthquakes and floods. They are the vectors of epidemic typhus (*Rickettsia prowazekii*) and epidemic relapsing fever (*Borrelia recurrentis*).

Transmission of body lice is directly from person to person and from shared clothing and blankets. Control is with 0.5% malathion lotion or 5% carbaryl dust and treatment of clothing, blankets, etc., with methyl bromide fumigation. washing in hot water at 60 °C or higher by heating in a domestic tumble drier for at least 5 min.

PTHIRUS PUBIS (THE CRAB OR PUBIC LOUSE)

Pth. pubis has a distinctive appearance and is usually found in the pubic region of humans only. It may also be found tightly attached to the hairs of the leg, the axilla or the beard (Fig. 28.92). Eggs are laid attached to hairs or even eyelashes (Fig. 28.93). It is usually transmitted during sexual intercourse and because of this, it is mostly found infesting

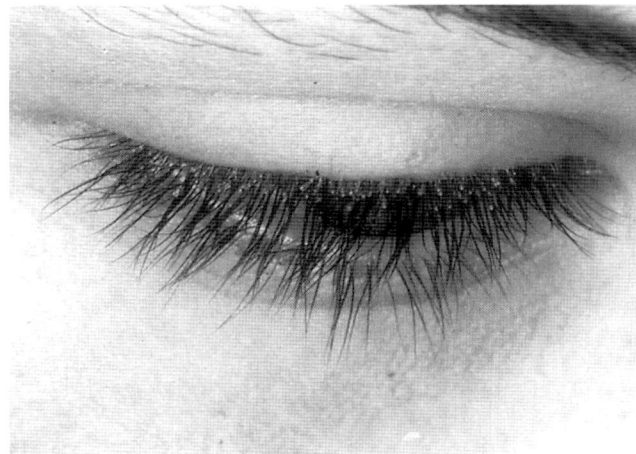

Fig. 28.93 Eggs of pubic louse on eyelashes.

adults. However, children can harbor the lice and even young children may become infected from heavily infested parents through close nonsexual contact. Thus, toddlers are at times found to have phthiriasis, the lice being found attached to the eyelashes and even the hair of the forehead. The lice can survive for 9–44 h off the host, and infestation from clothing and toilet seats is thus feasible, although unlikely.

Heavy infestations may result in itching and, rarely, *maculae cerulae* or bluish spots due to repeated biting may be found.

Treatment is similar to that for head lice, using insecticides such as gamma-benzene hexachloride (lindane) as a lotion, shampoo or powder. This insecticide is toxic and treatment needs to be repeated, as it is not ovicidal. 0.5% malathion or carbaryl are safer and, being ovicidal, are more effective, but spirit base preparations should not be used. Pyrethroids are also effective and are widely used.

When on the eyelashes (Fig. 28.93), *Pth. pubis* should be dealt with by removal of individual lice or by treating each egg individually with a paint brush dipped in an ovicidal insecticide. Alternatively, the thick application of Vaseline twice daily for 8 days may be effective.[1014] Laundering of clothing, sheets, etc., in hot water is advisable to prevent spread.

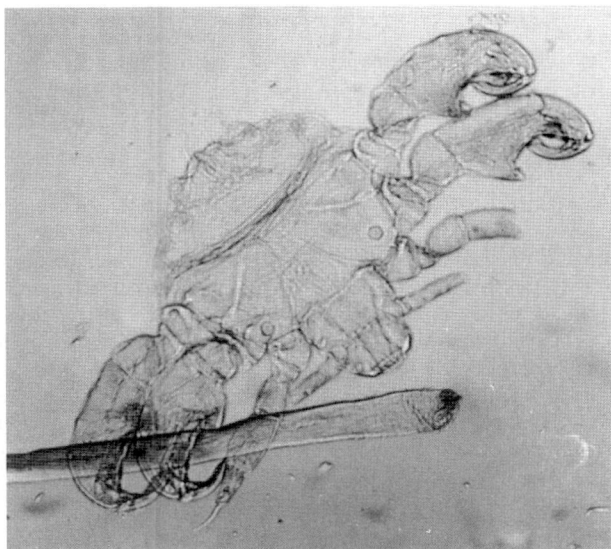

Fig. 28.92 Photomicrograph of nymph of *Pthirus pubis* tightly attached to hair (approx. × 100).

DISEASES TRANSMITTED BY ANIMALS

These are summarized in Table 28.48.[1029]

CAT-SCRATCH DISEASE (CSD)

Cat-scratch disease is a relatively benign, widely encountered infection characterized by malaise, low grade fever and lymphadenopathy. About half of the patients with CSD develop a nonpruritic, erythematous primary lesion 3–30 days after getting a scratch. This lesion may form a small pustule but overall the infection usually resolves spontaneously in a few weeks. Rarely, complications can occur such as encephalitis, conjunctivitis (Parinaud's oculoglandular syndrome), neuroretinitis and thrombocytopenic purpura.[1029-1031] Contact with cats followed by skin lesions associated with a scratch or bite are found in the majority of cases. There may be a maculopapular rash. Chronic lymphadenitis may occur with the cervical lymph nodes frequently involved. Murano et al[1032] reported a giant hepatic granuloma as associated with *Bartonella henselae* infection and suggested that this infection should be considered in the differential diagnosis of a large hepatic mass. Overall, systemic symptoms are unusual in CSD, but severe disease may occur in HIV positive patients. Isada et al[1033] reported that in the USA, 22 000 cases of CSD occur annually with 10% requiring hospitalization.

Table 28.48   Diseases transmitted/harbored by dogs, cats and rodents*

Dogs	Cats	Rodents
Rabies	Rabies	Lassa fever
Ringworm	Cat-scratch fever (*Bartonella henselae*)	Hantavirus disease
Scabies	Ringworm	S. American arenavirus hemorrhagic fevers
Echinococcus granulosus infection	Scabies	Omsk hemorrhagic fever
Toxocara canis infection (larva migrans)	*Toxocara cati* (larva migrans)	Kyasanur forest disease
Leptospirosis	Pasteurellosis (*Pasteurella multocida*)	Group C virus disease
Canicola fever (*Leptospira canicola*)	Cutaneous larva migrans	E. Hemisphere sandfly fever
Leishmaniasis	Toxoplasmosis	Vesicular stomatitis fever
Dipylidium caninum	*Bartonella clarridgeiae*	Venezuelan equine encephalitis
Cutaneous larva migrans	*Capillaria aerophila*	Lymphocytic choriomeningitis
Dirofilaria immitis	Cutaneous dirofilariasis	Rat bite fever (*Spirillum minor*)
Capnocytophaga canimorsus (DF-2)	Paragonimiasis	Haverhill fever (*Streptobacillus moniliformis*)
Bartonella clarridgeiae	Q fever	Bubonic plague (*Yersinia pestis*)
Bartonella vinsonii	Ctenocephalides felis	Campylobacteriosis
Spotted fever (some forms)	Salmonellosis (gastroenteritis)	Salmonellosis (gastroenteritis)
Ehrlichiosis	Giardiasis	Leptospirosis (e.g. Weil disease)
Cutaneous dirofilariasis	*Strongyloides* sp.	Endemic relapsing fever
Paragonimiasis	*Tunga penetrans*	Scrub typhus
Q fever		Murine typhus
Salmonellosis (gastroenteritis)		Rickettsialpox
Ctenocephalides canis		Spotted fever (some forms)
Giardiasis		Q fever
Diphyllobothrium latum		*Bartonella* spp.
Fasciola hepatica		*Babesia microti*
Lyme disease		Toxoplasmosis (where rodents are eaten)
Trichuris vulpis		Cutaneous leishmaniasis (some forms)
Strongyloides sp.		Clonorchis sinensis
Tunga penetrans		*Schistosoma japonicum*
Eosinophilic enteritis		Multilocular hydatid
		Hymenolepis nana
		Hymenolepis diminuta
		Inermicapsifer madagascariensis
		Angiostrongyliasis
		Capillaria hepatica
		Moniliformis moniliformis
		Cordylobia anthropophaga
		Xenopsylla cheopis
		Tunga penetrans
		Dermanyssid mites
		Trombiculid mites

*Not all of these infections are directly transmissible to humans from the animal reservoir and in some cases the animal may only be an occasional reservoir for the infection. For details of these and other infectious diseases relating especially to control, the reference edited by Chin[1029] is strongly recommended.

ETIOLOGY

The bacterium *Bartonella* (formerly *Rochalimaea*) *henselae* is considered the cause of CSD and the role of *Afipia felis* in the causation of CSD (if it has one) is small.[1029,1034,1035] Kordick et al,[1036] however, have described *B. clarridgeiae* as causing a cat-scratch disease-like syndrome.

Other species of the genus *Bartonella* can infect humans but are not involved in causing CSD. The species of *Bartonella* and their disease associations are summarized in Table 28.49.

DIAGNOSIS

The diagnosis of CSD is confirmed if the history of cat contact and a primary skin lesion is associated with typical silver-staining bacteria identified on histopathological sections of lymph nodes, skin or eye lesions. A skin test for cat-scratch disease is available, but this is being superseded by serology using an indirect fluorescent antibody test for *B. henselae* which is said to be more sensitive.

TREATMENT

As most patients with this disease are not ill and spontaneous recovery is common, treatment is usually symptomatic. Antibiotics should be reserved for patients with severe disease. The most commonly used antibiotics are not effective and a recent review indicated that only four antimicrobial drugs are useful, with the oral drugs in decreasing order of efficacy being rifampicin (87%), ciprofloxacin (84%) and trimethoprim–sulfamethoxazole (58%). Intramuscular gentamicin was 73% effective.[1037] Isada et al,[1033] while admitting that no controlled trials have been carried out in the treatment of CSD, report that erythromycin, doxycycline or co-trimoxazole, in that order, might be effective.

CAT-SCRATCH ENCEPHALOPATHY

CNS complications may develop from a few days to some weeks after the first evidence of illness, usually a mildly tender lymphadenopathy. Fever is not characteristic and may occur in only 50% of cases. Convulsions

Table 28.49 Disease associations in the genus *Bartonella* in humans

Species	Disease association	Comments
B. henselae	Cat-scratch disease (CSD) Bacillary angiomatosis	From cat bite/lick
B. quintana	Trench fever Bacillary angiomatosis	From body lice
B. bacilliformis	Oroya fever, verruga peruana	*Lutzomyia* flies
B. elizabethae	Subacute endocarditis Neuroretinitis	
B. clarridgeiae	Subacute endocarditis CSD-like syndrome	From cats/dogs
B. vinsonii	Subacute endocarditis	Various subspecies From cats, dogs, rodents

of varying severity will also affect about 50% of the children with encephalopathy, and they may remain lethargic or even comatose for several weeks. In the recovery phase, 'transient combative behavior' seems to be a characteristic feature of this particular type of encephalopathy. Changes in the CSF are neither consistent nor characteristic and peripheral blood counts are not helpful. In addition to the control of convulsions and supportive measures, the most important aspect is to establish the diagnosis and differentiate it from other causes of encephalopathy as quickly as possible to avoid extensive and invasive investigations. The prognosis is excellent with no evidence of lasting neurological impairment.[1038]

RAT-BITE FEVERS

Rat-bite fevers comprise two separate and distinct infections, both of which are characterized by a relapsing fever usually following a rat bite. They are particularly prevalent in rat-infested communities of low socioeconomic status. Children living in such areas are at especial risk and may even be bitten by rats while asleep. Children may also become infected following a bite from a pet mouse or rat. *Streptobacillus moniliformis* (streptobacillary rat-bite fever; Haverhill fever; erythema arthriticum epidemicum) has been recorded worldwide, including from Europe and the USA; *Spirillum minus* (spirillary rat-bite fever; sodoku or sokosha) has also been reported worldwide, but mostly from Japan.[1029] Streptobacillary rat-bite fever is a more common cause of fever following a rat bite than is the spirillary form.

STREPTOBACILLUS MONILIFORMIS (STREPTOBACILLOSIS)

Streptobacillus moniliformis is a commensal in the rat nasopharynx and has also occasionally been recorded from other small mammal species such as squirrels, weasels and gerbils.[1029,1031,1039] While transmission is usually through a rat bite, epidemic outbreaks in humans are believed to have resulted from ingestion of raw milk or water contaminated with rat urine or saliva.[1029,1031] The incubation period is usually 3–10 days,

occasionally longer, during which a gastroenteritis may be present. The infected bite usually heals rapidly but a fever develops which is often relapsing and, although usually subsiding within 10 days or so, may continue for months if untreated. A generalized erythematous, morbilliform or even purpuric rash, particularly on the hands and feet, may develop and arthralgia (especially of the large joints) and sore throat, extreme prostration and headache may occur. Complications may include infective endocarditis, pericarditis and abscesses of soft tissue or brain.[1029,1040,1041] The fatality rate may reach 10% if untreated.

Streptobacillary rat-bite fever needs to be differentiated from coxsackie infections, meningococcal septicemia and erythema multiforme but infection can be confirmed by isolation of *S. moniliformis* from blood, infected joint fluid, abscesses or pustules. Serological diagnosis using an agglutination test is available and becomes positive in the second to third week of the infection. Penicillin, given as soon as possible after the bite, is effective,[1031] as are cephalosporins, but strains resistant to penicillin, streptomycin and erythromycin have been recorded.

SPIRILLUM MINUS (SPIRILLOSIS)

Transmission of *Spirillum minus* is most commonly via the bite of an infected rat but can occur following the bite from other mammals including cats, which can serve as healthy reservoirs. Food contaminated by infected rat urine may also presumably cause infection.

The incubation period varies from 7 to 28 (mean 8) days after the bite, which may heal or become necrotic and chancre-like. Recurrent fevers occur at 5–10 day intervals, sometimes continuing for weeks in untreated patients, and may be accompanied by profuse sweating, often with a marked flare up of inflammation at the site of the bite. Regional lymphadenopathy usually develops and a characteristic purplish, papular (or sometimes nodular) rash or urticaria may be present, especially on the chest and arms. Muscle pains, but rarely joint pains and arthritis, hyperesthesia and localized edema are additional signs. In severe cases, a meningoencephalitis with delirium may develop, as may endocarditis and involvement of other organs. In untreated cases, the mortality may reach 10%, being associated with neuronal degeneration of the brain and degenerative changes in the liver and kidneys.

The differential diagnosis should consider other febrile infections, including those caused by spirochetes (such as relapsing fever), viruses, rickettsiae (such as the spotted fevers), bacterial infections (such as plague), tularemia and also malaria, in endemic regions. A puffiness of the face may suggest nephritis and children may present with persistent diarrhea and weight loss, which may further confuse the correct diagnosis. During febrile paroxysms there may be a leukocytosis and occasionally eosinophilia and anemia may be present. CSF pressure may be raised.

Diagnosis of spirillosis can be confirmed by detecting *S. minus* in lesion/tissue exudates, in an enlarged lymph node or, during a febrile episode, in peripheral blood by dark ground microscopy or by inoculation of guinea pigs, mice or laboratory rats. No specific serological tests are available.

Penicillin is the treatment of choice for spirillosis[965,1031] but streptomycin, erythromycin, chloramphenicol and tetracyclines (not during pregnancy or for children under 7–8 years of age) are also effective.

REFERENCES (* Level 1 evidence)

Mortality and Morbidity in Infectious Disease

1. World Bank. Investing in health. World Development Report. Oxford: Oxford University Press; 1993.
2. The United Nations Children's Fund. The state of the world's children 2007. New York: United Nations Children's Fund (UNICEF); 2006.
3. UNAIDS and WHO. AIDS epidemic update 2006. Geneva: United Nations AIDS Program (UNAIDS); 2006.

4. Murray CJL, Lopez AD, Chin B, et al. Estimation of potential global pandemic influenza mortality on the basis of vital registry data from the 1918–20 pandemic: a quantitative analysis. Lancet 2006; 368:2211–2218.
5. Fleming D, Smith GE, Charlton J, et al. Impact of infections on primary care – greater than expected. Commun Dis Public Health 2002; 5:7–12.
6. Murray CJL. Quantifying the burden of disease: the technical basis for disability-adjusted life years. In:

Murray CJL, Lopez AD, eds. Global comparative assessments in the health sector. Geneva: WHO; 1994:3–19.
7. Cliffe S, Tookey P, Nicoll A. Antenatal detection of HIV: national surveillance and unlinked anonymous surveys. BMJ 2001; 325:376–377.
8. The UK Collaborative Group for HIV and STI Surveillance. A complex picture. HIV and other sexually transmitted infections in the United Kingdom: 2006. London: Health Protection Agency, Centre for Infections; 2006.

9. Trotter CL, Ramsay ME, Slack MP. Rising incidence of *Haemophilus influenza* type b disease in England indicates a need for second catch-up vaccination campaign. Commun Dis Public Health 2003; 6:55–58.

10. Miller E, Salisbury D, Ramsay ME. Planning, registration and implementation of an immunization campaign against meningococcal C disease in the UK: a success story. Vaccine 2002; 20 Suppl 1:S8–S67.

11. Ramsay M, Gay N, Miller E, et al. The epidemiology of measles in England and Wales: rationale for the 1994 national vaccination campaign. CDR Rev 1994; 4:R141–R146.

12. Communicable Disease Surveillance Centre (CDSC). The national measles and rubella campaign – one year on. CDR Rev 1995; 5:237.

13. Health Protection Agency. Protecting the health of England's children: the benefit of vaccines. First national report of the current status of the national universal vaccination programmes from the Centre for Infections. London: Health Protection Agency Centre for Infections; 2005.

14. Ramsay ME, Yarwood, Lewis D, et al. Parental confidence in measles, mumps and rubella vaccine: evidence from vaccine coverage and attitudinal surveys. Br J Gen Pract 2002; 52:912–916.

15. Gangarosa EJ, Galazka AM, Wolfe CR, et al. Impact of anti-vaccine movements on pertussis control. Lancet 1998; 351:356–361.

16. Nicoll A. Benefits, safety and risks of immunisation programmes. Interdisc Sci Rev 2001; 26:20–30.

17. Colditz GA, Brewer TF, Berkey JCS, et al. Efficacy of BCG vaccine in the prevention of tuberculosis. JAMA 1994; 271:698–702.

18. Elliott EJ, Robins-Browne RM, O'Loughlin EV, et al. Contributors to the Australian Paediatric Surveillance Unit. Nationwide study of haemolytic uraemic syndrome: clinical, microbiological, and epidemiological features. Arch Dis Child 2001; 5:125–131.

19. Nicoll A, Catchpole M, Cliffe S, et al. Sexual health of teenagers in England and Wales. BMJ 1999; 318:1321–1322.

20. National Chlamydia Screening Steering Group. New frontiers: Annual report of the National Chlamydia Screening Programme in England 2005/6. London: Health Protection Agency; 2006.

21. Harling R, Twisselmann B, Asgari-Jihandeh N, et al, for the Deliberate Release Team. Deliberate releases of biological agents: initial lessons for Europe from events in the United States. Euro Surveill 2001; 6:166–171.

22. World Health Organization, International Health Regulations 2005. http://www.who.int/csr/ihr/en/

23. Satcher D. Emerging infections: getting ahead of the curve. Emerg Infect Dis 1997; 1:1–6.

24. Verity CM, Nicoll A, Will RG, et al. Variant Creutzfeldt–Jakob disease in UK children: a national surveillance study. Lancet 2000; 356:1224–1227.

25. Morse SS. Factors in the emergence of infectious diseases. Emerg Infect Dis 1995; 1:7–15.

26. Begg N, Nicoll A. Myths in medicine, Immunisation. BMJ 1994; 309:1073–1075.

27. Gill ON, Sockett PN, Bartlett CLR, et al. Outbreak of *Salmonella napoli* caused by contaminated chocolate bars. Lancet 1983; 2:544–547.

28. Bell BP, Goldoft M, Griffin PM, et al. A multistate outbreak of *E. coli* O157: H7-associated bloody diarrhea and hemolytic uremic syndrome from hamburgers. JAMA 1994; 272:1349–1353.

29. Wasserheit JN. Effect of changes in human ecology and behaviour on patterns of sexually transmitted diseases, including immunodeficiency virus infection. Proc Natl Acad Sci USA 1994; 91:2430–2435.

30. Bobadilla J-L, Cowley P, Musgrove P, et al. Design, content and financing of an essential national package of health services. In: Murray CJL, Lopez AD, eds. Global comparative assessments in the health sector. Geneva: WHO; 1994:171–192.

31. Hull HF, Ward NA, Hull BF, et al. Paralytic poliomyelitis: seasoned strategies, disappearing disease. Lancet 1994; 343:1331–1337.

32. Grassly NC, Fraser C, Wenger J, et al. New strategies for the elimination of polio from India. Science 2006; 314:1150–1153.

33. Nicoll A, Lynn R, Rahi J, et al. Public health outputs from the British Paediatric Surveillance Unit and similar clinician-based systems. J Roy Soc Med 2000; 93:580–585.

34. Rowland D. Mapping communicable disease control administration in the UK: between devolution and Europe. London: Nuffield Trust; 2006.

The Child with Fever

35. Wailoo MP, Petersen SA, Whitaker H, et al. Sleeping body temperatures in 3–4 month old infants. Arch Dis Child 1989; 64:596–599.

36. Morley CJ, Hewson PH, Thornton AJ, et al. Axillary and rectal temperature measurements in infants. Arch Dis Child 1992; 67:122–125.

37. Davies EG, Elliman DAC, Hart CA, et al. Manual of childhood infections. London: WB Saunders; 2001.

38. Weinberg GA, D'Angio CT. Laboratory aids for diagnosis of neonatal sepsis. In: Remington J, Klein J, eds. Infectious diseases of the fetus and newborn infant. 6th edn. Philadelphia: Elsevier; 2006:1207–1222.

39. Bonadio WA, Hegenbarth M, Zachamason M. Correlating reported fever in young infants with subsequent temperature patterns and risk of serious bacterial infections. Pediatr Infect Dis J 1990; 9:158–160.

40. Bass JW, Steele R, Wittler R, et al. Antimicrobial treatment of occult bacteremia: a multicentre cooperative study. Pediatr Infect Dis J 1993; 12:466–473.

41. Baraff LJ, Oslund SA, Schriger DL, et al. Probability of bacterial infections in febrile infants less than three months of age: a meta-analysis. Pediatr Infect Dis J 1992; 11:257–265.

42 National Institute for Clinical Excellence. Feverish illness in children. http://guidance.nice.org.uk/CG47

Clinical Problems: Suspected Meningitis

43. Hargreaves RM, Slack MP, Howard AJ, et al. Changing patterns of invasive *Haemophilus influenzae* disease in England and Wales after introduction of the Hib vaccination programme. BMJ 1996; 312:160–161.

44. Garg RK. Tuberculosis of the central nervous system. Postgrad Med J 1999; 75:133–140.

45. Carrol ED, Latif AH, Misbah SA, et al. Lesson of the week: Recurrent bacterial meningitis: the need for sensitive imaging. BMJ 2001; 323:501–503.

46. van Furth AM, Roord JJ, van Furth R. Roles of proinflammatory and anti-inflammatory cytokines in pathophysiology of bacterial meningitis and effect of adjunctive therapy. Infect Immun 1996; 64:4883–4890.

47. Heyderman RS, Klein NJ. Emergency management of meningitis. J R Soc Med 2000; 93:225–229.

48. Tauber MG. To tap or not to tap? Clin Infect Dis 1997; 25:289–291.

49. Reacher MH, Shah A, Livermore DM, et al. Bacteraemia and antibiotic resistance of its pathogens reported in England and Wales between 1990 and 1998: trend analysis. BMJ 2000; 320:213–216.

50. Trends in Antimicrobial Resistance in England and Wales, 2004–2005. Health Protection Agency, 2006.

51. Bradley JS, Scheld WM. The challenge of penicillin-resistant *Streptococcus pneumoniae* meningitis: current antibiotic therapy in the 1990s. Clin Infect Dis 1997; 24:S213–S221.

52. Tauber MG, Moser B. Cytokines and chemokines in meningeal inflammation: biology and clinical implications. Clin Infect Dis 1999; 28:1–11.

53. McIntyre PB, Berkey CS, King SM, et al. Dexamethasone as adjunctive therapy in bacterial meningitis. A meta-analysis of randomized clinical trials since 1988. JAMA 1997; 278:925–931.

54. van de Beek D, de Gans J, McIntyre P, et al. Corticosteroids for acute bacterial meningitis. Cochrane Database Syst Rev 2007; (1): CD004405.

55. Powell KR, Sugarman LI, Eskenazi AE, et al. Normalization of plasma arginine vasopressin concentrations when children with meningitis are given maintenance plus replacement fluid therapy. J Pediatr 1990; 117:515–522.

56. Bedford H, de Louvois J, Halket S et al. Meningitis in infancy in England and Wales: follow up at age 5 years. BMJ 2001; 323:533–536.

Septic Shock

57. Sprung CL, Bernard GR, Dellinger RP. Guidelines for the management of severe sepsis and septic shock. Intensive Care Med 2001; 27(suppl 1).

58. Docke WD, Randow F, Syrbe U, et al. Monocyte deactivation in septic patients: restoration by IFN-gamma treatment. Nat Med 1997; 3:678–681.

59. Levin M, Klein N. Shock in the febrile child. In: Isaacs D, Moxon ER, eds. A practical approach to pediatric infections. New York: Churchill Livingstone; 1996:4425–4444.

60. Novelli V, Peters M, Dobson S. Infectious disease. In: Macnab A, Macrae D, Henning R, eds. Care of the critically ill child. London: Churchill Livingstone; 1999:281–298.

61. Minneci PC, Deans KJ, Banks SM, et al. Meta-analysis: the effect of steroids on survival and shock during sepsis depends on the dose. Ann Intern Med 2004; 141:47–56.

62. Alejandria MM, Lansang MA, Dans LF, et al. Intravenous immunoglobulin for treating sepsis and septic shock. Cochrane Database Syst Rev 2002;(1):CD001090.

63. Bernard GR, Vincent J-L, Laterre P-F, et al. Efficacy and safety of recombinant human activated protein C for severe sepsis. N Engl J Med 2001; 344:699–709.

64. Van Den Berghe G, Wouters P, Weekers F, et al. Intensive insulin therapy in critically ill patients. N Engl J Med 2001; 345:1359–1367.

Congenital and Neonatal Infections

65. Gregg NM. Congenital cataract following German measles in the mother. Trans Ophthalmol Soc Aust 1941; 3:35–46.

66. Tookey PA, Peckham CS. Surveillance of congenital rubella in Great Britain, 1971–1996. BMJ 1999; 318:769–770.

67. Rahi J, Adams G, Russell-Eggit I, et al. Epidemiological surveillance of rubella must continue. BMJ 2001; 323:112.

68. Miller E, Cradock-Watson JE, Pollock TM. Consequences of confirmed maternal rubella at successive stages of pregnancy. Lancet 1982; 2:781–784.

69. Best JM, Banatvala JE, Morgan-Capner P, et al. Fetal infection after maternal reinfection with rubella: criteria for defining reinfection. BMJ 1989; 299:773–775.

70. Best JM, Castillo-Solorzano C, Spika JS, et al. Reducing the global burden of congenital rubella syndrome: report of the World Health Organization Steering Committee On Research Related To Measles and Rubella Vaccines and Vaccination, June 2004. J Infect Dis 2005; 192:1890–1897.

71. MMWR 2005; 54:279–282.

72. Boppana SB, Fowler KB, Britt WJ, et al. Symptomatic congenital cytomegalovirus infection in infants born to mothers with pre-existing immunity to cytomegalovirus. Pediatrics 1999; 104:55–60.

73. Boppana SB, Rivera LB, Fowler KB, et al. Intrauterine transmission of cytomegalovirus to infants of women with pre-conceptional immunity. N Engl J Med 2001; 344:1366–1371.

74. Ross SA, Folwer KB, Ashrith G, et al. Hearing loss in children with congenital cytomegalovirus infection born to mothers with pre-existing immunity. J Pediatr 2006; 148:332–336.

75. Noyola DE, Demmler GJ, Nelson CT, et al. Early predictors of neurodevelopmental outcome in symptomatic congenital cytomegalovirus infection. J Pediatr 2001; 138:325–331.

76. Fowler KB, McCollister FP, Dahle AJ, et al. Progressive and fluctuating sensorineural hearing loss in children with asymptomatic congenital cytomegalovirus infection. J Pediatr 1997; 130:624–630.

77. Kylat RI, Kelly EN, Ford-Jones EL. Clinical findings and adverse outcomes in neonates with symptomatic congenital cytomegalovirus (SCCMV) infection. Eur J Pediatr 2006; 165:773–778.

78. Lanari M, Lassarotto T, Venturi V, et al. Neonatal cytomegalovirus blood load and risk of sequelae in symptomatic and asymptomatic congenitally infected newborns. Pediatr 2006; 117:76–83.

79. Paryani SG, Yeager AS, Hosford-Dunn H, et al. Sequelae of acquired cytomegalovirus infection in premature and sick term infants. J Pediatr 1985; 107:451–456.

80. Whitley RJ, Cloud G, Gruber W, et al. Ganciclovir treatment of symptomatic congenital cytomegalovirus infection: results of a phase II study. National Institute of Allergy and Infectious Diseases Collaborative Antiviral Study Group. J Infect 1997; 175:1080–1086.

81. Nigro G, Krzysztofiak A, Bartmann U, et al. Ganciclovir therapy for cytomegalovirus-associated liver disease in immunocompetent or immunocompromised children. Arch Virol 1997; 142:573–580.

82. Smets K, De Coen K, Dhooge I, et al. Selecting neonates with congenital cytomegalovirus infection for ganciclovir therapy. Eur J Pediatr 2006; 165:885–890.

83. Rojo P, Ramos JT. Ganciclovir treatment of children with congenital cytomegalovirus infection. Pediatr Infect Dis J 2004; 23:88–89.

84. Nigro G, Adler SP, La Torre R, et al. Passive immunization during pregnancy for congenital cytomegalovirus infection. N Engl J Med 2005; 353:1350–1362.

85. Enders G, Miller E, Cradock-Watson J, et al. Consequences of varicella and herpes zoster in pregnancy: prospective study of 1739 cases. Lancet 1994; 343:1548–1551.

86. Chant KG, Sullivan EA, Burgess MA, et al. Varicella-zoster virus infection in Australia. Aust N Z J Public Health 1998; 22:413–418.

87. Heuchan AM, Isaacs D. The management of varicella-zoster virus exposure and infection in pregnancy and the newborn period. Australasian Subgroup in Paediatric Infectious Diseases of the Australasian Society for Infectious Diseases. Med J Aust 2001; 174:288–292.

88. Reynolds L, Struik S, Nadel S. Neonatal varicella: varicella zoster immunoglobulin (VZIG) does not prevent disease. Arch Dis Child Fetal Neonatal Ed 1999; 81:F69–F70.

89. Gutierrez KM, Falkovitz HM, Maldonado Y, et al. The epidemiology of neonatal herpes simplex virus infections in California from 1985 to 1995. J Infect Dis 1999; 180:199–202.

90. Tookey P, Peckham CS. Neonatal herpes simplex virus infection in the British Isles. Paediatr Perinat Epidemiol 1996; 10:432–442.

91. Brown ZA, Selke S, Zeh J, et al. The acquisition of herpes simplex virus during pregnancy. N Engl J Med 1997; 337:509–515.

92. Whitley RJ. Herpes simplex virus infections of the central nervous system. A review. Am J Med 1988; 85(suppl 2A):61–67.

93. American Academy of Pediatrics. Herpes simplex. In: Pickering L, ed. Red book report of the Committee on Infectious Diseases, 25th edn. Elk Grove Village: American Academy of Pediatrics; 2000:309–318.

*94 Stanberry LR, Spruance SL, Cunningham AL, et al. Glycoprotein-D-adjuvant vaccine to prevent genital herpes. N Engl J Med 2002; 347:1652–1661.

95. Fowler SL, Dickey M, Kern P, et al. Perceptions of parents seeking an experimental herpes simplex vaccine for their adolescent and preadolescent daughters. Pediatr Infect Dis J 2006; 25:747–748.

96. Sheffield JS, Hill JB, Hollier LM, et al. Valacyclovir prophylaxis to prevent recurrent herpes at delivery: a randomized clinical trial. Obstet Gynecol 2006; 108:141–147.

97. Kurt-Jones EA, Belko J, Yu C, et al. The role of toll-like receptors in herpes simplex infection in neonates. J Infect Dis 2005; 191:746–748.

98. Dunn D, Wallon M, Peyron F, et al. Mother-to-child transmission of toxoplasmosis: risk estimates for clinical counselling. Lancet 1999; 353:1829–1833.

99. Gilbert R, Tan HK, Cliffe S, et al. Symptomatic toxoplasma infection due to congenital and postnatally acquired infection. Arch Dis Child 2006; 91:495–498.

100. Vogel N, Kirisits M, Michael E, et al. Congenital toxoplasmosis transmitted from an immunologically competent mother infected before conception. Clin Infect Dis 1996; 23:1055–1060.

101. Dunn D, Gilbert R, Newell ML, et al. Low incidence of congenital toxoplasmosis in children born to women infected with human immunodeficiency virus. European Collaborative Study and Research Network on Congenital Toxoplasmosis. Eur J Obstet Gynecol Reprod Biol 1996; 68:93–96.

102. McAuley J, Boyer KM, Patel D, et al. Early and longitudinal evaluations of treated infants and children and untreated historical patients with congenital toxoplasmosis: the Chicago Collaborative Treatment Trial. Clin Infect Dis J 1994; 18:38–72.

*103. Peyron F, Wallon M, Liou C, et al. Treatments for toxoplasmosis in pregnancy (Cochrane Review). In: The Cochrane Library, 2. Oxford: Update Software; 2000.

104. McMinn P, Stratov I, Nagarajan L, et al. Neurological manifestations of enterovirus 71 infection in children during an outbreak of hand, foot, and mouth disease in Western Australia. Clin Infect Dis J 2001; 32:236–242.

105. Ho M, Chen ER, Hsu KH, et al. An epidemic of enterovirus 71 infection in Taiwan. Taiwan Enterovirus Epidemic Working Group. N Engl J Med 1999; 341:929–935.

106. Rotbart HA, Webster AD. Treatment of potentially life-threatening enterovirus infections with pleconaril. Clin Infect Dis J 2001; 32:228–235.

Hospital Infection Control

107. Huskins WC, Goldman DA. Nosocomial infections. In: Feigin R, Cherry J, Demmler G, et al, eds. Textbook of pediatric infectious disease, 5th edn. Philadelphia: Saunders; 2004.

108. Centers for Disease Control. Guidelines for hand hygiene in health care settings. MMWR 2002; 51:1–44.

109. Edmond MB, Wenzel RP. Isolation. In: Mandell G, Bennett J, Dolin R, eds. Principles and practice of infectious diseases, 6th edn. Philadelphia: Elsevier; 2005.

110. Tablan OC, Boyyard EA, Shapiro CN, et al. Personnel health services. In: Bennett JV, Brachman PS. Hospital infections, 4th edn. Philadelphia: Lippincott-Raven; 1998.

111. Chamberland ME, Bell DM. Human immunodeficiency virus. In: Bennett JV, Brachman PS. Hospital infections, 4th edn. Philadelphia: Lippincott-Raven; 1998.

112. MacDougall C, Polk RE. Antimicrobial stewardship programs in health care systems. Clin Microbiol Rev 2005; 18:638–656.

113. Jarvis WR. Investigating endemic and epidemic nosocomial infections. In: Bennett JV, Brachman PS. Hospital infections, 4th edn. Philadelphia: Lippincott-Raven; 1998.

The Use of the Bacteriology Laboratory by the Pediatrician

114. Peterson LR, Hamilton JD, Baron EJ, et al. Role of the microbiology laboratory in the management and control of infectious diseases and the delivery of health care. Clin Infect Dis 2001; 32:605–611.

115. O'Grady NP, Alexander M, Delinger P, et al. Guidelines for the prevention of intravascular catheter-related infections. Clin Infect Dis 2002; 35:1281–1307.

116. Bisno AL, Gerbe MA, Gwaltney Jr JM, et al. Practice Guidelines for the Diagnosis and Management of Group A Streptococcal Pharyngitis. Clin Infect Dis 2002; 35:113–125.

117. Carroll KC. Laboratory diagnosis of lower respiratory tract infections: controversy and conundrums. J Clin Microbiol 2002; 40:3115–3120.

118. Thompson RB, Bertram H. Laboratory diagnosis of central nervous system infections. Infect Dis Clin North Am 2001; 15:1047–1071.

119. Hayden R, Pershing DH. Diagnostic molecular microbiology. Curr Clin Top Infect Dis 2001; 21:323–348.

120. Hines J, Nachamkin I. Effective use of the clinical microbiology laboratory for the diagnosis of diarrhoeal diseases. Clin Infect Dis 1996; 23(Supp):S97–S101.

Principles of Antimicrobial Therapy

121 Muller M, delaPena A, Derendorf H. Issues in pharmacokinetic and pharmacodynamics of anti-infective agents: Distribution in tissue. Antimicrob Agents Chemother 2004; 48:1441–1453.

122. Lowy FD. Staphylococcus aureus infections. N Engl J Med 1998; 339:520–532.

123. Jacoby GA, Munoz-Price LS. The new β-lactamases. N Engl J Med 2005; 352:380–391.

124. Bradford PA. Extended spectrum β-lactamases in the 21st century; characterisation, epidemiology and detection of this important resistance threat. Clin Microbiol Rev 2001; 14:933–951.

125. Paterson DL, Bronomo RA. Extended-spectrum β-lactamases: a clinical update. Clin Microbiol Rev 2005; 18:657–686.

126. Philippon A, Arlert G, Jacoby GA. Plasmid-determined AmpC-type β-lactamases. Antimicrob Agents Chemother 2002; 46:1–11.

127. Kotra LP, Haddad J, Mobashery S. Aminoglycosides: Perspectives of action and resistance and strategies to counter resistance. Antimicrob Agents Chemother 2000; 44:3249–3256.

128. Gruchalla RS, Pirmoharmed M. Antibiotic allergy. N Engl J Med 2006; 254:601–609.

129. Kessler RE. Cefapime microbiologic profile and update. Pediatr Infect Dis J 2001; 20:331–336.

130. Kucers A. Vancomycin. In: Kucers A, Crowe S, Grayson ML, et al, eds. The use of antibiotics, 5th edn. Oxford: Butterworth-Heinemann; 1997.

131. Vakulenko SB, Mobashery S. Versatility of aminoglycosides and prospects for their future. Clin Microbiol Rev 2003; 16:430–450.

132. Ruuskanen O. Safety and tolerability of azithromycin in pediatric infectious diseases: 2003 update. Pediatr Infect Dis J 2004; 23:S135–S139.

133. Kucers A, Crowe S, Grayson M, et al. The use of antibiotics. Part IV and part V, 5th edn. Oxford: Butterworth-Heinemann; 1997:1245–1881.

134. Groll AH, Walsh TJ. Antifungal agents. In: Feigin R, Cherry J, Demmler G, et al, eds. Textbook of pediatric infectious disease, 5th edn. Philadelphia: Saunders; 2004.

135. Demmler GJ. Antiviral agents. In: Feigin R, Cherry J, Demmler G, et al, eds. Textbook of pediatric infectious disease, 5th edn. Philadelphia: Saunders; 2004.

Bacterial Infections: Botulism

136. Thomas DG. Infant botulism: a review in South Australia (1980–1989). J Paediatr Child Health 1993; 29:24–26.

137. Spika JS, Shaffer N, Hargrett-Bean N, et al. Risk factors for infant botulism in the United States. Am J Dis Child 1989; 143:828–832.

138. Schreiner MS, Field E, Ruddy R. Infant botulism: a review of 12 years' experience at The Children's Hospital of Philadelphia. Pediatrics 1991; 87:59–165.

139. Frankovich TL, Arnon SS. Clinical trial of botulism immune globulin for infant botulism. West J Med 1991; 154:103.

140. Thompson JA, Filloux FM, Van Orman CB, et al. Infant botulism in the age of botulism immune globulin. Neurology 2005; 64:2029–2032.

141. Tacket CO, Shandera WX, Mann JM, et al. Equine antitoxin use and other factors that predict outcome in type A foodborne botulism. Am J Med 1984; 76:794–798.

142. Arnon SS, Schechter R, Maslanka SE, et al. Human botulism immune globulin for the treatment of infant botulism. N Engl J Med 2006; 354:462–471.

Bacterial Infections: Brucellosis; Undulant Fever
*143. Lubani MM, Dudkin KI, Sharda DC, et al. A multicenter therapeutic study of 1100 children with brucellosis. Pediatr Infect Dis J 1989; 8:75–78.

Bacterial Infections: Cholera
144. World Health Organization. Guidelines for cholera control. Geneva: World Health Organization; 1993.

145. Kalluri P, Naheed A, Rahman S, et al. Evaluation of three rapid diagnostic tests for cholera: does the skill level of the technician matter? Trop Med Int Health 2006; 11:49–55.

146. CHOICE Study Group. Multicenter, randomized, double-blind clinical trial to evaluate the efficacy and safety of a reduced osmolarity oral rehydration salts solution in children with acute watery diarrhea. Pediatrics 2001; 107:613–618.

147. Murphy C, Hahn S, Volmink J. Reduced osmolarity oral rehydration solution for treating cholera. Cochrane Database Syst Rev 2004; 4:CD003754.

148. World Health Organization. Implementing the new recommendations on the clinical management of diarrhoea: guidelines for policy makers and programme managers. Geneva: World Health Organization; 2006.

149. Trach DD, Clemens JD, Ke NT, et al. Field trial of locally produced, killed, oral cholera vaccine in Vietnam. Lancet 1997; 349:231–235.

150. Lucas ME, Deen JL, von Seidlein L, et al. Effectiveness of mass oral cholera vaccination in Beira, Mozambique. N Engl J Med 2005; 352:757–767.

151. Ali M, Emch M, von Seidlen L, et al. Herd immunity conferred by killed oral cholera vaccines in Bangladesh: a reanalysis. Lancet 2005; 366:7–9.

152. Thiem VD, Deen JL, von Seidlein L, et al. Long-term effectiveness against cholera of oral killed whole-cell vaccine produced in Vietnam. Vaccine 2006; 24:4297–4303.

Bacterial Infections: Diphtheria
153. Galazka AM, Robertson SE, Oblapenko GP. Resurgence of diphtheria. Eur J Epidemiol 1995; 11:95–105.

154. Dittmann S, Wharton M, Vitek C, et al. Successful control of epidemic diphtheria in the states of the Former Union of Soviet Socialist Republics: lessons learned. J Infect Dis 2000; 181 Suppl 1: S10–S22.

155. WHO. The World Health Report 2004 – changing history. Geneva: World Health Organization; 2004.

156. Bowler IC, Mandal BK, Schlecht B, et al. Diphtheria – the continuing hazard. Arch Dis Child 1988; 63:194–195.

157. PHLS. A case of diphtheria from Pakistan. CDR Weekly 1994; 4:173.

158. Nuorti P. Fatal case of diphtheria in an unvaccinated infant, Finland 2001. Eurosurveill Weekly 2002; 6:4.

159. Efstratiou A, Engler KH, Mazurova IK, et al. Current approaches to the laboratory diagnosis of diphtheria. J Infect Dis 2000; 181 Suppl 1: S138–S145.

160. Engler KH, Efstratiou A. Rapid enzyme immunoassay for determination of toxigenicity among clinical isolates of corynebacteria. J Clin Microbiol 2000; 38:1385–1389.

161. Mothershed EA, Cassiday PK, Pierson K, et al. Development of a real-time fluorescence PCR assay for rapid detection of the diphtheria toxin gene. J Clin Microbiol 2002; 40:4713–4719.

162. Pappenheimer AM, Jr. Diphtheria toxin. Annu Rev Biochem 1977; 46:69–94.

163. Zuber PL, Gruner E, Altwegg M, et al. Invasive infection with non-toxigenic Corynebacterium diphtheriae among drug users. Lancet 1992; 339:1359.

164. Tiley SM, Kociuba KR, Heron LG, et al. Infective endocarditis due to nontoxigenic Corynebacterium diphtheriae: report of seven cases and review. Clin Infect Dis 1993; 16:271–275.

165. MMWR. Respiratory diphtheria caused by Corynebacterium ulcerans – Terre Haute, Indiana, 1996. Morb Mortal Wkly Rep 1997; 46:330–332.

166. Wagner J, Ignatius R, Voss S, et al. Infection of the skin caused by Corynebacterium ulcerans and mimicking classical cutaneous diphtheria. Clin Infect Dis 2001; 33:1598–1600.

167. Harnisch JP, Tronca E, Nolan CM, et al. Diphtheria among alcoholic urban adults. A decade of experience in Seattle. Ann Intern Med 1989; 111:71–82.

168. de Benoist AC, White JM, Efstratiou A, et al. Imported cutaneous diphtheria, United Kingdom. Emerg Infect Dis 2004; 10:511–513.

169. Loukoushkina EF, Bobko PV, Kolbasova EV, et al. The clinical picture and diagnosis of diphtheritic carditis in children. Eur J Pediatr 1998; 157:528–533.

170. Kneen R, Nguyen MD, Solomon T, et al. Clinical features and predictors of diphtheritic cardiomyopathy in Vietnamese children. Clin Infect Dis 2004; 39:1591–1598.

171. Lumio JT, Groundstroem KW, Melnick OB, et al. Electrocardiographic abnormalities in patients with diphtheria: a prospective study. Am J Med 2004; 116:78–83.

172. Logina I, Donaghy M. Diphtheritic polyneuropathy: a clinical study and comparison with Guillain-Barré syndrome. J Neurol Neurosurg Psychiatry 1999; 67:433–438.

173. Solders G, Nennesmo I, Persson A. Diphtheritic neuropathy, an analysis based on muscle and nerve biopsy and repeated neurophysiological and autonomic function tests. J Neurol Neurosurg Psychiatry 1989; 52:876–880.

174. Bonnet JM, Begg NT. Control of diphtheria: guidance for consultants in communicable disease control. World Health Organization. Commun Dis Public Health 1999; 2:242–249.

175. Kneen R, Pham NG, Solomon T, et al. Penicillin vs. erythromycin in the treatment of diphtheria. Clin Infect Dis 1998; 27:845–850.

176. Bethell DB, Nguyen Minh D, Ha Thi L, et al. Prognostic value of electrocardiographic monitoring of patients with severe diphtheria. Clin Infect Dis 1995; 20:1259–1265.

177. Thisyakorn U, Wongvanich J, Kumpeng V. Failure of corticosteroid therapy to prevent diphtheritic myocarditis or neuritis. Pediatr Infect Dis 1984; 3:126–128.

178. Stockins BA, Lanas FT, Saavedra JG, et al. Prognosis in patients with diphtheric myocarditis and bradyarrhythmias: assessment of results of ventricular pacing. Br Heart J 1994; 72:190–191.

179. Dung NM, Kneen R, Kiem N, et al. Treatment of severe diphtheritic myocarditis by temporary insertion of a cardiac pacemaker. Clin Infect Dis 2002; 35:1425–1429.

180. Quick ML, Sutter RW, Kobaidze K, et al. Epidemic diphtheria in the Republic of Georgia, 1993–1996: risk factors for fatal outcome among hospitalized patients. J Infect Dis 2000; 181 Suppl 1: S130–S137.

181. Galazka A. The changing epidemiology of diphtheria in the vaccine era. J Infect Dis 2000; 181Suppl 1:S2–S9.

Bacterial Infections: Escherichia coli
182. Blattner FR, Plunkett G, Bloch CA, et al. The complete genome sequence of Escherichia coli K12. Science 1997; 277:1453–1474.

183. Perna NT, Plunkett G, Burland V, et al. Genome sequence of enterohaemorrhagic Escherichia coli O157: H7. Nature 2001; 409:529–533.

184. Reid SD, Herbelin CJ, Bumbaugh AC, et al. Parallel evolution of virulence in pathogenic Escherichia coli. Nature 2000; 406:64–67.

185. Whitfield C, Roberts IS. Structure, assembly and regulation of expression of capsules in Escherichia coli. Mol Microbiol 1999; 31:1307–1319.

186. Kariuki S, Gilks C, Kimari J, et al. Genotypic analysis of Escherichia coli strains isolated from children and chickens living in close priority. Appl Environ Microbiol 1999; 65:472–476.

187. Clermont O, Bonacorsi S, Bingen E. Rapid and simple determination of the Escherichia coli phylogenetic group. Appl Environ Microbiol 2000; 66:4555–4558.

188. Martindale J, Stroud D, Moxon ER, et al. Genetic analysis of Escherichia coli K1 gastrointestinal colonization. Mol Microbiol 2000; 37:1293–1305.

189. Kariuki S, Hart CA. Global aspects of antimicrobial resistant enteric bacteria. Curr Opin Infect Dis 2001; 14:579–586

Bacterial Infections: Haemophilus influenzae
190. Pitmann M. Variation and type specificity in bacterial species of Haemophilus influenzae. J Exp Med 1931; 53:471–492.

*191. Booy R, Hodgson SA, Slack MPE, et al. Invasive Haemophilus-influenzae-type-b disease in the Oxford region (1985–91). Arch Dis Child 1993; 69:225–228.

*192. Kilpi T, Herva E, Kaijalainen T, et al. Bacteriology of acute otitis media in a cohort of Finnish children followed for the first two years of life. Pediatr Infect Dis J 2001; 20:654–662.

*193. Heath PT, Booy R, Azzopardi HJ, et al. Non-type b Haemophilus influenzae disease: clinical and epidemiologic characteristics in the Haemophilus influenzae type b vaccine era. Pediatr Infect Dis J 2001; 20:300–305.

*194. Shann F, Gratten M, Germer S, et al. Aetiology of pneumonia in children in Goroka hospital, Papua, New Guinea. Lancet 1984; 2:537–541.

*195. Farley MM, Stephens DS, Harvey RC, et al and the CDC Meningitis Surveillance Group. Incidence and clinical characteristics of invasive Haemophilus influenzae disease in adults J Infect Dis 1992; 165(suppl 1):S42–S43.

196. Moxon ER, Zwahlen A, Rubin LB. Pathogenesis of Haemophilus influenzae meningitis: use of a rat model for studying microbial determinants of virulence. In: Sande M, Smith A, Root R, eds. Bacterial meningitis. Edinburgh: Churchill Livingstone; 1985:23–36.

197. Kauppi M, Saarinen L, Kayhty H. Anti-capsular polysaccharide antibodies reduce nasopharyngeal colonization by Haemophilus influenzae type b in infant rats. J Infect Dis 1993; 167:365–371.

*198. Fernandez J, Levine OS, Sanchez J, et al. Prevention of Haemophilus influenzae type b colonization by vaccination: correlation with serum anti-capsular IgG concentration. J Infect Dis 2000; 182:1553–1556.

*199. Heath PT, Booy R, Griffiths H, et al. Clinical and immunological risk factors associated with *Haemophilus influenzae* type b conjugate vaccine failure in childhood. Clin Infect Dis 2000; 31:973–980.

*200. Schaad U, Lips U, Gnehm H, et al. Dexamethasone therapy for bacterial meningitis. Lancet 1993; 342:457–461.

*201. Peltola H, Kayhty H, Virtanen M, et al. Prevention of *Haemophilus influenzae* type b bacteremic infections with the capsular polysaccharide vaccine. N Engl J Med 1984; 310:1561–1566.

*202. Booy R, Hodgson S, Carpenter L, et al. Efficacy of *Haemophilus-influenzae* type b conjugate vaccine PRP-T. Lancet 1994; 344:362–366.

*203. Adegbola RA, Secka O, Lahai G, et al. Elimination of *Haemophilus influenzae* type b (Hib) disease from The Gambia after the introduction of routine immunisation with a Hib conjugate vaccine: a prospective study. Lancet 2005; 366:144–150.

*204. Cowgill KD, Ndiritu M, Nyiro J, et al. Effectiveness of *Haemophilus influenzae* type b conjugate vaccine introduction into routine childhood immunization in Kenya. JAMA 2006; 296:671–678.

*205. Prymula R, Peeters P, Chrobok V, et al. Pneumococcal capsular polysaccharides conjugated to protein D for prevention of acute otitis media caused by both Streptococcus pneumoniae and non-typable Haemophilus influenzae: a randomised double-blind efficacy study. Lancet 2006; 367:740–748.

Bacterial Infections: Leprosy

206. Selvasekar A, Geetha J, Nisha K, et al. Childhood leprosy in an endemic area. Lepr Rev 1999; 70:21–27.

207. Lockwood DNJ, Reid AJC. The diagnosis of leprosy is delayed in the United Kingdom. Q J Med 2001; 94:207–212.

208. WHO Technical Report Series. WHO Expert Committee on Leprosy. Geneva: World Health Organization; 1998.

209. Jain S, Reddy RG, Osmani SN, et al. Childhood leprosy in an urban clinic-Hyderabad, India: clinical presentation and the role of household contacts. Leprosy review 2002; 73:248–253.

210. Hammond PJ, Rao PS. The tragedy of deformity in childhood leprosy. Lepr Rev 1999; 70:217–220.

211. Department of Health and the Welsh Office. Memorandum on leprosy. London: The Stationery Office; 1997.

Bacterial Infections: Lyme Disease

212. Schmid GP. The global distribution of Lyme disease. Rev Infect Dis 1985; 7:41–50.

213. Steere AC, Hardin JA, Malawista SE. Erythema chronicum migrans and Lyme arthritis. Cryoimmunoglobulins and clinical activity of skin and joints. Science 1977; 196:1121.

214. Muhlemann MF, Wright DJM. Emerging pattern of Lyme disease in the United Kingdom and Irish Republic. Lancet 1987; 1:260–263.

215. Berglund J, Eitrem R, Orristein K, et al. An epidemiological study of Lyme disease in Southern Sweden. N Engl J Med 1995; 333:1319–1324.

216. Anderson JF. Epizootiology of *Borellia* in *Ixodes* tick vectors and reservoir hosts. Rev Infect Dis 1989; 11(suppl 6):S1451–S1459.

217. Steere AC, Dwyer E, Winchester R. Association of chronic Lyme arthritis with HLA-DR4 and HLA-DR2 alleles. N Engl J Med 1990; 323:219–223.

218. Steere AC, Gibofsky A, Patarroyo M, et al. Chronic Lyme arthritis. Ann Intern Med 1979; 90:896–901.

219. Steere AC, Bartenhagen NH, Craft JE, et al. The early clinical manifestations of Lyme disease. Ann Intern Med 1983; 99:76–82.

220. Shapiro ED, Gerber MA. Lyme disease in children study group: Lyme disease in children. Sixth International Conference of Lyme Borreliosis, Bologna, Italy, 1994.

221. O'Neill PM, Wright DJM. Lyme disease. Br J Hosp Med 1988; 40:284–289.

222. Garcia-Monoco JC, Benach JI. Lyme neuroborelliosis. Ann Neurol 1995; 37:691–702.

223. Steere AC, Schoen RT, Taylor E. The clinical evolution of Lyme disease arthritis. Ann Intern Med 1987; 107:725–731.

224. Shapiro ED. Lyme disease in children. Am J Med 1995; 98(suppl 4A):695–735.

225. Feder HM, Hunt MS. Pitfalls in the diagnosis and treatment of Lyme disease in children. JAMA 1995; 274:66–68.

226. Dressler F, Whalen JA, Reinhardt BN, et al. Western blotting in the serodiagnosis of Lyme disease. J Infect Dis 1993; 167:392–400.

227. Steere AC. Lyme disease. N Engl J Med 1989; 321:586–596.

228. Gardner P. Editorial. JAMA 2000; 283:658–659.

229. Lufti BJ, Gardener R, Lightfoot RW JR. Empiric antibiotic treatment of patients who are seropositive for Lyme disease but lack classic features. Clin Infect Dis 1994; 18:112.

230. Steere AC, Hutchinson DJ, Rahn DW, et al. Treatment of the early manifestations of Lyme disease. Ann Intern Med 1983; 99:22.

231. Pal GA, Baker JT, Wright DJM. Penicillin resistant borrelia encephalitis responding to cefotaxime. Lancet 1988; 1:50–51.

Bacterial Infections: Meningococcemia

232. Invasive meningococcal infections, England and Wales: Commun Dis Rep CDR Wkly [serial online] 2001 [cited 22 November] 2001; 11(2).

233. van Deuren M, Brandtzaeg P, van der Meer JW. Update on meningococcal disease with emphasis on pathogenesis and clinical management. Clin Microbiol Rev 2000; 13:144–166.

234. Thompson MJ, Ninis N, Perera R, et al. Clinical recognition of meningococcal disease in children and adolescents. Lancet 2006; 367:397–403.

235. Lala HM, Mills GD, Barratt K, et al. Meningococcal disease deaths and the frequency of antibiotic administration delays. J Infect 2007; 54:551–557.

236. Peters MJ, Ross-Russell RI, White D, et al. Early severe neutropenia and thrombocytopenia identifies the highest risk cases of severe meningococcal disease. Paediatr Crit Care Med 2001; 2:225–231.

Bacterial Infections: *Mycobacterium tuberculosis*

237. Wilkins EGL. Antibody detection in tuberculosis. In: Davies PDO, ed. Clinical tuberculosis. London: Chapman & Hall; 1998:367–380.

238. Pfyffer GE. Nucleic acid amplification for mycobacterial diagnosis. J Infect 1999; 39:21–26.

239. Delacourt C, Poueda J-D, Chureau C, et al. Use of polymerase chain reaction for improved diagnosis of tuberculosis in children. J Pediatr 1995; 126:703–709.

240. Gomez-Pastrana D, Torronteras R, Caro P, et al. Comparison of ampiclor, in-house polymerase chain reaction, and conventional culture for the diagnosis of tuberculosis in children. Clin Infect Dis 2001; 32:17–22.

241. Nelson LJ, Wells CD. Global epidemiology of childhood tuberculosis. Int J Tuberc Lung Dis 2004; 8:636–647.

242. Beyers N, Gie RP, Zietsman H, et al. The use of a geographical information system (GIS) to evaluate the distribution of tuberculosis in a high incidence community. S Afr Med J 1996; 86:40–44.

243. Balasegaram S, Watson JM, Rose AMC, et al. A decade of change: tuberculosis in England and Wales. Arch Dis Child 2003; 88:772–777.

244. American Thoracic Society/Centers for Disease Control and Prevention/Infectious Diseases Society of America: controlling tuberculosis in the United States. Am J Respir Crit Care Med 2005; 172:1169–2227.

245. Sharp D. Bovine tuberculosis and badger blame. Lancet 2006; 367:631–632.

246. Miller FJW. Tuberculosis in children. Edinburgh: Churchill Livingstone; 1982.

247. Dannenberg AM. Immune mechanism in the pathogenesis of pulmonary tuberculosis. Rev Infect Dis 1989; II(suppl 2):369–378.

248. Spellberg B, Edwards JE. Type 1/type 2 immunity in infectious diseases. Clin Infect Dis 2001; 32:76–102.

249. Rook GAW, Hernandez-Pando R. The pathogenesis of tuberculosis. Ann Rev Microbiol 1996; 50:259–284.

250. Smith DW, Wiegeshaus EH. What animal models can teach us about the pathogenesis of tuberculosis in humans. Rev Infect Dis 1989; II(suppl 2):385–393.

251. Steiner P, Rao M, Victoria MS, et al. Persistently negative tuberculin reactions. Am J Dis Child 1980; 134:747–750.

252. Pai M, Riley LW, Colford Jr JM. Interferon-γ assays in the immunodiagnosis of tuberculosis: a systematic review. Lancet Infect Dis 2004; 4:761–776.

253. Liebeschuetz S, Bamber S, Ewer K, et al. Diagnosis of tuberculosis in South African children with a T-cell-based assay: a prospective study. Lancet 2004; 364:2196–2203.

254. Department of Health (DoH). Immunization against infectious disease. London: HMSO; 2006.

255. Moss WJ, Clements CJ, Halsey NA. Immunisation of children at risk of infection with human immunodeficiency virus. Bull World Health Org 2003; 81:61–70.

256. Hesseling AC, Rabie H, Marais BJ, et al. Bacille Calmette-Guerin vaccine-induced disease in HIV-infected and HIV-uninfected children. Clin Infect Dis 2006; 42:548–558.

257. Casanova JL, Blanche S, Emile JF, et al. Idiopathic disseminated Bacille Calmette-Guerin infection: a French national retrospective study. Pediatrics 1996; 98:774–778.

258. Kroger L, Korppi M, Brander E, et al. Osteitis caused by Bacille Calmette-Guérin vaccinations: a retrospective analysis of 222 cases. J Infect Dis 1995; 172:574–576.

259. Rodrigues LC, Diwan VK, Wheeler JG. Protective effect of BCG against tuberculous meningitis and miliary tuberculosis: a meta analysis. Int J Epidemiol 1993; 22:1154–1158.

260. Colditz GA, Berkey CS, Mosteller F, et al. The efficacy of Bacillus Calmette-Guérin vaccination of newborns and infants in the prevention of tuberculosis: meta-analyses of the published literature. Pediatrics 1995; 96:29–35.

261. Boudin Trunz B, Fine PEM, Dye C. Effect of BCG vaccination on childhood tuberculous meningitis and miliary tuberculosis worldwide: a meta-analysis and assessment of cost-effectiveness. Lancet 2006; 367:1173–1180.

262. Fine PEM. Variation in protection by BCG: implications of and for heterologous immunity. Lancet 1995; ii:1339–1345.

263. Sutherland I, Springett VH. Effectiveness of BCG vaccination in England and Wales in 1983. Tubercle 1987; 68:81–92.

264. Ormerod LP, Garnett JM. Tuberculin skin reactivity four years after neonatal BCG vaccination. Arch Dis Child 1992; 67:530–531.

265. Teale C, Cundall DB, Pearson SB. Heaf status 12 years after BCG vaccination. Tuber Lung Dis 1992; 73:210–212.

266. Menzies D. What does tuberculin reactivity after Bacille Calmette-Guérin vaccination tell us. Clin Infect Dis 2000; 31(suppl 3):S71–S74.

267. Haile M, Kallenius G. Recent developments in tuberculosis vaccines. Curr Opin Infect Dis 2005; 18:211–215.

268. NICE guideline. Tuberculosis: clinical diagnosis and management of tuberculosis, and measures for its prevention and control. www.nice.org.uk/CGO33NICEguideline

269. Swanson DS, Starke JR. Drug-resistant tuberculosis in pediatrics. Pediatr Clin North Am 1995; 42:553–581.

270. Miller FJW. The natural history of primary tuberculosis. WHO/TB/84.144. Geneva: World Health Organization; 1984.

271. Delacourt C, Mani TM, Bonnerot V, et al. Computed tomography with normal chest radiograph in tuberculous infection. Arch Dis Child 1993; 69:430–432.

272. Khan EA, Starke JR. Diagnosis of tuberculosis in children: increased need for better methods. Emerg Infect Dis 1995; 1:115–122.

273. Vallejo JG, Ong LT, Starke JR. Clinical features, diagnosis and treatment of tuberculosis in infants. Pediatrics 1994; 84:1–7.

274. Graham SM, Gie RP, Schaaf HS, et al. Childhood tuberculosis: clinical research needs. Int J Tuberc Lung Dis 2004:8:648–657.

275. Thakur A, Coulter JBS, Zutshi K, et al. Laryngeal swabs for diagnosing tuberculosis. Ann Trop Paediatr 1999; 19:333–336.

276. Franchi LM, Cama RI, Gilman RH, et al. Detection of Mycobacterium tuberculosis in nasopharyngeal aspirate samples in children. Lancet 1998; 352:1681–1682.

277. Montenegro SH, Gilman RH, Sheen P, et al. Improved detection of Mycobacterium tuberculosis in Peruvian children by use of a heminested polymerase chain reaction assay. Clin Infect Dis 2003; 36:16–23.

278. Shata AMA, Coulter JBS, Parry CM, et al. Sputum induction for the diagnosis of tuberculosis. Arch Dis Child 1996; 74:535–536.

279. Zar HJ, Hanslo D, Apolles P, et al. Induced sputum versus gastric lavage for microbiological confirmation of pulmonary tuberculosis in infants and young children: a prospective study. Lancet 2005; 365:130–134.

280. Abadco DL, Steiner P. Gastric lavage is better than bronchoalveolar lavage for isolation of Mycobacterium tuberculosis in childhood pulmonary tuberculosis. Pediatr Infect Dis J 1992; 11:735–738.

281. Somu N, Swaminathan S, Paramasivan CN, et al. Value of bronchoalveolar lavage and gastric lavage in the diagnosis of pulmonary tuberculosis in children. Tuber Lung Dis 1995; 76:295–299.

282. American Thoracic Society. Treatment of tuberculosis and tuberculosis infection in adults and children. Am J Respir Crit Care Med 1994; 149:1359–1374.

*283. Matchaba PT, Volmink J. Steroids for treating tuberculous pleurisy. Cochrane Database Syst Rev 2000; (1):CD001876.

284. Hugo-Hamman CT, Scher H, De Moor MMA. Tuberculous pericarditis in children: a review of 44 cases. Pediatr Infect Dis J 1994; 13:13–18.

*285. Mayosi BM, Ntsekhe M, Volmink JA, et al. Interventions for treating tuberculous pericarditis. Cochrane Database Syst Rev 2002; (4):CD000526.

286. Strang JI, Nunn AJ, Johnson DA, et al. Management of tuberculous constrictive pericarditis and tuberculous pericardial effusion in Transkei: results at 10 years follow-up. QJM 2004; 97:525–535.

287. Hussey G, Chisholm T, Kibel M. Miliary tuberculosis in children: a review of 94 cases. Pediatr Infect Dis J 1991; 10:832–836.

288. Starke JR. Tuberculosis of the central nervous system in children. Semin Pediatr Neurol 1999; 6:318–331.

289. Donald PR, Schoeman JF, Cotton MF, et al. Cerebrospinal fluid investigations in tuberculous meningitis. Ann Trop Paediatr 1991; 11:241–246.

290. Hejazi N, Hassler W. Multiple intracranial tuberculomas with atypical response to tuberculostatic chemotherapy: literature review and a case report. Infection 1997; 25:233–239.

291. Ravenscroft A, Schoeman JF, Donald PR. Tuberculous granulomas in childhood tuberculous meningitis: radiological features and course. J Trop Pediatr 2001; 47:5–12.

292. Jacobs RF, Sunakorn P, Chotpitayasunonah T, et al. Intensive short course chemotherapy for tuberculous meningitis. Pediatr Infect Dis J 1992; 11:194–198.

293. Donald PR, Schoeman JF, Van Zyl LE, et al. Intensive short course chemotherapy in the management of tuberculous meningitis. Int J Tuber Lung Dis 1998; 2:704–711.

294. Donald PR, Seifart HI. Cerebrospinal fluid concentration of ethionamide in children with tuberculous meningitis. J Pediatr 1989; 115:483–486.

295. Humphries M. The management of tuberculous meningitis. Thorax 1992; 47:577–581.

296. Ellard GA, Humphries MJ, Allen BW. Cerebrospinal drug concentrations and the treatment of tuberculous meningitis. Am Rev Respir Dis 1993; 148:650–655.

297. Girgis NI, Farid Z, Kilpatrick ME, et al. Dexamethasone adjunctive treatment for tuberculous meningitis. Pediatr Infect Dis J 1991; 10:179–183.

298. Schoeman JF, Van Zyl LE, Laubscher JA, et al. Effect of corticosteroids on intracranial pressure, computed tomographic findings, and clinical outcome in young children with tuberculous meningitis. Pediatrics 1997; 99:226–231.

299. Prasad K, Volmink J, Menon GR. Steroids for treating tuberculous meningitis (Cochrane Review). In: The Cochrane Library, 3. Oxford: Update Software; 2000.

300. Humphries MJ, Teoh R, Lau J, et al. Factors of prognostic significance in Chinese children with tuberculous meningitis. Tubercle 1990; 71:161–168.

301. Starke J, Correa AG. Management of mycobacterial infection and disease in children. Pediatr Infect Dis J 1995; 14:455–470.

302. Shribman JH, Eastwood JBJ, Uff J. Immune complex nephritis complicating miliary tuberculosis. BMJ 1983; 287:1593–1594.

303. Lancet Editorial. Perinatal prophylaxis of tuberculosis. Lancet 1990; ii:1479–1480.

304. Connolly Smith K. Congenital tuberculosis: a rare manifestation of a common infection. Curr Opin Infect Dis 2002;15:269–274.

305. Thomas P, Bornschlegel K, Singh TP, et al. Tuberculosis in human immunodeficiency virus-infected and human immunodeficiency virus-exposed children in New York City. Pediatr Infect Dis J 2000; 19:700–706.

306. Graham SM, Coulter JBS, Gilks CF. Pulmonary disease in HIV-infected African children. Int J Tuber Lung Dis 2000; 15:12–23.

307. Cotton MF, Schaaf HS, Hesseling AC, et al. HIV and childhood tuberculosis: the way forward. Int J Tuberc Lung Dis 2004; 8:675–682.

308. Hesseling AC, Westra AE, Werschkull H, et al. Outcome of HIV-infected children with culture confirmed tuberculosis. Arch Dis Child 2005; 90:1171–1174.

*309. Woldehanna S, Volmink J. Treatment of latent tuberculous infection in HIV infected persons. Cochrane Database Syst Rev 2004; (1):CD000171.

310. British Thoracic Society: Joint Tuberculosis Committee. Chemotherapy and management of tuberculosis in the United Kingdom. Thorax 1998; 53:536–548.

311. Frieden TR, Sterling TR, Munsiff SS, et al. Tuberculosis. Lancet 2003; 362:887–899.

*312. Volmink J, Garner P. Directly observed therapy for treating tuberculosis. Cochrane Database of Syst Rev 2006; (2):CD003343.

313. Reed MD, Blumer JL. Clinical pharmacology of antitubercular drugs. Pediatr Clin North Am 1983; 30:177–193.

314. Ormerod LP, Skinner C, Wales J. Hepatotoxicity of antituberculosis drugs. Thorax 1996; 51:111–113.

315. Dooley DP, Carpenter JL, Rademacher S. Adjunctive corticosteroid therapy for tuberculosis: a critical reappraisal of the literature. Clin Infect Dis 1997; 25:872–887.

Bacterial Infections: Mycobacteria – Environmental

316. Grange JM. Mycobacteria and human disease. London: Edward Arnold; 1988.

317. Coulter JBS, Lloyd DA, Jones M, et al. Nontuberculous mycobacterial adenitis: effectiveness of chemotherapy following incomplete excision. Acta Paediatr 2006; 95:182–188.

318. Starke JR. Nontuberculous mycobacterial infections in children. Adv Pediatr Infect Dis 1992; 7:123–159.

319. Wolinsky E. Mycobacterial diseases other than tuberculosis. Clin Infect Dis 1992; 15:1–12.

320. Romanus V, Hallander HO, Wahten P, et al. Atypical mycobacteria in extrapulmonary disease among children. Incidence in Sweden from 1969 to 1990 related to changing BCG vaccination coverage. Tuber Lung Dis 1995; 76:300–310.

321. Jindal N, Devi B, Aggarwal A. Mycobacterial cervical lymphadenitis in childhood. Ind J Med Sci 2003; 57:12–15.

322. Nylen O, Berg-Kelly K, Andersson B. Cervical lymph node infections with non-tuberculous mycobacteria in preschool children: interferon gamma deficiency as a possible cause of clinical infection. Acta Paediatr 2000; 89:1322–1325.

323. Wolinsky E. Mycobacterial lymphadenitis in children: a prospective study of 105 non-tuberculous cases with long-term follow-up. Clin Infect Dis 1995; 20:954–963.

324. Starke JR, Correa AG. Management of mycobacterial infection and disease in children. Pediatr Infect Dis J 1995; 14:455–470.

325. Wansbrough-Jones M, Phillips R. Buruli ulcer: emerging from obscurity. Lancet 2006; 367:1849–1858.

326. Dore ND, Le Sou'f PN, Masters B. Atypical mycobacterial pulmonary disease and bronchial obstruction in HIV-negative children. Pediatr Pulmonol 1997; 26:380–388.

327. Oliver KN, Yankaskas JR, Knowles MR. Non-tuberculous mycobacterial pulmonary disease in cystic fibrosis. Semin Respir Infect 1996; 11:272–284.

*328. British Thoracic Society. Management of opportunist mycobacterial infections: Joint Tuberculosis Committee Guidelines 1999. Thorax 2000; 55:210–218.

329. Lammas DA, Casanova JL, Kumararatne DS. Clinical consequences of defects in the IL-12-dependent interferon-gamma (IFN-gamma) pathway. Clin Exp Immunol 2000; 121:417–425.

*330. Gordin FM, Sullam PM, Shafran SD, et al. A randomised placebo-controlled study of rifabutin added to a regimen of clarithromycin and ethambutol for treatment of disseminated infection with Mycobacterium avium complex. Clin Infect Dis 1999; 28:1080–1085.

Bacterial Infections: Pertussis (Whooping Cough)

331. Olin P, Rasmussen F, Gustafsson L, et al. Randomised controlled trial of two-component, three-component and five-component acellular pertussis vaccines compared with whole-cell vaccine. Lancet 1997; 350:1569–1577.

Bacterial Infections: Pneumococcus

332. Gray BM, Dillon HC. Natural history of pneumococcal infections. Pediatr Infect Dis J 1989; 8 (suppl):S23–S25.

333.   Hussain M, Melegaro A, Pebody RG, et al. A longitudinal household study of *Streptococcus pneumoniae* nasopharyngeal carriage in a UK setting. Epidemiol Infect 2005; 133:891–898.

334.   Obaro SK, Monteil MA, Henderson DC. The pneumococcal problem. BMJ 1996; 312:1521–1525.

335.   Earley A, Richman S, Ansell BM. Pneumococcal arthritis mimicking juvenile chronic arthritis. Arch Dis Child 1988; 63:1089–1090.

336.   Lister PD. Multiply-resistant pneumococcus: therapeutic problems in the management of serious infections. Eur J Clin Microbiol Infect Dis 1995; 14(suppl 1):18–25.

337.   Ada G, Isaacs D. Vaccination: the facts, the fears, the future. Sydney: Allen & Unwin; 2000.

*338.   Black S, Shinefield H, Fireman B, et al. Efficacy, safety and immunogenicity of heptavalent pneumococcal conjugate vaccine in children. Pediatr Infect Dis J 2000; 19:187–195.

*339.   Whitney CG, Farley MM, Hadler J, et al. Decline in invasive pneumococcal disease after the introduction of protein-polysaccharide conjugate vaccine. N Engl J Med 2003; 348:1737–1746.

340.   Klugman KP, Madhi SA, Huebner RE, et al. A trial of a 9-valent pneumococcal conjugate vaccine in children with and those without HIV infection. N Engl J Med 2003; 349:1341–1348.

341.   Black S, Shinefield H, Baxter R, et al. Impact of the use of heptavalent pneumococcal conjugate vaccine on disease epidemiology in children and adults. Vaccine 2006; 24Suppl 2:S2–79–80.

*342.   Whitney CG, Pilishvili T, Farley MM, et al. Effectiveness of seven-valent pneumococcal conjugate vaccine against invasive pneumococcal disease: a matched case-control study. Lancet 2006; 368: 1495–1502.

*343.   Grijalva CG, Nuorti JP, Arbogast PJ, et al. Decline in pneumonia admissions after routine childhood immunisation with pneumococcal conjugate vaccine in the USA: a time-series analysis. Lancet 2007; 369:1179–1186.

344.   Centers for Disease Control and Prevention (CDC). Direct and indirect effects of routine vaccination of children with 7-valent pneumococcal conjugate vaccine on incidence of invasive pneumococcal disease – United States, 1998–2003. MMWR Morb Mortal Wkly Rep 2005; 54:893–897.

345.   Poehling KA, Talbot TR, Griffin MR, et al. Invasive pneumococcal disease among infants before and after introduction of pneumococcal conjugate vaccine. JAMA 2006; 295:1668–1674.

346.   Abzug MJ, Pelton SI, Song LY, et al. Immunogenicity, safety, and predictors of response after a pneumococcal conjugate and pneumococcal polysaccharide vaccine series in human immunodeficiency virus-infected children receiving highly active antiretroviral therapy. Pediatr Infect Dis J 2006; 25:920–929.

347.   Gaston MH, Verter JI, Woods G, et al. Prophylaxis with oral penicillin in children with sickle cell anemia: a randomized trial. N Engl J Med 1986; 314:1593–1599.

Bacterial Infections: Pseudomonas

*348.   Boisseau AM, Sarlangue J, Perel Y, et al. Perineal ecthyma gangrenosum in infancy and early childhood: septicaemic and nonsepticaemic forms. J Am Acad Dermatol 1992; 27:415–418.

*349.   Henwood CJ, Livermore DM, James D, et al. Antimicrobial susceptibility of *Pseudomonas aeruginosa*: results of a UK survey and evaluation of the British Society for Antimicrobial Chemotherapy disc susceptibility test. J Antimicrob Chemother 2001; 47:789–799.

*350.   Mahenthiralingam E, Baldwin A, Vandamme P. *burkholderia cepacia* complex in patients with cystic fibrosis. J Med Microbial 2002; 51:533–538.

*351.   Chaowagul W. Recent advances in the treatment of severe melioidosis. Acta Trop 2000; 74:133–137.

Bacterial Infections: Relapsing Fever

352.   Mekasha A, Mehari S. Outbreak of louse-borne relapsing fever in Jimma, south Western Ethiopia. East Afr Med J 1996; 73:54–58.

353.   Southern PM, Sanford JP. Relapsing fever; Clinical and microbiological review. Medicine 1969; 48:12–49.

354.   Mekasha A. Louse-borne relapsing fever in children. J Trop Med Hyg 1992; 95:206–209.

355.   Hodes R. Relapsing fever. In: Zein AZ, Kloos H, eds. The ecology of health and disease in Ethiopia. Addis Ababa: Ministry of Health; 1988:177–183.

356.   Fekade D, Knox K, Hussein K, et al. Prevention of Jarisch–Herxheimer reaction by treatment with antibodies against tumor necrosis factor alpha. N Engl J Med 1996; 335:311–315.

357.   Cox RE, Fekade D, Knox K, et al. The effect of TNFα on cytokine response in Jarisch–Herxheimer reactions of louse-borne relapsing fever. Q J Med 1997; 90:213–221.

358.   Daniel E, Beyene H, Tessema T. Relapsing fever in children – demographic, social and clinical features. Ethiop Med J 1992; 30:207–214.

359.   Bryceson ADM, Parry EHO, Perine PL, et al. Louse-borne relapsing fever: A clinical and laboratory study of 62 cases in Ethiopia and reconsideration of the literature. Q J Med 1970; 39:129–170.

360.   Salih SY, Mustafa D. Louse-borne relapsing fever. II Combined penicillin and tetracycline therapy in 160 Sudanese patients. Trans R Soc Trop Med Hyg 1977; 71:49–50.

361.   Teklu B, Habte-michael A, Warrell DA, et al. Meptazinol diminishes the Jarisch–Herxheimer reaction of relapsing fever. Lancet 1983; 1:835–839.

362.   Barclay AJG, Coulter JBS. Tick-borne relapsing fever in central Tanzania. Trans R Soc Trop Med Hyg 1990; 84:852–856.

363.   Ramos JM, Malmierca E, Reyes F, et al. Characteristics of louse-borne relapsing fever in Ethiopian children and adults. Ann Trop Med Parasitol 2004; 98:191–196.

364.   Mitiku K, Mengistu G. Relapsing fever in Gondar, Ethiopia. East Afr Med J 2002; 79:85–87.

Bacterial Infections: Salmonellosis

365.   Graham SM. Salmonellosis in children in developing and developed countries and populations. Curr Opin Infect Dis 2002; 15:507–512.

366.   Weinberger M, Keller N. Recent trends in the epidemiology of non-typhoid Salmonella and antimicrobial resistance: the Israeli experience and worldwide review. Curr Opin Infect Dis 2005; 18:513–521.

367.   Graham SM, Molyneux EM, Walsh AL, et al. Nontyphoidal Salmonella infections of children in tropical Africa. Pediatr Infect Dis J 2000; 19:1189–1196.

368.   Brent A, Oundo JO, Mwangi I, et al. Salmonella bacteremia in Kenyan children. Pediatr Infect Dis J 2006; 25:230–236.

369.   Saha SK, Baqui AH, Hanif M, et al. Typhoid fever in Bangladesh: implications for vaccination policy. Pediatr Infect Dis J 2001; 20:521–524.

*370.   Sirinavin S, Garner P. Antibiotics for treating salmonella gut infections (Cochrane Review). In: The Cochrane Library, 4. Oxford: Update Software; 2001.

*371.   Sirinavin S, Thavornuth J, Sakchainanont B, et al. Norfloxacin and azithromycin for treatment of nontyphoidal salmonella carriers. Clin Infect Dis 2003; 37:685–691.

372.   St Geme JW, Hodes HL, Marcy SM, et al. Consensus management of *Salmonella* infection in the first year of life. Pediatr Infect Dis J 1988; 7:615–621.

Bacterial Infections: Typhoid Fever

373.   Health Protection Agency. Accessed at www. hpa.org.uk/infections/default.htm

374.   World Health Organization background document. The diagnosis, treatment and prevention of typhoid fever. WHO/V&B/03.07. Accessed at www. who.int/entity/vaccine-_research/documents/en/ typhoid-diagnosis.pdf on 26.04.07

375.   Parry CM. Typhoid fever. Curr Infect Dis Rep 2004; 6:27–33.

376.   Mahle WT, Levine MM. *Salmonella typhi* infections in children younger than five years of age. Pediatr Infect Dis J 1993; 12:627–631.

*377.   Parry CM, Ho VA, Phuong LT, et al. Randomized controlled comparison of ofloxacin, azithromycin, and an ofloxacin-azithromycin combination for treatment of multidrug-resistant and nalidixic acid-resistant typhoid fever. Antimicrob Agents Chemother 2007; 51:819–825.

378.   Cooke FJ, Wain J, Threlfall EJ. Fluoroquinolone resistance in *Salmonella* typhi. BMJ 2006; 33: 353–354.

379.   Schaad UB. Pediatric use of quinolones. Pediatr Infect Dis J 1999; 18:469–470.

*380.   Punjabi NH, Hoffman SL, Edman DC, et al. Treatment of severe typhoid fever in children with high dose dexamethasone. Pediatr Infect Dis J 1988; 7:598–600.

*381.   Engels EA, Lau J. Vaccines for preventing typhoid fever (Cochrane Review). In: The Cochrane Library, 4. Oxford: Update Software; 2001.

382.   Lin FYC, Ho VA, Khiem HB, et al. The efficacy of a *Salmonella typhi* Vi conjugate vaccine in two-to-five year-old children. N Engl J Med 2001; 344: 1263–1269.

Bacterial Infections: *Shigella* (Bacillary Dysentery)

383   Kotloff KL, Winickoff JP, Ivanoff B, et al. Global burden of Shigella infections: Implications for vaccine development and implementation. Bull WHO 1999; 77:651–656.

384.   Goma Epidemiology Group. Public health impact of Rwandan refugee crisis: what happened in Goma, Zaire, in July, 1994? Goma Epidemiology Group. Lancet 1995; 345:339–344.

385.   Clemens JD, Stanton B, Stoll B, et al. Breast feeding as a determinant of severity in shigellosis. Evidence for protection throughout the first three years of life in Bangladeshi children. Am J Epidemiol 1986; 123:710–720.

386.   Tacket CO, Binion SB, Bostwick E, et al. Efficacy of bovine milk immunoglobulin concentrate in preventing illness after *Shigella flexneri* challenge. Am J Trop Med Hyg 1992; 47:276–283.

387.   Levine MM, Kotloff KL, Barry EM, et al. Clinical trials of Shigella vaccines: Two steps forward and one step back on a long, hard road. Nat Rev Microbiol In press 2007.

Bacterial Infections: Staphylococcus

388.   Yamasaki O, Yamaguchi T, Sugai M, et al. Clinical manifestations of staphylococcal scalded-skin syndrome depend on serotypes of exfoliative toxins. J Clin Microbiol 2005; 43:1890–1893.

389.   Gillet Y, Issartel B, Vanhems P, et al. Association between *Staphylococcus aureus* strains carrying gene for Panton-Valentine leukocidin and highly lethal necrotising pneumonia in young immunocompetent patients. Lancet 2002; 359:753–759.

390.   Hiramatsu K. Vancomycin-resistant *Staphylococcus aureus*: a new model of antibiotic resistance. Lancet Infect Dis 2001; 1:147–155.

Bacterial Infections: *Streptococcus and Enterococcus*

391.   Stevens DL. Invasive group A streptococcus infections. Clin Infect Dis 1992; 14:2–11.

392.   Zirakzadeh A, Patel R. Vancomycin-resistant enterococci: colonization, infection, detection, and treatment. Mayo Clin Proc 2006; 81:529–536.

Bacterial Infections: Tetanus

393.   Farrar JJ, Yen LM, Cook T, et al. Tetanus. J Neurol Neurosurg Psych 2000; 69:292–301.

394. Whitman C, Belgharbi L, Gasse F, et al. Progress towards the global elimination of neonatal tetanus. World Health Stat Q 1992; 45:248–256.

395. Silveira CM, Caceres VM, Dutra MG, et al. Safety of tetanus toxoid in pregnant women: a hospital-based case control study of congenital anomalies. Bull WHO 1995; 73:605–608.

396. Thwaites CL, Yen LM, Loan HT, et al. Magnesium sulphate for treatment of severe tetanus: a randomised controlled trial. Lancet 2006; 368:1436–1443.

397. Anlar B, Yalaz K, Dizmen R. Long-term prognosis after neonatal tetanus. Develop Med Child Neurol 1989; 31:76–80.

Bacterial Infections: Tularemia

398. Johansson A, Ibrahim A, Goransson I, et al. Evaluation of PCR-based methods for discrimination of *Francisella* species and subspecies and development of a specific PCR that distinguishes the two major subspecies of *Francisella tularensis*. J Clin Microbiol 2000; 38:4180–4185.

*****399.** Staples JE, Kubota KA, Chalcraft LG, et al. Epidemiologic and molecular analysis of human tularemia, United States, 1964–2004. Emerg Infect Dis 2006; 12:1113–1118.

400. Payne L, Arneborn M, Tegnell A, et al. Endemic tularemia, Sweden, 2003. Emerg Infect Dis 2005; 11:1440–1442.

401. Oyston PC, Sjostedt A, Titball RW. Tularaemia: bioterrorism defence renews interest in Francisella tularensis. Nat Rev Microbiol 2004; 2:967–978.

402. Jacobs RF, Condrey YM, Yamauchi T. Tularemia in adults and children: a changing presentation. Pediatrics 1985; 76:818–822.

403. Enderlin G, Morales L, Jacobs RF, et al. Streptomycin and alternative agents for the treatment of tularemia: review of the literature. Clin Infect Dis 1994; 19:42–47.

404. Johansson A, Berglund L, Gothefors L, et al. Ciprofloxacin for treatment of tularemia in children. Pediatr Infect Dis J 2000; 19:449–453.

405. American Academy of Pediatrics. Tularemia. In: Pickering LK, ed. Red book: Report of the Committee on Infectious Diseases, 25th edn. Elk Grove Village: American Academy of Pediatrics; 2000:618–620.

Bacterial Infections: Yersiniosis and Plague

406. Cover TL, Aber RC. *Yersinia enterocolitica*. N Engl J Med 1989; 321:16–24.

407. Naktin J, Beavis KG. *Yersinia enterocolitica* and *Yersinia pseudotuberculosis*. Clin Lab Med 1999; 19:523–536.

408. Fredriksson-Ahomaa M, Stolle A, Korkeala H. Molecular epidemiology of *Yersinia enterocolitica* infections. FEMS Immunol Med Microbiol 2006; 47:315–329.

409. Larson JH. The spectrum of clinical manifestations of infections with *Yersinia enterocolitica* and their pathogenesis. Contrib Microbiol Immunol 1979; 5:257–269.

410. Abdel-Haq NM, Papadopol R, Asmar BI, et al. Antibiotic susceptibilities of *Yersinia enterocolitica* recovered from children over a 12-year period. Int J Antimicrob Agents 2006; 27:449–452.

411. Perry RD, Fetherston JD. *Yersinia pestis* – etiologic agent of plague. Clin Microbiol Rev 1997; 10:35–66.

412. Smego RA, Frean J, Koornhof HJ. Yersiniosis I: microbiological and clinicoepidemiological aspects of plague and non-plague Yersinia infections. Eur J Clin Microbiol Infect Dis 1999; 18:1–15.

*****413.** Mwengee W, Butler T, Mgema S, et al. Treatment of plague with gentamicin or doxycycline in a randomized clinical trial in Tanzania. Clin Infect Dis 2006; 42:614–621.

Use of the Virology Laboratory by The Clinician

414. Fong C, Lee M, Griffith B. Evaluation of R-mix fresh cells in shell vials for detection of respiratory viruses. J Clin Microbiol 2000; 38:4660–4662.

415. Liolios L, Jenney A, Spelman D, et al. Comparison of a multiplex reverse transcription-PCR-enzyme hybridization assay with conventional viral culture and immunofluorescence techniques for the detection of seven viral respiratory pathogens. J Clin Microbiol 2001; 39:2779–2783.

416. Mancini A. Exanthems in childhood: an update. Pediatr Ann 1998; 27:163–170.

417. Sawyer MH. Enterovirus infections; Diagnosis and treatment. Curr Opin Paediatr 2001; 13:65–69.

418. Gubler DJ. Resurgent vector-born diseases as a global health problem. Emerg Infect Dis 1998; 4:442–450.

419. Levy J. Three new human herpes viruses (HHV-6, 7 and 8). Lancet 1997; 349:558–562.

420. Yan SS, Fedoroko DP. Recent advances in laboratory diagnosis of human cytomegalovirus infection. Clin Appl Immunol Rev 2002; 2:155–167.

421. Berger C, Day P, Meier G, et al. Dynamics of Epstein-Barr virus DNA levels in serum during EBV-associated disease. J Med Virol 2001; 64:505–512.

422. Fong IW, Britton CB, Luinstra KL, et al. Diagnostic value of detecting JC virus DNA in cerebrospinal fluid of patients with progressive multifocal leukoencephalopathy. J Clin Microbiol 1995; 33:484–486.

423. van den Hoogen BG, de Jong JC, Groen J, et al. A newly discovered human pneumovirus isolated from young children with respiratory tract disease. Nat Med 2001; 7:719–724.

424. Ksiazek TG, Erdman D, Goldsmith CS, et al. A novel coronavirus associated with severe acute respiratory syndrome. N Engl J Med 2003; 348:1953–1966.

HIV Infection

425. Palella FJ Jr, Delaney KM, Moorman AC, et al. Declining morbidity and mortality among patients with advanced human immunodeficiency virus infection. HIV outpatient study investigators. N Engl J Med 1998; 338:853–860.

426. Gibb DM, Duong T, Tookey PA et al. Decline in mortality, AIDS, and hospital admissions in perinatally HIV-1 infected children in the United Kingdom and Ireland. BMJ 2003; 327:1019–1021.

427. European Collaborative Study. HIV-infected pregnant women and vertical transmission in Europe since 1986. AIDS 2001; 15:761–770.

428. Duong T, Ades AE, Gibb DM, et al. HIV vertical transmission in the British Isles: estimates based on surveillance data. BMJ 1999; 319:1227–1229.

429. Joint United Nations Programme on HIV/AIDS. Report on the global HIV/AIDS epidemic. UNAIDS 2006. Available: http://www.unaids.org.

430. Pedraza MA, del Romero J, Roldan F, et al. Heterosexual transmission of HIV-1 is associated with high plasma viral load levels and a positive viral isolation in the infected partner. J Acquir Immune Defic Syndr 1999; 21:120–125.

431. Struick S, Tudor-Williams G, Taylor GP, et al. 4 Cases of infant HIV due to seroconversion in pregnancy; Should partner screening and/or repeat 3rd trimester HIV screening be recommended in the UK? BHIVA 12th Annual Conference, April 2006, p.68.

432. Judd A, Doerholt K, Sharland M, et al. Morbidity, mortality, and response to treatment in perinatally HIV-infected children in the UK and Ireland, 1996–2006: planning for teenage and adult care. In press BMJ 2007

433. European Collaborative Study. The mother-to-child HIV transmission epidemic in Europe: evolving in the East and established in the West. AIDS 2006; 20:1419–1427.

434. Ades AE, Walker J, Botting B, et al. Effect of the worldwide epidemic on HIV prevalence in the United Kingdom: record linkage in anonymous neonatal seroprevalence surveys. AIDS 1999; 13:2437–2443.

435. Cliffe S, Tookey PA, Nicoll A. Antenatal detection of HIV: national surveillance and unlinked anonymous survey. BMJ 2001; 323:376–377.

436. Supplementary data tables: Unlinked Anonymous Prevalence surveys of Pregnant Women: data to the end of 2004 Surveillance Update: 2005 HPA.

437. Melvin D, Jungmann E, Foster C, et al. Guidance on transition and long term follow up services for adolescents with HIV infection acquired in infancy. CHIVA Guidelines 2005 (updated Feb 2007) Available: http://www.BHIVA.org

438. Peckham C, Gibb DM. Mother-to-child transmission of the human immunodeficiency virus. N Engl J Med 1995; 333:298–302.

439. Dunn DT, Newell ML, Ades AE, et al. Risk of human immunodeficiency virus type 1 transmission through breastfeeding. Lancet 1992; 340:585–588.

440. Fowler MC, Simonds RJ, Roonsgpisuthipong A. Update on perinatal HIV transmission. Pediatr Clin North Am 2000; 47:21–38.

441. Mandelbrot L, Le Chenadec J, Berrebi A, et al. Perinatal HIV-1 transmission. Interaction between zidovudine prophylaxis and mode of delivery in the French perinatal cohort. JAMA 1998; 280:55–60.

442. Connor EM, Mofenson LM. Zidovudine for the reduction of perinatal human immunodeficiency virus transmission: Pediatric AIDS Clinical Trials Group Protocol 076 – results and treatment recommendations. Pediatr Infect Dis J 1995; 14:536–541.

443. Fiscus SA, Adimora AA, Schoenbach VJ, et al. Perinatal HIV infection and the effect of zidovudine therapy on transmission in rural and urban countries. JAMA 1996; 275:1483–1488.

444. Mandelbroot L, Landreau-Mascaro A, Rekacewicz C, et al. Lamivudine-zidovudine combination for prevention of maternal-infant transmission of HIV-1. JAMA 2001; 285:2083–2093.

445. Cooper ER, Charurat M, Mofenson L, et al. Combination antiretroviral strategies for the treatment of pregnant HIV-1-infected women and prevention of perinatal HIV-1 transmission. J Acquir Immune Defic Syndr 2002; 29:484–494.

446. Mofenson LM, Lambert JS, Stiehm ER, et al. Risk factors for perinatal transmission of human immunodeficiency virus type 1 in women treated with zidovudine. Pediatric AIDS Clinical Trials Group Study 185 Team. N Engl J Med 1999; 341:385–393.

447. Ioannidis JP, Abrams EJ, Ammann A, et al. Perinatal transmission of human immunodeficiency virus type 1 by pregnant women with RNA virus loads 1000 copies/ml. J Infect Dis 2001; 183:539–545.

448. Guay LA, Musoke P, Fleming T, et al. Intrapartum and neonatal single-dose nevirapine compared with zidovudine for prevention of mother-to-child transmission of HIV-1 in Kampala, Uganda; HIVNET 012 randomized trial. Lancet 1999; 354:795–802.

449. British HIV Association (BHIVA). Guidelines for the management of HIV infection in pregnant women and the prevention of mother-to-child transmission. 2005. Available: http://www.BHIVA.org

450. Live document a. Public Health Service Task Force recommendations for the use of antiretroviral drugs in pregnant women infected with HIV-1 for maternal health and interventions to reduce perinatal HIV-1 transmission in the United States. 12 October 2006 Available: http://www.hivatis.org.

451. Schaffer N, Chuachoowong R, Mock PA, et al. Short-course zidovudine for perinatal HIV-1 transmission in Bangkok. Collaborative Oriental HIV Transmission Study group. Lancet 1999; 353:773–780.

452. Lallemant M, Jourdain G, Le Coeur S, et al. A trial of shortened zidovudine regimens to prevent mother-to-child transmission of human immunodeficiency virus type 1. N Engl J Med 2000; 343:982–991.

453. The PETRA Study Team. Efficacy of three short-course regimens of zidovudine and lamivudine in preventing early and late transmission of HIV-1 from mother to child in Tanzania, South Africa, and Uganda (Petra Study): a randomised, double-blind, placebo-controlled trial. Lancet 2002; 359:1178–1186.

454. Muro E, Droste JA, Hofstede HT, et al. Nevirapine plasma concentrations are still detectable after more than 2 weeks in the majority of women receiving single-dose nevirapine: implications for intervention studies. J Acquir Immune Defic Syndr 2005; 39:419–421.

455. Johnson JA, Li JF, Morris L, et al. Emergence of drug-resistant HIV-1 after intrapartum administration of single-dose nevirapine is substantially under-estimated. J Infect Dis 2005; 192:16–23.

456. Flys T, Nissley DV, Claasen CW, et al. Sensitive drug-resistance assays reveal long-term persistence of HIV-1 variants with the K103N nevirapine (NVP) resistance mutation in some women and infants after the administration of single-dose NVP: HIVNET 012. J Infect Dis 2005; 192:24–29.

457. Jourdian G, Ngo-Giang-Huong N, et al. Perinatal HIV Prevention Trial Group. Intrapartum exposure to nevirapine and subsequent maternal responses to nevirapine-based antiretroviral therapy. N Engl J Med 2004; 351:229–240.

458. Martinson NA, Morris L, Gray G, et al. Selection and persistence of viral resistance in HIV-infected children after exposure to single-dose nevirapine. J Acquir Immune Defic Syndr 2007; 44:148–153.

459. McIntyre J, Martinson N, Boltz V, et al. Addition of short course Combivir (CBV) to single dose Viramune (sdNVP) for prevention of mother-to-child transmission of HIV-1 can significantly decrease the subsequent development of maternal NNRTI-resistant virus. XV Intl AIDS Conference, Bangkok. LbOrB09.

460. McIntyre JA, Martinson N, Gray GE, et al. Single dose nevirapine combined with a short course of Combivir for prevention of mother to child transmission of HIV-1 can significantly decrease the subsequent development of maternal and infant resistant virus. 14th International HIV Drug Resistance Workshop Quebec June 2005. Abstract 2.

461. Eshleman SH, Hoover DR, Hudelson SE, et al. Development of nevirapine resistance in infants is reduced by use of infant-only single-dose nevirapine plus zidovudine postexposure prophylaxis for the prevention of mother-to-child transmission of HIV-1. J Infect Dis 2006; 193:479–481.

462. Lockman S, Shapiro RL, Smeaton LM, et al. Response to antiretroviral therapy after a single, peripartum dose of nevirapine. N Engl J Med 2007; 356:135–147.

463. European Collaborative Study. Mother-to-child transmission of HIV infection in the era of highly active antiretroviral therapy. Clin Infect Dis 2005; 40:458–465.

464. Suy A, Coll O, Martinez E, et al. Increased risk of pre-eclampsia and foetal death in HIV-infected pregnant women receiving highly active antiretroviral therapy. XV International AIDS Conference, Bangkok, 2004 Abs ThOrB1359.

465. Thorne C, Patel D, Newell ML. Increased risk of adverse pregnancy outcomes in HIV-infected women treated with highly active antiretroviral therapy in Europe. AIDS 2004; 18:2337–2339.

466. Tuomala RE, Shapiro DE, Mofenson LM, et al. Antiretroviral therapy during pregnancy and the risk of an adverse outcome. N Engl J Med 2002; 346:1863–1870.

467. Blanche S, Tardieu M, Rustin P, et al. Persistent mitochondrial dysfunction and perinatal exposure to antiretroviral nucleoside analogues. Lancet 1999; 354:1084–1089.

468. Dominguez K, Bertolli J, Fowler M, et al. Lack of definitive severe mitochondrial signs or symptoms among deceased HIV uninfected and HIV indeterminate children < 5 years of age, Pediatric Spectrum of Disease Project (PSD), USA. Ann N Y Acad Sci 2000; 918:236–246.

469. Le Chenadec J, Mayaux MJ, Guihenneuc-Jouyaux C, et al; Enquete Perinatale Francaise Study Group. Perinatal antiretroviral treatment and hematopoiesis in HIV-uninfected infants. AIDS 2003; 17:2053–2061.

470. International Perinatal HIV Group. Duration of ruptured membranes and vertical transmission of HIV-1: a meta-analysis from 15 prospective cohort studies. AIDS 2001; 15:357–368.

471. European Mode of Delivery Collaboration. Elective caesarean-section versus vaginal delivery in prevention of vertical HIV-1 transmission: a randomised clinical trial. Lancet 1999; 353:1035–1039.

472. International Perinatal HIV Group. Mode of delivery and the risk of vertical transmission of human immunodeficiency virus type 1. A meta-analysis of fifteen prospective cohort studies. N Engl J Med 1999; 340:977–987.

473. Read JS. Caesarean section delivery to prevent vertical transmission of human immunodeficiency virus type 1. Associated risks and other considerations. Ann N Y Acad Sci 2000; 918:115–121.

474. Leroy V, Newell ML, Dabis F, et al. International multicentre pooled analysis of late postnatal mother-to-child transmission of HIV-1 infection. Ghent International Working Group on Mother-to-Child Transmission of HIV. Lancet 1998; 352:597–600.

475. Nduati R, John G, Mhori-Ngacha D, et al. Effect of breast-feeding and formula feeding on transmission of HIV-1: a randomized clinical trial. JAMA 2000; 283:1167–1174.

476. WHO Collaborative Study Team on the role of Breastfeeding on the Prevention of Infant Mortality. Effect of breastfeeding on infant and child mortality due to infectious diseases in less developed countries: a pooled analysis. Lancet 2000; 355:451–455.

477. Coutsoudis A, Pillay K, Kuhn L, et al. Method of feeding and transmission of HIV-1 from mothers to children by 15 months of age: prospective cohort study from Durban, South Africa. AIDS 2001; 15:379–387.

478. Giuliano M, Guidotti G, Andreotti M, et al. Triple antiretroviral prophylaxis administered during pregnancy and after delivery significantly reduces breast milk viral load: a study within the Drug Resource Enhancement Against AIDS and Malnutrition Program. J Acquir Immune Defic Syndr 2007; 44:286–291.

479. Gaillard P, Mwanyumba F, Verhofstede C, et al. Vaginal lavage with chlorhexidine during labour to reduce mother-to-child HIV transmission: clinical trial in Mombasa, Kenya. AIDS 2001; 15:389–396.

480. Read JS, Bethel J, Harris DR, et al. Serum vitamin A concentrations in a North American cohort of human immunodeficiency virus type 1-infected children. National Institute of Child Health and Human Development Intravenous Immunoglobulin Clinical Trial Study Group. Pediatr Infect Dis J 1999; 18:134–142.

481. Fawzi WW, Msamanga G, Hunter D, et al. Randomized trial of vitamin supplements in relation to vertical transmission of HIV-1 in Tanzania. J Acquir Immune Defic Syndr 2000; 23:246–254.

482. Ades AE, Sculpher MJ, Gibb DM, et al. Cost-effectiveness of antenatal HIV screening in the UK. BMJ 1999; 319:1230–1234.

483. Williams AJ, Gibb DM. Pneumocystis carinii pneumonia and CMV infection in HIV infected infants. HIV and AIDS, Current Trends March; 2002:1–5.5.

484. De Cock KM, Fowler MG, Mercier E, et al. Prevention of mother-to-child HIV transmission in resource-poor countries: translating research into policy and practice. JAMA 2002; 283:1175–1182.

485. O'Brien SJ, Moore JP. The effect of genetic variation in chemokines and their receptors on HIV transmission and progression to AIDS. Immunol Rev 2000; 177:99–111.

486. Wasik TJ, Bratosiewicz J, Wierzbicki A, et al. Protective role of beta-chemokines associated with HIV-specific Th responses against perinatal HIV transmission. J Immunol 1999; 162:4355–4364.

487. Hogan CM, Hammer SM. Host determinants in HIV infection and disease. Part 1: cellular and humoral immune responses. Ann Intern Med 2001; 134:761–776.

488. Soudeyns H, Pantaleo G. The moving target: mechanisms of HIV persistence during primary infection. Immunol Today 1999; 20:446–450.

489. Feeney ME, Roosevelt KA, Tang Y, et al. Comprehensive screening reveals strong and broadly directed human immunodeficiency virus type 1-specific CD8 responses in perinatally infected children. J Virol 2003; 77:7492–7501.

490. Sandberg JK, Fast NM, Jordan KA. HIV-specific CD8+ T cell function in children with vertically acquired HIV-1 infection is critically influenced by age and the state of the CD4+ T cell compartment. J Immunol 2003; 170:4403–4410.

491. Shearer WT, Quinn TC, LaRussa P, et al. Viral load and disease progression in infants infected with human immunodeficiency virus type 1. Women and Infants Transmission Study Group. N Engl J Med 1997; 336:1337–1342.

492. Gibb DM, Newberry A, de Rossi A, et al. HIV-1 viral load and CD4 count in untreated children with vertically acquired asymptomatic or mild disease – PENTA 1 Virology. AIDS 1998; 12:F1–F8.

493. De Rossi A, Walker AS, De Forni D, et al. for PENTA. Relationship between changes in thymic emigrants and cell associated HIV-1 DNA in HIV-1-infected children initiating antiretroviral therapy. Antivir Ther 2005; 10:63–71.

494. Honeyborne I, Prendergast A, Pereyra F, et al. Control of HIV-1 is associated with HLA-B9913 and targeting of multiple GAG-specific CD8+ T cell epitopes. J Virol 2007; [Epub ahead of print]

495. Ho DD. Perspectives series: host/pathogen interactions. Dynamics of HIV-1 replication in vivo. J Clin Invest 1997; 99:2565–2567.

496. Zhang L, Ramratnam B, Tenner-Racz K, et al. Quantifying residual HIV-1 replication in patients receiving combination antiretroviral therapy. N Engl J Med 1999; 340:1605–1613.

497. Wade AM, Ades AE. Age-related reference ranges: significance tests for models and confidence intervals for centiles. Stat Med 1994; 13:2359–2367.

498. HIV Paediatric Prognostic Markers Collaborative Study (writing committee Dunn DT, Gibb DM, Duong T et al). Short-term risk of disease progression in HIV-1-infected children receiving no antiretroviral therapy or zidovudine monotherapy: a meta-analysis. Lancet 2003; 362:1605–1611.

499. HIV Paediatric Prognostic Markers Collaborative Study (writing committee Dunn DT, Gibb DM, Duong T et al). Use of total lymphocyte count for informing when to start antiretroviral therapy in HIV-infected children: a meta-analysis of longitudinal data. Lancet 2005; 366:1868–1874.

500. HIV Paediatric Prognostic Markers Collaborative Study (writing committee Dunn DT, Gibb DM, Duong T et al). Predictive value of absolute CD4 cell count for disease progression in untreated HIV-1 infected children. AIDS 2006; 20:1289–1294.

501. WHO case definitions of HIV for surveillance and revised clinical staging and immunological classification of HIV-related disease in adults and children. 7 August 2006. www.who. int/hiv/pub/guidelines.

502. Dunn D, Newell ML, Peckham C, et al. (for the European Collaborative Study Group). CD4 T cell count as a predictor of Pneumocystis carinii pneumonia in children born to mothers infected with HIV. BMJ 1994; 308:437–440.

503.   Galli L, de Martino M, Tovo PA, et al. Predictive value of the HIV paediatric classification system for the long term course of perinatally infected children. Int J Epidemiol 2000; 29:573–578.

504.   CDC. 1994 Revised classification system for human immunodeficiency virus infection in children <13 years of age. MMWR 1994; 43(RR-12).

505.   Dunn DT, Brandt CD, Krivine A, et al. The sensitivity of HIV-1 DNA polymerase chain reaction in the neonatal period and the relative contributions of intra-uterine and intra-partum transmission. AIDS 1995; 9:F7–11.

506.   Tovo PA, De Marino M, Gabiano C, et al. Prognostic factors and survival in children with perinatal HIV-1 infection. Lancet 1992; 339:1249–1253.

507.   Blanche S, Newell ML, Mayaux MJ, et al. Morbidity and mortality in European children vertically infected by HIV-1. The French Pediatric HIV Infection Study Group and European Collaborative Study. J Acquir Immune Defic Syndr 1998; 14:442–450.

508.   Diaz C, Hanson C, Cooper ER, et al. Disease progression in a cohort of infants with vertically acquired HIV infection observed from birth: the Women and Infants Transmission Study (WITS). J Acquir Immune Defic Syndr 1998; 18:221–228.

509.   Gona P, Van Dyke R, Williams P, et al. Incidence of opportunistic and other infections in HIV-infected children in the HAART era. JAMA 2006; 296:292–300.

510.   Dankner WM, Lindsey JC, Levin MJ and the Pediatric AIDS Clinical Trials Group 2001. Correlates of opportunistic infections in children infected with the human immunodeficiency virus managed before highly active antiretroviral therapy. Pediatr Infect Dis J 2001; 20:40–48.

511.   Simonds RJ, Oxtoby MJ, Caldwell MB, et al. Pneumocystis carinii pneumonia among US children with perinatally acquired HIV infection. JAMA 1993; 270:470–473.

512.   Williams AJ, Duong T, McNally LM, et al. Pneumocystis carinii pneumonia and cytomegalovirus infection in children with vertically acquired HIV infection. AIDS 2001; 15:335–339.

513.   Chintu C, Bhat GJ, Walker AS, et al. on behalf of the CHAP Trial team. A randomized placebo-controlled trial of cotrimoxazole as prophylaxis against opportunistic infections in HIV-infected Zambian children: the CHAP (Children With HIV Antibiotic Prophylaxis) Trial. Lancet 2004; 364:1865–1871.

514.   Chandwani S, Kaul A, Bebenroth D, et al. Cytomegalovirus infection in human immuno-deficiency virus type 1-infected children. Pediatr Infect Dis J 1996; 15:310–314.

515.   Gibb DM, Giacomelli A, Masters J, et al. Persistence of antibody responses to Haemophilus influenzae type b polysaccharide conjugate vaccine in children with vertically acquired human immunodeficiency virus infection. Pediatr Infect Dis J 1996; 15:1097–1101.

516.   Sharland M, Gibb DM, Holland F. Respiratory morbidity from lymphocytic interstitial pneumonitis (LIP) in vertically acquired HIV-1 infection. Arch Dis Child 1997; 76:334–337.

517.   Shanbhag MC, Rutstein RM, Zaoutis T, et al. Neurocognitive functioning in pediatric human immunodeficiency virus infection: effects of combined therapy. Arch Pediatr Adolesc Med 2005; 159:651–656.

518.   Chiriboga CA, Fleishman S, Champion S, et al. Incidence and prevalence of HIV encephalopathy in children with HIV infection receiving highly active anti-retroviral therapy (HAART). J Pediatr 2005; 146:402–407.

519.   Foster C, Biggs R, Melvin D, et al. Neurodevelopmental outcomes in children with HIV infection under 3 years of age. Dev Med Child Neurol 2006; 48:677–682.

520.   Gifford GM, Polesel J, Rickenbach M, et al. Cancer risk in the Swiss HIV Cohort Study: associations with immunodeficiency, smoking, and highly active antiretroviral therapy. J Natl Cancer Inst 2005; 97:407–409.

521.   Evans JA, Gibb DM, Holland FJ, et al. Malignancies in children with HIV infection acquired from mother-to-child transmission in the United Kingdom. Arch Dis Child 1997; 76:330–334.

522.   Rabkin CS. AIDS and cancer in the era of highly active antiretroviral therapy (HAART). Eur J Cancer 2001; 37:1316–1319.

523.   Kest H, Brogly S, McSherry G, et al. Malignancy in perinatally human immunodeficiency virus-infected children in the United States. Pediatr Infect Dis J 2005; 24:237–242.

524.   Krishnan A, Molina A, Zaia J, et al. Durable remissions with autologous stem cell transplantation for high-risk HIV-associated lymphomas. Blood 2005; 105:874–878.

525.   McCarthy GA, Kampmann G, Novelli V, et al. Vertical transmission of Kaposi's sarcoma. Arch Dis Child 1996; 76:455–457.

526.   Walker AS, Mulenga V, Sinyinza F, et al. and the CHAP Trial Team. Determinants of survival without antiretroviral therapy after infancy in HIV-1 infected African children in the CHAP Trial. J Acquir Immune Defic Syndr 2006; 42:637–645.

527.   Kinghorn G. A sexual health and HIV strategy for England. BMJ 2001; 323:243–244.

528.   British HIV Association Guidelines (BHIVA) for the treatment of HIV-infected adults with antiretroviral therapy 2005. Available: http://www.bhiva.org.

529.   Guidelines for the use of antiretroviral agents in HIV infected adults and adolescents Available: http://www.aidsinfo.nih.gov/Guidelines2006

530.   Sharland M, Blanche S, Castelli G, et al; PENTA Steering Committee PENTA guidelines for the use of antiretroviral therapy, 2004. HIV Med 2004;5 Suppl 2:61–86. Available: http://www.bhiva.org and www.pentatrials.org

531.   Guidelines for the use of antiretroviral agents in pediatric HIV infection. Working Group on Antiretroviral Therapy and Medical Management of HIV-Infected Children 3rd November 2005. Available: http://AIDSinfo.nih.gov.

532.   American Academy of Pediatrics. Committee on Pediatric AIDS, Section on International Child Health. Increasing antiretroviral drug access for children with HIV infection. Policy statement 2007. Pediatrics 2007; 119:838–845.

533.   Gortmaker SL, Hughes M, Cervia J, et al. for the PACTG 219 team. Effect of combination therapy including protease inhibitors on mortality among children and adolescents infected with HIV-1. N Engl J Med 2001; 345:1522–1528.

534.   Mulenga V, Ford D, Walker AS, et al. and the CHAP Trial Team. Effect of cotrimoxizole on causes of death, hospital admissions and antibiotic use in HIV-infected children in the CHAP trial. AIDS 2007; 21:77–84.

535.   Paediatric European Network for Treatment of AIDS (PENTA). Comparison of dual nucleoside-analogue reverse-transcriptase inhibitor regimens with and without nelfinavir in children with HIV-1 who have not previously been treated: the PENTA 5 randomised trial. Lancet 2002; 359:733–739.

536.   Walker AS, Doerhalt K, Sharland M, et al. Collaborative HIV Paediatric Study (CHIPS) Steering Committee. Response to highly active antiretroviral therapy varies with age: the UK and Ireland Collaborative HIV Paediatric Study. AIDS 2004: 18:1915–1924.

537.   Melvin AJ, Rodrigo AG, Mohan KM, et al. HIV dynamics in children. AIDS 1999; 20:468–473.

538.   De Rossi A, Walker AS, Klein N, et al. Increased thymic output after initiation of antiretroviral therapy in human immunodeficiency virus type 1-infected children in the Paediatric European Network for Treatment of AIDS (PENTA) 5 Trial. J Infect Dis 2002; 186:312–320.

539.   Lindsey JC, Hughes MD, McKinney RE, et al. Treatment mediated changes in human immunodeficiency virus (HIV) type 1 RNA and CD4 cell counts as predictors of weight growth failure, cognitive decline, and survival in HIV infected children. J Infect Dis 2000; 182:1385–1393.

540.   Menson EN, Walker AS, Sharland M, et al. Underdosing of antiretrovirals in UK and Irish children with HIV as an example of problems of prescribing medicines to children, 1997–2005:cohort study. BMJ 2006; 332:1183–1187.

541.   Foster C, Mackie N, Seery P, et al. Emerging multi-drug resistance in children with perinatally acquired HIV-1. Eighth International Congress on Drug Therapy in HIV Infection, Glasgow, November 2006 [P360].

542.   Paediatric European Network for Treatment of AIDS (PENTA). Five-year follow-up of vertically HIV infected children in a randomised double blind controlled trial of immediate versus deferred zidovudine: the PENTA 1 trial. Arch Dis Child 2001; 84:230–236.

543.   Strategies for Management of Antiretroviral Therapy (SMART) Study Group; El-Sadr WM, Lundgren JD, Neaton JD, et al. CD4+ count-guided interruption of antiretroviral treatment. N Engl J Med 2006; 355:2359–2361.

544.   Doerholt K, Duong T, Tookey P, et al. Collaborative HIV Paediatric Study. Outcomes for human immunodeficiency virus-1-infected infants in the United Kingdom and Republic of Ireland in the era of effective antiretroviral therapy. Pediatr Infect Dis J 2006; 25:420–426.

545.   Luzuriaga K, McManus M, Catalina M, et al. Early therapy of vertical human immunodeficiency virus type-1 (HIV-1) infection: control of viral replication and absence of persistent HIV-1 specific immune responses. J Virol 2000; 74:6984–6991.

546.   Aboulker JP, Babiker A, Chaix ML, et al. Highly active antiretroviral therapy started in infants under 3 months of age: 72 week follow-up for CD4 count, viral load and drug resistance outcome. AIDS 2004; 18:237–245.

547.   Newell ML, Patel D, Goetghebuer T, et al. European Collaborative Study. CD4 cell response to antiretroviral therapy in children with vertically acquired HIV infection: is it associated with age at initiation? J Infect Dis 2006; 193:954–962.

548.   Litalein C, Faye A, Compacnucci A, et al. on behalf of PENTA. Pharmacokinetics of nelfinavir and its active metabolite, hydroxy-tert-butylamide, in infants perinatally infected with HIV-1. Pediatr Infect Dis J 2003; 22:48–55.

549.   WHO Antiretroviral therapy of HIV infection in infants and children in resource-limited settings: towards universal access: Recommendations for a public health approach. 7 August 2006. www.who.int/hiv/pub/guidelines.

550.   Bergshoeff A, Burger D, Verweij C, et al. PENTA-13 Study Group. Plasma pharmacokinetics of once- versus twice-daily lamivudine and abacavir: simplification of combination treatment in HIV-1-infected children (PENTA-13). Antivir Ther 2005; 10:239–246.

551.   LePrevost M, Green H, Flynn J, et al: Pediatric European Network for the Treatment of AIDS 13 Study Group. Adherence and acceptability of once daily Lamivudine and abacavir in human immunodeficiency virus type-1 infected children. Pediatr Infect Dis J 2006; 25:533–537.

552.   Bergshoeff A, Burger D, Verweij C, et al, on behalf of the PENTA-13 Study Group. Pharmacokinetics of once versus twice daily lamivudine and abacavir; Simplification of combination treatment in HIV-1 infected children (Penta 13). Antivir Ther 2005; 10:239–246.

553. Reddington C, Cohen J, Baldillo A, et al. Adherence to medication regimens among young children with human immunodeficiency virus infection. Pediatr Infect Dis J 2000; 19:1148–1153.

554. Duong T, McGee L, Sharland M, et al, on behalf of CHIPS. Effects of antiretroviral therapy (ART) on morbidity and mortality of UK and Irish HIV infected children. Arch Dis Child 2002; 86(suppl 1):A69.

555. Martinez J, Bell D, Camacho R, et al. Adherence to antiretroviral drug regimens in HIV-infected adolescent patients engaged in care in a comprehensive adolescent young adult clinic. J Nat Med Assoc 2000; 92:55–61.

556. Cohan D, Feakins C, Wara D et al. Perinatal transmission of multi-drug resistant HIV-1 despite viral suppression on an enfuvirtide based regimen. AIDS 2005; 19:989–990.

557. Giaquinto C, Green H, De Rossi A, et al, on behalf of the PENTA 8 Study Group. A randomised trial of resistance testing versus no resistance testing in children with virological failure: the PERA (PENTA 8) trial. IAS 2005 Abstract no. WeOa0106.

558. European Paediatric Lipodystrophy Group. Antiretroviral therapy, fat redistribution and hyperlipidaemia in HIV-infected children in Europe. AIDS 2004; 18:1443–1451.

559. Beregszaszi M, Dollfus C, Levine M, et al. Longitudinal evaluation and risk factors of lipodystrophy and associated metabolic changes in HIV-infected children. J Acquir Immune Defic Syndr 2005; 40:161–168.

560. Hartman K, Verweel G, de Groot R, et al. Detection of lipoatrophy in human immunodeficiency virus-1-infected children treated with highly active antiretroviral therapy. Pediatr Infect Dis J 2006; 25:427–431.

561. Beregszaszi M, Dollfus C, Levine M et al. Longitudinal evaluation and risk factors of lipodystrophy and associated metabolic changes in HIV-infected children. J Acquir Immune Defic Syndr 2005; 40:161–168.

562. Charakida M, Donald AE, Green H, et al. Early structural and functional changes of the vasculature in HIV-infected children: impact of disease and antiretroviral therapy. Circulation 2005; 112:103–109.

563. Mora S, Zamproni I, Beccio S, et al. Longitudinal changes of bone mineral density and metabolism in antiretroviral-treated human immunodeficiency virus-infected children. J Clin Endocrinol Metab 2004; 89:24–28.

564. Rosso R, Vignolo M, Parodi A, et al. Bone quality in perinatally HIV-infected children: role of age, sex, growth, HIV infection, and antiretroviral therapy. AIDS Res Hum Retroviruses 2005; 21:927–932.

565. Rey C, Prieto S, Medina A, et al. Fatal lactic acidosis during antiretroviral therapy. Pediatr Crit Care Med 2003; 4:485–487.

566. Desai N, Mathur M, Weedon J. Lactate levels in children with HIV/AIDS on highly active antiretroviral therapy. AIDS 2003; 17:1565–1568.

567. Centers for Disease Control and Prevention. Revised guidelines for prophylaxis against Pneumocystis carinii pneumonia for children infected with or perinatally exposed to human immunodeficiency virus. MMWR 1995; 44(RR-4):1–11.

568. Urschel S, Schuster T, Dunsch D, et al. Discontinuation of primary Pneumocystis carinii prophylaxis after reconstitution of CD4 cell counts in HIV-infected children. AIDS 2001; 15:1589–1591.

569. Nachman S, Philimon G, Dankner W, et al. The rate of serious bacterial infections among HIV-infected children with immune reconstitution who have discontinued opportunistic infection prophylaxis. Paediatrics 2005; 115:488–494.

570. Gibb DM, Masters J, Shingadia D, et al. A family clinic – optimising care for HIV infected children and their families. Arch Dis Child 1997; 77:478–482.

Exanthemata

571. Rice AL, Sacco L, Hyder A, et al. Malnutrition as an underlying cause of childhood deaths associated with infectious diseases in developing countries. Bull World Health Organ 2000; 78:1207–1221.

572. Karp CL, Wysocka M, Wahl LM, et al. Mechanism of suppression of cell-mediated immunity by measles virus. Science 1996; 273:228–231.

573. Krugman S, Ward R. Infectious diseases of children. St Louis: Mosby; 1968.

574. Ozanne G, d'Halewyn MA. Performance and reliability of the Enzygnost measles enzyme-linked immuno-sorbent assay for detection of measles virus-specific immunoglobulin M antibody during a large measles epidemic. J Clin Microbiol 1992; 30:564–569.

575. Permar SR, Moss WJ, Ryon JJ, et al. Prolonged measles virus shedding in human immunodeficiency virus-infected children, detected by reverse transcriptase-polymerase chain reaction. J Infect Dis 2001; 183:532–538.

576. Mustafa MM, Weitman SD, Winick NJ, et al. Subacute measles encephalitis in the young immunocompromized host: report of two cases diagnosed by polymerase chain reaction and treated with ribavirin and review of the literature. Clin Infect Dis J 1993; 16:654–660.

*577. Shann F, D'Souza RM, D'Souza R. Antibiotics for preventing pneumonia in children with measles (Cochrane Review). In: The Cochrane Library, 4. Oxford: Update Software; 2001.

578. Noah ND. What can we do about measles? BMJ 1984; 289:1476.

579. Aickin R, Hill D, Kemp A. Measles immunisation in children with allergy to egg. BMJ 1994; 309:223–225.

580. Mulholland EK. Measles in the United States, 2006. N Engl J Med 2006; 355:440–443.

581. Asaria P, MacMahon E. Measles in the United Kingdom: can we eradicate it by 2010? BMJ 2006; 333:890–895.

582. Wildig J, Michon P, Siba P, et al. Parvovirus B19 infection contributes to severe anemia in young children in Papua New Guinea. J Infect Dis 2006; 194:146–153.

583. Smith-Whitley K, Zhao H, Hodinka RL, et al. Epidemiology of human parvovirus B19 in children with sickle cell disease. Blood 2004; 103:422–427.

584. Anand A, Gray ES, Brown T, et al. Human parvovirus infection in pregnancy and hydrops fetalis. N Engl J Med 1987; 316:183–186.

585. Yamanishi K, Okuno T, Shiraki K, et al. Identification of human herpesvirus-6 as a causal agent for exanthem subitum. Lancet 1988; i:1065–1067.

586. Jones CA, Isaacs D. Human herpesvirus-6 infections. Arch Dis Child 1996; 74:98–100.

587. Torigoe S, Kumamoto T, Koide W, et al. Clinical manifestations associated with human herpesvirus 7 infection. Arch Dis Child 1995; 72:518–519.

588. Zerr DM, Meier AS, Selke SS, et al. L. A population-based study of primary human herpesvirus 6 infection. N Engl J Med 2005; 352:768–776.

589. Ward KN, Andrews SJ, Verity CM, et al. Human herpesviruses-6 and -7 each cause significant neurological morbidity in Britain and Ireland. Arch Dis Child 2005; 90:619–623.

Herpesviruses

590. Meyer PA, Seward JF, Jumaan AO, et al. Varicella mortality: trends before vaccine licensure in the United States, 1970–1994. J Infect Dis 2000; 182:383–390.

591. Lopez AS, Guris D, Zimmerman L, et al. One dose of varicella vaccine does not prevent school outbreaks: is it time for a second dose? Pediatrics 2006; 117:1070–1077.

592. Heuchan AM, Isaacs D. The management of varicella-zoster virus exposure and infection in pregnancy and the newborn period. Australasian Subgroup in Paediatric Infectious Diseases of the Australasian. Med J Aust 2001; 174:288–292.

593. Reynolds L, Struik S, Nadel S. Neonatal varicella: varicella zoster immunoglobulin (VZIG) does not prevent disease. Arch Dis Child Fetal Neonatal Ed 1999; 8:F69–70.

594. Vazquez M, LaRussa PS, Gershon AA, et al. The effectiveness of the varicella vaccine in clinical practice. N Engl J Med 2001; 344:955–960.

*595. Weinberg A, Horslen SP, Kaufman SS, et al. Safety and immunogenicity of varicella-zoster virus vaccine in pediatric liver and intestine transplant recipients. Am J Transplant 2006; 6:565–568.

*596. Levin MJ, Gershon AA, Weinberg A, et al. Administration of live varicella vaccine to HIV-infected children with current or past significant depression of CD4(+) T cells. J Infect Dis 2006; 194:247–255.

597. Asano Y, Yoshikawa T, Suga S, et al. Postexposure prophylaxis of varicella in family contact by oral acyclovir. Pediatrics 1993; 92:219–222.

598. Huang YC, Lin TY, Chiu CH. Acyclovir prophylaxis of varicella after household exposure. Pediatr Infect Dis J 1995; 14:152–154.

599. Goldstein SL, Somers MJ, Lande MB, et al. Acyclovir prophylaxis of varicella in children with renal disease receiving steroids. Pediatr Nephrol 2000; 14:305–308.

600. Ogilvie MM. Antiviral prophylaxis and treatment in chickenpox. A review prepared for the UK Advisory Group on chickenpox on behalf of the British Society for the Study of Infection. J Infect Dis 1998; 36(suppl 1):31–38.

601. Watson B, Seward J, Yang A, et al. Postexposure effectiveness of varicella vaccine. Pediatrics 2000; 105:84–88.

*602. Oxman MN, Levin MJ, Johnson GR, et al. A vaccine to prevent herpes zoster and postherpetic neuralgia in older adults. N Engl J Med 2005; 352:2271–2284.

603. Lafferty WE, Coombs RW, Benedetti J, et al. Recurrences after oral and genital herpes simplex virus infection. Influence of site of infection and viral type. N Engl J Med 1987; 316:1444–1449.

604. Thomas J, Rouse BT. Immunopathogenesis of herpetic ocular disease. Immunol Res 1997; 16:375–386.

605. Casrouge A, Zhang SY, Eidenschenk C, et al. Herpes simplex virus encephalitis in human UNC-93B deficiency. Science 2006; 314:308–312.

606. Schwartz GS, Holland EJ. Oral acyclovir for the management of herpes simplex virus keratitis in children. Ophthalmology 2000; 107:278–282.

607. Kovacs A, Schluchter M, Easley K, et al. Cytomegalovirus infection and HIV-1 disease progression in infants born to HIV-1-infected women. Pediatric Pulmonary and Cardiovascular Complications of Vertically Transmitted HIV Infection Study Group. N Engl J Med 1999; 341:77–84.

608. Sia IG, Wilson JA, Groettum CM, et al. Cytomegalovirus (CMV) DNA load predicts relapsing CMV infection after solid organ transplantation. J Infect Dis 2000; 181:717–720.

609. Meyers JD. Management of cytomegalovirus infection. Am J Med 1988; 85(suppl 2A):102–106.

*610. Hodson EM, Jones CA, Webster AC, et al. Antiviral medications to prevent cytomegalovirus disease and early death in recipients of solid-organ transplants: a systematic review of randomised controlled trials. Lancet 2005; 365:2105–2115.

611. Pondarre C, Kebaili K, Dijoud F, et al. Epstein-Barr virus-related lymphoproliferative disease complicating childhood acute lymphoblastic leukemia: no recurrence after unrelated donor bone marrow transplantation. Bone Marrow Transplant 2001; 27:93–95.

Viral and Allied Infections of the Respiratory Tract

612. World Health Organization. Memorandum: a revision of the system of nomenclature for influenza viruses. Bull World Health Organ 1980; 58:585–591.

613. Beigel JH, Farrar J, Han AM, et al. Avian influenza A (H5N1) infection in humans. N Engl J Med 2005; 353:1374–1385.

614. Lancet Editorial. Reinfection with influenza. Lancet 1986; i:1017–1018.

615. Poehling KA, Edwards KM, Weinberg GA, et al. The underrecognized burden of influenza in young children. N Engl J Med 2006; 355:31–40.

616. Keren R, Zaoutis TE, Bridges CB, et al. Neurological and neuromuscular disease as a risk factor for respiratory failure in children hospitalized with influenza infection. JAMA 2005; 294:2188–2194.

*617. Hayden FG, Treanor JJ, Fritz RS, et al. Use of the oral neuraminidase inhibitor oseltamivir in experimental human influenza: randomized controlled trials for prevention and treatment. JAMA 1999; 282:1240–1246.

*618. Lalezari J, Campion K, Keene O, et al. Zanamivir for the treatment of influenza A and B infection in high-risk patients: a pooled analysis of randomized controlled trials. Arch Int Med 2001; 161:212–217.

*619. Advisory Committee on Immunization Practices. Prevention and control of influenza: recommendations of the Advisory Committee on Immunization Practices (ACIP). MMWR Recomm Rep 2006; 55(RR-10):1–42.

*620. Madhi SA, Cutland C, Zhu Y, et al. Transmissibility, infectivity and immunogenicity of a live human parainfluenza type 3 virus vaccine (HPIV3cp45) among susceptible infants and toddlers. Vaccine 2006; 24:2432–2439.

621. Broughton S, Bhat R, Roberts A, et al. Diminished lung function, RSV infection, and respiratory morbidity in prematurely born infants. Arch Dis Child 2006; 91:26–30.

622. DeVincenzo JP, El Saleeby CM, Bush AJ. Respiratory syncytial virus load predicts disease severity in previously healthy infants. J Infect Dis 2005; 191:1861–1868.

623. Tal G, Mandelberg A, Dalal I, et al. Association between common Toll-like receptor 4 mutations and severe respiratory syncytial virus disease. J Infect Dis 2004; 189:2057–2063.

624. MacDonald NE, Hall CB, Suffin SC, et al. Respiratory syncytial virus infection in infants with congenital heart disease. N Engl J Med 1982; 307:397–400.

625. Hall CB, Powell KR, McDonald NE, et al. Respiratory syncytial virus infection in children with compromised immune function. N Engl J Med 1986; 315:77–80.

626. Isaacs D, Moxon ER, Harvey D, et al. Ribavirin in respiratory syncytial virus infection. Arch Dis Child 1988; 63:986–990.

*627. The PREVENT Study Group. Reduction of respiratory syncytial virus hospitalization among premature infants and infants with bronchopulmonary dysplasia using respiratory syncytial virus immune globulin prophylaxis. Pediatrics 1997; 99:93–99.

628. The IMpact-RSV Study Group. Palivizumab, a humanized respiratory syncytial virus monoclonal antibody, reduces hospitalization from respiratory syncytial virus infection in high-risk infants. Pediatrics 1998; 102:531–537.

*629. Wang EEL, Tang NK. Immunoglobulin for preventing respiratory syncytial virus infection (Cochrane Review). In: The Cochrane Library, 3. Oxford: Update Software; 2001.

630. Thomas M, Bedford-Russell A, Sharland M. Hospitalisation for RSV infection in ex-preterm infants – implications for use of RSV immune globulin. Arch Dis Child 2000; 83:122–127.

631. van den Hoogen BG, de Jong JC, Groen J, et al. A newly discovered human pneumovirus isolated from young children with respiratory tract disease. Nat Med 2001; 7:719–724.

632. van den Hoogen BG, van Doornum GJ, Fockens JC, et al. Prevalence and clinical symptoms of human metapneumovirus infection in hospitalized patients. J Infect Dis 2003; 188:1571–1577.

633. Williams JV, Harris PA, Tollefson SJ, et al. Human metapneumovirus and lower respiratory tract disease in otherwise healthy infants and children. N Engl J Med 2004; 350:443–450.

634. Sloots TP, Mackay IM, Bialasiewicz S, et al. Human metapneumovirus, Australia, 2001–2004. Emerg Infect Dis 2006; 12:1263–1266.

635. Klein MI, Coviello S, Bauer G, et al. The impact of infection with human metapneumovirus and other respiratory viruses in young infants and children at high risk for severe pulmonary disease. J Infect Dis 2006; 193:1544–1551.

636. Debiaggi M, Canducci F, Sampaolo M, et al. Persistent symptomless human metapneumovirus infection in hematopoietic stem cell transplant recipients. J Infect Dis 2006; 194:474–478.

637. Madhi SA, Ludewick H, Kuwanda L, et al. Pneumococcal coinfection with human metapneumovirus. J Infect Dis 2006; 193:1236–1243.

638. Pham TT, Burchette JLJr, Hale LP. Fatal disseminated adenovirus infections in immunocompromised patients. Am J Clin Pathol 2003; 120:575–583.

639. Peled N, Nakar C, Huberman H, et al. Adenovirus infection in hospitalized immuno-competent children. Clin Pediatr (Phila) 2004; 43:223–229.

640. Brandt CD, Kim HW, Rodriguez WJ, et al. Adenoviruses and pediatric gastroenteritis. J Infect Dis 1985; 151:437–443.

641. Legrand F, Berrebi D, Houhou N, et al. Early diagnosis of adenovirus infection and treatment with cidofovir after bone marrow transplantation in children. Bone Marrow Transplant 2001; 27:621–626.

642. Bloom S, Wharton M. Mumps outbreak among young adults in UK. BMJ 2005: 331:E363–E364.

643. Lemanske RF Jr, Jackson DJ, Gangnon RE, et al. Rhinovirus illnesses during infancy predict subsequent childhood wheezing. J Allergy Clin Immunol 2005; 116:571–577.

644. McIntosh K. Coronavirus. In: Mandell GL, Bennett JE, Dolin R, eds. Principles and practice of infectious diseases. New York: John Wiley; 1995.

645. Isaacs D, Flowers D, Clarke JR, et al. Epidemiology of coronavirus respiratory infections. Arch Dis Child 1983; 58:500–503.

646. WHO. Severe acute respiratory syndrome (SARS). Wkly Epidemiol Rec 2003; 78:81–83.

647. WHO. Severe acute respiratory syndrome (SARS). Wkly Epidemiol Rec 2003; 78:86.

648. Peiris JSM, Lai ST, Poon LLM, et al. Coronavirus as a possible cause of severe acute respiratory distress. Lancet 2003; 362:1–8.

649. Kuiken T, Fouchier RA, Schutten M, et al. Newly discovered coronavirus as the primary cause of severe acute respiratory syndrome. Lancet 2003; 362:263–270.

650. Tai JH, Williams JV, Edwards KM, et al. Prevalence of reovirus-specific antibodies in young children in Nashville, Tennessee. J Infect Dis 2005; 191:1221–1224.

651. Corsaro D, Valassina M, Venditti D. Increasing diversity within Chlamydiae. Crit Rev Microbiol 2003; 29:37–78.

652. Bas S, Muzzin P, Ninet B, et al. Chlamydial serology: comparative diagnostic value of immunoblotting, microimmunofluorescence test, and immunoassays using different recombinant proteins as antigens. J Clin Microbiol 2001; 39:1368–1377.

653. Hammerschlag MR. Chlamydia trachomatis and Chlamydia pneumoniae infections in children and adolescents. Pediatr Rev 2004; 25:43–51.

Viral Infections of the CNS

654. Biggar RJ, Woodall JP, Walter PD, et al. Lymphocytic choriomeningitis outbreak associated with pet hamsters. Fifty-seven cases from New York State. JAMA 1975; 232:494–500.

655. Fishbein DB, Robinson LE. Rabies. N Engl J Med 1993; 329:1632–1638.

656. Bahmanyar M, Fayaz A, Nour-Salehi S, et al. Successful protection of humans exposed to rabies infection: postexposure treatment with the new diploid cell rabies vaccine and antirabies serum. JAMA 1976; 236:2751–2754.

657. Pruisner S. Novel proteinaceous infectious particles cause scrapie. Science 1982; 216:134–144.

658. Whitley RJ, MacDonald N, Asher DM. American Academy of Pediatrics. Technical report: transmissible spongiform encephalopathies: a review for pediatricians. Committee on Infectious Disease. Pediatrics 2000; 106:1160–1165.

659. Will RG, Ironside JW, Zeidler M, et al. A new variant of Creutzfeldt–Jakob disease in the UK. Lancet 1996; 347:921–925.

660. Hill AF, Desbruslais M, Joiner S, et al. The same prion strain causes vCJD and BSE. Nature 1997; 389:448–450, 526.

661. Scott MR, Will R, Ironside J, et al. Compelling transgenetic evidence for transmission of bovine spongiform encephalopathy prions to humans. Proc Natl Acad Sci USA 1999; 96:1537–1542.

662. Cousens S, Smith PG, Ward H, et al. Geographical distribution of variant Creutzfeldt–Jakob disease in Great Britain, 1994–2000. Lancet 2001; 357:1002–1007.

663. Centers for Disease Control and Prevention (CDC). Update on vaccine-derived polioviruses. MMWR Morb Mortal Wkly Rep 2006; 55:1093–1097.

664. Halsey NA, Abramson JS, Chesney PJ, et al. Poliomyelitis prevention: revised recommendations for use of inactivated and live oral poliovirus vaccines. American Academy of Pediatrics Committee on Infectious Diseases. Pediatrics 1999; 103:171–172.

665. Burgess M, McIntyre PB. Vaccine-associated paralytic poliomyelitis. Commun Dis Intel 1999; 23:80–81.

666. Rotbart HA, Webster AD. Treatment of potentially life-threatening enterovirus infections with pleconaril. Clin Infect Dis J 2001; 32:228–235.

Viruses and the Gastrointestinal Tract

667. Isaacs D, Day D, Crook S. Child gastroenteritis: a population study. BMJ 1986 293:545–546.

668. Morbidity and Mortality Weekly Report. Intussusception among recipients of rotavirus vaccine – United States, 1998–1999. Morbid Mortal Wkly Rep 1999; 48:577–581.

669. Bines JE, Liem NT, Justice FA, et al. Risk factors for intussusception in Vietnam and Australia: adenovirus implicated, but not rotavirus. J Pediatr 2006; 149:452–460.

670. Storch GA. Diagnostic virology. Clin Infect Dis J 2000; 31:739–751.

Viral Infection of the Liver

671. Goilav C, Zuckerman J, Lafrenz M, et al. Immunogenicity and safety of a new inactivated hepatitis A vaccine in a comparative study. J Med Virol 1995; 46:287–292.

672. Boxall EH, Sira J, Standish RA, et al. Natural history of hepatitis B in perinatally infected carriers. Arch Dis Child Fetal Neonatal Ed 2004; 89:F456–F460.

673. Wen WH, Chang ME, Hsu HY, et al. The development of hepatocellular carcinoma among prospectively followed children with chronic hepatitis B virus infection. J Pediatr 2004; 144:397–399.

674. Marx G, Martin SR, Chicoine JF, et al. Long-term follow-up of chronic hepatitis B virus infection in children of different ethnic origins. J Infect Dis 2002; 186:295–301.

*675.   Lee C, Gong Y, Brok J, et al. Effect of hepatitis B immunisation in newborn infants of mothers positive for hepatitis B surface antigen: systematic review and meta-analysis. BMJ 2006; 332:328–336.

676.   Papatheodoridis GV, Hadziyannis SJ. Diagnosis and management of pre-core mutant chronic hepatitis B. J Viral Hepatol 2001; 8:311–321.

677.   Lau GK, Piratvisuth T, Luo KX, et al. Peginterferon Alfa-2a, lamivudine, and the combination for HBeAg-positive chronic hepatitis B. N Engl J Med 2005; 352:2682–2695.

678.   Kazim SN, Wakil SM, Khan LA, et al. Vertical transmission of hepatitis B virus despite maternal lamivudine therapy. Lancet 2002; 359:1488–1489.

679.   Hartman C, Berkowitz D, Eshach-Adiv O, et al. Long-term lamivudine therapy for chronic hepatitis B infection in children unresponsive to interferon. J Pediatr Gastroenterol Nutr 2006; 43:494–498.

680.   Resti M, Azzari C, Mannelli F, et al. Mother to child transmission of hepatitis C virus: prospective study of risk factors and timing of infection in children born to women seronegative for HIV-1. Tuscany Study Group on Hepatitis C Virus Infection. BMJ 1998; 317:437–441.

681.   Mast EE, Hwang LY, Seto DS, et al. Risk factors for perinatal transmission of hepatitis C virus (HCV) and the natural history of HCV infection acquired in infancy. J Infect Dis 2005; 192:1880–1889.

682.   European Paediatric Hepatitis C Virus Network. A significant sex – but not elective cesarean section – effect on mother-to-child transmission of hepatitis C virus infection. J Infect Dis 2005; 192:1872–1879.

683.   Ogasawara S, Kage M, Kosai K, et al. Hepatitis C virus RNA in saliva and breastmilk of hepatitis C carrier mothers. Lancet 1993; 341:561.

684.   Jones CA. Maternal transmission of infectious pathogens in breast milk. J Paediatr Child Health 2001; 37:576–582.

685.   Dunn D, Gibb DM, Healy M, et al. Timing and interpretation of tests for diagnosing perinatally acquired hepatitis C virus infection. Pediatr Infect Dis J 2001; 20:716–717.

686.   England K, Pembrey L, Tovo PA, et al, European Paediatric Hcv Network. Growth in the first 5 years of life is unaffected in children with perinatally-acquired hepatitis C infection. J Pediatr 2005; 147:227–232.

687.   Bortolotti F, Resti M, Marcellini M, et al. Hepatitis C virus (HCV) genotypes in 373 Italian children with HCV infection: changing distribution and correlation with clinical features and outcome. Gut 2005; 54:852–857.

688.   Jhaveri R, Grant W, Kauf TL, et al. The burden of hepatitis C virus infection in children: estimated direct medical costs over a 10-year period. J Pediatr 2006; 148:353–358.

689.   Jonas MM. Treatment of chronic hepatitis C in pediatric patients. Clin Liver Dis 1999; 3:855–867.

690.   Hardikar W, Moaven LD, Bowden DS, et al. Hepatitis G: viroprevalence and seroconversion in a high-risk group of children. Viral Hepat 1999; 6:337–341.

Miscellaneous Viral Infections

691.   Nishizawa T, Okamoto H, Konishi K, et al. A novel DNA virus (TTV) associated with elevated transaminase levels in posttransfusion hepatitis of unknown etiology. Biochem Biophys Res Commun 1997; 241:92–97.

692.   Gerner P, Oettinger R, Gerner W, et al. Mother-to-infant transmission of TT virus: prevalence, extent and mechanism of vertical transmission. Pediatr Infect Dis J 2000; 19:1074–1077.

693.   Mostashari F, Bunning ML, Kitsutani PT, et al. Epidemic West Nile encephalitis, New York, 1999: results of a household-based seroepidemiological survey. Lancet 2001; 358:261–264.

694.   Monath TP. Yellow fever. In: Warren KA, Mahmoud AA, eds. Tropical and geographical medicine. New York: McGraw Hill; 1984.

695.   World Health Organization. Haemorrhagic fever with renal syndrome. Bull World Health Organ 1983; 61:269–275.

Protozoal Infections: Amebic Infections

696.   Stanley SL Jr. Amoebiasis. Lancet 2003; 361:1025–1034.

697.   Haque R, Huston CD, Hughes M, et al. Amebiasis. N Engl J Med 2003; 348:1565–1573.

698.   Stauffer W, Ravdin JI. Entamoeba histolytica. Curr Opin Infect Dis 2003; 16:479–485.

699.   Hanna RM, Dahniya MH, Badr SS, et al. Percutaneous catheter drainage in drug-resistant amoebic liver abscess. Trop Med Int Health 2000; 5:578–581.

700.   Ma P, Visvesvara GS, Martinez AJ, et al. Naegleria and Acanthamoeba infections: review. Rev Infect Dis 1990; 12:490–513.

701.   Singhal T, Bajpai A, Kabra V, et al. Successful treatment of Acanthamoeba meningitis with combination oral antimicrobials. Pediatr Infect Dis J 2001; 20:623–627.

702.   Kumar R, Lloyd D. Recent advances in the treatment of Acanthamoeba keratitis. Clin Infect Dis 2002; 35:434–439.

Cryptosporidiosis

703.   Nime FA, Burek JD, Page DA, et al. Acute enterocolitis in a human being infected with the protozoon Cryptosporidium. Gastroenterology 1976; 70:592–593.

704.   Meisel JC, Perera DA, Meligro C, et al. Overwhelming watery diarrhea associated with Cryptosporidium in an immunosuppressed patient. Gastroenterology 1976; 70:1156–1160.

705.   Hart CA. Cryptosporidiosis. In: Gilles HM, ed. Protozoal disease. London: Arnold; 1999: 592–606.

706.   Xaio L, Ryan UM. Cryptosporidiosis an update in molecular epidemiology. Curr Opin Infect Dis 2004; 17:483–490.

707.   Baxby D, Hart CA, Taylor CJ. Human Cryptosporidiosis: a possible case of hospital cross-infection. Br Med J 1983; 287:1760–1761.

708.   Rosales MJ, Cordon GP, Moreno MS, et al. Extracellular gregarine-like stages of Cryptosporidium parvum. Acta Trop 2005; 95:74–78.

709.   Xu P, Widmer G, Wang Y, et al. The genome of Cryptosporidium hominis. Nature 2004; 431:1107–1112.

710.   Current WL, Garcia LS. Cryptosporidiosis. Clin Microbiol Rev 1991; 4:325–358.

711.   Mackenzie WR, Hoxie NJ, Proctor ME, et al. A massive outbreak in Milwaukee of cryptosporidium infection transmitted through public water supply. N Engl J Med 1997; 331:161–167.

712.   Gatei W, Wamae CN, Mbae C, et al. Cryptosporidiosis: prevalence, genotype analysis and symptoms associated with infection in children in Kenya. Am J Trop Med Hyg 2006; 75:78–82.

713.   Tumwine JK, Kekitiinwa A, Bakeera-Kitaka S, et al. Cryptosporidiosis and microsporidiosis in Uganda children with persistent diarrhea with and without concurrent infection with human immunodeficiency virus. Am J Trop Med Hyg 2005; 73:921–925.

714.   Gatei W, Greensill J, Ashford RW, et al. Molecular analysis of the 18S rRNA gene of Cryptosporidium parasites from patients with or without human immunodeficiency virus living in Kenya, Malawi, Brazil and the United Kingdom. J Clin Microbiol 2003; 41:1458–1462.

715.   Gatei W, Ashford RW, Beeching NJ, et al. Cryptosporidium muris infection in an HIV-infected adult. Emerg Infect Dis 2002; 8:204–206.

716.   Ungar BLP. Cryptosporidiosis in humans (Homo sapiens). In: Dubey JP, Speer CA, Fayer R, eds. Cryptosporidiosis of man and animals. Boca Raton, USA: CRC Press; 1990:59–82.

717.   Sallon S, El Showaa R, El Masri M, et al. Cryptosporidiosis in children in Gaza. Ann Trop Paed 1991; 11:277–281.

718.   Hojlyng N, Holten-Anderson W, Jepson S. Cryptosporidiosis: a case of airborne transmission. Lancet 1987; 2:271–272.

719.   Lahdevirta J, Jokipii AMM, Sammalkoysi K, et al. Perinatal infection with Cryptosporidium and failure to thrive. Lancet 1987; 1:48–49.

720.   Jokipii L, Jokipii AMM. Timing of symptoms and oocysts excretion in human cryptosporidiosis. N Engl J Med 1986; 315:1643–1647.

721.   Chen XM, Keithly JS, Pava CV, et al. Cryptosporidiosis. N Engl J Med 2002; 346:1723–1731.

722.   Baxby D, Hart CA. The incidence of cryptosporidiosis: a two year prospective study in a children's hospital. J Hyg 1985; 96:107–111.

723.   Hart CA, Baxby D, Blundell N. Gastroenteritis due to Cryptosporidium: a prospective survey in a children's hospital. J Infect 1984; 9:264–270.

724.   Baxby D, Hart CA, Blundell N. Shedding of oocyst by immunocompetent individuals with cryptosporidiosis. J Hyg 1985; 95:705–709.

725.   MacFarlane DE, Homer-Bryce J. Cryptosporidiosis in well nourished and malnourished children. Acta Paediatr Scand 1987; 76:474–477.

726.   Leav BA, Mackay M, Ward HD. Cryptosporidium species: New insights and old challenges. Clin Infect Dis 2003; 36:903–908.

727.   Rossignol JF, Kabil SM, el-Gohary Y et al. Effect of nitozoxonide in diarrhea and enteritis caused by Cryptosporidium species. Clin Gastroenterol Hepatol 2006; 4:320–324.

728.   Molbak K, Hojlyng N, Ingholt L, et al. Cryptosporidiosis in infancy and childhood mortality in Guinea Bissau. Br Med J 1993; 307:417–420.

Giardiasis

729.   Thompson RCA, Hopkins RM, Homan WL. Nomenclature and genetic groupings of Giardia infecting mammals. Parasitol Today 2000; 16:210–213.

730.   Adam RD. Biology of Giardia lamblia. Clin Microbiol Rev 2001; 14:447–475.

731.   World Health Organization (WHO). The World Health Report: Fighting disease, fostering development. Geneva: WHO; 1996.

732.   Warburton ARE, Jones PH, Bruce J. Zoonotic transmission of giardiasis: a case control study. Commun Dis Rep 1994; 4:R33–R36.

733.   Homan WL, Monk TG. Human giardiasis: genotype linked differences in clinical symptomatology. Int J Parasitol 2001; 31:822–826.

734.   Farthing MJG. Giardiasis. In: Gilles HM, ed. Protozoal diseases. London: Arnold; 1999:562–584.

735.   Eichinger D. Encystation in parasitic protozoa. Curr Opin Microbiol 2001; 4:421–426.

736.   Weiland MEL, McArthur AG, Morrison HG, et al. Annexin-like alphas giardins: a new cytoskeletal gene family in Giardia lamblia. Int J Parasitol 2005; 35:617–626.

737.   Aziz H, Beck CE, Lux MF, et al. A comparison study of different methods used in the detection of Giardia lamblia. Clin Lab Sci 2001; 14:150–154.

738.   Sharp SE, Suarez CA, Duncan Y, et al. Evaluation of the Triage Micro Parasite Panel for detection of Giardia lamblia, Entamoeba histolytica/Entamoeba dispar and Cryptosporidium parvum in patient stool samples. J Clin Microbiol 2003; 39:332–334.

*739.   Zaat JO, Monk T, Assendelft WJ. Drugs for treating giardiasis (Cochrane Review). In: The Cochrane Library, 2. Oxford: Update Software; 2000.

740.   Olson ME, Ceri H, Morck DW. Giardia vaccination. Parasitol Today 2000; 16:213–217.

Leishmaniasis

741.   Lainson R, Shaw JJ. The role of animals in the epidemiology of South American leishmaniasis. In:

Lumsden WHR, Evans DA, eds. The biology of the Kinetoplastida. London: Academic Press; 1979: vol 2:1–116.

742.   Lainson R, Shaw JJ. Evolution classification and geographical distribution. In: Peters W, Killick-Kendrick R, eds. The leishmaniases in biology and medicine, biology and epidemiology. London: Academic Press; 1987: vol 1:1–20.

743.   Chance ML. The biochemical and immunological taxonomy of leishmania. In: Chang KP, Bray RS, eds. Human parasitic diseases, vol 1. Leishmaniasis. Amsterdam: Elsevier; 1985:93–110.

744.   Berman JD. Human leishmaniasis: clinical, diagnostic, and chemotherapeutic developments in the last 10 years. Clin Infect Dis 1997; 24:684–703.

745.   Herwaldt BL. Leishmaniasis. Lancet 1999; 354:1191–1199.

746.   Aronson NE, Wortmann GW, Johnson SC, et al. Safety and efficacy of intravenous sodium stibogluconate in the treatment of leishmaniasis: recent U.S. military experience. Clin Infect Dis 1998; 27:1457–1464.

747.   Maltezou HC, Siafas C, Mavrikou M, et al. Visceral leishmaniasis during childhood in southern Greece. Clin Infect Dis 2000; 31:1139–1143.

748.   Cascio A, di Martino L, Occorsio P, et al. A 6 day course of liposomal amphotericin B in the treatment of infantile visceral leishmaniasis: the Italian experience. J Antimicrob Chemother 2004; 54:217–220.

749.   Sundar S, Jha TK, Sindermann H, et al. Oral miltefosine treatment in children with mild to moderate Indian visceral leishmaniasis. Pediatr Infect Dis J 2003; 22:434–438.

750.   Bhattacharya SK, Jha TK, Sundar S, et al. Efficacy and tolerability of miltefosine for childhood visceral leishmaniasis in India. Clin Infect Dis 2004; 38:217–221.

751.   Murray HW, Berman JD, Davies CR, et al. Advances in leishmaniasis. Lancet 2005; 366:1561–1577.

752.   Uzun S, Uslular C, Yucel A, et al. Cutaneous leishmaniasis: evaluation of 3,074 cases in the Cukurova region of Turkey. Br J Dermatol 1999; 140:347–350.

753.   Soto J, Toledo J, Gutierrez P, et al. Treatment of American cutaneous leishmaniasis with miltefosine, an oral agent. Clin Infect Dis 2001; 33:57–61.

754.   Palacios R, Osorio LE, Grajalew LF, et al. Treatment failure in children in a randomized clinical trial with 10 and 20 days of meglumine antimonate for cutaneous leishmaniasis due to Leishmania viannia species. Am J Trop Med Hyg 2001; 64:187–193.

755.   Bern C, Joshi AB, Jha SN, et al. Factors associated with visceral leishmaniasis in Nepal: bed-net use is strongly protective. Am J Trop Med Hyg 2000; 63:184–188.

Malaria

756.   Garnham PCC. Malaria parasites of man: life cycles and morphology (excluding ultrastructure). In: Wernsdorfer WH, McGregor IA, eds. Malaria. The principles and practice of malariology, vol 1. Edinburgh: Churchill Livingstone; 1988:61–96.

757.   Breman JG. The ears of the hippopotamus: manifestations, determinants and estimates of the malaria burden. Am J Trop Med Hyg 2001; 64:1–11.

758.   Snow RW, Guerra CA, Noor AM, et al. The global distribution of clinical episodes of Plasmodium falciparum malaria. Nature 2005; 434:214–217.

759.   Snow RW, Craig M, Deichmann U, et al. Estimating mortality, morbidity and disability due to malaria among Africa's non-pregnant population. Bull World Health Organ 1999; 77:624–640.

760.   Trape JF. The public health impact of chloroquine resistance in Africa. Am J Trop Med Hyg 2001; 64(1–2 Suppl):12–17.

761.   Molineaux L. The epidemiology of human malaria as an explanation of its distribution, including some implications for its control. In: Wernsdorfer WH, McGregor IA, eds. Malaria. The principles and practice of malariology, vol. II. Edinburgh: Churchill Livingstone; 1988:913–998.

762.   Miller LH. Genetically determined human resistance factors. In: Wernsdorfer WH, McGregor IA, eds. Malaria. The principles and practice of malariology. Vol. I. Edinburgh: Churchill Livingstone; 1988:487–500.

763.   McGregor IA, Wilson RJM. Specific immunity acquired in man. In: Wernsdorfer WH, McGregor IA, eds. Malaria. The principles and practice of malariology. Vol. I. Edinburgh: Churchill Livingstone; 1988:559–619.

764.   Allison AC. The role of cell-mediated immune responses in protection against plasmodia and in the pathogenesis of malaria. In: Wernsdorfer WH, McGregor IA, eds. Malaria. The principles and practice of malariology. Vol. I. Edinburgh: Churchill Livingstone; 1988: 501–513.

765.   Weatherall DJ. The anaemia of malaria. In: Wernsdorfer WH, McGregor IA, eds. Malaria. The principles and practice of malariology. Vol. I. Edinburgh: Churchill Livingstone; 1988:735–751.

766.   Boonpucknavig V, Boonpucknavig S. The histopathology of malaria. In: Wernsdorfer WH, McGregor IA, eds. Malaria. The principles and practice of malariology. Vol. I. Edinburgh: Churchill Livingstone; 1988:673–734.

767.   Berendt AR, Ferguson DJP, Gardner J, et al. Molecular mechanisms of sequestration in malaria. Parasitology 1994; 108 (suppl): S19–S28.

*768.   Baruch DI, Pasloske BL, Singh HB, et al. Cloning the P. falciparum gene encoding PfEMP-1, a malarial variant antigen and adherence receptor on the surface of parasitised human erythrocytes. Cell 1995; 82:77–87.

*769.   Pain A, Ferguson DJP, Kai O, et al. Platelet-mediated clumping of P. falciparum-infected erythrocytes is a common adhesive phenotype and is associated with severe malaria. Proc Natl Acad Sci USA 2001; 98:1805–1810.

770.   Clark IA. Monokines and lymphokines in malarial pathology. Ann Trop Med Parasitol 1987; 81:577–585.

771.   Grau GE, Mackenzie CD, Carr RA, et al. Platelet accumulation in brain microvessels in fatal paediatric cerebral malaria. J Infect Dis 2003; 187:461–466.

*772.   Molyneux ME, Taylor TE, Wirima JJ, et al. Clinical features and prognostic indicators in pediatric cerebral malaria: a study of 131 comatose Malawian children. Q J Med 1989; 71:441–459.

773.   Taylor TE, Fu WN, Carr RA, et al. Differentiating the pathologies of cerebral malaria by post mortem parasite counts. Nat Med 2004; 10:143–145.

*774.   Croft A. Malaria: prevention in travellers. Clinical evidence issue 5. BMJ 2001; 505–519.

775.   Kublin JG, Patnaik P, Jere CJ, et al. Effect of Plasmodium falciparum malaria on HIV-1 RNA blood concentration in a cohort of adults in rural Malawi. Lancet 2005; 365:233–240.

776.   Chintu C, Bhat GJ, Walker AS, et al; CHAP trial team. Co-trimoxazole as prophylaxis against opportunistic infections in HIV-infected Zambian children (CHAP): a double-blind randomised placebo-controlled trial. Lancet 2004; 364:1865–1871.

777.   Alonso PL, Sacarlal J, Aponte JJ, et al. Efficacy of the RTS,S/AS02A vaccine against Plasmodium falciparum infection and disease in young African children: randomised controlled trial. Lancet 2004; 364:1411–1420.

778.   Alonso PL, Sacarlal J, Aponte JJ, et al. Duration of protection with RTS,S/AS02A malaria vaccine in prevention of Plasmodium falciparum disease in Mozambican children: single-blind extended follow-up of a randomised controlled trial. Lancet 2005; 366:2012–2018.

779.   Quinn TC, Jacobs RF, Mertz GJ, et al. Congenital malaria: a report of four cases and a review. J Pediatr 1982; 101:229–232.

*780.   Marsh K, Foster D, Waruiru C, et al. Indicators of life-threatening malaria in African children. N Engl J Med 1995; 332:1399–1404.

781.   Planche T, Krishna S. Severe malaria: metabolic complications. Curr Mol Med 2006; 6:141–153.

*782.   Taylor TE, Molyneux ME, Wirima JJ, et al. Blood glucose levels in Malawian children before and during the administration of intravenous quinine for severe falciparum malaria. N Engl J Med 1988; 319:1040–1047.

*783.   Lewallen S, Bakker H, Taylor TE, et al. Retinal findings predictive of outcome in cerebral malaria. Trans R Soc Trop Med Hyg 1996; 90:144–146.

784.   Lewallen S, Harding SP, Ajewole J, et al. A review of the spectrum of clinical ocular fundus findings in P. falciparum malaria in African children with a proposed classification and grading system. Trans R Soc Trop Med Hyg 1999; 93:619–622.

785.   Beare NA, Southern C, Chalira C, et al. Prognostic significance and course of retinopathy in children with severe malaria. Arch Ophthalmol 2004; 122:1141–1147.

*786.   Newton CRJC, Crawley J, Sowumni A, et al. Intracranial hypertension in Africans with cerebral malaria. Arch Dis Child 1997; 76:219–226.

*787.   Waller D, Krishna S, Crawley J, et al. Clinical features and outcome of severe malaria in Gambian children. Clin Infect Dis 1995; 21:577–587.

788.   White NJ, Miller KD, Marsh K, et al. Hypoglycaemia in African children with severe malaria. Lancet 1987; 1:708–711.

*789.   Newton CRJC, Peshu N, Kendall B, et al. Brain swelling and ischaemia in Kenyans with cerebral malaria. Arch Dis Child 1994; 70:281–287.

790.   Kihara M, Carter JA, Newton CR. The effect of Plasmodium falciparum on cognition: a systematic review. Trop Med Internat Health 2006; 11:386–397.

791.   Casals-Pascual C, Roberts DJ. Severe malarial anaemia. Curr Mol Med 2006; 6:155–168.

*792.   English M, Sauerwein R, Waruiru C, et al. Acidosis in severe childhood malaria. Q J Med 1997; 90:263–270.

793.   Bates I. Splenomegaly in the tropics. In: Gill G, Beeching N, eds. Tropical medicine, 5th edn. Oxford: Blackwell Science; 2004.

*794.   Berkley J, Mwarumba S, Bramham K, et al. Bacteraemia complicating severe malaria in children. Trans R Soc Trop Med Hyg 1999; 93:283–286.

795.   World Health Organization. Guidelines for the treatment of malaria. Geneva: WHO/HTM/MAL; 2006.

*796.   Meremikwu M, Logan E, Garner P. Antipyretic measures for treating fever in malaria (Cochrane Review). In: The Cochrane Library, 4. Oxford: Update Software; 2001.

*797.   Lackritz EM, Campbell CC, Ruebush TKII, et al. Effect of blood transfusion on survival among children in a Kenya hospital. Lancet 1992; 340:524–528.

798.   Maitland K, Pamba A, English M, et al. Randomised trial of volume expansion with albumin or saline in children with severe malaria: preliminary evidence of albumin benefit. Clin Infect Dis 2005; 40:538–545.

799.   World Health Organization. Severe and complicated malaria. Report of an informal technical meeting in Geneva, 1985. Trans R Soc Trop Med Hyg 1986; 80(suppl):1–50.

800.   Dondorp A, Nosten F, Stepniewska K, et al. Artesunate versus quinine for treatment of severe falciparum malaria: a randomised trial. Lancet 2005; 366:717–725.

801.   Carrara VI, Sirilak S, Thonglairuam J, et al. Deployment of early diagnosis and mefloquine-artesunate treatment of falciparum malaria in Thailand: the Tak Malaria Initiative. PLoS Medicine 2006; 3:e183.

802. Marsh VM, Mutemi WM, Willetts A. Improving malaria home treatment by training drug retailers in rural Kenya. Trop Med Internat Health 2004; 9:451–460.

803. Barnes KI, Mwenechanya J, Tembo M, et al. Efficacy of artesunate administered by suppository in the initial treatment of moderately severe malaria in African children and adults. Lancet 2004; 363:1598–1605.

*804. Lengeler C. Insecticide-treated bednets and curtains for preventing malaria (Cochrane Review). In: The Cochrane Library, 1. Oxford: Update Software; 2001.

*805. Armstrong Schellenberg JRM, Abdulla S, Nathan R. Effect of large-scale social marketing of insecticide-treated nets on child survival in rural Tanzania. Lancet 2001; 357:1241–1247.

*806. Garner P, Gulmezoglu AM. Prevention versus treatment for malaria in pregnant women (Cochrane Review). In: The Cochrane Library, 3. Oxford: Update Software; 2000.

*807. Schellenberg D, Menendez C, Kahigwa E, et al. Intermittent treatment for malaria and anaemia control at time of routine vaccinations in Tanzanian infants: a randomised, placebo-controlled trial. Lancet 2001; 357:1471–1477.

Toxoplasmosis

*808. Dunn D, Wallon M, Peyron F, et al. Mother-to-child transmission of toxoplasmosis: risk estimates for clinical counselling. Lancet 1999; 353:1829–1833.

809. Dubey JP. Sources of *Toxoplasma gondii* infection in pregnancy. Until rates of congenital toxoplasmosis fall, control measures are essential. BMJ 2000; 321:127–128.

810. Cook AJ, Gilbert RE, Buffolano W, et al. Sources of toxoplasma infection in pregnant women: European multicentre case-control study. European Research Network on Congenital Toxoplasmosis. BMJ 2000; 321:142–147.

811. Michaels MG, Wald ER, Fricker FJ, et al. Toxoplasmosis in pediatric recipients of heart transplants. Clin Infect Dis 1992; 14:847–851.

812. Derouin F, Devergie A, Auber P, et al. Toxoplasmosis in bone marrow-transplant recipients: report of seven cases and review. Clin Infect Dis 1992; 15:267–270.

813. Bonametti AM, Passos JN, Koga da Silva EM, et al. Probable transmission of acute toxoplasmosis through breast feeding. J Trop Pediatr 1997; 43:116.

814. Montoya JG, Remington JS. Toxoplasmic chorioretinitis in the setting of acute acquired toxoplasmosis. Clin Infect Dis 1996; 23:277–282.

815. Petersen E, Pollak A, Reiter-Owona I. Recent trends in research on congenital toxoplasmosis. Int J Parasitol 2001; 31:115–144.

*816. Peyron F, Wallon M, Liou C, et al. Treatments for toxoplasmosis in pregnancy (Cochrane Review). In: The Cochrane Library, 2. Oxford: Update Software; 2000.

Trypanosomiasis

817. Triolo N, Trova P, Fusco C, et al. Report on 17 years of studies of human African trypanosomiasis caused by *T. gambiense* in children 0–6 years of age. Med Trop (Mars) 1985; 45:251–257.

818. Blum J, Schmid C, Burri C. Clinical aspects of 2541 patients with second stage human African trypanosomiasis. Acta Trop 2006; 97:55–64.

819. Chappuis F, Loutan L, Simarro P, et al. Options for field diagnosis of human African trypanosomiasis. Clin Microbiol Rev 2005; 18:133–146.

820. Bailey JW, Smith DH. The use of the acridine orange QBC technique in the diagnosis of African trypanosomiasis. Trans R Soc Trop Med Hyg 1992; 86:630.

821. Lumsden WHR, Kimber CD, Evans DA, et al. *Trypanosoma brucei*: miniature anion-exchange centrifugation technique for detection of low parasitaemias: adaptation for field use. Trans R Soc Trop Med Hyg 1979; 73:312–317.

822. Inojosa WO, Augusto I, Bisoffi Z, et al. Diagnosing human African trypanosomiasis in Angola using a card agglutination test: observational study of active and passive case finding strategies. BMJ 2006; 332:1479.

823. Asonganyi T, Doua F, Kibona SN, et al. A multi-centre evaluation of the card indirect agglutination test for trypanosomiasis (TrypTect CIATT). Ann Trop Med Parasitol 1998; 92:837–844.

824. World Health Organization. Control and surveillance of African trypanosomiasis. Technical Report Series No 881. Geneva: World Health Organization; 1998.

825. Burri C, Nkunku S, Merolle A, et al. Efficacy of new, concise schedule for melarsoprol in treatment of sleeping sickness caused by *Trypanosoma brucei gambiense*: a randomised trial. Lancet 2000; 355:1419–1425.

826. Pepin J, Mpia B. Randomized controlled trial of three regimens of melarsoprol in the treatment of *Trypanosoma brucei gambiense* trypanosomiasis. Trans R Soc Trop Med Hyg 2006; 100:437–441.

827. Pepin J, Milord F, Guern C, et al. Trial of prednisolone for prevention of melarsoprol-induced encephalopathy in gambiense sleeping sickness. Lancet 1989; 1:1246–1250.

*828. Balasegaram M, Harris S, Checchi F, et al. Melarsoprol versus eflornithine for treating late-stage Gambian trypanosomiasis in the Republic of the Congo. Bull World Health Organ 2006; 84:783–791.

*829. Chappuis F, Udayraj N, Stietenroth K, et al. Eflornithine is safer than melarsoprol for the treatment of second-stage *Trypanosoma brucei gambiense* human African trypanosomiasis. Clin Infect Dis 2005; 41:748–751.

*830. Bisser S, N'siesi FX, Lejon V, et al. Equivalence trial of melarsoprol and nifurtimox monotherapy and combination therapy for the treatment of second-stage *Trypanosoma brucei gambiense* sleeping sickness. J Infect Dis 2007; 195:322–329.

831. Kierszenbaum F. Chagas' disease and the autoimmunity hypothesis. Clin Microbiol Rev 1999; 12:210–223.

832. Riarte A, Luna C, Sabatiello R, et al. Chagas' disease in patients with kidney transplants: 7 years of experience 1989–1996. Clin Infect Dis 1999; 29:561–567.

833. Russomando G, de Tomassone MM, de Guillen I, et al. Treatment of congenital Chagas' disease diagnosed and followed up by the polymerase chain reaction. Am J Trop Med Hyg 1998; 59:487–491.

834. Solari A, Ortiz S, Soto A, et al. Treatment of *Trypanosoma cruzi*-infected children with nifurtimox: a 3 year follow-up by PCR. J Antimicrob Chemother 2001; 48:515–519.

*835. Villar JC, Marin-Neto JA, Ebrahim S, et al. Trypanocidal drugs for chronic asymptomatic *Trypanosoma cruzi* infection. Cochrane Database Syst Rev 2002;(1):CD003463.

836. Viotti R, Vigliano C, Lococo B, et al. Long-term cardiac outcomes of treating chronic Chagas disease with benznidazole versus no treatment: a nonrandomized trial. Ann Intern Med 2006; 144:724–734.

837. Apt W, Aguilera X, Arribada A, et al. Treatment of chronic Chagas' disease with itraconazole and allopurinol. Am J Trop Med Hyg 1998; 59:133–138.

838. Apt W, Arribada A, Zulantay I, et al. Itraconazole or allopurinol in the treatment of chronic American trypanosomiasis: the regression and prevention of electrocardiographic abnormalities during 9 years of follow-up. Ann Trop Med Parasitol 2003; 97:23–29.

839. Blanco SB, Segura EL, Cura EN, et al. Congenital transmission of *Trypanosoma cruzi*: an operational outline for detecting and treating infected infants in north-western Argentina. Trop Med Int Health 2000; 5:293–301.

840. Moncayo A. Progress towards interruption of transmission of Chagas disease. Mem Inst Oswaldo Cruz 1999; 94 Suppl 1:401–404.

Fungal Infections

841. Drake DP, Holt RJ. Childhood actinomycosis. Report of 3 recent cases. Arch Dis Child 1976; 51:979–981.

842. Schmidt P, Koltai JL, Weltzien A. Actinomycosis of the appendix in childhood. Pediatr Surg Int 1999; 15:63–65.

843. Hilfiker ML. Disseminated actinomycosis presenting as a renal tumor with metastases. J Pediatr Surg 2001; 36:1577–1578.

844. Goussard P, Gie R, Kling S, et al. Thoracic actinomycosis mimicking primary tuberculosis. Pediatr Infect Dis J 1999; 18:473–475.

845. Rosenberg M, Patterson R, Mintzer R, et al. Clinical and immunological criteria for the diagnosis of allergic bronchopulmonary aspergillosis. Ann Intern Med 1977; 86:405–414.

846. Cunningham S, Madge SL, Dinwiddie R. Survey of criteria used to diagnose allergic bronchopulmonary aspergillosis in cystic fibrosis. Arch Dis Child 2001; 84:89.

847. Baddley JW, Thomas P, Stroud D, et al. Invasive mold infections in allogeneic bone marrow transplant recipients. Clin Infect Dis 2001; 32:1319–1324.

848. Wong-Beringer A, Jacobs RA, Guglielmo BJ. Lipid formulations of amphotericin B: clinical efficacy and toxicities. Clin Infect Dis 1998; 27:603–618.

849. Smith CE, Beard RR, Whiting EG, et al. Variation of coccidioidal infection in relation to the epidemiology and control of the disease. Am J Public Health 1946; 36:1394–1402.

850. Rollot F, Bossi P, Tubiana R, et al. Discontinuation of secondary prophylaxis against cryptococcosis in patients with AIDS receiving highly active antiretroviral therapy. AIDS 2001; 15:1448–1449.

851. Kasuga T, Taylor JW, White TJ. Phylogenetic relationships of varieties and geographical groups of the human pathogenic fungus *Histoplasma capsulatum* Darling. J Clin Microbiol 1999; 37:653–663.

852. Deepe GS. Immune response to early and late *Histoplasma capsulatum* infections. Curr Opin Microbiol 2000; 3:359–362.

853. Kügler S, Sebghati TS, Eissenberg LG, et al. Phenotypic variation and intracellular parasitism by *Histoplasma capsulatum*. Proc Natl Acad Sci USA 2000; 97:8794–8798.

854. Odio CM, Navarrete M, Carrillo JM, et al. Disseminated histoplasmosis in infants. Pediatr Infect Dis J 1999; 18:1065–1068.

855. Fahal AH, Hassan MA. Mycetoma. Br J Surg 1992; 79:1138–1141.

856. Hamid ME, Maldonado L, Eldin S, et al. *Nocardia africana* spp. nov., a new pathogen isolated from patients with pulmonary infections. J Clin Microbiol 2001; 39:625–630.

857. Spargo BJ, Crowe LM, Ioneda T, et al. Cord factor (a,a-trehalose 6,6'-dimycolate) inhibits fusion between phospholipid vesicles. Proc Natl Acad Sci U S A 1991; 88:737–740.

858. Black CM, Palieschesckey M, Beaman BL, et al. Acidification of phagosomes in murine macrophages: blockage by *Norcardia asteroides*. J Infect Dis 1986; 54:917–919.

859. Fergie JE, Purcell K. Nocardiosis in South Texas children. Pediatr Infect Dis J 2001; 20:711–714.

860. Duong TA. Infection due to *Penicillium marneffei*, an emerging pathogen: review of 155 reported cases. Clin Infect Dis 1996; 23:125–130.

861. Lopez-Martinez R, Neumann L, Gonzalez-Mendoza A. Case report: cutaneous penicilliosis

due to *Penicillium chrysogenum*. Mycoses 1999; 42:347–349.

862. Bustamante B, Campos PE. Endemic sporotrichosis. Curr Opin Infect Dis 2001; 14:145–149.

863. Fleury RN, Taborda PR, Gupta AK, et al. Zoonotic sporotrichosis. Transmission to humans by infected domestic cat scratching: report of four cases in Sao Paulo, Brazil. Int J Dermatol 2001; 40:318–322.

864. de Lima Barros MB, Schubach TMP, Galhardo MCG, et al. Sporotrichosis: an emergent zoonosis in Rio de Janeiro. Mem Inst Oswaldo Cruz, Rio de Janeiro 2001; 96:777–779.

865. Lortholary O, Denning DW, Dupont B. Endemic mycoses: a treatment update. J Antimicrob Chemother 1999; 43:321–331.

866. Lee JW, Siebel NC, Amantea M, et al. Safety and pharmacokinetics of fluconazole in children with neoplastic diseases. J Pediatr 1992; 120:987–993.

867. Spanakis EK, Aperis G, Mylonakis E. New agents for the treatment of fungal infections: Clinical efficacy and gaps in coverage. Clin Infect Dis 2006; 43:1060–1068.

Helminth Infection

868. McCarthy J, Moore TA. Emerging helminth zoonoses. Int J Parasitol 2000; 30:1351–1360.

869. Rim H-J, Forag HF, Sormani S, et al. Food-borne trematodes: ignored or emerging. Parasitol Today 1994; 10:207–209.

870. Goldsmid JM, Speare R. The parasitology of foods. In: Hocking AD, ed. Foodborne microorganisms of public health significance, 6th edn. Sydney: AIFST; 2003.

871. Goldsmid JM. The deadly legacy. Sydney: University of NSW Press; 1988.

872. Nokes C, Bundy DP. Does helminth infection affect mental processing and educational achievement? Parasitol Today 1994; 10:14–18.

*873. Dickson R, Awasthi S, Demellweek C, et al. Antihelmintic drugs for treating worms in children; effects on growth and cognitive performance (Cochrane Review). In: The Cochrane Library, 4. Oxford: Update Software; 2005.

874. Bettiol S, Goldsmid JM. A case of probable imported *Moniliformis moniliformis* infection in Tasmania. J Travel Med 2000; 7:336–337.

875. Maizels R, Blaxter M, Kennedy M. Parasitic helminths: genomes to vaccines. Parasitol Today 1998; 14:131–132.

876. Flores A, Esteban J-G, Anler R, et al. Soil-transmitted helminth infections at very high altitudes. Trans R Soc Trop Med Hyg 2001; 95:272–277.

877. Janssens PG. Chemotherapy of gastrointestinal nematodiasis in man. In: Vanden Bossche H, Thienpont D, Janssens PG, eds. Chemotherapy of gastrointestinal helminths. Berlin: Springer; 1985:183–406.

878. Lancet Editorial. Ascariasis. Lancet 1989; i:997–998.

879. Crompton D. Chronic ascariasis and malnutrition. Parasitol Today 1985; 1:47–52.

880. Pawlowski ZS. Ascariasis. In: Pawlowski ZS, ed. Baillière's Clinical tropical medicine and communicable diseases. Vol 2.3. London: Baillière Tindall; 1987:595–615.

881. Crompton D. The prevalence of ascariasis. Parasitol Today 1988; 4:162–165.

882. Santra A, Bhattacharya T, Chowdhury A, et al. Serodiagnosis of ascariasis with a specific IgG 4 antibody and its use in an epidemiological study. Trans R Soc Trop Med Hyg 2001; 95:289–292.

883. Schneider J, Hughes J, Henderson A. Infectious diseases: prophylaxis and chemotherapy. Australia: Appleton & Lange; 1990.

884. Lengeler C. Insecticide – treated bed nets and curtains for preventing malaria. *Cochrane Database of Systematic Reviews* 2004, Issue 2. Art. No: CD000363.

885. Gustafsson LL, Beerman B, Abdi YA. Handbook of drugs for tropical parasitic infections. London: Taylor & Francis; 1987.

886. James SL, Gilles HM. Human antiparasitic drugs. Chichester: Wiley; 1985.

887. World Bank. Investing in health, World Development Report. Oxford: Oxford University Press; 1993.

888. Guyatt HL. Mass chemotherapy and school-based anthelmintic delivery. Trans R Soc Trop Med Hyg 1999; 93:12–13.

889. Gillespie SH. The epidemiology of *Toxocara canis*. Parasitol Today 1988; 4:180–182.

890. Shorey M, Walker J, Biggs B-A. Clinical parasitology. Melbourne: Melbourne University Press; 2000.

891. Milstein T, Goldsmid JM. The presence of Giardia and other zoonotic parasites of urban dogs in Hobart, Tasmania. Aust Vet J 1995; 72:154–155.

892. Rochette F. Chemotherapy of gastrointestinal nematodiasis in carnivores. In: Vanden Bossche H, Thienpont D, Janssens PG, eds. Chemotherapy of gastrointestinal helminths. Berlin: Springer; 1985:487–504.

893. Hungerford TG. Hazards from domestic pets. Aust Fam Phys 1977; 6:1503–1507.

894. Pawlowski ZS. Enterobiasis. In: Pawlowski ZS, ed. Baillière's Clinical tropical medicine and communicable diseases. Vol 2.3. London: Baillière Tindall; 1987:667–676.

895. Mills A, Goldsmid JM. Intestinal protozoa. In: Doerr WS, Siefert G, eds. Tropical pathology. Vol. 8. Berlin: Springer; 1995:477–556.

896. Marty AM, Andersen EM. Helminthology. In: Doerr WS, Siefert G, eds. Tropical pathology. Vol. 8. Berlin: Springer; 1995:801–982.

897. Smyth JD. Rare, new and emerging helminth zoonoses. Adv Parasitol 1995; 36:1–47.

898. Crompton DH. Hookworm disease: current status and new directions. Parasitol Today 1989; 5:1–2.

899. Behnke JM. Do hookworms elicit protective immunity in man? Parasitol Today 1987; 3:200–206.

900. Pritchard DI. The survival strategies of hookworms. Parasitol Today 1995; 11:255–259.

901. Goldsmid JM. The African hookworm problem: an overview. In: Macpherson C, Craig P, eds. Parasitic helminths and zoonoses in Africa. London: Unwin & Hyman; 1991.

902. Reynolds JEF, ed. Martindale, the extra pharmacopoeia. London: The Pharmaceutical Press; 1996.

903. Quinell RJ, Griffin J, Nowell MA, et al. Predisposition to hookworm infection in Papua New Guinea. Trans R Soc Trop Med Hyg 2001; 95:139–142.

904. Hotez PJ, Le Trang N, Cerami A. Hookworm antigens: a potential for vaccination. Parasitol Today 1987; 3:247–249.

905. Cooper ES, Bundy D. Trichuriasis. In: Pawlowski ZS, ed. Baillière's Clinical tropical medicine and communicable diseases. Vol 2.3. London: Baillière Tindall; 1987:629–643.

906. Cooper ES, Bundy D. Trichuris is not trivial. Parasitol Today 1988; 4:301–306.

907. Ashford RW, Barnish G. Strongyloidiasis in Papua New Guinea. In: Pawlowski ZS, ed. Baillière's Clinical tropical medicine and communicable diseases. Vol 2.3. London: Baillière Tindall; 1987:765–773.

908. Ashford RW, Barnish G, Viney ME. *Strongyloides fuelleborni*: infection and disease in Papua New Guinea. Parasitol Today 1992; 8:314–318.

909. Genta RM. *Strongyloides stercoralis*. In: Guerrant RL, Walker DH, Weller PF, eds. Essentials of tropical infectious diseases. New York: Churchill Livingstone; 2001:464–468.

910. Oliver NW, Rowbottom DJ, Sexton P, et al. Chronic strongyloidiasis in Tasmanian veterans – clinical diagnosis by use of a screening index. Aust N Z J Med 1990; 19:458–462.

911. Smallman LA, Young JA, Shortland-Webb WR, et al. *Strongyloides stercoralis* hyper-infestation syndrome with *Escherichia coli* meningitis: report of two cases. J Clin Pathol 1986; 39:366–370.

912. Pagliuca A, Layton D, Allen S, et al. Hyperinfection with strongyloides after treatment for adult T-cell leukaemia-lymphoma in an African immigrant. BMJ 1988; 297:1456–1457.

913. Pearson RL, et al. Chemotherapy of tropical infectious diseases. In: Guerrant RL, Walker DH, Weller PF, eds. Essentials of tropical infectious diseases. New York: Churchill Livingstone; 2001:613–637.

914. Grove D. Human strongyloidiasis. Adv Parasitol 1996; 38:252–309.

915. Cross JH. Public health importance of *Angiostrongylus cantonensis* and its relatives. Parasitol Today 1987; 3:367–369.

916. Chin J, ed. Control of communicable diseases manual, 17th edn. Washington: APHA; 2000.

917. Morera P. Abdominal angiostrongyliasis: intestinal helminthic infections. In: Pawlowski ZS, ed. Baillière's Clinical tropical medicine and communicable diseases. Vol 2.3. London: Baillière Tindall; 1987:747–753.

918. Polderman AM, Blotkamp J. *Oesophagostomum* infections in humans. Parasitol Today 1995; 11:451–456.

919. Jozefzoon LM, Oostburg BF. Detection of hookworm and hookworm-like larvae in human fecocultures in Suriname. Am J Trop Med Hyg 1994; 51:501–505.

920. Hemsrichart V. *Ternidens* infection – first pathological report of a human case in Asia. J Med Assoc Thailand 2005; 88:1140–1143.

921. Moore DAJ, Girdwood RWA, Chiodini PL. Treatment of anisakiasis with albendazole. Lancet 2002; 360:54.

922. Bier JW, Deardorff TL, Jackson GJ, et al. Human anisakiasis. In: Pawlowski ZS, ed. Baillière's Clinical tropical medicine and communicable diseases. Vol 2.3. London: Baillière Tindall; 1987:723–733.

923. Oshima T. Anisakis – is the sushi bar guilty? Parasitol Today 1987; 3:44–48.

924. Anonymous. Trichinosis outbreak associated with horsemeat. Parasitol Today 1986; 2:295.

925. Campbell WC. Trichinosis revisited – another look at modes of transmission. Parasitol Today 1988; 4:83–86.

926. Kociecka W. Intestinal trichinellosis. In: Pawlowski ZS, ed. Baillière's Clinical tropical medicine and communicable diseases. Vol 2.3. London: Baillière Tindall; 1987:755–763.

927. Cross JH, Basaca-Sevilla V. Intestinal capillariasis. In: Pawlowski ZS, ed. Baillière's Clinical tropical medicine and communicable diseases. Vol 2.3. London: Baillière Tindall; 1987:735–744.

928. Goldsmid JM. More than meets the eye: artefacts and pseudoparasites in faeces. Aust Microbiol 1995; 16:87–89.

929. Muller R. Guineaworm eradication – the end of another disease? Parasitol Today 1985; 1:39.

930. Nelson GS. Lymphatic filaria. In: Gilles HM, ed. Clinics in tropical medicine and communicable disease. Vol 1, no. 3. London: Saunders; 1986: 671–683.

931. Shelley M, Maia-Herzog M, Calvao-Brito R. The specificity of an ELISA for detection of *Onchocerca volvulus* in Brazil in an area endemic for Mansonella. Trans R Soc Trop Med Hyg 2001; 95:171–173.

932. Cupp EW. Treatment of onchocerciasis with ivermectin in Central America. Parasitol Today 1992; 8:212–214.

933. Whitworth J. Treatment of onchocerciasis with ivermectin in Sierra Leone. Parasitol Today 1992; 8:138–140.

934. Chodakewitz J. Ivermectin and lymphatic filariasis: a clinical update. Parasitol Today 1995; 11:233–235.

935. Gardon J, Boussinesq M, Kamgno J, et al. Effects of standard and high doses of ivermectin on adult worms of *Onchocerca volvulus*: a randomized controlled trial. Lancet 2002; 360:203–210.

936. Unnasch TR. River blindness. Lancet 2002; 360:182.

937. Hoerauf A, Mand S, Adjei O, et al. Depletion of Wolbachia endobacteria in *Onchocerca volvulus* by doxycycline and microfilaria after ivermectin treatment. Lancet 2001; 357:1415–1416.

938. Lockwood D. Dermatology. In: Eddleston M, Davidson R, Wilkinson R, et al, eds. Oxford Handbook of tropical medicine, 2nd edn. Oxford: Oxford University Press; 2005:487–514.

939. Pinder M. *Loa loa* – a neglected filaria. Parasitol Today 1988; 4:279–284.

940. Klion AD, Nutman TB. Loiasis and *Mansonella* infections. In: Guerrant RL, Walker DL, Weller PF, eds. Essentials of tropical infectious diseases. New York: Churchill Livingstone; 2001:404–411.

941. Dreyer G, Medeiros Z, Netto M, et al. Acute attacks in the extremeties of persons living in an area endemic to bancroftian filariasis: differentiation of two syndromes. Trans R Soc Trop Med Hyg 1999; 93:413–417.

942. Hightower AW, Lamine PJ, Eberhard MC. Maternal filarial infections – a persistent risk factor for microfilaraemia in offspring? Parasitol Today 1993; 9:418–419.

943. Partono F. Diagnosis and treatment of lymphatic filariasis. Parasitol Today 1985; 1:52–57.

944. Ganesh B, Kader A, Agarwal G, et al. A simple and inexpensive dot-blot assay using a 66-kDa *Brugia malayi* microfilarial protein antigen for diagnosis of bancroftian filariasis in an endemic area. Trans R Soc Trop Med Hyg 2001; 95:168–169.

945. Kluber S, Supali T, Williams S, et al. Rapid PCR-based detection of *Brugia malayi* DNA from blood spots by DNA detection test. Trans R Soc Trop Med Hyg 2001; 95:169–170.

946. Rahmah N, Lim B, Anuar AK, et al. A recombinant antigen-based IgG4 ELISA for the specific and sensitive detection of *Brugia malayi* infection. Trans R Soc Trop Med Hyg 2001; 95:280–284.

947. Ottesen EA, Vijayasekaran V, Kumaraswami V, et al. A controlled trial of ivermectin and diethylcarbamazine in lymphatic filariasis. N Engl J Med 1990; 322:1113–1117.

948. Molyneaux D, Neira M, Liese B, et al. Elimination of lymphatic filariasis as a public health problem. Trans R Soc Trop Med Hyg 2000; 94:589–591.

949. Alexander N, Bockarie M, Dimber Z, et al. Migration and dispersal of lymphatic filariasis in Papua New Guinea. Trans R Soc Trop Med Hyg 2001; 5:277–279.

950. Molyneaux D. Vector-borne infections in the tropics and health policy issues in the twenty-first century. Trans R Soc Trop Med Hyg 2001; 95:233–238.

951. Muller R. *Dipetalonema* by any other name. Parasitol Today 1987; 3:358.

952. Ito A. Cysticercosis in the Asian-Pacific regions. Parasitol Today 1992; 8:182–183.

953. McManus DP, Bowles J. Asian (Taiwan) *Taenia*: species or strain? Parasitol Today 1994; 10:273–275.

954. McKelvie P, Goldsmid JM. Childhood central nervous system cysticercosis in Australia. Med J Aust 1988; 149:42–44.

955. Jaroonvesama N. Differential diagnosis of eosinophilic meningitis. Parasitol Today 1988; 4:262–264.

956. Tillez-Giron E, Ramos MC, Dufour I. Detection of *Cysticercus cellulosae* antigens in cerebrospinal fluid by DOT enzyme-linked immunosorbent assay (DOT-ELISA) and standard ELISA. Am J Trop Med Hyg 1987; 37:169–173.

957. Hughes AJ, Biggs BA. Parasitic worms of the central nervous system: an Australian perspective. Int Med J 2002; 32:541–553.

958. Craig PS, Rogers M, Alfan J. Detection, screening and community epidemiology of taeniid and cestode zoonoses. Adv Parasitol 1996; 38:169–250.

959. Kociecka W. Intestinal cestodiasis. In: Pawlowski ZS, ed. Baillière's Clinical tropical medicine and communicable diseases. Vol 2.3. London: Baillière Tindall; 1987:677–694.

960. Kammerer WS. Chemotherapy of tapeworm infections in man. In: Vanden Bossche H, Thienpont D, Janssens PG, eds. Chemotherapy of gastrointestinal helminths. Berlin: Springer; 1985.

961. Moodley M, Moosa A. Treatment of neurocysticercosis: is praziquantel the new hope? Lancet 1989; 1:262.

*962. Salinas R, Prasad K. Drugs for treating neurocysticercosis (tapeworm infection of the brain) (Cochrane Review). In: The Cochrane Library, 4. Oxford: Update Software; 2001.

963. Goldsmid JM, Rogers S, Parsons GS, et al. The intestinal protozoa and helminths infecting Africans in the Gatooma region of Rhodesia. Cent Afr J Med 1976; 22:91–95.

964. Schenone H. Praziquantel in the treatment of *Hymenolepis nana* infections in children. Am J Trop Med Hyg 1980; 19:320–321.

965. Bartlett JG. Pocket book of infectious disease therapy. Philadelphia: Lippincott Williams and Wilkins; 2002:184.

966. McManus DP, Smyth JD. Hydatidosis: changing concepts in epidemiology and speciation. Parasitol Today 1986; 2:163–167.

967. Craig PS, Desham L, Zhaoxun D. Hydatid disease in China. Parasitol Today 1991; 7:46–50.

968. Lucius R, Frosch M, Kern P. Alveolar echinococcosis: immunogenics and epidemiology. Parasitol Today 1995; 11:4–5.

969. Goldsmid JM, Pickmere J. Hydatid eradication in Tasmania – point of no return? Aust Fam Phys 1987; 16:1672–1674.

970. Gemmell MA, Lawson JR, Roberts MG. Towards global control of cystic and alveolar hydatid disease. Parasitol Today 1987; 3:144–151.

971. Goldsmid JM, Fleming F. The tapeworm infections of children in Rhodesia. Cent Afr J Med 1977; 23:7–10.

972. Frean J, Dini L. Unusual anoplocephalid tapeworm infections in South Africa. Annals of the ACTM 2004; 5:8–11.

973. Warren KS, Mahmoud AAF. Algorithms in the diagnosis and management of exotic diseases. I. Schistosomiasis. J Infect Dis 1975; 131:614–620.

974. Mahmoud AAF. ed. Baillière's Clinical tropical medicine and communicable diseases: schistosomiasis. Vol. 2.2. London: Baillière Tindall; 1987.

975. Woolhouse MEJ. International Conference on Schistosomiasis. Parasitol Today 1993; 9:235–236.

976. Lancet Editorial. Immunity to schistosomiasis. Lancet 1987; i:1015–1016.

977. Hagan P, Williams HA. Concomitant immunity in schistosomiasis. Parasitol Today 1993; 9:1–6.

978. Terry RJ. Concomitant immunity in schistosomiasis. Parasitol Today 1994; 10:377–378.

979. Butterworth AE. Human immunity to schistosomiasis: some questions. Parasitol Today 1994; 10:378–380.

980. Greyseels B. Human resistance to schistosome infections. Parasitol Today 1994; 10:380–384.

981. Anderson RM. Determinants of infection in human schistosomiasis. In: Mahmoud AAF, ed. Baillière's Clinical tropical medicine and communicable diseases. Vol 2.2. London: Baillière Tindall; 1987:279–300.

982. Colley DG. Dynamics of the human immune response to schistosomes. In: Mahmoud AAF, ed. Baillière's Clinical tropical medicine and communicable diseases. Vol 2.2. London: Baillière Tindall; 1987:315–332.

983. Warren KS. Determinants of disease in human schistosomiasis. In: Mahmoud AAF, ed. Baillière's

Clinical tropical medicine and communicable diseases. Vol 2.2. London: Baillière Tindall; 1987:301–313.

984. Wyler DJ. Why does liver fibrosis occur in schistosomiasis? Parasitol Today 1992; 8:277–279.

985. Phillips SM, Lammie PJ. Immunopathology of granuloma formation and fibrosis in schistosomiasis. Parasitol Today 1986; 3:296–302.

986. Peters PAS, Kazura JW. Update on diagnostic methods for schistosomiasis. In: Mahmoud AAF, ed. Baillière's Clinical tropical medicine and communicable diseases. Vol 2.2. London: Baillière Tindall; 1987:419–433.

987. Webster LT. Update on chemotherapy of schistosomiasis. In: Mahmoud AAF, ed. Baillière's Clinical tropical medicine and communicable diseases. Vol 2.2. London: Baillière Tindall; 1987:435–447.

*988. Saconato H, Atalhah A. Interventions for treating *Schistosomiasis mansoni* (Cochrane Review). In: The Cochrane Library, Issue 2. Chichester: Wiley and Sons: Update 2006.

989. Squares N. Interventions for treating *Schistosomiasis haematobium* (Cochrane Review). In: The Cochrane Library. Issue 2. Chichester: Wiley and Sons; 2006.

990. Jong EC, McMullin R. The tropical and travel medicine manual. Philadelphia: Saunders; 1995.

991. Tchuente LAT, Southgate VR, Webster BL, et al. Impact of installation of a water pump on schistosomiasis transmission in a focus in Cameroon. Trans R Soc Trop Med Hyg 2001; 95:255–256.

992. Capron A. Schistosomiasis: Forty years war on the worm. Parasitol Today 1998; 14:379–384.

993. James SL, Sher A. Prospects for a non-living vaccine against schistosomiasis. Parasitol Today 1986; 2:134–137.

994. Butterworth AE. Potential for vaccines against human schistosomes. In: Mahmoud AAF, ed. Baillière's Clinical tropical medicine and communicable diseases. Vol 2.2. London: Baillière Tindall; 1987:465–483.

995. Butterworth AE, Wilkins HA, Capron A, et al. The control of schistosomiasis – is a vaccine necessary? Parasitol Today 1987; 3:1–3.

996. Coulson P. The radiation-attenuated vaccine against schistosomiasis in animal models. Adv Parasitol 1997; 39:272–336.

997. Haswell-Elkins MR, Sithithawarn P, Elkins D. *Opisthorchis viverrini* and cholangiocarcinoma in northwest Thailand. Parasitol Today 1992; 8:86–89.

998. Gillett JD. The behaviour of *Homo sapiens*, the forgotten factor in the transmission of tropical disease. Trans R Soc Trop Med Hyg 1985; 79:12–20.

999. Harinasuta T, Bunnag D, Radomyos P. Intestinal flukes. In: Pawlowski ZS, ed. Baillière's Clinical tropical medicine and communicable diseases. Vol 2.3. London: Baillière Tindall; 1987:695–721.

1000. Butcher AR, Graham AT, Norton RE, et al. Locally acquired *Brachylaima* sp. (Digenia: Brachylaimidae) intestinal fluke infection in two South Australian infants. Med J Aust 1996; 164:475–478.

Flies, Fleas, Mites and Lice

1001. Hall M, Wall R. Myiasis of humans and domestic animals. Adv Parasitol 1995; 35:257–334.

1002. Alexander JO'D. Arthropods and human skin. Berlin: Springer; 1984.

1003. Goldsmid JM. The deadly legacy. Sydney: University of NSW Press; 1988.

1004. Dominey A, Rosen T, Tschen J. Papulonodular demodicidosis associated with acquired immuno-deficiency syndrome. J Am Acad Dermatol 1989; 20:197–201.

1005. Christopherson J. Epidemiology of scabies. Parasitol Today 1986; 2:247–248.

1006. Chosidow O. Scabies. N Engl J Med 2006; 354:1718–1726.

1007. Robinson J. Fight the mite, ditch the itch. Parasitol Today 1985; 1:140–142.

1008.   Commens CA. The treatment of scabies. Aust Prescriber 2000; 23:33–35.

1009.   Burgess I. *Sarcoptes scabiei* and scabies. Adv Parasitol 1994; 33:235–292.

1010.   Commens CA. We can get rid of scabies: new treatment available soon. Med J Aust 1994; 160:317–318.

1011.   Chin J, ed. Control of communicable diseases manual, 17th edn. Washington: APHA; 2000.

1012.   Goldsmid JM. Unusual arthropod ectoparasitic infestations of man. Aust Fam Physician 1985; 14:386–388.

*1013.   Walker GJ, Johnstone PW. Interventions for treating scabies (Cochrane Review). In: The Cochrane Library, Issue 2. Chichester; 2006.

1014.   Burgess I. Human lice. Adv Parasitol 1995; 36:271–342.

1015.   Vander Stichele RH, Gyssels L, Bracke C, et al. Wet combing for head lice: feasibility in mass screening, treatment preference and outcome. J Roy Soc Med 2002; 95:348–350.

1016.   Counahan M, Andrews R, Buttner P, et al. Head lice prevalence in primary schools in Victoria, Australia. J Paediatr Child Hlth 2004; 40:616–619.

1017.   Meinking TL, Taplin D. Advances in pediculosis, scabies and other mite infestations. Adv Dermatol 1990; 5:131–152.

*1018.   Vander Steichele RH, Dezeure EM, Bogaert MG. Systematic review of clinical efficacy of topical treatments for head lice. BMJ 1995; 311:604–608.

1019.   Burgess I. Malathion lotions for head lice – a less reliable treatment than commonly believed. Pharmaceutical J 1991; (Nov 9):630–632.

*1020.   Dodd CS. Interventions for treating headlice. (Cochrane review). In: The Cochrane Library, Issue 2. Chichester: Wiley and Sons; 2006.

1021.   Goldsmid JM. The treatment and control of head lice: a review. Aust J Pharm 1989; 70:1021–1024.

1022.   Goldsmid JM, Langley J, Naylor P, et al. Further studies on head lice and their control in Tasmania. Aust Fam Physician 1989; 18:253–255.

1023.   Burgess I, Peock S, Brown CM, et al. Headlice resistant to pyrethroid insecticides in Britain. BMJ 1995; 311:752.

1024.   Wargon O. Treating head lice. Austr Prescriber 2000; 23:62–63.

1025.   Namazi MR. Levamisole: a safe and economical weapon against pediculosis. Int J Dermatol 2001; 40:292–294.

1026.   Roberts RJ, Casey D, Morgan DA, et al. Comparison of wet combing with malathion for treatment of head lice in the UK. Lancet 2000; 356:540–544.

1027.   Roberts RJ. Clinical practice: Head lice. N Engl J Med 2002; 346:1645–1650.

1028.   Hill N, Moor G, Cameron MM, et al. The Bug Buster Kit was better than single dose pediculicide for head lice. Evid Based Med 2006; 11:17.

Diseases Transmitted by Animals

1029.   Chin J, ed. Control of communicable diseases manual, 17th edn. Washington: APHA; 2000.

1030.   Margileth AM. Cat scratch disease. Adv Pediatr Infect Dis 1993; 8:1–21.

1031.   Wilks CR, Humble MW. Zoonoses in New Zealand. Palmeston North: Veterinary Continuing Education; 1997.

1032.   Murano I, Yoshii H, Kurashige H, et al. Giant hepatic granuloma caused by *Bartonella henselae*. Pediatr Infect Dis J 2001; 20:319–320.

1033.   Isada CM, Kasten BL, Goldman MP, et al. Infectious diseases handbook, 3rd edn. Hudson: American Pharmaceutical Association, Lexi-Comp; 1999.

1034.   Brenner DJ, Hollis DG, Moss CW, et al. Proposal of *Afipia* gen. nov., with *Afipia felis* sp. nov. (formerly cat scratch disease bacillus), *Afipia clevelandensis* sp. nov. (formerly the Cleveland Clinic Foundation strain), *Afipia broomeae* sp. nov., and three unnamed genospecies. J Clin Microbiol 1991; 29:2450–2460.

1035.   Adal KA, Cockerell CJ, Petri WAJr. Cat scratch disease, bacillary angiomatosis, and other infections due to *Rochalimaec*. N Engl J Med 1994; 330:1509–1515.

1036.   Kordick DL, Hilyard EJ, Hadfield TL, et al. *Bartonella clarridgeiae*, a newly recognized zoonotic pathogen causing inoculation papules, fever and lymphadenopathy (cat scratch disease). J Clin Microbiol 1997; 35:1813–1818.

1037.   Margileth AM. Antibiotic therapy for cat-scratch disease: clinical study of therapeutic outcome in 268 patients and a review of the literature. Pediatr Infect Dis J 1992; 11:474–478.

1038.   Carithers HA, Margileth AM. Cat scratch disease: acute encephalopathy and other neurologic manifestations. Am J Dis Child 1991; 145:98–101.

1039.   Stevenson WJ, Hughes KL. Synopsis of zoonoses in Australia. 2nd edn. Canberra: Commonwealth Dept of Community Services; 1988.

1040.   Hockman DE, Pence CD, Whittler RR, et al. Septic arthritis of the hip secondary to rat bite fever: a case report. Clin Orthop 2000; 380:173–176.

1041.   Rordorf T, Zuger C, Zbinden R, et al. *Streptobacillus moniliformis* endocarditis in an HIV-positive patient. Infection 2000; 28:393–394.

29

Disorders of bones, joints and connective tissues

Joyce Davidson, Andrew Gavin Cleary, Colin Bruce

Musculoskeletal symptoms are common in children and frequently present to pediatricians. A comprehensive review of all conditions affecting the musculoskeletal system in childhood would not be possible within the scope of a single chapter. We have tried to cover in some detail those conditions most commonly seen in pediatrics while also giving sufficient information to enable consideration of many of the more unusual conditions that may be encountered. We have also endeavoured to highlight areas of recent progress.

ASSESSMENT OF THE MUSCULOSKELETAL SYSTEM

Clinical assessment of the musculoskeletal system should be part of the routine pediatric examination. A few simple screening questions and assessments can be used to determine whether or not an abnormality is likely. If a child has no pain, swelling or stiffness of the joints, walks with a normal gait, and is able to keep up with his or her peers in normal activities then it is unlikely that a significant problem exists. Any suggestion of a musculoskeletal problem merits detailed assessment. It must be remembered that some rheumatic conditions may present with constitutional symptoms such as a rash, fever or fatigue before the development of any musculoskeletal problems. This section describes a general approach to the examination of the musculoskeletal system. The more detailed assessment of individual problems is described in the relevant sections of the chapter.

A meticulous history and clinical examination will lead to the correct diagnosis in the majority of cases. Investigations may be diagnostically helpful but are more usually used to confirm the clinically suspected diagnosis.

When assessing the musculoskeletal system in a child, knowledge of normal development is clearly important as normal findings vary considerably at different ages. For example a significant degree of joint laxity is normal in the young child and should not be confused with abnormal hypermobility.

HISTORY

As with many areas of pediatric practice the clinical history is often the most informative part of the assessment. Information must be gleaned from both the parents/carers and the child, even the very young child contributing to the history when age-appropriate questions are used. Questions must be asked about musculoskeletal symptoms such as joint pain or swelling, muscle pain; functional difficulties and about relevant non-articular symptoms.

Non-articular symptoms

Children with musculoskeletal or rheumatic conditions frequently have prominent constitutional symptoms. Fever, fatigue, anorexia and weight loss are common to many inflammatory conditions but may also occur in infection and malignancy. Rashes may be characteristic of individual conditions and may be helpful diagnostically.

Pain

Pain is the most frequently reported musculoskeletal symptom, and musculoskeletal pain is a frequent cause of presentation in both primary care and pediatric practice.[1] Detailed enquiry should be made into its location and characteristics including severity, precipitating and relieving factors, radiation and diurnal variation. It must be remembered that joint pain (arthralgia) is common in children and that most do not have serious pathology (Table 29.1). It should also be noted that not all children with a significant musculoskeletal problem will complain of pain.

Based on the history of the pain, its characteristics and associated features, musculoskeletal problems can be usefully divided into three broad categories: inflammatory, mechanical and idiopathic.

Inflammatory

Inflammatory pain is characteristic of arthritis but also occurs in other conditions such as myositis, the hallmark being a relationship to immobility. The affected child is frequently worst first thing in the morning (morning stiffness) or after periods of inactivity ('gelling'). A young child with arthritis may be unable to walk first thing in the morning but be running around later in the day. Exercise will generally relieve the pain which is usually described as aching or uncomfortable rather than severe. Occasionally children with acute exacerbations of arthritis experience severe pain, sufficient to disturb sleep.

Table 29.1 The differential diagnosis of joint pain in children

1. **Arthritis**
   Infective and reactive
   Juvenile idiopathic arthritis
   Other: autoimmune rheumatic disorders (e.g. systemic lupus erythematosus, dermatomyositis); vasculitis; miscellaneous

2. **Mechanical/degenerative**
   Trauma: accidental and non-accidental
   Hypermobility
   Avascular necrosis, osteochondritis and apophysitis, including Perthes, Osgood–Schlatter and Scheurmann
   Slipped capital femoral epiphysis
   Anterior knee pain

3. **Non-organic/idiopathic**
   Idiopathic pain syndromes – localized and diffuse
   Benign idiopathic limb pains (growing pains)
   Psychogenic

4. **Other**
   Osteomyelitis
   Tumors:
       Malignant: leukemia, neuroblastoma
       Benign: osteoid osteoma, pigmented villonodular synovitis
   Metabolic abnormalities: rickets, diabetes, hypophosphatemic rickets, hypo/hyperthyroidism
   Genetic disorders: skeletal dysplasias, mucopolysaccharidoses, collagen disorders

Inflammatory pain in arthritis is almost universally accompanied by objective evidence of persistent joint swelling without which the diagnosis of arthritis should not be made.

Mechanical

By contrast, mechanical pain is generally exacerbated by exercise and relieved by rest. It is frequently intermittent rather than persistent and tends to be described as more severe than that associated with arthritis. Mechanical problems are more common in older children and adolescents and frequently affect the joints of the lower limb and the back.

Associated symptoms are common. Joint 'locking' is frequently described. True joint locking, where there is a block to extension, is uncommon and may indicate a meniscal problem or patellar dislocation. Joint instability may occur with ligamentous laxity and a complaint of the knee 'giving way' is common with anterior knee pain. Joint swelling may occur with mechanical problems but is usually intermittent rather than persistent.

Idiopathic

Children and adolescents with the most severe pain frequently fall into this category where there is no identifiable organic pathology. Their pain is severe, unremitting and frequently associated with fatigue, poor sleep and significant functional impairment.[2] Complaints of intermittent joint swelling are common but seldom corroborated on clinical examination, which is usually normal.

Functional difficulties

It is important to enquire about the ability of the child to function normally both in activities of day-to-day living such as dressing and toileting and in more physically demanding activities such as sports. Such questions are informative in determining both the type of problem and its severity. It must be remembered that young children are particularly good at compensating for loss of function in one area by using another and absence of functional impairment does not imply absence of pathology. Conversely, the most functionally disabled children may be those with idiopathic or non-organic problems.

Discriminating questions of function are useful in determining progress of disease and are important in assessing response to treatment in conditions such as juvenile idiopathic arthritis. There are a variety of validated quantitative functional assessment tools available for use in children with rheumatic disorders.[3] The Childhood Health Assessment Questionnaire (CHAQ) is the most widely used and has been validated for use in both juvenile arthritis and dermatomyositis[4] in a number of different countries and languages.

EXAMINATION

As with any system, examination of the musculoskeletal system of a child must be age appropriate.[5] Much information can be gained particularly in the younger child by observing the child at play before attempting any more formal examination. Observing the child's general demeanour, gait and ability to get up and down off the floor is informative. Ideally the musculoskeletal system should be examined in detail, with assessment of all joints and muscle groups. This is frequently impractical in the very young or the child who is in a lot of pain. The examination may need to be opportunistic, focusing initially on problem areas which will have been identified by initial observation of the child.

A simple screening examination (Table 29.2) may be appropriately used to identify children who merit more detailed assessment and can be incorporated into the routine physical examination of any child.

General systemic examination

The child should be examined for evidence of any systemic features that may be relevant to musculoskeletal disorders. Rashes may be useful diagnostically. Growth impairment is common in many chronic disorders and documentation of height and weight is mandatory. Temperature, blood pressure and urinalysis should be measured where systemic involvement may occur.

Gait

Observation of the gait may help identify the nature and site of the problem, particularly in the younger child who may find it difficult to localize pain.

A child who is unable to weight bear may have a serious disorder such as septic arthritis or a malignancy. A child with fixed flexion deformities at the hips will adopt an exaggerated lordosis to compensate. Weak hip and pelvic muscles will result in a waddling gait, while a painful hip or knee will result in an antalgic gait, where the child walks in such a way as to spend as little time as possible on the affected leg.

Examination of joints

Joints should be inspected, palpated and their range of movement determined. Preprinted tables or cartoon figures are available to aid systematic documentation of the results.

Inspection of joints yields useful information. The position of the joint and any limb deformity should be documented. The limb should be inspected for evidence of wasting of surrounding muscles or limb length discrepancy, resulting from overgrowth at an inflamed joint. Erythema or unusual laxity of the skin overlying the joint should be noted. Joint swelling is frequently obvious on inspection.

Table 29.2 The screening musculoskeletal examination in a child

1. Extend the arms straight out in front then make a fist
2. Place palms and fingers together with wrists extended to 90°: 'prayer position'
3. Raise arms straight above the head
4. Turn neck to look over each shoulder
5. Walk normally, on tip-toe and on the heels
6. Sit cross-legged on the floor then jump up

A child who can perform all these actions without difficulty is unlikely to have a significant musculoskeletal problem

Following inspection the joint should be palpated for warmth, swelling or tenderness. Documenting the presence of joint effusions is important in assessing and diagnosing arthritis. It must be remembered that in some joints, e.g. the hips, effusions can not be detected clinically and must be sought in other ways, e.g. using ultrasound (Fig. 29.1).

In many musculoskeletal conditions loss of joint range is one of the earliest objective signs of a problem. Examining for this requires experience, patience and a knowledge of the normal range of movement of the joints. Where the problem is clearly localized to a particular joint, the examination may focus on this area. If the child has evidence of a condition that may affect more than one area, e.g. a polyarthritis, a meticulous assessment of all joints should be made. Arthritis in children is usually asymmetrical enabling the contralateral joint to be used for comparison.

Range of movement should be assessed both actively and passively. Assessment of active joint range involves observing the child moving the joints. Passive range is assessed by the examiner moving the joints through their full range. A useful sign of early arthritis in a joint is pain at the end of the range of passive movement. The child may deny pain but withdraw the limb consistently when pushed to the end of its range.

Joints frequently forgotten, but important in the overall assessment of the child, are the sacroiliac joints, the temporomandibular joint and the cervical spine.

Examination of muscles

Assessment of muscles is also an essential part of the musculoskeletal examination. Muscle tenderness may indicate an underlying inflammatory process, while wasting and weakness may indicate a disorder of the muscle itself, of the surrounding joints or of the nervous system. Gait abnormalities, or an inability to get up off the floor easily, may be indicative of muscle weakness. The well-known Gower sign, where the child uses his/her hands to push off the body when attempting to stand is an indicator of proximal muscle weakness and not specific to any one group of disorders.

Muscle strength should be formally assessed using a standard scale for grading muscle strength. This requires experience in young children ensuring that clear, understandable instructions are given and taking care not to underestimate the strength of the younger child. A five-point scale for grading muscle strength is familiar to most clinicians. A ten-point scale may be more precise and is equally simple to use (Table 29.3).[6]

In children with inflammatory myositis the childhood myositis assessment scale (CMAS)[7] is a validated method of quantitating muscle strength by scoring the child's ability to perform a variety of maneuvers. Its use in conjunction with manual testing of muscle strength gives reproducible scores which can be used to assess a child's response to treatment.

CONGENITAL AND DEVELOPMENTAL PROBLEMS

In broad terms congenital abnormalities can be classified into:
1. failure of formation (transverse or longitudinal);
2. failure of differentiation;
3. duplication;
4. overgrowth (or gigantism);
5. undergrowth (or hypoplasia);
6. congenital constriction band syndrome;
7. generalized skeletal abnormalities.

It is important to bear in mind that, although congenital abnormalities may be isolated, they may also occur in association with other abnormalities, sometimes as part of a recognized syndrome.

SPINAL PROBLEMS
Congenital spinal problems

The child with a vertebral anomaly must be fully assessed for associated abnormalities as in the VATER (Vertebral, Anorectal, Tracheo-Esophageal, Renal, Radial) and VACTERL (Vertebral, Anorectal, Cardiac,

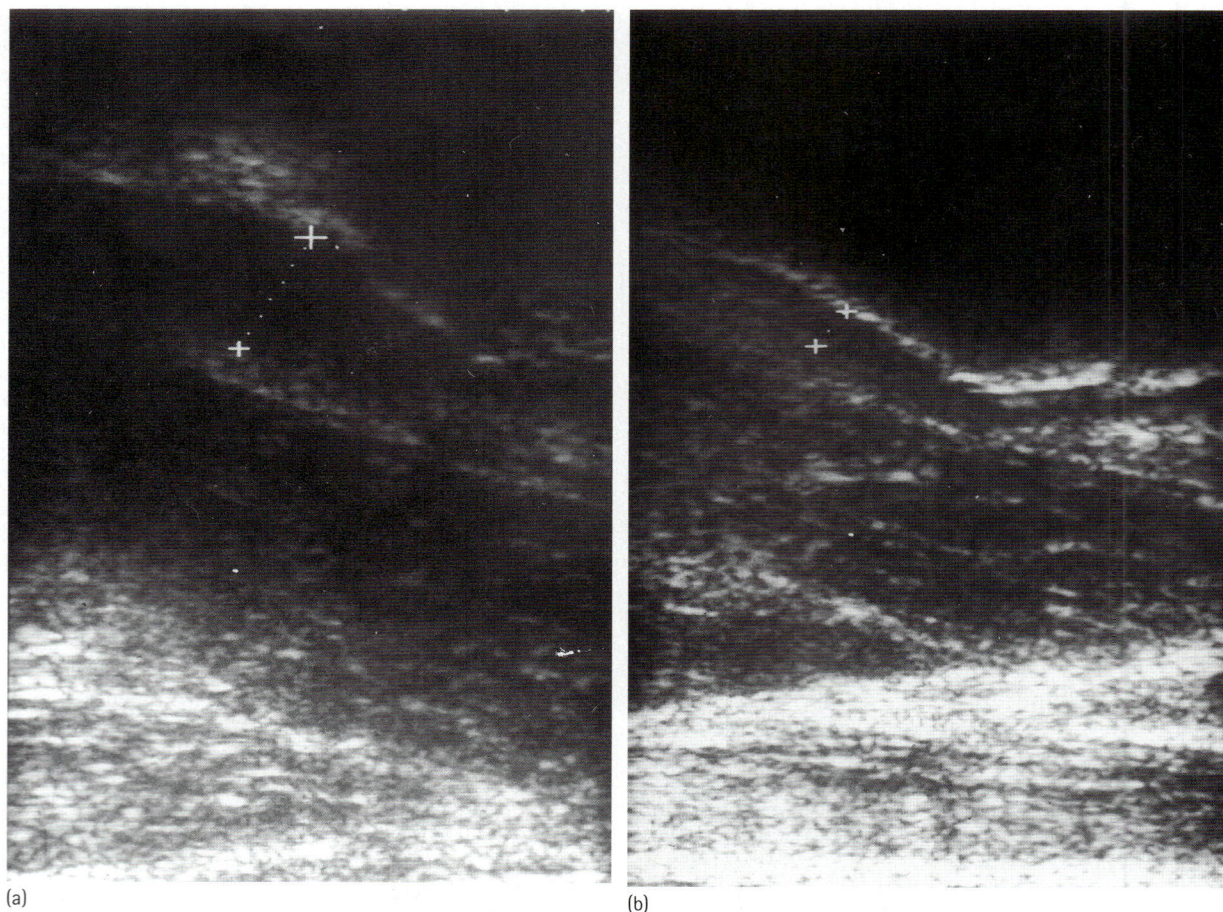

Fig. 29.1   (a) Hip ultrasound showing effusion; (b) normal hip for comparison.

Tracheo-Esophageal, Renal, Limb) syndromes. Deformities occurring as result of vertebral anomalies include scoliosis, kyphosis and lordosis.

Congenital spinal anomalies are classified into failure of formation or failure of separation of individual vertebrae or parts of vertebrae. Failure of separation is termed an unsegmented bar, the position of such a bar determining the deformity. With a lateral unsegmented bar the growth of the spinal column is tethered on that side, continued growth on the opposite side leading to a progressive scoliosis. Failure of formation may involve the anterior, posterior or lateral side of a vertebra and once again the site will dictate the deformity. A hemivertebra on one side of the spinal column leads to extra growth on that side versus the side with the absent segment and a scoliosis may result (Fig. 29.2).

Treatment of the vertebral anomaly depends on its potential to lead to progressive deformity. Some abnormalities have only modest potential and two separate abnormalities may cancel each other out. Other anomalies or combinations have significant potential to progress and will need careful management to prevent progressive deformity.

Idiopathic infantile scoliosis

This usually presents during the first 3 years of life and is distinguished from congenital scoliosis by the absence of a spinal malformation. In contradistinction to adolescent idiopathic scoliosis the condition is more common in boys and the convexity of the thoracic scoliosis is to the left in 90%. The condition is often self-limiting but some cases do progress leading to poor cardiopulmonary development. Prolonged molded plaster jacket treatment is often successful although some may require surgery.

Congenital muscular torticollis

Congenital muscular torticollis, resulting from a contracture of the sternocleidomastoid muscle, is the most common cause of torticollis in the infant. The etiology is unknown. Theories include in-utero crowding and muscle fibrosis following a compartment syndrome within the muscle as a result of compression of the neck during a difficult delivery. Clinically a nontender 'tumor' or swelling can be palpated in the sternocleidomastoid muscle in the first 4–6 weeks, but subsequently regresses. Radiographs of the cervical region should be obtained if there is any suspicion of an underlying cervical abnormality.

Left untreated, plagiocephaly and facial asymmetry may develop. Treatment initially consists of passive stretching exercises together with encouragement of head rotation in the restricted direction

Table 29.3   Manual muscle testing: 5- and 10-point scales for grading of muscle strength

5-point scale	10-point scale	
0	0	No evidence of muscle function
1	1	Slight flicker of contractility; no effective function
2	2	Movement with gravity eliminated
3	3	Movement against gravity
	4	Movement against gravity: unable to hold position
	5	Movement against gravity: able to hold position
4	6	Resists slight pressure
	7	Resists slight/moderate pressure
	8	Resists moderate pressure
	9	Resists moderate/strong pressure
5	10	Full power

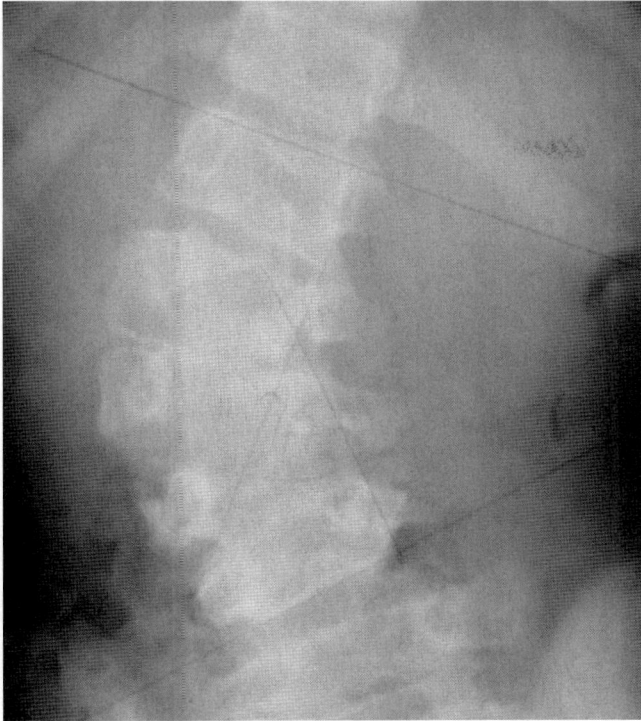

Fig. 29.2   Congenital hemivertebra resulting in scoliosis.

by placing objects of interest toward that side. Passive stretching begun early is successful in 90%.[8] After the age of 1 year surgical treatment may be necessary. This involves division of the tight tendon and is best done before 4 years of age. Established facial deformity or a limitation of more than 30° of rotation usually precludes good results.

Klippel–Feil syndrome

Klippel–Feil syndrome results from failure of the normal segmentation of the cervical vertebrae so that two or more are joined forming block vertebrae. The etiology is unknown. The most consistent clinical finding is limitation of neck motion. Shortening of the neck is subtle.

Associated anomalies include facial asymmetry, torticollis or webbing of the neck in 20%. Sprengel shoulder (a high riding scapula) occurs in up to one third and other associated abnormalities occasionally include ptosis of the eyelid, lateral rectus muscle palsy of the eye, facial nerve palsy, a cleft or high arched palate and abnormalities of the upper limbs including supernumery digits, hypoplasia of the thumb or even the entire upper limb. Abnormalities of the lower limbs are infrequent.[9] Affected patients should be screened for other abnormalities which include scoliosis or kyphosis in up to 60%, renal abnormalities in 30%, cardiovascular abnormalities in 14%, deafness or hearing impairment in 30%. Twenty percent of patients demonstrate mirror motions (synkinesia) or involuntary paired movement of the hands.

UPPER LIMB PROBLEMS

Sprengel shoulder

The scapula develops within the upper limb bud and descends to overlie the second to seventh thoracic vertebrae and ribs. Failure to descend fully gives rise to congenital elevation of the scapula – Sprengel deformity. The condition is usually sporadic but occasionally inherited in an autosomal dominant fashion. It is commoner on the left but can be bilateral. Radiographs of the chest and the cervical spine should be taken to rule out associated rib abnormalities and anomalies of the cervical vertebrae such as Klippel–Feil syndrome.

Shoulder elevation is usually only modestly limited and significant functional problems are rare. Treatment is directed toward maintaining the existing range of movement. Surgical procedures to remove the prominent superomedial tip of the scapula are cosmetic and do not improve shoulder function. Procedures to bring about descent of the whole scapula are associated with significant potential complications and long, sometimes ugly scarring.

Pseudarthrosis of the clavicle

This rare condition presents as a nontender lump at about the midpoint of clavicle. When identified soon after birth it may be mistaken for a fracture, but should be distinguished by the absence of rapid callus formation and persistence of the pseudoarthrosis (Fig. 29.3). It should also be differentiated from cleidocranio-dysostosis where parts of both clavicles are deficient and associated anomalies are found in the skull, facial bones and pelvis. The clavicle develops from medial and lateral ossification centers and the condition may represent a failure of these centers to fuse. Pseudoarthrosis of the clavicle is almost always seen on the right, thought to be a consequence of pressure attrition from the somewhat higher right-sided subclavian vessels.

Shoulder and upper limb function is normally good but the prominent lump is unsightly, and overhead activity may become uncomfortable in maturity. Unlike congenital pseudoarthrosis of the tibia and radius, the condition is not associated with neurofibromatosis and readily unites after excision and bone grafting. Surgery is best performed around the age of 4 years.

Radial club hand (preaxial absence)

Radial dysplasia is the commonest of the major longitudinal failures of formation (Fig. 29.4). It may present as partial or complete absence, bilateral or unilateral. When sporadic the etiology is unknown. The abnormality was seen previously in association with thalidomide when two thirds of cases were bilateral.

Radial dysplasia is always associated with thumb hypoplasia. The spectrum of clinical abnormality can range from mild radial deviation of the wrist and minimal thumb hypoplasia, to complete absence of the preaxial structures including the thumb, the carpal and metacarpal bones and the radius with associated shortening of the ulna and a stiff elbow joint. The deformity is characterized by a weak, radially deviated wrist and a short forearm which grows to only one half to two thirds of normal length. The hand is usually correctable upon the wrist after birth and the elbow lies extended with reduced active and passive flexion.

Early passive stretching and splinting is indicated and should continue until a decision is made regarding surgical treatment. The standard surgical management is centralization of the carpus over the third metacarpal with subsequent pollicization of the index finger.

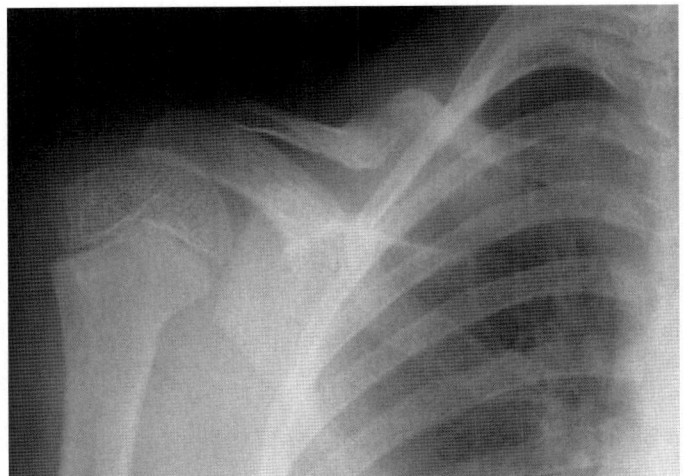

Fig. 29.3   Pseudoarthrosis of the clavicle.

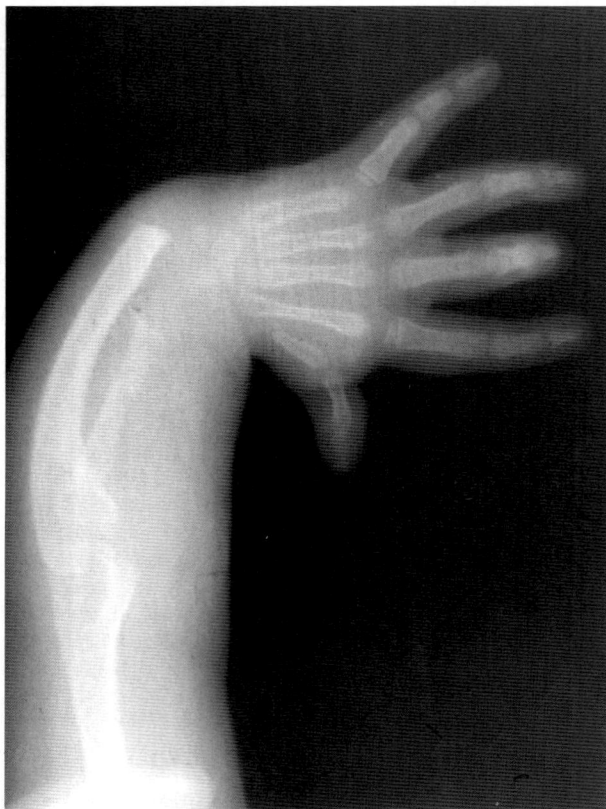

Fig. 29.4   Radial club hand.

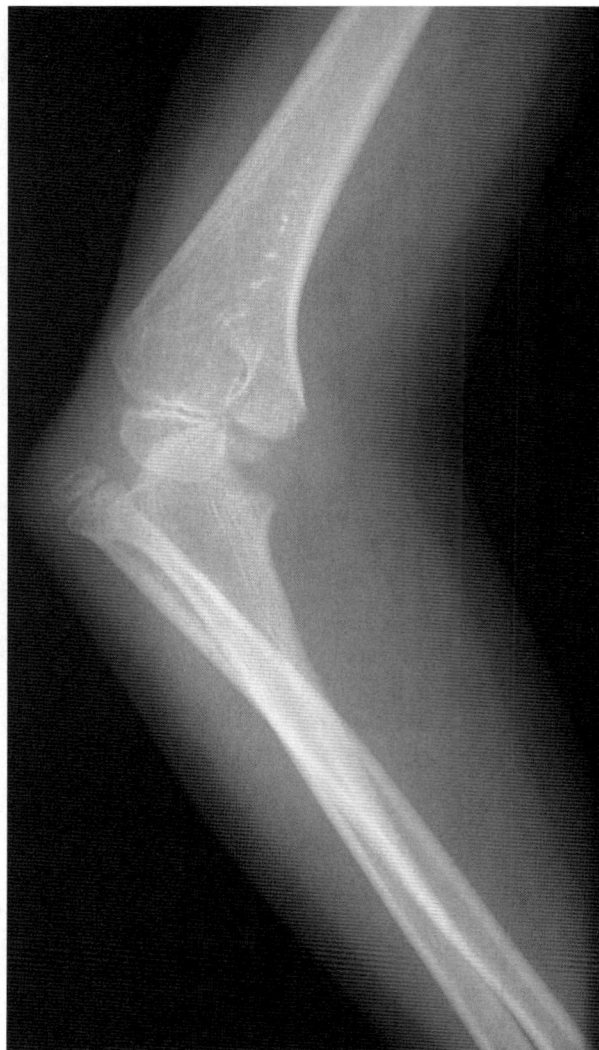

Fig. 29.5   Congenital dislocation of the radial head.

Pollicization is the surgical shortening and rotation of an index finger to allow opposition with the other digits, so compensating for the absent thumb. Elbow mobility is a prerequisite for centralization procedures to ensure that hand to mouth movement is possible.

Radial deficiency may occur in isolation. Forty percent of patients with unilateral and 27% with bilateral radial club hand have associated malformations including those of the cardiac, genitourinary, respiratory, skeletal and neurological systems.[10] Syndromes associated with longitudinal radial deficiency include the VATER syndrome; the Holt–Oram syndrome (an autosomal dominantly inherited condition characterized by upper limb and cardiac malformations); thrombocytopenia absent radius (TAR) syndrome (a recessively inherited disorder where thrombocytopenia is present at birth and usually improves with growth); and Fanconi anemia.

Ulna club hand (postaxial absence)

This condition is about ten times less common than absence of the radius. It is usually a partial absence of the lower two thirds of the ulna and sometimes the postaxial rays. The absent bone may be represented by a fibrous remnant which becomes a deforming force during growth, leading to progressive ulnar deviation of the wrist and secondary curvature of the radius. As the forearm grows, the radial bowing increases and the radial head may subluxate or dislocate proximally at the elbow joint.

Complete absence of the ulna is usually associated with a severe flexion contraction of the elbow and surgery has little to offer. In partial absence the deforming fibrous band can be excised to prevent progressive deformity. Other treatment strategies include ulna lengthening procedures as well as procedures to construct a so-called 'one bone forearm' where the proximal ulna is fused to the distal radius.

Congenital dislocation of the radial head

Congenital dislocation of the radial head is rare and usually occurs in isolation (Fig. 29.5). It frequently presents late, often not until school age, and may be difficult to distinguish from an overlooked post-traumatic dislocation. Radial head dislocation may also be acquired as a result of differential growth disturbance between the radius and ulna or secondary to conditions such as Madelung deformity or familial osteochondromatosis. Features that suggest congenital dislocation include a positive family history, bilateral involvement and the absence of a history of trauma. Radiographic features more typical of congenital dislocation include a small dome-shaped radial head, a hypoplastic capitellum and ulnar bowing.

Children present during school years with limited elbow extension, a palpable mass (the radial head) or pain with athletic activities. The radial head is most commonly dislocated posterolaterally and can be palpated at the lateral side of the elbow joint.

If identified under 2 years, consideration may be given to open surgical reduction of the radial head and anular ligament reconstruction. Though some promise is reported following this procedure the indications are yet to be properly defined, particularly the upper age limit at which surgery might be helpful.[11] Most children present beyond infancy and are best managed conservatively. If significant discomfort occurs, management may include the removal of degenerate fragments of bone or excision of the entire radial head, a procedure to be approached with caution in the immature skeleton because of its association with progressive valgus deformity at the elbow and subsequent elbow, wrist and ulnar nerve problems.

Congenital radioulnar synostosis

Congenital synostosis of the proximal radius and ulna is a rare congenital abnormality caused by a failure of separation (Fig. 29.6). Forearm rotation is therefore prevented and the hand fixed in a degree of pronation. Many children present late because of their ability to compensate for the absent rotation of the affected forearm with rotational hypermobility of the wrist and compensating shoulder movement. If the fixed pronation is more than 60°, or if the condition is bilateral, children may present earlier with functional problems related to manual dexterity.

In the absence of functional limitation no treatment is required. Functional difficulties may lead to consideration of surgery to remove the abnormal fusion between radius and ulna, but this has generally proved disappointing.

Congenital pseudarthrosis of the forearm

Congenital pseudoarthrosis of the forearm is very rare but affects the ulna more commonly than the radius. Like its more common counterpart in the tibia it is associated with neurofibromatosis and nonunion after attempted reconstruction precludes successful treatment.

Madelung deformity

This wrist deformity results from an unexplained premature growth arrest of the ulnar aspect of the distal radial physis (or growth plate). Continued normal growth of the ulnar physis and the radial and dorsal aspects of the distal radial physis leads to progressive deformity. The distal ulna becomes more prominent and the distal radial articular surface becomes angulated toward the ulna. The carpus sinks into the developing gap between the radial and ulnar styloids.

Madelung deformity usually occurs in girls and is most often bilateral. It is usually sporadic but may be inherited as part of dyschondrosteosis (Leri–Weill disease), and has been associated with a variety of conditions including Hurler syndrome, Turner syndrome, multiple hereditary exostoses and Olliers disease. Damage to the growth plate from trauma or infection can also give rise to Madelung-like deformities.

Most patients do not present until adolescence when deformity and discomfort with activity are often marked. Treatment strategies include corrective radial osteotomy and ulnar shortening or other procedures to remove or stabilize the distal ulna, which is frequently the site of pain and wrist degeneration.

Syndactyly

Syndactyly is classified as simple, if the failure of separation involves only skin, and complex, if other structures such as nail, bone, tendon, nerve or blood vessels are involved. It is complete if the skin bridge is present to the distal tip of the finger. The interspace between the third and fourth fingers is most commonly affected, with that between the first and second less frequently involved. Treatment depends upon the site and complexity, border digits being separated early to prevent progressive angulation. The separation of simple syndactyly gives excellent results.

Polydactyly

Polydactyly is classified as preaxial (thumb), central (index, middle) or postaxial (ring, little). Genetic transmission of polydactyly is common especially in native Africans, where postaxial duplication is predominant. The extra digit may be fully formed or vestigial. Before embarking on surgical correction it is important to determine which digit has the majority of intact parts and is therefore most suitable for reconstruction.

Camptodactyly

This is a flexion deformity affecting the proximal interphalangeal joint of the fingers and often inherited as an autosomal dominant trait. The precise etiology is unknown but it usually presents during periods of rapid growth, i.e. infancy and adolescence. In infants there is an equal sex distribution and any finger can be affected. Adolescent cases are more common and invariably affect the little finger, usually in girls. Treatment in infancy involves passive stretching and splintage and occasionally surgical release of soft tissues. In adolescence dynamic splintage may lead to modest improvement.

Clinodactyly

This is angulation of a digit in the radial or ulnar direction. Radial angulation of the tip of the little finger is the most common and often inherited as an autosomal dominant trait. Treatment is seldom necessary.

Trigger thumb

This is the commonest hand anomaly in infants and small children. It is something of a misnomer because the thumb does not really 'trigger' with sudden extension, as does the adult trigger finger, but is usually stuck in a flexed position. Clinically there is a palpable swelling in the thumb flexor tendon and flexor sheath on the volar aspect of the base of the thumb. About one third of cases resolve spontaneously in the first year but later persistence makes spontaneous resolution unlikely. Surgical treatment to divide the entrance to the flexor sheath is simple and gives excellent results. It should be done before 4 years of age.

Hypoplastic thumb

Thumb hypoplasia is a form of preaxial longitudinal failure of formation and like radial club hand is associated with congenital anomalies in other systems (e.g. VATER, VACTERL syndromes). It ranges from a mild anomaly where the thumb is fully formed but small, to complete absence of the thumb. In mild hypoplasia no treatment is necessary but if function is impaired by a tight thumb–index finger web space or thenar muscle hypoplasia, reconstructive surgery can be helpful. If the thumb is absent or unreconstructable pollicization of the index finger can be considered.

Constriction band syndrome

This condition occurs sporadically and is alternatively known as Streeter dysplasia or amniotic band syndrome (Fig. 29.7). The etiology remains uncertain: hypotheses include constriction by intrauterine amniotic bands and localized failures of formation. Bands can be multiple and are asymmetric. Structures proximal to the band are normal but distally may be deformed or even amputated. Tight bands can cause severe distal edema and vascular compromise with urgent 'Z'-plasty release required in the neonatal period.

LOWER LIMB PROBLEMS

Congenital abnormalities of the femur

Congenital abnormalities of the femur fall into two main groups: proportional hypoplasia of the whole femur and a deficiency of part or all of the bone. Both can be associated with more distal abnormalities, including absence of the anterior cruciate ligament at the knee and congenital abnormalities of the lower leg and foot.

Children present with a limb length discrepancy either at birth or during early development. The femoral head and neck are radiolucent for the first 6 months of life even when no abnormality is present and ultrasonography provides a more reliable assessment.

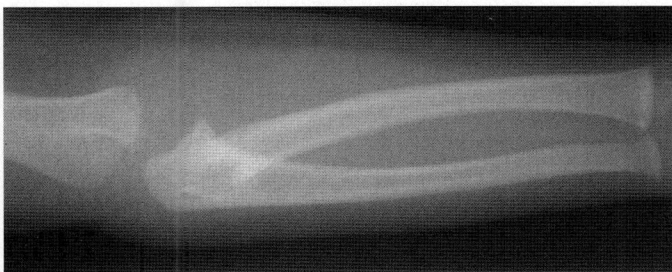

Fig. 29.6 Congenital radioulnar synostosis.

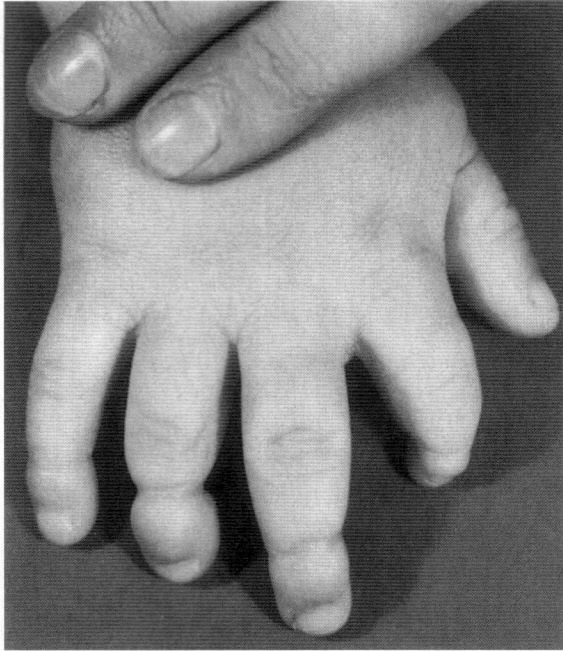

Fig. 29.7   Constriction band syndrome.

Proximal femoral focal deficiency (PFFD)

PFFD or deficiency of the proximal part of the femur varies in severity (Fig. 29.8). Clinical examination typically reveals a position of flexion at the hip and the knee. Management of these children is complex and depends not only upon the potential limb length discrepancy, but also upon the stability of the hip joint and the presence of associated limb problems.

Developmental coxa vara

The neck-shaft angle of the proximal femur measures a mean 144° in the first years of life, gradually falling to a mean 125° at maturity. Coxa vara is present when the neck-shaft angle falls below these parameters.

Coxa vara can be congenital, developmental or acquired as a consequence of a variety of conditions including developmental dislocation of the hip, slipped upper femoral epiphysis, Perthes disease, infection, trauma, tumors and metabolic disorders.

Congenital coxa vara is present at birth and commonly associated with other congenital musculoskeletal abnormalities.

Developmental coxa vara is a specific entity of unknown etiology and an incidence of 1 in 25 000 births. There is an equal sex ratio and 30–50% of patients have bilateral disease. Most patients present between 1 and 6 years of age with a progressively deteriorating, but painless, Trendelenburg gait. Radiographs classically reveal coxa vara often with a neck-shaft angle of 90° or less and a vertically orientated physis (growth plate). A triangular piece of metaphysis outlined by an inverted 'Y' formed by the physis on one side and radiolucent dystrophic bone on the other, is pathognomonic of the condition (Fig. 29.9). If left untreated the condition will lead to progressive degeneration, disability and pain. Valgus osteotomy to correct the deformity has been shown to be effective.[12]

Developmental dysplasia of the hip (DDH) and congenital dislocation of the hip (CDH)

The term developmental dysplasia of the hip (DDH) encompasses the located hip with a shallow acetabulum (dysplasia), through subluxation to frank dislocation. DDH is a more accurate term than congenital dislocation of the hip (CDH) and was introduced in recognition of the concept that a hip, located at birth, can become dislocated postnatally. When dislocation of the hip presents at birth or in the neonatal period it is termed an early presentation. Dislocation presenting beyond this period, commonly after 6 months, is termed a late presentation. The term 'missed dislocation' should be avoided because it can be inaccurate. The term teratological dislocation is used to describe a dislocated hip in association with underlying problems such as arthrogryposis multiplex congenita or neuromuscular conditions.

One in 60 neonates have hip instability demonstrable at birth, although most of these hips stabilize spontaneously within the first weeks of life. Before the introduction of routine clinical screening in the UK the incidence of late dislocation was about 1–2/1000 live births. Screening has reduced but not eradicated late presentation in the UK, a recent MRC trial showing the incidence to be at least 0.78/1000 live births.[13] There is considerable racial variation in the incidence of DDH. The incidence is very high in Navajo Native Americans, in the order of 50/1000 live births, but very low in peoples of Chinese and African descent. DDH is six times more common in females than males, and more common in first-born infants. It can present bilaterally but is usually unilateral and twice as common on the left.

Environmental factors both in utero and after delivery can influence hip development. The most common fetal lie places the infant's left hip adducted against the maternal sacrum and it is thought that this might be the explanation for the predilection for the left side. Breech position in utero is a significant risk factor, as is oligohydramnios which limits fetal movement. Other conditions considered to be a result of intrauterine molding, including metatarsus adductus and torticollis, are associated with DDH. Postnatal influences include nursing habits such as swaddling. The infant hip and knee joints in utero are in a flexed position and normally have modest flexion contractures at birth. An attempt

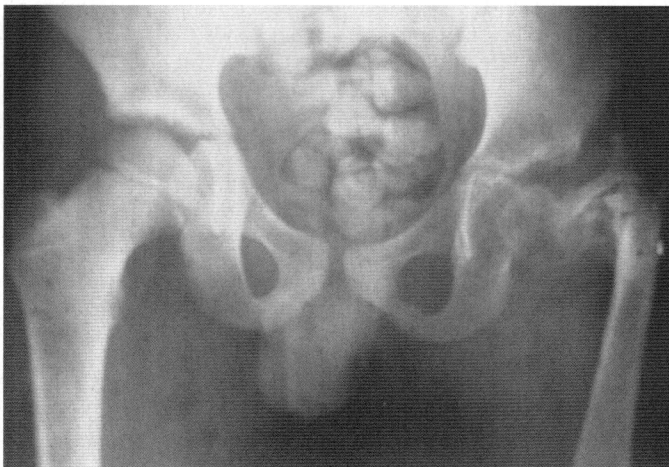

Fig. 29.8   Proximal femoral focal deficiency.

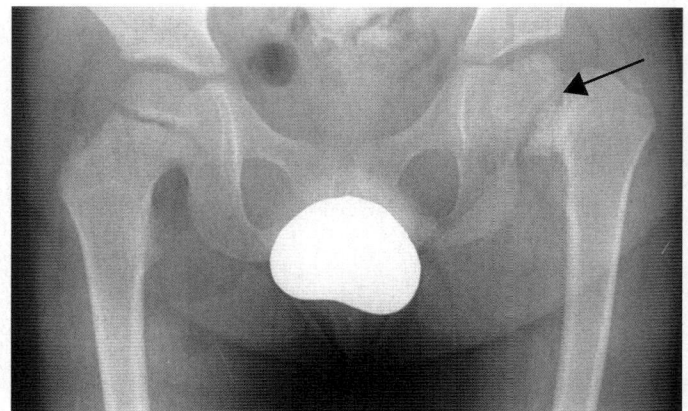

Fig. 29.9   Developmental coxa vara.

to straighten and adduct the limbs prematurely results in compression forces along the shaft of the femur, pushing the femoral head postero-superiorly, where it is unstable. Cultural swaddling may in part explain the differing incidence of DDH between races. The hips are best allowed to rest in flexion and abduction, the position most infants naturally adopt. Early diagnosis gives the best chance of a satisfactory outcome.

Clinical examination to identify DDH is based on the observations of Ortolani and Barlow. The first part of clinical examination is to determine whether the hip is in or out of joint. Clinical signs sugges-tive of dislocation include limited abduction, limb length asymmetry and asymmetrical skin creases (Fig. 29.10). If the hip is considered to be in joint, its stability is evaluated with a Barlow maneuver. The hip is first placed in a vulnerable position of slight extension and adduction before longitudinal compression is applied along the shaft of the femur (Fig. 29.11a) (the positioning is important because the hip is more sta-ble and resists subluxation or dislocation if held incorrectly in a position of flexion and abduction). If the hip is unstable there is a palpable sen-sation of the femoral head riding posteriorly over the posterior rim of the acetabulum, the so-called 'clunk'. There is a similar sensation when compression is released and the femoral head returns to the acetabu-lum or if an Ortolani maneuver is used to reduce the joint. If the hip is considered to be dislocated, a gentle attempt can be made to return it to the acetabulum using an Ortolani maneuver. Once again positioning is important. The hip is held in 90 degrees of flexion so that the femoral head is directly posterior to the acetabulum. Gentle traction is applied to the leg and the long fingers of the examiner's hand are placed on the greater trochanter where they gently lift the femoral head (Fig. 29.11b). If the dislocation is reducible, the femoral head can be felt passing across the posterior lip of the acetabulum and into the joint. Once in joint, the hip can be gently abducted and flexed to a more stable position so that the reduction can be maintained.

These examinations are difficult and the introduction of clinical screening has not eradicated late presenting dislocations. The sensa-tion of dislocation or reduction is difficult to elicit in the conscious child over about 3–4 months of age and thereafter limited abduction, or limb asymmetry are more reliable. After walking age the child with a uni-lateral dislocated hip stands either with the 'long' leg flexed at the knee or with the 'short' leg standing tiptoe to compensate for the length dis-crepancy. The child will walk with a limp, which can be a simple short leg gait, sometimes with a classic waddle or Trendelenburg gait pattern. Symmetry in bilateral dislocation can make these signs less easily iden-tifiable. Radiographs reveal a subluxed or dislocated femoral head with a small ossific nucleus and a dysplastic acetabulum (Fig. 29.12).

The limitations of clinical examination and the inability of radio-graphs to image the cartilaginous infant hip has led to the development of ultrasound screening. Population ultrasound screening has been intro-duced in Germany and parts of Europe but remains sporadic in the UK.

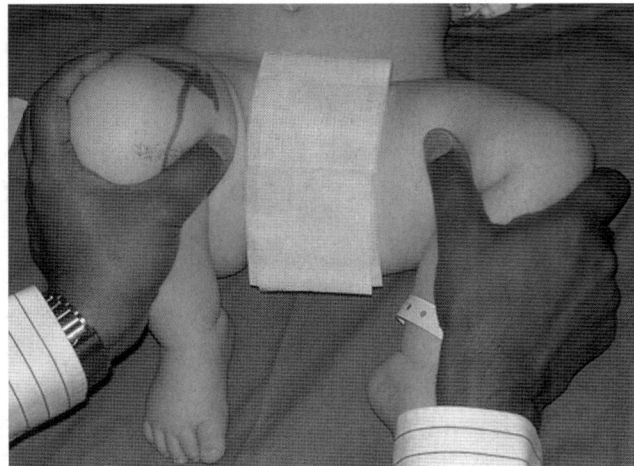
(a)

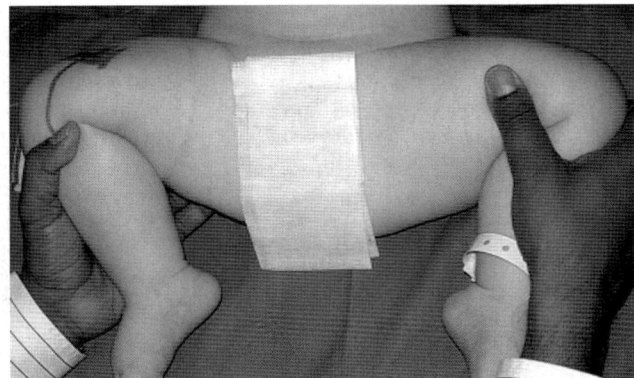
(b)

Fig. 29.11   (a) Barlow and (b) Ortolani maneuvers.

Many units practice selective screening of higher risk infants, i.e. those with a family history, a breech position in utero, a suspicious hip exami-nation or who exhibit other structural examination abnormalities such as metatarsus adductus or torticollis. The investigation can result in false negatives and especially false positives, revealing 'abnormalities' of uncertain significance and resulting in high treatment rates. While it is acknowledged that ultrasound examination is an unequivocally useful tool to evaluate the progress of unstable and dislocated hips, its role as a screening tool for DDH in the UK remains controversial and its cost

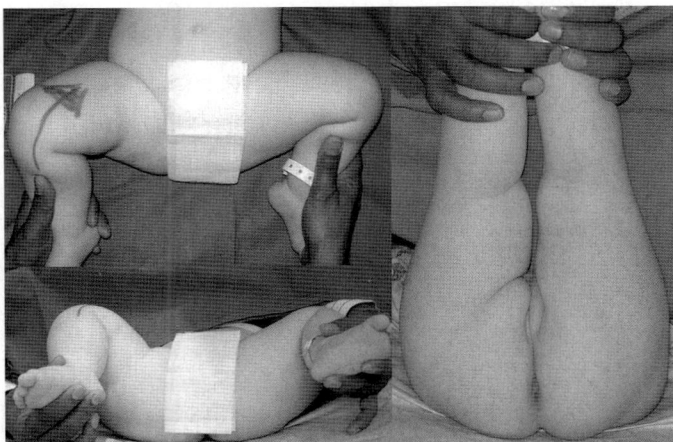

Fig. 29.10   Dislocated right hip showing limited abduction, asymmetrical skin creases and short limb.

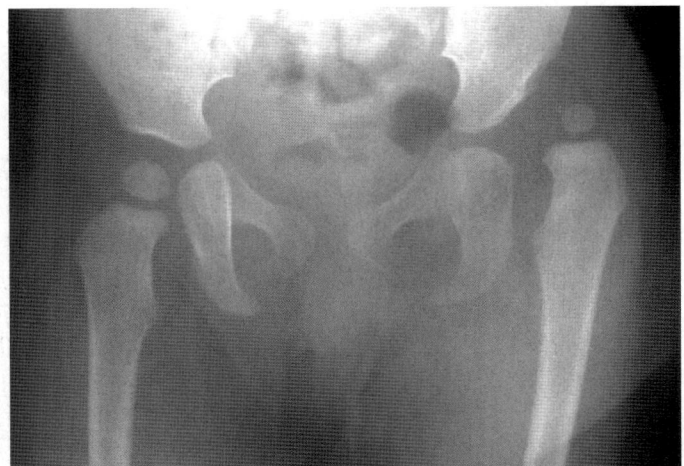

Fig. 29.12   Dislocated left hip with dysplastic acetabulum and small ossific nucleus.

effectiveness is questioned.[14] The National Screening Committee (NSC) in the UK currently recommends that every child should have a clinical examination based on the Ortolani Barlow maneuver within the first week of life and again at 6 weeks.[15] Those with a positive clinical examination should have an ultrasound. In July 2006 the NSC determined that population ultrasound screening should not be offered unless part of an ethically approved and externally funded research project (http://www.library.nhs.uk/screening).

In general terms, reduction of a dislocated hip becomes progressively more difficult the longer it has been dislocated. Treatment involves first reducing the hip and then keeping it in joint until it becomes stable. The chief complications of any treatment are re-dislocation and avascular necrosis (AVN) of the femoral head. The circulation of the femoral head is vulnerable and especially sensitive to pressure. It is known that forceful reduction or positioning of the hip in extreme flexion, abduction or internal rotation can apply excessive pressure to the femoral head and disturb the blood supply leading to AVN. In spite of avoiding these known causes, AVN remains a troublesome complication in the management of hip dislocation (Fig. 29.13).

From birth to about 3–4 months the dislocated or subluxed hip will often reduce with a gentle Ortolani maneuver and should then be maintained in a position of gentle flexion and abduction until it becomes stable when released. There are a wide variety of splints available to maintain this position but the Pavlik harness (Fig. 29.14), a dynamic splint affording the infant some movement within a safe arc, is probably the most widely used. The harness is worn 23–24 hours a day and requires regular scrutiny to ensure proper fitting. Hip development can be followed by repeated ultrasound examination at 2- or 4-weekly intervals until normal with a clinically stable hip. Harness treatment typically lasts 12–16 weeks if the dislocation is identified early. The Pavlik harness is not practical in children older than about 5 months.

When children present between 4 and 6 months of age it can be difficult to be certain of an adequate reduction, in the conscious patient, and these infants are often examined under anaesthesia. Radio-paque contrast is introduced into the hip joint during the examination and the resulting arthrogram outlines the cartilaginous femoral head and acetabulum so that a satisfactory reduction can be confirmed (Fig. 29.15). If there is any obstruction to proper location or extreme force or positioning is required to maintain satisfactory location, closed (nonsurgical) reduction is best abandoned in favor of later open (surgical) reduction when the obstruction or resistance to location can be addressed operatively. If closed reduction is possible, immobilization in a stable position of gentle flexion and abduction can be achieved by a plaster of Paris hip spica cast, once again avoiding extreme or forced positions. The reduction should be confirmed by a later CT scan of the hips in the spica cast. Typically such children remain immobilized for 6–9 months.

When children present after about 12–18 months successful closed reduction becomes unlikely. The later a child presents the more likely they are to require a surgical open reduction and further secondary operations either to the femur or to the acetabulum to correct secondary problems especially persistent acetabular shallowness (dysplasia). Late presentation increases the chance of secondary surgery and complications reducing the chance of a perfect outcome.

Congenital dislocation of the knee

This presents at birth with the knee severely hyperextended instead of in the normal flexed position (Fig. 29.16). The etiology is unknown, but there is a high incidence of breech delivery indicating a role for intrauterine positioning. Associated musculoskeletal abnormalities, especially subluxation or dislocation of the hip, are present in approximately 50%. Plain lateral radiographs reveal anterior subluxation or dislocation of the tibia on the femur.

Treatment begins soon after birth with serial casting to gradually flex the knee and is often successful within a few weeks of birth. If conservative treatment fails, there may be some underlying fibrosis of the quadriceps mechanism and open surgical release early in life can give good long term results.

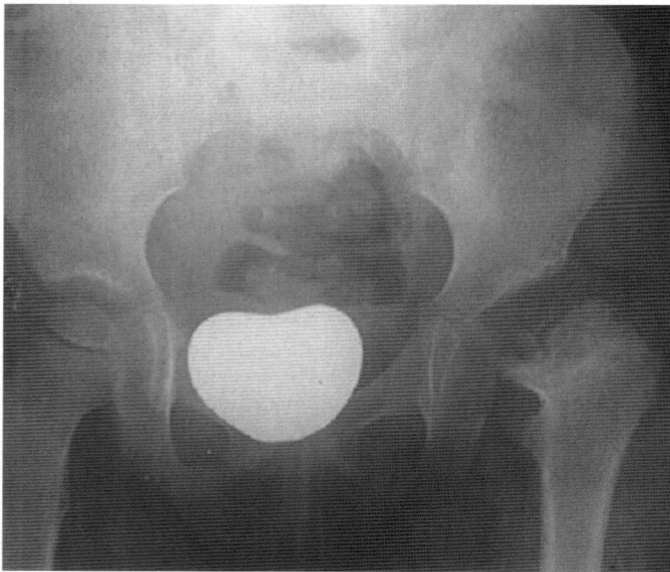

Fig. 29.13   Avascular necrosis after treatment for developmental dislocation of the hip.

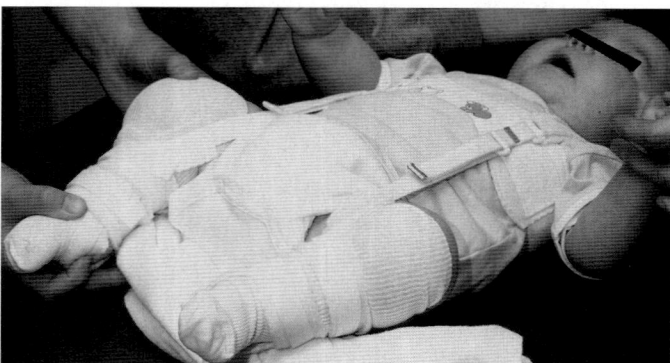

Fig. 29.14   Infant in Pavlik harness.

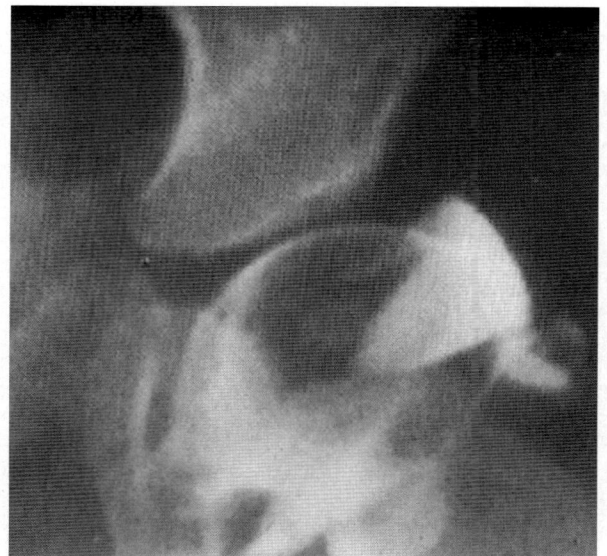

Fig. 29.15   Arthrogram showing a satisfactory closed reduction of a dislocated hip.

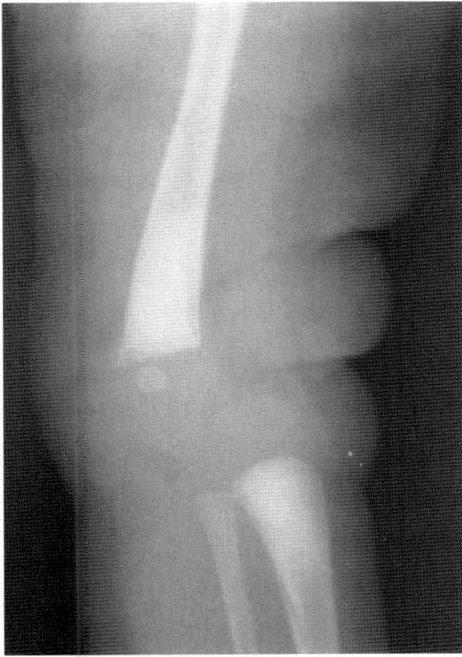

Fig. 29.16 Congenital dislocation of the knee.

Tibial bowing

Tibial bowing at birth can take four characteristic forms. Broadly speaking the convexity of the bow points to the four points of the compass namely anteromedial, anterolateral, posterolateral and posteromedial. The first three directions are associated with relatively severe problems namely fibula hemimelia, pseudoarthrosis of the tibia and tibia hemimelia respectively. Posteromedial bowing of the tibia is relatively benign.

Posteromedial bowing of the tibia

Posteromedial bowing of the tibia is associated with a severe calcaneovalgus deformity of the foot.[16] The appearance can be alarming at birth. Initial treatment is directed toward passive stretching of the foot deformity, sometimes with the addition of serial casting. The tibial bowing generally corrects in the first year of life, although tibial length inequality may persist and require later orthopedic intervention.

Congenital fibula deficiency (fibula hemimelia)

The fibula is the most frequently congenitally deficient long bone. The deficiency can be modest and isolated. Severe fibula deficiency is more common and is associated with a generally dysplastic limb and other deformities.

The choice of appropriate management can be extremely difficult. Modern prosthetics make amputation more acceptable and new methods of limb reconstruction, especially with the Ilizarov external fixator, make reconstruction more feasible. Amputation is recommended if the foot is nonfunctional, regardless of limb length, and if the length discrepancy is more than 30% even with a functional foot. Application of the appropriate management requires considerable clinical experience and should be tailored to the individual patient.

Congenital tibial deficiency (tibia hemimelia)

The child presents at birth with shortening of the tibia and a rigid equinovarus foot. The leg is bowed convex laterally. Other congenital limb abnormalities occur in up to 75%.[17] The tibia can be completely absent (Type I); absent in its distal portion but with a proximal portion remaining to form an articulation at the knee (Type II) (Fig. 29.17); or present but forming an abnormal distal tibiofibula diastasis or separation at the ankle (Type III).[18]

Management strategies range from prosthetics to reconstruction and once again, as in fibula hemimelia, considerable clinical experience is required to chart an appropriate course for each individual patient.

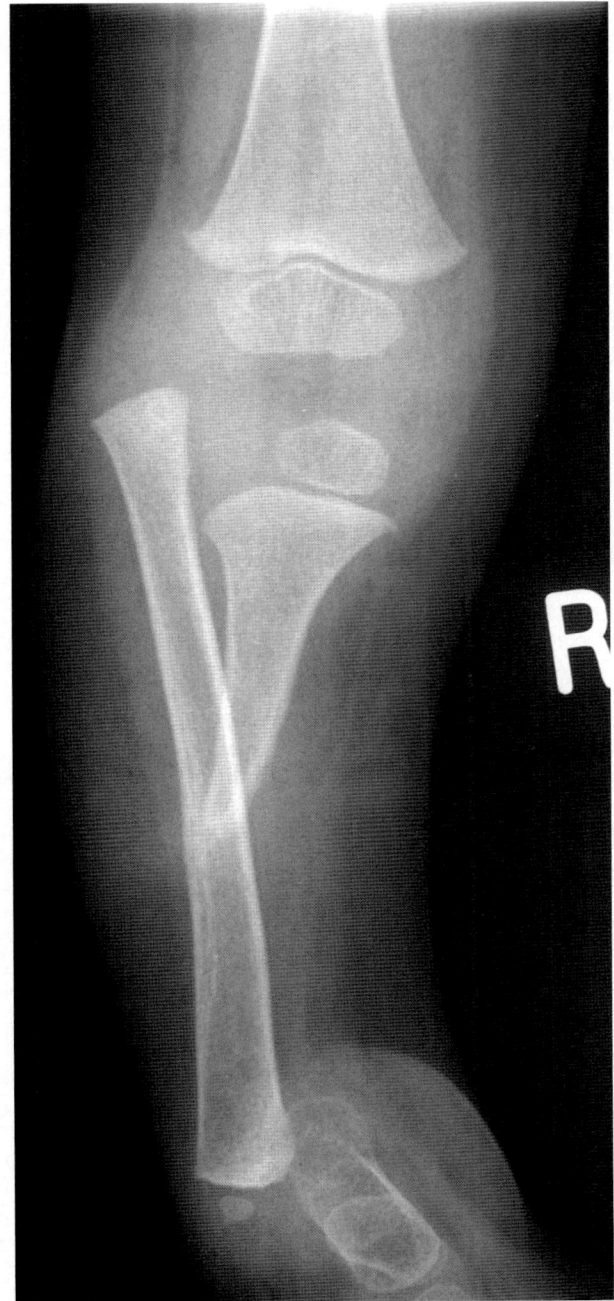

Fig. 29.17 Congenital tibial deficiency.

Congenital pseudoarthrosis of the tibia

Congenital pseudoarthrosis of the tibia presents with anterior or anterolateral bowing at the junction of the proximal two thirds and the distal one third of the tibia. Up to 80% of cases are associated with neurofibromatosis.[19] The bone and its covering periosteum are abnormal at the site of the bowing and the fibula may also be involved in the pathology. Spontaneous fracture at the abnormality can occur and subsequently leads to persistent nonunion or pseudoarthrosis.

Management should include the avoidance of fracture for as long as possible by the use of protective orthoses. Numerous methods have been used to encourage union at the fracture site with modest success. A Syme amputation of the foot followed by a below knee prosthesis remains a satisfactory long term solution, although modern reconstructive techniques especially using the Ilizarov external fixator offer new solutions. The abnormal bone and periosteum at the site of the pathology can be excised and the remaining healthy bone lengthened.

Metatarsus varus

See section on 'Common orthopedic problems in childhood', page 1415.

Congenital talipes calcaneovalgus

This foot posture is frequent in newborns and in the majority of children is within the spectrum of normality. The foot is dorsiflexed so that the dorsum touches the shin. If the foot can be fully plantarflexed the condition is termed postural, requires no treatment and will resolve spontaneously. Occasionally the foot cannot be fully plantarflexed. Physiotherapy and/or splintage should be commenced promptly to stretch the tight anterior structures and should be successful in most cases. In resistant cases, the possibility of an underlying neurological or skeletal abnormality should be considered.

Congenital talipes equinovarus (CTEV; congenital club foot)

Congenital talipes equinovarus is a common foot abnormality with an incidence of 1–2/1000 live births (Fig. 29.18). It is twice as common in boys, bilateral in up to 50% and has a familial predisposition. Unaffected parents with an affected son have a 1:40 chance of having another son with the disorder. The pathogenesis is unknown.

Clinically the hindfoot is in equinus and varus (inversion) and the heel is difficult to feel. The forefoot is adducted and plantarflexed on the hindfoot giving a cavus or high arched appearance, and there is a deep transverse skin crease on the medial border of the foot. Internal tibial torsion is present and the foot and calf are often smaller than the opposite side. The navicular is medially displaced on the head of the talus. Passive correction to a neutral position is not possible.

A complete examination of the child is indicated to rule out potential neurological causes and associated conditions including DDH. Assessment of the severity and rigidity of the deformity at birth is difficult but helpful in determining the likely success of nonoperative treatment such as serial manipulation or casting versus the need for operative surgical correction. According to Harrold and Walker in 1983, if the foot can be passively returned to neutral, conservative treatment can be expected to be successful in 90%.[20] If fixed equinus is 0–20°degrees conservative treatment can be expected to succeed in 50% of cases; but if fixed equinus is more than 20° conservative treatment can only be expected to be successful in 10%.[20]

More recently a serial manipulation and casting technique described by Ignacio Ponseti[21] has become the preferred method of management in many centers. Results indicate a higher success rate for this nonoperative management technique, even in feet that are quite stiff from the outset. Children should be referred soon after delivery so that treatment can begin early. The technique involves a specific series of manipulative maneuvers to correct the underlying deformity followed by the application of a series of holding casts which are changed weekly. Typically after about six cast changes the forefoot and hindfoot are corrected but the foot remains in equinus. A percutanous Achilles tenotomy is often necessary at this stage to allow correction of the equinus, followed by the application of the final cast which holds the position. The final cast is usually removed about 3–6 weeks later and thereafter the child must wear 'Denis Browne' boots and bar . This consists of boots that are connected by an adjustable bar holding the feet in external rotation, eversion and dorsiflexion. It is important for the success of the method that the patient and family comply with the proper use of this holding device. In the typical program the patient must wear the boots and bar continuously for 3 months following removal of the last holding cast and then for night time and naps for a further 3–4 years.

Although the Ponseti technique has changed the management of CTEV, some cases do not respond favorably and require surgical intervention although this is often less invasive than previously. It is important to warn parents of this potential from the outset and also to explain that some very resistant cases still require a more traditional surgical management. Recurrence of deformity is always a concern during the management of CTEV treated by any means and secondary surgery to correct recurring deformity, especially forefoot varus is not uncommon. Sometimes repeated recurrence occurs in spite of secondary operations: this can be successfully managed using Ilizarov external fixator techniques.

Congenital vertical talus

This is a rigid foot deformity that presents clinically as a 'rocker bottom' foot. In about 50%[22] the condition is associated with other congenital neuromuscular and genetic disorders like neural tube defects and arthrogryposis. The head of the talus is dislocated from its normal articulation with the navicular and takes on a more vertical position. Diagnosis is made with a lateral radiograph and the foot stressed into maximal plantarflexion. If the navicular remains dorsally dislocated on the talus, the diagnosis is confirmed (Fig. 29.19).

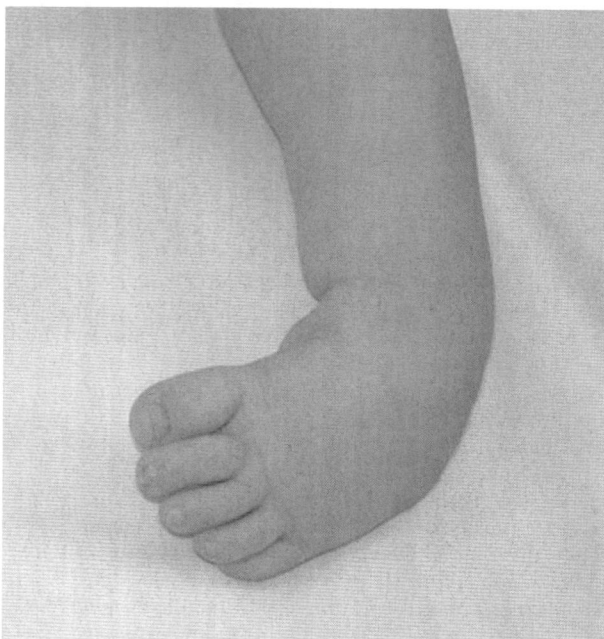

Fig. 29.18   Congenital talipes equinovarus.

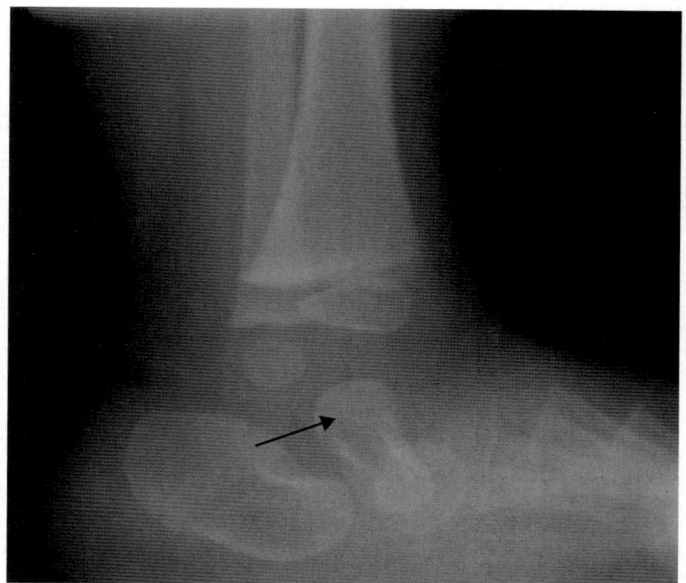

Fig. 29.19   Congenital vertical talus.

In addition to the vertical position of the talus and the tight anterior structures causing dorsal dislocation of the forefoot, the posterior structures are also tight resulting in fixed equinus of the hindfoot as in CTEV. The hindfoot and forefoot are therefore essentially broken over the vertically disposed talus giving the foot the characteristic 'rocker bottom' in severe cases.

Initial treatment is directed toward passive stretching and splinting of the foot into plantarflexion to stretch the tight anterior structures. Surgery is frequently necessary later to lengthen the tight anterior and posterior structures and to restore the normal alignment and relationship of the talus with the other bones of the foot. Favorable results are emerging with a modification of the Ponseti technique used in CTEV.[23]

INHERITED DISORDERS OF BONES AND JOINTS

Inherited disorders of bones and joints are a rare but important source of diagnostic confusion for the unwary as they may be easily confused with other disorders such as juvenile arthritis and Perthes disease. Most present with some combination of joint swelling or deformity; joint hypermobility or stiffness; and short stature. An awareness of these conditions will enable the correct diagnosis to be made, ensuring appropriate advice and genetic counseling is given.

This section is not intended to be an exhaustive review of a very complex area but describes some of the more common primary genetic disorders of bones and connective tissues, as well as identifying other genetic disorders in which bone and joint problems are a dominant feature. Many of these primary disorders of bones and connective tissues have been associated with identifiable genetic defects, particularly of the collagen genes. As these genetic defects are increasingly delineated it seems likely that the classification of these conditions will continually be updated and improved.[24,25]

HYPERMOBILITY

Joint mobility follows a normal distribution in the population and is influenced by factors including age, sex and ethnicity. Infants and young children have joints that are more mobile than older children and adults but there are no good studies defining normal joint ranges in the very young. Females have a greater degree of joint laxity than males and hypermobile joints are much more common in certain ethnic groups, e.g. oriental. Hypermobility of the joints may be generalized or affect only one or two joints. Generalized joint hypermobility may occur as an isolated entity or as part of a number of well-recognized genetic syndromes.

The definition of hypermobility is based on clinical assessment. The criteria most frequently used are those defined by Beighton[26] which assess joint laxity based on a number of clinical maneuvers:

1. passive dorsiflexion of the 5th metacarpophalangeal joint to 90°;
2. apposition of the thumb to the flexor aspect of the forearm (Fig. 29.20a);
3. hyperextension of the elbow to greater than 10° (Fig. 29.20b);
4. hyperextension of the knee to greater than 10°;
5. forward flexion of the trunk to place the palms of the hands flat on the floor with the knees extended.

Those experienced in examining children will immediately realize that these measurements are not appropriate in the very young in whom these degrees of joint laxity are normal. There is a need to define age-related normal values but the Beighton scoring system has been shown to be valid in children over the age of 4 years when interpreted correctly.[27] More recently revised criteria have been developed[28] but have not been extensively used or validated in pediatric practice.

Benign hypermobility syndrome

Joint hypermobility is a normal variant and causes no symptoms in most individuals. In others it is associated with a variety of musculoskeletal symptoms as part of the 'benign joint hypermobility syndrome'(BJHS).[29] Although labeled 'benign', affected individuals may have troublesome symptoms with significant morbidity and it may be impossible to differentiate from the milder variants of some of the genetic disorders such as Ehlers–Danlos syndrome.

BJHS occurs more commonly in females than in males and appears to have an autosomal dominant mode of inheritance. Affected children may have a variety of symptoms including arthralgia, joint effusions, widespread muscle pain, low back pain, flat feet and recurrent dislocations with many reporting significant functional difficulties.[30] Young children with hypermobility should be carefully assessed for associated coordination or proprioceptive difficulties which may contribute to their symptoms. Recurrent sports injuries, back pain and an increase in chronic musculoskeletal pain are reported in older children and adolescents with BJHS.

Despite much interest, the association between hypermobility and symptoms remains poorly understood.[31] Many hypermobile individuals remain asymptomatic while others have significant symptoms. Management consists of explanation of the condition, multidisciplinary input from physiotherapy, occupational therapy and podiatry together with appropriate pain management if required.

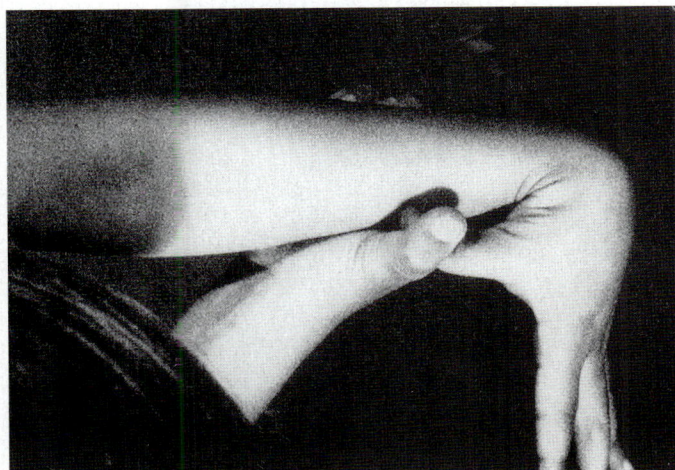

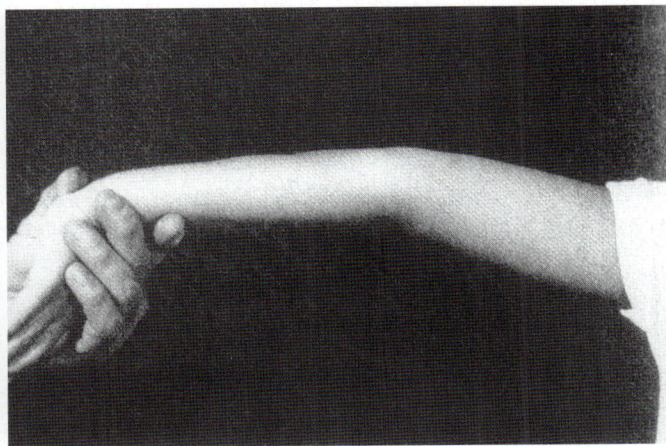

(a)   (b)

Fig. 29.20   Hypermobility: (a) apposition of the thumb to the flexor aspect of the forearm; (b) hyperextension of the elbow to greater than 10°.

INHERITED SYNDROMES WITH SIGNIFICANT HYPERMOBILITY

Ehlers–Danlos syndrome

Ehlers–Danlos syndrome (EDS) consists of a group of disorders of connective tissue characterized by joint hypermobility plus fragility and laxity of the skin and other tissues. These conditions are characterized by abnormalities in collagen genes resulting in the production of abnormal collagens III and V and consequent tissue fragility. They vary both in severity and mode of inheritance and an accurate diagnosis is essential if patients are to be offered appropriate advice and counseling.

Over the years, 11 different types of Ehlers–Danlos syndrome have been described. A revised, simplified classification was agreed in 1997[32] with three major types being defined clinically. Although further refinement will occur this classification has been widely accepted and is helpful clinically and prognostically in clearly distinguishing between the vascular, potentially catastrophic, form of the condition and the others. The three major types are defined as follows.

1. 'Classical' EDS (previously types I and II): characterized by the classical skin hyperextensibility and associated joint hypermobility. In many cases this results from abnormalities of the COL5A1 and A2 genes.
2. Hypermobility EDS (previously type III): characterized predominantly by joint hypermobility and very difficult to distinguish from BJHS.
3. Vascular EDS (previously type IV): associated with vascular, intestinal and uterine rupture. This results from mutations in the COL3A1 gene which causes production of abnormal type III collagen. Although the inheritance is autosomal dominant, approximately one third are new mutations. The diagnosis can be confirmed by collagen studies of cultured dermal fibroblasts.

Marfan syndrome

Marfan syndrome, also an inherited disorder of connective tissue, affects approximately 1 in 10 000 of the population. Inherited as an autosomal dominant trait it results from mutations in the genes encoding for the glycoprotein fibrillin, a component of elastin fibrils in the extracellular matrix.[33]

Marfan syndrome is characterized by tall stature, long extremities, fingers and feet, chest deformities, high arched palate and ocular abnormalities including lens dislocation. Joint hypermobility, although not diagnostic, is recognized frequently and there is a high incidence of spinal problems with the development of both scolioses and kyphoses. Mitral valve prolapse is common. Aortic valve disease and a tendency to sudden aortic rupture are of major concern.

Many individuals are only mildly affected and the diagnosis can be difficult. Diagnostic criteria are currently based on clinical features[34] but recent reports suggest that this can now be supported by molecular analysis.[35]

Individuals with type 1 homocystinuria may have tall stature, a high arched palate and resemble Marfan syndrome. Hypotonia occurs but the joints are stiff rather than hypermobile. Severe osteoporosis and mental retardation are characteristic.

Osteogenesis imperfecta

Osteogenesis imperfecta (OI) is a group of autosomal dominantly inherited collagen gene disorders typified by bone fragility and often associated with joint hypermobility.[36] The underlying defect in these conditions lies in the genes COL1A1 and COL1A2[37] which encode the peptide chains of type I collagen, the major structural protein of bone, ligament and tendon. Clinically the important features are those of an inherited osteoporosis. Radiological appearances range from mild osteoporosis with occasional fractures to a widespread skeletal abnormality with multiple fractures. In its most severe form, OI may be lethal in utero.

Types I and IV OI are the mildest forms of the condition, presenting with recurrent fractures in infancy and childhood (Fig. 29.21). Spinal involvement results in short stature which may be marked. There is a

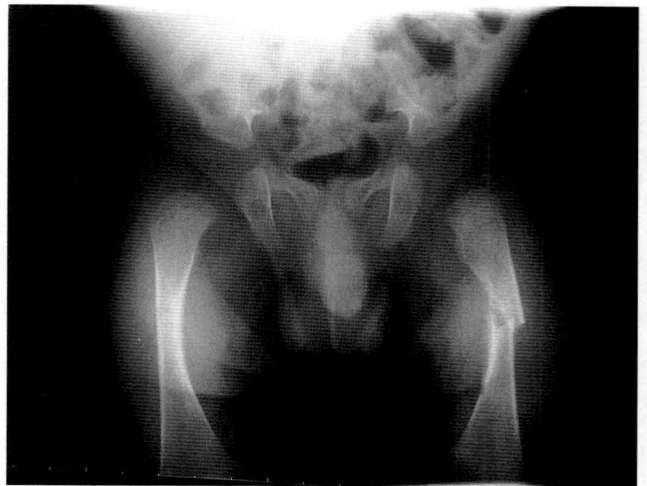

Fig. 29.21   Osteogenesis imperfecta type I.

tendency for the fracture rate to reduce after adolescence but become more severe again in later adult life. Type I is distinguished by the presence of the characteristic blue sclerae. Associated dentinogenesis imperfecta and joint laxity occur with variable frequency.

Type II OI is a severe, crippling and frequently lethal disease. Multiple intrauterine fractures occur and early death results from chest infections and pulmonary restriction caused by the widespread fractures. Type III (Fig. 29.22) is the most severe nonlethal form causing severe bone fragility with marked joint hypermobility. Survivors of infancy are usually significantly disabled.

Until recently there has been no treatment for individuals with OI other than appropriate orthopedic management of fractures and supportive care. Expert physiotherapy and orthopedic input remain critical to optimal management of these children. The development of the bisphosphonate group of drugs offers new possibilities for treatment. Cyclical treatment with intravenous pamidronate has been shown to result in reduced bone pain, a significant increase in bone density, a

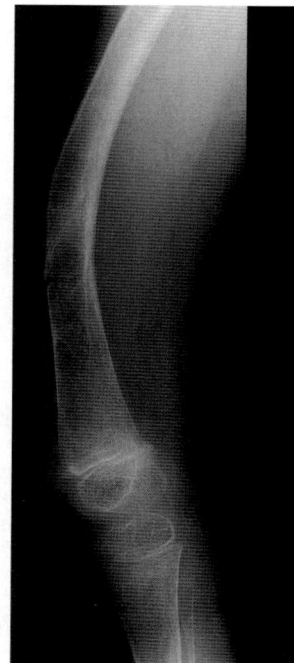

Fig. 29.22   Osteogenesis imperfecta type III showing recent fracture, severe osteoporosis and femoral deformity.

decreased number of fractures and an improved quality of life in many.[38] The role of oral bisphosphates remains unclear.

Stickler syndrome

Stickler syndrome is an inherited disorder of connective tissues characterized by a typical facies with midface hypoplasia, high myopia with early onset, progressive hearing loss and arthropathy. Joint problems include both generalized joint hypermobility and early degenerative joint disease. Retinal detachment is a serious complication. Type I Stickler syndrome, the majority, has been associated with mutations in the COL2A1 gene encoding type II collagen and diagnostic criteria based on clinical features plus genetic confirmation have been developed.[39]

INHERITED SKELETAL DYSPLASIAS

Spondyloepiphyseal dysplasia (SED)

The spondyloepiphyseal dysplasias consist of a group of heritable disorders principally involving the spine and the epiphyses of the long bones. Several forms are described of varying severity. Type II collagen is the main protein component of articular cartilage and mutations of the COL2A1 gene are thought to result not only in the already mentioned Stickler syndrome but also in a number of other disorders including the spondyloepiphyseal dysplasias.

SED congenita is an autosomal dominant condition with its onset at birth. Affected children may have delay in walking, a waddling gait and short stature. Limitation of range of motion affects elbows, knees and hips. Radiological investigation shows flattening of the vertebrae (Fig. 29.23) and coxa vara.

SED tarda results in symptoms which seldom present before adolescence. Although usually X-linked recessive, autosomal recessive and dominant forms have also been described. Spinal and hip involvement occur and the course is usually benign. Early onset of osteoarthritis occurs in adult life.

Progressive pseudorheumatoid arthropathy is a variant of SED (Fig. 29.24) which presents between 3 and 11 years of age with painful, swollen joints especially affecting the hands. Progressive joint contractures and short stature develop and the condition is unresponsive to standard antiinflammatory medication.

Multiple epiphyseal dysplasia

This is one of the more common skeletal dysplasias and is inherited as an autosomal dominant trait. It presents in childhood with pain and stiffness, usually progressing to joint contractures and associated short stature. At first sight it may be confused with juvenile arthritis, but the absence of signs and symptoms of inflammation can distinguish the two. Radiology demonstrates irregularities of the end-plates of the mid-thoracic vertebral bodies, shortening of the metacarpals and flattening, sclerosis and fragmentation of the epiphyses at the hips and knees (Fig. 29.25).

Achondroplasia and hypochondroplasia

These disorders result from mutations of fibroblast growth factor receptor 3 (FGFR3) genes. Although inherited as an autosomal dominant trait, most cases of achondroplasia occur as new mutations. The classic form of achondroplasia causes severe disproportionate short stature. Affected individuals have normal or large heads with shortening of the limbs and an increased lumbar lordosis. The pedicles of the vertebrae are short which may lead to symptomatic spinal stenosis in adult life. Hypochondroplasia is a milder form resulting from different mutations in the FGFR3 gene.

Trichorhinophalangeal dysplasia

This autosomal dominant disorder results from the deletion of multiple genes on chromosome 8. It is characterized by enlargement of the interphalangeal joints with characteristic facial features: a bulbous nose, hyperplastic nares, sparse, brittle hair and short stature.

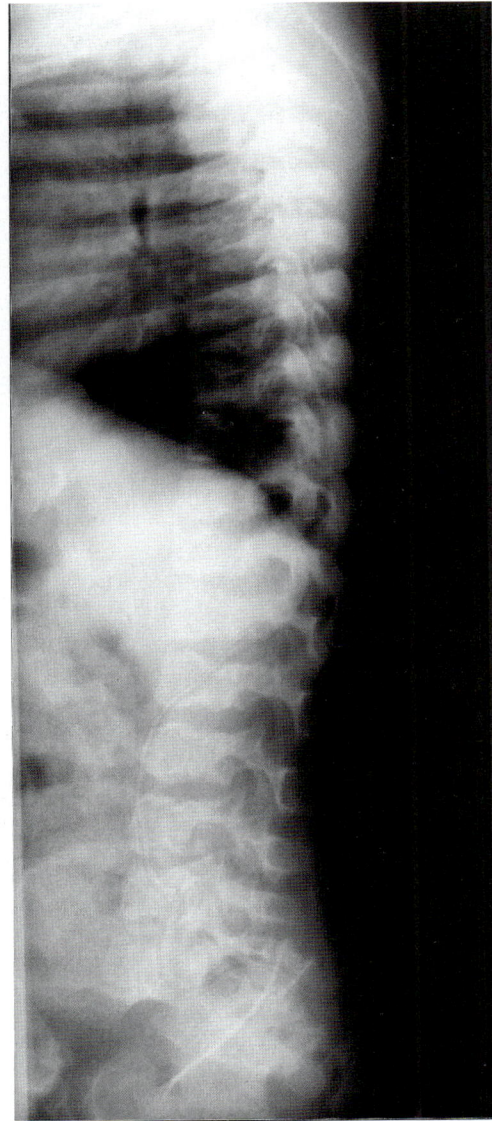

Fig. 29.23   Spondyloepiphyseal dysplasia congenita showing abnormal vertebrae.

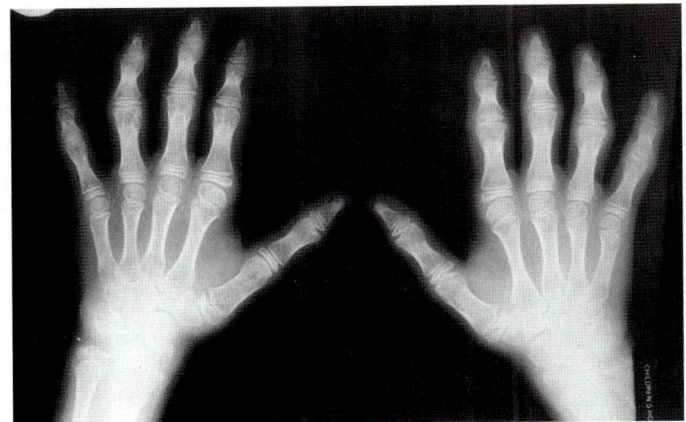

Fig. 29.24   Spondyloepiphyseal dysplasia tarda (progressive pseudorheumatoid arthropathy) affecting hands with obvious swelling of joints and bulbous ends to the phalanges.

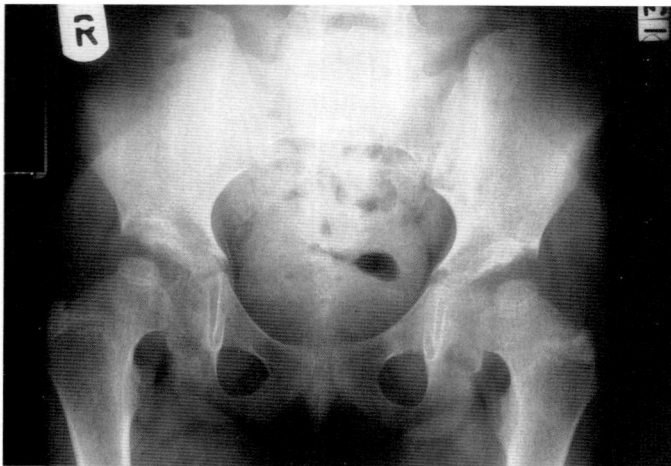

Fig. 29.25 Multiple epiphyseal dysplasia with bilateral hip involvement.

Radiographic features include cone-shaped epiphyses with short metacarpals and metatarsals plus fragmentation of the epiphyses. Fragmentation of the femoral epiphyses may cause confusion with Perthes disease.

Storage disorders: the mucopolysaccharidoses (MPS)

The MPS are genetically determined deficiencies of enzymes involved in the metabolism of glycosaminoglycans. All are inherited as autosomal dominant conditions and a prominent feature of most is a skeletal dysplasia affecting particularly the hands, feet and vertebrae and which may be the presenting feature. In the milder forms such as Scheie and Morquio syndromes the joint problems may dominate the clinical picture. In the more severe forms such as Hurler syndrome the characteristic coarsening of the facial features is striking but may be preceded by flexion deformities of the fingers.

An awareness that these conditions may present with skeletal symptoms will enable their early recognition, allowing appropriate genetic advice and counseling. For more detail see Chapter 26.

OTHER INHERITED DISORDERS PRIMARILY AFFECTING THE MUSCULOSKELETAL SYSTEM

There are many other inherited disorders that primarily affect the musculoskeletal system and are currently difficult to categorize.

Osteopetrosis

This is a rare disorder resulting in frontal bossing, hypertelorism, exophthalmos and nasal obstruction which may be present from birth. It progresses during early childhood resulting in severe bleeding problems, recurrent fractures and early death. The disease is characterized by an increased density of the bones with metaphyseal flaring. Bone marrow transplantation may offer a cure.

Arthrogryposis

This refers to a number of disorders characterized by multiple congenital contractures.

Ollier disease

Ollier disease or multiple enchondromatosis becomes apparent during childhood when it presents with multiple juxta-articular outgrowths.

Idiopathic acro-osteolysis

This is inherited as an autosomal dominant trait and generally presents around 3 years with bony lysis which may affect the carpus or tarsus alone or occur in a more widespread pattern. The condition may mimic juvenile arthritis in that affected areas are warm and swollen. Radiographs show progressive bone lysis and destruction of affected joints.

Fibrodysplasia ossificans progressiva (FOP)

FOP is a rare autosomal dominant condition now known to result from dysregulation of the BMP-4 signaling pathway.[40] Painful inflammation of muscles and fascia, often triggered by minor trauma, is rapidly followed by fibrosis and calcification and the child presents with swelling in a muscle or the development of a contracture. Radiographs will show calcification in, and eventually ossification of, the muscles (Fig. 29.26a). The condition is characterized by congenitally short great toes (Fig. 29.26b), and sometimes thumbs, which may be diagnostic. The disease progresses to severe disability and to date no treatment has been shown to influence the natural disease progression.

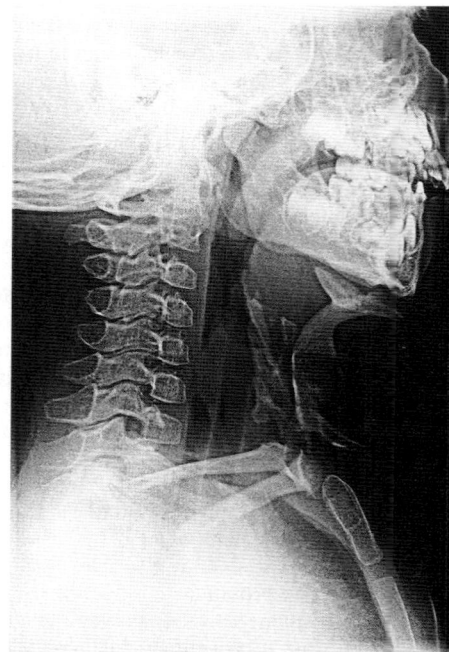

(a)

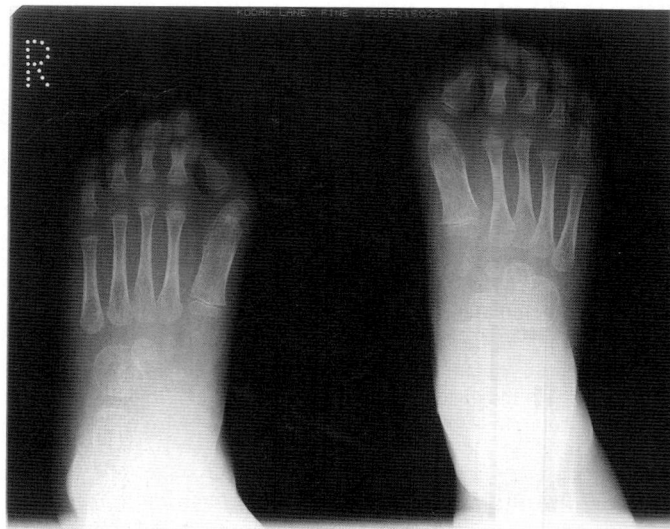

(b)

Fig. 29.26 Fibrodysplasia ossificans progressiva showing (a) ossification of anterior neck muscles and (b) dysplastic great toes.

OTHER INHERITED DISORDERS ASSOCIATED WITH MUSCULOSKELETAL PROBLEMS

Many inherited conditions may result in musculoskeletal problems. Some of the more important are outlined here. All are covered in more detail in other relevant chapters.

Down syndrome (trisomy 21)

Down syndrome is associated with a variety of musculoskeletal problems. In infancy generalized muscular hypotonicity may be striking and many affected individuals remain significantly hypermobile with associated symptoms. Atlantoaxial instability is of major concern. An inflammatory arthropathy of unknown cause is well recognized in affected children.

Velocardiofacial syndrome (22q11 deletion syndrome)

This syndrome is a common cause of congenital cardiac malformations and is associated with a variety of immunological abnormalities, particularly impairment of T cell function. Perhaps as a consequence of this it is now known to be associated with an inflammatory arthritis.[41]

Cystic fibrosis (CF)

Many individuals with CF have arthralgias which may be troublesome but are not associated with any serious joint pathology. A few develop a recurrent acute arthropathy which can be extremely painful and distressing. Although the exact pathology is unclear it seems likely that this results from immune complex deposition and the cutaneous vasculitis that may occur is presumed to have a similar mechanism. Nonsteroidal anti-inflammatory drugs may be inadequate to control these acute symptoms and short courses of oral steroids may be helpful. In severe longstanding cystic fibrosis, hypertrophic pulmonary osteoarthropathy may develop as a cause for joint pain and swelling and should be considered in an individual with marked clubbing of the fingers and severe pulmonary disease. Plain radiography will demonstrate the characteristic periosteal reaction.

Hemophilia

Hemophilia has previously been complicated by a destructive arthritis occurring as a consequence of recurrent intraarticular bleeds. It is a tribute to advances in care in hemophilia and the use of prophylactic factor VIII that chronic hemophilic arthropathy is now seldom seen in resource rich countries. Hemophilia must still be remembered in the differential diagnosis of a young boy presenting for the first time with a tense joint effusion. Joint aspiration demonstrates blood and abnormal coagulation will be found.

Metabolic bone disease

Rickets usually presents with bone pain and bowing of the long bones. The most common cause is vitamin D deficiency (Fig. 29.27), but rickets may also result from a number of inherited disorders. Hypophosphatemic or vitamin D resistant rickets may be inherited as either an X-linked recessive or an autosomal disorder and is characterized by impaired parathormone-dependent proximal renal tubular reabsorption of phosphate. Hypophosphatasia is a rare autosomal recessive disorder characterized by severe rickets and reduced serum levels of alkaline phosphatase.

Gout

Gout may result from either an increased production or a decreased excretion of urate and is extremely rare in childhood. It may result from a number of inherited disorders of purine metabolism; of these, familial juvenile hyperuricemic nephropathy is the most common.[42]

Periodic fever syndromes

Familial Mediterranean fever (FMF) and other periodic fever syndromes may result in musculoskeletal symptoms including myalgia, arthralgia

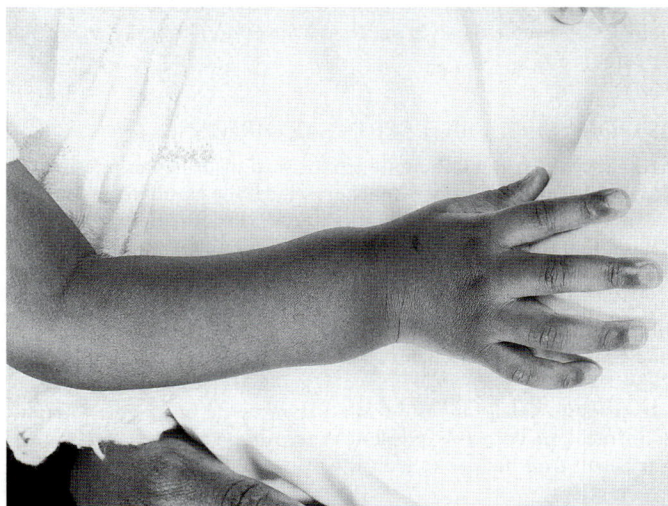

(a)

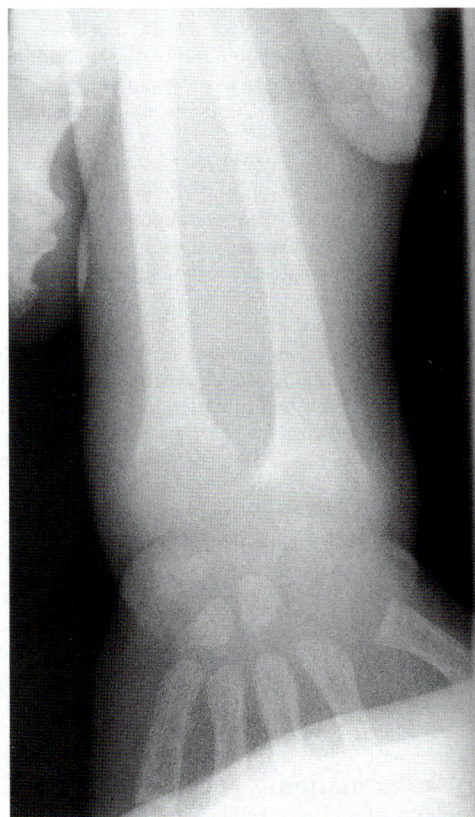

(b)

Fig. 29.27 Dietary rickets in a breast-fed toddler: (a) clinical appearance; (b) radiological features with characteristic metaphyseal fraying.

and arthritis. These conditions are described in more detail in the section on the 'The differential diagnosis of systemic inflammatory disorders' (see p. 1434).

INFECTION IN BONES AND JOINTS

Bone and joint infections are relatively rare disorders in children, but may be associated with considerable skeletal morbidity and potential mortality unless rapidly recognized and adequately treated. A multidisciplinary approach to diagnosis and management, with close collaboration between physician, orthopedic surgeon, microbiologist and radiologist, is necessary for optimal management and outcome.

OSTEOMYELITIS AND SEPTIC ARTHRITIS

Frequently the result of hematogenous seeding of bacteria, osteomyelitis may also result from extension of local sepsis, iatrogenic inoculation (rare) or trauma. In osteomyelitis the vascular-rich metaphyses of long bones or vertebral bodies are the commonest sites involved. Fever and pain are frequent symptoms and the differential diagnosis includes trauma, rheumatic fever, septic arthritis, soft tissue infection, rheumatic disease (e.g. juvenile idiopathic arthritis), bone infarction secondary to hemoglobinopathy, leukemia and bony neoplasm.[43] Osteomyelitis may be acute, subacute or chronic. Subacute osteomyelitis has a longer duration than acute and tends to result from infection with less virulent organisms. Chronic osteomyelitis may result from failure to identify or ineffective treatment of acute osteomyelitis.

In neonates the clinical features may be nonspecific and include poor feeding, irritability and poor temperature control. An affected limb may become erythematous, tender and swollen, and there may be a paucity of spontaneous movement ('pseudo-paralysis'). Concomitant septicemia is commoner in this age group. In older children the features tend to be more localized when the peripheral skeleton is affected, but less so in the pelvis or spine.

As with osteomyelitis, the majority of cases of septic arthritis occur as a result of hematogenous seeding of the synovium during an episode of bacteraemia. Septic arthritis occasionally arises from contiguous spread from adjacent osteomyelitis, especially in the younger child in whom the metaphyseal–epiphyseal junction lies adjacent to the joint space.[44]

A septic joint will exhibit the classic features of inflammation: swelling, pain, warmth and erythema. An affected hip is held in flexion and external rotation for comfort; a knee in flexion. All passive movement will be resisted. The hip warrants specific consideration, as increased intracapsular pressure arising from septic arthritis may interrupt blood supply and lead to avascular necrosis of the femoral head.

Fever, malaise and anorexia are usually seen, and progression of symptoms is often rapid. In neonates, as with osteomyelitis, features may be nonspecific. Children with immunodeficiency states, including those on systemic corticosteroid therapy, should be evaluated with great care as clinical signs of inflammation may be masked.

The differential diagnosis includes traumatic effusion, hemarthrosis, transient synovitis, reactive arthritis, JIA, Lyme arthritis, malignant disease, slipper upper femoral epiphysis and Perthes disease. Local spread of infection may result in pyomyositis.

Laboratory investigations

The full blood count may reveal thrombocytosis and neutrophil leucocytosis. Erythrocyte sedimentation rate (ESR) and C-reactive protein (CRP) are both likely to be elevated, the CRP tending to mirror the course of the infection more closely.[45]

Radiological investigations

Plain radiographs remain the primary initial imaging modality for suspected skeletal infections. In osteomyelitis soft tissue swelling and a periosteal reaction may be seen within a few days. Bony changes develop later (Fig. 29.28). In septic arthritis the early features are osteopenia of the epiphysis, increased joint space and soft tissue swelling (Fig. 29.29). Later in the disease destructive changes occur (Fig. 29.30).

Radionuclide bone scanning is sensitive at detecting areas of increased uptake, and may reveal multiple foci within the skeleton. However the specificity of this method is low and the features may not distinguish septic from nonseptic inflammatory lesions.

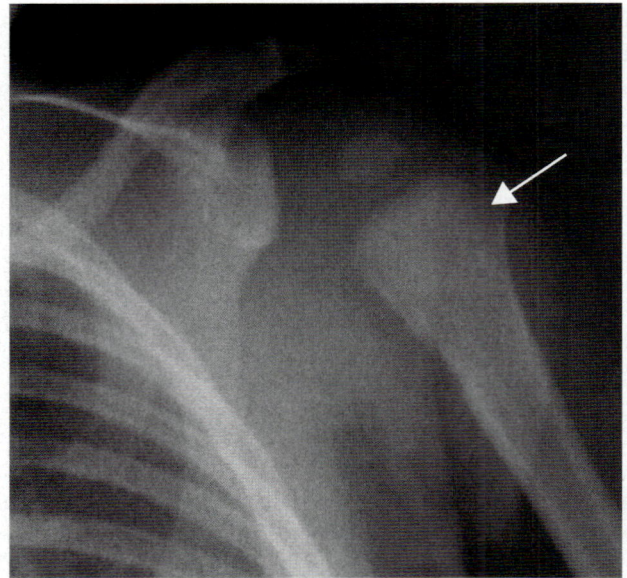

Fig. 29.28   Osteomyelitis of proximal humerus – 'moth eaten' appearance of bone and periosteal reaction.

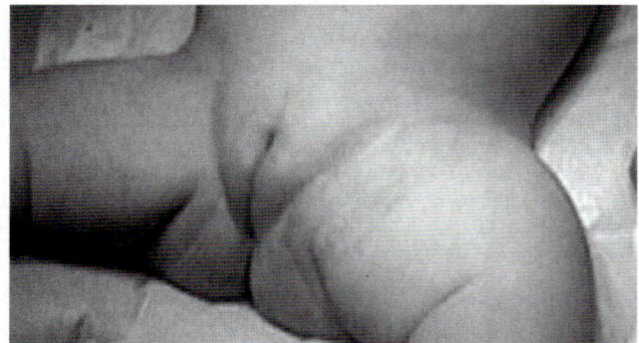

(a)

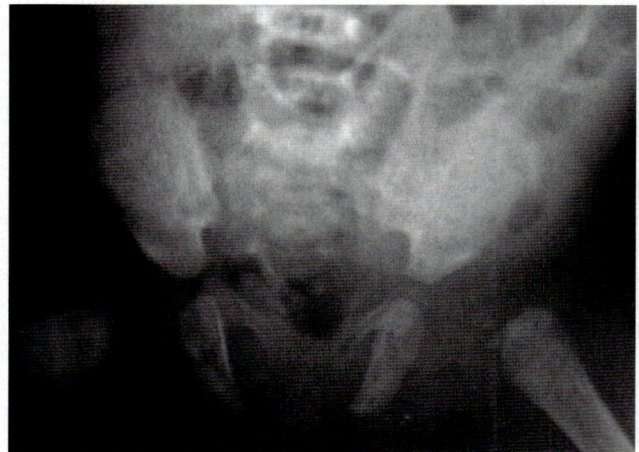

(b)

Fig. 29.29   Septic arthritis of the hip: (a) soft tissue swelling of thigh; (b) subluxation of the hip.

Ultrasound (US) is a rapidly available and sensitive method for detecting effusions in the hip. Magnetic resonance (MR) imaging plays a particular role because of excellent delineation of anatomy including soft tissues and bone. T1-weighted fat-suppressed postcontrast images are recommended in both osteomyelitis and septic arthritis.

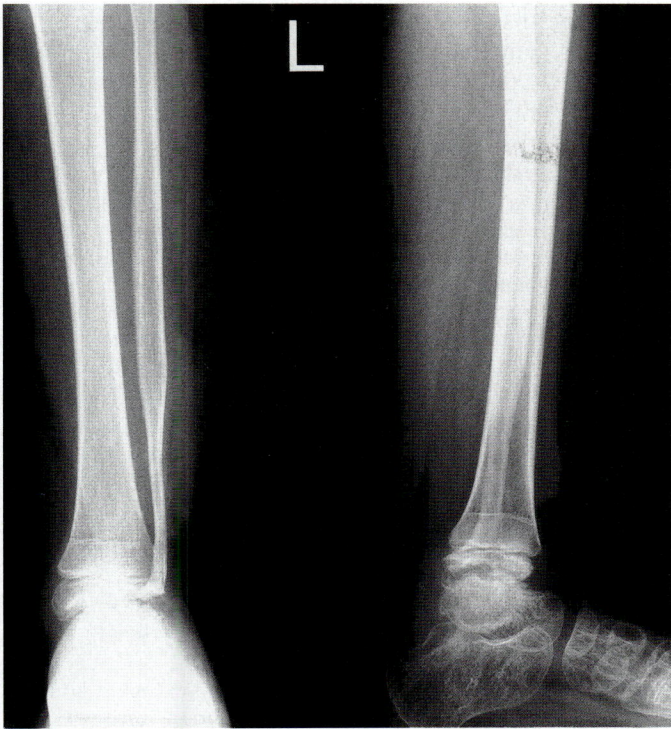

Fig. 29.30 Damage to ankle joint and distal fibula following disseminated staphylococcal sepsis with septic arthritis and osteomyelitis.

Microbiological investigations

Isolation of the infecting organism will allow targetting of appropriate antibiotic therapy, so vigorous microbiological investigation is mandatory. Peripheral blood cultures must be taken. The suspicion of septic arthritis should prompt microbiological analysis of synovial fluid, with joint aspiration also helping to relieve pain. Typical synovial fluid features on microscopy and a comparison with noninfective inflammatory arthritis are shown in Table 29.4.[46] Bone biopsy may reveal the organism in osteomyelitis.

Approximately 75% of bone and joint infection in resource rich countries is currently caused by *Staphylococcus aureus*[47] and the primary source of the infection is rarely clear. The introduction of vaccination against *Haemophilus influenzae* type b (Hib) has virtually eliminated the incidence of septic arthritis caused by this organism in countries where the vaccination is available. In neonates Group B *Streptococcus* and Gram negative enteric bacteria are relatively common cause of skeletal infection. Group A beta-hemolytic streptococci (*Streptococcus pyogenes*) and *Streptococcus pneumoniae* are important causes at all ages. *Kingella kingae* skeletal infections are increasingly recognized and reported, especially in younger children and frequently after upper respiratory tract infections.[48]

Table 29.4 Comparison of synovial fluid analysis in children with infective and inflammatory arthritis. (Adapted from Shetty & Gedalia 1998[46])

Characteristic	Normal	Juvenile idiopathic arthritis	Septic arthritis
Color	Yellow	Yellow	Serosanguinous
Clarity	Clear	Cloudy	Turbid
WBC count/mm³	< 200	$15–20 \times 10^3$	$40–300\,000 \times 10^3$
PMN count (%)	< 25	60–75	> 75

PMN, polymorphic neutrophil; WBC, white blood cell

Tuberculous arthritis is insidious in onset, and there is a tendency to sinus formation. If tuberculosis is suspected, synovial fluid and biopsy of synovial tissue should be sent for specific culture and also for analysis by the polymerase chain reaction (PCR). A Mantoux test should be performed. Gonococcal arthritis must be considered in the adolescent presenting systemically unwell with a very acute arthropathy. Brucellosis and infection with *Mycoplasma pneumoniae* may both cause a low grade septic arthritis.

In the immunocompromised, Gram negative organisms, fungi or atypical mycobacteria need to be considered. Children with hemoglobinopathies are at increased risk of acute recurrent osteomyelitis with Gram negative bacteria such as *Salmonella*, *Shigella sonnei*, *Escherichia coli* and *Serratia* species.

Treatment

Initial therapy is with empirical intravenous antibiotics for both osteomyelitis and septic arthritis. With concomitant septicemia supportive management on the neonatal or pediatric intensive care unit may be necessary.

The septic hip should be drained surgically to relieve pressure in the joint and minimize the risk of subsequent avascular necrosis. Surgical intervention is not always necessary in osteomyelitis[47] but may facilitate microbiological diagnosis. Subperiosteal or soft tissue abscesses and necrotic bone sequestra may need drainage.

The choice of antibiotic will depend upon the clinical context and local guidelines, but in the child with previously normal immune function must include adequate staphylococcal cover. Local incidence of methicillin-resistant *S. aureus* (MRSA) will determine whether antibiotic therapy should cover this possibility, and guidance from an expert microbiologist should be sought. Cefotaxime should be added if the child is not immunized against *Haemophilus influenzae*. A summary of empirical antibiotic therapy, by age, in an immunocompetent child is shown in Table 29.5.

In the immunocompromised, flucloxacillin plus cefotaxime are first line agents to provide adequate Gram positive and Gram negative cover. In the penicillin-allergic child cefradine is an alternative; with cephalosporin allergy vancomycin should be considered. Cefotaxime or ciprofloxacin may be used in *Salmonella* osteomyelitis.[47]

The duration of antibiotic therapy is controversial. There has been a move toward greater use of oral antibiotics beyond the initial stages of treatment in recent years. Intravenous antibiotic therapy should be continued for a minimum of 3 days, and then switched to oral for 3–4 weeks if fever has settled.[49] Switch to oral antibiotics should only be when the clinical condition of the child has improved, the fever has settled and the CRP is falling. Intravenous administration of antibiotics for longer periods is necessary in the immunocompromised or neonate.

Outcome

With early recognition of the diagnosis and prompt treatment, the long term outcome of skeletal sepsis in children is good. Growth disturbance may follow if the epiphysis has been involved and these children will require prolonged follow-up. In the minority with articular damage permanent impairment of joint function and early osteoarthritis may ensue (Fig. 29.30). Inadequate or ineffective treatment of acute osteomyelitis may result in chronic osteomyelitis with necrosis and sequestration of the bone.

DISCITIS

Infection in the intervertebral disc is a condition related to osteomyelitis, with infection arising from the vertebral end-plates, but without resulting in osteomyelitis of the vertebral body. The condition is believed by many to be secondary to infection,[50] the organism most commonly responsible being *S. aureus*. It is considered by others to have a non-infective inflammatory pathogenesis.

Table 29.5 Guidelines for empirical parenteral antibiotic treatment of acute bacterial skeletal sepsis by age

Age	Antibiotic	Notes
Neonate	Cefotaxime and flucloxacillin	Alternative: flucloxacillin with gentamicin
Child < 5 years	Cefotaxime and flucloxacillin or cefuroxime	MRSA* use vancomycin and consider clindamycin if sensitive – beware resistance developing during treatment Flucloxacillin or cefradine monotherapy if methicillin sensitive Staph. aureus
Child > 5 years	Cefuroxime or flucloxacillin	MRSA* use vancomycin and consider clindamycin if sensitive – beware resistance developing during treatment Flucloxacillin or cefradine monotherapy if methicillin sensitive Staph. aureus

* MRSA: Expert microbiologist advice should be sought

The condition is more common in preschool age children and any disc may be involved. The most striking clinical feature is the refusal of the patient to flex the lumbar spine. The older child may have difficulty walking or limp, will have a stiff back and will complain of back pain associated with constitutional upset. The younger child will frequently refuse to walk, often spontaneously adopting a prone position with extension of the lumbar spine for comfort. Discomfort may be reported when the child is traveling in an infant car seat.

The blood picture reveals a leucocytosis and raised ESR. Blood culture is usually negative although Staph. aureus may be identified in some. Culture of disc tissue is rarely indicated and frequently negative. Radionuclide bone scanning may highlight a 'hot' spot in the region of a disc space. MRI will demonstrate clearly the inflammatory lesion within the disc (Fig. 29.31a). Plain radiographs eventually reveal disc space narrowing and varying vertebral end-plate damage (Fig. 29.31b).

Most children respond quickly to antibiotic therapy, initially intravenous and then oral, without the need for surgical intervention. Pain is managed symptomatically with analgesics and sometimes a short term removable brace to unload the involved disc. Therapy is usually continued for 6 weeks. Failure to respond after a week or deterioration in spite of treatment should raise concerns regarding the potential of an abscess requiring surgical drainage or an unusual organism such as tuberculosis. The prognosis of juvenile discitis is generally good with no significant long term sequelae in the majority.

VIRAL INFECTION AND ARTHRITIS

Arthralgia is a common symptom of viral infection. In some cases a true septic arthritis results, with virus particles being isolated in the joint fluid. In others arthritis occurs as a reactive process with no evidence of infection in the joint. Rubella, particularly 'natural infection' but also post vaccination, is associated with arthritis.[51] Parvovirus B19 (slapped cheek syndrome or Fifth disease) is occasionally associated with arthritis similar to that of rubella. Varicella may be associated with a benign reactive arthritis, but is occasionally complicated by a potentially fatal syndrome of necrotizing fasciitis and toxic shock syndrome as a sequelae of concomitant Group A streptococcus infection.[52] Paromyxovirus (mumps), adenovirus, ECHO virus and Coxsackie B virus may all be associated with arthritis.

Infection with the human immunodeficiency virus may be associated with a variety of rheumatological problems. These include arthralgias, septic arthritis (frequently fungal in origin), reactive arthritis, Reiter syndrome and a seronegative spondyloarthropathy.

REACTIVE ARTHRITIS

Transient synovitis of the hip

See section on 'Common orthopedic problems in childhood', page 1434.

Reactive arthritis associated with bowel and genitourinary infections

In children, as in adults, a reactive arthritis may develop after enteric infections with Salmonella, Shigella, Yersinia and Campylobacter, and posturethritis with Chlamydia in sexually active adolescents. The HLA-B27 antigen is commonly identified. There is usually a peripheral, asymmetrical lower limb arthritis. There may be associated dactylitis ('sausage digit' resulting from inflammation of both joints and tendon sheaths), tenosynovitis and involvement of the sacroiliac joints. There is usually a history of enteritis or urethritis within the preceding 4 weeks. Reiter syndrome, a triad of arthritis, conjunctivitis and urethritis, is uncommon in children.

Treatment requires nonsteroidal anti-inflammatory drugs in adequate doses. Occasionally systemic steroids are required to settle an acute arthritis. If the arthritis becomes chronic, intra-articular steroids and second-line agents including sulphasalazine and methotrexate may be considered.

Rheumatic fever and poststreptococcal arthritis
(see Ch. 21)

Acute rheumatic fever remains prevalent in developing areas of the world. The disease arises as a complication of infection (pharyngotonsillitis) with Group A beta-hemolytic Streptococcus pyogenes. The modified Jones criteria are the basis for the diagnosis (Table 29.6).

Inflammation in various tissues may result in arthritis, carditis, a typical rash (erythema marginatum), subcutaneous nodules and a characteristic neurological syndrome, Sydenham chorea. Arthritis is a common clinical feature, tends to affect large joints and is flitting and self-limiting in nature. Erythema marginatum is an erythematous macular and nonpruritic lesion with serpiginous margins surrounding areas of normal skin. Sydenham chorea (also known as St Vitus dance) is caused by inflammation of the basal ganglia of the brain. It presents with involuntary movements of the extremities, muscular incoordination and emotional lability. Subcutaneous nodules may be seen on extensor surfaces of joints in the chronic phase of rheumatic heart disease. Rheumatic heart disease is discussed in more detail in Chapter 21.

Arthritis following Group A streptococcal infection is recognized in some children who do not fulfill the criteria for acute rheumatic fever. This poststreptococcal reactive arthritis differs from that of rheumatic fever in that it is nonmigratory and more persistent. As with rheumatic fever recurrent episodes are recognized.

Treatment of both rheumatic fever and poststreptococcal reactive arthritis involves antibiotics to eradicate the streptococcus. Penicillin V is the antibiotic of choice, and should be given as a 10-day course. In penicillin-allergic individuals, erythromycin is a suitable alternative. In rheumatic fever prophylaxis against streptococcal infection is indicated for at least 5 years after the initial attack, and into adulthood in patients with carditis.[53] There is no consensus regarding the use of prophylactic penicillin in those with poststreptococcal arthritis but if attacks are recurrent antibiotic prophylaxis may prove beneficial. Additional prophylaxis for surgical or dental procedures is necessary in the chronic stage of rheumatic heart disease (see Ch. 21).

In the acute illness nonsteroidal anti-inflammatory drugs (NSAIDs) may provide symptomatic relief from the arthritis. Steroids are reserved for patients with pancarditis associated with congestive cardiac failure.

Lyme disease

The infectious spirochaete Borrelia burgdorferi, transmitted by the tick Ixodes, is responsible for Lyme disease. The regions where Lyme

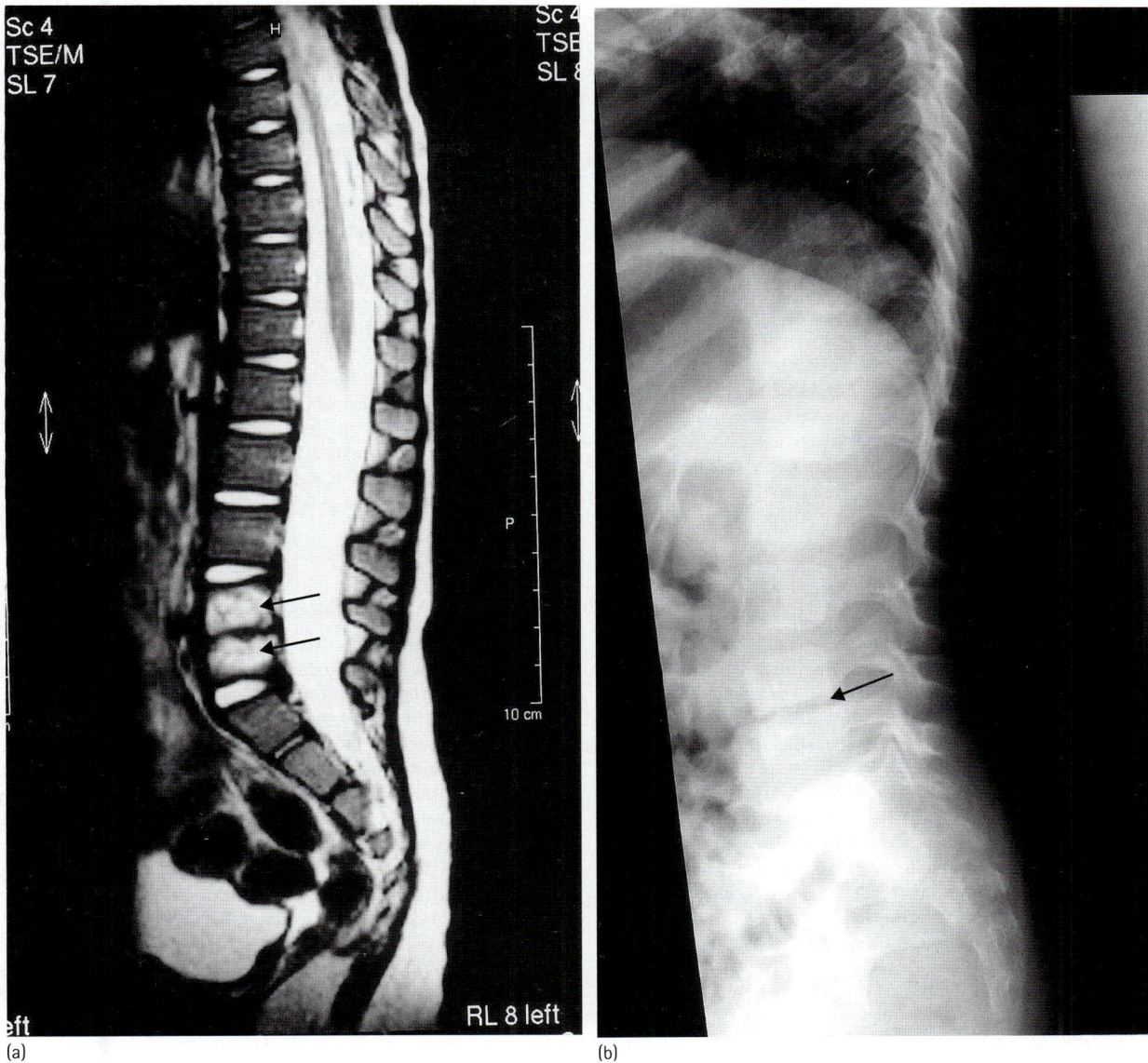

Fig. 29.31   (a) MFI in discitis – abnormal signal in the L4 and L5 vertebral bodies with destruction of the intervening disc space; (b) plain radiograph showing narrowing of L4/5 disc space following resolution of acute illness.

Table 29.6   Modified Jones criteria for the diagnosis of rheumatic fever

Major criteria	Minor criteria
Polyarthritis common: flitting, large joints	Fever
Carditis common: pancarditis	Arthralgia
Chorea (Sydenham) uncommon: persistent	Prolonged P-R interval
Erythema marginatum uncommon: macules evolving to serpiginous	Elevated ESR/CRP, leucocytosis
Subcutaneous nodules uncommon: extensor surfaces	Previous rheumatic fever

The diagnosis of rheumatic fever is made in the presence of either two major criteria or one major plus two minor criteria together with evidence of recent group A streptococcal infection (positive throat swab, elevated antistreptolysin O titer (ASOT) or other antistreptococcal antibodies).

disease is seen most frequently are central Europe and northeastern United States. The disease is manifest by cutaneous, articular, neurological and other systemic features. The most typical skin manifestation is erythema chronicum migrans. Early lymphocytic meningitis is commoner in children than in adults. The arthritis typically appears months to years after the original infection, and becomes chronic in up to 16%. In the majority there is an episodic monoarthritis, but occasionally polyarthritis develops. Treatment with antibiotics is necessary, with ceftriaxone recommended at a dose of 50 mg/kg/day for 14–28 days.[54] Amoxicillin at a dose of 50 mg/kg/day for 28 days is an alternative, but compliance may be poorer due to the dosage regimen. Some authors recommend doxycycline, but not in children below the age of 8 years. Intra-articular steroids should be avoided until completion of antibiotic therapy.

Arthritis associated with meningococcal infection

Meningococcal disease may be associated with both a true septic arthritis occurring in association with the acute septicemic illness or a reactive arthritis seen in the post-acute phase. With improved survival rates from severe meningococcal septicemia a post-infectious, immune complex mediated arthritis is seen with increasing frequency, often in association with a recrudescence of fever and the development of a vasculitic rash.

JUVENILE IDIOPATHIC ARTHRITIS

Juvenile idiopathic arthritis (JIA) is not a single disease entity, rather a collection of heterogeneous diseases. JIA may be associated with significant morbidity, both articular and extra-articular, and may place a significant burden on child and carers alike. Mortality is rare and largely confined to the systemic onset subtype.

JIA is diagnosed according to a constellation of clinical features supported by the judicious use of relevant investigations (frequently to exclude other causes of arthritis). At the current time there are no pathognomic diagnostic tests for JIA. A number of children with JIA will attain spontaneous remission, although rates vary according to disease subtype. Packham reported follow-up data on 246 adults with all subtypes of JIA and found that 43% had clinically active disease.[55] There is now a realistic expectation of disease control with modern therapeutic regimens delivered by an experienced multidisciplinary team. Future studies reporting the outcome of children treated since the advent of these newer therapeutic approaches are awaited, with an expectation that results will be improved. Nonetheless patients, families and professionals must remain realistic that no fundamental cure yet exists.

Significant advances made during the final decade of the 20th century and beyond include:

- Development and subsequent revision of a new classification system of JIA.
- Preliminary definition of improvement measures to evaluate outcome in drug studies (core set criteria).
- Further understanding of immunogenetic pathways.
- Drug studies exploring both optimal doses and routes of administration for conventional drug therapies such as methotrexate, and the new products of the biotechnology revolution, the so-called 'biologic' agents.
- Online resources: the British Society for Paediatric and Adolescent Rheumatology (BSPAR; www.bspar.org.uk); Paediatric Rheumatology European Society (PReS; www.pres.org); and the Pediatric Rheumatology International Trials Organization (PRINTO;www.printo.it) have all developed websites providing useful sources of information for professionals, patients and parents on childhood rheumatic diseases of childhood with links to other relevant websites.

DEFINITION AND CLASSIFICATION

JIA is defined as arthritis of unknown etiology that begins before the 16th birthday and persists for at least 6 weeks. Other known conditions must be excluded. For the purposes of defining arthritis, an inflamed joint is swollen, or limited in range of joint movement with joint pain or tenderness, which is not due to a primary mechanical disorder or to other identifiable cause.

In the final decade of the 20th century the International League of Associations for Rheumatology (ILAR) proposed and subsequently revised consensus guidelines for the classification of JIA.[56] The goal of this major work was to replace and unify previous historical classification criteria, namely juvenile rheumatoid arthritis and juvenile chronic arthritis. Although the ILAR criteria were proposed with the primary aim of defining and classifying clinically homogeneous subgroups within JIA for research purposes, they have been widely embraced and incorporated into clinical practice and are now in mainstream use as clinical diagnostic criteria despite awaiting full validation in further studies. The ILAR criteria define subtypes according to the onset pattern of the disease and associated clinical features. A summary of the clinical features of the JIA classification system is given in Table 29.7.

DIFFERENTIAL DIAGNOSIS

Juvenile idiopathic arthritis must always be considered a diagnosis of exclusion. Musculoskeletal symptoms are common in childhood, and in many cases are related to simple trauma. It should be possible to make a clinical distinction between inflammatory arthritis and arthralgia. If doubt exists, an expert pediatric rheumatology opinion should be consided before embarking on investigations that may be unpleasant for the child and potentially delay the diagnosis of JIA. As the nature of the differential diagnosis of inflammatory arthritis includes potentially life threatening disorders such as sepsis, malignancy and non-accidental injury, any child presenting requires careful assessment by means of thorough history taking, meticulous clinical examination and prompt, judicious use of appropriate investigations. Etiologies can be considered as follows: infection, trauma, autoimmune, neoplasia,

Table 29.7   Clinical features of juvenile idiopathic arthritis

JIA subtype	Clinical features	Alerts
Systemic arthritis	Arthritis with or preceded by daily ('quotidian') fever for at least 3 days, accompanied by one or more of: evanescent erythematosus rash; lymphadenopathy; hepatomegaly and/or splenomegaly; serositis	Arthritis may not be present early in course Mandatory exclusion of infective and malignant conditions

Oligoarthritis:
    Persistent
 	
    Extended
	Arthritis of four or fewer joints within the first 6 months
	Affecting not more than four joints throughout the disease process. Frequently children below the age of 5 years
	Affecting more than four joints after the first 6 months
		High risk of associated uveitis, especially if ANA positive

Polyarthritis
    RF positive
    RF negative
	Arthritis of five or more joints within the first 6 months. Subdivided according to presence of RF	RF positive disease rare but equivalent to 'adult' rheumatoid arthritis

Psoriatic arthritis	Arthritis and psoriasis OR arthritis with at least two of dactylitis, nail pitting or onycholysis, psoriasis in first degree relative	Psoriasis and arthritis may not co-exist for many years
Enthesitis-related arthritis	Arthritis and enthesitis OR arthritis or enthesitis with two of: SI joint tenderness or inflammatory lumbosacral pain, HLA B27 antigen, onset after age 6 years in a male, acute (symptomatic) anterior uveitis, history of HLA B27 associated disease in a first degree relative	
Undifferentiated arthritis	Arthritis that fulfils criteria in no or more than two of the above categories	

Abbreviations: ANA, antinuclear antibody; RA, rheumatoid arthritis; RF, rheumatoid factor; SI, sacro-iliac.

hematological, metabolic, genetic, drug reactions, trauma (including non-accidental), mechanical/orthopedic. Such an approach should allow distinction of the many possible causes of arthritis, as shown in Table 29.8.

CORE SET CRITERIA

To facilitate standardization of clinical measures of change in JIA, a core set of criteria have been developed by consensus primarily for the purposes of clinical trials,[57] although they may be useful within routine clinical practice. These criteria comprise:

- physician global assessment of disease activity (10-cm visual analogue scale);
- parent/patient assessment of overall well-being (10-cm visual analogue scale);
- functional ability (Childhood Health Assessment Questionnaire – CHAQ (www.rheumatology.org/sections/pediatric/chaq);
- number of joints with active arthritis;
- number of joints with limited range of movement;
- erythrocyte sedimentation rate.

Table 29.8 Differential diagnosis of inflammatory arthritis in childhood

Infection:
    Acute septic arthritis
    Viral arthritis
    Reactive/post-infectious arthritis

Juvenile idiopathic arthritis.
Arthritis associated with inflammatory bowel disease
Other autoimmune rheumatic disorders:
    Systemic lupus erythematosus
    Juvenile dermatomyositis
    Systemic sclerosis
    Mixed connective tissue disease

Systemic vasculitis
    Henoch–Schönlein purpura
    Kawasaki disease
    Polyarteritis nodosa

Malignancy:
    Leukemia
    Neuroblastoma

Hematological:
    Sickle cell anemia
    Hemophilia

Immune deficiency syndromes
Genetic disorders:
    Cystic fibrosis
    Velocardiofacial syndrome
    CINCA syndrome
    Down syndrome
    Stickler syndrome

Drug reactions
Trauma including non-accidental injury
Orthopedic:
    Perthe disease
    Pigmented villonodular synovitis
Miscellaneous:
    Sarcoidosis
    SAPHO syndrome
    Familial Mediterranean fever

Abbreviations. SAPHO, synovitis, acne, pustulosis, hyperostosis and osteitis syndrome; CINCA, chronic infantile neurological cutaneous and articular syndrome.

EPIDEMIOLOGY

Data describing incidence and prevalence of JIA are confusing and unclear. A detailed review of 34 studies beginning in 1966 showed the reported prevalence of JIA to vary from 0.07 to 4.01 per 100 000 children, while the reported incidence for JIA over the same period ranged from 0.008 to 0.226 per 1000 children.[58] This study highlights the need for standardization of diagnostic criteria, case definition, and case ascertainment and also the need to consider the clinical qualification and experience of participating researchers, health resources available within the study population, expectation of health and the size of the study cohort. Despite methodological differences between studies there does appear to be a true variability in disease occurrence according to geographical factors.

Overall, girls with JIA outnumber boys by approximately 2:1. There are important variations within disease subtypes with girls outnumbering boys in oligoarthritis, polyarthritis and psoriatic arthritis, but a more even sex distribution in systemic JIA[59] and boys outnumbering girls in the enthesitis-related arthritis subtype. In those with uveitis the ratio of girls to boys is higher, up to 6.6:1.[60]

ETIOLOGY AND PATHOGENESIS

As with all autoimmune disease there is a complex interplay between genetic risk factors and environmental triggers. JIA has been referred to as a 'complex genetic trait', albeit one in which there are now several consistent and strong associations.[61]

Studies of genetic polymorphisms in both adult and childhood chronic arthritis have frequently, but not exclusively, involved the major histocompatibility complex (MHC). The MHC class II loci DR, DQ and DP are particularly associated with JIA. Age-related genetic susceptibility is suggested by the association of early childhood onset oligoarthritis with HLA A2, DR5, DR8 and DPB1*0201.[62] Oligoarthritis in older boys is associated with HLA-B27, and to date this remains the only HLA association with any major relevance to routine clinical practice. Polyarticular JIA with a positive rheumatoid factor is associated with HLA DR4, as in adults with rheumatoid arthritis.

The British Paediatric Rheumatology Study Group demonstrated in a large multicenter study of 521 Caucasian patients with JIA the presence of multiple HLA class II associations. Differences were demonstrated between the seven subtypes defined by the ILAR classification criteria, which encouragingly lends support to this classification approach.[63]

There is growing evidence to support an etiological role for polymorphisms within individual genes coding for pro- and anti-inflammatory cytokines. In studies of synovial tissue from adults with rheumatoid arthritis, proinflammatory cytokines such as interleukin (IL)-1 and tumor necrosis factor (TNF)-alpha are elevated, and induce the release of tissue-destroying metalloproteinases.[64] There has been great interest in the role of cytokines as mediators of the inflammatory response in JIA, both to further the understanding of the pathogenesis of the disease and also as potential targets for biological therapies.

The pro-inflammatory cytokine TNF-alpha (TNFα) occupies a central position in the cytokine network. TNFα is produced by several cells throughout the body, including synovial cells, T lymphocytes and mononuclear phagocytes, but in inflammatory arthritis it is mostly derived from activated macrophages. TNFα, with lymphotoxin-alpha (a related cytokine), is detected in synovial tissue in JIA and may amplify local inflammation and contribute to joint destruction.[65] TNFα stimulates further proinflammatory cytokine production including IL-1 and IL-6.

JIA is a heterogeneous disease. It is not surprising then that studies have revealed differences in cytokine profiles between JIA subtypes. Rooney et al demonstrated an imbalance between TNFα and its soluble receptor (sTNFR) in JIA, with different ratios in different subtypes, which may explain variations in disease patterns and resulting joint damage.[66]

CLINICAL FEATURES

Systemic arthritis

The systemic onset subtype accounts for 11% of all cases of juvenile arthritis, often occurring in younger children with a median age of onset of 4.3 years and a male to female ratio of 1:1.2 (data on percentages of each subclass is taken from Symmons 1996 which uses the historical classification, JCA;[59] percentages using the ILAR classification JIA may differ slightly from these, but data is not yet available).

Systemic JIA is defined as arthritis in one or more joints with or preceded by fever of at least 2 weeks' duration that is documented to be daily ('quotidian') for at least 3 days, and is accompanied by one or more of the following:

- evanescent (nonfixed) erythematous rash;
- generalized lymph node enlargement;
- hepatomegaly and/or splenomegaly;
- serositis.

The systemic features may precede the onset of arthritis. In toddlers, the arthritis may be subtle and difficult to confirm. Many will therefore require detailed workup to exclude sepsis and hematological malignant diseases.

The associated systemic manifestations of the disease are often much worse during the periods of fever, and the children are intensely miserable during these periods, with significant improvement when the fever settles. The rash is pale pink, macular (evanescent) and flitting in nature. It often occurs in linear streaks and it exhibits the Koebner phenomenon (Fig. 29.32). It most commonly occurs on the trunk, but can be generalized. Generalized lymphadenopathy occurs in the majority, and enlarged nodes are painless, rubbery and mobile. Hepatomegaly is common and splenomegaly occurs in approximately 50%. Serum transaminases are frequently elevated, and there is often hypoalbuminemia. Pericardial effusion on echocardiogram is common and usually asymptomatic, but a useful feature to aid diagnosis. Pleural effusion may co-exist with pericardial effusion, and either may occasionally require surgical drainage.

The pattern of arthritis associated with systemic JIA is variable. Approximately one third develop a polyarticular course with joint destruction within 2 years of disease onset (Fig. 29.33). Hepatosplenomegaly, serositis and low serum albumin are recognized as risk factors at disease onset, while later risk factors for an adverse outcome in systemic JIA are thrombocytosis, persistent fever or steroid dependency at 6 months.[67]

Three patterns of disease progression have been described:
1. monocyclic (systemic disease with a single episode);
2. intermittent (recurrent fever and arthritis interspersed with periods of remission);
3. persistent disease activity with systemic and polyarticular phases.

Functional outcome is largely dependent on the course of the arthritis rather than on the systemic features.

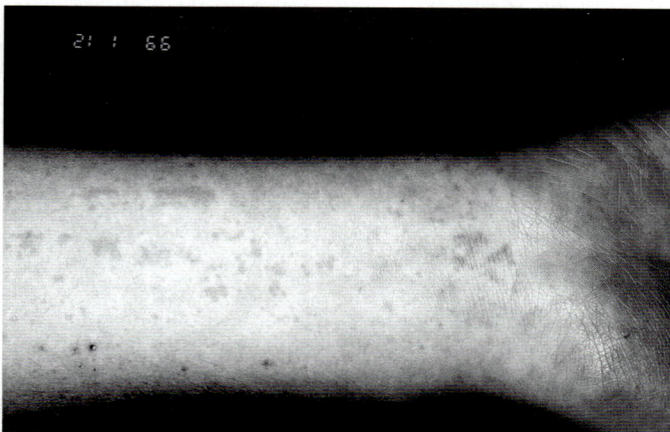

Fig. 29.32 Rash of systemic juvenile idiopathic arthritis.

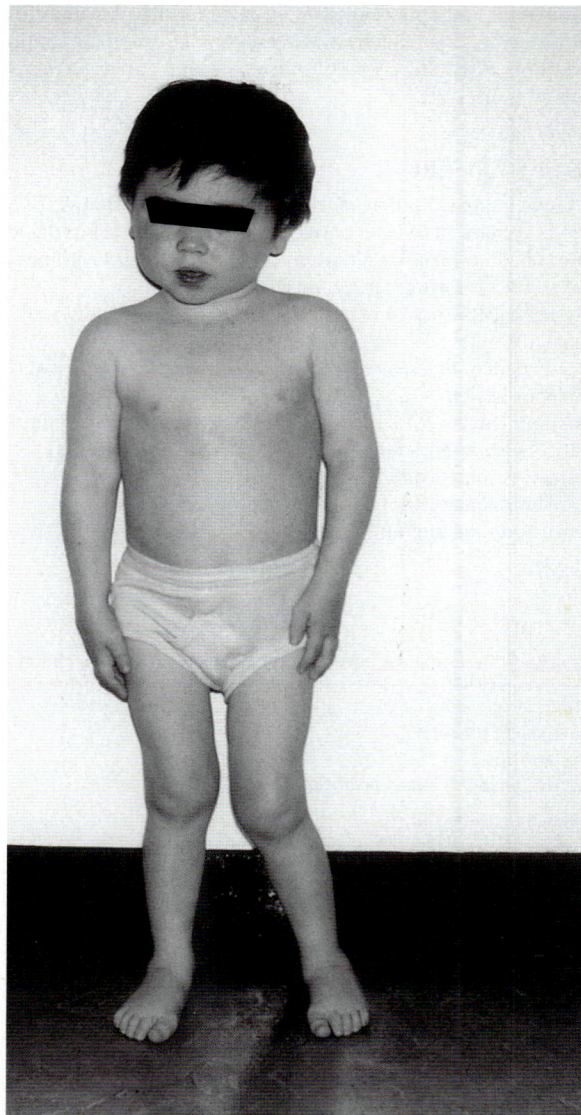

Fig. 29.33 Systemic juvenile idiopathic arthritis with polyarticular course – involvement of knees, ankles, hips, wrists and cervical spine.

Oligoarthritis

This is defined as arthritis affecting between one and four joints during the first 6 months of disease and further subdivided into:

- persistent oligoarthritis: affects no more than four joints throughout the disease course;
- extended oligoarthritis: affects a cumulative total of five joints or more after the first 6 months of disease.

Oligoarthritis is the commonest onset pattern of JIA in Caucasian populations, accounting for approximately 50% of affected children.[59] Persistent oligoarthritis is commonest in preschool age girls (although does occur in boys) and in this age group is frequently associated with positive antinuclear antibodies (ANA) and an increased risk of silent, potentially blinding, uveitis.

Oligoarthritis most frequently develops asymmetrically in large lower limb joints, especially the knee (Fig. 29.34) and the ankle, and occasionally in the upper limb.

Oligoarthritis in preschool children is often insidious, but occasionally manifests acutely. The child may limp, especially after rest. The joint appears swollen and is warm, but rarely painful until passively moved through its full range. Examination of the knee may reveal a palpable effusion. With time, if unrecognized, flexion contractures may occur.

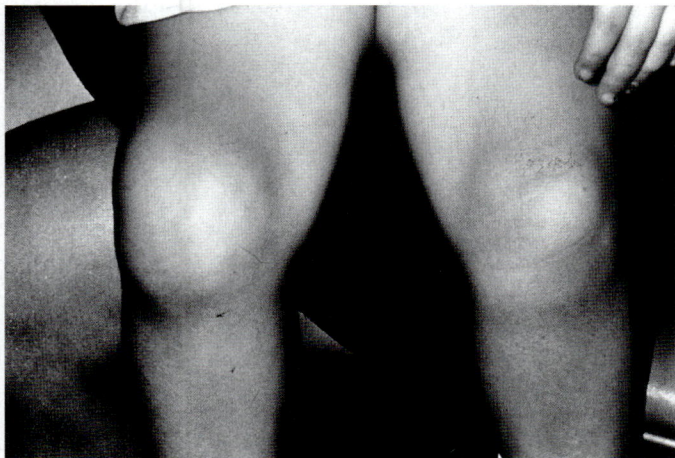

Fig. 29.34   Oligoarthritis showing marked swelling of R knee.

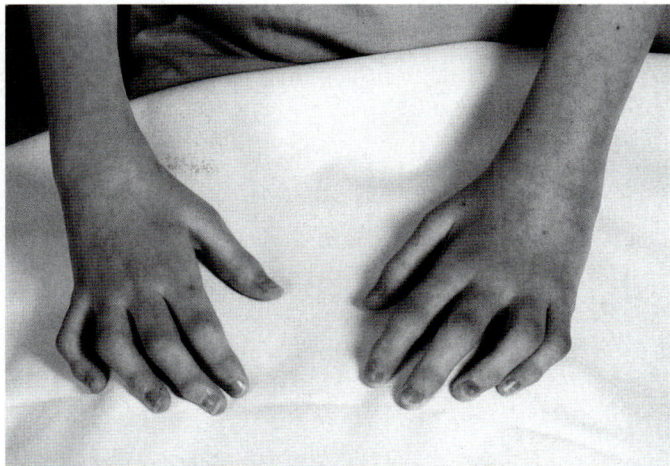

Fig. 29.36   Polyarthritis affecting wrists and the small joints of the hands.

Bony overgrowth of the joint may be seen with leg length discrepancy (Fig. 29.35). Prompt recognition and treatment will prevent the development of such complications.

In a proportion of children with an oligoarticular onset there is an 'adding on' of involved joints beyond 6 months of disease – so-called extended oligoarthritis.

Polyarthritis

This is defined as arthritis affecting five or more joints during the first 6 months of disease. This subtype is further subdivided on the basis of testing for IgM rheumatoid factor into:

- rheumatoid factor positive (seropositive);
- rheumatoid factor negative (seronegative).

Seronegative polyarthritis (Fig. 29.36) has a variable clinical expression ranging from low grade grumbling disease to an aggressive polyarthritis. An early peak age of onset is seen around 2 years, with a later peak around 8 years.[60] It varies in clinical expression ranging from low grade grumbling disease to an aggressive polyarthritis. Joints may be hot and swollen or simply tender with loss of function, without gross synovial swelling or palpable effusions (so-called 'dry synovitis'). Onset may be insidious but joint deformities, of both large and small joints, may develop rapidly.

Seropositive polyarthritis is rare, accounting for 3% of all children with JIA, compared to 17% for seronegative polyarthritis.[59] Children with seropositive polyarthritis typically are girls and develop disease in late childhood and adolescence. The arthritis is usually symmetrical affecting upper and lower limbs, in particular the small joints of the hands and feet. The test for IgM rheumatoid factor should be positive on at least two occasions 3 months apart.

Psoriatic arthritis

Psoriatic arthritis is defined as arthritis and psoriasis (Fig. 29.37), or arthritis and at least two of the following:

- dactylitis;
- nail pitting and onycholysis;
- psoriasis in a first-degree relative.

In the UK, psoriatic arthritis accounts for 7% of all cases of JIA, is commoner in girls (male:female ratio 1:1.6) with a median age of onset 10.1 years.[59] Oligoarticular onset (asymmetrical involvement of large and small joints) is frequent and dactylitis (diffuse swelling of a finger or toe joint and periarticular tissues is a hallmark feature (Fig. 29.38). The arthritis can be highly erosive. Nail abnormalities may be seen, including nail pitting and nail dystrophy (onycholysis). The arthritis precedes the psoriasis in as many as 75% of cases, and 45% of children develop psoriasis within 5 years of onset of arthritis.[68] The outcome in psoriatic arthritis is variable, with both oligo- and polyarticular courses described.

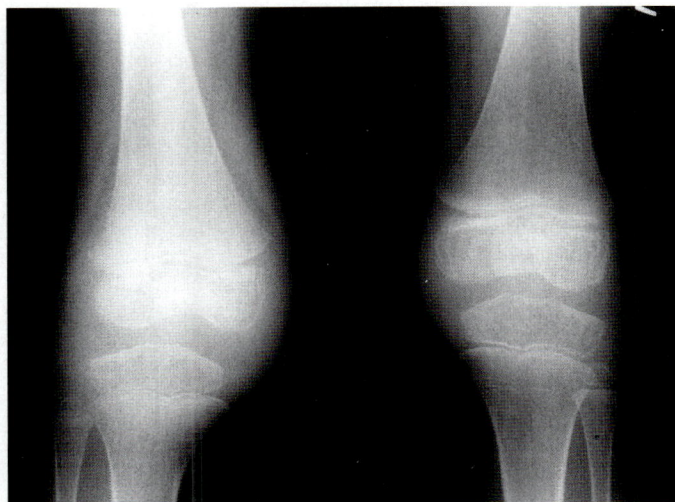

Fig. 29.35   Oligoarthritis – plain radiograph showing overgrowth of right knee.

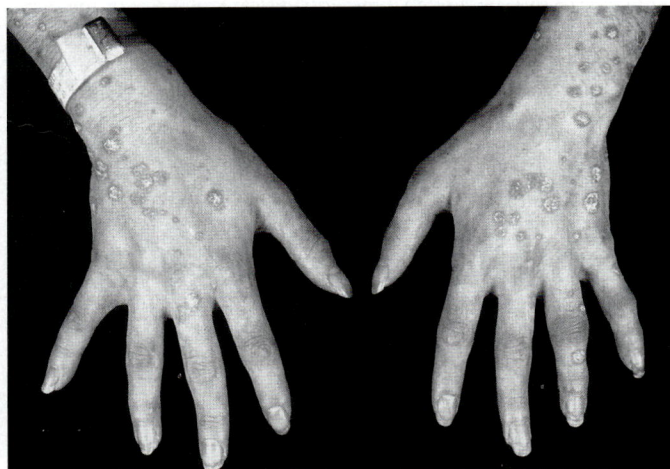

Fig. 29.37   Psoriatic arthritis.

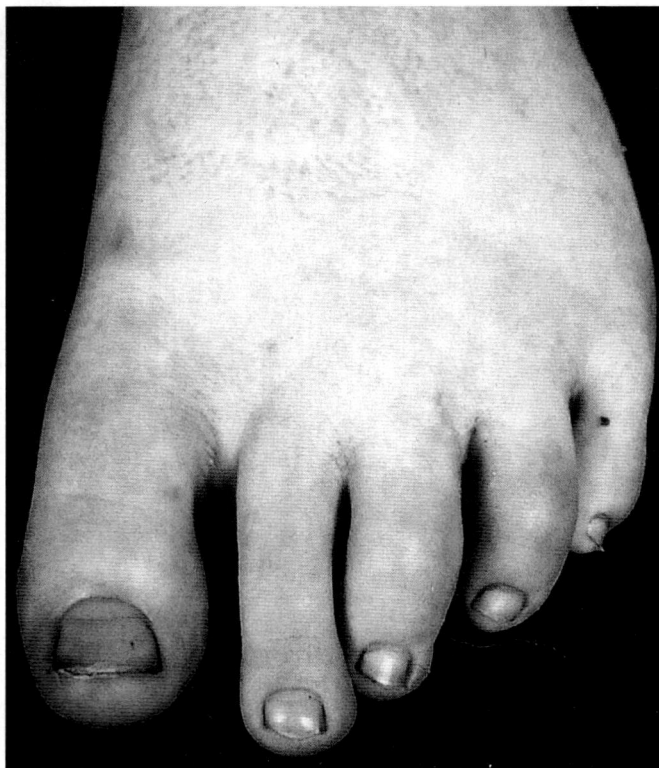

Fig. 29.38 Dactylitis – swelling of third and fourth toes.

Enthesitis–related arthritis

This is defined as arthritis and enthesitis (inflammation of tendon insertion into bone), or arthritis or enthesitis with at least two of the following:

- sacroiliac joint tenderness and/or inflammatory lumbosacral pain;
- presence of the HLA-B27 antigen;
- onset of arthritis in a male over 6 years of age;
- acute (symptomatic) anterior uveitis;
- history of ankylosing spondylitis, enthesitis-related arthritis, sacroiliitis with inflammatory bowel disease, Reiter syndrome or acute anterior uveitis in a first-degree relative.

This subtype defines those with disease related to the HLA-B27 antigen, and avoids the term juvenile spondyloarthropathy, inaccurate because of the rarity of spinal involvement in children. The commonest joints involved are the peripheral large joints of the lower limb, in an asymmetrical distribution. It is rare for children to present with axial skeleton symptoms or signs, although a minority develops arthritis of the sacroiliac joints in teenage years (Fig. 29.39) and subsequently ankylosing spondylitis in adulthood. There is a marked predominance of boys in this group, presenting after the age of 6 years. Enthesitis is a characteristic feature, often affecting the insertion of the Achilles tendon into the calcaneum, and may be distressingly painful resulting in significant functional impairment. The eye disease associated with enthesitis-related arthritis is an acute painful iritis (in contrast to the asymptomatic uveitis associated with other subtypes of JIA), and occurs in less than 20% of children.

Undifferentiated arthritis

At present children who either fulfill criteria for no category, or who fulfill criteria for more than one of the other categories, are defined as undifferentiated.

INVESTIGATIONS

Judicious investigation may serve to support the diagnosis of JIA. At presentation as a minimum full blood count, liver chemistry and a disease

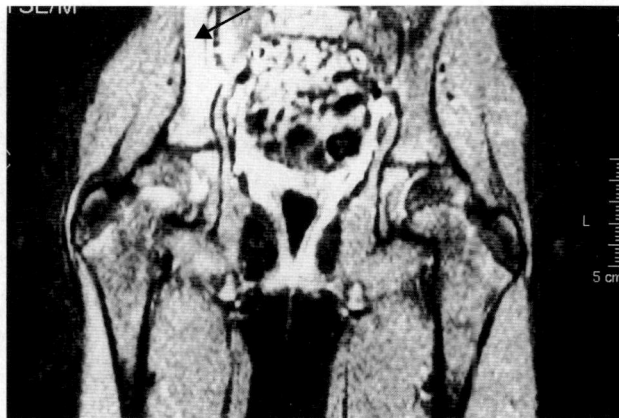

Fig. 29.39 Gadolinium enhanced MRI showing right-sided sacroiliitis (note high signal on right compared to left).

activity measure, preferably erythrocyte sedimentation rate (ESR), are recommended for all JIA subtypes. A positive antinuclear antibody in oligoarthritis is a risk factor for silent uveitis and will help to guide the ophthalmology screening program. Rheumatoid factor is only of clinical significance in the context of those children with a polyarthritis. Serum ferritin may be disproportionately high in systemic JIA. Nonspecific hyperimmunoglobulinemia is often seen in polyarticular and systemic JIA. Hypoalbuminemia is common in systemic JIA along with elevations of liver enzymes.[67]

Radiological investigations

All imaging modalities may have a potential role in JIA:

- to aid diagnosis – particularly to exclude other musculoskeletal conditions;
- to document and define evidence of joint damage;
- to aid the assessment of complex joints, e.g. hip, subtalar, shoulder and temporomandibular joints;
- to detect subclinical or very early synovitis – magnetic resonance scanning with gadolinium contrast is a very sensitive technique;
- to distinguish synovitis from tenosynovitis;
- to facilitate intra-articular steroid injection.

Three stages of radiographic changes are seen on plain radiographs in JIA.[69]

- Early: soft tissue swelling, e.g. blurring of the infrapatellar fat pad on lateral knee radiograph and periarticular osteopenia.
- Intermediate: cortical erosions, joint space narrowing and subchondral cysts.
- Late: destructive joint changes with ankylosis, joint contractures, metaphyseal and diaphyseal changes and growth anomalies (Fig. 29.40).

Radionuclide bone scanning is sensitive in detecting areas of increased uptake within the skeleton, but will not differentiate between inflammation, infection or malignant disease. Ultrasound is a reliable method for detecting effusions, especially in the hip, guiding intra-articular injections and confirmation of popliteal cysts. In expert hands it is also increasingly useful as a method of documenting synovitis of joints and tendons. Intravenous contrast (gadolinium-DPTA) enhanced magnetic resonance sequences are exquisitely sensitive at detecting inflamed synovium and particularly valuable in the assessment of inaccessible joints such as the hip, and complex joints such as the ankle, where it may be difficult to distinguish clinically between the tibiotalar and subtalar joint. T1-weighted images with fat suppression are particularly recommended for demonstrating synovitis (Fig. 29.41).

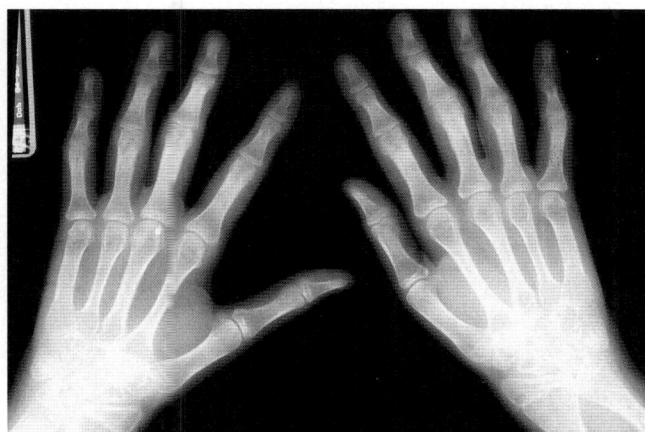

(a)

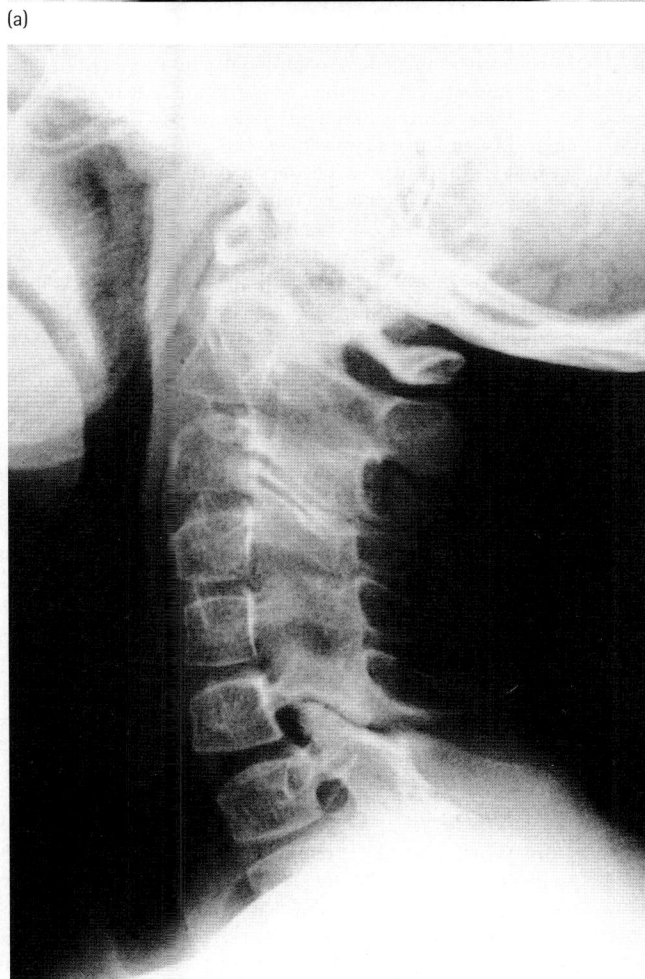

(b)

Fig. 29.40 Plain radiographs in juvenile idiopathic arthritis: (a) destructive changes of wrists with crowding of carpal bones; periarticular osteopenia and loss of joint space at proximal interphalangeal joints; (b) fusion in block of posterior elements of C2–C7.

COMPLICATIONS: ARTICULAR

Articular complications are a direct result of synovial inflammation and can generally be minimized or prevented by optimizing control of the inflammatory process. Flexion contractures occur commonly and at a very early stage in JIA and if not treated intensively may become permanent. Overgrowth of affected limbs (Fig. 29.35) is a particular problem of oligoarthritis which may have serious long term complications

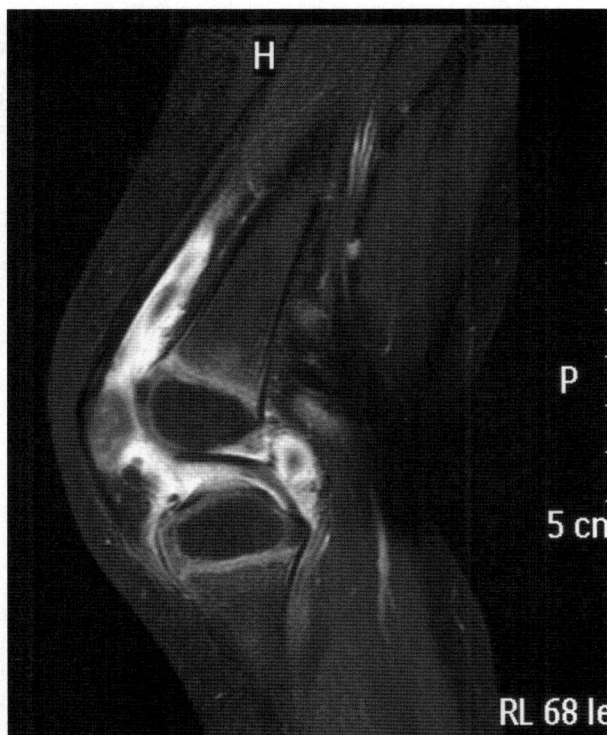

Fig. 29.41 MR scan of left knee with fat suppression and gadolinium contrast. There is a small effusion with synovial thickening and enhancement.

e.g. a discrepancy in lower limb length resulting in a pelvic tilt and scoliosis in adult life. The temporomandibular joint (TMJ) may be involved in polyarthritis and specific features such as asymmetrical mouth opening and micrognathia may be noted during clinical examination. TMJ involvement may result in both cosmetic and functional difficulties and appropriate advice from an interested maxillofacial surgeon should be sought.

COMPLICATIONS: EXTRA–ARTICULAR

Uveitis

The incidence of uveitis in JIA overall is approximately 10%, although it is commoner in ANA (antinuclear antibody) positive oligoarthritis.[70] Two patterns of ocular inflammation are seen in JIA. An acute, painful iritis is seen in children with enthesitis-related arthritis, and usually resolves rapidly with topical corticosteroid therapy. Chronic, asymptomatic anterior uveitis that may become sight threatening if not recognized and treated is especially common in preschool age girls with oligoarthritis. It is strongly associated with positive antinuclear antibodies. The diagnosis requires slit-lamp examination by an ophthalmologist.

To date no prospective randomized controlled data exist comparing immunosuppressive therapy in childhood uveitis. Visual complications (synechiae, band keratopathy, cataract or glaucoma) may develop in up to 30%, and significant visual loss has been reported in 11%,[70] highlighting the need for aggressive treatment.

In many cases uveitis in children with JIA can be controlled with topical corticosteroids and short-acting mydriatics. Early steroid-sparing therapy, to reduce the risk of steroid-related complications such as cataract and glaucoma, is indicated if it proves impossible to taper local steroid therapy because of persistent disease activity. Methotrexate is the commonest second line agent in use, with significant reduction in uveitis activity and steroid dependency being shown in a retrospective study.[71] If control cannot be achieved with oral methotrexate alone, parenteral administration of methotrexate, or methotrexate in combination with ciclosporin, should be considered. Data from uncontrolled studies suggest benefit from infliximab in therapy-resistant uveitis.[72] Relapses and first presentation uveitis have been reported in patients receiving etanercept therapy, indicating more studies are needed to define any potential role for the biological agents in treating uveitis.

Nutritional status and growth

Nutritional impairment and growth failure is a recognized complication of all subtypes of JIA. The etiology of nutritional impairment in JIA is not fully understood, nor is it clear how frequently it occurs. It may affect the general well-being of the child and contributes to the growth disturbance that is a serious consequence of JIA in some children.

Osteoporosis

Osteoporosis is a significant long term complication of a variety of rheumatological disorders including JIA and occurs as a consequence of the underlying inflammatory process; of inactivity; and of steroid therapy.

Psychosocial

Long term outcome studies have demonstrated a significant incidence of psychosocial difficulty in young adults with JIA. Attention to rehabilitation and early return to normal activities where possible is essential to minimize this. Families and schools must be encouraged to treat the child as normal and all should be in mainstream schooling. Good transitional care with an early focus on independence and career counseling is essential.

Macrophage activation syndrome (MAS)/secondary hemophagocytic lymphohistiocytosis (HLH)

MAS/HLH is a rare but potentially life threatening complication of systemic JIA. Features in a child raising suspicion of MAS/HLH are fever, lymphadenopathy and hepatosplenomegaly, pancytopenia, low ESR, elevated liver enzymes and coagulopathy.[73] MAS/HLH may be triggered by an intercurrent infection or change in drug therapy. The pathognomic feature, macrophages actively phagocytosing hematopoietic elements, may be seen on the bone marrow aspirate but it must be noted that false negative bone marrow examinations may occur. Other laboratory features include hypertriglyceridemia and hyperferritinemia. Treatment of MAS/HLH consists of high dose corticosteroids and ciclosporin with good supportive care and vigorous treatment of concomitant sepsis. Such patients may require management in a pediatric intensive care setting.

MANAGEMENT

As with all pediatric chronic diseases, optimal management of JIA is delivered by an experienced multidisciplinary team (Table 29.9). Adequate education of the child and family about the disease and possible therapeutic strategies is essential from the outset. The impact of JIA on patient and family may be significant and good results depend on considerable commitment from all. Information and encouragement will empower patients and families to be involved in and committed to their treatment with improved compliance and better results. The provision of appropriate written information is helpful; directing families to appropriate online resources is increasingly important.

Physiotherapy and occupational therapy

The aim of physiotherapy is to maintain and restore joint function, and to increase muscle strength. This can only be achieved in association with medical therapy to control synovitis. An occupational therapist may provide adaptations at home or school. Many different strategies are available, but there is consensus that physical and occupational therapy early in the disease is associated with an improved outcome.[74]

Table 29.9 Members of the multidisciplinary team involved in the care of a child with juvenile idiopathic arthritis

Medical	Professions allied to medicine	Community
Pediatric rheumatologist	Physiotherapist	Family
Pediatrician	Occupational therapist	Friends
Ophthalmologist	Psychologist	School teacher
General practitioner	Social worker	Parental employer
Orthopedic surgeon	Dietitian	
Dental practitioner	Orthotist	
Radiologist	Podiatrist	

Medical management

The pharmacological management of JIA continues to evolve, in terms of specific drugs and strategies for their deployment. Early use of methotrexate (MTX) in polyarthritis, frequently at diagnosis or shortly after, is now standard practice in order to achieve and maintain disease remission. MTX is now regularly used in oligoarthritis resistant to local intra-articular corticosteroid injection therapy. MTX and other systemic immunosuppressive agents are frequently used in uveitis whether or not associated with JIA. Biological agents are now licensed therapies and appear effective and to date safe in treating JIA. There is the likelihood of further advances and new experimental therapies likely to follow rapidly. An algorithm showing an approach to pharmacological management of JIA is shown in Table 29.10.

Nonsteroidal anti-inflammatory drugs (NSAIDs)

NSAIDs are widely used at diagnosis, provide good symptomatic relief and contribute to the control of the inflammatory process although this takes time to achieve. Table 29.11 lists the commonly used NSAIDs and the doses required to achieve anti-inflammatory effect. Drugs with once or twice daily regimens are likely to have better compliance particularly in older children.

Side-effects are uncommon in children. Gastrointestinal upset is uncommon and may be relieved by the addition of a H_2 antagonist or proton pump inhibitor. Naproxen (and occasionally other NSAIDs) may be associated with scarring pseudoporphyria affecting the face and care should be taken in fair skinned children. Mood and behavior disturbances are occasionally reported by parents of young children on NSAIDs.

Corticosteroid therapy

The early use of effective disease-modifying anti-rheumatic drugs (DMARDs), historically methotrexate and more recently anti TNFα agents, has dramatically reduced the dependency upon, and toxicity associated with chronic administration of systemic corticosteroids. Corticosteroids still have a role in the management of JIA, in particular for remission induction, and may be administered systemically by the intravenous and oral route, or locally by intra-articular injection.

Local corticosteroid therapy. Intra-articular steroid injections are effective, with a low risk of complications, in all subtypes of JIA, particularly oligoarthritis.[75] In polyarthritis, multiple intra-articular injections may be used simultaneously with the initiation of methotrexate therapy. The early use of intra-articular steroid injections and rapid resolution of synovitis relieves pain and facilitates early physiotherapy and rehabilitation thus preventing joint contractures. When used early, and if necessary repeatedly, intra-articular steroids may prevent leg length discrepancy in oligoarthritis.[76] Triamcinolone hexacetonide (TH) is the drug of choice for intra-articular injection in JIA, as shown in a randomized controlled trial with the alternative agent triamcinolone acetonide.[77]

A typical regimen for dosage of triamcinolone hexacetonide is 1 mg/kg for large joints (knees, hips and shoulders) to a maximum

Table 29.10   Algorithm for the medical treatment of JIA by onset pattern

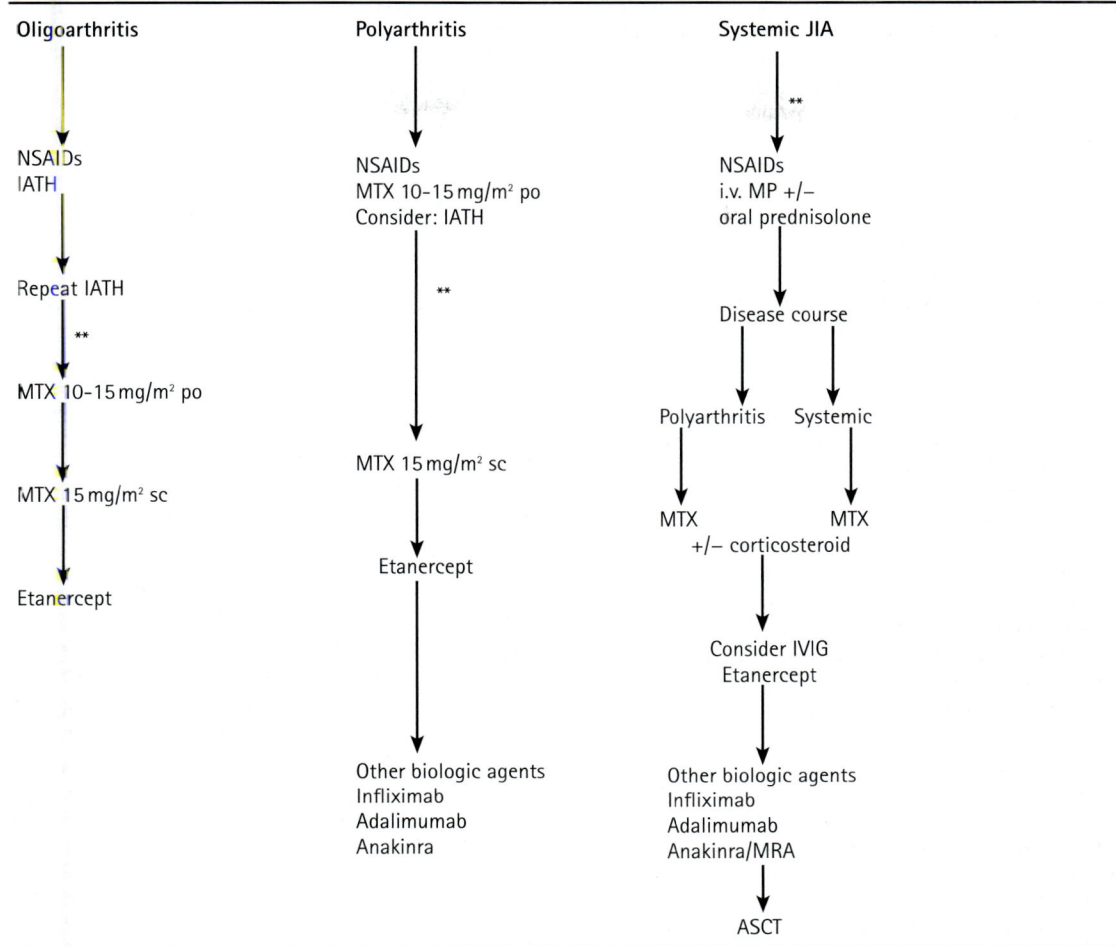

Key to algorithm: po—oral, sc—subcutaneous, NSAIDs—nonsteroidal anti-inflammatory drugs, iv MP—iv methylprednisolone, IATH—intra-articular triamcinolone hexacetonide, MTX TNFα methotrexate, IVIG—intravenous immunoglobulin; ASCT—autologous stem cell transplant.
** Indicates stage requiring management in conjunction with regional pediatric rheumatology center.

Table 29.11   Nonsteroidal anti-inflammatory drugs commonly used in children with juvenile idiopathic arthritis

Drug	Dose	Times daily	Notes
Diclofenac sodium	1 mg/kg	2–3	Max 150 mg/day *SR available*
Naproxen	5–10 mg/kg	2	Max 1 g/day
Ibuprofen	10 mg/kg	3–4	
Indometacin	0.5–1 mg/kg	2	Max 200 mg/day *SR available*
Piroxicam	<15 kg 5 mg 16–25 kg 10 mg 26–45 kg 15 mg >46 kg 20 mg	Once daily	Sublingual preparation available

SR, slow release.

of 40 mg, 0.5 mg/kg in smaller joints (ankles, wrists and elbows) and 2–4 mg/joint for the small joints of the hands and feet. The dose of triamcinolone acetonide is typically double that of triamcinolone hexacetonide. In young children with JIA or if multiple joints are to be injected, intra-articular injection will be performed using general anesthesia. In older children the procedure can be safely and effectively carried out using a 50/50 mix of nitrous oxide and oxygen (Entonox). Subcutaneous atrophy at the injection site is the only common adverse effect, with the highest incidence in a single study of 8.3% of patients.[78] A transient cushingoid state is reported with the use of triamcinolone acetonide, including occasionally after injection of a single joint.[79]

Systemic corticosteroids.   Systemic corticosteroids, administered either as intravenous high dose 'pulses' (methylprednisolone 30 mg/kg usually for 3 consecutive days and repeated as necessary) or oral prednisolone may be considered as an adjunct in a defined course during the 'lag' phase while MTX becomes effective or may be used to control acute disease flares, again in strictly limited courses.

Methotrexate

Methotrexate (MTX) is currently the disease modifying agent of first choice in JIA. MTX is a dihydrofolate reductase inhibitor, although its mechanism of action as an anti-inflammatory agent is not fully understood. In a double-blind placebo-controlled trial, MTX at a dose of 10 mg/m² was effective in polyarthritis (significant response in 63% of patients).[80] MTX is effective in extended oligoarthritis and systemic JIA.[81] Ruperto and colleagues for PRINTO reported in a randomized controlled trial that 28% of patients failed to respond to an oral dose of 8–12.5 mg/m². Of those, a further 62.5% achieved a clinical response to subcutaneous administration at 15 mg/m²/week, but no additional benefit was seen at 30 mg/m²/week.[82]

Subcutaneous administration should be considered if oral administration fails to produce effective control, or is not tolerated. This can be self-administered at home by patients or carers. In the UK the Royal College of Nursing have produced guidelines regarding subcutaneous administration of MTX (http://www.rcn.org.uk/publications/pdf/administering-methotrexate.pdf).

Common side-effects of weekly low dose methotrexate include nausea and vomiting, which in some cases can be overcome by giving the MTX in two doses over 24 hours, use of an antiemetic agent or regular administration of folic acid. Mouth ulcers may also respond to folic acid supplementation. Transient elevations in liver enzymes are common, frequently associated with intercurrent viral infections, and resolving with temporary withdrawal of MTX. Significant liver toxicity and bone marrow suppression is rare.[83] Blood monitoring is mandatory while children take MTX. Monthly full blood count (FBC) and liver function tests (LFTs) initially, reduced to 2–3 monthly thereafter is satisfactory. There is no consensus on the use of folic acid to minimize adverse effects in children on weekly low dose MTX, although weekly administration in doses of 2.5–5 mg per week is standard in some centers.

Immunization with live vaccines is contraindicated during treatment with MTX. If circumstances permit, children known to be varicella zoster (VZ) susceptible should be immunised with VZ vaccine 2 weeks prior to starting MTX. Children known to be VZ susceptible and in contact with VZ, should be treated with either VZ specific immunoglobulin or prophylactic oral aciclovir according to local guidelines. A best practice statement on the immunization of the immunocompromised child is available.[84]

Methotrexate is teratogenic and liver toxicity may be increased with concomitant alcohol ingestion. Adolescents need specific counseling in these areas. A checklist prior to administration of MTX is given in Table 29.12.

Biological therapies

Following publication of the previous edition of this text, there has been rapid growth in this form of therapy in JIA. Acute infection of any type mandates temporary interruption of therapy, and all live vaccines are contraindicated. A summary of anti-TNF agents used to treat JIA is given in Table 29.13.

Etanercept. In a multicenter clinical trial of children with polyarticular JIA who had previously failed to respond to therapy with low dose methotrexate, 74% improved with etanercept.[85] Adverse effects were similar to those in the placebo group, and included injection site

Table 29.12 Information to be discussed prior to commencing methotrexate for JIA

Blood monitoring – FBC and LFTs monthly until dose stable and 2–3 monthly thereafter

Avoid all live vaccines

Miss a dose if acutely unwell with intercurrent infection – contact rheumatology team for advice

Ensure adequate contraception if sexually active

Limit alcohol intake to 5 units per week, and highlight the alcohol content of popular brands

reactions, headaches, minor upper respiratory tract infections, rhinitis, urticarial reactions, nausea and vomiting. Follow-on data have demonstrated safety and efficacy over a 4-year period, with the rate of serious adverse events being 0.13 per patient-year. The rate of serious infections was 0.04 per patient-year, in a total etanercept exposure of 225 patient-years.[86]

Infliximab. Efficacy similar to etanercept has been shown in an open label prospective pilot study of 24 patients.[87] In a randomized controlled trial, comparing infliximab at doses of 3 mg/kg vs 6 mg/kg, 75% of JIA patients responded to a dose of 6 mg/kg. Antibodies to infliximab were higher with the lower dose resulting in a higher incidence of allergic type infusion reactions and serious adverse events in the 3 mg/kg group compared to 6 mg/kg group (19% vs 9% respectively at weeks 14–52 of treatment).[88] Co-administration with weekly methotrexate is recommended to limit autoantibody production.

Adalimumab. Adalimumab is a recombinant human IgG1 monoclonal antibody, specific to human TNF. Theoretically there should be less risk of immunogenic reactions than with infliximab. Efficacy has been demonstrated in in adult rheumatoid arthritis. At the time of writing JIA data are only available in abstract form, albeit with encouraging efficacy and safety at 1-year follow up.[89]

Adverse effects of anti TNF agents. Anti TNF agents have been shown to induce production of antinuclear antibodies, although the incidence of a lupus-like state remains low.[90] There have been reports of lymphoproliferative disease in adult patients with rheumatoid arthritis and Crohn disease treated with anti TNF agents,[91] although a causal link remains to be established. This highlights the need for further long term surveillance studies in JIA and a biologics registry has been established in the UK for this purpose (British Society for Paediatric and Adolescent Rheumatology Biologics and New Drugs Registry: www.bsparreg.org).

At the time of writing, etanercept is the only biological agent licensed for use in JIA in the UK. The National Institute for Health and Clinical Excellence (NICE: www.nice.org.uk) has recommended etanercept for children with active JIA in at least five joints, with inadequate response to MTX, or intolerable side-effects from MTX.

Other biologic agents

Preliminary data suggests a role for two other agents in JIA. IL-1 is now known to play a role in systemic JIA.[92] Anakinra, an IL-1 receptor ana-

Table 29.13 Biologic anti TNF agents for the treatment of JIA

Biologic agent	Structure	Mechanism of action	Administration	Red flags
Etanercept	Soluble fusion molecule of two human p75 TNF receptors	Binds and blocks TNFα and lymphotoxin α	0.4 mg/kg twice weekly s.c. injection, maximum 25 mg per dose	Injection site reactions, infections
Infliximab	Chimeric human-mouse anti TNFα monoclonal antibody	Binds TNFα	6 mg/kg at 0, 2 and 6 weeks, then 8 weekly thereafter by intravenous infusion	Infusion reactions, infection, TB reactivation, ANA and anti-dsDNA antibody formation
Adalimumab	Recombinant human IgG1 anti-TNFα mononclonal antibody	Binds TNFα	24 mg/m² fortnightly by subcutaneous injection	Injection site reactions, infections

tagonist, has been used in adult RA and anecdotal evidence suggests that it may be effective in systemic JIA. An open label phase II clinical trial of anti-IL-6 receptor monoclonal antibody (MRA) has also shown promise in systemic JIA.[93]

Other therapies

Intravenous immunoglobulin may be used in systemic arthritis[94] unresponsive to more conventional therapies. Dose regimens vary between 1 g/kg/day for 2 consecutive days and 400 mg/kg/day for 5 consecutive days, repeated monthly. Hydroxychloroquine may be of benefit in some seropositive patients. Sulphasalazine may be used in enthesitis-related arthritis. Leflunomide, an oral dihydrooratate dehydrogenase inhibitor, has shown efficacy in adults with rheumatoid arthritis. There is anecdotal evidence of benefit in JIA[95] but no controlled studies.

Autologous hemopoietic stem cell transplantation (ASCT) may be a possible option for patients with JIA refractory to conventional treatment and in whom the burden of drug toxicity is unacceptable. Early results have shown the potential for prolonged drug free remission, but a mortality rate of 9% was reported in a preliminary case series highlighting the importance of developing future protocols through collaborative multicenter studies.[96]

Surgical management

Orthopedic surgery has an increasingly limited role in JIA. Joint replacement may ultimately be required in some cases, but should be deferred as long as possible. Newer techniques such as hip resurfacing may have a role in some, but detailed discussion is beyond the scope of this text.

Transitional care

Young people with JIA entering transition into adulthood have specific medical and psychosocial needs, and many advocate that this process should be pro-actively managed. A multicenter study of a coordinated, evidence-based program of transitional care reported encouraging results.[97]

OTHER ARTHROPATHIES IN CHILDHOOD

Infections and JIA are the only common causes of arthritis in childhood. The differential diagnosis of inflammatory arthritis in children (Table 29.8) is wide and other causes must be excluded as necessary. Many of these conditions are described elsewhere in the chapter.

COMMON ORTHOPEDIC PROBLEMS IN CHILDHOOD

Children present to the clinician with a wide spectrum of problems ranging from complaints relating to form, posture and gait to complaints of localized pain at various sites. This section covers the more common orthopedic explanations for such presentations.

COMMON PAINLESS COMPLAINTS

Normal variants

The shape and form of the lower limbs in children cause a great deal of parental anxiety. In spite of such concern, the majority of these children are normal and sound knowledge of normal variation cannot be overemphasized. The most common causes for parental concern are flat feet, bow legs, knock knees, and in-toe gait. The chief objective when presented with such children is to exclude a pathological explanation. In broad terms unilateral 'deformities' are more suspicious of pathology than bilateral which frequently reflect normal physiological variation.

Toe walking

The commonest explanation for this presentation is habitual or idiopathic toe walking although more serious explanations should be considered and excluded. A thorough neuromuscular evaluation is mandatory since toe walking may be a feature of muscular dystrophy, cerebral palsy, a tethered cord or indeed any neuromuscular disorder. Children with habitual or idiopathic toe walking persistently walk on the toes, but can be encouraged to adopt a more normal heel strike. They should be able to stand still with the heels to the ground. Treatment is directed toward constant encouragement to reinforce the normal heel–toe gait pattern, but occasionally serial casting is helpful to break a persistent habit or if true tendo-Achilles shortening develops.

Flat feet

Most children who are brought for assessment of flat feet are normal. The clinician's responsibility is to exclude potential pathological causes such as congenital vertical talus, tarsal coalition or juvenile idiopathic arthritis.

The clinical assessment aims to determine if the flat appearance is flexible or rigid. Rigid flat feet are never normal; flexible flat feet usually are. The feet should be observed weightbearing and walking. Many infants have 'fat feet' rather than flat feet, a pad of fat in the sole of the foot hiding the normal arch. Jack's test should be done. This requires the great toe to be dorsiflexed. As this is done a windlass mechanism tightens the planter fascia and draws the flexible flat foot up into a normal arch (Fig. 29.42). The child should be asked to stand on tiptoe while the foot is observed both from behind and from the medial side. When standing, the heel of the flat foot is in valgus if viewed from behind. On tip toe the heel and hindfoot should swing into a varus posture and when viewed from the medial side an arch should develop. The flexible flat foot has a normal or even an increased range of movement as a result of a degree of ligamentous laxity. Limitation suggests pathology. Radiographs are not necessary in the evaluation of the flexible flat foot but should be included if there is any suspicion of inflexibility or symptoms of pain.

Flexible flat feet are rarely symptomatic and in most individuals represent an anatomical variant. They are occasionally associated with conditions where ligamentous laxity is a feature, such as Ehlers–Danlos and Marfan syndromes when they may persist into adult life. Treatment is rarely necessary. Footwear modifications do not alter the development of the foot although a simple arch support or a heel cup, to prevent the heel collapsing into valgus, can help to reduce symptoms of foot ache or minimize rapid shoe wear. In the rare cases where symptomatic flat foot persists into maturity, surgical correction can be considered.

Bow legs and knock knees

Whilst the majority of children who present with bow legs or knock knees are physiologically normal, both presentations can be a manifestation of metabolic bone disease and consideration of such conditions is important.

Bow legs (genu varum)

Figure 29.43 charts the development of the tibiofemoral angle during growth. Varus angulation is normal in infants but usually resolves by 18–24 months.[98] Valgus angulation is normal in 3- to 5-year-olds, usually resolving by age 7–8 years. Clinical assessment should be made with

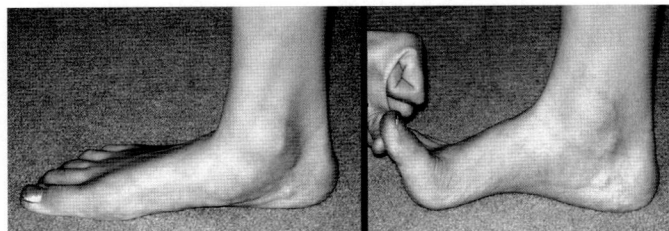

Fig. 29.42   Flexible flat foot – Jack's test.

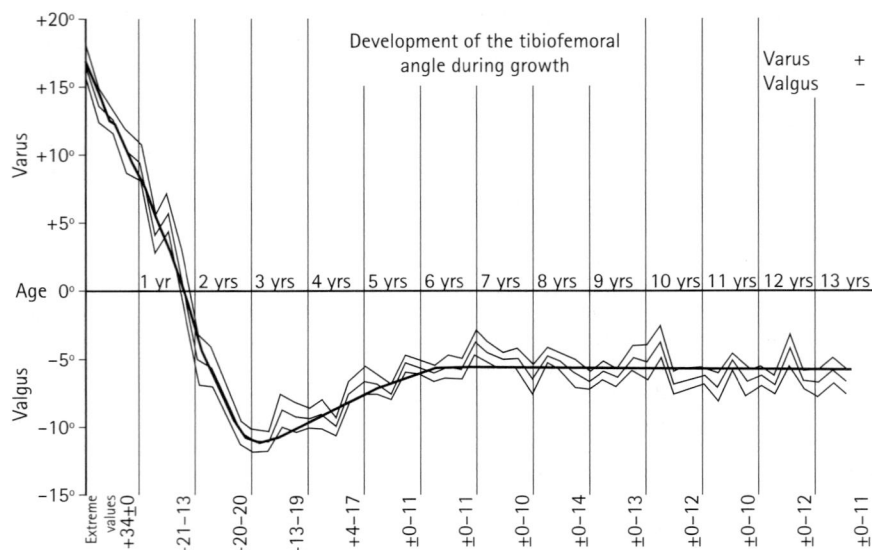

Fig. 29.43   The tibiofemoral angle curing growth. (Adapted from Salenius and Vankka 1975[98].)

the child standing, if possible, and both patellae pointing forwards. The tibiofemoral angle can then be measured with a goniometer. This assessment is relatively crude but measurements more than two standard deviations from normal suggest further evaluation, to exclude a pathological explanation.

The principal pathological explanations for bow legs are metabolic bone disease, Blount disease and skeletal dysplasias. Radiographs are not usually helpful under 18 months of age but should be taken if there is a suspicion of pathology. Typical feature of rickets with widening and irregularity of the growth plate and trumpet-like flaring of the metaphysis (Fig. 29.27), or features of Blount disease or some skeletal dysplasia may be seen.

Infantile Blount disease can be difficult to distinguish from physiological bowing but is suggested by bowing that is severe or persisting beyond 24 months. Blount disease is the result of an idiopathic growth disturbance in the posteromedial part of the proximal tibial physis and is most common in people of Scandinavian or West Indian descent. Affected infants are often heavy and walk early and it is thought that increased pressure across the growth plate may play a role in the etiology. Differentiation from physiological bowing can be difficult and it is possible that the two conditions are part of a continuum. Radiographs can be helpful. In physiological bowing there is varus of the whole leg, both the distal femur and the proximal tibia, whereas in Blount disease bowing is principally at the proximal tibia, often with a sharp angulation in the medial metaphyseal region (Fig. 29.44). Early brace treatment may be effective in children under 3 years old.[99] A knee ankle foot orthosis (KAFO) is used to keep the knee in extension for 23 out of 24 hours a day in order to unload the posteromedial physis, but if the deformity continues to progress tibial osteotomy may become necessary.

Knock knees (genu valgum)
As can be seen from Figure 29.43 genu valgum of around 8–10° is normal in 3- to 5-year-old children and gradually returns to adult values of 5–7° by around 7 years of age. Normal children, by definition, fall within two standard deviations of the mean and the normal distribution of the tibiofemoral angle is wide. Treatment of physiological knock knees is not necessary. The underlying cause of pathological cases should be addressed before attending to the limb deformity. Brace treatment is of little benefit and treatment often involves osteotomy or asymmetrical growth plate epiphyseodesis or stapling.

In-toe and out-toe gait
We walk along a straight, imaginary line of progression, which stretches out before us. When the foot is placed on the ground, the line

of its long axis forms an angle with the line of progression and this angle is termed the foot progression angle. In-toe gait (internal foot progression angle) where the toes of each foot point inwards is a common cause for parental concern. Most patients who present with rotational problems in the lower limbs are normal. Occasionally rotational

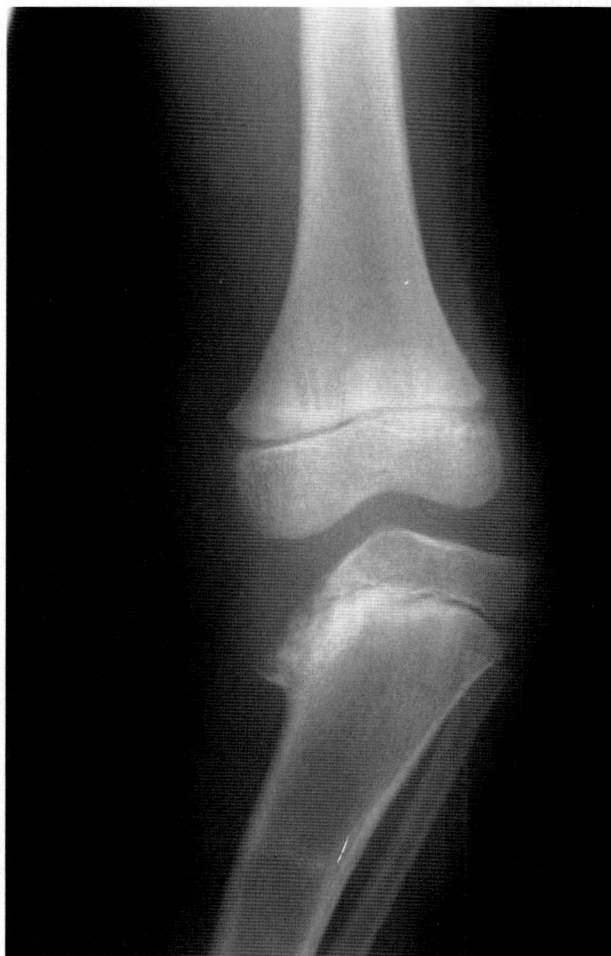

Fig. 29.44   Blount disease.

problems may be pathological, representing part of a bone, joint or neuromuscular disorder.

The foot is at the end of the limb and an in-toe or out-toe gait may result from a twist or torsion in the femur, the tibia or the foot itself. Initial assessment of these children involves determining the site and magnitude of the torsion, by examining the rotational profile of the limb. The child should stand and walk so that the foot progression angle can be estimated. This is very variable in early childhood: most children under 4 years have a degree of in-toeing while most adults have a degree of out-toeing.

The rotational profile of the lower limbs should be evaluated (Fig. 29.45). The hips should be examined with the child prone on the examination couch and the knees flexed to 90°. External and internal rotation at the hip can then be assessed (Fig. 29.45AB,). This gives some indication of torsion within the femur but is also influenced by soft tissue tension about the hip capsule. With the child still prone and the knees flexed to 90° the limb can be viewed from above. The thigh–foot angle is the angle between the long axis of the thigh and the long axis of the foot (Fig. 29.45C). It gives some indication of torsion within the tibia. Care should be taken to encourage the patient to relax the foot for the examination while the examiner gently holds the foot in slight dorsiflexion. Soft tissue laxity about the knee can allow the foot to be twisted into internal or external rotation giving a spurious assessment. The sole of the foot should now be viewed from above. A line bisecting the center of the calcaneum should pass through the second toe or the second web interspace. This assessment helps to determine if deformity in the foot is contributing to the gait pattern.

Femoral torsion

The long axis of the femoral neck is aligned slightly forwards of the transcondylar axis (or coronal plane) of the femur. The angle between the femoral neck axis and the transcondylar axis is the angle of femoral anteversion. At birth, femoral anteversion measures about 40° gradually falling to adult values of 10–15° during development. Infants have the greatest degree of anteversion but do not normally demonstrate an excessive range of internal rotation at the hips because of soft tissue external rotation contracture which is normal in this age range. Femoral anteversion is the most common explanation for in-toe gait in children over 3–4 years and persistence of immature degrees of femoral anteversion is a frequent cause of in-toe gait in early adolescence particularly in girls. Patients present with various complaints especially awkwardness of gait and tripping. They sit in the 'W' position both because they can and because they find it comfortable.

Treatment is rarely necessary since most cases resolve during development. If the problem persists into late adolescence and is sufficiently severe, derotation osteotomy is effective. Sometimes especially in adolescent girls external tibial torsion coexists: this compensates for the internal femoral torsion so that the feet point forwards but the patellae are left 'squinting' medially toward each other (Fig. 29.46). If treatment proves to be necessary in such patients, it will involve bilateral femoral and tibial osteotomies. This is a considerable undertaking, not to be approached lightly.

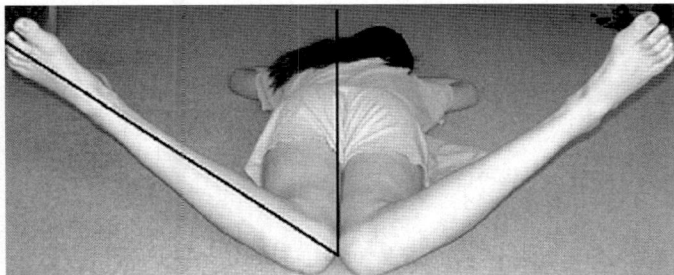

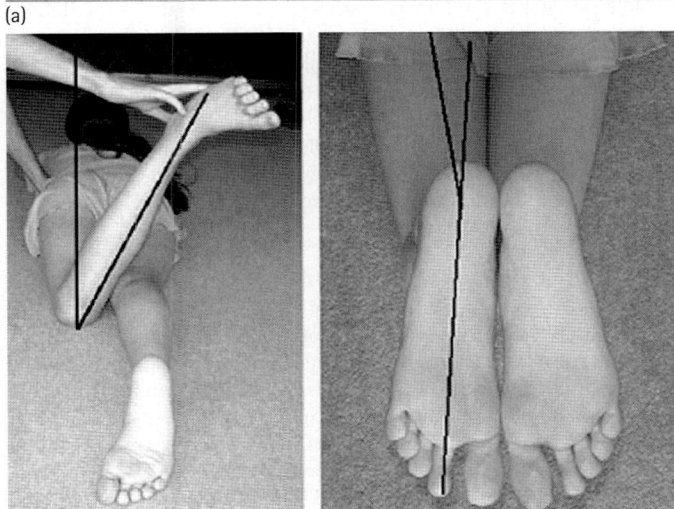

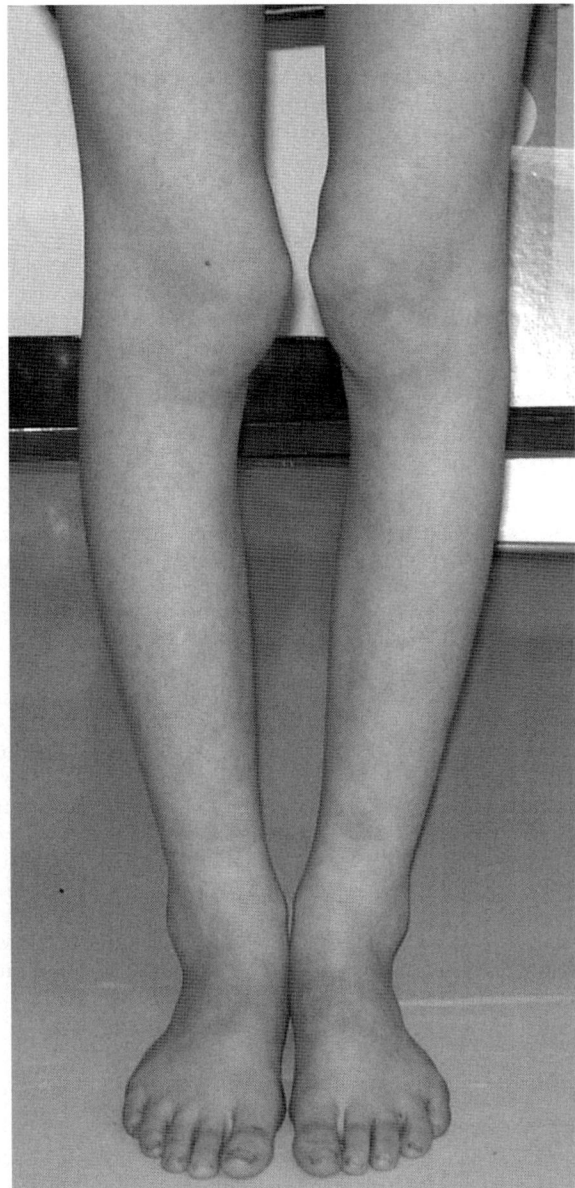

Fig. 29.45 Assessment of the rotational profile of the lower limbs.

Fig. 29.46 'Squinting' patellae.

Tibial torsion

Internal tibial torsion is a common explanation for in-toe gait in the toddler age range. The degree of tibial torsion is assessed by measuring the thigh–foot axis, as already described, or by measuring the angle between the coronal (or transcondylar) plane and a line joining the tips of medial and lateral malleoli at the ankle. In the term infant at birth, the medial malleolus usually lies behind the lateral malleolus. By walking age the malleoli are level on the coronal plane and by the time walking is well established the lateral malleolus is behind the medial. In other words the infant normally has relative internal tibial torsion, which gradually rotates externally with growth. Internal tibial torsion often coexists with bowing of the legs in infants and young children and may exaggerate the appearance of the bowing. No treatment is necessary or effective for physiological internal tibial torsion.

Excessive external tibial torsion is less common than internal tibial torsion and more likely to persist into adolescence.[100] Once again the only effective treatment for tibial rotational abnormalities is tibial osteotomy. Serious thought needs to be given before offering operative solutions as neither internal nor external tibial torsion have been shown to be risk factors for later degenerative change.

Metatarsus varus

Metatarsus varus or metatarsus adductus is medial deviation of the forefoot on the hindfoot. The subtalar and ankle joints are normal and the hindfoot is in neutral or slight valgus. This distinguishes the condition from clubfoot deformity where the hindfoot is stiff and in varus and equinus. The foot has a concave medial border which can be the cause of, or at least contribute to, an in-toe gait appearance.

The severity of the condition can be classified using the heel bisector as previously described. The condition is described as flexible if the forefoot can be passively overcorrected, partly flexible if it can be passively corrected to the midline and rigid if it cannot be returned to the midline. The natural history is of progressive spontaneous resolution. Consideration can be given to treatment if the deformity is rigid or partly flexible and serial casting has been shown to be effective.[101]

COMMON ORTHOPEDIC EXPLANATIONS FOR MUSCULOSKELETAL PAIN IN CHILDHOOD

Growing pains

Musculoskeletal pain in children is relatively common and usually benign. In evaluating children it is wise to remember that infection and neoplasia are amongst the myriad of potential explanations. Both commonly present in childhood as localized bone pain and must be given due consideration in the differential diagnosis.

The syndrome of benign 'growing pains' is common; usually presenting in children between 4 and 8 years. It can occur in the upper but more frequently the lower limbs. The typical history is of a child who, after a busy day, complains of aching pains in the limbs, frequently in the thighs, shins or around the front or the back of the knees. The pain can be severe, even disturbing sleep, and usually settles after a variable period of parental rubbing of the affected limbs. The next day the child is fine and there are no sequelae. The natural history is of resolution after 18–24 months but the course may be more protracted. The cause remains unknown but growth seems to have little to do with the symptoms. The likely explanation is muscle fatigue or cramp.[102] Treatment is primarily reassurance but can include stretching exercises if muscle fatigue is thought to be a factor.

Neck and back pain

See later section, page 1437.

The painful or irritable hip

The term irritable hip is not a diagnosis but the clinical presentation of hip pathology. The patient may present with symptoms ranging from severe pain with complete inability to weightbear to modest pain, localized to the hip or referred to the knee, with virtually no limp.

The most sensitive sign of hip joint pathology is subtle limitation of internal rotation, which should be carefully sought. Clinical examination of the hip is equally important when patients present with localized hip pain or with isolated thigh or knee pain. The potential for knee pain to be referred from the hip is frequently overlooked.

The commonest cause for an irritable hip in childhood is transient synovitis, but the differential is wide and includes infections, acute and chronic, including septic arthritis and osteomyelitis, Perthes disease and slipped capital femoral epiphysis (SCFE). Less common causes include the inflammatory arthritides such as juvenile idiopathic arthritis, idiopathic chondrolysis and neoplasms. Transient synovitis, Perthes disease, SCFE and chondrolysis will be discussed here. The other disorders are discussed elsewhere in the chapter.

Transient synovitis

This is the commonest cause for hip pain in children: it is estimated that about 3% of children will have at least one episode.[103] It is twice as common in boys and usually occurs between 3 and 8 years with a peak incidence around 6.[104] It is characterized by a transient period of hip joint irritability in a systemically well child. The etiology is unknown but hypotheses include trauma, allergic hypersensitivity or infection. In up to 70% of cases there is a history of either current or antecedent nonspecific upper respiratory infection, and the most widely accepted explanation is that the condition represents a transient reactive synovitis.

Hip joint ultrasonography is the most useful investigation, confirming that the hip joint is the source of complaint. The findings are nonspecific and do not necessarily exclude other causes of an irritable hip. Radiographs and laboratory tests are normal or nonspecific. Transient synovitis is essentially a diagnosis of exclusion and investigations are aimed at excluding other diagnoses. Pyogenic septic arthritis is the most important alternative diagnosis. The child with septic arthritis is usually systemically unwell with a high fever, a high white cell count and ESR and fails to improve with rest. The patient with an effusion due to transient synovitis may have a modest fever and mildly elevated ESR and improves with rest.

Treatment is symptomatic. Skin traction has been popular but is not now recommended because positioning the hip in extension increases intracapsular pressure and pain. If traction is to be used, the leg should be supported with the hip flexed. In practice it is more practical to let the child rest the limb in a position of flexion and external rotation for comfort, provided symptoms settle promptly.

Most cases resolve progressively over 5–10 days. Deterioration is more characteristic of septic arthritis and persistence of moderate or modest symptoms should raise suspicion of alternative explanations such as Perthes disease. Isotope bone scanning can be helpful in these circumstances to distinguish Perthes disease, characterized by reduced uptake, from transient synovitis and other inflammatory conditions where increased uptake is usual. A relationship between transient synovitis and the development of Perthes disease has been suggested but no direct causal correlation has ever been shown. It is safest to conclude that the only relationship is a similar mode of presentation, with an irritable hip.

Perthes disease (Legg–Calvé–Perthes disease)

Perthes disease is avascular necrosis of the femoral head epiphysis due to a disturbance of the epiphyseal blood supply. The disturbance can affect part or all of the femoral epiphysis and the extent of involvement is related to the ultimate prognosis. Despite enthusiasm for the notion that thrombophilia or hypofibrinolysis may be involved in the pathogenesis, more recent work has proved less than encouraging and Perthes disease remains a condition of unknown etiology.[105] Eighty percent of cases occur between the ages of 4 and 9 years and the condition is five times more common in boys.[106] Children present insidiously with an irritable hip syndrome which persists and may deteriorate.

Initial radiographs may be normal. Radionuclide bone scanning shows decreased uptake, distinguishing Perthes from other causes of an irritable hip. MRI can reveal epiphyseal necrosis earlier than plain radiographs as well as defining the extent of involvement. Radiographs will ultimately reveal progressive changes in the hip joint and the femoral epiphysis.

The pathogenesis is reflected in sequential radiological stages. In the initial phase there is increased epiphyseal density which gives way to the fragmentation phase (Fig. 29.47a), sometimes heralded by the appearance of a subchondral radiolucent line or 'crescent sign' (Fig. 29.47b) and eventually characterized by the appearance of lucent areas fragmenting the epiphysis. The reparative or reossification phase supervenes and normal bone density slowly substitutes areas of previous lucency. The process continues from the periphery of the epiphysis to the center until the healed phase is reached. The bony epiphysis once again has the consistency of normal bone but may have become deformed to a greater or lesser degree.

Although Perthes disease can be bilateral in 10–12% of cases[107] radiographs characteristically reveal different stages of disease in the two sides. A similar appearance in both hips is very unusual and should raise suspicion of skeletal dysplasias such as multiple epiphyseal dysplasia (MED) (Fig. 29.25) and spondyloepiphyseal dysplasia (SED).

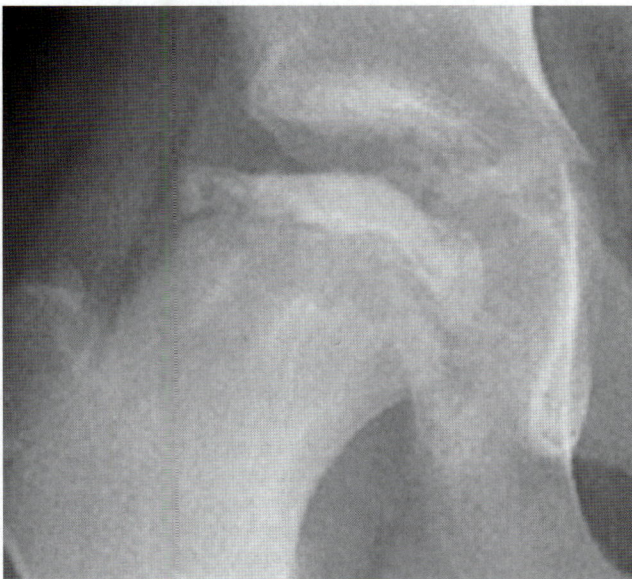

(a)

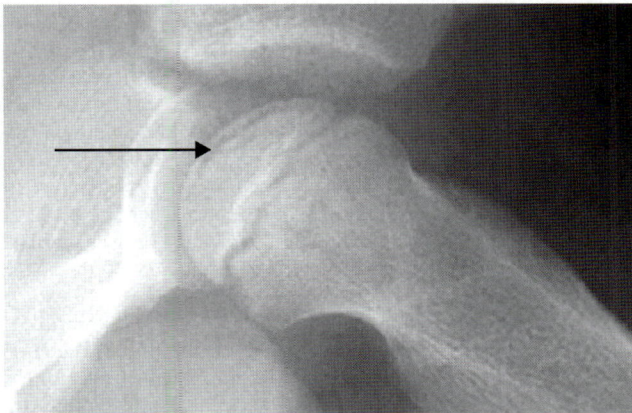

(b)

Fig. 29.47   Perthes disease: (a) stage of fragmentation and collapse; (b) crescent sign.

The progression from the initial phase to the end of the healed phase can take several years. During this time, especially during the fragmentation phase, the cartilaginous femoral head loses the support of its internal bony skeleton and becomes plastic, or able to change shape. The shape the femoral head becomes is determined by the extent of loss of support (or epiphyseal necrosis), and by the mechanical environment in which the plastic femoral head finds itself. The long term prognosis depends on how spherical the femoral head remains and how congruently it fits the acetabulum.

In early Perthes disease, when the femoral head remains plastic, the principle of treatment is the principle of 'containment'. The patient's own acetabulum is used as a template or mold to keep the femoral head spherical, or at least congruent. This can be achieved by the patient themselves if a good range of movement, especially abduction, is maintained. Alternatively, 'containment' treatment with an abduction brace or femoral or pelvic osteotomy is used to position the plastic part of the femoral epiphysis within the acetabulum. Clinical examination is a crucial part of patient assessment. If the patient maintains a good range of movement the soft femoral epiphysis will be constantly moving in and out of the acetabulum during day-to-day activity and will remain congruent. If, on the other hand, range of movement is limited especially abduction, the femoral epiphysis will not be contained within the acetabulum and weightbearing forces will lead to flattening of the epiphysis and incongruity. Loss of range of movement is therefore a sinister clinical sign.

Radiological evaluation is easiest using the Herring grading system. Herring divided the epiphysis as seen on an anteroposterior (AP) radiograph into medial, middle and lateral columns. Only the lateral column is evaluated. The hip is classified as Herring A if there is no necrosis involving the lateral column, Herring B if the lateral column is involved but retains more than 50% of its original height and Herring C if it has lost more than 50% of its original height. The prognosis deteriorates from grades A to C. In concept if the lateral column is intact, the remainder of the femoral head is protected from weightbearing forces, but if the lateral column fails the whole femoral head is exposed to forces from above and will flatten.

Patients under 5 years at the onset of Perthes disease have a good prognosis. In this age group patients frequently maintain an excellent range of movement, even in the face of extensive epiphyseal necrosis on radiographs, and they essentially contain their own femoral head. They rarely require intervention, but should be constantly reviewed to ensure that a good range of movement is maintained. The good prognosis in this age range is also a reflection of the immature acetabulum with much growth remaining. If the femoral head does become aspherical as a result of the Perthes process, the acetabulum will grow to match.

In older children the acetabulum has less growth remaining, is less able to accommodate an aspherical femoral head and incongruity becomes progressively more likely. Clinical signs reflect the radiological extent of epiphyseal necrosis. If there is clinical loss of range of movement in this age group radiographs will usually reveal Herring grade C or B lateral column involvement. These findings usually dictate 'containment' treatment. In the past a wide range of abduction braces have been used but more recent reports question their efficacy.[108] There is a growing inclination to offer surgical containment because of emerging evidence of improved outcome. Surgical containment is usually in the form of a varus femoral or pelvic osteotomy. It is common practice for surgical candidates to undergo an examination of the joint under anesthetic and hip joint arthrography, to ensure that the epiphysis is containable before embarking on surgical treatment. Patients should be followed to maturity, mainly to ensure a significant leg length discrepancy does not develop. A modest leg length discrepancy is common; one requiring treatment unusual.

Once the Perthes disease is over and the femoral epiphysis healed, it is no longer plastic. Hip pain can result if incongruity has developed. The objective of treatment now is restoration of functional congruity. Once again assessment commonly includes examination under anesthesia and arthrography. The principal problem encountered in a deformed incongruent joint is 'hinge abduction'. Because the femoral head is too big to enter the acetabulum during abduction, it levers itself out of the joint with the 'hinge' at the lateral lip of the acetabulum. This limits the patient's functional abduction. The problem can sometimes be helped with a valgus femoral osteotomy.[109]

Slipped capital femoral epiphysis (SCFE)

Slipped capital femoral epiphysis (SCFE) or slipped upper femoral epiphysis (SUFE) is the commonest hip disorder in the adolescent age range and is frequently the subject of medical negligence claims because of delay in diagnosis with potentially disabling consequences for the patient.

The capital femoral epiphysis is fixed to the femoral metaphysis by the proximal femoral growth plate or physis. If the cartilaginous physis is subjected to shear forces it can fail, usually through its hypertrophic zone, and the femoral epiphysis will then 'slip' posteriorly on the metaphysis, either progressively or suddenly. A SCFE occurs when the load applied exceeds the resistance of the physis to slip. This can occur because the load is too great, because the physis is vulnerable or, most often, because of a combination of these factors.

Hormonal events during normal adolescence lead to relative widening of the physis and its hypertrophic zone during periods of rapid growth. The threshold at which the widened physis fails is lower than a normal physis, making the adolescent vulnerable to SCFE. Any condition that widens the growth plate either because of increased growth or decreased ossification predisposes to SCFE and it has been associated with a variety of endocrine abnormalities including hypothyroidism, panhypopituitarism and hypogonadal conditions and treatment of short stature with growth hormone.[110,111] If a vulnerable physis is subjected to increased load, such as might occur in obesity, the risk of SCFE is further increased. Sixty-three percent of affected individuals are over the 90th percentile for weight.

The incidence of SCFE is around 2:100 000 and its peak presentation is 9–15 years in girls and 10–16 years in boys, i.e. during the adolescent growth spurt. The condition is more common in boys than girls in a ratio of 1.5:1.0. If a case presents in a child outside the expected age range or in a child with an unusual body habitus, more serious consideration should be given to an underlying endocrine or metabolic abnormality.

Careful radiographic interpretation is important for early detection. The AP radiograph is insufficiently sensitive and where a slip is considered possible a lateral radiograph should be obtained. Signs on the AP radiograph include subtle blurring and irregularity of the physis and slight loss of epiphyseal height. When the epiphysis slips a little further it is more obvious. A line, Klein's line,[112] drawn along the superior aspect of the femoral neck should cut off the lateral edge of the epiphysis but does not if the epiphysis has slipped. Minor degrees of slip are more easily seen on the lateral radiograph because the epiphysis primarily slips posteriorly (Fig. 29.48).

SCFE is classified into unstable (acute) or stable (chronic).[113] A third category of a stable slip suddenly becoming unstable also exists (acute on chronic). The distinction between the different types of slip is important because the clinical presentation and the prognosis differ significantly.

In the stable slip the femoral epiphysis gradually and progressively slips posteriorly on the femoral metaphysis. The patient may have a limp but can weightbear and the presentation is essentially that of an irritable hip. Referred knee pain may be the patient's only complaint and a futile search for a local explanation at the knee is a common cause for delayed diagnosis. Pain, discomfort or reluctance when the hip is internally rotated is a subtle indicator of hip pathology and should prompt further radiographic evaluation. Stable slips rarely if ever suffer the serious complication of avascular necrosis but can lead to significant proximal femoral deformity, limited range of movement, limb length discrepancy and premature degenerative change. If a stable slip remains undetected an unstable slip may supervene and seriously affect the

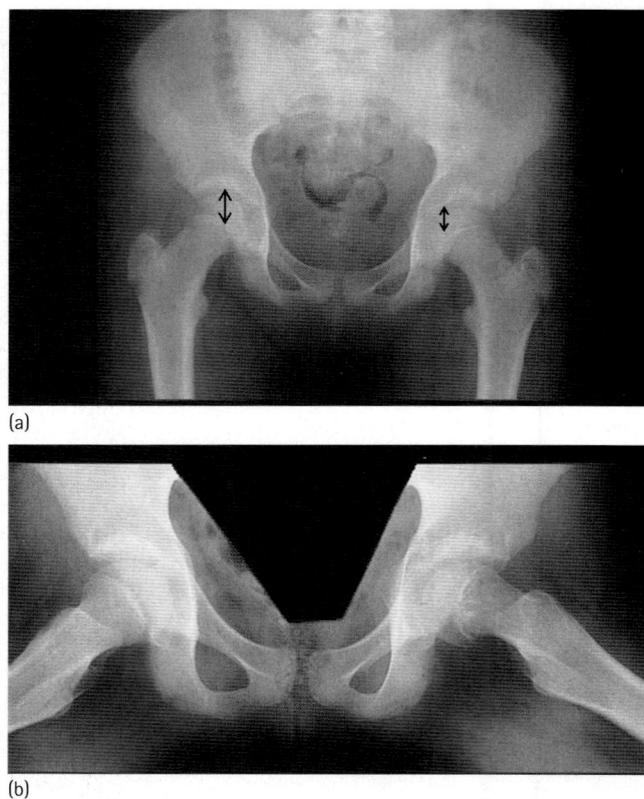

(a)

(b)

Fig. 29.48   Slipped capital femoral epiphysis: (a) AP radiograph; (b) frog lateral radiograph. Note the relative insensitivity of the AP radiograph – arrows demonstrate subtle difference in epiphyseal height.

prognosis. The keystone of management is early detection followed in most cases by fixation in situ with a cannulated screw. The principle of this treatment is to promote fusion of the growth plate to prevent further slippage and deformity. Osteotomies to correct deformity are controversial and are usually, though not always, deferred for 18–24 months to allow for remodeling. Persistent difficulties are unlikely to improve spontaneously thereafter.

There is usually no difficulty in diagnosing the unstable slip which occurs when the femoral epiphysis suddenly slips posteriorly off the femoral metaphysis. The patient presents in severe pain, unable to weightbear and the leg is held in external rotation. The rate of avascular necrosis in the unstable slip is around 47%.[113] The blood supply to the femoral epiphysis is vulnerable in the immature hip and the vessels passing along the femoral neck to the epiphysis are suddenly torn or stretched in the unstable slip. The avascular necrosis that follows may not be seen radiographically for some months, but if it occurs it is a devastating complication with no satisfactory treatment. The management of the unstable slip once again involves fixing the slipped epiphysis in situ to promote physeal fusion and to prevent further slippage and damage to the epiphyseal blood supply. No attempt is made to deliberately correct the unstable slip, for fear of further damage to the epiphyseal blood supply, but inadvertent reduction does take place during positioning for fixation in unstable slips and can be accepted. Once again the role of femoral osteotomies in the management of unstable slips is controversial.

The incidence of symptomatic bilateral SCFE averages around 25%, most contralateral slips occurring within 12 months of the original slip. Prophylactic fixation of the opposite side should be considered, especially in the child with an underlying endocrine or metabolic abnormality or some years of growth remaining. If the contralateral hip is not fixed the patient should be warned to return urgently at the first sign of hip or knee symptoms.

Idiopathic chondrolysis

This uncommon condition is characterized by the rapid and progressive destruction of articular cartilage from both sides of the affected joint with subsequent pain and stiffness. It is five times more common in girls than boys and is typically a condition of adolescents. Radiographs reveal narrowing of the affected joint space. Chondrolysis of the hip is of unknown etiology in most cases but has been reported in association with SCFE,[114] trauma, prolonged immobilization and severe burns of the extremities.[115]

The natural history of chondrolysis includes an acute stage lasting 6–18 months with pain, inflammation, loss of range of motion and destruction of articular cartilage. Eventually the chronic stage emerges and can last from 3 to 5 years. During the chronic stage the hip may continue to deteriorate. Ultimately the hip may become pain free but stiff in a poor position, or pain free with partial or rarely complete return of motion and some restoration of the joint space.

The principles of treatment include control of any inflammation with therapeutic doses of NSAIDs and maintenance of motion with an aggressive physiotherapy program. Surgical release of persistent tendon contractures may be necessary in some patients and there are some encouraging results reported following aggressive subtotal capsulotomy and tendon release.[116] Some patients may ultimately come to hip arthrodesis in a functional position for the relief of pain.

Knee pain

Complaints of knee swelling, mechanical symptoms (giving way and locking) or pain are common in both children and adolescents. A knee joint effusion indicates intra-articular pathology and mechanical symptoms often indicate joint instability, loose bodies or meniscal pathology. Pain is either localized or diffuse. There are numerous explanations for localized knee pain in children including a variety of overuse and sport-related problems (see later section, p. 1440). Referred knee pain is common and clinical examination of the hip is important in any patient presenting with unexplained knee pain.

Anterior knee pain (patellofemoral pain syndrome and chondromalacia)

Anterior knee pain is a descriptive term for diffuse pain at the front of the knee. It is a very common complaint in the adolescent age range, typically affecting girls. The complaint is of a diffuse ache around the front of the knee at the patellofemoral joint (patellofemoral pain syndrome), which is worse after activity, after climbing up or down stairs and after sitting for prolonged periods with the knees in a flexed position. Chondromalacia is a term often used to describe this syndrome, but is really a pathological description of cartilage softening and degeneration, rarely present in young patients complaining of anterior knee pain.

The presentation of patellofemoral pain syndrome is fairly typical but evaluation should include reasonable steps to exclude other potential sources of pain. Lateral maltracking or subluxation of the patella is highly correlated with patellofemoral pain syndrome. Because the line of the quadriceps from the anterior superior spine to the tibial tuberosity passes to the lateral side of the knee joint, there is an inherent tendency for the patella to track to the lateral side of the trochlear sulcus in the anterior femur of the patellofemoral articulation. There are mechanisms to prevent such lateral maltracking, but these are sometimes inadequate. Pain at the lateral part of the articular surface of the patella can be a subtle consequence as can more overt subluxation or dislocation. Rotational malalignment also contributes to the problem and many patients will be found to have persistent femoral anteversion in association with compensatory external tibial torsion so that the feet point forwards but the patellae squint medially, the so-called 'miserable malalignment'.[117]

The natural history of anterior knee pain is of slow resolution and most cases respond to non-operative treatment.[118] For many, reassurance is all that is necessary. Physiotherapy is helpful and activity modification, especially the avoidance of provoking sports, may be necessary.

If there is evidence of maltracking some patients find a knee brace with a patella cut out, to hold the patella medially, is useful. An experienced physiotherapist can help with medial taping of the patella in combination with a program to stretch and strengthen quadriceps muscles. If symptoms are persistent and very troublesome in a patient with convincing maltracking, surgical intervention in the form of a lateral retinacular release can be successful in 75% of cases.[119]

Discoid lateral meniscus

This is a congenital abnormality of the meniscus, which is the shape of a disc rather than the usual crescent. The discoid shape can be either complete, covering the whole lateral tibial plateau, or partial forming a rather wider crescent than usual. Children present with mechanical symptoms of giving way, locking or snapping similar to patients with a meniscal tear. Radiographs of the knee sometimes reveal a lateral joint space that is wider than usual, but MRI is the investigation of choice to demonstrate the extensive and thickened meniscus. Asymptomatic discoid menisci found incidentally should be left undisturbed. Symptomatic menisci can be successfully trimmed arthroscopically into a more normal crescent shape.[120]

Popliteal cyst

This common condition presents as a fluctuant transilluminable swelling in the popliteal fossa. The usual reason for referral is parental concern. The cysts are asymptomatic although they may ache with activity and fluctuate in size. They are typically found subcutaneously along the medial side of the popliteal fossa and are simple synovial lined cysts arising from the semimembranosus sheath.

Plain X-rays of the knee are normal and the cyst is best confirmed by ultrasound scan examination. No treatment is required; spontaneous resolution over months or years is usual.

Occasionally, usually in association with an inflammatory arthropathy, popliteal cysts may rupture presenting with calf pain and swelling, the ruptured 'Baker cyst'. Ultrasound and MRI (Fig. 29.49) will distinguish this from other rare causes of calf pain and swelling in children.

Osteochondritis dissecans (OCD)

Osteochondritis dissecans most commonly involves the knee joint, but can affect the articular surface of any joint. For reasons that remain unclear an area of subchondral bone undergoes avascular necrosis. Etiological theories include trauma, ischemia, a genetic predisposition or a combination of these. Symptoms are usually vague and develop insidiously over several months. The overlying cartilage is initially intact but may subsequently develop degenerative change and break into a flap or a loose body causing the onset of mechanical joint symptoms, including locking, snapping or giving way. The most commonly affected part of the knee is the lateral part of the medial femoral condyle, although it can affect any part of the articular surface including the patella.

Radiographs usually reveal a lucent fragmented area in the subchondral bone (Fig. 29.50). In addition to the routine anteroposterior and lateral views of the knee, a tunnel view is useful because it visualizes the intercondylar notch region and the lateral part of the medial femoral condyle where the condition is most common. Magnetic resonance imaging is the investigation of choice and not only delineates the bony abnormality but also provides some indication of whether the overlying cartilage is intact.

The prognosis of the condition is relatively good in young patients when the growth plate remains open but in adults and adolescents with a closed growth plate the prognosis is more guarded. Treatment should include activity modification to limit aggressive sporting activity, which may cause intact overlying cartilage to become loose. If there are no mechanical symptoms and MRI suggests that the overlying cartilage is intact, activity modification to limit symptoms is recommended until resolution which may take months or even years. If there are mechanical symptoms or the MRI suggests the possibility of a breach or flap of the overlying cartilage, arthroscopic examination is recommended. Large flaps, especially on the weightbearing

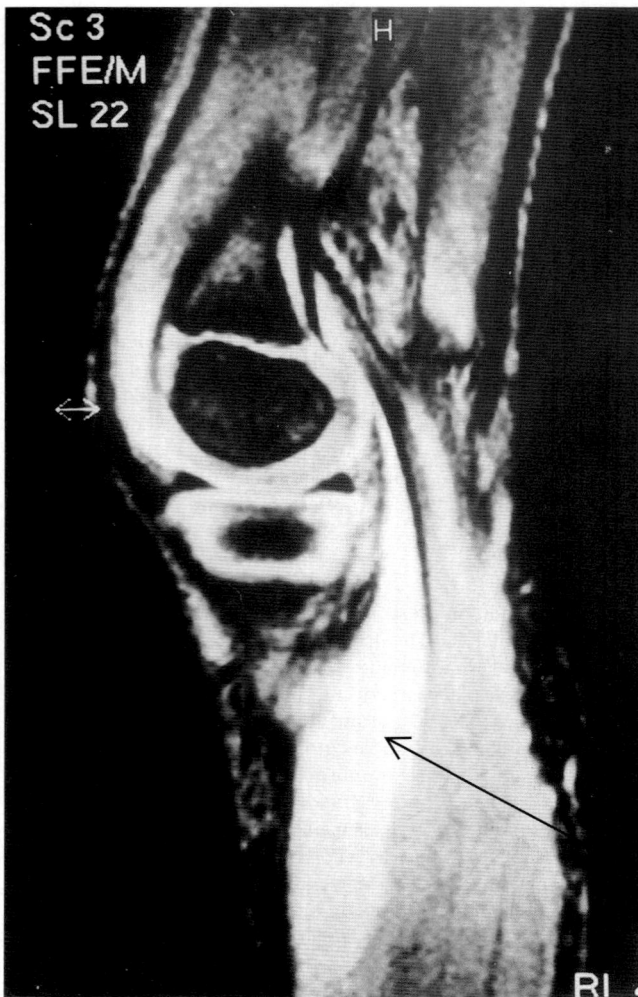

Fig. 29.49 MRI showing ruptured Baker cyst – arrow indicates inflammatory fluid collection extending from the popliteal fossa into the calf.

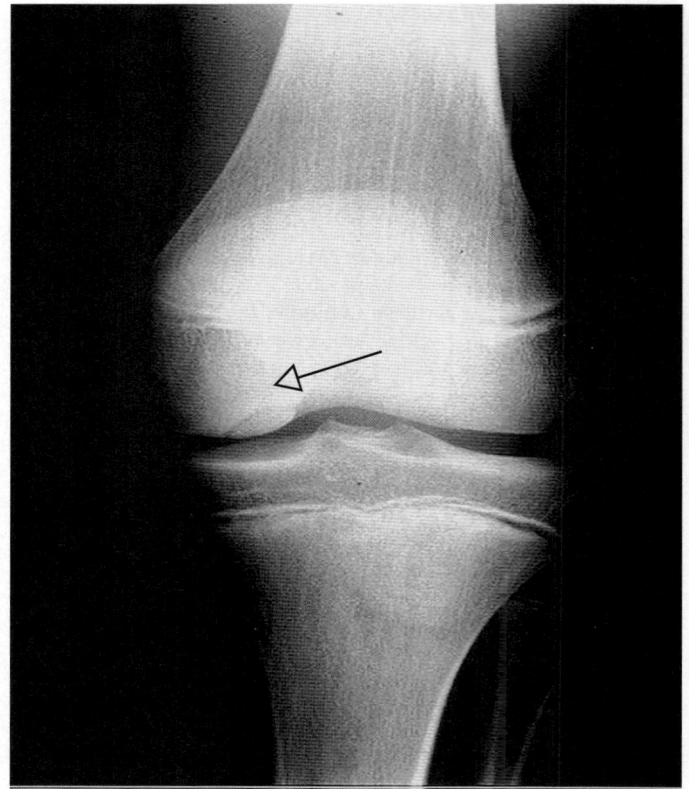

Fig. 29.50 Osteochondritis dissecans of the knee.

surface, should be fixed into position, although loose flaps are usually trimmed flush with the articular surface to prevent further mechanical symptoms and the base of the defect drilled to promote healing with fibrocartilage.

Kohler disease

Kohler disease or osteochondritis of the navicular presents in children around the age of 6 years. The radiographic appearance is that of fragmentation and flattening of the navicular (Fig. 29.51) but this radiological appearance may be a normal variant. The appearance is only considered pathological if there are associated symptoms of localized pain over the bone. Treatment of Kohler disease is symptomatic. There is no evidence of any long term sequelae.

Freiberg disease

Freiberg disease or osteochondritis of the metatarsal head is most common in the second metatarsal. It usually presents in adolescence with localized pain. Radiographs reveal flattening and fragmentation of the metatarsal head. It is believed to be an avascular necrosis developing in a stress fracture and is associated with local trauma as might occur in sport or in dancing. The condition is much commoner in girls. Treatment is initially conservative but persistent local pain and limited dorsiflexion of the metatarsophalangeal joint may necessitate surgical debridement.

Tarsal coalition

Tarsal coalition is an abnormal cartilaginous, fibrous or bony connection between two or more tarsal bones. It is surprisingly common with a reported incidence of 2%. The condition is inherited as an autosomal dominant trait and the incidence in first-degree relatives is 39%.[121] Fortunately the majority of coalitions are asymptomatic. If symptoms develop they usually present during the late juvenile or early adolescent years when the coalition, initially cartilaginous, begins to ossify. The condition is characterized by a painful, rigid valgus foot and peroneal muscle spasm which may be continuous or intermittent, exacerbated by activity and relieved by rest.[122]

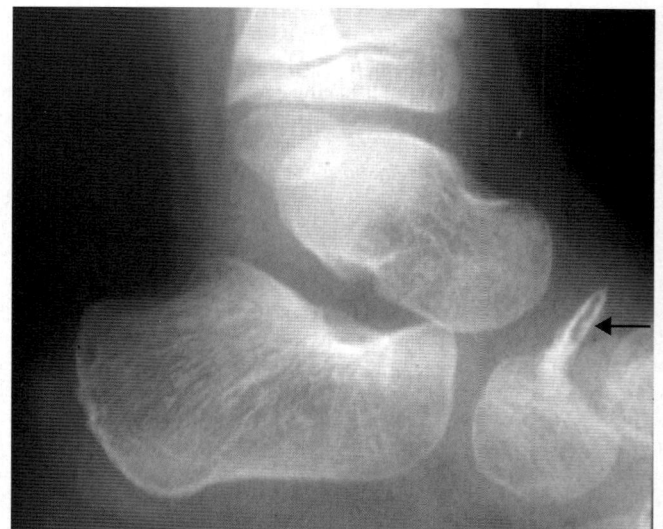

Fig. 29.51 Kohler disease.

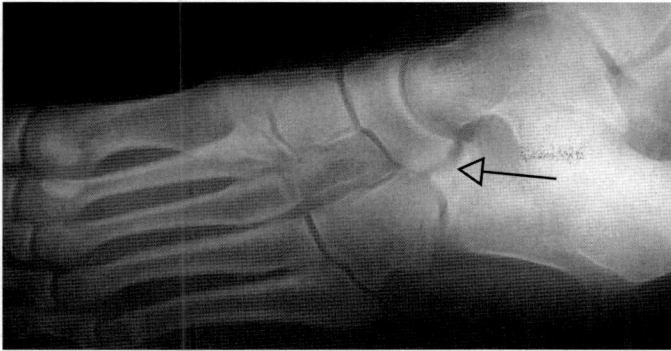

Fig. 29.52   Calcaneonavicular coalition.

The two commonest sites of coalition are between the calcaneus and the navicular (Fig. 29.52) and between the calcaneus and the talus, at the middle facet of the subtalar joint. Sixty percent of calcaneonavicular and 50% of talocalcaneal coalitions are bilateral.[123] Multiple coalitions can rarely coexist in the same foot. Calcaneonavicular coalitions begin to ossify between 8 and 12 years and talocalcaneal coalitions between 12 and 16 years.

Calcaneonavicular coalitions are most easily demonstrated radiographically with a 45° oblique radiograph of the foot. CT best demonstrates talocalcaneal coalitions. Secondary radiographic findings such as talar beaking should suggest the possibility of a tarsal coalition. Treatment is initially symptomatic with analgesia and immobilization. If conservative treatment fails, surgical resection of the abnormal coalition and interposition of fat or muscle to prevent recoalition has been shown to be successful in both calcaneonavicular[124] and talocalcaneal [125] coalitions. Generally, results are less satisfactory after talocalcaneal coalition resection and ultimately some patients come to a triple arthrodesis of the subtalar joint.

Adolescent hallus valgus

Hallux valgus or 'bunions' in adolescents is usually familial rather than the result of poor footwear. It is girls that usually present because of the appearance rather than because of functional problems or pain. There is often an associated bunionette of the fifth toe and patients often have a characteristically broad forefoot with varus of the first metatarsal (metatarsus primus varus). Surgery is best deferred until skeletal maturity is reached. Surgical treatment gives good results for symptomatic feet with a painful bunion but caution should be exercised in the pain free patient who may be disappointed if surgery leaves a better looking but painful foot.

VASCULITIS

Vasculitis is characterized by inflammation and necrosis of vessel walls. This may occur as a primary disorder, where the etiology remains unknown, or as a secondary phenomenon. Within the group of disorders known as the systemic vasculitides there are a variety of different conditions. Categorization of these conditions in childhood has been problematic and it is only recently that a specific pediatric classification system has been proposed[126] (Table 29.14). This is essentially a modification of the Chapel Hill criteria used in adults which classifies the systemic vasculitides based on vessel size.[127] Specific criteria are included for the diagnosis of the main childhood vasculitides.

There remain many children with a systemic vasculitis in whom categorization is difficult due to overlapping clinical features. The importance of attempting to classify these conditions relates to their variable prognosis. While some are self-limiting, others require aggressive immunosuppressive therapy to minimize morbidity and even mortality.

Table 29.14   Classification of childhood vasculitis. (Adapted from Ozen et al 2006[126])

I   **Large vessels**
    Takayasu arteritis

II **Medium sized vessels**
    Childhood polyarteritis nodosa
    Cutaneous polyarteritis
    Kawasaki disease

III **Small vessels**
    a. Granulomatous:
       Wegener granulomatosus
       Churg–Strauss syndrome
    b. Nongranulomatous:
       Microscopic polyangiitis
       Henoch–Schönlein purpura
       Other (isolated cutaneous leucocytoclastic vasculitis; hypocomplementemic urticarial vasculitis)

IV **Other**
    Behçet disease
    Secondary vasculitis:
       Infection
       Connective tissue disease
    Isolated CNS vasculitis
    Cogan syndrome
    Unclassified

Prompt recognition of those requiring such treatment is perhaps more important than an exact diagnostic label.

PRIMARY VASCULITIS

The only primary vasculitides seen with any frequency in childhood are Henoch–Schönlein purpura and Kawasaki disease.

Henoch–Schönlein purpura

Henoch–Schönlein purpura (HSP) is the most common of the childhood vasculitides with an estimated incidence of 20.4:100 000[128] peaking at around the age of 5. In the majority of affected individuals it is a benign, self-limiting condition but it can be associated with significant morbidity and occasionally mortality if serious organ involvement occurs. It has been estimated that approximately 1% of children with HSP develop persistent renal disease with less than 0.1% having serious disease.[129]

Pathologically HSP causes a leukocytoclastic vasculitis. The etiology remains uncertain but an infectious trigger is postulated in many cases. Although the pathology is poorly understood, there is much interest in the role of IgA. An elevated serum IgA may occur and the renal pathology overlaps with that seen in IgA nephropathy. Abnormalities in glycosylation of IgA1 have been identified in HSP and appear to be associated with renal involvement.[130]

HSP typically involves the skin, joints, GI tract and kidneys. The rash, characteristically a palpable purpura, affects the lower limbs (Fig. 29.53), buttocks, scrotum and elbows. More extensive involvement including rash affecting the face is not uncommon especially in younger children in whom the rash may be atypical.

Arthralgia and an acute, self-limiting arthritis are common. Gastrointestinal involvement with abdominal pain is one of the more troublesome symptoms of HSP and may be complicated by serious gastrointestinal bleeding, intussusception and rarely perforation of the bowel. Renal involvement occurs in around 50%[131] and ranges from mild asymptomatic hematuria and proteinuria to a nephrotic/nephritic picture with hypertension and a rapidly progressive glomerulonephritis. The importance of HSP lies in its potential for long term renal disease, and children with persisting urinary abnormalities require long term follow-up.

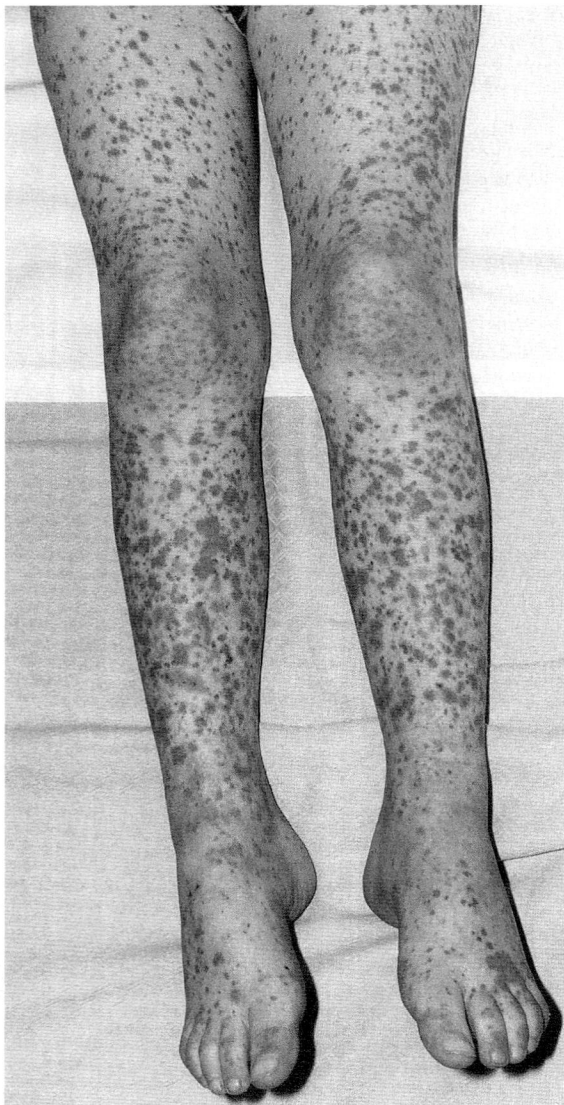

Fig. 29.53   Rash of Henoch–Schönlein purpura.

The diagnosis of HSP is clinical and usually straightforward. With an atypical course, the possibility of some other systemic vasculitis must be considered. Urinalysis should be monitored throughout in all affected children to identify nephritis. Other laboratory investigation is unhelpful and unnecessary in most cases. Abdominal ultrasound may be useful in the assessment of gastrointestinal involvement: characteristic thickening of the bowel wall can be seen and intussusception ruled out where necessary. Evidence of serious or persistent renal involvement may be an indication for renal biopsy to assess the pathology and guide appropriate therapy.

Management of HSP depends on its severity and the particular organ involvement in an individual. In most children it is mild and self-limiting although it may take a few weeks to settle. Recurrent attacks may be seen over a period of a few weeks or months. Most can be managed as outpatients with the parents being taught to test the urine for signs of renal involvement. Simple analgesia such as paracetamol may be adequate for joint and abdominal pain. More significant arthritis may require the use of NSAIDs although these must be used with caution if there is gastrointestinal or renal involvement. There is much anecdotal evidence to support the use of corticoteroids for severe abdominal pain in HSP but no controlled trials. Management of renal involvement depends on its severity. Asymptomatic renal disease requires monitoring but no active

therapy. There is uncontrolled evidence supporting the use of high dose steroids and immunosuppressive therapy where there is a rapidly progressive glomerulonephritis.[132,133] Debate continues around the issue of whether the incidence of serious renal sequelae can be reduced by the earlier administration of steroids. One recent controlled study suggests that in more severe disease early prednisolone therapy while not preventing renal involvement , may shorten its course.[134]

Kawasaki disease

Kawasaki disease or Kawasaki syndrome, first described in Japan in 1967 by Tomisaku Kawasaki, is the other systemic vasculitis seen commonly in childhood, affecting medium sized vessels and with a particular predilection for involvement of the coronary arteries. This may lead to long term sequelae: Kawasaki disease has replaced rheumatic fever as the most common cause of acquired heart disease in children in the resource rich world.[135] Kawasaki disease predominantly affects children under 5 years with most serious sequelae affecting the under twos.

As with all forms of primary vasculitis Kawasaki syndrome is poorly understood and its etiology unclear. Susceptibility to the disease appears to vary with race, children of Asian origin having a higher incidence than Caucasian populations. Recurrence is unusual but reported in around 3%.[136] It occurs in mini-epidemics, its epidemiology suggesting a role for an infectious trigger but no single agent has been consistently associated with Kawasaki disease. There has been interest in the possible role of superantigens in view of clinical similarities to toxic-shock syndrome and the identification of superantigen positive bacteria (both *Staphylococcus aureus* and *Streptococcus*) from a number of individuals with the syndrome.[137] This theory remains unproven. Although the trigger remains uncertain, immunological abnormalities are well documented in Kawasaki disease. Elevated levels of pro-inflammatory cytokines (TNF-α and -β, IL-1 and IL-6); upregulation of adhesion molecules (ELAM-1, ICAM-1 and VCAM-1) and elevated serum levels of macrophage colony-stimulating factor have all been demonstrated.[138]

The diagnosis is based on well-established clinical criteria (Table 29.15). The problem lies with those children, commonly the youngest, who have 'atypical' or 'incomplete' Kawasaki syndrome[139] and are at high risk of coronary artery involvement. The current criteria are insufficiently sensitive for diagnosis in this group and more comprehensive criteria are required.[140] A high index of suspicion is required to ensure that Kawasaki is not missed in the very young child.

The rash in Kawasaki syndrome is polymorphous, usually occurring early in the disease course. Crusting, petechiae and vesicle formation should prompt a search for an alternative diagnosis. An erythematous rash affecting the groin and perineal area and which peels within 48 hours is characteristic (Fig. 29.54a). Involvement of the hands and feet consists of diffuse swelling and/or erythema of the palms and soles. Peeling of the digits (Fig. 29.54b) is well known as a feature of Kawasaki but occurs relatively late in the subacute phase and is not diagnostically helpful. Kawasaki is a multisystem disease and can affect many organ systems. Extreme irritability is very typical of the younger child.

As with most of the vasculitides, laboratory features are nonspecific. Elevation of acute phase reactants, a mild hepatitis and sterile pyuria are common. Thrombocytosis may be marked in the subacute phase.

Table 29.15   Diagnostic criteria for Kawasaki disease

Fever persisting for at least 5 days plus four of the following features:
Changes in peripheral extremities or perineal area
Polymorphous exanthema
Bilateral conjunctival injection
Changes of lips and oral/pharyngeal mucosa
Cervical lymphadenopathy
In the presence of confirmed coronary artery involvement and fever, less than four of the remaining criteria are sufficient to make the diagnosist

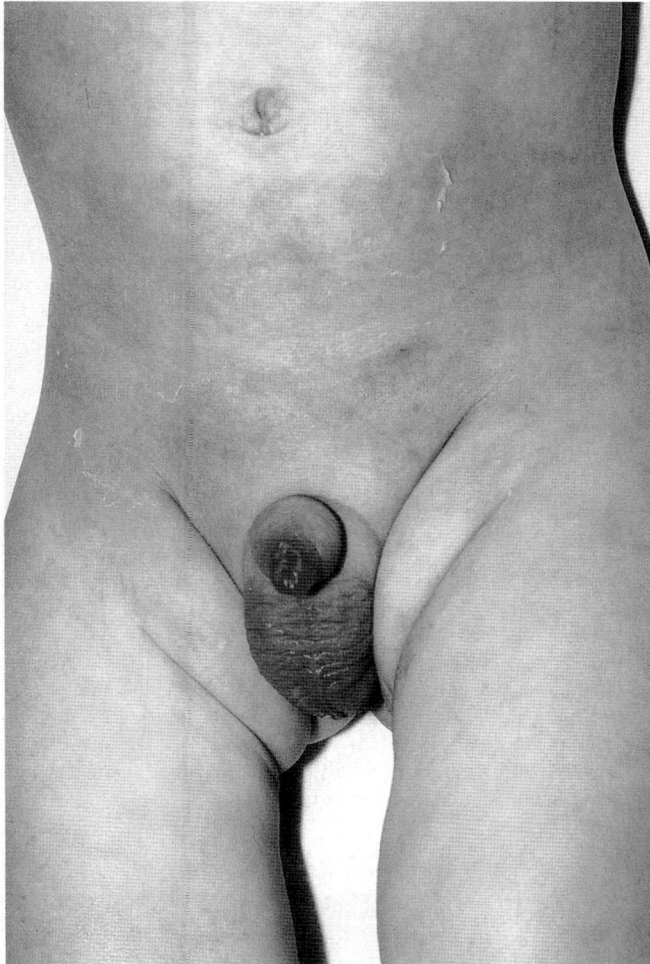

(a)

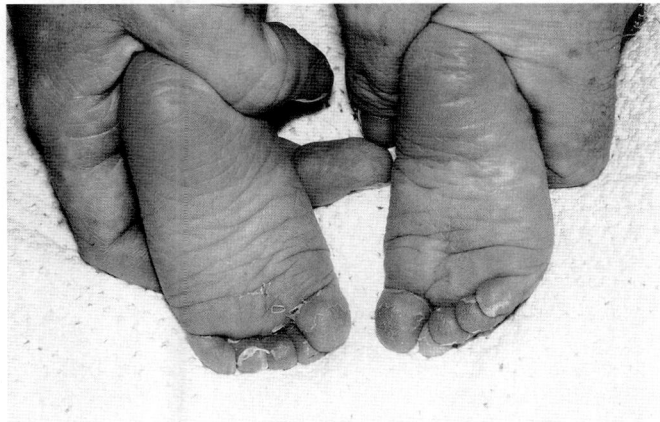

(b)

Fig. 29.54 Kawasaki disease: (a) typical erythematous groin rash with peeling; (b) peeling of digits

phase Kawasaki disease with intravenous immunoglobulin has been clearly shown to reduce coronary artery involvement and hence mortality and morbidity.[141] A single infusion of 2 g/kg is now known to be the optimal regimen.[142,143] This is given with aspirin in high doses initially with reduction to an antiplatelet dose once defervescence occurs. Up to 20% of children with Kawasaki disease fail to settle following a first dose of intravenous immunoglobulin. Those refractory to a repeat dose are likely to benefit from treatment with high dose steroids.[144] The place of steroids earlier in the therapeutic regimen remains unclear.[145]

All children with a definite diagnosis of Kawasaki disease require cardiac assessment to look for evidence of coronary artery involvement which will necessitate long term cardiology follow-up. Guidelines are available for cardiac assessment and follow-up [146] and the reader is referred to Chapter 21 for further information.

Polyarteritis nodosa

The other primary systemic vasculitides are rare in childhood. Polyarteritis nodosa (PAN) is the least uncommon.

Childhood PAN affects predominantly medium sized arteries. Involved vessels are affected by a necrotizing vasculitis with the formation of aneurysmal nodules in the vessel walls. It frequently presents very nonspecifically and a high index of suspicion is required to make the diagnosis. Presenting symptoms include unexplained malaise and fever, skin rash, abdominal pain, arthropathy and myalgia. Laboratory features are nonspecific with the presence of anemia and raised inflammatory markers. Antineutrophil cytoplasmic antibodies (ANCA) are not associated with classic PAN.

The diagnosis is based on the presence of typical clinical features plus either characteristic abnormalities on biopsy of an affected tissue or abnormal angiography.

Even with correct diagnosis and treatment this condition may have a significant mortality, although this varies considerably in reported series. Prompt treatment is essential in order to minimize damage from the vasculitic process (Fig. 29.55) and improve outcome. Unfortunately the rarity of this condition in childhood means that there are no controlled studies. A combination of high dose steroids plus some other immunosuppressive drug, usually cyclophosphamide, is required. Cyclophosphamide is the drug of choice in most cases and can be used either orally or via intravenous pulses. Once remission has been attained, azathioprine has been shown to be as effective as cyclophosphamide for maintenance and is associated with less long term toxicity. For those children who fail to respond to standard therapy with steroids and cyclophosphamide, anecdotal evidence supports the use of alternatives such as plasmapheresis, new immunosuppressants such as mycophenolate mofetil and biologics (anti-TNFs and rituximab).[147]

Microscopic polyangiitis (MPA)

The microscopic variant of polyarteritis affects the smaller arteries and is less common than classic PAN in childhood. In adults this has a worse prognosis and outcome than classic PAN. It is not clear whether

A lumbar puncture may be indicated in the febrile, irritable child and will show a mononuclear pleocytosis.

Untreated Kawasaki disease goes through three phases, acute, subacute and convalescent, the whole process lasting 6–8 weeks. Mortality from coronary artery involvement is 2%. With treatment the process can be switched off in the acute phase and the mortality reduced to 0.3%.

The recognition that the clinical features of Kawasaki disease were the result of an immunologically driven process led to the use of immunoglobulin in treatment with dramatic benefit. Treatment of acute

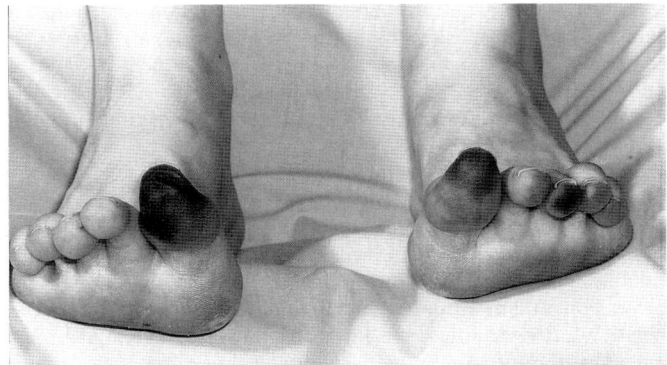

Fig. 29.55 Gangrene of several toes in polyarteritis nodosa.

this applies to pediatric cases. Renal involvement dominates the clinical presentation and course of this condition. As with other small vessel vasculitides, ANCA may be detectable. Management is similar to that of classic PAN.

Cutaneous polyarteritis

There are a group of children who present with a rash identical to that seen in PAN, sometimes associated with systemic upset, but with no evidence of major organ involvement. There is frequently evidence of previous streptococcal infection[148] and this is thought to play a role in the etiology. There is no evidence that this progresses to full blown PAN and it appears to be a separate entity. Prophylaxis with long term penicillin may prevent relapses.

Wegener granulomatosis

Wegener granulomatosis is rare in childhood. Pathologically this is a necrotizing granulomatous vasculitis that affects the small vessels with a predilection for the upper and lower respiratory tract and kidneys. Although the exact pathophysiology is unclear, Wegener granulomatosis is strongly associated with the presence of autoantibodies directed against proteinase 3 (c-ANCA). Whether or not these antibodies play a pathogenic role in the condition remains unclear. Wegener granulomatosis may cause either localized or generalized disease. Steroids and cyclophosphamide are the mainstay of treatment in those with severe disease. With less serious involvement there may be a role for drugs such as methotrexate.

Churg–Strauss syndrome

This vasculitis is exceptionally rare in childhood. The clinical picture is of variable vasculitic features associated with asthma, eosinophilia and infiltrates on chest X-ray.

Takayasu arteritis

Takayasu arteritis, also known as 'pulseless disease', is rare in the UK but worldwide is one of the more common forms of systemic vasculitis affecting younger people. Pathologically it is a chronic giant cell arteritis which segmentally affects the large vessels particularly the aorta and its major branches. Following the initial inflammatory phase, stenosis of vessels leading to ischemia occurs.

During the active inflammatory phase of the disease, affected children may present with features of systemic upset such as fever, weight loss and myalgia. Often the disease presents with evidence of organ ischemia or hypertension.

The etiology of Takayasu arteritis is unclear but genetic factors are important with evidence of racial variations in both incidence and disease expression. Infections and especially tuberculosis have been thought to play a role in triggering the disease but this remains unproven. Management is difficult. Steroids and methotrexate have a role in the active inflammatory phase. Once stricture formation has occurred, angioplasty and reconstructive surgery may be necessary.

Behçet syndrome

Behçet syndrome is an uncommon, poorly understood inflammatory condition in which at least some of the clinical features are the result of a vasculitis which can affect both arteries and veins. Behçet syndrome is characterized by aphthous oral ulceration, genital ulcers and uveitis. Rare in the UK, Behçet syndrome occurs much more commonly in eastern Mediterranean regions.

Behçet syndrome most commonly presents in early adult life and is rare in childhood. The diagnosis is based on clinical features. In children, recurrent oral ulceration may be the only manifestation for some years and until other features become apparent, it may not be possible to confirm the diagnosis. Painful oral ulcers occur in crops lasting up to 2 weeks. Genital ulceration occurs frequently. Uveitis, although common in affected adults, occurs less frequently in children. Arthralgia and arthritis are common in childhood Behçet syndrome as is recurrent fever. Skin lesions seen most frequently in children are folliculitis

and erythema nodosum. Gastrointestinal involvement may cause abdominal pain and diarrhea and is reported in approximately a fifth of affected children. CNS involvement, particularly meningoencephalitis, occurs in approximately 25%. Vascular involvement, which includes both venous and arterial thromboses and aneurysm formation, is potentially the most serious complication of Behçet syndrome. Pulmonary vasculitis, although rare in affected children, is associated with a high mortality.

Significant vascular involvement is associated with a poor outcome and merits treatment with systemic immunosuppressive agents.[149] Colchicine[150] and thalidomide[151] have been shown to be effective for Behçet syndrome where mucocutaneous lesions predominate.

Cogan's syndrome

This systemic vasculitis is extremely rare. It is characterized by the association of vasculitic features with interstitial keratitis and vestibulo-auditory dysfunction.

SECONDARY VASCULITIS

Secondary vasculitis occurs quite commonly in children. It may be seen in the context of a child known to have some other autoimmune rheumatic disorder such as juvenile idiopathic arthritis or systemic lupus erythematosus (Fig. 29.56). Treatment is that of the underlying disorder.

Vasculitis may also occur in association with a variety of infections. These include bacterial infections, viruses such as Epstein–Barr virus and infections such as tuberculosis. Vasculitis is seen not uncommonly in association with meningococcal disease.

Drugs may also be associated with vasculitis which usually remits when the offending agent is withdrawn.

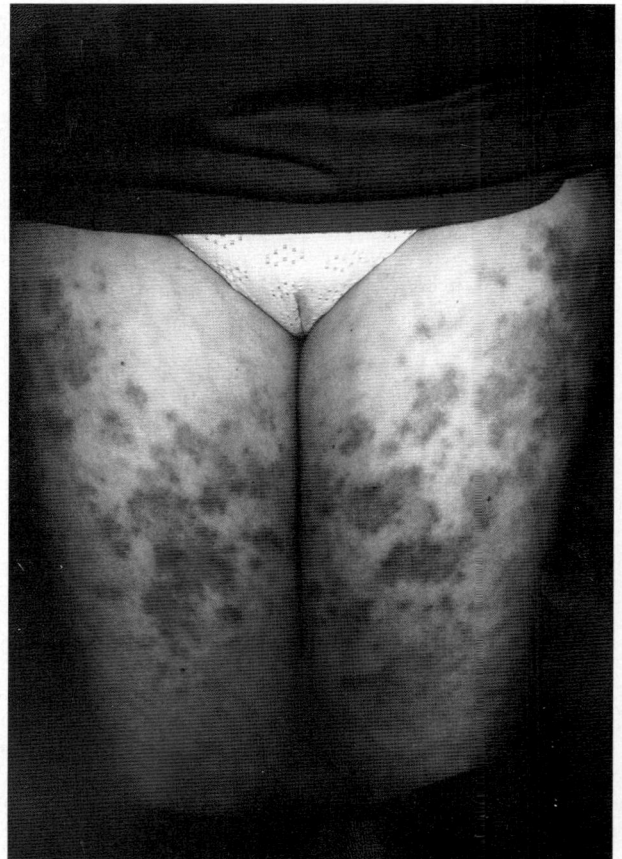

Fig. 29.56   Secondary vasculitis in a child with systemic lupus erythematosus.

ANTINEUTROPHIL CYTOPLASMIC ANTIBODIES (ANCA)

Antineutrophil cytoplasmic antibodies (ANCA) were first described in association with Wegener granulomatosis in 1985 and subsequently with MPA and Churg–Strauss syndrome. Cytoplasmic or c-ANCA gives coarse granular staining of the cytoplasm, is strongly associated with proteinase-3 and is characteristically found in Wegener granulomatosis. Perinuclear or p-ANCA gives staining of the nucleus and perinuclear area, is associated with antimyeloperoxidase and is more commonly seen in MPA. Atypical ANCA staining patterns are seen nonspecifically in many inflammatory conditions. Measurement of these antibodies has become part of the routine workup of a patient with suspected systemic vasculitis. Nonetheless these are not diagnostic tests and results must be interpreted with care. A strongly positive c-ANCA may support the clinical suspicion of a diagnosis of Wegener granulomatosis. A negative ANCA does not rule out the possibility of a systemic vasculitis.

OTHER AUTOIMMUNE RHEUMATIC DISORDERS

SYSTEMIC LUPUS ERYTHEMATOSUS

Systemic lupus erythematosus (SLE) is a multisystem systemic inflammatory disorder most commonly seen in young adult women but well recognized in the pediatric age group. Rare in prepubertal children it occurs more commonly in the teenage years. Most pediatric series show a peak at 11–14 years but this may reflect referral bias, with older teenagers being referred direct to adult clinics. Females predominate in adult series, making up 85–90% of all cases. In childhood males make up a larger percentage of cases with a male to female ratio of 1:4.5. There are no good epidemiological studies of lupus in children: estimates of incidence are in the region of 10–20 per 100 000 children (under 18 years) but vary widely depending on the ethnic mix of the population. Lupus is more common in non-Caucasian races.

SLE has been regarded as the prototype autoimmune disorder with the recognition that one of the hallmarks of the disease is the production of a variety of autoantibodies. The presence of antinuclear antibodies (ANA) is virtually universal in children with lupus, a fact which can aid in making the diagnosis. Despite this recognition, the pathophysiology of lupus remains poorly understood. The presence of antibodies against double-stranded DNA is associated with the development of glomerulonephritis in lupus and the deposition of DNA–anti-DNA immune complexes may play a pathologic role. The role of other autoantibodies remains unclear.

Abnormalities in the functioning of many areas of the immune system have been documented in lupus, with recent interest in the role of dendritic cells[152] and abnormal apoptosis. A genetic predisposition to the development of lupus exists[153] and environmental triggers, including viruses, are thought to be important. Despite progress in our understanding of the widespread immune dysregulation seen in SLE its cause remains unknown. Nonetheless such progress is beginning to open up new therapeutic possibilities.[154]

Lupus is a multisystem disorder which can present in many different ways and with many different features making diagnosis difficult unless a high level of awareness of the condition exists. Delays in making the diagnosis are common, with the mean time to diagnosis being estimated at over a year in most pediatric series. The diagnosis is based on a combination of clinical and laboratory features (Table 29.16). Diagnostic criteria developed for use in adult patients[155] have been validated in a pediatric population.[156]

Lupus is extremely variable in both its clinical presentation and its severity, ranging from a relatively mild condition characterized by a facial rash, joint pains and fatigue to a severe life threatening illness. A wide variety of systems may be affected. General systemic symptoms such as fevers, weight loss, fatigue, arthralgia and general malaise are common throughout the disease course. The fatigue may be profound, disabling and difficult to treat. The characteristic skin rash is the facial butterfly rash which crosses the bridge of the nose and spares the nasolabial folds (Fig. 29.57). Other rashes (e.g. vasculitic)

Table 29.16 Revised American College of Rheumatology criteria for the classification of systemic lupus erythematosus. (Adapted from Hochberg 1997[155])

1. Malar rash
2. Discoid rash
3. Photosensitivity
4. Oral ulceration
5. Arthritis
6. Serositis:
   a. Pleuritis
   b. Pericarditis
7. Renal disorder:
   a. Proteinuria >0.5 g/24 h
   b. Cellular casts
8. Neurological disorder:
   a. Seizures
   b. Psychosis (other causes excluded)
9. Hematological disorders:
   a. Hemolytic anemia
   b. Leukopenia $< 4 \times 10^9$/L (two or more occasions)
   c. Lymphopenia $< 1.510^9$/L (two or more occasions)
   d. Thrombocytopenia $< 100 \times 10^9$/L
10. Immunological disorders:
    a. Raised antinative DNA antibody binding
    b. Anti-Sm antibody
    c. Antiphospholipid antibodies:
       i. Abnormal serum levels of IgG or IgM anticardiolipin antibodies
       ii. Positive test for lupus anticoagulant
       iii. False positive serological test for syphilis present for at least 3 months
11. Antinuclear antibody present in raised titer

A person shall be said to have SLE if four or more of the 11 criteria are present (serially or simultaneously).

may occur in SLE and many children with lupus exhibit marked photosensitivity. Alopecia is usually mild but can be severe with scarring. Raynaud phenomenon is common. Hematological involvement is frequent in pediatric lupus which may present initially with what appears to be idiopathic thrombocytopenic purpura. CNS lupus is a cause of long term morbidity and may manifest as seizure activity, psychosis, aseptic meningitis or headaches. Mood alteration is common and it

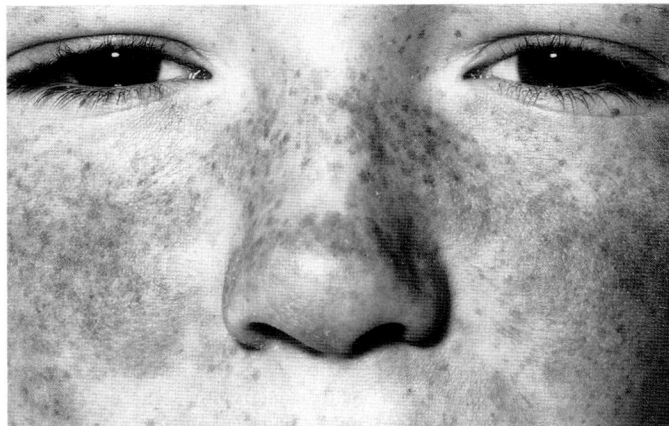

Fig. 29.57 Typical facial rash in systemic lupus erythematosus – crossing the bridge of the nose and sparing the nasolabial folds.

may be difficult to separate organic CNS involvement from reactive symptoms due to coping with a chronic illness. Renal involvement is frequent in childhood lupus and one of the major causes of morbidity. When present it tends to dominate the clinical picture. It may present as asymptomatic hematuria and proteinuria, hypertension, nephrotic syndrome or a rapidly progressing glomerulonephritis. Renal biopsy has an important role to play in determining the severity and therefore the likely outcome of the renal disease. Children with lupus are at particular risk from infection which is now the most common cause of death. This is a result both of the disease process itself and of immunosuppressive treatment regimens. Pneumococcal sepsis is a particular risk and pneumococcal vaccination is recommended.

Laboratory investigations are helpful both in the diagnosis and monitoring of SLE. Anemia occurs as a result of chronic disease or hemolysis. Thrombocytopenia and leukopenia are common. Characteristically the ESR is elevated while the CRP remains normal. Renal function should be monitored in those with renal involvement. A mild transaminitis is common but serious liver abnormalities are rare. Serum complement levels are reduced in most patients while serum immunoglobulin levels are nonspecifically elevated. A positive antinuclear antibody (ANA) is found in virtually all patients and is a useful diagnostic tool. The ANA result must be interpreted in the light of the clinical picture as the specificity for lupus is low and children may have a positive ANA for many reasons. Antibodies against double-stranded DNA and Sm (Smith antigen) are of greater specificity. Other autoantibodies such as anti-Ro, La and RNP may occur.

Management of lupus requires regular monitoring and attention to detail. Optimal management is in a multidisciplinary team setting with input from both a pediatric rheumatologist and a pediatric nephrologist. Drug therapy depends on disease severity and organs involved. Mild lupus can be managed with NSAIDs, hydroxychloroquine and low dose methotrexate. Avoidance of sun exposure and the use of sunblock are important. Thalidomide has been used for severe mucocutaneous disease. More significant organ involvement will require the use of moderate doses of steroids while severe disease which is life or organ threatening will require treatment with high dose steroids and immunosuppressive agents such as azathioprine and cyclophosphamide. Controlled studies in adults have shown the superiority of combinations of steroids and immunosuppressants over steroids alone[157,158] but there are no controlled studies in pediatric SLE. Treatment must be sufficient to suppress disease activity but aim to minimize toxicity. The long term toxicity particularly of high dose steroid regimens is very significant and steroid side-effects are particularly unacceptable to teenage girls who are the group most affected by lupus. Recently there has been interest in the use of mycophenolate mofetil a potentially less toxic alternative to cyclophosphamide.[159] Rituximab, a biologic drug which targets B cells, has been shown to be effective in individuals with disease resistant to more conventional therapies.[160] There are no pediatric studies to date and concern from some anecdotal reports regarding the frequency of side-effects.[161]

The ESR, urine protein level, levels of C3 and C4 and ds-DNA titer may all be used in monitoring disease activity and response to treatment but clinical assessment of disease activity remains the gold standard. A variety of assessment tools have been developed to allow quantitative assessment of disease activity in lupus and have been validated for pediatric use.[162] PRINTO (The Pediatric Rheumatology International Trials Organization) has developed and validated both a disease activity core set and a definition of improvement for use in pediatric lupus.[163,164]

SLE is a serious disease and those who present in childhood have a high incidence of major organ involvement. Current treatment has markedly reduced the mortality but the long term morbidity remains high. Infection is the most common cause of death but renal death with the consequent need for dialysis and transplantation continues to occur in those with aggressive nephritis. Early diagnosis and optimal management should reduce this but the need for improved treatment protocols remains.

As survival rates from childhood lupus have improved it is clear that there is a high incidence of serious long term morbidity.[165] CNS disease results in long term psychological sequelae in many. Osteoporosis results both from the disease and its treatment. Lupus is known to cause a dyslipoproteinemia[166] and early onset coronary artery disease is a major complication of childhood lupus. Whether this can be altered by treatment of the lipid abnormalities is unknown.

Drug-induced lupus

A number of drugs are well known to cause a lupus-like syndrome. The best known in children are the antiepileptic drugs phenytoin and carbamazepine and the antihypertensives hydralazine and captopril. An addition to the list, of importance in teenagers, is minocycline commonly prescribed for acne.[167]

Antiphospholipid syndrome

As with other autoantibodies such as ANA, low titer antiphospholipid antibodies are seen not uncommonly in children, and are frequently thought to be epiphenomena of no clinical significance. Low titer antiphospholipid antibodies occur in around 30% of children with SLE but are of dubious clinical significance. The antiphospholipid syndrome occurs where higher titers of antibodies are associated with coagulation abnormalities and thromboembolic events.

Antiphospholipid syndromes are usually secondary, frequently in association with SLE. Primary antiphospholipid syndromes have been described in childhood but are rare.

These antibodies should be looked for in any child presenting with unexplained thromboembolic phenomena. Anticoagulation is required where there is evidence of an associated thrombotic problem. The role of prophylaxis, with either low dose anticoagulation or aspirin, in children is unclear.

Neonatal lupus erythematosus

The neonatal lupus syndrome is defined by the presence of maternal autoantibodies to Ro and La which cross the placenta causing clinical abnormalities in the fetus and neonate. The characteristic skin rash, thrombocytopenia and hepatic abnormalities are usually self limiting. The importance of the syndrome lies in its association with congenital heart block which may cause intrauterine bradycardia, cardiac failure and death. This syndrome usually affects pregnancies of women with only mild lupus or of healthy women subsequently found to have anti-Ro and La antibodies.

JUVENILE DERMATOMYOSITIS AND POLYMYOSITIS

The idiopathic inflammatory myopathies comprise a group of conditions characterized by unexplained inflammation of the muscles. In childhood, dermatomyositis is ten times more common than polymyositis.

Juvenile dermatomyositis (JDM) is a rare condition with an incidence of 1.9 per million children under 16 years in the UK.[168] Juvenile dermatomyositis occurs at all ages throughout childhood but with two peaks of presentation at 5–9 years and at 11–14 years. The condition is more common in females than males.

The etiology of JDM remains unknown. In children, unlike adults, there is no association with malignancy. Studies have shown a strong association with HLA-DQ1*0501[169] confirming a role for genetic factors. There has been interest in the role of TNF in the inflammatory myopathies and an overrepresentation of TNF-α-308A allele has been demonstrated in a population of children with JDM.[170] A number of epidemiological studies have documented clustering of onset of cases, stimulating interest in the role of infectious agents as triggers. No single agent has been identified.

Once established, a variety of immunological abnormalities occur in children with JDM. Antinuclear antibodies are found in approximately 60%. Their specificity is for the most part unknown and in contrast to adults, myositis-specific antibodies (e.g. Jo-1; Mi) are seldom present. Active disease is associated with elevation of serum immunoglobulin levels, evidence of complement activation, lymphopenia and an increase in the percentage of B lymphocytes.

The diagnosis of JDM is based on criteria published by Bohan and Peters in 1975.[171] A child is considered to have JDM if, having excluded other known causes, they have a characteristic rash plus three of the following four criteria: symmetrical proximal muscle weakness, elevated muscle enzymes, abnormal muscle histology and EMG changes. The increasing use of modalities such as MRI to demonstrate inflammatory muscle changes is replacing more invasive investigations in many patients and there is a need for a revision of these diagnostic criteria.[172]

The rash in JDM is the first symptom in approximately 50%. A further 25% report a simultaneous onset of the rash and weakness while in the last 25% weakness precedes the rash. The typical rash affects the eyelids, knuckles and extensor aspects of the knees and elbows (Fig. 29.58). Erythema affecting the face and upper trunk may also be seen. The eyelid rash is violaceous in hue, while the lesions over the knuckles may have a hypertrophic appearance (Gottron papules) (Fig. 29.59). Marked nailfold erythema occurs and is indicative of the vasculopathy that characterizes JDM. Examination of the nail fold capillaries will show typical changes with capillary dilatation and areas of thrombosis (Fig. 29.59).

The other major feature of JDM is an inflammatory myopathy. This affects the proximal limb muscles, often first noticed by difficulty with climbing stairs or brushing hair. Muscle weakness may be severe and involvement of the neck flexors and abdominal muscles occurs in addition to those in the limbs. Weakness is frequently associated with complaints of muscle pain and tenderness. Myositis is confirmed by documenting abnormalities of muscle enzymes such as creatine kinase, aspartate aminotransferase (AST), alanine aminotransferase (ALT), aldolase and lactate dehydrogenase (LDH). It should be remembered that muscle enzymes may be normal despite active disease. EMG,

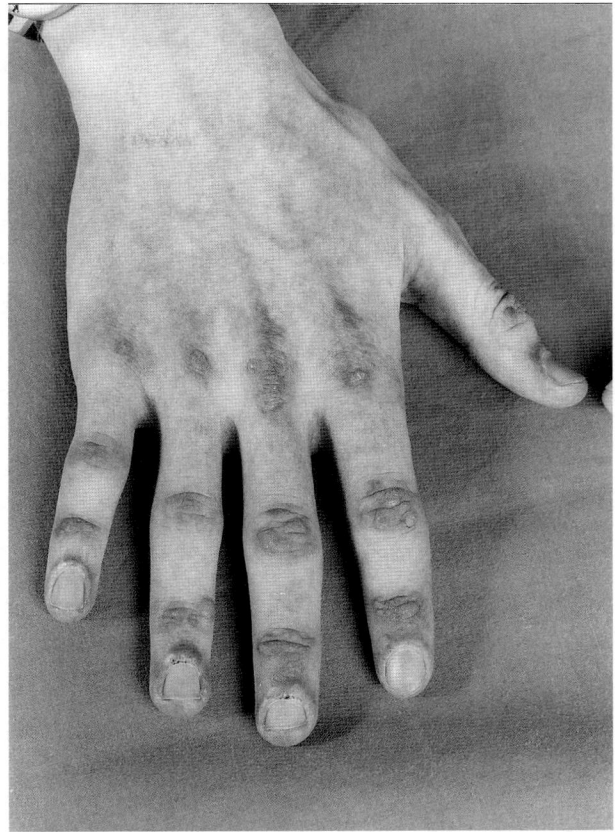

Fig. 29.59 Juvenile dermatomyositis showing Gottron papules and typical nailfold changes.

muscle biopsy and MRI will show characteristic inflammatory change (Fig. 29.60).

JDM is a multisystem disease and although the main features are of skin and muscle involvement, many organ systems can be affected by the widespread vasculopathy. Dysphagia occurs as a result of disease affecting the esophagus, while dysphonia results from involvement of the soft palate. Cardiac abnormalities are reported in up to 50%. Most are minor but cardiomyopathy can occur. Interstitial lung disease is uncommon but carries a poor prognosis.

Before the advent of steroids, JDM had a very poor prognosis. Thirty percent of affected children died, 30% had severe chronic disease and

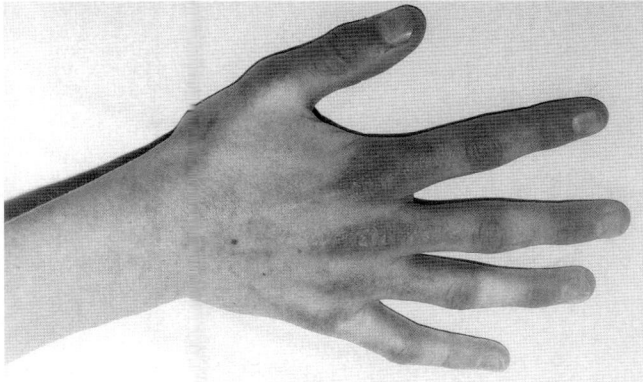

(a)

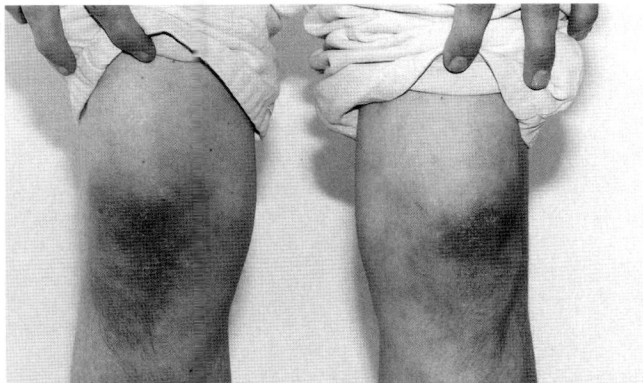

(b)

Fig. 29.58 Typical rash of juvenile dermatomyositis with erythema over: (a) extensor aspects of metacarpophalangeal and proximal interphalangeal joints; (b) knees.

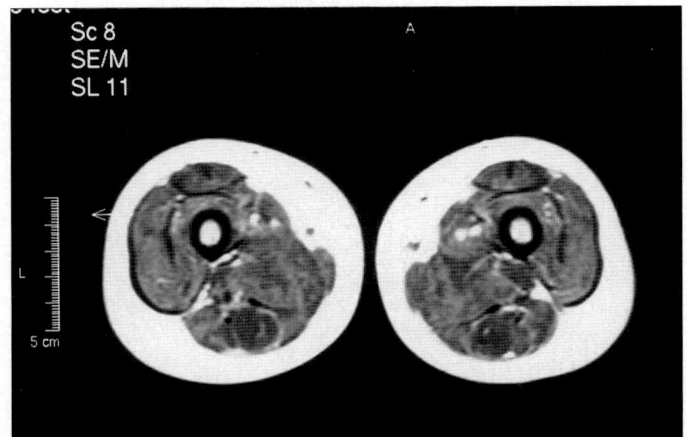

Fig. 29.60 Muscle MRI in juvenile dermatomyositis showing patchy, heterogeneous texture of the muscles typical of an inflammatory myopathy.

only 30% recovered. Steroids and more recent developments in therapy have dramatically changed the outlook but this is still a disease with an associated mortality and significant morbidity. Three characteristic disease courses are recognized. Some children have an acute monocyclic course which resolves with treatment; others a relapsing, remitting course while a third group have severe, unremitting chronic disease. In addition it is now recognized that there is a wide variety of clinical patterns seen within the overall label of JDM. Some children have predominantly muscle disease, others cutaneous. Some have both while a further group have evidence of a widespread vasculopathy with cutaneous ulceration (Fig. 29.61) and serious organ involvement.

Calcinosis of the muscle is a well-recognized complication of JDM (Fig. 29.62). It is at least in part related to disease severity and duration and its incidence can be reduced by prompt and appropriate treatment. Lipodystrophy may complicate JDM (Fig. 29.63) and in some is associated with the development of insulin resistance. As with lupus, osteoporosis is a complication both of the disease and its therapy.

Treatment of JDM remains controversial. There is no consensus on the type, route of administration and duration of treatment and there are no randomized controlled trials. In uncomplicated JDM, oral prednisolone is the most commonly used treatment in a dose of 1–2 mg/kg/day, tapering over 12–18 months. In an attempt to get more rapid disease control and minimize toxicity from oral steroids, many now advocate initial treatment with pulsed intravenous methylprednisolone. Other drugs were traditionally reserved for those with severe or steroid resistant disease but it is now recognized that early use of an additional drug, usually methotrexate,[173] results in reduced morbidity and a reduction

in the total steroid dosage required. Intravenous immunoglobulin may play a role in some patients and cyclophosphamide may be indicated in refractory disease.[174] There is interest in the use of new therapeutic options such as mycophenolate mofetil, the anti-TNF drugs or stem cell transplantation in children who fail to respond to other therapies but these must still be regarded as experimental.

Treatment is adjusted depending on the clinical response but monitoring may be difficult. Levels of muscle enzymes are not a good guide to activity and should not be used to plan treatment. Clinical assessment is the gold standard and there have been various attempts to try and improve methods of doing this. The childhood myositis assessment scale[7] is a useful method for objectively assessing muscle strength, serial scores then being used to quantify changes in the disease process. MRI is being used as a non-invasive method of assessing muscle inflammation and again may be used serially to document progress. A core set of criteria for the assessment of disease activity has been proposed by PRINTO but remains to be validated.[175]

SCLERODERMA IN CHILDHOOD

The scleroderma group of disorders is characterized clinically by thickening of the skin. This can occur in both localized and systemic forms, the former occurring much more commonly in pediatric practice.

Localized scleroderma
Localized scleroderma may be subdivided into morphea and linear scleroderma. Morphea lesions most commonly occur on the trunk

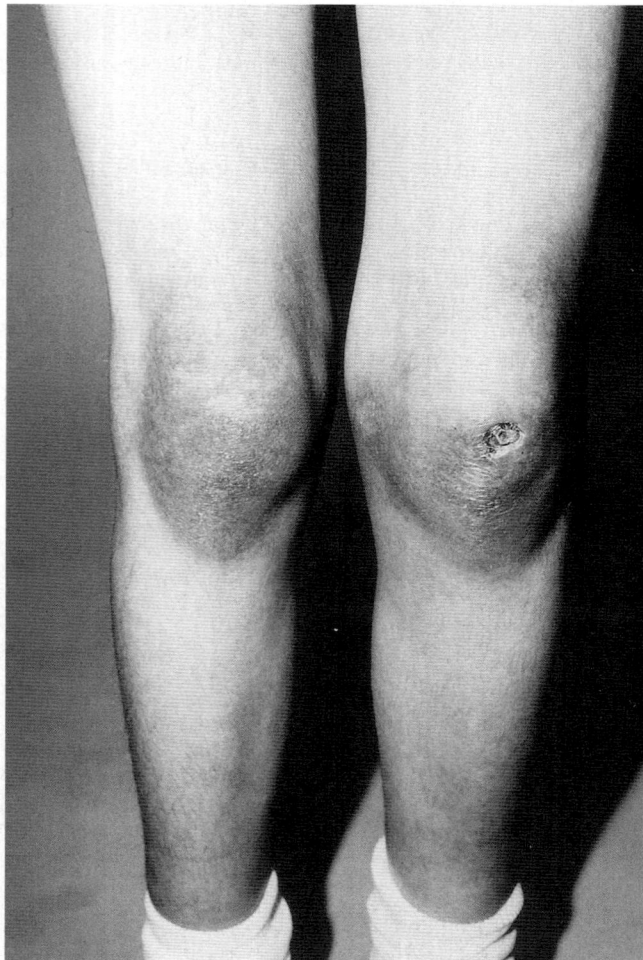
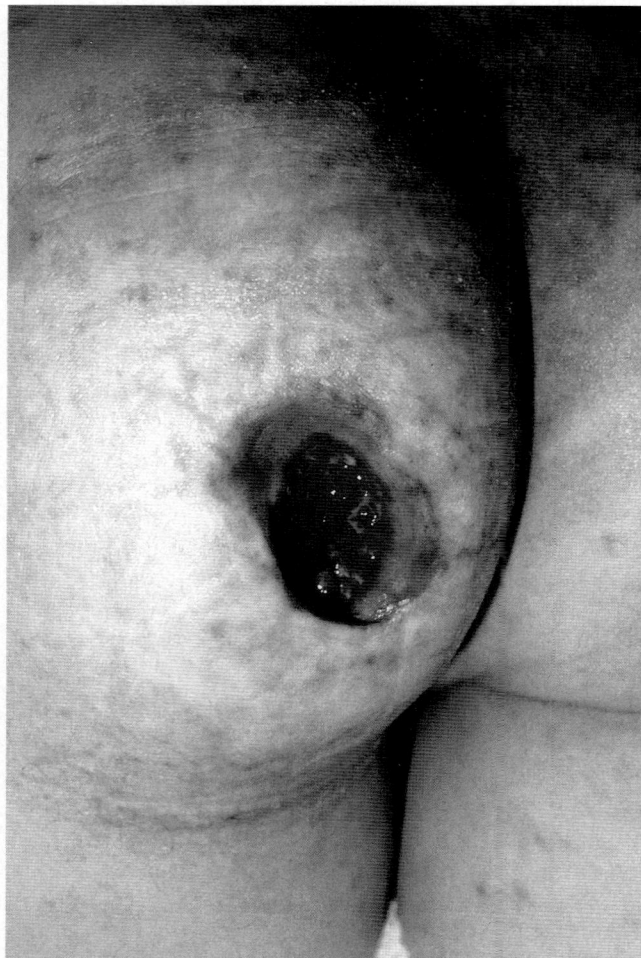

(a)   (b)

Fig. 29.61   (a,b) Ulcerative vasculopathy in juvenile dermatomyositis.

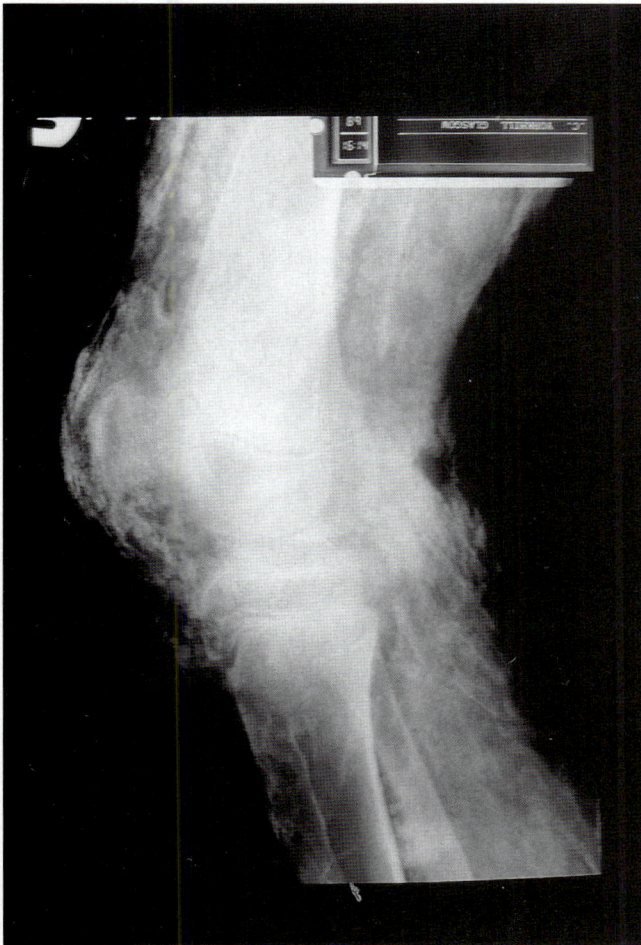

(a)

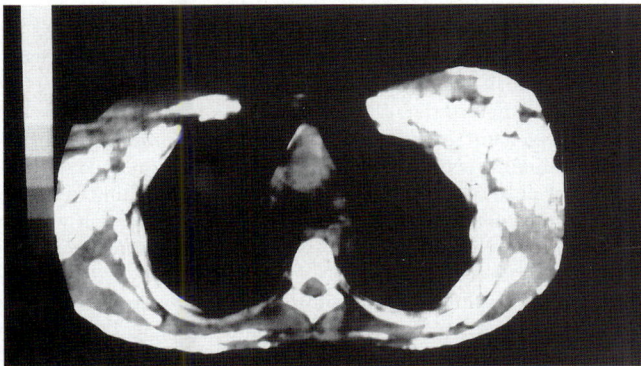

(b)

Fig. 29.62   Juvenile dermatomyositis with extensive calcinosis affecting: (a) lower limb (plain radiograph); (b) chest wall (CT scan).

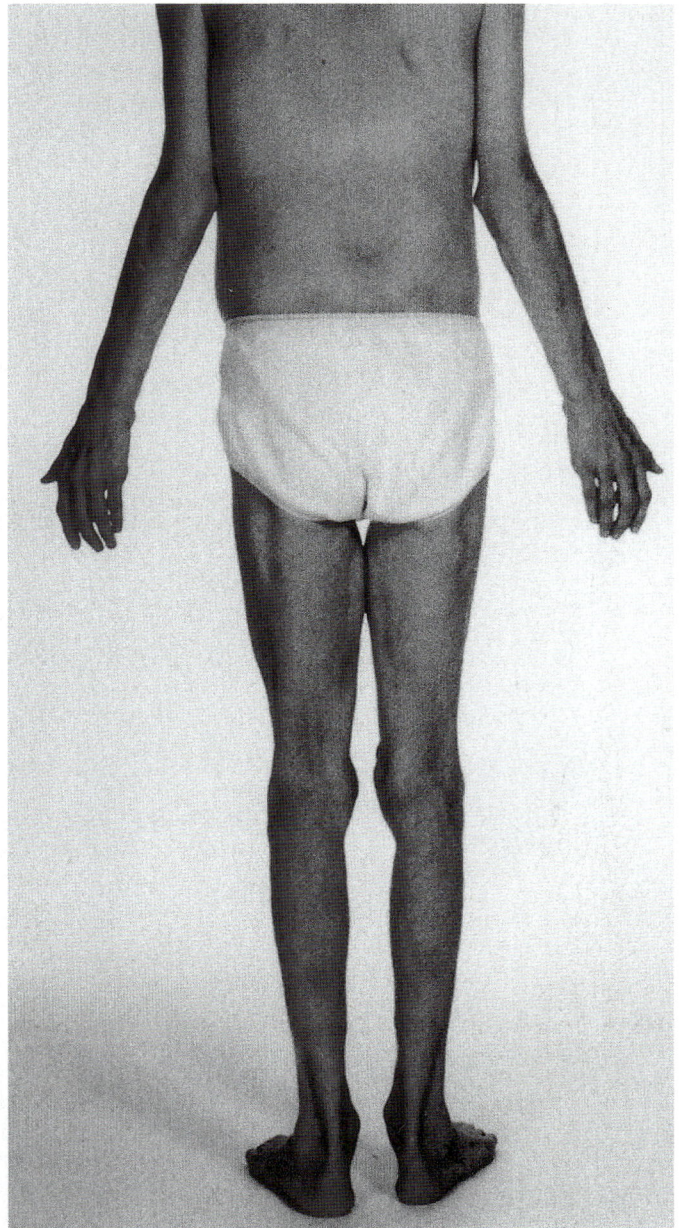

Fig. 29.63   Lipodystrophy in juvenile dermatomyositis – absence of subcutaneous fat in lower limbs.

and present as pale patches of thickened skin. When active there may be surrounding erythema and with time they become hyperpigmented (Fig. 29.64). They usually occur as isolated lesions and, although they may be cosmetically unpleasant, seldom cause other problems.

Linear scleroderma is of much greater concern. In this condition the child or parent may notice a band of skin discoloration in a linear distribution on a limb or on the face/scalp (when it is known as 'en coup de sabre'; Fig. 29.65). These lesions do not follow a dermatomal distribution and they are poorly understood. As with morphea, an erythematous color may indicate an active lesion: with time they become hyperpig-

mented. These lesions may be associated with atrophy and undergrowth of surrounding structures or the affected limb (Fig. 29.66) causing significant cosmetic and functional difficulties.

In a large collaborative data collection, 40% of children with localized scleroderma were found to be ANA positive. In a percentage of affected children extracutaneous manifestations (e.g. arthritis, neurological) occur but progression to systemic sclerosis does not.[176]

Our lack of understanding of the underlying process in these conditions makes treatment difficult. Methotrexate is now widely used to treat active lesions[177] and there is anecdotal evidence supporting the use of steroids and methotrexate in combination. Where a band of scleroderma crosses a joint, vigorous physiotherapy is helpful in maintaining joint range.

Systemic sclerosis

The systemic sclerosis disorders are extremely uncommon in pediatric practice. In adults, systemic sclerosis can be subdivided into

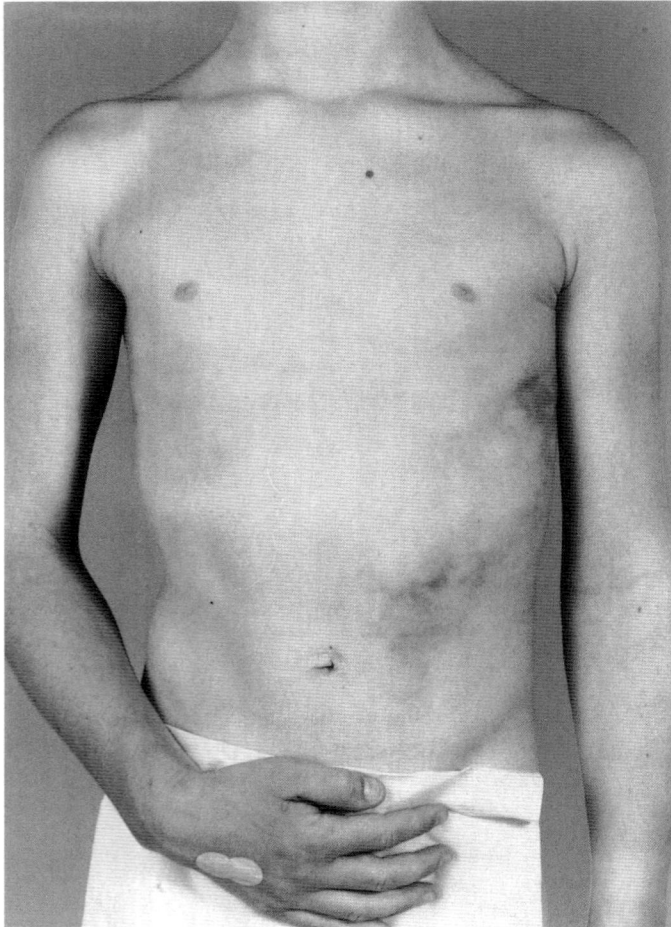

Fig. 29.64   Morphea.

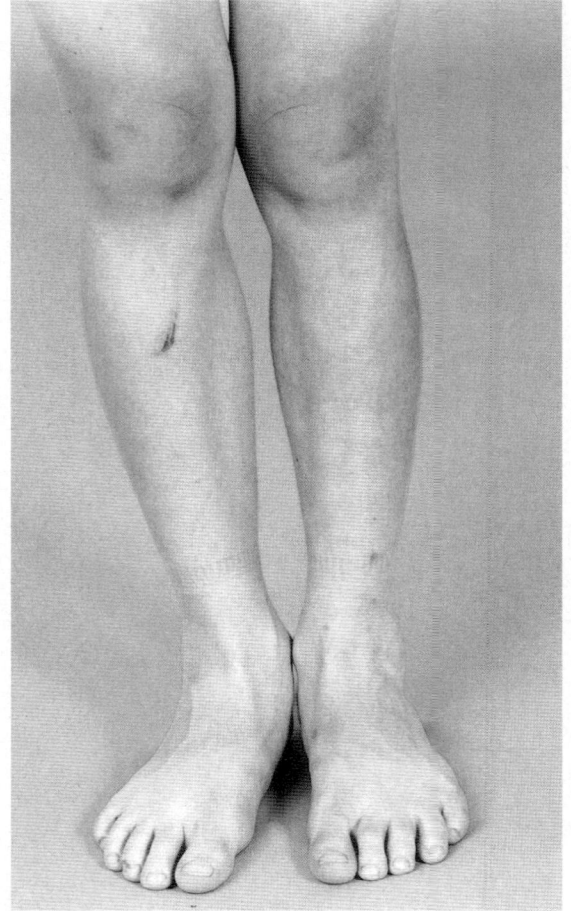

Fig. 29.66   Limb atrophy in linear scleroderma.

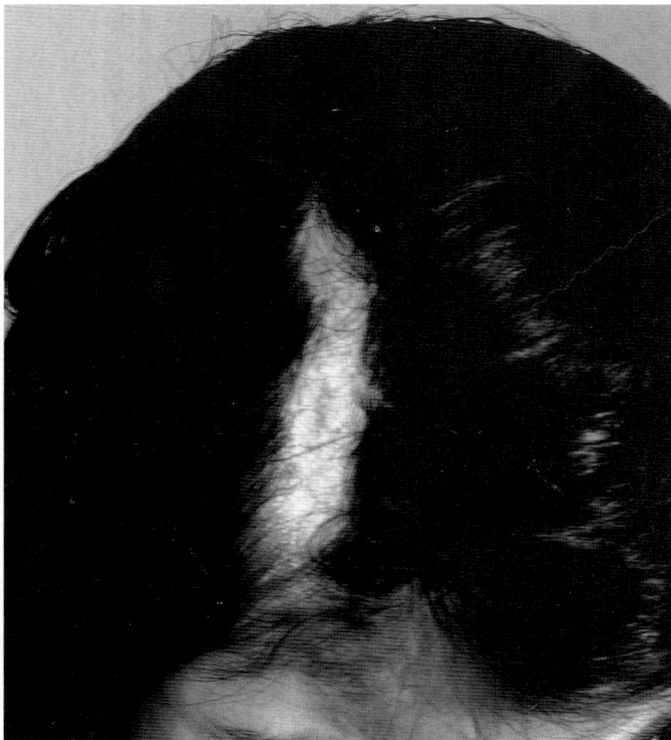

Fig. 29.65   En coup de sabre lesion.

diffuse cutaneous sytemic sclerosis (formerly known as progressive systemic sclerosis) and limited cutaneous systemic sclerosis (formerly CREST syndrome). Diffuse disease, characterized by cutaneous involvement extending to the proximal limbs and trunk, progresses rapidly over the first few years and is associated with the presence of anti-Scl 70 antibodies. The hallmark of limited disease is skin involvement of the distal extremities and face only. These categories appear less clearcut in childhood, many having features that overlap between the two

Raynaud phenomenon is usually the first feature of these conditions and if not present the diagnosis is unlikely. A history of Raynaud phenomenon may be difficult to obtain in a young child. The earliest clinical finding is cutaneous edema usually affecting the hands which consequently feel firm on palpation Biopsy at this stage will show inflammatory change in the subcutaneous tissue which becomes thicker and tighter. This results in stiffness of the extremities and the characteristic pinched appearance of the face. Joint contractures develop and the skin is very susceptible to minor trauma. Ischemia results in loss of the finger pulp and the typical digital pitting scarring (Fig. 29.67). Severe ischemia may result in the loss of digits. Subcutaneous calcification, pulmonary hypertension and esophageal disease are common in the limited form of the disease. Diffuse disease is characterized by early interstitial lung disease, gastrointestinal involvement, cardiac abnormalities due to small vessel obliteration and renal disease. The scleroderma renal 'crisis' which results from a critical reduction in renal blood flow causing cortical ischemia, activation of the renin–angiotensin system and malignant hypertension, was previously a fatal event but can now be treated with angiotensin converting enzyme (ACE) inhibitors.

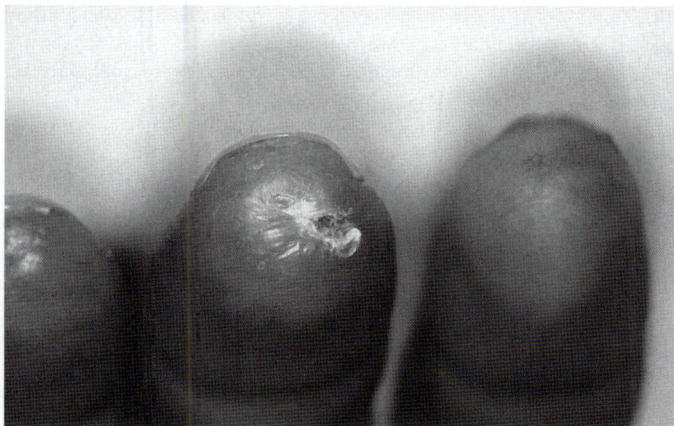

Fig. 29.67   Digital pitting scars in systemic sclerosis.

Renal disease is less common in the childhood form of the disease and the outcome is generally better than in adults.[178] Cardiac disease is the most common cause of death in affected children.

Management requires meticulous attention to detail. Protective measures (avoidance of cold exposure, use of warm mittens and avoidance of smoking) are important in reducing ischemia of the digits. Nifedipine, in a long-acting preparation, is the drug of choice. Occasional patients with severe digital ischemia and impending gangrene will benefit, often impressively, from the use of intravenous prostaglandin. Emollients are helpful for dry skin while physiotherapy and splinting may benefit joint disease. Gastrointestinal symptoms may be helped by the use of omeprazole together with a prokinetic agent such as cisapride. Broad-spectrum antibiotics may help malabsorption secondary to bacterial overgrowth. ACE inhibitors given where there is any evidence of renal involvement will reduce the risk of a scleroderma crisis.

Immunosuppressive therapy is used early where there is evidence of serious organ involvement and may influence the course of the disease. Once fibrosis is well established it is likely to be irreversible. Monitoring to detect signs of early organ involvement is therefore essential. Traditionally, treatment was with d-penicillamine but there is no evidence of benefit and the drug is associated with significant toxicity. Interest now lies in the use of powerful immunosuppressive regimens. Steroids, methotrexate, ciclosporin, cyclophosphamide, mycophenolate mofetil and antithymocyte globulin may all have a role. There is some anecdotal evidence suggesting that if used early, steroids and cyclophosphamide will halt progression of the lung disease which is one of the major determinants of mortality. There are no controlled studies to date and little hard evidence on which to base treatment plans.

MIXED CONNECTIVE TISSUE DISEASE

Mixed connective tissue disease (MCTD) is an entity characterized by Raynaud disease, swollen fingers and hands, myositis and a strongly positive antibody against RNP. Whether this is truly a separate disease or a subset of some other condition such as SLE is a matter of continuing debate. Many individuals with MCTD would also fulfill diagnostic criteria for the diagnosis of SLE.

OVERLAP SYNDROMES

A number of patients are seen with features of more than one autoimmune disorder and are classed as having overlap syndromes. The most commonly seen in pediatric practice are overlaps between JDM or polymyositis and scleroderma.

UNDIFFERENTIATED CONNECTIVE TISSUE DISORDERS

A number of children and adolescents will present with some features of this group of conditions, often associated with a positive antinuclear antibody, but insufficient to be defined as one of the well-characterized conditions already described. Some will evolve with time into one of the clearly defined conditions while others will remain undifferentiated.

SJÖGREN SYNDROME

Sjögren syndrome is a chronic inflammatory disorder characterized by lymphocytic infiltration of the exocrine glands and resulting in sicca symptoms, i.e. dry eyes and dry mouth. Sjögren syndrome may be primary or secondary, occurring in association with some other autoimmune rheumatic disorder. Conditions known to be associated with Sjögren syndrome include SLE, rheumatoid arthritis, MCTD, systemic sclerosis, dermatomyositis and primary biliary cirrhosis. Recognition is important as there is a significant risk of a lymphoid malignancy developing in the affected glands.

Although uncommon in pediatric practice, Sjögren syndrome does occur. Secondary Sjögren syndrome is more common than primary and usually develops in the context of a patient with a known autoimmune rheumatic disorder. Sjögren syndrome in childhood generally presents with parotid swelling which may be troublesome, recurrent and painful (Fig. 29.68a). The most important differential diagnosis is viral sialedinitis. If the problem is recurrent then Sjögren syndrome should be considered.

Although there are established criteria for the diagnosis of Sjögren syndrome in adults these are difficult to apply in children. Parotid imaging may be difficult to interpret. Ultrasound may be the most useful imaging procedure as it is inexpensive, well tolerated and shows characteristic abnormalities (Fig. 29.68b). For the diagnosis to be made the parotid swelling should be accompanied by evidence of dry eyes, dry mouth and the presence of autoantibodies.

Management of Sjögren syndrome consists firstly of management of the underlying disorder. Artificial tears are used for dry eyes and a variety of preparations are available to relieve the dry mouth. Dental care must be meticulous as the lack of saliva predisposes to severe dental caries. Monitoring for the development of malignancy in the salivary glands is important.

RAYNAUD PHENOMENON

Raynaud phenomenon was first described in 1862 as episodic digital ischemia provoked by factors such as cold or emotion. Classically in Raynaud syndrome there is a triphasic color change. The digits initially blanche followed by cyanosis and then erythema on rewarming. For the diagnosis to be considered at least two of these phases must be present. In addition to the digits, changes may be seen in the ear lobes, tip of the nose and around the mouth.

Primary Raynaud syndrome, where the phenomenon occurs in isolation in an otherwise healthy individual, is common in young women and frequently familial. Secondary Raynaud syndrome occurs in conditions such as SLE, systemic sclerosis and MCTD and may be the presenting feature of such illnesses. All young people presenting with Raynaud syndrome should have a careful evaluation to exclude an underlying disorder. Any atypical features (year-round symptoms, digital ulceration) or the presence of antinuclear antibodies raise the possibility of secondary Raynaud syndrome and the child or teenager should be followed up to ensure no further problems develop.

Primary Raynaud syndrome will usually be controlled by symptomatic measures and protection from the cold. Unfortunately the use of warm gloves or mittens is unpopular in teenage years when primary Raynaud syndrome may be troublesome. Nifedipine will often improve symptoms, the dose being titrated to clinical response and the development of side-effects.

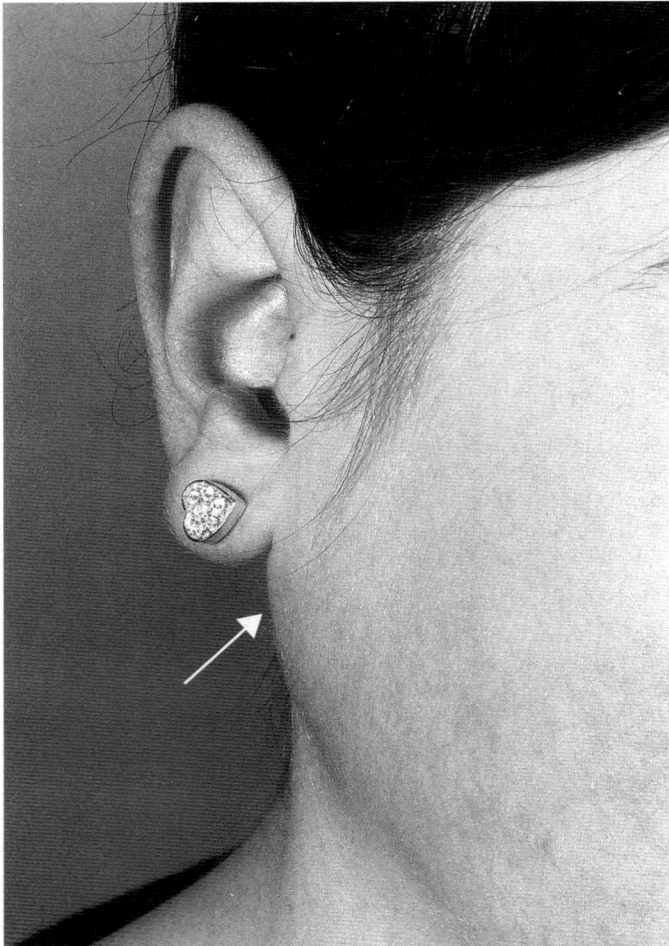

(a)

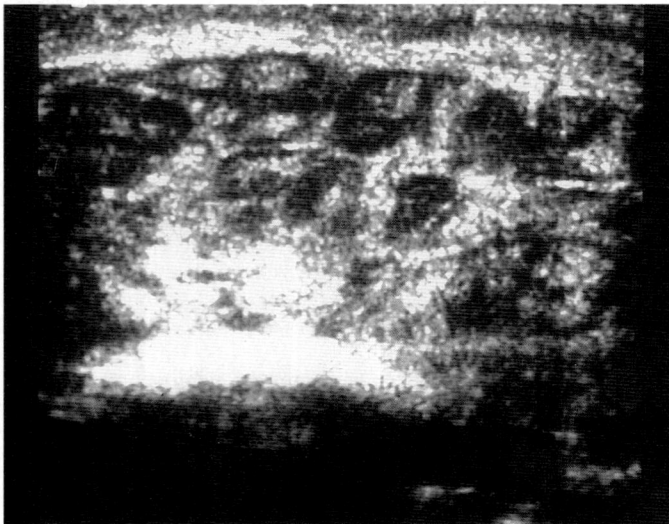

(b)

Fig. 29.68 Sjögren syndrome: (a) parotid swelling; (b) abnormal echogenicity on ultrasound.

ERYTHEMA NODOSUM

Erythema nodosum is seen not infrequently in children. The typical story is of the sudden onset of one or more tender, erythematous raised nodules or plaques on the anterior surface of the tibia. Pathologically this represents a septal panniculitis (inflammation within the subcutaneous fat). The nodules lie deep and may be easier to feel than to see. As they resolve they develop an ecchymotic appearance and lesions at varying stages of development are frequently seen. Resolution usually occurs over a 4-to 6-week period.

In the majority of cases, erythema nodosum is an acute process occurring in response to an infectious trigger. Recurrent or chronic erythema nodosum merits investigation for some underlying cause.

Most cases in children occur as a post-streptococcal phenomenon and are associated with markedly raised ASO titers. Other infections such as mycoplasma, viruses and tuberculosis must be remembered. Drugs including antibiotics and oral contraceptive pills may cause erythema nodosum. Rarely, but importantly, it may be the presenting feature of some systemic disorder such as inflammatory bowel disease, sarcoidosis or an autoimmune rheumatic disorder.

THE DIFFERENTIAL DIAGNOSIS OF SYSTEMIC INFLAMMATORY DISORDERS

A chronic systemic inflammatory process in a child may result from chronic infection, malignancy or a rheumatological disorder such as systemic onset juvenile idiopathic arthritis, SLE, JDM or a systemic vasculitis. There are a number of unusual conditions of unknown etiology that may present in this fashion and must be remembered in the differential diagnosis. Some are outlined in this section.

Familial Mediterranean fever and other periodic fever syndromes

The periodic fever syndromes are a group of disorders characterized by unprovoked inflammation. Many have now been associated with gene mutations affecting the IL-1 and TNFα pathways enabling both genetic diagnosis and possible therapeutic options.[179]

Familial Mediterranean fever (FMF) principally affects individuals of eastern Mediterranean origin especially Sephardic and Iraqi Jews, Armenians and Levantine Arabs and is inherited as an autosomal recessive trait. It results from mutations of a gene on chromosome 16 that influences the production of a protein known as pyrin or marenostrum.[180] It is characterized by recurrent episodes of fever, serositis, arthralgia and synovitis of the large joints. Between attacks the joints return to normal. Untreated, it is associated with a high incidence of amyloidosis, the risk of which can be minimized by treating with colchicine.

Other periodic fever syndromes include the hyper-IgD syndrome which is characterized by recurrent fevers and an elevated immunoglobulin-D level. Mutations of the gene encoding mevalonate kinase have been identified in this condition.[181] An autosomal dominant syndrome characterized by periodic fever has been found to result from a mutation of the TNF receptor 1.[182]

Chronic infantile neurological, cutaneous and articular (CINCA) syndrome

This syndrome is characterized by the triad of rash, joint abnormalities and CNS involvement.[183] The rash which is urticarial and migratory appears in the first few months of life. Joint manifestations result from a disordered growth of cartilage (Fig. 29.69) and range from arthralgia and intermittent swelling to severe overgrowth of the epiphyses with loss of range of motion. Severe overgrowth of the patella is characteristic. Abnormalities of the CNS are universal and include chronic meningeal irritation, impairment of cognition and sensorineural deafness. Laboratory examination shows nonspecific elevation of inflammatory markers. Affected individuals have a characteristic facial appearance with frontal bossing, a hypoplastic midface and blond hair. This rare disorder is now known to be associated with dominantly inherited mutations in the CIAS1 gene, involved in the processing of IL-1β.[184] This has led to the therapeutic use of IL-1 blockade in the form of anakinra with dramatic benefit in many patients.

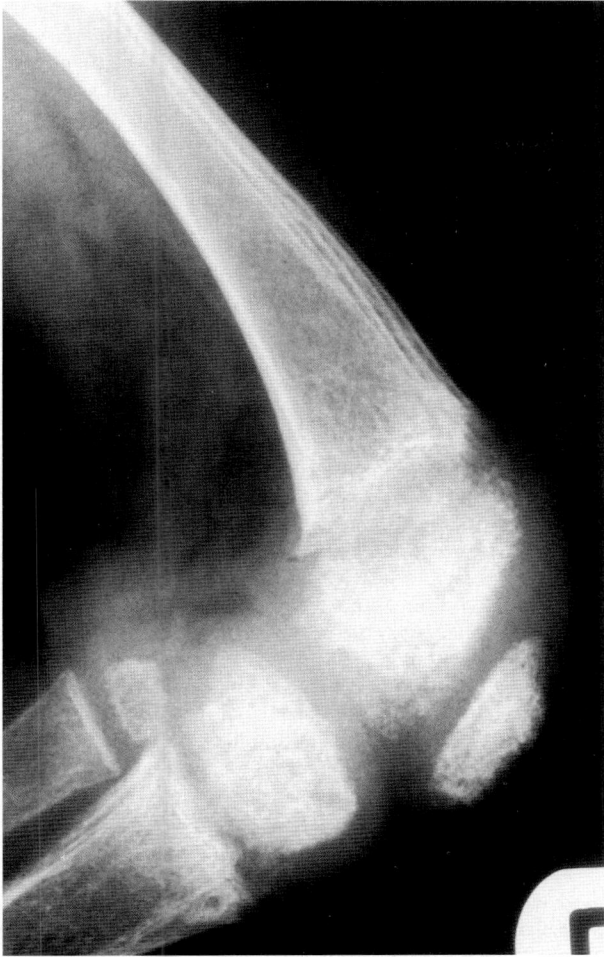

Fig. 29.69   Chronic infantile neurologic cutaneous and articular syndrome showing abnormal bone development.

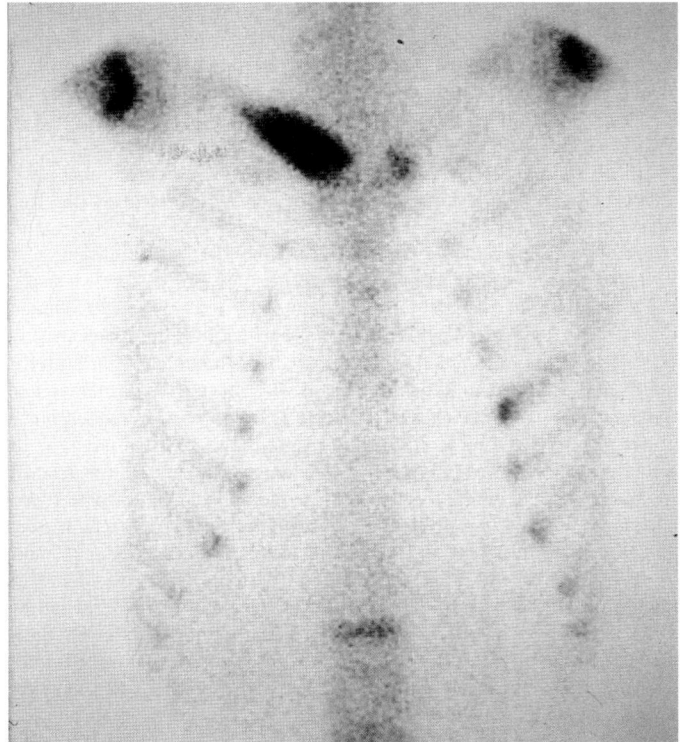
(a)

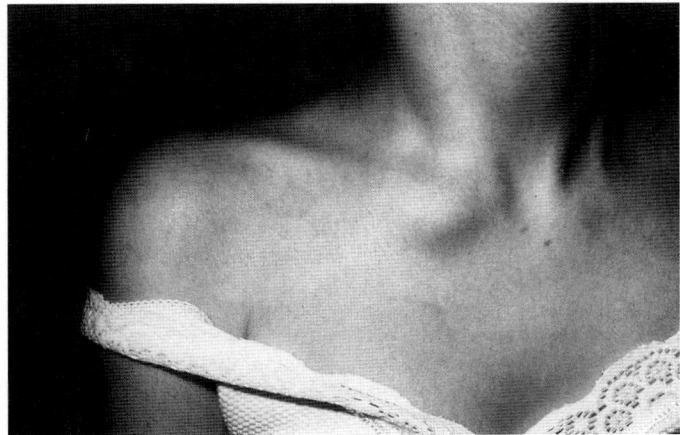
(b)

Fig. 29.70   SAPHO syndrome: (a) radionuclide bone scan demonstrating lesions in clavicle, rib and vertebra; (b) hyperostotic lesion of right clavicle.

Sarcoidosis

Sarcoidosis is an uncommon disorder in children and is characterized by a multisystem inflammatory process of unknown etiology. Two distinct disease patterns are seen although there are many cases where features overlap. In older children the pattern is very similar to that seen in adults with constitutional symptoms, lymphadenopathy and lung disease. In infants and young children a different pattern of disease is described with cutaneous involvement, arthropathy and uveiitis. Histologically the disease may result in the formation of granulomata. There is no single diagnostic test: serum levels of angiotensin converting enzyme are elevated in 80% but it should be remembered that levels are higher in normal children than in adults and pediatric standards are required. The Kveim test is no longer used.

SAPHO syndrome and chronic recurrent multifocal osteomylelitis (CRMO)

The SAPHO syndrome is an inflammatory disorder of unknown etiology characterized by synovitis, acne, pustulosis, hyperostosis and osteitis. Many cases only have a few of these features and CRMO, which is characterized by multifocal osteitic lesions, is thought to be part of the same spectrum of disease. The etiology is unknown. A family history of psoriasis is associated with SAPHO and an infectious trigger has been postulated, although no infecting organism is identified in most individuals. Radionuclide bone scanning is useful for demonstrating the multifocal nature of the problem (Fig. 29.70a). Biopsy may be necessary to exclude infection or malignancy. The hyperostostic clavicular lesions (Fig. 29.70b) may be both painful and cosmetically unsightly. Laboratory investigations may show mildly elevated inflammatory markers. Steroids and methotrexate are used to suppress the inflammatory process and bisphosphonates may also have a role.

CHRONIC PAIN SYNDROMES

Musculoskeletal pain is common in children and adolescents but generally shortlived and easily explained. A small group will develop unexplained disabling chronic musculoskeletal pain which poses a challenging diagnostic and management problem.

Pain is a universal phenomenon and in most cases a useful symptom, alerting the individual to tissue damage. Chronic pain differs in serving no useful function. Chronic pain occurring with no underlying physical disorder, or disproportionate chronic pain where the pain is out of all proportion to any known disease (the idiopathic pain syndromes), are perplexing conditions. Pain is by definition subjective and must therefore be accepted at face value.[185] The International Association for the Study of Pain[186] defines pain as 'an unpleasant sensory and emotional experience associated with actual or potential tissue damage, or described in terms of such damage ... It is unquestionably a sensation in part of the body but is always unpleasant and therefore also an emotional experience.'

In all reported series, idiopathic pain syndromes predominantly affect girls. The age of onset peaks in the early adolescent years and these conditions are uncommon under 8 years.[187] Recent data suggest that the prevalence of these conditions in childhood is increasing.[188]

Children with idiopathic pain syndromes are among the most disabled children seen in pediatric rheumatology and orthopedic clinics. They complain of severe pain unresponsive to standard therapies and frequently have major functional limitations. It is often difficult for both the family and pediatrician to accept that there is no organic pathology and the diagnosis is often delayed while a prolonged series of investigations is undertaken. With the correct diagnosis and management many will do well and it is therefore important to recognize these conditions as early as possible. The diagnosis is by definition one of exclusion of underlying pathology. In most cases this can be done on the basis of a careful history and clinical examination and few investigations are necessary or helpful.

The terminology and classification system used to define the idiopathic pain syndromes in the literature is confusing and generally unhelpful in children. Pain syndromes in children differ in many respects from those described in adults and frequently fail to meet criteria required for clearly defined syndromes. Children with pain syndromes seem to divide into two distinct groups: those with localized pain and those with diffuse or generalized pain.[189]

LOCALIZED IDIOPATHIC PAIN SYNDROMES

The best example of a localized pain syndrome in children is reflex sympathetic dystrophy (RSD) also known as complex regional pain syndrome type 1, reflex neurovascular dystrophy, algodystrophy and Sudeck atrophy. RSD is characterized by localized pain associated with evidence of autonomic dysfunction. In adults this syndrome usually follows immobilization of a limb following trauma. In children any preceding trauma is usually insignificant. It is presumed that the child stops using the limb in response to minor trauma and that subsequent changes are secondary to immobility, but the condition is poorly understood. Psychological factors are thought to be significant in the majority of children with the condition.[190] The child develops severe pain in the affected limb and rapidly becomes unable to use it. Hyperesthesia (an increased sensitivity to stimulation), allodynia (pain due to a stimulus that does not usually cause pain) and dysesthesia (an unpleasant abnormal sensation) are characteristic. The limb becomes cold, blue, diffusely swollen and at times may adopt bizarre postures (Fig. 29.71). Rarely, wasting and trophic changes occur.

The diagnosis in most cases is straightforward as long as the physician is aware of the condition and considers it. The child presents with a single cold, extremely painful limb and complains of severe pain on even light touch. Frequently they are unable to tolerate even a sock on the affected foot. Despite their predicament many seem remarkably unconcerned (la belle indifference) unless asked to touch or use the painful limb. With an atypical history or a younger child, care must be taken to ensure that no underlying pathology (particularly malignancy) is missed. A blood count, ESR, plain radiograph and radionuclide bone scan are usually sufficient, the typical bone scan in established RSD showing reduced uptake in the affected limb (Fig. 29.72).

The management of these children depends on establishing trust. Many have seen multiple health professionals before a diagnosis has been reached;[191] this frequently leads to increasing psychosocial difficulty and a loss of faith in the medical profession. It is essential to successfully reassure both child and family that there is no underlying organic pathology while accepting their pain at face value. Once the diagnosis is made a simple explanation of the effect of immobilization on a limb is usually easily accepted and the role of 'stress' in contributing to this condition can be discussed. A combination of an individualized program of physiotherapy together with attention to psychological factors leads to full recovery in the majority.[187,192] Sympathetic blockade and other treatment modalities used in affected adults are neither necessary nor helpful in the management of children and young people with RSD.

RSD is only one form of localized pain syndrome. Other individuals may have chronic musculoskeletal pain localized to one area of the body but without associated autonomic dysfunction. These syndromes are not clear cut and there is an overlap between such groups of patients.

DIFFUSE CHRONIC PAIN SYNDROMES

Widespread musculoskeletal pain affects a further group of young people, again predominantly female. The mean age tends to be slightly older than those with RSD with a peak at around 15 years. These patients can be subdivided into those with multiple tender points who meet criteria for the diagnosis of fibromyalgia and those without specific tender points. In our experience it is unhelpful to differentiate between

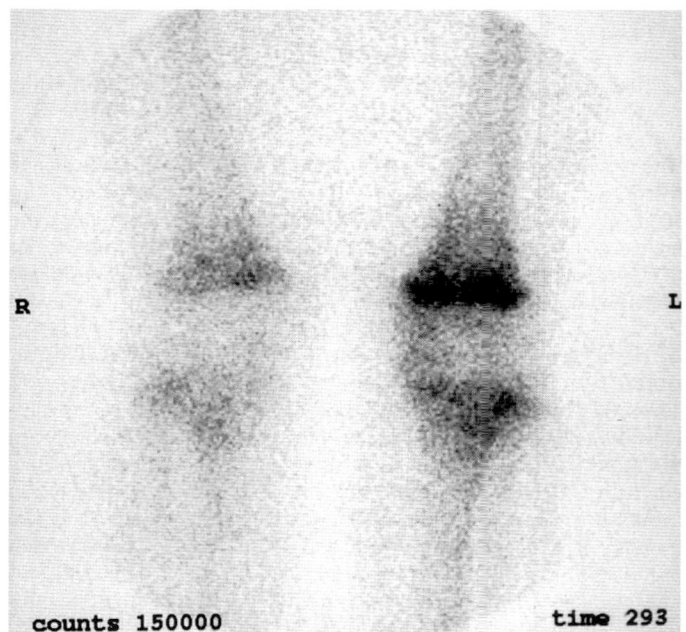

Fig. 29.71 Bizarre posturing of the hand in reflex sympathetic dystrophy.

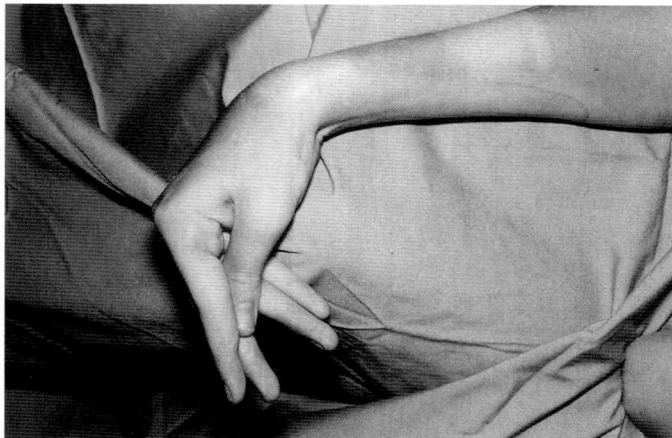

counts 150000   time 293

Fig. 29.72 Radionuclide bone scan in reflex sympathetic dystrophy showing reduced uptake in (R) affected compared to the (L) normal limb.

the two groups. There are no significant differences between them and they differ in many ways from adults with fibromyalgia. It is more helpful to class all as simply having a diffuse chronic pain syndrome.

In association with their pain many of these young people complain of fatigue, poor sleep and, in some, feelings of depression. There appears to be an overlap between this group of teenagers and those with chronic fatigue syndrome, the exact diagnosis depending on whether the pain or the fatigue predominates.

The etiology of this group of disorders is unknown. An association with hypermobility has been noted and psychosocial factors are contributory.[193,194] Management of these young people is similar to those with localized pain, although the outcome is generally less good with a higher incidence of relapse. An exercise regimen will often result in significant improvement but relapse when this is withdrawn is frequent. Attention to psychological factors is essential. In some, particularly those with poor sleep, the use of drugs such as tricyclic antidepressants may be helpful. Recent interest has focussed on improving methods and developing tools for assessing the impact of chronic pain on these young people.[195]

BACK PROBLEMS IN CHILDHOOD AND ADOLESCENCE

Neck or back pain is unusual in the young child and must be taken seriously. Persistent or deteriorating pain is an important complaint and tumors and infections should always be considered in the differential diagnosis. Localized pain is usually more suggestive of significant pathology than ill-defined pain, but young children are often unable to give a history of local pain and some conditions such as discitis may present with odd symptoms such as a gait abnormality or even abdominal pain.

In the adolescent population complaints of ill-defined pain without pathological explanation are common.[196] Nevertheless careful evaluation is important. Additional signs and symptoms such as torticollis, scoliosis or neurological radicular symptoms will direct the approach to appropriate investigations.

As a rule of thumb, while pain, or pain provoking pathology, may cause abnormal spinal postures like torticollis or scoliosis, it is unusual for congenital or developmental explanations for spinal deformity to be responsible for pain.

TUMORS

Malignant neoplasms, primary or secondary, though rare, are a potential source of back pain in children. Primary tumors can arise from the bone, such as Ewing sarcoma; from the hemopoietic tissue, such as the leukemias; or from the contained neurological tissue or its coverings. Only 3% of primary bone tumors occur in the axial skeleton and in children 60% of these are benign.[197] The most common benign lesions include osteoid osteoma or osteoblastoma, eosinophilic granuloma and aneurysmal bone cysts.

Osteoid osteomas typically involve the posterior elements and characteristically present with pain, especially night pain classically relieved by NSAIDs. Radiographs may show an area of sclerosis; radionuclide bone scanning will reveal intense focal uptake in the lesion. Subsequent CT scanning will identify a discrete lesion with a thick sclerotic rim and a lucent nidus of osteoid material at the center. Osteoblastoma is similar histologically to osteoid osteoma but larger. Aneurysmal bone cysts are typically expansile lytic lesions with a thin rim of cortical bone. Once again they usually occur in the posterior elements but may involve the adjacent pedicle or body. Eosinophilic granuloma usually affects the body of the vertebra which subsequently flattens, giving the characteristic vertebra plana of Calvé disease.

INFECTION

See section on 'Infection in bones and joints', page 1401.

TORTICOLLIS

Torticollis secondary to congenital and developmental problems is not usually accompanied by pain. In practice the commonest cause of painful torticollis in children is atlantoaxial rotatory displacement, but it is important to bear in mind that there are other explanations including infections, tumors, CNS abnormalities like syringomyelia, and ocular dysfunction.[198]

Atlantoaxial rotatory displacement

Typically the child awakes with a 'wryneck'. This commonly resolves without treatment over the course of a week but occasionally the posture persists when it is best described as atlantoaxial rotatory fixation. There is often associated muscle spasm of the long sternocleidomastoid muscle because of its attempts to correct the deformity, unlike congenital muscular torticollis where the contracted muscle is responsible for the deformity.

In most cases the etiology is not apparent although the condition can be caused by trauma or occur in association with recent upper respiratory tract infection. When subluxation occurs in association with inflammation of adjacent neck tissues or upper respiratory tract infection it is known as Grisel syndrome. It is postulated that hyperemia of the atlantoaxial joints leads to variable ligament laxity and synovitis. Thickened synovial folds may subsequently impinge during rotation and lead to fixation.

Diagnosis in the acute stage is based on the history. Radiological assessment is difficult because of the head posture, but in the anteroposterior film the anteriorly rotated lateral mass of C1 appears wider and closer to the midline than the posteriorly rotated lateral mass. Because of the difficulty in interpretation of plain radiographs, CT scanning or dynamic MRI is usually of more value for definitive diagnosis.

Atlantoaxial rotatory displacement with minimal subluxation and no encroachment of the vertebral canal is relatively benign. Greater degrees of subluxation are rare but do have potentially serious neurological complications because of increasing encroachment of the vertebral canal. Most cases resolve spontaneously with simple analgesia and a soft collar for support. If persistent the patient should be admitted for halter traction with analgesia and muscle relaxation. Halo traction is occasionally required, especially if presentation is delayed. If the displacement is fixed and significant there is potential compromise of the vertebral canal and surgical fusion is a consideration.

Paroxysmal torticollis of infancy

Paroxysmal torticollis of infancy is a rare episodic torticollis of unknown etiology. Episodes last for minutes to days with eventual spontaneous recovery. Two thirds of affected children are girls, with an average age of onset of 3 months. Attacks usually occur in the morning, occurring 1–4 times each month and can be associated with trunk curvature, eye deviations and torticollis which may alternate sides on different episodes. The condition usually resolves over 12–24 months and requires no treatment.

Sandifer syndrome

This syndrome is the association of infant gastroesophageal reflux with posturing of the neck and trunk. It is believed that the torticollis is the child's attempt to decrease the discomfort resulting from reflux.

JUVENILE DISCITIS

See previous section on 'Infection in bones and joints', page 1401.

Calcific discitis

This condition occurs in children with an average age of onset of 8 years. It is most common in the cervical spine and usually presents with the acute onset of neck pain and sometimes torticollis. Radiographs reveal calcified deposits in the affected nucleus pulposus. The etiology of the condition is unknown and treatment is symptomatic. The calcific deposits disappear in most patients by 6 months.

SCHEUERMANN KYPHOSIS

This condition can be responsible for a painful kyphosis. Patients present either with pain or an increasing round back deformity during adolescence (Fig. 29.73). The condition is more frequent in the thoracic but can also occur in the lumbar spine. There is usually a clear apex to the spinal deformity, which is relatively rigid distinguishing the condition from benign postural round back, which is flexible on extension. Lateral radiographs show vertebral wedging, end-plate irregularity and Schmorl node formation (herniation of intervertebral disc into the end-plate of an adjacent vertebra).

Treatment of the deformity with extension exercises and ocasionally extension bracing is usually successful. Surgical intervention for severe deformities is seldom required.

SPONDYLOLISTHESIS AND SPONDYLOLYSIS

Spondylolisthesis is the slipping forward of a vertebra on its neighbor below. It is classified into five types. Isthmic and dysplastic types are most common in children; degenerative, traumatic and pathological types are unusual.

Isthmic spondylolisthesis occurs when a defect or lysis develops in the pars interarticularis (spondylolysis) and is most common in L5 and L4 (Fig. 29.74). This defect is usually the result of a stress fracture at the pars. Affected patients often give a history of sporting activity. The vertebra concerned, having lost its 'bony hook' on the vertebra below, is able to slip forward, although this probably only occurs in about 20% of cases of spondylolysis. Clinical examination of a significant slip reveals a step on palpation of the lumbar spine and so-called 'heart shaped buttocks' because of the deformity.

Neurological radicular symptoms are rare but there is often associated hamstring spasm. The defect can be seen on oblique radiographs (the classic 'collar on the Scottie dog') but is best seen on reverse gantry CT scanning. If the slip is translated less than 50% symptoms can be treated by activity modification, analgesia and bracing. If symptoms settle the patient can be observed. Persistent symptoms, a slip of more than 50% or progressive slippage are all indications for surgical intervention. There are various surgical techniques but the principle is to fuse the unstable vertebra to its neighbor below.

Dysplastic (or congenital) spondylolisthesis is due to hypoplasia of the L5/S1 facet joint. This leads to instability of the L5 vertebra, which may subsequently slip.

ADOLESCENT DISC PROLAPSE

Disc prolapse is infrequent in children but occurs occasionally in adolescents when its presentation is somewhat different from adults. Stiffness is a more common symptom than back pain. There is commonly severe hamstring spasm with very limited straight leg raising and a spinal list (or tilt) is often present. The majority resolve without need for surgical intervention. If MRI shows a large sequestered fragment of disc material with significant symptoms, surgical excision may be considered.

OSTEOPOROSIS

Osteoporosis is a major health problem in the modern world and of major consequence in terms of its associated morbidity, mortality and health economics. The formation of bone structure occurs primarily during childhood and adolescence, with 90% of the peak bone mass being accumulated during the years of longitudinal growth. At any given age,

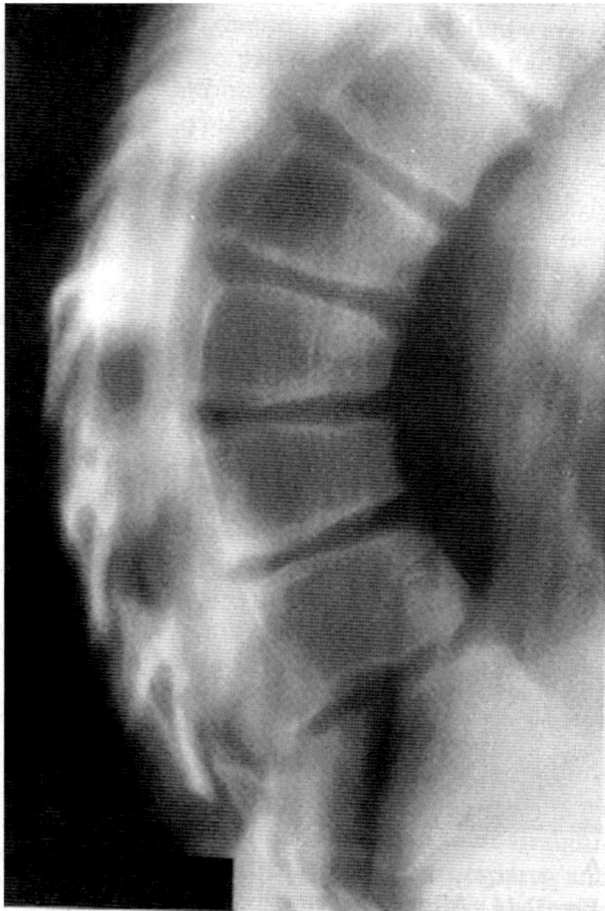

Fig. 29.73   Scheuermann kyphosis.

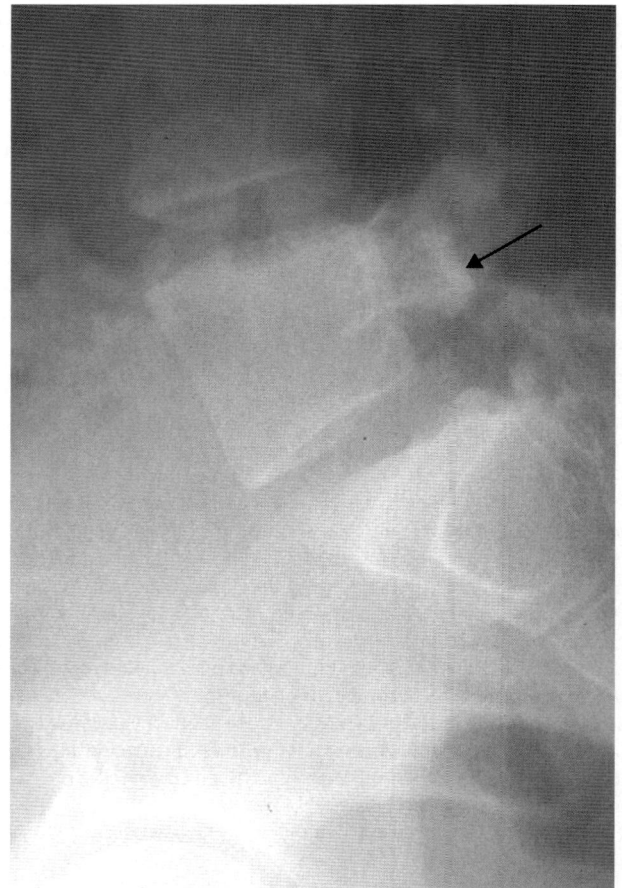

Fig. 29.74   Spondylolysis of L5.

bone mass is the result of both the peak bone mass, i.e. that acquired during the growth years, and the rate of age-related loss which starts from around 30 years and accelerates in women after the menopause. Optimization of skeletal development during childhood and adolescence therefore has a role in the longer term reduction in osteoporosis. This becomes particularly important when caring for children with chronic diseases which may adversely influence bone formation.

Bone exists in a constant state of remodeling during which old bone is removed and replaced by new bone. Bone gain during childhood and adolescence, and bone loss in later life, is therefore the result of a positive or negative balance between these two processes. This balance can be altered or disrupted by a variety of other factors. Bone structure is influenced by both genetic and lifestyle factors. It has been estimated that up to 80% of bone mineral density (BMD) can be accounted for by genetic factors, with gender, race and body size being important determinants. A number of candidate gene polymorphisms have been identified that are significant in relation to bone mass. Of particular importance appear to be polymorphisms of the vitamin D receptor, estrogen receptor and collagen type 1 alpha-1 genes. Other polymorphic genes encoding for bone proteins, hormones and cytokines may prove significant and it seems likely that a great variety of genes are involved in determining bone mass and strength. Lifestyle factors have an important contribution to make, with diet and physical activity being particularly important. There is a relationship between the amounts of muscle and fat in the body and the amount of bone: any dieting that results in an excessive weight loss will be associated with bone loss. Nutritional factors such as dietary calcium and vitamin D are contributory and ensuring an adequate intake will optimize bone development. Physical activity has an importance influence on bone density and an adequate amount of weightbearing activity is essential for optimal bone growth.

The World Health Organization defines osteoporosis as 'a disease characterized by low bone mass and micro-architectural deterioration of bone tissue, leading to enhanced bone fragility and a consequent increased risk in fracture'. Categories of disease are based on the measurement of BMD, with osteoporosis being defined as BMD more than 2.5 SD below the young adult mean value. Severe or established osteoporosis is defined as more than 2.5 SD below the young adult mean value in the presence of one or more low-trauma or fragility fractures.

These diagnostic criteria for osteoporosis have limitations. It must be remembered that they were developed in postmenopausal women and their applicability to other groups such as males and younger patients remains unclear. For such groups the relationship between BMD and fracture risk may be different and it is the fracture risk that is ultimately of importance. There are also difficulties inherent in the measurement of BMD in the growing child (see below) which may make the use of such definitions inappropriate. The definition of osteoporosis where fractures have not yet occurred is therefore somewhat arbitrary at present in children and young people. Further work is needed in this area.

ASSESSMENT OF BONE DENSITY IN PEDIATRIC PRACTICE

Conventional radiography is a relatively insensitive method of assessing bone mass and significant osteoporosis can only be diagnosed confidently when associated with a typical fracture. There has been interest in the use of ultrasound to assess bone density[199] and its acceptibility in pediatric practice may lead to further interest in this method in the future. Quantitative methods of CT scanning can be used to assess bone density but the tool most frequently used now, and generally regarded as the gold standard, is DEXA (dual energy X-ray absorptiometry) scanning.

DEXA scanning can be used to assess muscle mass, total and percent body fat and bone mineral. DEXA measures both the bone mineral content and the bone mineral density. This has a number of pitfalls in pediatric practice and results must be interpreted with care.[200] The amount of bone mineral content is directly related to body size and it is necessary to correlate values with skeletal size. Reference standards for children in different populations are not widely available, while genetic and racial difference in bone density make population-based reference values essential. In addition, machines vary considerably and calibration is important. With these provisos DEXA appears at present to be the method of choice for the assessment of bone density. Measurements are generally taken from the lumbar spine and proximal femur. Results should be expressed in terms of the number of standard deviations above or below the mean of an age-related control population (Z-score). DEXA provides a quantitative method that can be repeated serially to monitor change and assess the effects of treatment, provided the results are interpreted with caution in the growing child or adolescent.

PRIMARY OR IDIOPATHIC JUVENILE OSTEOPOROSIS

Primary osteoporosis is rare in childhood. Juvenile osteoporosis occurs before or around puberty, affects both sexes and is of unknown pathophysiology. The child will present with pain in the back, hips and feet with evidence of fractures including vertebral crush fractures (Fig. 29.75). This is a self-limiting condition which resolves with puberty but treatment with pamidronate to reduce pain and increase bone density during the active phase may be helpful.

SECONDARY OSTEOPOROSIS IN CHILDHOOD

Osteoporosis in children usually occurs in relation to some underlying chronic disease or as a consequence of treatment with glucocorticoids.

Disease related

Osteoporosis is increasingly recognized as an important sequel of a number of chronic childhood disorders, contributing greatly to the long term morbidity. In the childhood rheumatic disorders such as

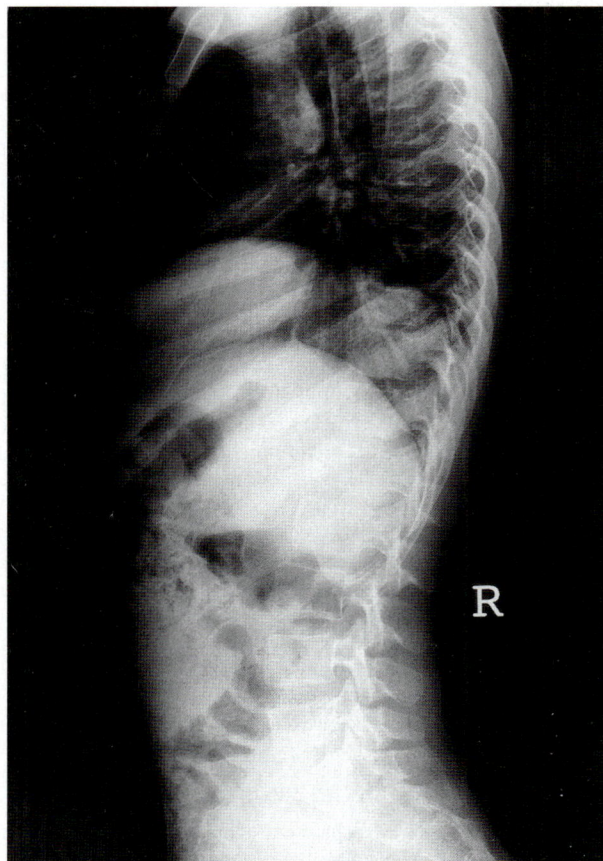

Fig. 29.75 Idiopathic juvenile osteoporosis – plain radiograph showing osteoporotic collapse of thoracic vertebrae.

juvenile idiopathic arthritis, dermatomyositis or systemic lupus erythematosus, osteoporosis occurs as a direct result of the underlying inflammatory process and prevention depends on optimal control of the disease process. Nutritional impairment, immobility or even relative inactivity in children with chronic ill-health are all contributory. Other unknown factors which are disease specific are clearly of importance, e.g. individuals with JDM or SLE appear more vulnerable than those with juvenile arthritis.

Drug related

Glucocorticosteroids are widely used in the treatment of a number of common diseases in childhood including the rheumatic disorders, inflammatory bowel disease, asthma and nephrotic syndrome. Although clearly necessary for treatment their effect on bone mineral density can be significant. The adverse effects of steroids on bone metabolism are well known and result from a variety of actions of these drugs. They are known to induce renal calcium efflux and inhibit calcium uptake from the intestine, leading to a fall in serum calcium and secondary hyperparathyroidism. This increases bone resorption and reduces bone formation and is well documented immediately after commencement of treatment. The increase in bone resorption does not usually continue but the amount of new bone formation is reduced as a result of increased apoptosis of osteoblasts and contributes to ongoing bone loss. The bulk of the bone loss in steroid-induced osteoporosis occurs in the first 6 months of treatment but overall the effect is related both to the total dose used and to the duration of therapy. There is considerable individual variation in the effect of steroids on bone density presumably as a result of genetic factors. Some individuals will tolerate a significant dose with no adverse effect whereas others will become significantly osteoporotic with minimal dosage regimens.

Other drugs such as methotrexate, heparin and thyroxine are known to reduce bone mineral density but none has been shown to have significant clinical effect in pediatric practice.

PROPHYLAXIS OF OSTEOPOROSIS IN CHILDHOOD

There is ongoing debate regarding the use of prophylactic measures to prevent osteoporosis in childhood. General advice regarding exercise and nutrition are important. Weightbearing exercise is clearly beneficial and with an increasingly sedentary lifestyle for many it is important to advise patients regarding this. The avoidance of severe weight loss is also important.

A diet with an adequate calcium intake is frequently lacking in adolescents. There has been much interest in the relationship between calcium intake and bone mineral acquisition and some evidence that calcium supplementation can increase bone mineral density. Any benefit shown in children and adolescents is transient and disappears when the supplementation is discontinued, making it seem unlikely that this is of any longer term benefit. Current evidence supports the use of calcium supplements to improve bone mineralization where the diet is deficient[201] but the benefits of supplementing above the normal dietary recommended intake are unproven.

Current recommendations for adults are that patients on steroids should receive prophylactic treatment for bone loss. There are no recommendations for children. A recent survey of pediatric rheumatology units in the UK (unpublished data) showed no consensus on the use of prophylactic measures in the prevention of steroid-induced osteoporosis. Some units advocate general advice only, some prescribe calcium supplements and others calcium and vitamin D for all children going on to long term steroids. At the moment there is no clear evidence on which to base a decision.

TREATMENT OF OSTEOPOROSIS IN CHILDHOOD

Until relatively recently, no specific treatments were available for osteoporosis. The advent of the bisphosphonates has altered our approach to the investigation and identification of at-risk children as there is now an effective treatment that can be used to reduce fracture risk.[202]

The bisphosphonates are synthetic compounds whose main action consists of the inhibition of osteoclastic bone resorption. The newer bisphosphonates are thought to act directly on the osteoclast to induce apoptosis. There were initial concerns about the use of these drugs in children with rapidly growing bones and in women of child-bearing potential. They are of low molecular weight and therefore likely to be able to cross the placenta. Fetal bone turnover is high and these drugs could potentially cause substantial effects on skeletal development. Nonetheless the cost of untreated osteoporosis is such that these drugs are now well established for use in pediatric practice.

The first generation bisphosphonates such as etidronate have been associated with bone mineralization defects and have generally been superseded in pediatric practice by the newer drugs such as pamidronate and alendronate. Pamidronate is the established treatment for osteoporosis in children and adolescents and is generally well tolerated. It has the disadvantage of requiring to be given by intravenous infusion and there is therefore increasing interest in the use of an oral alternative such as alendronate.[203]

Where there is established osteoporosis with evidence of a fracture there seems little doubt that the use of these drugs is appropriate. With reduced BMD but no fracture, there is no clear agreement as to when children should be treated as the relationship between BMD and fracture risk is not clearly established. Most clinicians would agree that a BMD measurement more than 3 SD below the mean is likely to represent an increased fracture risk and would therefore merit treatment.

OVERUSE AND SPORT-RELATED PROBLEMS IN CHILDREN

Active children frequently present with a variety of musculoskeletal symptoms that are a consequence of their activity. Such overuse syndromes can present in any child but become more common in the participants of organized competitive sport. While children are subject to the same injuries as adults, their immature musculoskeletal system responds somewhat differently. Submaximal loading of musculoskeletal structures leads to tissue damage, followed by repair. Repeated submaximal loading results in tissue hypertrophy. Overuse syndromes are characterized by the development of inflammatory pain when tissue damage exceeds the rate of tissue repair. The structures involved can be the bones, the soft tissues or, most commonly the junctions where they converge. In children these junctions are weaker than either the tendons or ligaments: apophysitis and avulsion fractures are therefore more common than ligament or tendon rupture. In children tendon rupture is also rare because overuse typically results in inflammation of the tendon sheath (tenosynovitis) rather than the tendon itself (tendonitis), and tendon degeneration is rare in the young.

STRESS FRACTURES

Stress fractures are undisplaced fatigue fractures, which develop as a result of repeated loading. The lower limbs are most frequently affected especially the metatarsals (march fractures) and the tibia.

Younger children and even toddlers can present with stress fractures but they are more common in adolescents where the proximal third of the tibia is the most frequent site, and running the most common explanation.[204] Symptoms of localized pain develop insidiously and are usually relieved by rest. Plain radiographs eventually show a localized periosteal reaction and increased density, but are frequently unhelpful at presentation. Radionuclide bone scanning is a more sensitive investigation. Infection and tumors can present with similar features and should always be considered in the differential diagnosis.

Treatment involves protection from further trauma, which sometimes involves immobilization and always involves abstinence from the causative stress, usually running. Once symptoms have resolved a gradual return to activity can be begun.

EPIPHYSEOLYSIS

Repeated traction, compression, torsion and angular stress on the growth plate (physis) can lead to stress injury resulting in localized peri-articular pain. Radiographs reveal widening of the growth plate and irregularity of the metaphyseal margin (Fig. 29.76). Involvement of the proximal humeral physis has been reported in baseball pitchers,[205] while female gymnasts have involvement of the distal radius.[206] Treatment involves modification of activity. Severe cases can be slow to resolve and premature physeal closure with subsequent wrist problems have been reported in gymnasts.[207]

OSTEOCHONDRITIS DISSECANS

See 'Common orthopedic problems in childhood', page 1415.

APOPHYSITIS

In the growing skeleton tendons join long bones at sites of ossification called apophyses. Apophysitis is inflammation at these junctions as a result of traction injury caused by the repeated pull of the attached tendon. Radiographs often reveal fragmentation and sclerosis of the apophysis with small, avulsed ossified fragments. Patients are usually in the adolescent age range from about 10 to 16 years. Symptoms usually begin insidiously, are made worse by activity and better by rest. Eponymous names are associated with the condition at some sites, but all are benign self-limiting conditions. The usual natural history is resolution by maturity. Treatment includes activity modification and symptomatic treatment. Occasionally in young athletes, explosive contraction of a muscle causes a tendon to pull off its whole attachment with a significant fragment of bone.

Pelvic apophysitis and avulsion fractures

The hip and pelvis can be the source of symptoms at the site of several apophyses. Sudden explosive contraction of the attached muscles can result in acute avulsion fractures of these apophyses and repeated submaximal trauma can result in the insidious development of symptoms. The iliac crest is the site of insertion of the abdominal muscles and can become painful as a result of trunk rotation such as when running. Other sites of apophysitis around the hip and pelvis include the insertion of sartorius at the anterior superior iliac spine (Fig. 29.77), the insertion of the rectus femoris at the anterior inferior iliac spine, the insertion of the gluteal muscles at the greater trochanter, the insertion of the psoas muscle at the lesser trochanter and the insertion of the hamstrings at the ischial tuberosity. Each of these conditions can explain pain in and around the hip region, but in the adolescent age range more serious explanations such as a slipped capital femoral epiphysis must be considered.

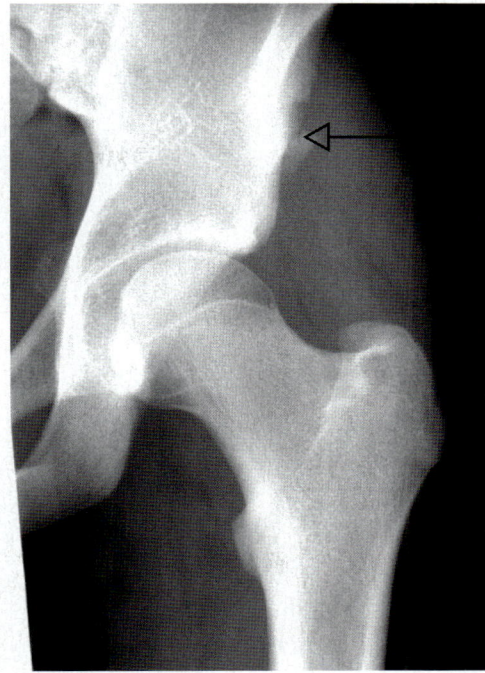

Fig. 29.77   Avulsion of anterior superior iliac spine.

Osgood–Schlatter disease

Osgood–Schlatter disease of the tibial tuberosity is the most common apophysitis, presenting in approximately 15% of teenage boys and 10% of teenage girls.[208] There is localized pain and swelling at the tibial tuberosity. Radiographs typically show fragmentation of the tibial tuberosity with avulsed fragments (Fig. 29.78). Symptoms usually respond to activity modification. In the enthusiastic young athlete sport need not be prevented but simply modified. Occasionally symptoms do persist after maturity with up to 20% of mature patients complaining of discomfort when kneeling.[209] Treatment is seldom required or helpful, except if a loose ossicle persists, when excision can be curative.

Sinding–Larsen–Johansson disease

Sinding–Larsen–Johansson disease is apophysitis at the lower pole of the patella. It is similar to Osgood–Schlatter disease and the two conditions can coexist (Fig. 29.78). Treatment follows a conservative activity modification approach.

Sever disease

Sever disease is inflammation of the calcaneal apophysis, at the insertion of the tendo-Achilles. Radiographs show increased density and fragmentation of the calcaneal apophysis, but this appearance is nonspecific and can be seen in asymptomatic subjects. Treatment is conservative and a heel lift is sometimes helpful.

Iselin disease

Iselin disease is apophysitis at the insertion of peroneus brevis at the base of the fifth metatarsal. It should not be confused with fractures in the vicinity, which can follow acute trauma.

VALGUS OVERLOAD OF THE ELBOW

Valgus overload of the elbow occurs in a variety of throwing and batting sports and in activities where the upper limb is required to bear heavy loads such as in gymnastics. Perhaps the best example is the

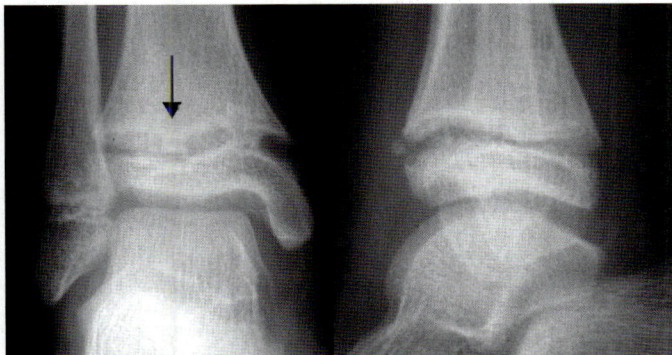

Fig. 29.76   Epiphyseolysis of distal tibia.

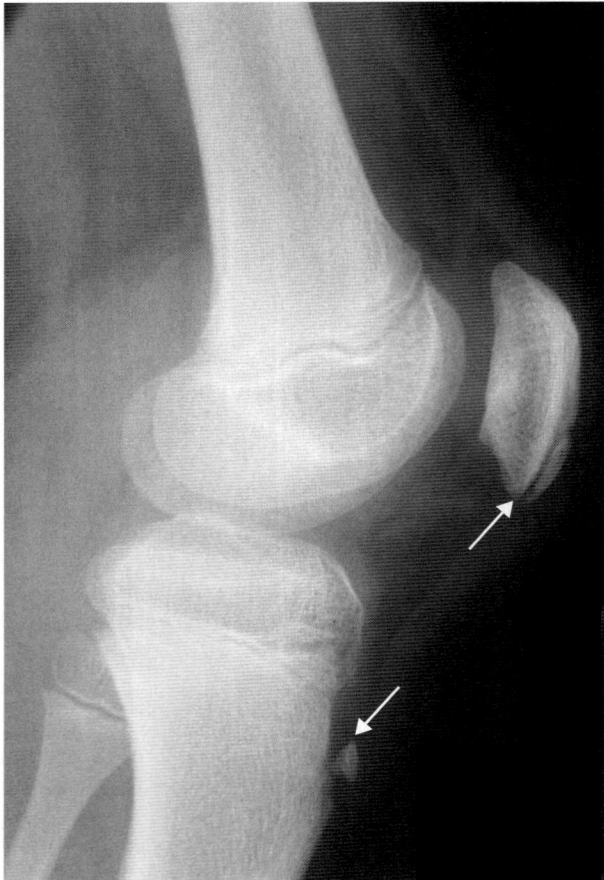

Fig. 29.78   Knee with coincidental Osgood–Schlatter and Sinding–Larsen–Johansson disease.

junior baseball pitcher – 'Little Leaguer's elbow'. Valgus stress of the elbow generates tension and distraction of the medial structures, including the medial collateral ligament and the medial epicondyle and compression of the lateral structures, namely the capitellum and the radial head. The young athlete can develop problems in any of these areas.[210] The medial epicondyle may become painful and prominent in a typical apophysitis-like presentation. Occasionally the medial epicondyle can be completely avulsed and if significantly displaced it should be reduced and fixed. The ossific nucleus of the capitellum may become fragmented with appearances similar to Perthes disease when the condition is referred to as Panner disease. If the patient is young the prognosis for complete resolution is good. Older and adolescent patients can also develop subchondral defects, which are considered to be a form of osteochondritis dissecans. Loose flaps or loose bodies can develop causing mechanical symptoms including elbow locking as well as pain. Treatment of the painful elbow usually involves activity modification but surgical debridement may be necessary if mechanical symptoms secondary to a loose body occur.

SNAPPING TENSOR FASCIA LATA SYNDROME

The iliotibial band is a broad condensation of the fascia on the lateral side of the leg running from the tensor fascia lata muscle at the iliac crest, across the greater trochanter of the hip and across the lateral side of the knee. When the leg is adducted at the hip and internally and externally rotated the iliotibial band can be pushed backward and forward by the passing greater trochanter beneath. The band is put under tension and then suddenly snaps back with a disconcerting clunk. If this occurs repeatedly a tender secondary trochanteric bursitis develops. The condition is more common in girls and the clunking is sometimes

voluntary. Management includes stretching exercises, avoidance of the provoking movements and reassurance because some patients believe that their hip is dislocating. The condition sometimes presents in runners and if refractory to conservative management the iliotibial band can be lengthened by 'Z' plasty.

ILIOTIBIAL BAND FRICTION SYNDROME

This condition is caused by rubbing of the iliotibial band against the lateral epicondyle at the distal femur during repetitive knee flexion and extension. It usually affects runners and most cases are associated with a recent increase in activity.[211] Activity modification sometimes including stretching exercises, is the mainstay of treatment.

ANTERIOR KNEE PAIN, PATELLOFEMORAL PAIN SYNDROME AND CHONDROMALACIA

See 'Common orthopedic problems in childhood', page 1415.

MENISCAL INJURIES OF THE KNEE

Meniscal tears are unusual in young children unless there is an underlying meniscal anomaly such as a discoid meniscus (see 'Common orthopedic problems in childhood', p. 1415). In adolescence the incidence of meniscal tears begins to increase and are usually related to sport. Meniscal tears usually result from a twisting injury when a 'pop' is sometimes heard or felt, followed by knee swelling. There are few specific and reliable clinical tests but the patient may give a history of giving way and 'true' knee locking. 'True' locking specifically implies a block to full extension. If a tear is suspected, MRI is a sensitive investigation. In young patients the meniscus is more vascular than in the adult and is more likely to heal following injury. In recent years the vital role of the meniscus in load distribution and proper knee function has become recognized and preservation or repair of the injured meniscus, especially in young patients, is important. Fortunately children and adolescents have a higher incidence of peripheral tears which, because of a good peripheral blood supply, are more amenable to successful repair.[212]

COLLATERAL AND CRUCIATE LIGAMENT INJURY OF THE KNEE

Ligament injury of the knee, and indeed of other joints, is rare in young children, becoming increasingly common as maturity is approached. Rupture of collateral and cruciate ligaments does sometimes occur, the mechanism of injury being similar to that in the adult. In the child ligaments are stronger than the bone to which they are attached, and mechanisms that would lead to rupture of a ligament in an adult lead to avulsion of the underlying bone. The best example is an avulsion fracture of the tibial eminence, the site of insertion of the anterior cruciate ligament. In general terms if avulsion fractures are significantly displaced from their origin, management includes reduction and sometimes fixation.

BREASTSTROKER'S KNEE

Competitive breaststrokers can develop medial knee pain along the medial collateral ligament. The 'whip kick' technique, a modified frog kick, has been associated with the problem. Rest and avoidance of the technique is helpful.

'SHIN SPLINTS'

'Shin splints' is a term that has emerged to describe exercise-induced shin pain in the athlete. It is a nonspecific clinical presentation with a number of underlying pathological explanations. Radiographs are important to exclude serious explanations for bone pain such as infection or tumor and may identify other explanations such as stress fractures.

Periostitis

Inflammation of the tibial periosteum or periostitis is a common cause for shin splints syndrome. It is characterized by pain along the postero-medial edge of the distal third of the tibia where the soleus muscle and its investing fascia originate. It is presumed to be a traction phenomenon and a variety of anatomical alignment variations such as forefoot pronation, genu valgum, femoral anteversion and external tibial torsion have been implicated as potential causes as well as poor footwear and training regimens.[213]

Radiographs sometimes show periosteal new bone along the postero-medial tibia and radionuclide bone scanning shows increased uptake in a longitudinal distribution in contradistinction to the transverse pattern of increased uptake seen in stress fractures.[214] Management should first involve an attempt to identify the underlying cause followed by conservative measures including footwear and activity modification to address the symptoms. Surgical treatment should only be considered as a last resort.

Chronic compartment syndrome

Chronic compartment syndrome develops when muscle volume increases as a result of increased blood flow during exercise. The relatively unexpandable osseofascial compartment cannot accommodate the extra volume, and pressure within the compartment increases. When the intracompartmental pressure exceeds capillary filling pressure the muscles within the compartment develop ischemic pain. This usually resolves a short time after exercise stops. Some patients may experience a transient foot drop. Chronic compartment syndrome can present with 'shin splints' symptoms indistinguishable from periostitis.[215] Diagnosis depends on measuring compartment pressures during exercise on a treadmill. All four compartments in the leg should be assessed although the most commonly affected is the anterior compartment. Initial treatment involves a conservative approach with footwear and activity modification. Surgical treatment in the form of fasciotomy is reported to be successful in 90%.[216]

Superficial peroneal nerve compression

Superficial peroneal nerve compression can also give rise to activity-related shin pain. The superficial peroneal nerve emerges from the fascia of the lower third of the anterolateral part of the leg to the subcutaneous plane where it travels distally, to supply sensory innervation to the dorsum of the foot. During exercise increased muscle pressure can compress the superficial peroneal nerve against the edge of the fascial hiatus where it emerges. This leads to exercise-induced leg pain, sometimes with associated local pain at the hiatus in the fascia and altered sensation on the dorsum of the foot. In troublesome cases limited fasciotomy at the fascial hiatus is effective.

REFERENCES (* Level 1 evidence)

1. De Inocencio J. Epidemiology of musculoskeletal pain in primary care. Arch Dis Child 2004; 89:431–434.
2. Konijnenberg AY, Uiterwaal CS, Kimpen JL, et al. Children with unexplained chronic pain: substantial impairment in everyday life. Arch Dis Child 2005; 90:680–686.
3. Duffy CM. Measurement of health status, functional status, and quality of life in children with juvenile idiopathic arthritis: clinical science for the pediatrician. Pediatr Clin North Am 2005; 52:359–372.
4. Huber AM, Hicks JE, Lachenbruch PA, et al. Validation of the Childhood Health Assessment Questionnaire in the juvenile idiopathic myopathies. Juvenile Dermatomyositis Disease Activity Collaborative Study Group. J Rheumatol 2001; 28:1106–1111.
5. Foster HE, Cabral DA. Is musculoskeletal history and examination so different in pediatrics? Best Pract Clin Rheumatol 2006; 20:242–262.
6. Miller FW, Rider LG, Chung YL, et al. Proposed preliminary core set measures for disease outcome assessment in adult and juvenile idiopathic inflammatory myopathies. Rheumatology 2001; 40:1262–1273.
7. Lovell DJ, Lindsley CB, Rennebohm RM, et al. Development of validated disease activity and damage indices in the juvenile idiopathic inflammatory myopathies. II The Childhood Myositis Assessment Scale (CMAS): a quantitative tool for the evaluation of muscle function. The Juvenile Dermatomyositis Disease Activity Collaborative Study Group. Arthritis Rheum 1999; 42:2213–2219.
8. Binder H, Eng GD, Gaiser JF, et al. Congenital muscular torticollis: results of conservative management with long-term follow up in 85 cases. Arch Phys Med Rehabil 1987; 68:222–225.
9. Hensinger RN, Lang JR, MacEwan GD. The Klippel–Feil syndrome: a constellation of related anomalies. J Bone Joint Surg 1974; 56A:1246–1253.
10. Goldberg MJ, Bartoshesky LE. Congenital hand anomaly: etiology and associated malformations. Hand Clin 1985; 1:405–415.
11. Sachar K Mih A. Congenital radial head dislocations. Hand Clin 1998; 14:39–47.

12. Weighill FJ. The treatment of developmental coxa vara by abduction subtrochanteric and intertrochanteric femoral osteotomy with special reference to the role of adductor tenotomy. Clin Orthop 1976; 116:116–124.
*13. Godward S, Dezateux C. Surgery for congenital dislocation of the hip in the UK as a measure of outcome of screening. MRC working party on congenital dislocation of the hip. Lancet 1998; 351:1149–1152.
14. Jones D. Topic for debate at the crossroads – neonatal detection of developmental dysplasia of the hip. J Bone Joint Surg 2000; 82B:160–164.
15. The National Screening Committee 2006. Online. Available at: http://www.library.nhs.uk/screening/View Resource.aspx?resID=57180&tabID= 288re
16. Hoffman A, Wenger DR. Posteromedial bowing of the tibia. Progression in leg lengths. J Bone Joint Surg 1981; 63:384–388.
17. Schoenecker PL, Capelli AM, Millar EA, et al. Congenital longitudinal deficiency of the tibia. J Bone Joint Surg 1989; 71A:278–287.
18. Kalamchi A, Dawe RV. Congenital deficiency of the tibia. J Bone Joint Surg 1985; 67B:581–584.
19. Jacobsen ST, Crawford AH, Millar EA, et al. The Symes amputation in patients with congenital pseudoarthrosis of the tibia. J Bone Joint Surg 1983; 65A:533–537.
20. Harrold AJ, Walker CJ. Treatment and prognosis in congenital clubfoot. J Bone Joint Surg 1983; 65B:8–11.
21. Ponseti IV. Congenital clubfoot. Fundamentals of treatment. Oxford: Oxford University Press; 1996.
22. Hamanishi C. Congenital vertical talus: classification with 69 cases and new measurement system. J Pediatr Orthop 1984; 4:318–326.
23. Dobbs MB, Purcell DB, Nunley R, et al. Early results of a new method of treatment for idiopathic congenital vertical talus. J Bone Joint Surg Am 2006; 88:1192–1200.
24. Savariryan R, Rimoin DL. The skeletal dysplasias. Best Pract Clin Endocrinol Metab 2002; 16:547–560.
25. European Skeletal Dysplasia Network. Online. Available at: http://www.esdn.org
26. Beighton P, Solomon L, Soskolne CL. Articular mobility in an African population. Ann Rheum Dis 1973; 32:413–418.

27. van der Giessen LJ, Lickens D, Rutgers KJ, et al. Validation of Beighton score and prevalence of connective tissue signs in 773 Dutch children. J Rheumatol 2001; 28:2726–2730.
28. Grahame R, Bird HA, Child A. The revised (Brighton 1998) criteria for the diagnosis of joint hypermobility syndrome. J Rheumatol 2000; 27:1777–1779.
29. Grahame R. Heritable disorders of connective tissue. Best Pract Res Clin Rheumatol 2000; 14:345–361.
30. Adib N, Davies K, Grahame R, et al. Joint hypermobility syndrome in childhood. A not so benign multisystem disorder? Rheumatol 2005; 44:744–750.
31. Murray KJ. Hypermobility disorders in children and adolescents. Best Pract Res Clin Rheumatol 2006; 20:329–351.
32. Beighton P, De Paepe A, Steinmann B, et al. Ehlers–Danlos syndromes: revised nosology, Villefrance, 1997. Ehlers–Danlos National Foundation (USA) and Ehlers–Danlos Support Group (UK). Am J Med Genet 1998; 77:31–37.
33. Le Parc JM, Molcard S, Tubach F, et al. Marfan syndrome and fibrillin disorders. Joint Bone Spine 2000; 67:401–407.
34. De Paepe A, Devereux RB, Dietz HC, et al. Revised diagnostic criteria for the Marfan syndrome. Am J Med Genet 1996; 62:417–426.
35. Sakai H, Visser R, Ikegawa S, et al. Comprehensive genetic analysis of relevant four genes in 49 patients with Marfan syndrome or Marfan-related phenotypes. Am J Med Genet 2006; 140:1719–1725.
36. Rauch F, Glorieux FH. Osteogenesis imperfecta. Lancet 2004; 363: 1377–1385.
37. Venturi G, Tedeschi E, Mottes M, et al. Osteogenesis imperfecta: clinical, biochemical and molecular findings. Clin Genet 2006; 70:131–139.
38. Rauch F, Glorieux FH. Osteogenesis imperfecta, current and future medical treatment. Am J Med Genet C Semin Med Genet 2005; 139:31–37.
39. Rose PS, Levy HP, Liberfarb RM, et al. Stickler syndrome: clinical characteristics and diagnostic criteria. Am J Med Genet 2005; 138:199–207.
40. Kaplan FS, Fiori J, De La Pena LS, et al. Dysregulation of the BMP-4 signaling pathway in fibrodysplasia ossificans progressiva. Ann NY Acad Sci 2006; 1068:54–65.

41. Davies K, Stiehm ER, Woo P, et al. Juvenile idiopathic polyarticular arthritis and IgA deficiency in the 22q11 deletion syndrome. J Rheumatol 2001; 28:2326–2334.

42. McBride MB, Rigden S, Haycock GB, et al. Presymptomatic detection of familial juvenile hyperuricaemic nephropathy in children. Pediatr Nephrol 1998; 12:357–364.

43. Sonnen GM, Henry NK. Pediatric bone and joint infections. Pediatr Clin North Am 1996; 43:933–947.

44. Dagan R. Management of acute hematogenous osteomyelitis and septic arthritis in the pediatric patient. Pediatr Infect Dis J 1993; 12:88–93.

45. Kallio MJT, Unkila-Kallio L, Aalto K, et al. Serum C-reactive protein, erythrocyte sedimentation rate and white blood cell count in septic arthritis. Pediatr Infect Dis J 1997; 16:411–413.

46. Shetty AK, Gedalia A. Septic arthritis in children. Rheum Dis Clin North Am 1998; 24:287–304.

47. Davies EG, Monsell F. Managing osteoarticular infection in children. Curr Pediatrics 2000; 10:42–48.

48. Frank G, Mahoney HM, Eppes SC. Musculoskeletal infections in children. Pediatr Clin North Am 2005; 52:1083–1106.

49. Peltola H, Kallio-Unkila L, Kallio MJT, et al. Simplified treatment of acute staphylococcal osteomyelitis of childhood. Pediatrics 1997; 99: 846–850.

50. Wenger DR, Bobechko WP, Gilday DL. Spectrum of intervertebal disc space infection in children. J Bone Joint Surg 1978; 60A:100–108.

51. Tingle AJ, Allen M, Petty RE, et al. Rubella-associated arthritis. I. Comparative study of joint manifestations associated with natural rubella infection and RA 27/3 rubella immunization. Ann Rheum Dis 1986; 45:110–114.

52. Wall EJ. Childhood osteomyelitis and septic arthritis. Curr Opin Pediatr 1998; 10:73–76.

53. Dajani A, Taubert K, Ferrieri P, et al. Treatment of acute streptococcal pharyngitis and prevention of rheumatic fever: a statement for health professionals. Pediatrics 1995; 96:758–764.

54. Huppertz HI. Lyme disease in children. Curr Opin Rheumatol 2001; 13:434–439.

55. Packham JC, Hall MA. Long-term follow-up of 246 adults with juvenile idiopathic arthritis: functional outcome. Rheumatology 2002; 41:1428–1435.

56. Petty RE, Southwood TR, Manners P, et al. International League of Associations for Rheumatology classification of juvenile idiopathic arthritis: second revision, Edmonton, 2001. J Rheumatol 2004; 31:390–392.

57. Giannini EH, Ruperto N, Ravelli A, et al. Preliminary definition of improvement in juvenile arthritis. Arthritis Rheum 1997; 40:1202–1209.

58. Manners PJ, Bower C. Worldwide prevalence of juvenile arthritis: why does it vary so much? J Rheumatol 2002; 29:1520–1530.

59. Symmons DM, Jones M, Osborne J, et al. Paediatric rheumatology in the United Kingdom: data from the British Paediatric Rheumatology Group National Diagnostic Register. J Rheumatol 1996; 23:1975–1980.

60. Cassidy JT, Petty RE. 2001 Juvenile rheumatoid arthritis. In: Cassidy JT, Petty RE, eds. Textbook of pediatric rheumatology, 4th edn. Philadelphia: WB Saunders; 2001; 218–322.

61. Glass DN, Giannini EH. Juvenile Rheumatoid Arthritis as a complex genetic trait. Arthritis Rheum 1999; 42:2261–2268.

62. Murray KJ, Moroldo MB, Donnelly P, et al. Age-specific effects of juvenile rheumatoid arthritis-associated alleles. Arthritis Rheum 1999; 42: 1843–1853.

63. Thompson W, Barrett JH, Donn RP, et al. Juvenile idiopathic arthritis classified by the ILAR criteria: HLA associations in UK patients. Rheumatol 2002; 41:1183–1189.

64. Choy ES, Panayi GS. Cytokine pathways and joint inflammation in rheumatoid arthritis. N Engl J Med 2001; 344:907–916.

65. Grom AA, Murray KJ, Luyrink L, et al. Patterns of expression of tumor necrosis factor α, tumor necrosis factor β, and their receptors in the synovia of patients with juvenile rheumatoid arthritis and juvenile spondyloarthropathy. Arthritis Rheum 1996; 39:1703–1710.

66. Rooney M, Varsani H, Martin K, et al. Tumour necrosis factor alpha and its soluble receptors in juvenile chronic arthritis. Rheumatology 2000; 39:432–438.

67. Schneider R, Laxer RM. Systemic onset juvenile rheumatoid arthritis. Ballière Clin Rheum 1998; 12:245–271.

68. Roberton DM, Cabral DA, Malleson PN, et al. Juvenile psoriatic arthritis: Follow up and evaluation of diagnostic criteria. J Rheumatol 1996; 23:166–170.

69. Cohen PA, Job-Deslandre CH, Lalande G, et al. Overview of the radiology of juvenile idiopathic arthritis (JIA). Eur J Radiol 2000; 33:94–101.

70. Chalom EC, Goldsmith DP, Koehler MA, et al. Prevalence and outcome of uveitis in a regional cohort of patients with juvenile rheumatoid arthritis. J Rheumatol 1997; 24:2031–2034.

71. Malik AR, Pavesio C. The use of low dose methotrexate in children with chronic anterior and intermediate uveitis. Br J Ophthalmol 2005; 89:806–808.

72. Khan P, Weiss M, Imundo LF, et al. Favorable response to high-dose infliximab for refractory childhood uveitis. Ophthalmology 2006; 113:864.

73. Sawhney S, Woo P, Murray KJ. Macrophage activation syndrome: a potentially fatal complication of rheumatic disorders. Arch Dis Child 2001; 85:421–426.

74. Hackett J, Johnson B, Parkin A, et al. Physiotherapy and occupational therapy for juvenile chronic arthritis: custom and practice in five centers in the UK, USA and Canada. Br J Rheumatol 1996; 35:695–699.

75. Breit W, Frosch M, Meyer U, et al. A sub-group specific evaluation of the efficacy of intra-articular triamcinolone hexacetonide in juvenile chronic arthritis. J Rheumatol 2000; 27:2696–2702.

76. Sherry DD, Stein LD, Reed AM, et al. Prevention of leg length discrepancy in young children with pauciarticular juvenile rheumatoid arthritis by treatment with intra-articular steroids. Arthritis Rheum 1999; 42:2330–2334.

*77. Zulian F, Martini G, Gobber D, et al. Triamcinolone acetonide and hexacetonide intra-articular treatment of symmetrical joints in juvenile idiopathic arthritis: a double blind trial. Rheumatology 2004; 43:1288–1291.

78. Job-Deslandre C, Menkes CJ. Complications of intra-articular injections of triamcinolone hexacetonide in chronic arthritis in children. Clin Exp Rheumatol 1990; 8:413–416.

79. Gondwe JS, Davidson JE, Deeley S, et al. Secondary Cushing's syndrome in children with juvenile idiopathic arthritis following intra-articular triamcinolone acetonide administration. Rheumatol 2005; 44:1457–1458.

*80. Giannini EH, Brewer EJ, Kuzmina N, et al. Methotrexate in resistant juvenile rheumatoid arthritis. N Engl J Med 1992; 326:1043–1049.

*81. Woo P, Southwood TR, Prieur AM, et al. Randomized, placebo-controlled, crossover trial of low-dose oral methotrexate in children with extended oligoarticular or systemic arthritis. Arthritis Rheum 2000; 43:1849–1857.

*82. Ruperto N, Murray KJ, Gerloni V, et al. A randomized trial of parenteral methotrexate comparing an intermediate dose with a higher dose in children with juvenile idiopathic arthritis who failed to respond to standard doses of methotrexate. Arthritis Rheum 2004; 50:2191–2201.

83. Martini G, Zulian F. Juvenile idiopathic arthritis: current and future treatment options. Expert Opin Pharmacother 2006; 7:387–399.

84. Royal College of Paediatrics and Child Health. Immunization of the Immunocompromised Child. Best Practice Statement. ; February 2002. London: Royal College of Paediatrics and Child Health.

*85. Lovell DJ, Giannini EH, Reiff A. Efficacy and safety of etanercept (tumor necrosis factor receptor p75Fc fusion protein; Enbrel) in children with polyarticular-course juvenile rheumatoid arthritis. N Engl J Med 2000; 342:763–759.

*86. Lovell DJ, Reiff A, Jones OY, et al. Pediatric Rheumatology Collaborative Study Group. Long term safety and efficacy of etanercept in children with polyarticular-course juvenile rheumatoid arthritis. Arthritis Rheum 2006; 54:1987–1994.

87. Gerloni V, Pontikaki I, Gattinara M, et al. Efficacy of repeated infusions of an anti tumor necrosis factor α monoclonal antibody. Infliximab, in persistently active, refractory juvenile idiopathic arthritis. Arthritis Rheum 2005; 52:548–553.

*88. Lovell DJ, Ruperto N, Cuttica R, et al. Comparison of safety, efficacy and pharmacokinetics for 3 and 6 mg/kg infliximab plus methotrexate therapy in JRA patients. Arthritis Rheum 2005 52:(suppl):S724.

89. Lovell DJ, Ruperto N. Goodman S, et al. Preliminary data from the study of adalimumab in children with juvenile idiopathic arthritis (JIA). Arthritis Rheum 2004; 50:(suppl):S436–S437.

90. De Rycke L, Baeten D, Kruithof E, et al. The effect of TNFalpha blockade on the antinuclear antibody profile in patients with chronic arthritis: biological and clinical implications. Lupus 2005; 14:931–937.

91. Brown SL, Greene MH, Gershon SK, et al. Tumor necrosis factor antagonist therapy and lymphoma development: twenty-six cases reported to the Food and Drug Administration. Arthritis Rheum 2002; 46:3151–3158.

92. Pascual V, Allantaz F, Arce E, et al. Role of interleukin-1 (IL-1) in the pathogenesis of systemic onset juvenile idiopathic arthritis and clinical response to IL-1 blockade. J Exp Med 2005; 201:1479–1486.

93. Woo P, Wilkinson N, Prieur AM, et al. Open label phase II trial of single, ascending doses of MRA in Caucasian children with severe systemic juvenile idiopathic arthritis: proof of principle of the efficacy of IL-6 receptor blockade in this type of arthritis and demonstration of prolonged clinical improvement. Arthritis Res Ther 2005; 7:R1281–R1288.

94. Uziel Y, Laxer RM, Schneider R, et al. Intravenous immunoglobulin therapy in systemic onset juvenile rheumatoid arthritis: a follow up study. J Rheumatol 1996; 23:910–918.

95. Silverman E, Spiegel L, Hawkins D, et al. Long-term open-label preliminary study of the safety and efficacy of leflunomide in patients with polyarticular-course juvenile rheumatoid arthritis. Arthritis Rheum 2005; 52:554–562.

96. De Kleer IM, Brinkman DM, Ferster A, et al. Autologous stem cell transplantation for refractory juvenile idiopathic arthritis: analysis of clinical effects, mortality, and transplant related morbidity. Ann Rheum Dis 2004; 63:1318–1326.

97. McDonagh JE, Southwood TR, Shaw KL, et al. The impact of a coordinated transitional care program on adolescents with juvenile idiopathic arthritis. Rheumatology 2006; 46:61–68 Jun 20; Epub ahead of print.

98. Salenius P, Vankka E. The development of the tibiofemoral angle in children. J Bone Joint Surg 1975; 57A:259–261.

99. Greene WB. Infantile tibia vara. J Bone Joint Surg 1993; 75A:130–143.

100. Kling TF, Hensinger RN. Angular and torsional deformities of the lower limbs in children. Clin Orthop Rel Res 1983; 176:136–147.

101. Bleck ED. Metatarsus adductus: classification and relationship to outcome of treatment. J Pediatr Orthop 1983; 3:2–9.

102. Goodyear-Smith F, Arroll B. Growing pains. BMJ 2006; 333:456–457.

103. Landin LA, Danielsson LG, Wattsgard C, et al. Transient synovitis of the hip. Its incidence, epidemiology and relation to Perthes disease. J Bone Joint Surg 1987; 59B:238–242.

104. Haueisen DC, Weiner DS, Weiner SD. The characterization of 'transient synovitis of the hip' in children. J Pediatr Orthop 1986; 6:11–17.

105. Thomas J, Morgan G, Tayton K. Perthes disease and the relevance of thrombophilia. J Bone Joint Surg 1999; 81B:691–695.

106. Barker DJP, Hall AJ. The epidemiology of Perthes disease. Clin Orthop 1986; 209:89–94.

107. Van Den Bogaert G, De Rosa E, Moens P. Bilateral Legg–Calvè–Perthes disease: different from unilateral. Pediatr Orthop 1999; 8B:165–168.

108. Meehan PL, Angel D, Nelson JM. The Scottish Rite abduction orthosis for the treatment of Legg–Perthes disease: a radiographic analysis. J Bone Joint Surg 1992; 74A:2–12.

109. Quain S, Catterall A. Hinge abduction of the hip: diagnosis and treatment. J Bone Joint Surg 1986; 68B:61–64.

110. Loder RT, Wittenberg B, DeSilva G. Slipped capital femoral epiphysis associated with endocrine disorders. J Pediatr Orthop 1995; 15:349–356.

111. Weiner D. Pathogenesis of slipped capital femoral epiphysis: current concepts. J Pediatr Orthop 1996; 5:67–73.

112. Klein A, Joplin RJ, Reidy JA, et al. Roentgenographic features of slipped capital femoral epiphysis. Am J Roentgenol 1951; 66:361–374.

113. Loder RT, Richards BS, Shapiro PS, et al. Acute slipped capital femoral epiphysis: the importance of physeal stability. J Bone Joint Surg 1993; 75A:1134–1140.

114. Heppenstall RB, Marvel JP, Chung SMK, et al. Chondrolysis of the hip joint. Clin Orthop Rel Res 1974; 103:136–142

115. Pellicci PM, Wilson PD. Chondrolysis of the hips associated with severe burns. J Bone and Joint Surg 1979; 61A:592–596.

116. Roy PR, Crawford AH. Idiopathic chondrolysis of the hip. Management by subtotal capsulectomy and aggressive rehabilitation. J Pediatr Orthop 1988; 8:203–207.

117. Boucher JP, King MA, Lefebvre R, et al. Quadriceps femoris muscle activity in patellofemoral pain syndrome. Am J Sport Med 1992; 20:527–532.

118. Yates CK, Granna WA. Patellofemoral pain in children. Clin Orthop Rel Res 1990; 255:36–43.

119. Granna WA, Hinkley B, Hollingsworth S. Arthroscopic evaluation and treatment of patellar malalignment. Clin Orthop Rel Res 1984; 186:122–128.

120. Fugikawa K, Ieki F, Mikura Y. Partial resection of the discoid meniscus in the child's knee. J Bone Joint Surg 1981; 63A:391–395.

121. Leonard MA. The inheritance of tarsal coalition and its relationship to spastic flat foot. J Bone Joint Surg 1974; 56B:520–526.

122. Mosier KM, Asher M. Tarsal coalitions and peroneal spastic flatfoot. J Bone Joint Surg 1984; 66A:976–984.

123. Cowell HR. Diagnosis and management of peroneal spastic flatfoot. In: Instructional course lectures, The American Academy of Orthopedic Surgeons. St Louis: Mosby; 1975; 24:94–103.

124. Gonzalez P, Kumar SJ. Calcaneonavicular coalition treated by resection and interposition of the extensor digitorum brevis muscle. J Bone Joint Surg 1990; 72A:71–77.

125. Kumar SJ, Guille JT, Lee MS, et al. Osseous and non osseous coalition of the middle facet of the talocalcaneal joint. J Bone Joint Surg 1992; 74A:529–535.

126. Ozen S, Ruperto N, Dillon MJ, et al. EULAR/PReS endorsed consensus criteria for the classification of childhood vasculitides. Ann Rheum Dis 2006; 65:936–941.

127. Jenette JC, Falk RJ, Andrassay K, et al. Nomenclature of systemic vasculitides. Proposal of an international consensus conference. Arthritis Rheum 1994; 37:187–192.

128. Gardner-Medwin JM, Dolezalova P, Cummins C, et al. Incidence of Henoch–Schönlein purpura, Kawasakai disease and rare vasculitides in children of different ethnic origins. Lancet 2002; 360:1197–1202.

129. Stewart M, Savage JM, Bell B, et al. Long term renal prognosis of Henoch–Schönlein purpura in an unselected childhood population. Eur J Pediatr 1988; 147:113–115.

130. Allen AC, Willis FR, Beattie TJ, et al. Abnormal IgA glycosylation in Henoch–Schönlein purpura restricted to patients with clinical nephritis. Nephrol Dial Transplant 1998; 13:930–934.

131. Trapani S, Micheli A, Grisolia F, et al. Henoch–Schönlein Purpura in childhood: epidemiological and clinical analysis of 150 cases over a 5-year period and review of literature. Semin Arthritis Rheum 2005; 35:143–153.

132. Flynn JT, Smoyer WE, Bunchman TE, et al. Treatment of Henoch–Schönlein purpura with high dose corticosteroids plus oral cyclophosphamide. Am J Nephrol 2001; 21:128–133.

133. Shin JI, Park JM, Shin YH, et al. Can azathioprine and steroids alter the prognosis of severe Henoch–Schönlein nephritis in children?. Pediatr Nephrol 2005; 20:1087–1092.

*134. Ronkainen J, Koskimies O, Ala-Houhala M, et al. Early prednisone therapy in Henoch–Schönlein purpura: a randomized, double-blind, placebo-controlled study. J Pediatr 2006; 149:241–247.

135. Fulton DR, Newburger JW. Long-term sequelae of Kawasaki disease. Curr Rheumatol Rep 2000; 2:324–329.

136. Yanagawa H, Nakamura Y, Yashiro M, et al. Update of the epidemiology of Kawasaki disease in Japan – from the results of the 1993–1994 nationwide survey. J Epidemiol 1996; 6:148–157.

137. Leung DYM, Meissner HC, Schlievert PM. The etiology and pathogenesis of Kawasaki disease – how close are we to an answer?. Curr Opin Infect Dis 1997; 10:226–232.

138. Igarashi H, Hatake K, Shiraishi H, et al. Elevated serum levels of macrophage colony-stimulating factor in patients with Kawasaki disease complicated by cardiac lesions. Clin Exp Rheumatol 2001; 19:751–756.

139. Chang FY, Hwang B, Chen SJ, et al. Characteristics of Kawasaki disease in infants younger than six months of age. Pediatr Infect Dis 2006; 25:241–244.

140. Simonini G, Rose CD, Vierucci A, et al. Diagnosing Kawasaki syndrome: the need for a new clinical tool. Rheumatology 2005; 44:959–961.

*141. Newburger JW, Takahashi M, Burns JC, et al. The treatment of Kawasaki syndrome with intravenous gamma globulin. N Engl J Med 1986; 315:341–347.

*142. Newburger JW, Takahashi M, Beiser AS, et al. A single intravenous infusion of gamma globulin as compared with four infusions in the treatment of acute Kawasaki syndrome. N Engl J Med 1991; 324:1633–1638.

*143. Oates-Whitehead RM, Baumer JH, Haines L, et al. Intraveous immunoglobuilin for the treatment of Kawasaki disease in children. Cochrane Database Syst Rev 2003; CD004000.

144. Lang BA, Yeung RS, Oen KG. Corticosteroid treatment of refractory Kawasaki disease. J Rheumatol 2006; 33:803–809.

145. Wooditch AC, Aronoff SC. Effect of initial corticosteroid therapy on coronary artery aneurym formation in Kawasaki disease: a meta-analysis of 862 children. Pediatrics 2005; 116:989–995.

146. Newburger JW, Takahashi M, Gerber MA, et al. Diagnosis, treatment, and long-term management of Kawasaki disease: a statement for health professionals from the Committee on Rheumatic Fever, Endocarditis and Kawasaki disease, Council on Cardiovascular Disease in the Young, American Heart Association. Pediatrics 2004; 114:1708–1733.

147. Feinstein J, Arroyo R. Successful treatment of childhood onset refractory polyarteritis nodosa with tumor necrosis factor alpha blockade. J Clin Rheumatol 2005; 11:219–222.

148. David J, Ansell BM, Woo P. Polyarteritis nodosa associated with streptococcus. Arch Dis Child 1993; 69:685–688.

149. Kaklamani VG, Kaklamanis PG. Treatment of Behçet's disease – an update. Semin Arthritis Rheum 2001; 30:299–312.

*150. Yurdakul S, Mat C, Tuzun Y, et al. A double-blind trial of colchicine in Behçet's syndrome. Arthritis Rheum 2001; 44:2686–2692.

*151. Hamuryudan V, Mat C, Saip S, et al. Thalidomide in the treatment of the mucocutaneous lesions of Behçet's syndrome: a randomized, placebo-controlled, double-blind trial. Ann Intern Med 1998; 128:443–450.

152. Pascual V, Banchereau J, Palucka AK. The central role of dendritic cells and interferon-alpha in SLE. Curr Opinion Rheumatol 2003; 15:548–556.

153. Smerdel-Ramoya A, Finholt C, Lilleby V, et al. Systemic lupus erythematosus and the extended major histocompatibility complex – evidence for several predisposing loci. Rheumatology 2005; 44:1368–1373.

154. Stichweh D, Pascual V. Autoimmune mechanisms in children with systemic lupus erythematosus. Curr Rheumatol Rep 2005; 7:421–426.

155. Hochberg MC. Updating the American College of Rheumatology revised criteria for the classification of systemic lupus erythematosus. Arthritis Rheum 1997; 9:1725.

156. Ferraz MB, Goldenberg J, Hilario MO, et al. Evaluation of the ARA lupus criteria data set in pediatric patients. Committees of Pediatric Rheumatology of the Brazilian Society of Pediatrics and the Brazilian Society of Rheumatology. Clin Exp Rheumatol 1994; 12:689–690.

*157. Gourley MF, Austin HA 3rd, Scott D, et al. Methylprednisolone and cyclophosphamide, alone or in combination, in patients with lupus nephritis. A randomized controlled trial. Ann Intern Med 1996; 125:549–557.

*158. Bansal VK, Beto JA. Treatment of lupus nephritis: a meta-analysis of clinical trials. Am J Kidney Dis 1997; 29:193–199.

159. Buratti S, Szer IS, Spencer CH, et al. Mycophenolate mofetil treatment of severe renal disease in pediatric onset systemic lupus erythematosus. J Rheumatol 2001; 28:2103–2108.

160. Leandro MJ, Cambridge G, Edwards JC, et al. B-cell depletion in the treatment of patients with systemic lupus erythematosus: a longitudinal analysis of 24 patients. Rheumatology 2005; 44:1542–1545.

161. Willems M, Haddad E, Niaudet P, et al. Rituximab therapy for childhood-onset systemic lupus erythematosus. J Pediatr 2006; 148:623–627.

162. Brunner HI, Feldman BM, Bombardier C, et al. Sensitivity of the Systemic Lupus Erythematosus Disease Activity Index, British Isles Lupus Assessment Group Index and Systemic Lupus Activity Measure in the evaluation of clinical change in childhood-onset systemic lupus erythematosus. Arthritis Rheum 1999; 42:1354–1360.

163. Ruperto N, Ravelli A, Cuttica R, et al. The Pediatric Rheumatology International Trials

Organization criteria for the evaluation of response to therapy in juvenile systemic lupus erythematosus: prospective validation of the disease activity core set. Arthritis Rheum 2005; 52:2854–2864.

164. Ruperto N, Ravelli A, Oliviera S, et al. The Pediatric Rheumatology International Trials Organization/American College of Rheumatology provisional criteria for the evaluation of response to therapy in juvenile systemic lupus erythematosus: prospective validation of the definition of improvement. Arthritis Rheum 2006; 55:355–363.

165. Ravelli A, Ruperto N, Martini A. Outcome in juvenile systemic lupus erythematosus. Curr Opin Rheumatol 2005; 17:568–573.

166. Sarkissian T, Beyenne J, Feldman B, et al. The complex nature of the interaction between disease activity and therapy on the lipid profile in patients with pediatric systemic lupus erythematosus. Arthritis Rheum 2006; 54:1283–1290.

167. Gough A, Chapman S, Wagstaff K, et al. Minocycline induced autoimmune hepatitis and systemic lupus erythematosus-like syndrome. BMJ 1996; 312:169–172.

168. Symmons DPM, Sills JA, Davis SM. The incidence of juvenile dermatomyositis: results of a nation-wide study. Br J Rheumatol 1995; 43: 732–735.

169. Wargula JC. Update on juvenile dermatomyositis: new advances in understanding its etiopathogenesis. Curr Opin Rheumatol 2003; 15:595–601.

170. Pachman LM, Liotta-Davis MR, Hong DK, et al. TNF alpha-308A allele in juvenile dermatomyositis. Association with increased production of tumour necrosis factor, disease duration and pathologic calcifications. Arthritis Rheum 2000; 43:2368–2377.

171. Bohan A. Peter JB. Polymyositis and dermatomyositis. N Engl J Med 1975; 292:344–347.

172. Brown VE, Pilkington CA, Feldman BM, et al. An international consensus survey of the diagnostic criteria for juvenile dermatomyositis. Rheumatology 2006; 45:990–993.

173. Ramanan AV, Campbell-Webster N, Ota S, et al. The effectiveness of treating juvenile dermatomyositis with methotrexate and aggressively tapered corticosteroids. Arthritis Rheum 2005; 52:3570–3578.

174. Riley P, Maillard SM, Wedderburn LR, et al. Intravenous cyclophosphamide pulse therapy in juvenile dermatomyositis. A review of efficacy and safety. Rheumatology 2004; 43:491–496.

175. Ruperto N, Ravelli A, Murray KJ, et al. Preliminary core sets of measures for disease activity and damage assessment in juvenile systemic lupus erythematosus and juvenile dermatomyositis. Rheumatology 2003; 42:1452–1459.

176. Zulian F, Vallongo C, Woo P, et al. Localized scleroderma in childhood is not just a skin disease. Arthritis Rheum 2005; 52:2873–2881.

177. Zulian F, Athreya BH, Laxer R, et al. Juvenile localised scleroderma: clinical and epidemiological features in 750 children. An international study. Rheumatology 2006; 45:614–620.

178. Scalapino K, Arkachaisri T, Lucas M, et al. Childhood onset systemic sclerosis: classification, clinical and serological features and survival in comparison with adult onset disease. J Rheumatol 2006; 33:1004–1013.

179. Samuels J, Ozen S. Familial Mediterranean fever and the other autoinflammatory syndromes: evaluation of the patient with recurrent fever. Curr Opin Rheumatol 2006; 18:108–117.

180. The French FMF Consortium. A candidate gene for familial Mediterranean fever. Nat Genet 1997; 17:25–31.

181. Houten SM, Kuis W, Duran M, et al. Mutations in the gene encoding mevalonate kinase cause hyperimmunoglobulinemia D and periodic fever syndrome. Nat Genet 1999; 22:175–177.

182. McDermott MF, Aksentijevich I, Galen J, et al. Germline mutations in the extracellular domains of the 55 kDa TNF receptor, TNFR1, define a family of dominantly inherited autoinflammatory syndromes. Cell 1999; 9:133–144.

183. Prieur AM, Griscelli C, Lampert F, et al. A chronic, infantile, neurological, articular and cutaneous (CINCA) syndrome. A specific entity analysed in 30 patients. Scand J Rheumatol 1978; 66:57–68.

184. Hawkins PN, Lachmann HJ, Aganna E, et al. Spectrum of clinical features in Muckle–Wells syndrome and response to anakinra. Arthritis Rheum 2004; 50:607–612.

185. Turk DC, Okifuji A. Assessment of patients' reporting of pain: an integrated perspective. Lancet 1999; 353:1784–1788.

186. Merskey H. Pain terms: a list with definitions and notes on usage recommended by the ISAP subcommittee on taxonomy. Pain 1979; 6:249–252.

187. Sherry DD. Diagnosis and treatment of amplified musculoskeletal pain in children. Clin Exp Rheumatol 2001; 19:617–620.

188. Connelly M, Schanberg L. Latest developments in the assessment and management of chronic musculoskeletal pain syndromes in children. Curr Opin Rheumatol 2006; 18:496–502.

189. Malleson PN, Al-Matar M, Petty RE. Idiopathic musculoskeletal pain syndromes in children. J Rheumatol 1992; 19:1786–1789.

190. Sherry DD, Weisman R. Psychologic aspects of childhood reflex neurovascular dystrophy. Pediatrics 1988; 81:572–578.

191. Murray CS, Cohen A, Perkins T, et al. Morbidity in childhood reflex sympathetic dystrophy. Arch Dis Child 2000; 82:231–233.

192. Cleary AG, Sills JA, Davidson JE, et al. Reflex sympathetic dystrophy. Rheumatology 2001; 40:590–591.

193. McBeth J, Macfarlane GJ, Benjamin S, et al. Features of somatization predict the onset of chronic widespread pain: results of a large population-based study. Arthritis Rheum 2001; 44:940–946.

194. Aasland A, Flato B, Vandvik IH. Psychosocial factors in children with idiopathic musculoskeletal pain: a prospective, longitudinal study. Acta Pediatr 1997; 86:740–746.

195. Eccleston C, Jordan A, McCracken LM, et al. The Bath Adolescent Pain Questionnaire (BAPQ); development and preliminary psychometric evaluation of an instrument to assess the impact of chronic pain on adolescents. Pain 2005; 118:263–270.

196. Krist J, Ans D, Ottir G. Prevalence of self-reported back pain in school children: a study of sociodemographic differences. Eur J Pediatr 1996; 155:984–986.

197. Dreghorn CR, Newman RJ, Hardy G, et al. Primary tumours of the axial skeleton; experience of the Leeds Regional Bone Tumour Registry. Proceedings of British Scoliosis Society Meeting. J Bone Joint Surg 1989; 72B:338–339.

198. Williams CRP, O'Flynn E, Clarke NMP, et al. Torticollis secondary to ocular pathology. J Bone Joint Surg 1996; 78B:620–624.

199. Njeh CK, Shaw N, Gardner-Medwin JM, et al. Use of quantitative ultrasound to assess bone status in children with juvenile idiopathic arthritis: a pilot study. J Clin Densitom 2000; 3:251–260.

200. Schonau E. Problems of bone analysis in childhood and adolescence. Pediatr Nephrol 1998; 12:420–429.

201. NIH. Consensus Development Panel on Osteoporosis Prevention, Diagnosis and Therapy. Osteoporosis prevention, diagnosis, and therapy. JAMA 2001; 285:785–795.

202. Thornton J, Ashcroft DM, Mughal MZ, et al. Systematic review of effectiveness of bisphosphonates in treatment of low bone mineral density and fragility fractures in juvenile idiopathic arthritis. Arch Dis Child 2006; 91:753–761.

203. Bianchi ML, Cimaz R, Bardare M, et al. Efficacy and safety of alendronate for the treatment of osteoporosis in diffuse connective tissue diseases in children: a prospective multicenter trial. Arthritis Rheum 2000; 43:1960–1966.

204. Orava S, Jormakka E, Hulkko A. Stress fractures in young athletes. Arch Orthop Trauma Surg 1981; 98:271.

205. Barnett LS. Little league shoulder syndrome: proximal humeral epiphyseolysis in adolescent baseball pitchers. J Bone Joint Surg 1985; 67A:495–496.

206. Roy S, Caine D, Singer FM. Stress changes of the distal radial epiphysis in young gymnasts. Am J Sports Med 1985; 13:301–308.

207. Albanese S, Palmer A, Kerr D. Wrist pain and growth plate closure of the radius in gymnasts. J Pediatr Orthop 1989; 9:23–28.

208. Kujala UM, Kvist M, Heinonen O. Osgood–Schlatter's disease in adolescent athletes. Am J Sports Med 1985; 13:236–241.

209. Krause BL, Williams JPR. Catterral A. Natural history of Osgood–Schlatter's disease. J Pediatr Orthop 1990; 10:65–68.

210. Brogden BG, Crow NE. Little leaguer's elbow. Am J Roentgenol 1960; 83:671–675.

211. Noble CA. Iliotibial band friction syndrome in runners. Am J Sports Med 1980; 8:232–234.

212. Cassidy RE, Schaffer AJ. Repair of peripheral meniscus tears: a preliminary report. Am J Sports Med 1981; 9:209–214.

213. Lutter LD. Runners knee injuries. AAOS Instr Course Lect 1984; 33:258–268

214. Michael RH, Holder LE. The soleus syndrome. Am J Sports Med 1985; 13:87–94.

215. Mubarak SJ. The medial tibial stress syndrome. Am J Sports Med 1982; 10:201–205.

216. Detmer DE. Chronic compartment syndrome: diagnosis, management and outcomes. Am J Sports Med 1985; 13:162–170.

30

Disorders of the skin

Nigel P Burrows

INTRODUCTION

The skin comprises roughly 15% of the body weight. It is a complex organ which undergoes constant repair. Its main functions are:

1. a barrier to absorption and loss of fluid and electrolytes;
2. a barrier to external injurious agents and mechanical stress;
3. protection against ultraviolet light;
4. protection against pathogenic microorganisms;
5. regulation of body temperature;
6. as a sensory organ;
7. synthesis of vitamin D;
8. social (and sexual) communication.

To perform these functions, the skin requires a complicated structure. It consists of three layers:

1. epidermis, derived from ectoderm;
2. dermis, derived from mesoderm;
3. subcutis, derived from mesoderm.

The main function of the outermost horny layer of the epidermis is to act as a barrier to fluid and electrolyte loss as well as to external injurious agents. Ninety five percent of the epidermis is made up of *keratinocytes* which originate from the basal layer of the epidermis and progress towards the exterior. *Melanocytes* are also found in the basal layer, and are differentiated from keratinocytes by darkly staining nuclei and clear cytoplasm: their main function is protection against ultraviolet radiation by distributing melanin throughout the basal layer. The amount of melanin determines the racial color. The *Langerhans' cell*, located in the mid epidermis, is a dendritic antigen-presenting cell that plays an important role in allergic contact eczema and forms part of the immune defense in the skin. The exact function of a fourth cell, the *Merkel cell*, has not been determined, but present evidence suggests a mechanoreceptor role.

The dermoepidermal junction is the interface between the epidermis and dermis. Its major component, the basement membrane zone, has many functions including adhesion, signaling and barrier.

The dermis is composed of collagen and elastic fibers within a matrix of ground substance. Blood vessels, sensory and autonomic nerves and nerve endings, hair follicles (pilosebaceous units) and sweat glands traverse the dermis. Temperature is regulated mainly by autonomic control of blood shunting between the superficial and deep arteriolar and venular plexuses. Secondary temperature regulation, which is particularly important where the ambient temperature exceeds 37 °C, depends on evaporation from the eccrine sweat glands which are under adrenergic control.

The subcutis consists mainly of adipose tissue, whose main function is insulation of the body. In sites such as the sole of the foot, fibrous bands within the subcutis have a buffering and protective effect.

The skin appendages such as hair and nails are largely vestigial in the human; loss of either does not constitute any threat to the survival of the individual.

MANAGEMENT OF A SKIN PROBLEM IN A CHILD

It is important to take a detailed history either from the child or from the parents. History taking is similar to that in internal medicine, though the emphasis is different. Of particular importance are the following:

1. family history – many skin diseases are hereditary;
2. past history of the skin disease – conditions such as psoriasis and atopic eczema tend to be intermittent;
3. general health – some diseases (e.g. connective tissue diseases) are multiorgan problems;
4. previous treatment – both oral and topical: treatment may have modified the clinical picture (for better or for worse).

Examination of the child

The child should be undressed completely to allow full assessment of the condition. A general medical examination should also be performed. If a rash is present, note should be taken of the following points: (1) color, nature and distribution; (2) relationship of the rash to skin appendages, such as hair follicles and sweat ducts; (3) mucous membranes: some skin diseases have a banal appearance in the skin, but a characteristic appearance in mucous membranes, e.g. lichen planus, congenital syphilis; (4) examination of the hair and nails, as changes may give a clue as to the diagnosis.

TREATMENT OF SKIN DISEASES

As the skin is so accessible, it is sensible where possible to treat skin diseases with topical preparations. It is also important to introduce the active agent (e.g. steroid, antibiotic) in a suitable form or vehicle:

1. Lotions (solutions) are very useful for exudative rashes as 'wet dressings', where ointments and creams would 'float off', e.g. potassium permanganate. They are also useful for hairy areas, e.g. scalp. Shake lotions contain insoluble powders. e.g. calamine lotion.
2. Creams (oil–water emulsions). Bases such as cetomacrogol or aqueous cream are very acceptable to the patient, e.g. topical steroid creams.
3. Ointments such as petrolatum have a greasy base. They are useful for dry skin conditions, such as atopic eczema, e.g. steroid and antibiotic ointments.
4. Gels (semicolloids in alcohol base, which dry on the skin). Useful for scalp conditions.
5. Pastes (ointments + 15–30% powdered solids). Used on linen dressings, e.g. tar paste.
6. Powders, e.g. antifungal foot powders, miticides.

Topical corticosteroids

These are useful for treatment of symptoms and signs of inflammatory dermatoses, in particular eczema. Factors to be considered when prescribing include age of child, site of application and type of preparation. The fingertip unit (FTU) technique provides guidance for the quantity of corticosteroid to be applied.[1] One FTU is the amount of topical steroid that is squeezed out from a standard tube along an adult's fingertip. One FTU is used to treat an area of skin on a child equivalent to twice the size of the flat of an adult's hand with the fingers together. The weakest corticosteroid that controls the skin condition should be used. Preparations should be applied no more than twice daily. In general the more potent corticosteroids are not recommended in infants under 1 year but can be used on the trunk and limbs in severe cases for up to 2 weeks.

NEVI AND OTHER DEVELOPMENTAL DEFECTS

MELANOCYTIC NEVI

Congenital melanocytic nevi (CMN)

These occur in 0.5–2% of the population (Figs 30.1 and 30.2). They are arbitrarily classified as small (less than 1.5 cm), medium (1.5–20 cm) or large/giant (greater than 20 cm or 5% or more of body surface), in estimated adult size. They occur at birth as raised verrucose or lobulated nodules or plaques of varying shades of brown to black, sometimes with blue or pink components. They have an irregular margin and often long dark hairs and may become increasingly lobulated and hairy with time. Giant-sized lesions may produce considerable redundancy of skin and often occur in a 'garment' or 'bathing trunk' distribution on the trunk and adjacent limbs. The very small CMN initially may be difficult to distinguish from café-au-lait macules. In patients with multiple large nevi an eruption of smaller ones (satellite nevi) may occur over the first year of life. Once established, the nevi increase in size in proportion to the patient's growth. Although rare, large CMN on the scalp or dorsal spine, especially with satellite nevi, may be associated with symptomatic leptomeningeal melanocytosis (neurocutaneous melanocytosis) with a median age of onset of neurological symptoms at 2 years.[2] Furthermore, magnetic resonance imaging (MRI) scans detect

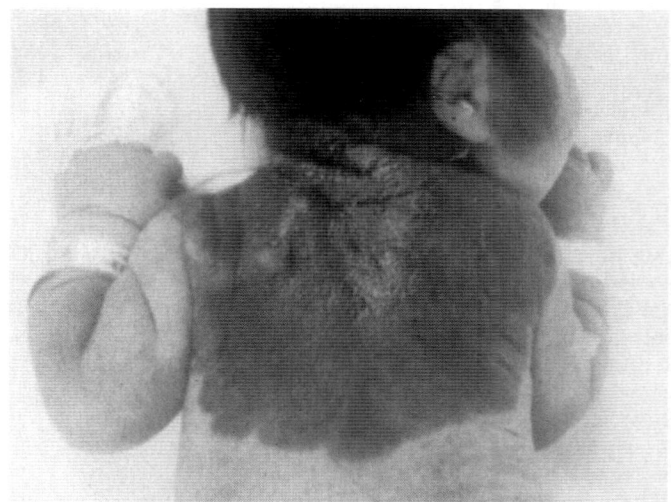

Fig. 30.1   Congenital melanocytic nevus.

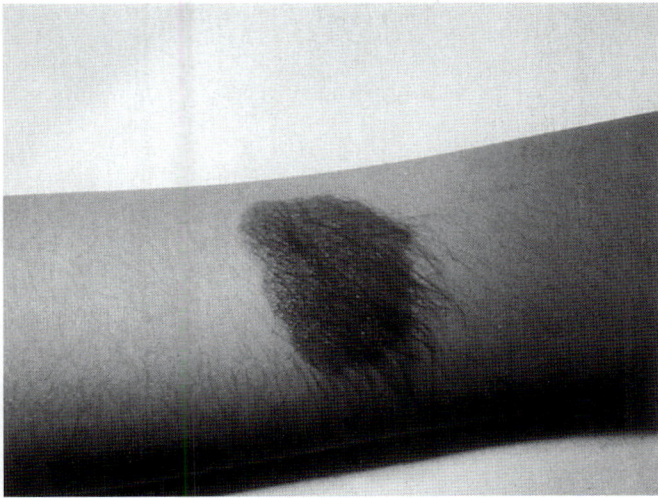

Fig. 30.2   Congenital melanocytic nevus.

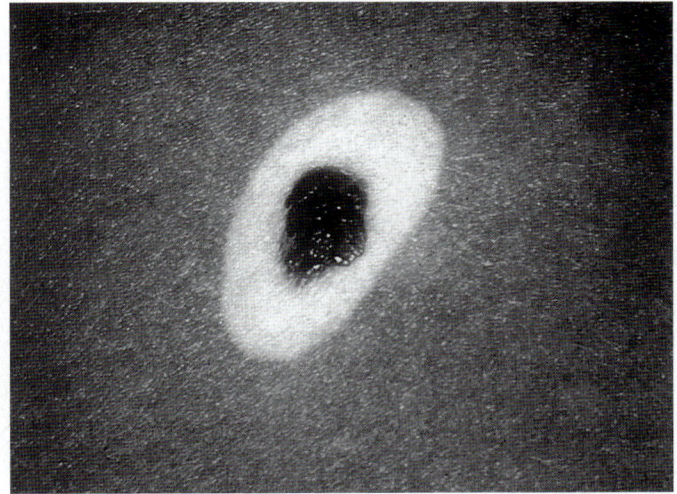

Fig. 30.3   Halo nevus.

leptomeningeal involvement in 5–30% of asymptomatic children with CMN in this distribution.[3–5]

Considerable controversy remains regarding the risk of development of malignant melanoma in CMN and hence the approach to management. Malignancy can arise from the dermal as well as the junctional component of CMN. The incidence of malignancy in large nevi has varied from 2 to 31% in different series but most studies have been retrospective and biased. A long term prospective study based on the Danish birth register is probably the most reliable and a lifetime risk of 4.6% is calculated from it.[6] In a retrospective study which included a review of the world literature primary cutaneous malignant melanoma was diagnosed within a large CMN before the age of 5 years in 50% of cases. No melanoma developed in the satellite nevi. Melanoma also occurs in medium-sized and small CMN[7,8] but the exact incidence for small lesions is not known, though it is definitely lower than for large nevi. A single follow-up study does not support the view of a significantly increased risk of melanoma in banal-appearing, medium-sized CMN, although median follow-up was short at 5.8 years.[9]

While small lesions, in which the malignancy risk is low and is usually postpubertal, can be easily excised, removal of large lesions in which the risk is much more significant is more difficult and with giant lesions may be impossible. In all cases the risk must be weighed against possible functional impairment and the morbidity of multiple operations. Many surgical procedures are available and are chosen depending on the site and extent of the lesions. Dermabrasion and laser therapy may improve the appearance of the nevus by removal of superficial pigment cells but the bulk of the lesion remains and the malignancy risk is not substantially reduced.

Acquired melanocytic nevi (AMN)

In a longitudinal study, 0.5% of babies had a CMN at birth and the number of melanocytic nevi in the same cohort at 1 year had risen to 35%.[10] These nevi continue to increase in number throughout childhood. They commence as brown or black macules, some of which become raised and enlarge laterally as they develop. They are usually of uniform color and well circumscribed. Histologically the flat lesions show clustering of nevus cells at the dermoepidermal junction (junctional nevus) and the raised ones also show intradermal nevus cells (compound nevus). Pure intradermal nevi are rare in children. The risk of melanoma arising from acquired melanocytic nevi is very low (less than 0.1%) and so their prophylactic removal in young patients is not justified.

Halo (Sutton's) nevi

A nevus may develop a depigmented halo (Fig. 30.3). The lesions are often multiple and are relatively common. The nevus may appear inflamed and often disappears leaving a white spot which may repigment years later. This is a completely benign change.

Atypical (dysplastic) nevi

Atypical nevi is the preferred term as dysplasia relates to histological features only. They are a subtype of acquired melanocytic nevi with characteristic clinicopathological features. They are a marker for the development of malignant melanoma, occurring in over 90% of patients with familial melanoma and over 10% of those with sporadic melanoma. These nevi differ from more typical AMNs by being larger (more than 5 mm diameter), having irregular and indistinct margins and irregular tan brown coloration, often with an erythematous component. They are predominantly macular, sometimes with a central elevated portion. They may appear in childhood as small typical appearing nevi which after puberty develop the atypical features. In adolescence and early adult life new atypical lesions may appear de novo. Atypical nevi may appear on the scalp in childhood. The final confirmation is based on the finding of some or all of a constellation of histopathological features of which the most important are nuclear atypia and a lymphocytic infiltrate. Familial atypical nevus syndrome is present when an individual has greater than 50 atypical nevi and a history of melanoma in a first or second degree relative.

Patients with multiple atypical nevi should be monitored with serial photography. Any mole showing significant alteration should be excised. Family members should be checked for the presence of atypical nevi or melanoma.

EPIDERMAL NEVI

Epidermal nevi are hamartomas arising from the basal layer of the embryonic epidermis that gives rise to skin appendages and keratinocytes. These nevi have been conventionally classified according to the main tissue of origin (keratinocytic, sebaceous and follicular) although this is somewhat arbitrary as more than one cell type may be present.

Epidermal nevi can involve any area of skin and may be present at birth (particularly those on the head) or appear in the first few years of life (or exceptionally later). They may simply grow with the patient or can extend well beyond their original distribution over months or years. Extension occurs less often with nevi on the head and with nevi present at birth, whatever their location. It is now clear that the linear and swirled patterns taken by epidermal nevi follow the lines of Blaschko, which define the tracks of clones of genetically identical cells. All epidermal nevi can be explained on the basis of genetic mosaicism[11] with each type of nevus representing the cutaneous manifestation of a different mosaic phenotype. In most patients the nevus is the only detectable manifestation but in some patients there are associated abnormalities in other organ systems, particularly skeletal, neurological and ocular.[12,13] This association has been called the 'epidermal nevus syndrome'.[11]

Keratinocyte nevi often start as lightly pigmented streaks that thicken and darken with time to become verrucous. They usually spare the face and scalp. Up to 10% may show histological features of epidermolytic hyperkeratosis and biopsy is therefore recommended, if possible, due to the risk of parenting a child with bullous ichthyosis. Inflammatory linear verrucous epidermal nevi (ILVEN) usually present after 6 months of age with a linear pruritic and inflamed lesion often on the lower limb.

Sebaceous and verrucous nevi are closely related. The former most commonly occur on the scalp and face and have a yellowish color due to prominent sebaceous glands. They present as a hairless, often solitary linear plaque, usually flat in infancy and childhood and becoming verrucose at puberty. Sebaceous nevi (Fig. 30.4) are rarely (< 5%) complicated in adult life by basal cell or squamous cell carcinoma.

The follicular or comedonal nevus presents as linear plaques with dilated follicular pores with comedones. The face is the commonest site but any involved site can be complicated in adolescence with acne-like cyst formation and scarring.

Skeletal abnormalities occur particularly with nevi of keratinocytic type on the limbs, and neurological and ocular abnormalities with nevi of sebaceous type on the head. The major clinical neurological features are seizures, developmental delay and hemiparesis. All patients with epidermal nevi should have a careful physical examination at presentation. Patients with linear nevi on the head who present in infancy and are normal on initial examination should be followed for several years. Most centers embark on imaging studies only in patients with clinical abnormalities.

Therapy of these lesions is difficult. Topical retinoic acid may temporarily flatten very thick areas. There are a few reports of improvement of gross lesions with oral retinoids but the effect depends on continued use of the drug. Recurrence is almost invariable following diathermy and cryotherapy. Carbon dioxide, argon and more recently erbium:YAG lasers have been used in some cases with good results though these may be temporary. Excision is appropriate for small and linear lesions and for irritating or cosmetically troubling areas of more widespread nevi.

VASCULAR NEVI

These can be divided into hemangiomas, which are proliferative vascular tumors, and vascular malformations which represent fixed collections of dilated abnormal vessels.[14]

Hemangiomas

Hemangiomas (Fig. 30.5) are usually not present at birth, undergo a fast growth phase and then, over a long period, tend to spontaneous

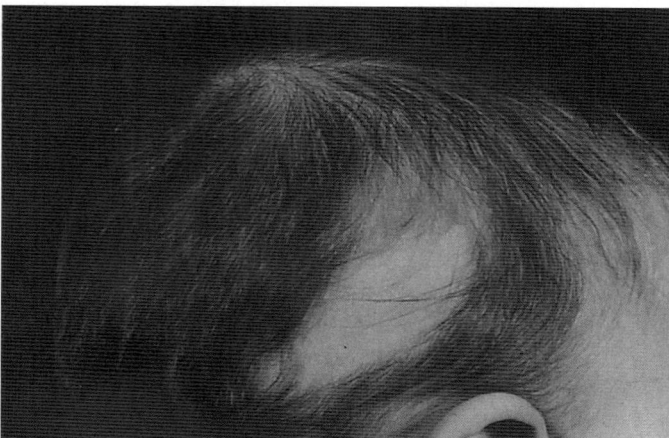

Fig. 30.5   Capillary (strawberry) hemangioma.

resolution. Emerging evidence shows that hemangiomas share unique tissue-specific markers (e.g. GLUT-1) with placental microvessels suggesting a possible common origin.[15] The terms capillary (strawberry), cavernous and capillary–cavernous are misleading and should be abandoned in favor of the simple term hemangioma.

Clinical features

Superficial hemangiomas are usually not present at birth but appear in the first weeks of life as an area of pallor followed by a telangiectatic patch. They then grow rapidly into a lobulated, well-demarcated, bright red tumor. Rapid growth continues over the first 6 months; the growth rate then slows and further growth after 10 months is unusual. After a stationary phase signs of involution appear with the appearance of gray areas which enlarge and coalesce. The tumor becomes softer and less bulky and then disappears in 90% of cases by 9 years of age.

Deeper hemangiomas may occur alone or beneath a superficial lesion. They also usually appear after birth and undergo a growth phase which however may be less striking than that of the more superficial lesions. The overlying skin is normal or bluish in color. As they resolve they soften and shrink and complete disappearance occurs in many cases; occasionally some redundant tissue remains in the place of large lesions. Apparent deep hemangiomas which show no sign of resolution are now recognized as vascular malformations, usually of venous type, and are not hemangiomas at all.

Complications

Ulceration may occur during the rapid growth phase of superficial hemangiomas. If secondary infection is controlled the ulcers usually heal in a few weeks but some scarring is inevitable. Ulceration of lesions on eyelids, lips or ala nasae can lead to full thickness tissue loss. Scarring following ulceration of lesions on or near the eyelids can result in a cicatricial ectropion and alopecia may be permanent after scalp ulceration.

Hemangiomas may encroach on vital structures. A hemangioma closing the eye for as little as 4 weeks in infancy can produce amblyopia. However, even without occluding the pupil an eyelid lesion, by pressing on the eye and producing a refractive error, can lead to failure of development of binocular vision and partial amblyopia. Large hemangiomas around the mouth may interfere with feeding and one blocking both nares can lead to respiratory difficulties while the child is being fed. A large deep hemangioma around the neck may displace the pharynx or trachea; the upper respiratory tract may also be directly involved with the hemangioma. The possibility of laryngeal involvement should be considered whenever there is a fast growing extensive lower face or neck hemangioma, particularly when there is accompanying intraoral involvement, and a lateral airways X-ray or MRI should be arranged. If there is stridor, an urgent laryngoscopy is mandatory. Even when traumatized, uncomplicated hemangiomas rarely bleed significantly.

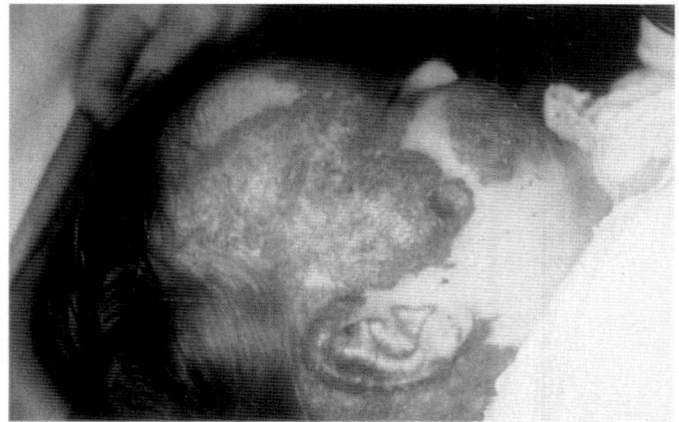

Fig. 30.4   Sebaceous nevus.

Management

Simple observation and reassurance while awaiting natural resolution is the ideal approach for most hemangiomas. Serial photography and showing photographs of other resolving lesions are encouraging. Indications for active intervention are: an alarming growth rate; threatening ulceration in areas where serious complications could ensue; interference with vital structures; and severe bleeding. Oral corticosteroids are the treatment of choice. The optimal dose is not known but a meta-analysis suggests that 3 mg/kg or more for 6–8 weeks may give the best response.[16] Repeated courses should be avoided wherever possible. Intralesional steroids may shrink localized hemangiomas which fail to respond to systemic steroids, and interferon-alpha has been effective in some life threatening cases although severe neurotoxicity, including spastic diplegia, has been reported.[17] Laser therapy became an increasingly popular treatment modality for uncomplicated hemangiomas but without good evidence for effectiveness. A randomized, controlled study of early pulsed dye laser treatment has shown no benefit of treatment at 1 year follow-up.[18] Life threatening hemangiomas have been treated with variable success with oral vincristine.[19] Cosmetic surgical procedures can improve the appearance when loose tissue remains.

Congenital hemangioma

Two types of this rare hemangioma are recognized.[20] Both are usually solitary lesions and account for about 3% of all hemangiomas. Rapidly involuting congenital hemangioma (RICH) is similar to infantile hemangioma but differs in that it is fully developed at birth, with subsequent rapid involution and regression. Non-involuting congenital hemangiomas (NICH) are usually plaque-like or bossed and as the name implies do not resolve spontaneously. Unlike infantile hemangiomas they are GLUT1 negative.

PHACE syndrome

PHACE is an acronym to describe a constellation of features: posterior fossa brain malformations, facial hemangioma, arterial anomalies, cardiac anomalies (including aortic coarctation) and eye abnormalities. If ventral developmental defects such as sternal clefting or supraumbilical raphe are present the association is referred to as PHACES. This syndrome should be considered in any infant presenting with an extensive facial hemangioma.[21]

Kasabach–Merritt syndrome (hemangioma – hemorrhage syndrome)

This is the rare association of thrombocytopenia with vascular tumors (Fig. 30.6). In children these are usually either large, deep hemangiomas, especially on limbs and around limb girdles, or diffuse hemangiomatosis. Thrombocytopenia is caused by entrapment of platelets within the lesions and is sometimes followed by disseminated intravascular coagulation (DIC). At first there may be bleeding into the

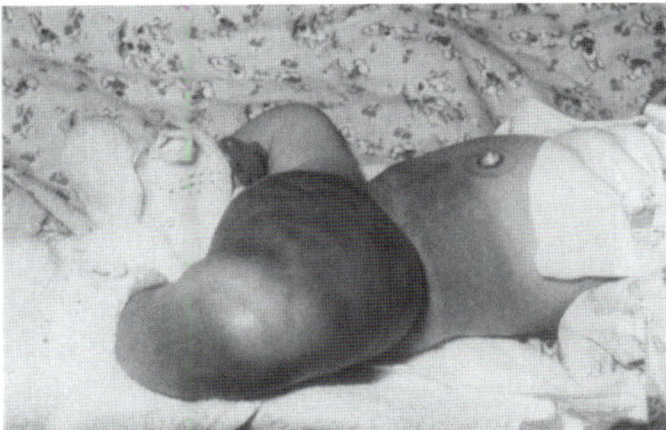

Fig. 30.6 Kasabach–Merritt syndrome.

hemangioma, which rapidly enlarges: widespread life threatening hemorrhage may follow. When bleeding is confined to the hemangiomas the approach should be conservative; in severe cases high dose systemic corticosteroids are indicated together with resuscitation, transfusion, and management of the DIC.

Diffuse infantile hemangiomatosis

This is a condition with multiple small hemangiomas in a widespread distribution. A benign form has lesions limited to the skin but a potentially serious systemic form may occur with lesions in many organs, particularly liver (64%), gastrointestinal tract (52%), lungs (52%) and central nervous system (52%) with or, rarely, without cutaneous lesions.[22] All patients with multiple cutaneous lesions should be carefully assessed with full blood count, chest X-ray, and examination for cardiac failure due to arteriovenous shunts and for bleeding from the gastrointestinal tract. An ultrasound or abdominal computerized tomography (CT) scan should be performed to exclude hepatic involvement and other organs may need to be further investigated. Angiography and technetium-labeled red blood cell scans can delineate further the extent of internal involvement.[23] With severe systemic involvement high dose corticosteroids are required along with management of cardiac failure and other complications, and active surgical intervention may be necessary in selected cases.

Vascular malformations

Vascular malformations are structural abnormalities and as such are present at birth, grow in proportion to the patient's growth and have no tendency at all to resolution. They can be further divided into fast flow, e.g. arteriovenous, or slow flow, e.g. venous, lymphatic or capillary malformations.

Capillary malformation (port-wine stain, nevus flammeus)

This is a vascular malformation composed of dilated mature capillaries. It is present at birth and shows no involution. Lesions may be unilateral or, less often, bilateral, and occur anywhere on the body, though they are most commonly found on the face. They are deep pink in infancy becoming more purple later. After puberty they may become raised and nodular. Good results can be achieved with the pulsed dye laser. Port-wine stains (PWS) must be distinguished from salmon patches at the nape of the neck (stork bite) and lesions on the eyelid or forehead (angel kiss). The vast majority of facial lesions resolve in months whilst the occipital ones persist.

It is important to be aware that, even in the absence of Sturge–Weber syndrome, ocular complications can occur. If the PWS encroaches the upper eyelid glaucoma may occur. The incidence increases to over 30% if the lower eyelid is also involved.[24]

Sturge–Weber syndrome

This is the association of a facial capillary malformation and a vascular malformation of the ipsilateral meninges and cerebral cortex. The cutaneous lesion always involves the skin in the distribution of the first division of the trigeminal nerve.[25] In 20% of infants the neurological manifestations of the syndrome include convulsions, hemiparesis and mental retardation.

Patients presenting with a capillary malformation in the appropriate distribution should have early neurological and ophthalmological consultation and continued close follow-up. A CT scan may demonstrate the intracranial malformations in the first few months of life. Parallel streaks of calcification may be demonstrated radiologically after about 2 years of age.

Vascular malformations with limb hypertrophy

Klippel–Trenaunay syndrome refers to a Parkes–Weber syndrome (PWS), associated with ipsilateral overgrowth of a limb, with soft tissue and/or bony hypertrophy and venous varicosities. The condition arises predominantly due to venous malformations whereas PWS, with similar clinical features, is caused by arteriovenous fistulae. In both instances, deeper lymphatic abnormalities may also be present. In 15% of cases of Klippel–Trenaunay syndrome involvement may be bilateral. Treatment is generally unsatisfactory with few cases being amenable to surgical correction. Compression bandaging may help to some extent with the increased girth of a limb.

CONGENITAL APLASIA CUTIS

Aplasia cutis congenita (ACC) is a congenital absence of skin and in 70% of patients is located as a solitary lesion on the scalp. The commonest form is a localized oval, stellate or linear area at or near the midline of the scalp which presents as an ulcerated area which crusts (Fig. 30.7). Resolution occurs after some months to leave a scar that is usually atrophic but is occasionally hypertrophic. There is permanent alopecia at the site. Rarely the lesion is already scarred at birth. The defect may involve not only skin but also subcutaneous fat and even bone. The bony defect will eventually heal but until it does there is a risk of meningitis. Deep aplasia may erode large vessels producing serious hemorrhage. A skull X-ray should be performed in all cases unless the lesion is obviously very superficial. Early management of scalp ACC is conservative with protection of the area and early treatment of secondary infection. Very deep lesions, however, may require skin and/or bone grafting. In later life scalp reduction techniques can be used to deal with the area of alopecia.

After the scalp the next commonest site is the lower limbs. When multiple lesions occur their distribution is often strikingly symmetrical and they may be covered with a shiny transparent membrane rather than being open erosions. Cases with extensive truncal and limb ACC are often associated with a fetus papyraceus at delivery, indicating the death of a twin early in the second trimester.

ACC-like lesions can occur on the lower limbs of patients with several types of epidermolysis bullosa probably resulting from intrauterine mechanical trauma. ACC may occur in a number of syndromes including trisomy 13, 4p-syndrome, 46XY gonadal dysgenesis and the Johanson–Blizzard syndrome. It may also be associated with a number of morphological abnormalities, particularly those involving the limbs.

DERMOID CYSTS

Congenital inclusion dermoid cysts typically present as asymptomatic subcutaneous swellings. Approximately 40% are present at birth with the rest appearing over the next 5 years. They arise due to entrapment of epithelium along embryonic fusion lines and occur particularly on the head and neck with predilection over the lateral eyebrow and dorsum of the nose. It is essential that adequate imaging investigations are performed prior to surgery as they may form deep tracts into underlying tissue.

HEREDITARY DISEASES

THE ICHTHYOSES

These are a group of inherited conditions with dry thickened skin of varying severity. The major ichthyoses comprise:
1. ichthyosis vulgaris (IV);
2. X-linked recessive ichthyosis (XLRI) (Fig. 30.8);
3. lamellar ichthyosis (LI);
4. congenital ichthyosiform erythroderma (CIE) (Fig. 30.9);
5. bullous ichthyosis (BI).

The histopathological and clinical features of the major ichthyoses are listed in Table 30.1. They are life-long disorders with little tendency to spontaneous improvement.

Management

Simple emollients such as aqueous cream may be adequate in IV. Keratolytics containing urea, propylene glycol or alpha-hydroxy acids may be more effective and useful in IV and XLRI but they may sting on fissured skin. The more severe ichthyoses often show little improvement with these topical agents. Oral retinoids may be very helpful in CIE but their effectiveness must always be weighed against their potential

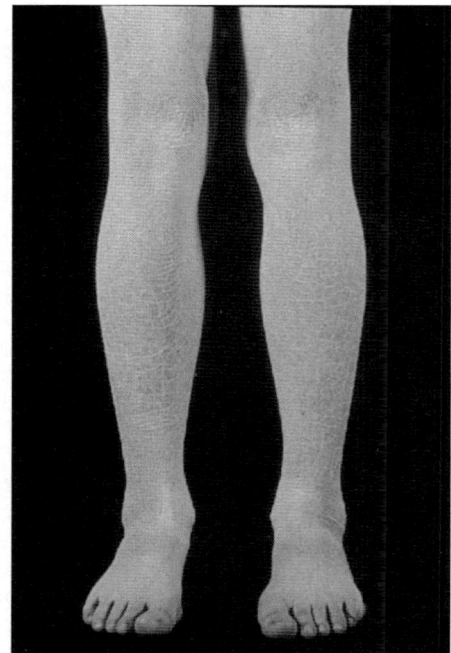

Fig. 30.8   X-linked ichthyosis.

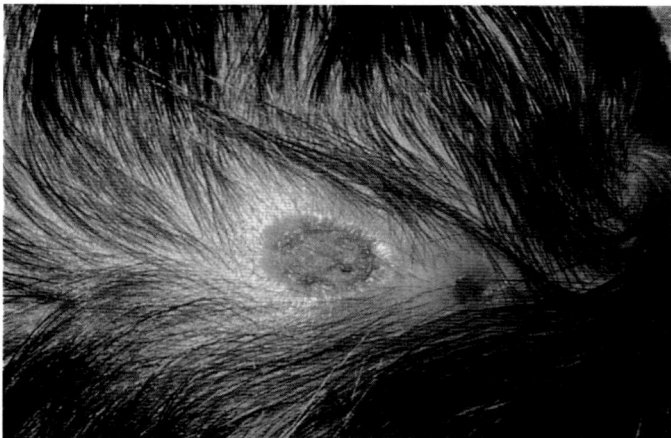

Fig. 30.7   Aplasia cutis.

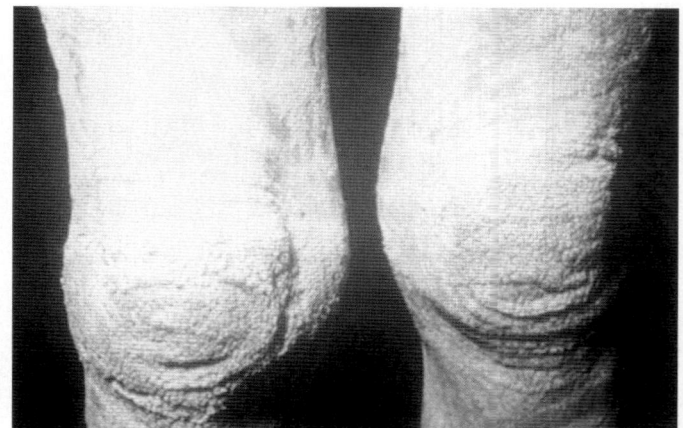

Fig. 30.9   Lamellar ichthyosis (congenital ichthyosiform erythroderma).

Table 30.1   Classification and features of the major ichthyoses

	Onset (and inheritance)	Clinical features	Complications and associations	Chromosomal/gene loci
Ichthyosis vulgaris	After birth but within the first year of life (AD)	Fine pale branny scales especially on extensor surfaces of limbs. Wide sparing of flexures of limbs. Trunk less severely involved. Face usually spared. Hyperlinear palms	Rarely corneal dystrophy, keratosis pilaris, atopy	Loss of function of filaggrin
Recessive X-linked ichthyosis	Appears within the first 3 months of life. Sometimes congenital with a thin shiny covering membrane (XLR)	Large dark adherent scales mainly on extensor surfaces of limbs. Scaling encroaches on limb flexures and axillae with narrow sparing. Trunk is diffusely involved. Sides of face often involved. Usually severe involvement of neck and thick scalp scaling. Palms and soles are uninvolved	Frequent corneal dystrophy (also in carriers). Cryptorchidism. Steroid sulfatase deficiency in most tissues including the amnion (which is derived from fetus). This placental steroid sulfatase deficiency may result in a failure of spontaneous onset of labor	Steroid sulfatase gene deletion (Xp22.3)
Lamellar ichthyosis	Usually at birth as 'collodion baby' (AR/AD)	Large dark plate-like scales. Mild to moderate erythroderma. The whole body surface is involved, including palms and soles	Ectropion. Blockage of external auditory meatus with scale resulting in hearing loss. Block of nares with scale. Pyrexia from sweat duct obstruction. Failure to thrive. Alopecia	TGM1 gene mutations (14q11.2); also 2q33–35, 19p12–q12
Congenital ichthyosiform erythroderma	Usually at birth as 'collodion baby' (AR)	Fine white scale in most areas, sometimes larger and darker on lower legs. Mild to very severe generalized erythroderma. Whole body surface is involved including palms and soles	Similar to those of lamellar ichthyosis but of lesser extent	TGM1 gene mutations (14q11.2); also 3p21
Bullous ichthyosis (epidermolytic hyperkeratosis)	At birth with erythroderma and widespread blistering. After a few days the redness subsides and over early months the blistering tendency reduces (AD)	Thick dark warty scales from time to time to leave denuded areas with a red base. Blistering is rare after 1 year. The condition may be localized to extensor surfaces but is usually widespread although the face is usually spared. Palm and sole involvement is variable	Bacterial superinfection is a recurrent problem. Heavy bacterial colonization is inevitable. Maceration and offensive odor are major problems	K2e gene mutations (12q11–13)

AD, autosomal dominant; AR, autosomal recessive; XLR, X-linked recessive.

side-effects, especially skeletal abnormalities and teratogenicity. In BI their usefulness is limited by their tendency to increase skin fragility. Detection and treatment of secondary bacterial infection is important in BI and topical disinfectants may reduce bacterial colonization and malodor.

Collodion baby

This is a descriptive term for the child who is encased at birth in a shiny tight membrane resembling collodion or plastic skin, producing ectropion and eclabium and fissuring (Fig. 30.10). The skin peels off in days or weeks. This may be a presentation of various conditions, particularly CIE (which overlaps with lamellar ichthyosis), chondrodysplasia punctata, trichothiodystrophy and rarely Netherton syndrome. In approximately 10% of collodion babies the membrane peels off to leave normal skin: this condition is called lamellar ichthyosis of the newborn. Collodion babies show temperature instability and excessive fluid loss. Corneal exposure may result if the eyes are not covered and the eclabium may necessitate squeeze bottle, tube or dropper feeding. As the fissures appear, secondary infection becomes a risk. The child should be nursed in a humidicrib with aseptic handling.

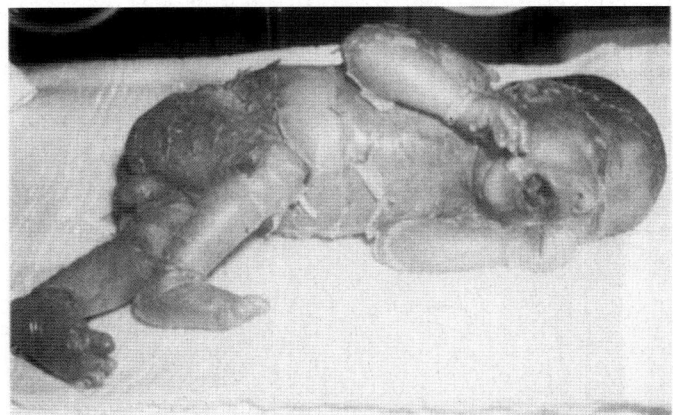

Fig. 30.10   Collodion baby.

Harlequin ichthyosis

This is a rare, potentially lethal, autosomal recesssive disorder. Causative mutations in the ABCA12 gene, which is a member of the ATP-binding (ABC) transporter family, have recently been identified.[26] ABCA12 is an epidermal lipid transporter and loss of the skin lipid barrier is thought to lead to abnormal keratinization.

At birth the child is covered in large dark plates of scale with deep fissures. Severe ectropion and eclabium, deformed ears and claw hands and feet are present. Most used to die as neonates due to secondary infection, anemia, circulatory disturbances or renal failure but the few who have survived have had a severe ichthyosiform erythroderma. (Note – this is different from the harlequin color change.)

Ichthyosis as part of other syndromes

Some of the syndromes of which ichthyosis is a part are listed in Table 30.2.

EPIDERMOLYSIS BULLOSA (EB)

This is a rare group of inherited diseases characterized by trauma-induced blistering of skin and mucosae. The prevalence is between 1/50000 and 1/2000000 for the more common and rarer forms, respectively. Over 20 types are now identified, separated on the basis of inheritance, clinical features, immunohistochemistry, electron microscopic (EM) and molecular pathology. The split may be within the epidermis, at the dermoepidermal junction in the lamina lucida (junctional; Figs 30.11 and 30.12) or in the upper dermis (sublamina densa; Fig. 30.13). A classification is given in Table 30.3. The structure of the cutaneous basement membrane zone and the gene defects in epidermolysis bullosa are shown in Figure 30.14.

A firm diagnosis should be established as soon as possible by EM and immunohistochemical analysis from an unaffected area of skin in which the split is induced by prior rubbing. This enables a prognosis to be given and a management plan to be established for present and future.

Epidermolysis bullosa simplex (EBS)
Localized EBS (Weber – Cockayne)
The blisters are often not noticed until the child starts to walk. It may be so mild that it does not present until adult life. However, morbidity can be such that daily activities are affected. Blisters develop on hands and feet and, as with all forms of EBS, they are often worse with increased temperatures in the summer months. Very occasionally other body sites are affected.

Generalized EBS (Koebner)
The onset of blisters is at birth or early infancy. They may be widespread but affect particularly areas of trauma such as hands, feet, knees and elbows. The oral mucosa is occasionally involved. Nails are not affected and there is no scarring. As with localized EB, secondary infection is the main complication. Life expectancy is normal.

Herpetiform EBS (Dowling – Meara)
Widespread blistering can be present at birth and severe cases may be mistaken for junctional EB. Transient milia develop at sites of grouped blisters. The hands and feet are especially affected, often leading to a palmoplantar keratoderma. Nail thickening is common. Oral, laryngeal and esophageal mucosal involvement is sometimes seen. Although blistering may persist through adult life the tendency is for considerable improvement.

Junctional EB
Generalized severe (Herlitz) EB
Blistering is present at birth and may be relatively minor at first. Slow wound healing is seen particularly on the face and around the nails. Typically affected babies have a hoarse cry due to mucosal involvement which is extensive and severe involving nasal, oral, esophageal as well as anogenital and urinary epithelium. Many infants die due to overwhelming sepsis. Survival to adolescence is rare but older children suffer from chronic sepsis, anemia and growth retardation.

Table 30.2 Syndromes associated with ichthyosis

Syndrome	Inheritance	Type of ichthyosis	Other major features	Molecular defects
Chondrodysplasia punctata	XLR	Onset may be as 'collodion baby'. Initially occurs as a diffuse redness and scaling. Later occurs in a whorled patchy distribution	Epiphyseal dysplasia, cataracts, follicular atrophoderma	XLR: Emopamil binding protein gene mutations
	XLD			XLD: Arylsulfatase E gene mutations
Sjögren–Larsson syndrome	AR	Generalized ichthyosis at birth. Later large dark scales most prominent in flexures	Mental retardation, spasticity	Aldehyde dehydrogenase family mutations
Chanarin–Dorfman syndrome (neutral lipid storage disease with ichthyosis)	AR	Ichthyosis simulating mild to moderate congenital ichthyosiform erythroderma	Lipid vacuoles in almost all cells. Normal serum lipids. Cataracts, deafness, developmental delay	Unknown
Refsum syndrome	AR	Delayed onset of ichthyosis of mild form, simulating ichthyosis vulgaris	Failure to degrade phytanic acid. Retinitis pigmentosa, peripheral neuropathy, cerebellar ataxia	Phytanoyl-CoA hydroxylase gene mutations
Netherton syndrome	AR	Erythroderma at birth. Late development of circinate migratory scaly lesions (ichthyosis linearis circumflexa) in widespread distribution. Some cases simulate congenital ichthyosiform erythroderma	Alopecia due to hair shaft abnormalities, especially trichorrhexis invaginata, atopic diathesis, developmental delay, generalized aminoaciduria	Serine proteinase inhibitor (SPINK 5) gene mutations

AR, autosomal recessive; XLD, X-linked dominant; XLR, X-linked recessive.

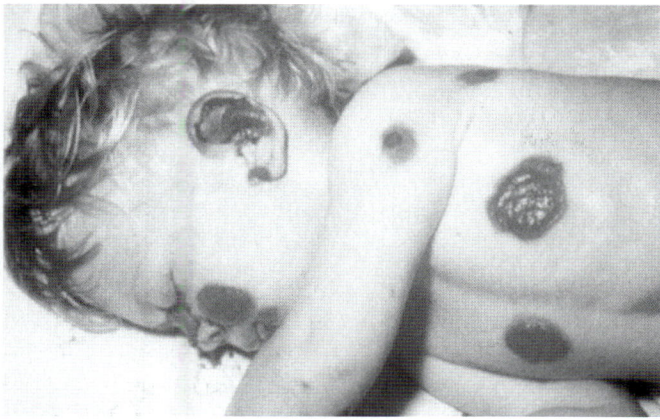

Fig. 30.11 Junctional epidermolysis bullosa.

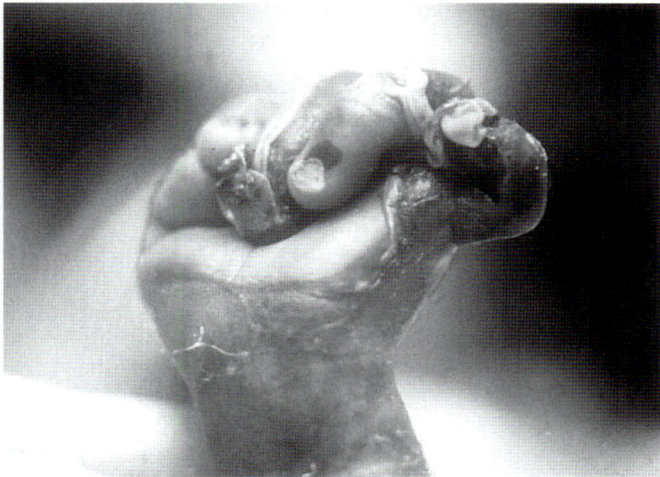

Fig. 30.12 Junctional epidermolysis bullosa.

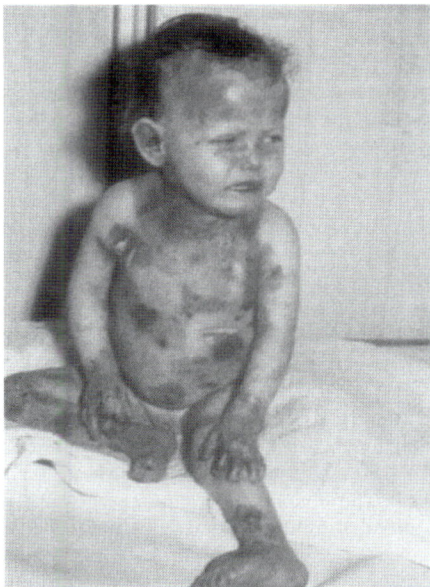

Fig. 30.13 Dystrophic epidermolysis bullosa.

Table 30.3 Classification of major types of hereditary epidermolysis bullosa

	Inheritance
Intraepidermal blister	
Epidermolysis bullosa simplex (EBS)	
Localized (hands and feet) EBS (Weber–Cockayne)	AD
Generalized EBS (Koebner)	AD
Herpetiform EBS (Dowling–Meara)	AD
EBS with muscular dystrophy	AR
Lamina lucida blister	
Junctional epidermolysis bullosa (JEB)	
Generalized severe (Herlitz)	AR
Generalized atrophic benign (GABEB)	AR
JEB with pyloric atresia	AR
Sublamina densa	
Dystrophic epidermolysis bullosa (DEB)	
Dominant DEB	AD
Recessive DEB (Hallopeau)	AR

AD, autosomal dominant; AR, autosomal recessive.

Generalized atrophic benign EB (GABEB)

Although in the initial stages the blistering has a similar pattern to Herlitz EB the child survives with a decreasing tendency to blister. Mucous membranes are involved but less so than the Herlitz form. The major feature of GABEB is alopecia which follows the blistering. Lesions may also heal with hyperpigmentation. The life span of the affected individual is normal.

Dystrophic EB

Dystrophic EB is characterized by skin fragility, blisters, scarring with milia formation and nail changes. The autosomal recessive form is more severe than the dominant disease with greater skin fragility and therefore more widespread blistering. Repeated blistering and scarring can lead to syndactyly of fingers and toes and club-like deformities of hands and feet with several digits encased together in a scar. Severe involvement of oral mucosa may lead to stricture formation in autosomal recessive patients. Laryngeal and tracheal involvement may threaten the airway. Hypoproteinemia is caused by constant loss of protein in blister fluid, malabsorption and malnutrition. In all cases the nails are thickened and often lost. Aggressive squamous cell carcinomas may arise in the scar tissues and metastatic disease is a major cause of death in adult patients with severe disease.

Management

In mild epidermolysis bullosa simplex and dominant dystrophic cases advice is required regarding avoidance of trauma, a reduction of friction, appropriate clothing and footwear. New blisters should be pricked to drain them but not deroofed and various dressings of non-stick material are appropriate. Secondary bacterial infection is treated with topical or oral antibiotics.

In the severe forms with extensive neonatal blistering extreme care is necessary to avoid further skin damage. The infant should initially be nursed naked in a humidicrib lying on non-adherent material with barrier nursing to prevent infection. Blisters should be drained and antibacterial creams such as silver sulfadiazine applied to large erosions. Vaseline gauze or non-adherent plastic dressings should be used as required, secured with tubular gauze or by other means but never taped to the skin with adhesive. A nasogastric tube should never be passed.

Severe complications may require a multidisciplinary approach. In the UK advice, both medical and nursing, should be sought whenever appropriate early in management from regional centers with a particular expertise in EB. Where possible, one physician should coordinate the entire management program to provide stability and continuity. The family should be directed towards support organizations, which can offer practical advice, emotional support and companionship. Finally, genetic counseling of the parents and later the patient should be arranged at an appropriate time.

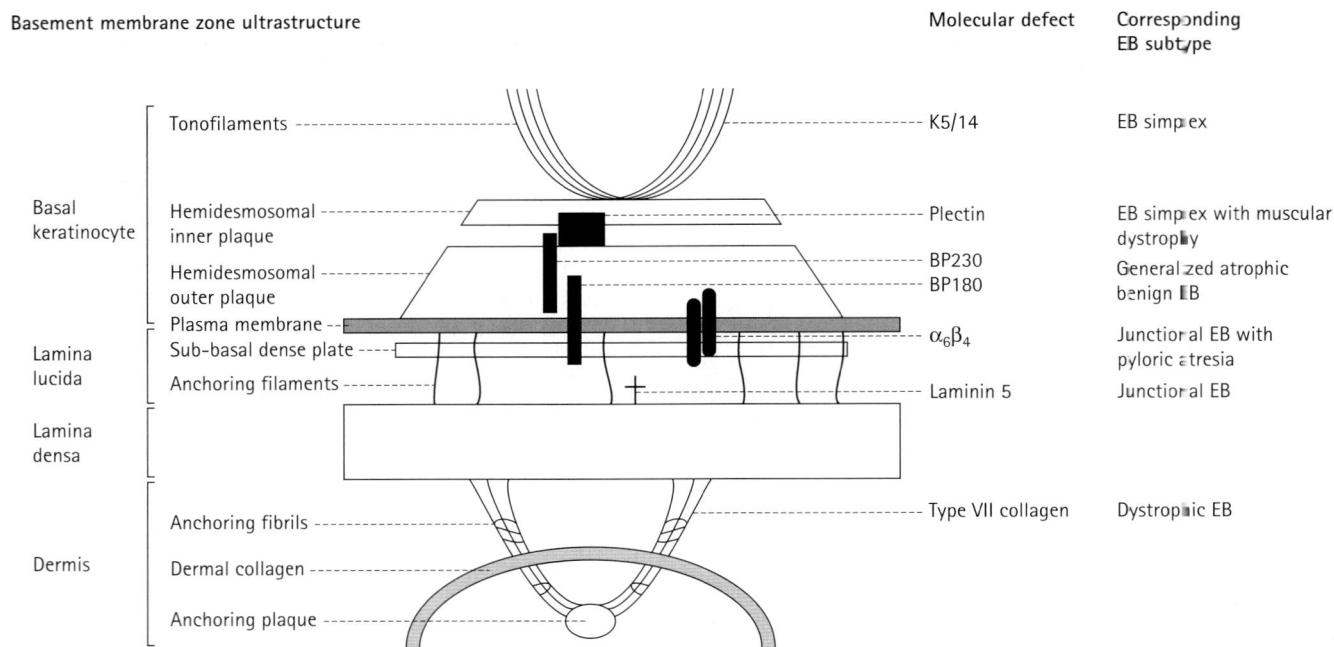

Fig. 30.14   Structure of cutaneous basement membrane zone and gene defects in epidermolysis bullosa.

ECTODERMAL DYSPLASIAS

The ectodermal dysplasias (Fig. 30.15) are a heterogeneous group of inherited conditions with a primary defect in two or more of the following: teeth, nails, hair, sweat glands or abnormalities in tissues of ectodermal origin, including eyes, ears, oral and nasal mucosa, melanocytes and central nervous system. Molecular genetics is increasingly yielding more insight into the abnormal regulatory mechanisms in ectodermal dysplasias and this is leading to revised classifications according to the function of the involved mutated genes.[27]

The major features of some of the more important ectodermal dysplasias are documented in Table 30.4.

Management

As these are disorders manifesting very diverse features, a multidisciplinary approach is essential.

If the scalp hair is very sparse the cosmetic benefit of a good wig may be invaluable. Primary and secondary dentitions can be assessed with dental X-rays in infancy in conjunction with a pediatric dentist experienced in these conditions. Early use of prostheses may prevent development of some of the structural facial abnormalities. Newer techniques include osseous implants into which prosthetic teeth can be fitted.

If hypohidrosis is extreme hyperthermia may result and may be severe and life threatening. Advice regarding activities, clothing and methods of cooling may be required.

Atopic eczema often accompanies hypohidrotic ectodermal dysplasia and will require the usual treatment. Many patients have dry skin and require emollients, and keratolytics may improve palmoplantar keratoderma.

All patients with eye abnormalities should be managed in conjunction with an ophthalmologist. Artificial tears are essential for dry eyes to prevent corneal damage. Reconstructive procedures will be required for atresia of nasolacrimal ducts and canaliculi. Severe respiratory infections complicate some of these syndromes and need antibiotics, physiotherapy and regular pediatric follow-up.

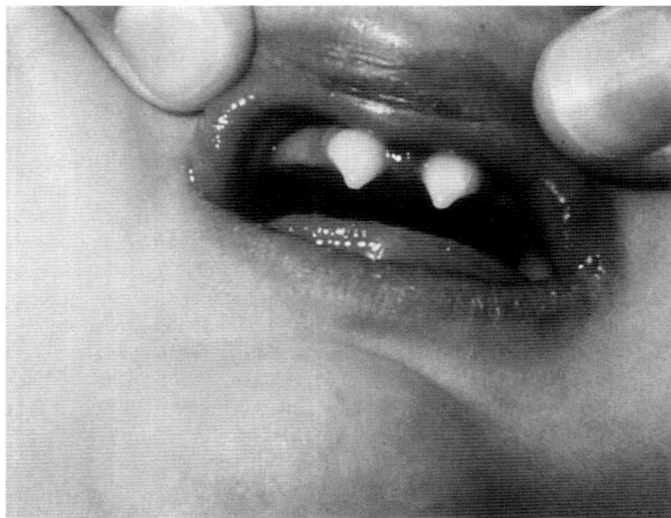

Fig. 30.15   Ectodermal dysplasia.

TUBEROUS SCLEROSIS

The tuberous sclerosis complex (TSC) is an autosomal dominant, neurocutaneous disorder characterized by the formation of hamartomata in many organs. Mutations in the hamartin gene (9q34) account for approximately half of the cases (TSC1) and the other half arise due to mutations in the tuberin gene (16p13) (TSC2).[28] Both act as tumor suppressor genes and around 60% arise due to spontaneous mutations. A small number of families are unlinked to either gene. Epilepsy occurs in 80% and mental retardation in 70%. Up to 20% of patients with infantile spasms will have TSC and should therefore have their skin examined. Other systemic abnormalities include retinal phacomata and a variety of hamartomata in renal tract, heart and other organs.

Dermatological features

The most pathognomonic features are angiofibromas (adenoma sebaceum), periungual fibromas, shagreen patches and ash leaf macules (Figs 30.16 and 30.17). The angiofibromas appear as 1–4 mm bright red papules in a centrofacial distribution. Sometimes they coalesce to form cauliflower-like masses. Their onset is usually between the ages of 3 and 10 years and they may become more extensive at puberty. Numbers vary from a few to several hundred. Periungual fibromas appear around puberty as

Table 30.4   The ectodermal dysplasias

	1. Hypohidrotic ectodermal dysplasia (Christ–Siemens–Touraine syndrome)	2. Hidrotic ectodermal dysplasia (Clouson syndrome)	3. Rapp–Hodgkin syndrome	4. EEC syndrome (ectrodactyly, ectodermal dysplasia and clefting)	5. AEC syndrome (ankyloblepharon, ectodermal dysplasia and clefting) (Hay–Wells syndrome)
Inheritance	X-linked recessive*	Autosomal dominant	Autosomal dominant	Autosomal dominant	Autosomal dominant
Hair	Hypotrichosis of scalp, body hair, eyebrows and lashes. Beard normal. Hair fine and fair	Hypotrichosis. Hair fine and dry	Sparse, coarse and stiff with hair shaft abnormalities	Sparse wiry hair	Severe hypotrichosis
Teeth	Hypodontia. Conical teeth	May be normal. Hypodontia, caries, widespaced teeth	Hypodontia, abnormally shaped teeth. Early caries	Hypodontia, abnormally shaped teeth	Variable hypodontia, abnormal shape, delayed eruption
Nails	Often normal. Sometimes fragile and occasionally dystrophic or absent	Thick, striated, discolored. Paronychia and nail loss. Rarely thin and brittle	Small and dysplastic	Thin, pitted and striated	Severe dystrophy. Short due to absence of distal nail plate
Sweating	Hypohidrosis often with hyperthermia	Normal	Hypohidrosis	Occasional hypohidrosis	Variable hypohidrosis
Skin	Smooth and dry, loss of dermatoglyphics, wrinkled and hyperpigmented around eyes, atopic dermatitis	Thick over finger joints, knees and elbows. Palmoplantar keratoderma	Dry and coarse. Thick over elbows and knees. Reduced dermatoglyphics	Dry and thin. Palmoplantar keratoderma	Large weeping areas at birth, later dry and scaly. May be recurrent scalp crusting. Palmoplantar keratoderma
Eyes	Hypoplasia of nasolacrimal duct, decreased lacrimal gland secretion, dry eyes, photophobia and corneal opacities	Usually normal. Occasionally premature cataracts	Atresia of lacrimal puncta producing epiphora, corneal opacities	Nasolacrimal duct stenosis, dacryocystitis, corneal scarring	Ankyloblepharon filiforme adnatum, nasolacrimal duct atresia
Facies	Variable. Thick lips, saddle nose, frontal bossing, maxillary hypoplasia. Occasionally abnormal ears	Normal	Cleft lip, hypoplastic maxilla. Microstomia. Prominent malformed ears	Cleft lip	Cleft lip often, microstomia, broad nasal bridge, sunken maxilla, abnormal pinnae
Mucosae	Poor development of mucous glands in gastrointestinal and respiratory tracts. Atrophic rhinitis, thick nasal secretion, recurrent chest infections, dysphagia. Dry mouth	Normal	Chronic rhinitis	Hoarseness due to abnormality of laryngeal mucosa	Filamentous bands in vagina, anal fissure
Miscellaneous	Absent or supernumerary nipples. Absent breast tissue in carriers. Asthma	Tufting of terminal phalanges with finger clubbing. Thickening of skull bones	Short stature. Cleft palate. Syndactyly	Cleft palate. Ectrodactyly (split hands and feet). Syndactyly	Cleft palate. Syndactyly

* Autosomal recessive variant is difficult to distinguish phenotypically.

firm smooth flesh-colored papules in a periungual or subungual location. The shagreen patch is a connective tissue nevus comprising an accumulation of collagen as an irregularly thickened yellow-white plaque, usually in the lumbosacral area. It develops between the ages of 2 and 5 years. Ash leaf macules are depigmented macules, usually 1–3 cm in diameter but occasionally much larger. They are usually oval in shape, with a minority truly ash leaf shaped. They may be present at birth or appear during the first year. Large numbers may be present and they are best visualized under Wood's (ultraviolet) light.

Other dermatological features include fibromatous plaques on brow or scalp, intraoral fibromas, multiple fibroepithelial polyps around the neck and in the axillae and a variety of other depigmented lesions including numerous guttate macules and large dermatomal lesions. Poliosis and canities may also occur.

Patients who present with these characteristic skin signs should be referred for neurological assessment and computerized axial tomography to demonstrate any intracranial lesions. Laser therapy may improve the cosmetic appearance of the angiofibromas.

INCONTINENTIA PIGMENTI

Incontinentia pigmenti (IP type 2) is a multisystem disorder inherited as an X-linked dominant trait and is usually prenatally lethal in males (Figs 30.18 and 30.19). It arises due to mutations (usually genomic

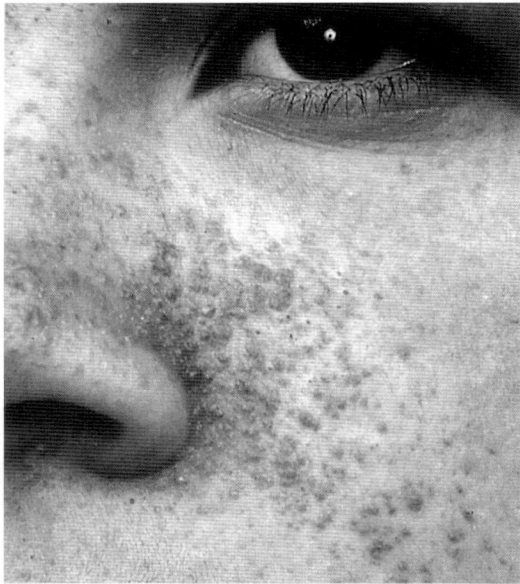

Fig. 30.16   Adenoma sebaceum: tuberous sclerosis.

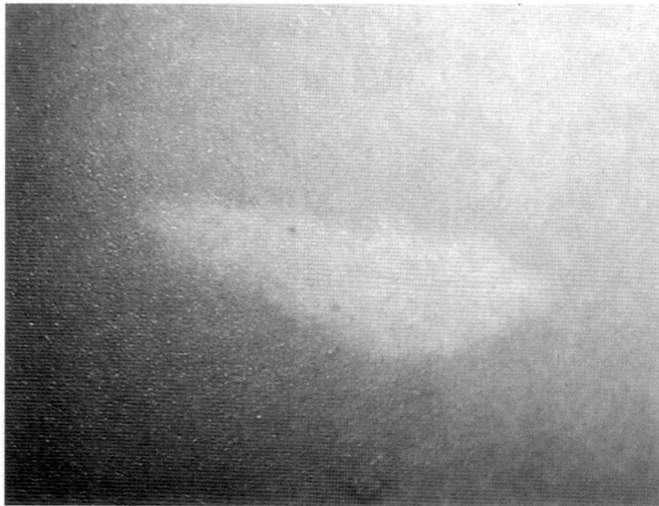

Fig. 30.18   Incontinentia pigmenti: pigmented stage.

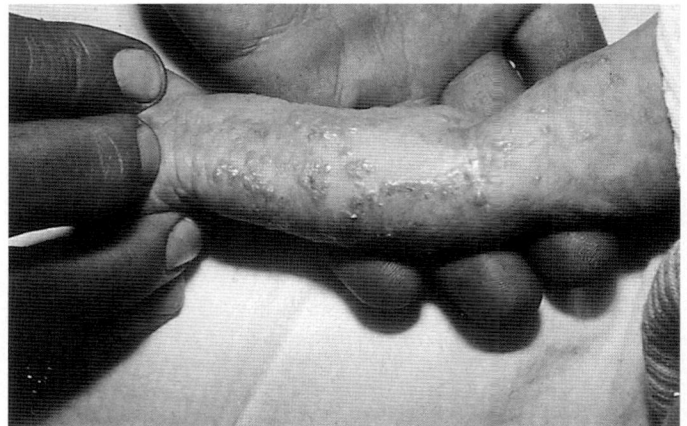

Fig. 30.17   Ash leaf patch: tuberous sclerosis.

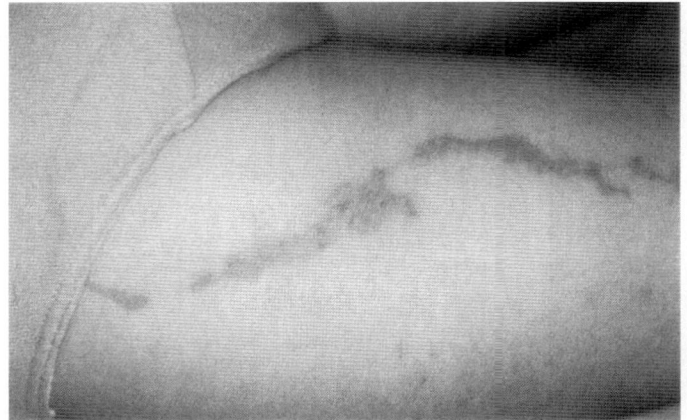

Fig. 30.19   Incontinentia pigmenti: vesicular stage.

weeks or months. Stage three comprises streaks and whorls and splattered patterns of macular hyperpigmentation which appear on both limbs and trunk at 12–24 months of age. Lesions persist to early adult life. Stage four is typically seen in affected female adults as linear, hypopigmented, atrophic streaks on the lower legs. These lesions are permanent.

Other dermatological features of incontinentia pigmenti are cicatricial alopecia over the vertex of the scalp and nail dystrophy in 40%.

rearrangement) in the NEMO gene (Xq28) and lesions probably occur through apoptosis of cells carrying the mutant gene.[29] There is increasing evidence that the 'sporadic type of IP' (IP type 1) represents a distinct disorder, hypomelanosis of Ito (q.v.), linked to Xp11. Neurological abnormalities occur in about 30% of cases and include epilepsy, mental retardation and spastic diplegia and tetraplegia. Ocular abnormalities are seen in 30% and include strabismus, cataracts, retinal vascular proliferation and retinal detachment. Over 80% of patients have dental abnormalities with partial anodontia and peg-shaped or conical teeth. A variety of skeletal abnormalities including limb reduction defects occur, and rarely cardiac abnormalities are seen.

Cutaneous lesions

The four cutaneous stages of this disease may follow each other in an orderly progression; however, overlap may occur, particularly in the earlier stages. Stage one comprises linear groups of vesicles which appear mainly on the limbs at birth or in the first days of life accompanied by a peripheral blood eosinophilia. They clear spontaneously over several weeks. Stage two is the verrucose stage with linear warty lesions appearing between 1 and 4 months of age: they occur particularly on the limbs, especially on dorsa of hands and feet, and resolve spontaneously after

ACRODERMATITIS ENTEROPATHICA AND NUTRITIONAL ZINC DEFICIENCY

Acrodermatitis enteropathica is an autosomal recessive condition in which there is a defective absorption of zinc, possibly due to the absence of a specific carrier protein. An identical condition occurs in infants with nutritional zinc deficiency. This may occur as a result of prematurity with low zinc stores, particularly in bottle-fed babies (as there is a lower bioavailability of zinc in bovine milk as compared to breast milk), or as a result of low breast milk zinc. Zinc deficiency also occurs in acquired immunodeficiency disease, cystic fibrosis and other causes of malabsorption and in infants on parenteral nutrition solutions not containing adequate zinc.

Clinical features

The onset in the primary form occurs usually when the child is weaned or in the first few weeks of life in a bottle-fed infant. In the children with nutritional zinc deficiency the onset is usually at the time of the first growth spurt. Erythematous and crusted, sometimes vesicular and pustular lesions appear in an acral distribution particularly around nose, mouth and eyes (Fig. 30.20) and sometimes on tips of digits and the paronychial areas. An anogenital rash (Fig. 30.21) is also common and psoriasiform

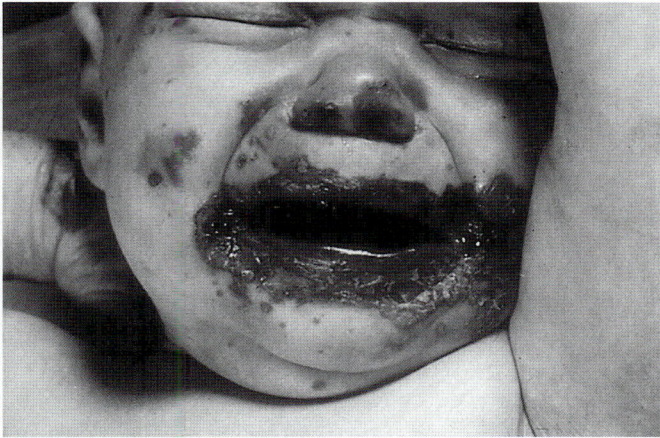

Fig. 30.20   Acrodermatitis enteropathica: mouth.

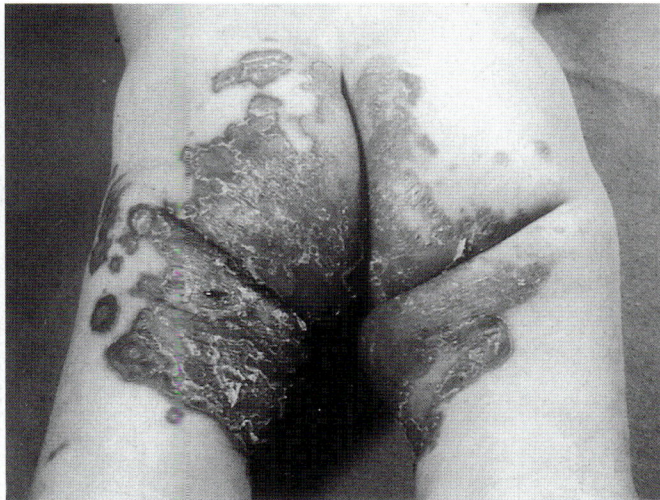

Fig. 30.21   Acrodermatitis enteropathica: buttocks.

lesions may occur on knees and elbows and occasionally elsewhere. Secondary bacterial and candidal infection is common. In the primary form mucosal involvement with glossitis, cheilitis and conjunctivitis may occur, a nail dystrophy is usual, and alopecia and diarrhea may occur.

The diagnosis is confirmed by finding a low serum zinc. The condition responds rapidly to the administration of high doses of oral zinc as either zinc gluconate or zinc sulfate. This is required life-long in the primary form but only for a few weeks in the secondary variety.

NEUROFIBROMATOSIS

Neurofibromatosis is a very variable multisystem disorder which is described in detail in Chapter 22. Only the dermatological features will be considered here.

Pigmented lesions

The café-au-lait macule is the most common of these: most prepubertal individuals with neurofibromatosis have at least six macules of greater than 0.5 cm in diameter increasing to at least 1.5 cm post puberty. Eventually hundreds of macules may be present.

In 20% of cases small freckle-like pigmented macules occur in the axillae. These occur only in the presence of café-au-lait macules and the combination is of great diagnostic significance. Similar small pigmented macules may occur in a widespread distribution, especially in patients with large numbers of café-au-lait spots. Larger pigmented patches 10 cm or more in diameter may overlie plexiform neuromas.

Neurofibromas (mollusca fibrosa)

These are soft pink or skin-colored tumors, often sessile or pedunculated and characteristically indentable. They usually develop after puberty. Their distribution is widespread and up to thousands of tumors half to several centimeters in diameter may occur. Small firmer discrete nodules occur along the course of peripheral nerves. The plexiform neuroma is a larger diffuse elongated neurofibroma along the course of a peripheral nerve. These may be present at birth or develop later. There may be an overgrowth of skin and subcutaneous tissue associated with these lesions producing gross disfigurement as a giant pendulous tumor with a wrinkled surface.

HEREDITARY PHOTOSENSITIVE DISORDERS (Table 30.5)

Photosensitivity is the cardinal feature of most of the porphyrias although some types may present with chronic nonspecific abdominal or musculoskeletal pain.[30] Photosensitivity occurs in other metabolic diseases such as phenylketonuria and Hartnup disease and severe photosensitivity also occurs in oculocutaneous albinism.

SKIN DISEASES OF THE NEONATE

ERYTHEMA TOXICUM NEONATORUM

This is a transient condition of unknown etiology occurring in up to 70% of neonates. The onset is from birth to 14 days but most cases start between day 1 and day 4. The commonest lesions are erythematous macules and papules but in some cases pustules appear. Lesions occur anywhere on the body surface except palms and soles but with a predilection for face and trunk. In cases present at birth, lesions are more acrally distributed and are often pustular. A peripheral blood eosinophilia is present and smears from pustules demonstrate sheets of eosinophils. The condition usually resolves in 2–3 days but, rarely, may persist for several weeks.

Recognition of this entity is important to avoid unnecessary investigations of serious neonatal infections.

TRANSIENT NEONATAL PUSTULAR DERMATOSIS

This is a benign condition in which superficial pustules are present at birth; it is rare for further lesions to develop postnatally. The pustules rupture within 24 h, developing a brown crust that separates after a few days to leave normal skin or a hyperpigmented macule in dark-skinned individuals. Lesions occur mainly on chin, upper anterior trunk, lower back and buttocks. They are asymptomatic and the infant is otherwise well. Lesions are sterile on culture enabling differentiation from important neonatal infections. If hyperpigmented macules occur, they resolve over 3–4 months.

ACROPUSTULOSIS OF INFANCY

This is a benign condition of unknown etiology occurring in otherwise healthy infants. The onset is usually in the neonatal period but may be delayed for some months. Recurrent crops of papules which quickly evolve into 2–4 mm vesicopustules occur, most commonly on the palms and soles and dorsa of hands and feet. Initially each crop takes 1–2 weeks to settle and new crops occur every 2–3 weeks. As time goes on the crops occur less frequently and the episodes are less severe and of shorter duration. Lesions are pruritic and finally resolve by 2–3 years.

The disease must be differentiated from other neonatal pustular conditions including herpes simplex, impetigo, scabies and candidiasis. Cultures of the lesions of infantile acropustulosis are sterile. A clinically identical condition can occur also as a postscabetic reaction in infants who have been successfully treated for scabies.

Topical therapy is usually ineffective. Oral antihistamines can be used if pruritus is severe.

MILIA

These represent retention cysts of the pilosebaceous follicles. They occur in approximately 50% of neonates as firm pearly white 1–2 mm

Table 30.5   Hereditary photosensitivity disorders

	Xeroderma pigmentosa	Bloom syndrome	Cockayne syndrome	Rothmund–Thomson syndrome	Erythropoietic protoporphyria	Congenital erythropoietic porphyria (Gunther disease)
Inheritance	AD	AR	AD	AR	AD	AR
Cutaneous features	Freckling initially, telangiectasia, spider nevi (angioma), subsequently atrophic hypopigmented guttate macules	Reticulate telangiectasia at sun-exposed sites. More than 50% have variable numbers of café-au-lait macules	Scaling and erythema at sun-exposed sites. Subsequently hyperpigmentation and atrophy	Mild photosensitivity only. Poikiloderma of cheeks and hands. Hyperkeratosis of palms and soles in adults	Relatively mild photosensitivity. Burning sensation after exposure to sunlight. Subsequently small scars on nose and cheeks	Severe photosensitivity in infancy. Blistering. Pink urine and brown discoloration of teeth. Hypertrichosis
Other features	Photophobia, conjunctivitis. Short stature, hypogonadism, microcephaly, mental retardation, deafness, ataxia	Dwarfism, hypogammaglobulinemia	Dwarfism. Disproportionately large limbs. Delayed psychomotor development. Optic atrophy, retinal degeneration and progressive deafness	Short stature. Sparse hair, cataracts, hypogonadism	Gallstones and hepatic cirrhosis	
Molecular defect	Defective DNA repair mechanisms	Chromosomal breakage disorder	Pathogenesis unknown	Mutations in RECQL4	Ferrochelatase deficiency	Uroporphyrinogen II synthase deficiency
Malignancy risk	Cutaneous melanoma and non-melanoma skin cancers	Cutaneous squamous cell carcinoma, leukemia, lymphoma, nephroblastoma		Cutaneous squamous cell carcinoma		
Other			Mean age of death 12 years due to renal failure, infections, neurological complications		Diagnosis confirmed by raised erythrocyte protoporphyrin. Beta-carotene may be helpful treatment	Diagnosis confirmed by elevated porphyrins in erythrocytes, urine and feces. Fatal outcome usually by second or third decade due to anemia, hepatic or renal failure. Successful cure following bone marrow/stem cell transplant

AD, autosomal dominant; AR, autosomal recessive.

papules particularly on the face. They usually disappear by 4 weeks of age. Epstein's pearls are epidermal cysts on the palate present in the majority of newborns. Persistent milia may be a marker for certain syndromes including Bazex syndrome, orofaciodigital syndrome type I and Marie – Unna hypotrichosis.

MILIARIA (PRICKLY HEAT)

This is a sweat retention phenomenon common in young infants. Unlike the equivalent condition in older persons it can occur in the absence of fever or significant occlusive factors. An obstruction of unknown etiology occurs within the intraepidermal portion of the eccrine sweat duct with retention of sweat behind the block. Lesions commence as red macules on which are superimposed 2–3 mm papules, vesicles or pustules (Fig. 30.22). Secondary infection can occur but most commonly these pustules are sterile. Characteristically the pattern and severity of the condition alter significantly from day to day enabling differentiation from infantile acne and infective conditions. Lesions occur most commonly on the face but scalp, neck and upper trunk are other common sites. The condition is also prone to occur under plastic napkins and napkin covers.

Management involves keeping the child as cool as practicable and avoidance of contact with non-porous materials such as nylon and plastic, and of occlusive topical agents. The parents should be reassured that this is a transient condition and is uncommon after 6 months of age.

SUBCUTANEOUS FAT NECROSIS OF THE NEWBORN

This is a necrosis of subcutaneous fat in the newborn probably induced by ischemia. It occurs usually in healthy full-term infants. Often, however, there is a history of a difficult labor and delivery with such complications as prolonged labor, fetal distress, perinatal asphyxia due to meconium aspiration or other cause and forceps delivery. The condition has also been reported in several cases following hypothermic cardiac surgery.

The lesions appear between the second and third weeks of life as non-tender, firm, skin-colored or red–purple nodules or plaques occurring particularly on buttocks, shoulders, upper back, proximal limbs and cheeks. New nodules may develop over several weeks. They usually disappear

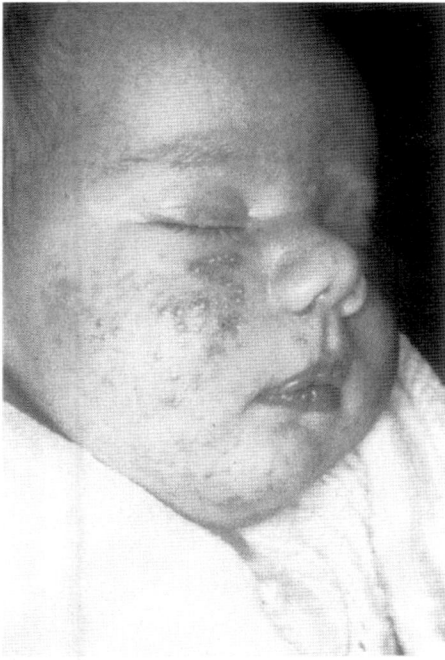

Fig. 30.22 Pustular miliaria (prickly heat).

spontaneously without complication in several months leaving no trace. However, sometimes they become fluctuant, ulcerate or calcify.

Metabolic complications include hypercalcemia, hypoglycemia, thrombocytopenia, anemia and hypertriglyceridemia. Fluctuant lesions should be aspirated, secondary infection should be dealt with if it complicates ulcerated lesions, and serum calcium levels should be monitored, particularly in the presence of calcified lesions, for up to 6 months. Otherwise management involves observation and reassurance.

CUTIS MARMORATA (CONGENITAL LIVEDO RETICULARIS)

This term usually refers to a transient benign physiological vascular reaction occurring in both premature and full-term infants as a response to minor cooling. A blue or purple discoloration in a marbled or reticulate pattern occurs on trunk and limbs. It lasts minutes to hours but reverses quickly on warming the infant. The tendency to the condition lasts for weeks or months.

There are a number of important conditions which may be associated with more severe and persistent cutis marmorata. These include Down syndrome, trisomy 18, homocystinuria, de Lange syndrome, neonatal lupus and congenital hypothyroidism. A nevoid vascular disorder, cutis marmorata telangiectatica congenita (CMTC), presents with reticulate purple lesions but the distribution is often segmental rather than generalized and atrophy and ulceration may occur in the affected areas. Musculoskeletal, neurological and vascular anomalies may be seen with CMTC.[31]

HARLEQUIN COLOR CHANGE

This vascular phenomenon is probably caused by an immature autonomic regulatory mechanism. It does not indicate any significant neural or vascular abnormality. When the neonate lies on one side the lower half of the body is red and the upper half is pale with a clear midline separation. This color change is transient and can be reversed by altering the infant's position. It is rarely seen after the first few days of life.

INFANTILE ACNE

This condition commences at about 3 months of age with lesions particularly on the cheeks. Open comedones predominate but closed comedones,

papules, pustules and even cysts can occur. Deeper lesions may produce significant scarring. Untreated the condition usually lasts 2–3 years. In patients with a strong family history of acne the condition may be more severe and there may be difficult acne at puberty. Hormonal abnormalities are rarely found in these patients and investigation is indicated only in cases which are unusually severe, prolonged or unresponsive to therapy. Most patients with mild acne respond well to topical therapies (benzoyl peroxide, erythromycin or retinoids). Oral antibiotics (erythromycin or trimethoprim) may be required for moderate/severe cases. Isotretinoin has also been successfully used in severe cases.

INFECTIONS AND INFESTATIONS OF THE SKIN

VIRUS INFECTIONS

Herpes simplex

Herpes simplex virus (HSV) infections are extremely common in children, and serological studies confirm that more than 90% of the population have been infected by adulthood (Fig. 30. 23). The commonest type is HSV1, though HSV2 is more important in adulthood, being the cause of genital herpes. Four distinct presentations are recognized in childhood.

Neonatal herpes simplex virus infection

This is a potentially devastating infection usually contracted during delivery from infected vaginal secretions (HSV2) (Fig. 30.24). However, intrauterine and postnatal infection may occur. Approximately 50% of infected infants have skin lesions which are manifested as grouped blisters localized initially on the presenting part, usually the head, with the onset usually between the 4th and 8th days of life. The eruption may

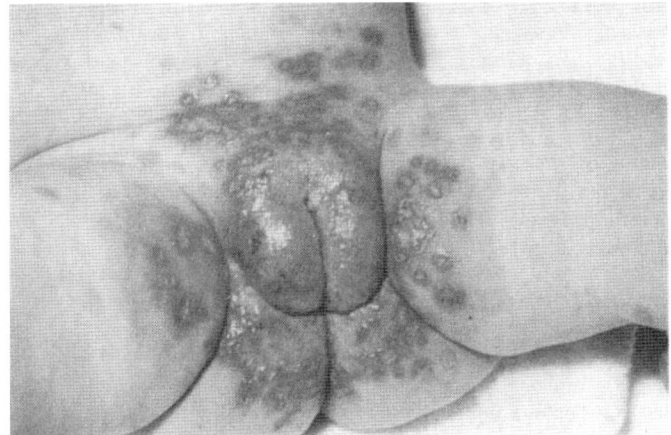

Fig. 30.23 Perineal herpes simplex.

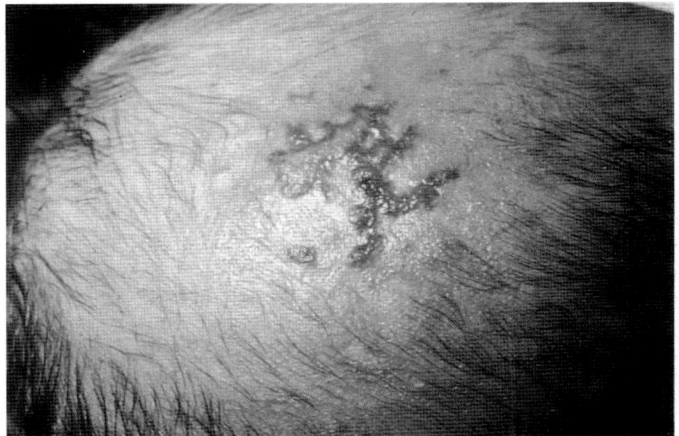

Fig. 30.24 Neonatal herpes on scalp.

become widespread with individual lesions a few millimeters across coalescing to produce large erosions. A rapid immunofluorescence test on material from the blister base enables a diagnosis within a few hours. Culture of the virus takes several days. A rising titer of complement-fixing antibodies can be demonstrated comparing acute and convalescent sera.

The child with cutaneous neonatal herpes should be assessed urgently for the presence and extent of other organ involvement. Immediate treatment with intravenous aciclovir is indicated.

Primary herpetic gingivostomatitis

This is a common presentation of HSV infection in children (Fig. 30.25). The child is systemically unwell with a high fever and there is severe swelling, erosion and bleeding of the gums and the anterior part of the buccal mucosa. Posterior spread is rare but anterior spread to the lips and the facial skin often occurs. There may be considerable soft tissue swelling and prominent lymphadenopathy. The condition is extremely painful and the child often refuses to eat or drink, necessitating parenteral fluids as the condition may take up to 2 weeks to resolve. Oral antibiotics may be required for secondary bacterial infection. Unless the condition is very severe systemic antiviral therapy is not usually required.

Recurrent herpes simplex (herpes labialis)

Recurrent herpes simplex of the face, particularly around the lips (herpes labialis), is common in childhood. As in adults various factors, including fever and sun exposure, may reactivate the virus. Saline bathing of the lesions speeds resolution and prevents secondary infection. Topical antiviral agents are of limited value.

Disseminated herpes simplex (eczema herpeticum)

This occurs as a complication of atopic eczema and in immunosuppressed patients (Fig. 30.26). It may originate from a primary or recurrent infection, or from external reinfection. Spread is both on the surface of the skin and also by hematogenous dissemination. The lesions are vesicles or pustules 2–4 mm across which may spread with alarming rapidity and have a tendency to coalescence to produce extensive punched-out lesions. Topical steroids should be avoided as their application may spread the virus. Secondary bacterial infection should be treated with oral antibiotics. In most cases systemic aciclovir is indicated. Minor recurrences of HSV infection are seen in up to 20% of cases.

Varicella (chickenpox)

Chickenpox (Ch. 28) is caused by the same herpes virus which produces herpes zoster/shingles (the varicella zoster virus). The incubation period is from 9 to 23 days (mean 14–17 days). After a prodrome of 2–3 days a vesicular eruption develops at the sites of erythematous papules. They appear in crops over 2–4 days, initially on the trunk then face and limbs. Vesicles are often seen in the mouth and occasionally affect other

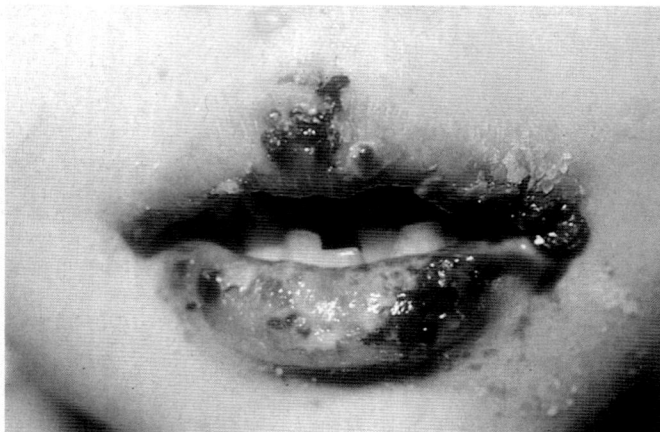

Fig. 30.26   Disseminated herpes simplex (eczema herpeticum).

mucous membranes. Pruritus and pyrexia are variable and resolution takes a little over 2 weeks. Complications (encephalitis, pneumonitis and hepatitis) are rare in otherwise healthy children and routine use of aciclovir is not recommended. A live attenuated vaccine is licensed for prophylactic use in North America.

Herpes zoster

This usually occurs when the virus, which has remained dormant in the cells of dorsal root or cranial nerve ganglia following an attack of chickenpox, reactivates, replicates and spreads along the nerves from these ganglia to infect areas of skin supplied by them (Fig. 30.27). Herpes zoster is much less common in children than in adults but it may occur as early as the first year of life. In children who develop zoster in the first 2 years of life there is rarely a history of previous chickenpox in the child but often a history of maternal chickenpox during pregnancy.

Herpes zoster presents as a segmental blistering eruption on an erythematous base. Usually a single dermatome is affected but spread to

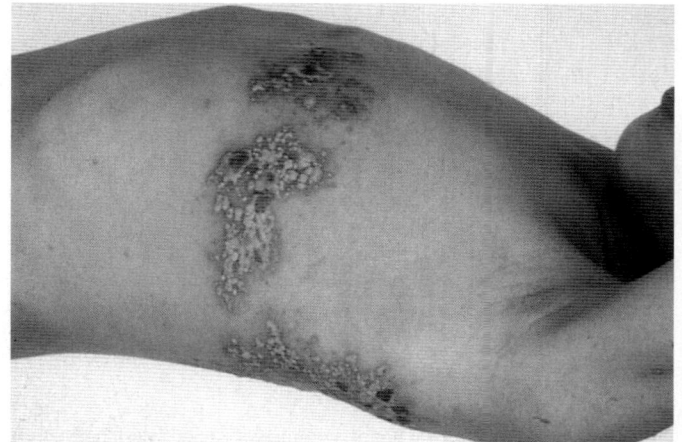

Fig. 30.25   Perioral herpes simplex.

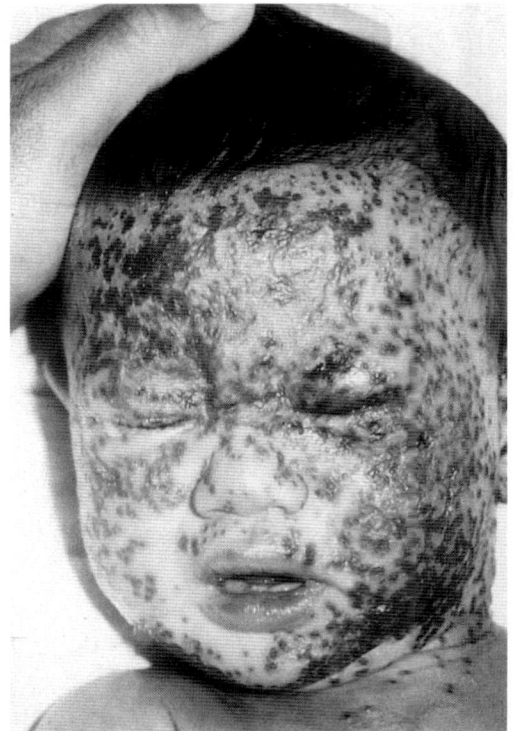

Fig. 30.27   Herpes zoster.

one or two adjoining dermatomes may occur. The eruption is essentially unilateral though there may be minor spread to the opposite side on the trunk or brow. Up to 20 or 30 scattered lesions identical to chickenpox commonly occur. Infection involving the ophthalmic division of the 5th cranial (trigeminal) nerve may produce keratitis and uveitis, threatening vision. An important cutaneous sign of potentially dangerous herpes zoster ophthalmicus is blisters on the nose indicating involvement of the nasociliary branch. Blisters in the oral cavity occur with involvement of maxillary and mandibular divisions of the trigeminal nerve. Anogenital blistering and sometimes disorders of urination and defecation occur with involvement of sacral nerves. Scarring and postherpetic neuralgia are rare complications in children.

Management

This is directed at providing symptomatic treatment with wet compresses and appropriate analgesia, and dealing with any secondary bacterial infection. Early ophthalmological consultation is essential for ophthalmic zoster patients. Intravenous aciclovir is indicated in very severe cases, particularly of ophthalmic zoster and for all immunosuppressed patients.

Molluscum contagiosum

This is a poxvirus infection which is rare under 1 year of age and occurs particularly in the 2–5-year age group (Fig. 30.28). Outbreaks may occur among children who bathe or swim together and in the adolescent age group sexual transmission becomes important. The typical lesion is spherical and pearly white with a central umbilication, but they may vary from tiny 1 mm papules to large nodules over 1 cm in diameter. They occur on any part of the skin surface with common sites being the axillae and sides of the trunk, the lower abdomen and anogenital area. Rarely they occur on the eyelids where they may cause conjunctivitis and punctate keratitis. A secondary eczema often occurs around lesions, particularly in atopics, and scratching of this spreads the mollusca. Hundreds of lesions may be present in an individual patient. Secondary bacterial infection may occur producing crusting, erythema and suppuration. However, these same changes may be seen during spontaneous resolution which occurs in most within 6–9 months leaving normal skin or small varicelliform scars.

Management

With multiple small lesions in a young child spontaneous resolution should be awaited. No controlled trials exist for treatment of mollusca in childhood. However cryotherapy after application of anesthetic cream, topical therapy with salicylic acid, podophyllotoxin, cantharidin and more recently imiquimod or cidofovir have all been reported with variable success. Physical extrusion of the contents of larger lesions can also be undertaken and is usually best after anesthetic cream application. Up to 10% of cases develop eczema around the lesions which resolves when the mollusca clear. Spontaneous regression may be associated with secondary bacterial infection requiring a topical antibiotic.

Warts

Warts are benign tumors caused by infection with a variety of human papilloma viruses. The common wart (verruca vulgaris) occurs particularly at sites of trauma such as hands, feet, knees and elbows. Plane or flat warts, 1–3 mm pink or brown barely raised papules, occur on the face and often spread along scratch marks or cuts. Plantar warts occur particularly over pressure points on the soles and can be differentiated from calluses by a loss of skin markings over the skin surface. Unlike corns or callosities they tend to be painful on lateral pressure. Warts at mucocutaneous junctions often have a filiform or fronded appearance. Anogenital warts may be acquired from maternal infection during delivery, but their presence should always raise the suspicion of sexual abuse (Fig. 30.29).

Management

Various forms of treatment are available: they depend on the area, the type of wart and the age of the patient. Because spontaneous disappearance is common, aggressive treatment is usually inappropriate. A Cochrane review[32] of local treatments for cutaneous warts shows that there is very little good evidence on which to determine best practice. The best available evidence was for the use of topical salicylic acid preparations. Perhaps surprisingly cryotherapy was not found to be superior. Other currently used topical agents include glutaraldehyde and formaldehyde preparations. Podophyllotoxin is less irritant than podophyllin but both can be used for isolated anogenital warts. Facial plane warts may respond to retinoic acid preparations. Cautery or diathermy is useful for lesions on the lips or anogenital area but elsewhere recurrence is fairly frequent following their use and there is also a risk of producing a painful scar. The initial favorable response to oral cimetidine has not been replicated in double-blind placebo-controlled trials.[33]

Papular acrodermatitis of childhood (Gianotti–Crosti syndrome)

Papular acrodermatitis of childhood was first described by Gianotti as an acrally distributed papular eruption occurring in young children due to the hepatitis B virus (Fig. 30.30). However, a similar eruption may occur with over a dozen different viruses and the condition is best regarded as a reaction pattern with multiple etiologies.[34]

This pattern of exanthem occurs particularly in children between 1 and 4 years of age. The rash comprises discrete firm red papules 1–5 mm in diameter, sometimes surmounted by vesicles. Pruritus is variable but not usually a significant feature. The lesions involve the limbs, particularly distally, and the face, with the trunk being essentially spared. The

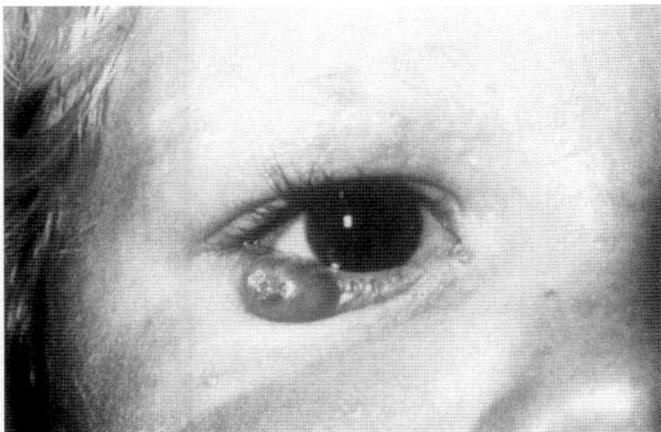

Fig. 30.28 Molluscum contagiosum.

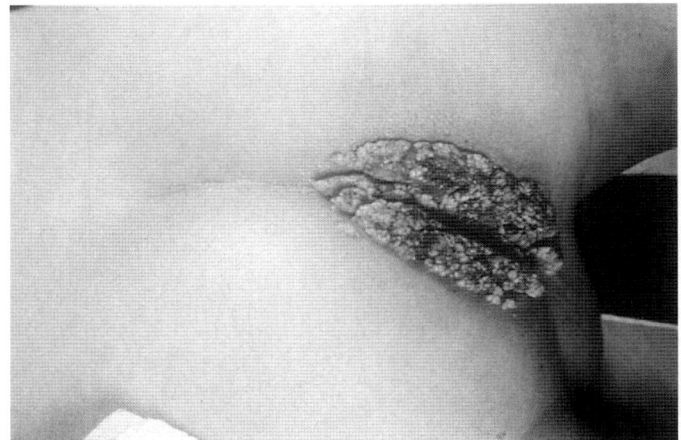

Fig. 30.29 Perianal warts.

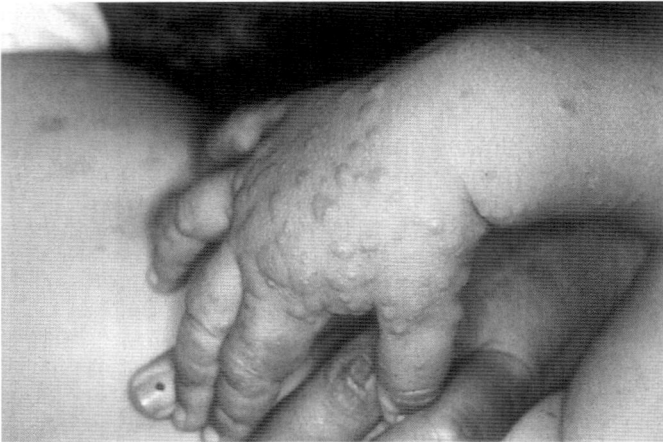

Fig. 30.30   Papular acrodermatitis of childhood.

rash fades within 3–4 weeks. Lymphadenopathy is usually present but the child is often otherwise remarkably well, leading to such misdiagnoses as insect bites and papular eczema.

Investigation should be aimed at excluding the more serious viral etiologies.

Pityriasis rosea

Epidemiological studies suggest a viral origin, now thought to be human herpes virus 7. It occurs in children and young adults and has no sexual or racial predilection (Fig. 30.31).

The eruption commences with the appearance of the so-called herald patch, typically a single round or oval scaly lesion 1–5 cm in diameter, flat or slightly raised with a tendency to clear in the center. It usually occurs on the trunk, neck or proximal limbs. Some 5–15 days later the secondary eruption appears comprising multiple, variably pruritic, dull pink, oval macules with a peripheral collarette of scale. The typical distribution is on trunk and proximal limbs but may be very extensive. The long axis of the lesions on the trunk runs parallel with the ribs giving

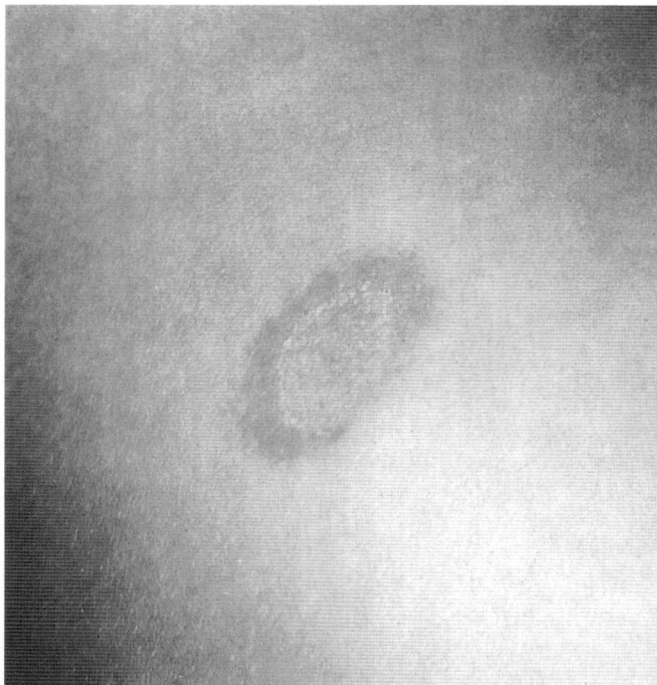

Fig. 30.31   Pityriasis rosea (herald patch).

a 'Christmas-tree' pattern. Rarer variants have lesions which are papular, urticarial, vesicular, purpuric or pustular but some of the typical lesions are usually intermingled. Lesions crop at 2–3 day intervals for 7–10 days and then spontaneous resolution occurs over several weeks. Sun exposure may speed this resolution and meanwhile symptomatic therapy can be used for the pruritus if this is troublesome.

BACTERIAL INFECTIONS

Staphylococcal and streptococcal infections of the skin are common in childhood. They take the following clinical forms:

Impetigo

This is a bacterial infection caused by *Staphylococcus aureus*, group A beta-hemolytic streptococcus (GABHS) or a combination of these organisms (Fig. 30.32). Recently there has been a worldwide increase in the predominance of staphylococci in the causation of impetigo.[35,36] An increasing proportion of *S. aureus* isolates are resistant to meticillin (MRSA).

Impetigo occurs in two forms, bullous and more commonly non-bullous (or crusted). Bullous impetigo (Fig. 30.33) is always due to staphylococci. Blisters arise on previously normal skin and increase rapidly in size and number, soon rupturing to produce superficial erosions with a peripheral brown crust. The erosions continue to expand, sometimes clearing centrally to produce annular lesions. The condition is usually neither itchy nor painful. Non-bullous impetigo may be due to either organism or to a combination. The lesions begin with a small transient vesicle on an erythematous base. The serum exuding from the ruptured

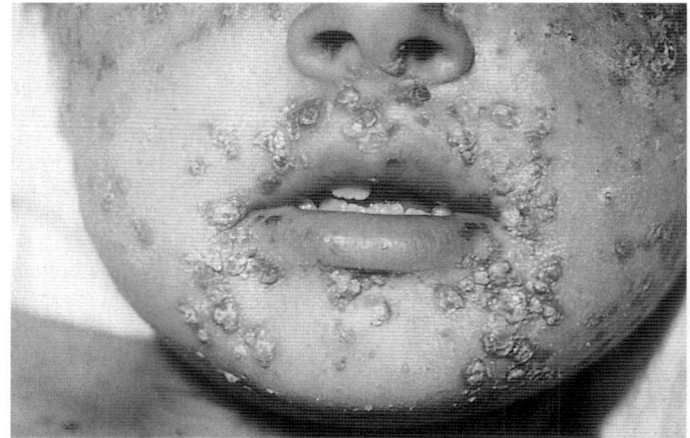

Fig. 30.32   Impetigo.

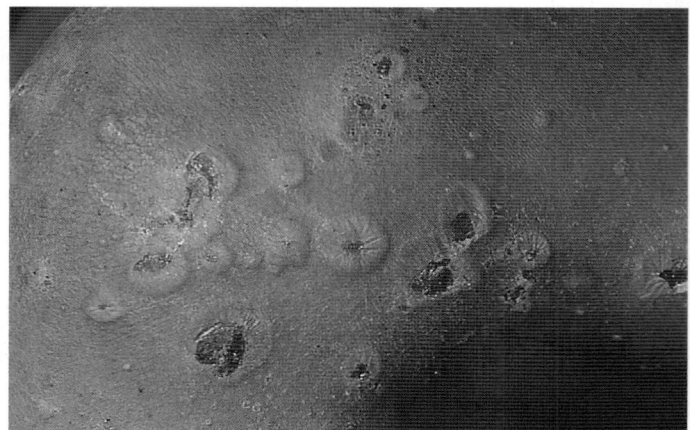

Fig. 30.33   Bullous impetigo.

vesicle produces a thick soft yellow crust, below which there is a moist superficial erosion. The lesions extend slowly and remain much smaller than those of bullous impetigo. Impetigo is often superimposed on other skin diseases such as insect bites, scabies, pediculosis and atopic eczema. As impetigo is an intraepidermal infection, the condition does not scar although postinflammatory pigmentation can occur, particularly in dark-skinned patients.

Management

Impetigo is very contagious and the patient should, if possible, be isolated. A swab for culture and sensitivity testing should always be taken. Topical mupirocin is as successful as oral erythromycin in eradicating both S. aureus and GABHS[37] and a double-blind study has shown hydrogen peroxide cream to be as effective as topical fusidic acid.[38] However, topical therapies will not eradicate bacteria on clinically uninvolved skin and therefore in general oral antibiotics should be used. Because of the rarity in most areas of pure streptococcal impetigo, a penicillinase-resistant penicillin or erythromycin is the treatment of choice while awaiting culture results. In many areas of the world there is an emergence of erythromycin-resistant staphylococci[35,39] and knowledge of the local situation is important in selecting the antibiotic of first choice while awaiting sensitivity testing. Underlying diseases should be sought and treated appropriately if the pattern of impetigo suggests them. If a group A streptococcus is isolated the patient should be watched for 8 weeks for signs of glomerulonephritis.

Folliculitis

Superficial bacterial folliculitis is common in children. It is characterized by inflammation confined to the opening of the hair follicle whereas furuncles or boils are cutaneous abscesses, centered around usually ruptured hair follicles. Both are caused by a wide variety of types and strains of S. aureus and predisposing factors are occlusion (e.g. overuse of very greasy emollients), friction, maceration and sweating. Patients with recurrent attacks are often found to carry the strains of S. aureus in their nose, axillae or perineum, or to be in close contact with another person who is a carrier. Folliculitis commences with perifollicular erythema with pustule formation that often ruptures to form a crust. Pruritus is common. Boils are larger, firm erythematous papules that evolve into fluctuant pus-filled nodules with central necrosis (pointing) and discharge.

Mild folliculitis is often self-limiting but can be treated with topical antiseptics. If the infection is persistent or recurrent, topical or oral antistaphylococcal antibiotics should be given. Swabs should first be taken for culture from affected as well as S. aureus carriage sites. If necessary, other carriers who are in close contact should be identified and treated.

Cellulitis

This is an acute bacterial infection involving the subcutis as well as the dermis. The lesion is erythematous sometimes with a purple or blue hue. It is warm and tender and has a less well-defined edge than erysipelas. Fever and malaise, leukocytosis and lymphadenopathy are usually present. When cellulitis follows a wound or other break in the skin, group A beta-hemolytic streptococcus is the commonest cause. Other organisms involved in cellulitis include Haemophilus influenzae, Streptococcus pneumoniae, S. aureus and Pseudomonas aeruginosa. Two special forms are discussed below.

Perianal streptococcal disease

This occurs in children between 1 and 10 years of age (Fig. 30.34). The child may complain of painful defecation or pruritus. Fresh blood is often found on the stool. There is a well-demarcated, very bright red erythema extending out several centimeters from the anus. The anal rim is often macerated and fissured. GABHS is grown from the skin and often also from the patient's throat. The condition may be surprisingly resistant to therapy, recurring after 5–10 days of oral penicillin therapy: an initial course of at least 14 days is advisable. The addition of topical mupirocin may further reduce the risk of recurrence.[40]

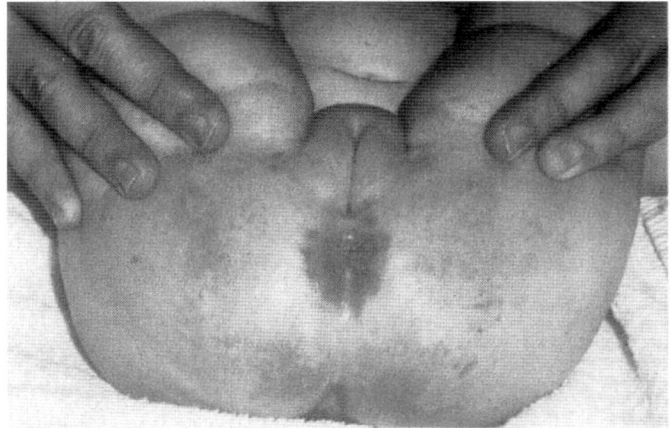

Fig. 30.34   Perianal streptococcal disease.

Facial cellulitis

Facial cellulitis in young children often occurs in the absence of any break in the skin and is due to H. influenzae or S. pneumoniae accompanying an upper respiratory tract infection or otitis media. Cellulitis due to these bacteria often has a lilac-blue color. The condition may be complicated by bacteremia, septicemia and meningitis. In all cases of facial cellulitis cultures should be taken from nasopharynx, ears, blood and, if indicated, cerebrospinal fluid. Needle aspiration from the lesion after saline injection may provide material from which the organism can be cultured.

Intravenous cefotaxime, a third generation cephalosporin, is the initial treatment of choice until an organism is identified and sensitivity tests performed.

Erysipelas

This is an acute bacterial infection of the dermal connective tissue and superficial lymphatics caused most often by GABHS but occasionally due to other streptococci, H. influenzae and S. aureus. A brightly erythematous, hot, tender area with a rapidly spreading distinct edge develops. Superimposed bullae may occur. There is accompanying fever and malaise and a leukocytosis. Predisposing factors include lymphatic obstruction and a break in the skin due, for example, to a wound, bite or tinea infection. The episode produces a lymphangitis which further damages the lymphatics, and chronic lymphedema may result from and further predispose to recurrent erysipelas. Treatment involves rest and high doses of the appropriate antibiotic, usually phenoxymethylpenicillin (penicillin V), orally or intravenously depending on the severity.

Staphylococcal scalded skin syndrome
Pathogenesis

The staphylococcal scalded skin syndrome (SSSS) is a widespread blistering disease caused by an epidermolytic toxin produced by certain strains of S. aureus, most often of phage group II, but occasionally phage group I or III (Figs 30.35 and 30.36). This toxin produces a superficial splitting of the skin with the level of split being high in the epidermis. Clinical disease occurs when there is sufficient toxin load produced from an infection with these organisms. The commonest sites of infection are the umbilicus (in neonates), the nose, nasopharynx or throat, the conjunctiva and deep wounds.

The condition commences with a macular erythema initially on the face and in the major flexures and then becoming generalized. The skin is exquisitely tender and the child draws back from contact. After 2 days flaccid bullae develop and the skin wrinkles and shears off. The exfoliation is most marked in the groin, neck fold and around the mouth and may involve the entire body surface but mucosae remain uninvolved. The child is usually febrile but because of the superficial level of the split fluid loss is rarely significant. The erosions crust and dry and heal with desquamation over the next 4–8 days leaving no sequelae.

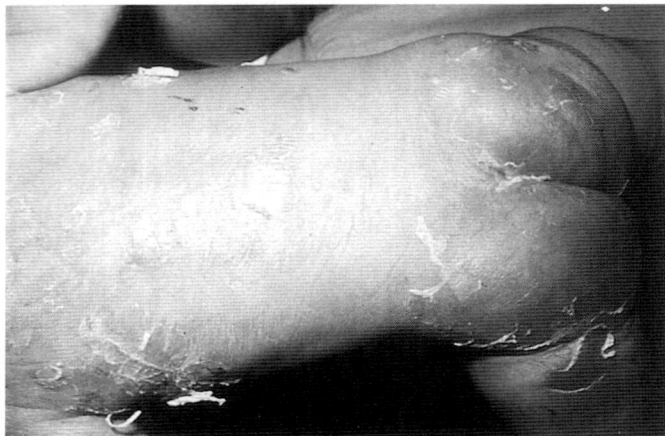

Fig. 30.35 Staphylococcal scalded skin syndrome.

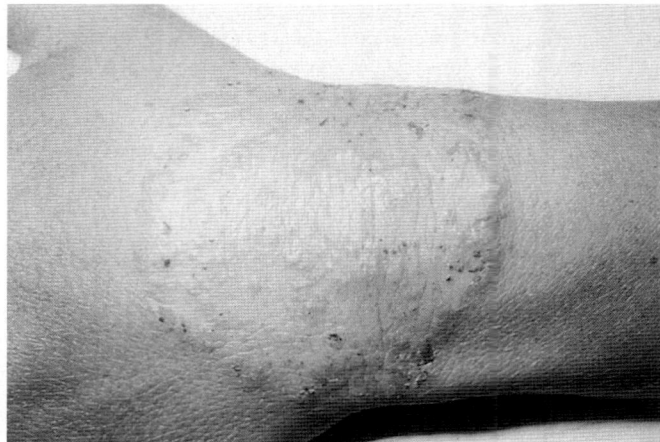

Fig. 30.37 Tinea.

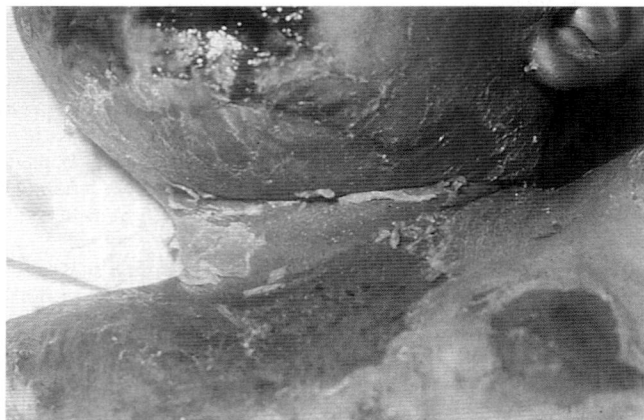

Fig. 30.36 Staphylococcal scalded skin syndrome.

Diagnosis

Cultures from skin and blister fluid are usually negative. Cultures should be obtained from any area of obvious infection but, if none is apparent, from nasopharynx and throat. The most important differential diagnosis is toxic epidermal necrolysis (TEN). In TEN the split is subepidermal and the blisters and erosions are usually hemorrhagic and mucosae are commonly involved. Microscopy of frozen or Giemsa-stained sections of the blister roof can detect the level of the split in the two conditions. Other conditions from which SSSS must be differentiated are scarlet fever, Kawasaki syndrome and toxic shock syndrome, all of which show mucosal involvement and rarely demonstrate frank blistering.

Management

The child should be nursed with as little handling as possible. No topical agents should be applied. A penicillinase-resistant penicillin is the treatment of choice and should be given orally if possible. Insertion and securing of an intravenous line is very painful in these patients and should be performed only if oral antibiotics are refused or if rehydration is required in a child refusing oral fluids. Analgesia is often necessary in the early stages. Emollients are useful once the skin dries and desquamation commences.

FUNGAL INFECTIONS

Tinea

This is an infection due to dermatophyte fungi: the source of the fungus is an animal (e.g. dog, cat, guinea pig, cattle), the soil or another human (Fig. 30.37). Tinea occurs on any part of the skin surface and can involve hair and nails.

The classical features of tinea on the skin are itch, erythema studded with papules or pustules, annular or geographical lesions ('ringworm') with a tendency to central clearing and a superficial scale. Family members or pets are the usual source of infection. On the palms and soles erythema and increased skin markings may be the only signs. Between the toes maceration with a thick white scale is the main finding and an annular lesion may extend onto the dorsum of the foot. On the soles there are deep seated blisters or pustules which dry to produce brown crusts. Tinea is often unilateral and always asymmetrical, whereas eczema and psoriasis, which it may resemble, are often symmetrical in distribution. Nail tinea (onychomycosis) is uncommon in children but increases with age.

In the UK the principal dermatophytes causing tinea capitis are *Microsporum canis* and *Trichophyton tonsurans*. Both cause a combination of alopecia and inflammation with the hair loss being due to breakage of hair shafts. The inflammation varies from mild erythema and a fine dandruff-like scale to a pustular carbuncle-like lesion (kerion), which occurs most commonly with *Trichophyton* species. Other causes of alopecia to be differentiated from tinea are trichotillomania (q.v.) and alopecia areata (q.v). Bright green fluorescence is seen under Wood's (ultraviolet) light in *Microsporum* infection of the scalp. Other varieties of scalp tinea produce no typical fluorescence and the Wood's light has no place in the diagnosis of tinea on the skin surface. The diagnosis of tinea is confirmed by plucking hairs or scraping scales. The fungus can be cultured on appropriate media.

Topical antifungals may be satisfactory for small localized patches of tinea on the skin. Griseofulvin is the only antifungal licensed for oral treatment in children. It is effective against dermatophytes but in general a 3 month course is used with longer courses for nail tinea. Terbinafine is not yet licensed for children but a number of published studies have shown it to be safe and effective for tinea capitis.[41]

Candidiasis (moniliasis)

This is due to a yeast, *Candida albicans*. It occurs on both skin and mucosal surfaces and certain factors predispose to its establishment (Fig. 30.38). General predisposing factors in children include drug therapy with broad spectrum antibiotics, corticosteroids and immunosuppressives, diabetes and any disease which interferes with immunological competence. Local predisposing factors are particularly those which create a warm moist environment. Flexural areas are susceptible, especially in the presence of sweating, obesity and other skin disease. The oral mucosa in infancy also has a particular susceptibility to this infection which is usually acquired during passage through an infected birth canal.

On the general body skin, where candidiasis rarely occurs except in the presence of immunodeficiency, the infection is manifested by small round erythematous lesions with a peripheral overhanging scale.

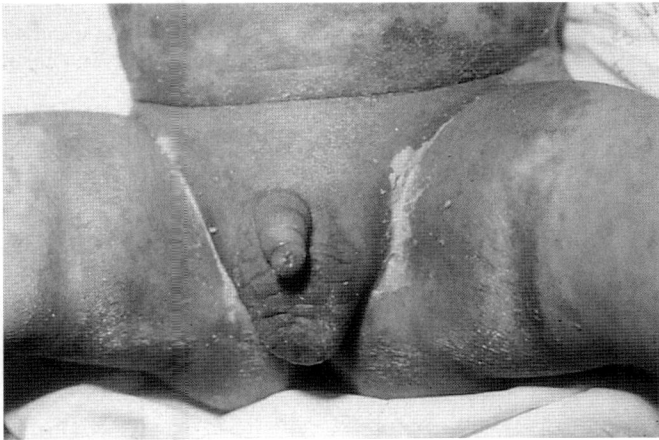

Fig. 30.38 Candidiasis.

Occasionally small papules or superficial pustules occur, especially in the neonate. In flexural areas the typical picture is of a cheesy white material deep in the folds and satellite lesions with the typical peripheral scale. On mucosae a curd-like white material is superimposed on a red base. Acute or chronic paronychia may be seen, particularly in children that suck their fingers.

Chronic mucocutaneous candidiasis is a progressive candidal infection occurring in patients who have an inability to destroy candida due to a severe general immunodeficiency or due to a specific immunological defect. A variety of endocrinopathies may be associated with this syndrome.

The diagnosis of candidiasis is usually a clinical one which may be confirmed by microscopy and culture. Candida is frequently a secondary invader rather than a primary cause of skin disease and local and general predisposing factors should be eliminated. Once predisposing factors have been eliminated most localized infections respond well to topical agents including polyene antibiotics, nystatin and imidazole derivatives. Reduction of intestinal carriage with oral preparations is rarely necessary. Oral ketoconazole is useful in chronic mucocutaneous candidiasis and other candidal infections in the immunosuppressed.

Pityriasis versicolor

This is an infection with *Malassezia* yeasts (*Pityrosporum* species) which are part of the normal skin flora. It occurs mainly in tropical and temperate zones and usually affects adolescents and young adults. It presents as well-demarcated, asymptomatic or slightly itchy macules with a fine branny scale which is often only obvious on light scratching of the lesions. Primary macules 1–10 mm in diameter coalesce into larger patches. They occur in two colors, red–brown especially in the fair skinned and hypopigmented in darker skinned. In a partially tanned individual, lesions of both colors may be found. In young children, unlike adults, approximately 30% present with only facial lesions.[42]

Diagnosis is confirmed by microscopic examination of skin scrapings to which 20% potassium hydroxide has been added. Grape-like clusters of spores and short fragments of thick mycelia are seen. In its hypopigmented forms the condition must be distinguished from: (a) vitiligo, where the depigmentation is total and scale absent; (b) pityriasis alba, where lesions are less well demarcated and some erythema may be seen; and (c) tuberculoid leprosy which is accompanied by anesthesia in the hypopigmented areas. The red-brown form has to be differentiated from seborrheic dermatitis, tinea and psoriasis, all of which lack the very fine branny type of scale.

Untreated the condition is persistent though some improvement may occur in winter. Various treatments are available. The treatment of choice is with topical imidazole creams. Alternatively two overnight applications of 2.5% selenium sulfide may be effective in the short term but relapse is frequent. With the depigmented form, whatever therapy is used, sun exposure is required for full repigmentation.

ECTOPARASITIC INFESTATIONS

Scabies

This is due to *Sarcoptes scabei*, an eight-legged, oval-shaped mite less than 0.5 mm in length. The disease is transmitted by close physical contact.

A small number of mites burrow into the skin in certain sites, particularly between the fingers, the ulnar border of the hand, around the wrists and elbows, the anterior axillary fold, nipples and penis and, in infants, the palms and soles. The pathognomonic primary lesion, a typical burrow, is a 2–3 mm long curved gray line with a vesicle at the anterior end. Other lesions which mark the sites of burrows are small blisters or papules, larger blisters on the palms and soles of infants, scratch marks, secondary eczema and secondary bacterial infection. Eczema or impetigo in the target areas for scabies should always raise suspicion of this disease as should blisters on the palms and soles of infants.

Often more prominent than the evidence of burrows is the so-called secondary eruption of scabies. This presents as multiple, very pruritic, urticarial papules which are soon excoriated (Fig. 30.39). They occur particularly on the abdomen, thighs and buttocks. Young children may show a striking dermographism in the areas of scratch marks. When dermographism occurs in the first year of life scabies should always be suspected. Large inflammatory nodules may form part of the secondary eruption, occurring particularly on covered areas especially axillae, scrotum, penis and buttocks. They may, however, be very widespread producing diagnostic difficulties. They may persist for months after effective scabies treatment.

The diagnosis of scabies is usually a clinical one but can be confirmed by demonstration of the mite. A burrow is scraped and the material smeared on a slide with potassium hydroxide for microscopic examination. Burrows may be more easily identified by rubbing a thick black marking pen over suspicious areas and wiping with an alcohol swab leaving a burrow outlined with ink.

Management

The patient and all close contacts should be treated simultaneously. The treatment of choice is 5% permethrin cream[43,44]: it should be applied to

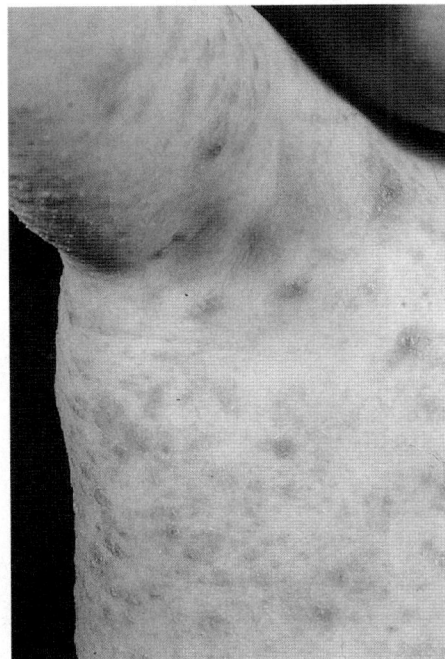

Fig. 30.39 Scabies.

all body surfaces from the neck down and left on overnight. A repeat application should be administered after 1 week. Bedclothes and clothing should be washed in the normal way. An irritant dermatitis may follow scabies treatment, particularly in atopics, and may require emollients and topical steroids once the miticide therapy is fully completed. Persistent nodules may respond to topical corticosteroids and families should be warned that it can take up to 3–4 weeks before the pruritus subsides.

Pediculosis (lice)

Human lice are ectoparasites dependent on man for survival. They are wingless six-legged insects, gray – white in color or red – brown when engorged with blood. The head louse (*Pediculus humanus capitis*) and the body louse (*Pediculus humanus humanus*) have a 24 mm long slim body and three similar pairs of legs. The pubic louse (*Pthirus pubis*, crab louse) has a wider, shorter body 12 mm long and the second and third pairs of legs are larger than the first, producing a crab-like appearance. The nits or ova are seen as oval gray – white 0.5 mm specks firmly attached by a chitinous ring to hairs or clothing.

Pediculosis capitis

This is a very common infection, occurring in epidemics amongst schoolchildren. The infestation is most severe in and may be confined to the occipital area. It is very itchy and excoriations are seen but secondary eczematization and bacterial infection may mask the condition. Nits may be differentiated from epidermal scales and hair casts by their firm attachment and by fluorescence with a Wood's light. Occasionally the head louse infects the eyelashes in children (Fig. 30.40).

Pediculosis corporis

This is rare in children except in conditions of overcrowding and poor hygiene. The louse infects bedding and seams of clothing and nits are not found on the human. With body warmth the pediculi hatch and puncture the skin to produce small urticarial papules with hemorrhagic puncta. Pruritus is extreme and scratch marks are the main clinical sign.

Pediculosis pubis

The pubic hairs are the normal habitat of *Pthirus pubis* but it may also infect facial hair, eyelashes, general body hair and rarely the frontal margin of the scalp. Pubic infestation is usually sexually transmitted but bedding and towels may be responsible. Clinical signs may be minimal, even with severe itching, but excoriated papules and flat blue macules containing altered blood pigment may be seen as may evidence of secondary infection or eczematization. Eyelash infestation in children may occur from innocent close contact with an infected adult but the possibility of sexual abuse must always be considered.

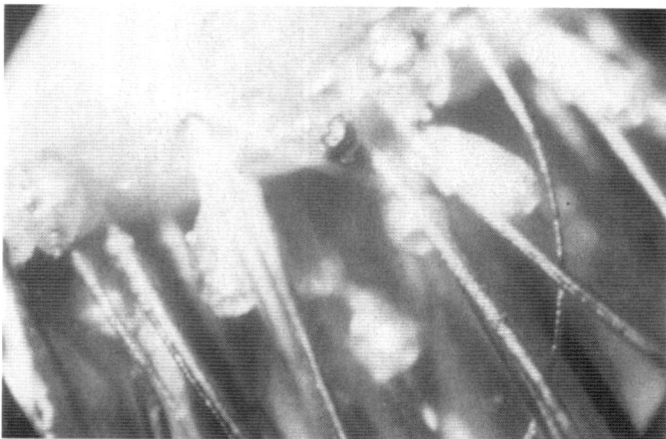

Fig. 30.40   Pediculosis of eyelid.

Management of pediculosis

The management of pediculosis corporis involves removing the infestation from clothing with hot water laundering, hot electric drying, hot ironing or dry cleaning.

Permethrin shampoo is an effective pediculocide for scalp infestations but the efficacy as an ovicide is less certain and repeat application after a few days is recommended. Removal of nits with a fine comb can be facilitated by prior wrapping of the scalp for 1–2 h in a towel soaked in vinegar which softens the chitin.

Pediculosis pubis is treated with 5% permethrin cream applied for 12 h to all hairy areas in the anogenital region, repeated after 1 week. Sexual contacts should be treated simultaneously and all underclothing appropriately laundered.

Pediculosis of eyelashes is best treated with petroleum jelly applied thickly twice a day for a week.

URTICARIA AND ERYTHEMAS

URTICARIA

The most characteristic feature of urticaria (nettle rash or hives) is its transience. Erythematous swellings develop in the skin and last for a few hours before disappearing. The urticarial wheals may be of variable size and may have an obvious annular configuration. Angioedema (giant urticaria) is a variant of urticaria which affects the face and genital region and mainly involves the subcutaneous tissues with resultant gross swelling of the tissues.

Urticaria is common in all age groups, and is particularly so in children. In children, widespread urticaria is often the presenting feature of a number of viral infections, when it is accompanied by fever and malaise. It is due to increased permeability of capillaries or other small vessels, with resultant transudation of fluid. Several chemical mediators are involved, which are mainly released from mast cells: these include histamine, prostaglandins and leukotrienes. Mast cell degranulation results from both immune (IgE, complement) and non-immune mechanisms.

IgE-mediated urticaria and angioedema

Urticaria and angioedema following ingestion of food allergens is quite common in children with atopic eczema and is often IgE mediated (confirmed by positive skin prick tests or radioallergosorbent tests). Swelling of the lips and tongue develops immediately after ingestion of the food, and contact urticaria may be seen if the food is in contact with the skin. If enough food allergen is ingested vomiting and diarrhea may occur, and the child may develop an asthmatic attack: generalized anaphylaxis may occur in a few children, especially with nuts. Widespread urticaria is common, usually occurring within 1 h of ingestion of the food, which may last for a few hours. Common foods involved in such reactions include hens' eggs, cows' milk, fish, nuts and soya. Food allergy is commonly outgrown by the age of 5 years although this is less likely for peanut and nut allergy.[45] IgE-mediated urticaria may also follow drug administration, particularly penicillin, and also insect stings, for example by bees or wasps.

Urticaria due to foods and drugs which is not apparently immunologically mediated

Certain foods such as strawberries, tomatoes and chocolate cause urticaria where no IgE-mediated mechanisms can be demonstrated. It seems likely that this is a direct effect on mast cells and is similar to that caused by tartrazine (a common coloring in foods), benzoates and salicylates. Aspirin and morphine also commonly cause urticaria by a non-immunological mechanism.

Chronic idiopathic urticaria

This type of urticaria is not very common in children. The urticaria may recur repeatedly for a period of years, with often daily exacerbations. It is now recognized that approximately one third of patients with chronic idiopathic urticaria have circulating histamine-releasing autoantibodies directed against the high affinity IgE receptor or less commonly against IgE.[46] The detection of these antibodies, however, is available in only a small number of research laboratories.

Papular urticaria

This is very common in children and results from insect, flea or mite bites. In Britain dog, cat and bird fleas are the usual cause, but human fleas, bed bugs, mosquitoes and dog lice may be implicated. The child presents with papules and blisters on exposed skin such as the legs and arms. Each lasts for about 7–10 days before resolving.

It often takes the parents quite a lot of convincing of the cause of the condition. The family pet should be inspected and treated if necessary.

Treatment of urticaria

The management of a child with urticaria depends on the cause. If a food is implicated, this is usually fairly obvious, except perhaps in infants where skin prick testing may be helpful. Any food implicated should be withdrawn from the diet, though it may be possible to reintroduce it when the child is older. In chronic idiopathic urticaria, by definition no cause is found but certain ingested chemicals in foods (e.g. salicylates, benzoates, food colorings) may make it worse. A non-sedating H1 antihistamine can be given.

MASTOCYTOSIS

This refers to a group of conditions whose signs and symptoms are due to the infiltration of tissues by mast cells and to the release of the chemical mediators contained in these cells. Local effects include erythema and swelling of lesions on rubbing (Darier's sign), dermographism, pruritus, hemorrhage and blistering. General effects include generalized pruritus, fever and flushing; tachycardia and hypotension; headache and irritability; vomiting, diarrhea, increased salivation and peptic ulceration; rhinorrhea and bronchospasm; increased lacrimation; and a generalized hemorrhagic diathesis.

Approximately 65% of patients with mastocytosis present in childhood. A retrospective review of 173 pediatric cases confirms that mastocytomas and urticaria pigmentosa are the commonest presentations in this age group.[47]

Mastocytoma

A round to oval flesh-colored to yellowish nodule or plaque usually presents at birth or appears in the first months of life (Fig. 30.41). Although it is usually solitary, some children develop a number of mastocytomas, particularly on arms or trunk. They usually regress spontaneously over a few years but while present they urticate on rubbing, and blisters, which may be hemorrhagic, often occur in infancy. These children commonly have attacks of generalized flushing but other symptoms and signs of mediator release are rare.

Urticaria pigmentosa

Pigmented multiple macules, with occasional papules, nodules or plaques, occur in a widespread distribution, particularly involving the trunk (Fig. 30.42). Urticaria pigmentosa is the most common form of mastocytosis with an onset usually between 1 and 9 months of age. The lesions erupt over 1–2 months, then become static and finally in most cases resolve by adolescence. They may be pruritic and individual lesions can urticate (Darier's sign) and occasionally blister. There may be dermographism in nearby clinically normal skin. Generalized pruritus and flushing may occur, and less frequently other signs of mediator release.

Diffuse cutaneous mastocytosis

This is a rare form of mastocytosis with the onset usually at birth. Massive mast cell infiltration into the skin produces a diffuse thickening with associated edema, erythema and blistering. The skin may have a leathergrain or peau d'orange appearance or be nodular or verrucose. The color is yellowish or red. Blistering is prominent and may be so severe that the presentation is that of a generalized bullous disease. The full spectrum of local and systemic symptoms and signs of mediator release may be seen. These are usually severe and disabling and may be life threatening. The cutaneous lesions tend to improve with time but some degree of infiltration usually remains.

Systemic mastocytosis

This is defined by infiltration of mast cells into organs other than the skin, and not simply systemic features due to the release of mediators from cutaneous mast cell infiltrates. It is extremely rare in childhood and is almost always associated with diffuse cutaneous involvement in this age group. Hepatosplenomegaly and lymphadenopathy may occur; the cells may infiltrate renal parenchyma and gastrointestinal mucosa; skeletal involvement produces both osteoporotic and osteosclerotic lesions. Mast cell leukemia is a very rare complication.

Management

In general, mastocytosis is a self-limiting disease. If an isolated lesion is producing generalized flushing, excision can be considered. The patient should carry a list of agents (i.e. aspirin, morphine, codeine, d-tubocurarine, scopolamine, quinine, thiamin, procaine, polymixin B, amphotericin B,

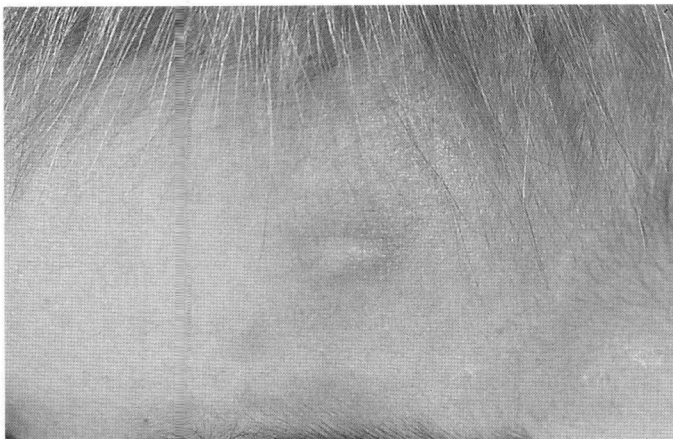

Fig. 30.41 Mastocytoma.

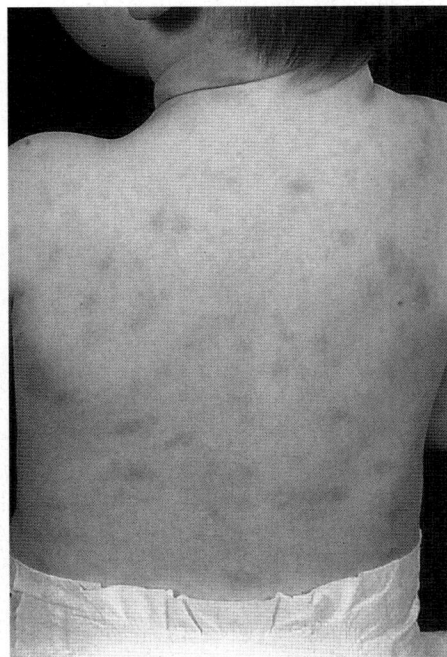

Fig. 30.42 Urticaria pigmentosa.

nonsteroidal anti-inflammatory drugs, and radiographic contrast media) which stimulate mast cell degranulation and avoid these where possible. Physical trauma to the lesions should be avoided.

H1 antihistamines are rarely effective in controlling symptoms and signs of mediator release but combined with H2 blockers they may be more effective. In more severe cases oral disodium cromoglicate, ketotifen and nifedipine may be tried.

A greater understanding of the underlying molecular abnormalities in the systemic mastocytoses is allowing patients to benefit from more specific therapy, for example 'kit-targeting' tyrosine kinase inhibitors.

ERYTHEMA MULTIFORME

This is an uncommon condition in children which tends to follow herpes simplex infection, mycoplasma pneumonia and sulfonamide ingestion (Figs 30.43 and 30.44). Clinically, it is characterized by the formation of circular target lesions on the limbs, with a red periphery and blue (often bullous) center. Stomatitis and genital involvement are common. The rash of erythema multiforme, unlike urticaria, for which it is often mistaken, is fixed with lesions lasting days as compared to hours in urticaria. The lesions may be widespread, and if extensive erosions are present at two or more mucosal sites the diagnosis of Stevens–Johnson syndrome (SJS) can be made. SJS in turn overlaps both clinically and histologically with toxic epidermal necrolysis. The rash of erythema multiforme usually fades within 10 days but may recur, particularly in the case of erythema multiforme following recurrent herpes simplex infections. No randomized controlled trials have been performed for treatment of childhood erythema multiforme and there is therefore no evidence to

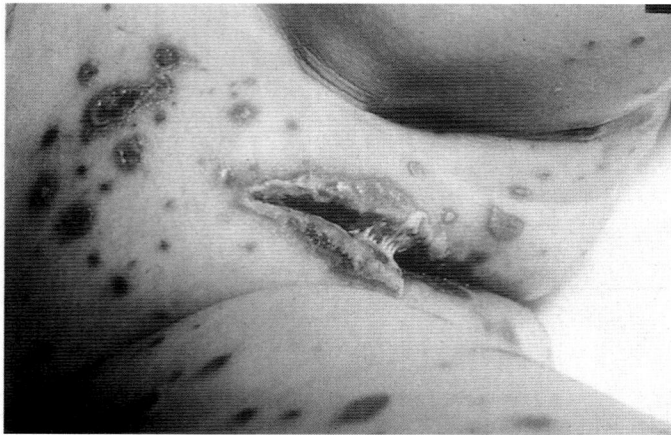

Fig. 30.43   Erythema multiforme, Stevens–Johnson: perineal.

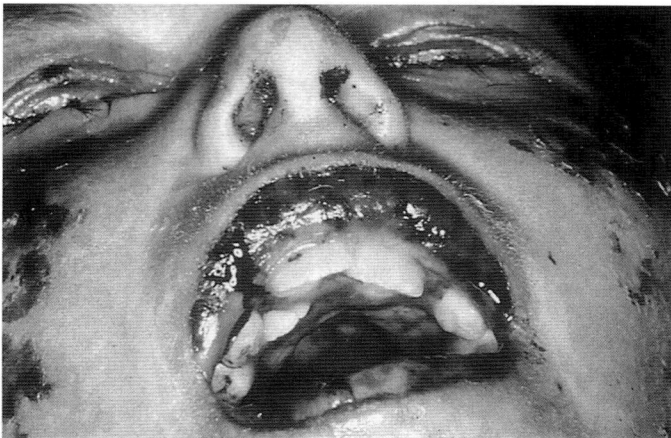

Fig. 30.44   Erythema multiforme, Stevens–Johnson: oral.

recommend oral steroids. However, one double-blind placebo-controlled study in adults found benefit with continuous aciclovir in recurrent erythema multiforme.[48]

VESICOBULLOUS DISORDERS

DERMATITIS HERPETIFORMIS

Dermatitis herpetiformis is associated with gluten-sensitive enteropathy (celiac disease), and in a study of 57 children only 3 (5%) had normal jejunal biopsies.[49] Deposition of IgA in the dermal papillae of skin is the hallmark of the disorder.

It is rare before the age of 2 years, and presents with small intensely itchy blisters symmetrically on the elbows, knees, shoulders and buttocks. The correct treatment is a gluten-free diet, when the blisters, and small bowel mucosa, should resolve (permanently) within 2 years; concomitant treatment with dapsone or sulfapyridine is usually required.

BULLOUS PEMPHIGOID

This rare blistering disease results from the formation of IgG antibodies to the basement membrane zone of the epidermis. The child presents with large and widespread blisters, which may (as in chronic bullous disease of childhood) be most marked on the face and around the genitalia. The hands and feet are more frequently involved in children 1 year or younger compared to older age groups. The diagnosis is confirmed by immunofluorescence of skin biopsy or serum (with appropriate substrate) to demonstrate anti basement membrane zone antibodies. Treatment is with oral steroids, which should be tapered off as the condition allows. In most the disease is self-limiting.

PEMPHIGUS

Pemphigus is also rare in children, the most common types being pemphigus vulgaris and foliaceus. The blistering is less evident than in pemphigoid, though there may be widespread plaques and erosions. Over 50% of children with pemphigus vulgaris present with erosive stomatitis. The diagnosis is confirmed by immunofluorescence studies of skin and serum, which demonstrate IgG antibodies to the intercellular substance of the keratinocytes in the epidermis. Treatment is with oral steroids, as in pemphigoid.

CHRONIC BULLOUS DISEASE OF CHILDHOOD

It is most commonly seen in young children, with blistering around the mouth, neck and genital regions (Fig. 30.45). Genital blistering may be mistaken for herpes simplex infection. Immunofluorescence studies of skin show linear IgA deposition along the basement membrane zone of the epidermis with evidence of circulating IgA antibodies in up to 80%.

Treatment with dapsone or sulfonamides usually clears the blisters very effectively. The disease is self-limiting, after months or years.

VASCULITIS

Vasculitis can be classified according to the size and nature of the vessel and the infiltrate.[50]

HENOCH–SCHÖNLEIN PURPURA

This is a distinct subset within the spectrum of leukocytoclastic (allergic) vasculitis that is relatively common in children (Fig. 30.46). The damage occurs to small blood vessels in the dermis, resulting in the development of purpura (often palpable) over the lower limbs, buttocks and forearms. Other organs involved in the vasculitis are the kidneys and intestinal vessels, resulting in proteinuria and hematuria, abdominal pain and gastrointestinal hemorrhage. In some arthralgia is also

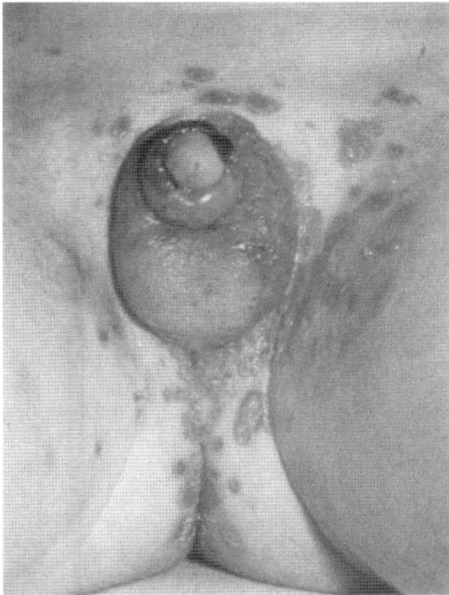

Fig. 30.45 Chronic bullous disease of childhood.

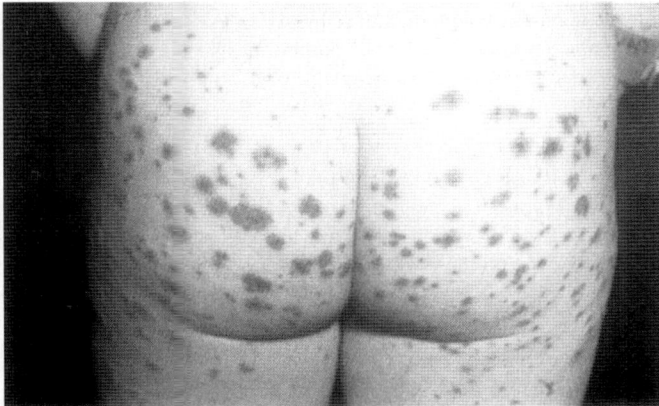

Fig. 30.46 Henoch–Schönlein purpura.

prominent. It usually follows a virus or respiratory infection, the vasculitis resulting from deposition of immune complexes in the vessels of the skin, kidneys and intestines, with complement activation and resultant polymorph infiltration. In Henoch–Schönlein purpura the immunoglobulin deposited is IgA, whereas in other types of vasculitis it is IgG.

The prognosis is very variable. In most children the condition is self-limiting; others may develop renal failure (usually treatable with dialysis or renal transplant) or may die of gastrointestinal hemorrhage.

URTICARIAL VASCULITIS

This is another variant of allergic vasculitis. The urticarial wheals last for several days, unlike those in 'classical' urticaria, where they last for a few hours. Urticarial vasculitis is often accompanied by arthralgia, and skin lesions may resolve with purpura. A skin biopsy shows leukocytoclastic vasculitis, and complement studies may reveal low CH50 and C3 levels. It may result from drug ingestion or viral infection, or may be a feature of lupus erythematosus.

ERYTHEMA NODOSUM

This is rare in young children. It is a type of vasculitis affecting initially deep, dermal venules with subsequent development of a septal panniculitis.

Clinically, erythematous nodules develop, usually on the shins though sometimes on the thighs and forearms. They last for about 2–3 weeks and are characteristically tender. They resolve leaving bruising, but then tend to recur in crops. Causes include streptococcal infections, sarcoidosis, tuberculosis and sulfonamide ingestion: often it occurs without obvious reason. Treatment is of the underlying cause. Usually it resolves spontaneously, but occasionally treatment with oral steroids is indicated.

ECZEMA, DERMATITIS AND PSORIASIS

Eczema and dermatitis are synonymous and are often used interchangeably. Eczema/dermatitis can be subdivided into atopic and non-atopic eczema, contact dermatitis (allergic and irritant) and other types (e.g. discoid, seborrheic, photosensitive).[51]

ATOPIC ECZEMA

Atopy is a genetically determined disorder with an increased tendency to form IgE antibody to inhalants and foods (see Ch. 33). There is increased susceptibility to asthma, allergic rhinitis and atopic eczema (Figs 30.47 and 30.48). Although eczema may begin at any age, in 75% of patients first signs are present by 6 months. Recent evidence has demonstrated that abnormality of the epidermal barrier is a major predisposing factor in atopic disease through loss of function of the epidermal barrier protein filaggrin.[52]

Clinical features

Diagnostic criteria have been defined for atopic eczema but the characteristic clinical features are erythema, generalized dryness and itching

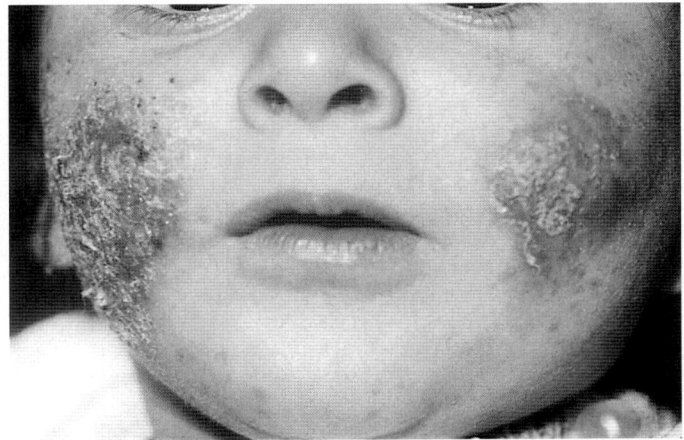

Fig. 30.47 Atopic eczema: facial in young infant.

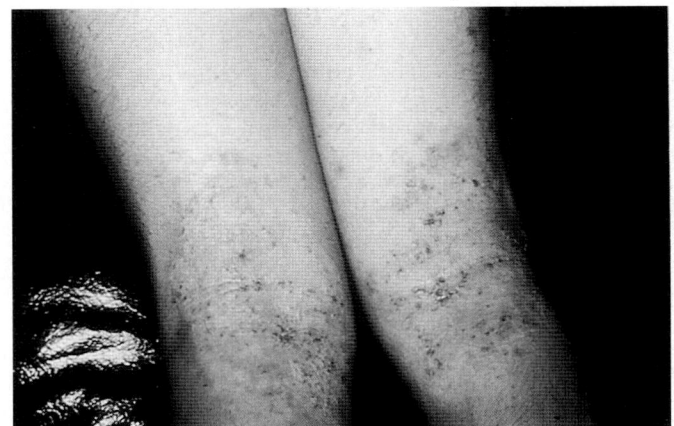

Fig. 30.48 Atopic eczema: flexural in older child.

which leads to excoriations and ultimately lichenification or thickening of the skin, particularly in children older than 2 years.[51] Involvement of the whole cutaneous surface may occur but the predominant areas are the face in infants, extensor aspects of the limbs as the child begins to crawl, and the limb flexures in older children. In severe cases the whole skin may be erythematous and in these patients white dermographism is often a prominent feature: this indicates that the condition is likely to be unstable and difficult.

Complications

Patients with atopic eczema may develop secondary bacterial infection which presents either as impetigo or folliculitis, or simply as worsening eczema. Mollusca contagiosa appear more common, although there are no prevalence studies to confirm this. Atopic patients are at risk of developing severe widespread herpes simplex infections. The usual childhood immunizations are quite safe.

Management

A comprehensive systematic review of all treatments for atopic eczema has been published.[53] This review summarizes the available data from all the randomized controlled trials. It is clear that although emollients and topical steroids are the mainstays of treatment there are very few objective data to recommend their use. Despite this, clinical practice suggests that they are very helpful in the management of atopic eczema.

Time should be taken in discussing factors that act as external irritants. Wool is a major irritant and should never be worn in direct contact with the skin. It is important to warn that wool contact may also occur with the parents' clothing, carpets, car seat and stroller covers, blankets and toys. Cotton material is always safe and cotton polyester combinations rarely irritate, but acrylic may be as troublesome as wool. Perfumed and medicated products, disinfectants and strong cleansers should be avoided. Soap in excess and bubble baths overdry the skin, so soap substitutes should be used.

It should be emphasized to parents that topical steroids are safe as long as these are used only where and when there is active eczema. In general, ointment bases, which are more emollient, are preferred. Only 1% hydrocortisone should be used on the face and in the groin but fluorinated steroids may be used elsewhere for short periods. Patients and parents should be educated regarding the quantities of creams necessary to apply and guidance has been published regarding amount and frequency of application.[1,54]

Second line therapy for severe cases or those not responding to routine treatment includes paste bandages or wet wraps. The latter involves applying two layers of tubular cotton bandages over topical steroids and emollients on the skin. The inner bandage is soaked in warm water prior to application. These dressings increase the hydration of the skin, physically prevent scratching, immediately reduce itching and enhance the penetration of topical steroids. In infants only weak steroids should be used because of the risk of absorption. The use of dressings should be adequately supervised and used for no more than a few days at a time with topical steroids.

Obvious secondary bacterial infection should be treated with oral antibiotics. However, these are indicated in most patients with severe weeping eczema even in the absence of clinically obvious infection. Although current randomized controlled trial evidence does not support the routine use of antihistamines in atopic eczema many parents say that their child appears to be more comfortable at night with less scratching after a nocturnal dose of a sedative antihistamine. Oral steroids should be avoided because a severe rebound can occur on withdrawal and after several courses the eczema is rendered very unstable.

Recently topical tacrolimus and topical pimecrolimus have received approval by the UK National Institute for Clinical Excellence (NICE) as second line treatments for patients greater than 2 years where topical corticosteroids have not worked or there is a serious risk of adverse effects with topical corticosteroids.[55] Concern has been raised about possible cancer risks based on information from animal studies, small numbers of post-marketing reports and how the drugs work. These drugs should therefore be prescribed only by doctors with experience in skin disease.

Third line treatments include phototherapy (narrow band UVB or psoralen plus UVA), ciclosporin (although not yet licensed in the UK for pediatric eczema)[56] and azathioprine. Small studies in children suggest montelukast might be beneficial[57] although a larger study in adults concluded that montelukast is not an effective treatment.[58] Further studies are required in children.

Chinese herbal medicine (CHM) has been evaluated and 1 year follow-up of children treated with CHM showed good, sustained improvement in nearly 50% although 1 out of 37 developed abnormal liver function tests and 14 withdrew due to lack of efficacy or unpalatability.[59]

In the absence of a clear history of worsening of eczema relating to food, no alteration to the child's diet should be considered unless the eczema has failed to respond to conventional topical therapy. Dietary manipulation in the management of refractory eczema is covered in Chapter 33. The role of the dust mite in these severe cases is covered in the same section.

There is increasing interest in the primary prevention of atopic disease. Probiotics are cultures of potentially beneficial bacteria and a randomized controlled trial of *Lactobacillus* GG was effective in reducing the frequency, but not severity, of atopic eczema.[60] At present, evidence is lacking to show the benefit of probiotics in established eczema.

As a child becomes older discussion about future careers is important as certain occupations are likely to aggravate the skin, such as hairdressing or car mechanics. It is important to develop a trusting and cooperative relationship with the patient and his parents as they will require much encouragement to help them cope with this distressing condition.

DISCOID ECZEMA (NUMMULAR ECZEMA)

In children this is often a manifestation of the atopic state. Well-defined patches of acute eczema occur in a strikingly symmetrical distribution (Fig. 30.49). In infants the commonest sites are the upper back and the tops of the shoulders; in older patients the extensor aspects of the limbs are particularly involved. The lesions may be very thick and exudative and they are very itchy. They have to be distinguished from tinea and impetigo which are less symmetrical and psoriasis which is rarely moist. The management involves emollients and topical steroids as for atopic dermatitis, with the continued use of emollient helping to prevent recurrences.

PITYRIASIS ALBA

This condition appears as poorly defined, slightly scaly, hypopigmented patches occurring particularly on the face and the upper

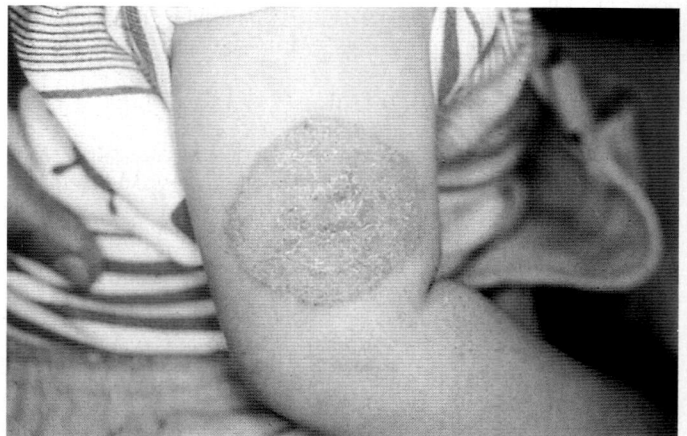

Fig. 30.49   Discoid eczema.

arms. It probably represents a very mild eczema which, however, produces a striking postinflammatory hypopigmentation. Occasionally some areas will show erythema and more definite eczematous changes. The condition is more common in atopics. The mild irritation and signs of mild eczema respond to emollients and weak topical corticosteroids but the hypopigmentation may be very persistent and require sun exposure over a prolonged period before repigmentation is complete. Most lesions clear by puberty. The condition should be differentiated from vitiligo where there is total depigmentation and no scale and from tinea versicolor which has very well demarcated lesions with very fine branny scaling.

SEBORRHEIC DERMATITIS

This condition usually presents between weeks 2 and 6 of infancy with a second peak in adult life; whilst in adults the dermatitis relates to sites of greatest sebum production, this relationship is less clear in infants.

The rash has an erythematous background and a greasy yellow scale. In the proximal flexures the scale may be absent and a glazed erythema the only sign. Scaling is particularly prominent on the scalp, producing the so-called 'cradle cap'. The main areas of involvement are scalp, glabella, behind and inside the ears, nasolabial folds, axillae and groin and in infants the neck and limb flexures. In the flexural areas candidiasis is commonly superimposed. The rash is usually asymptomatic.

Various conditions mimic seborrheic dermatitis including drug reactions (in children particularly due to phenytoin sodium), early psoriasis and Langerhans' cell histiocytosis. These should be considered when what appears to be a seborrheic dermatitis occurs at an unexpected age or fails to respond to therapy.

Seborrheic dermatitis usually responds quickly to weak topical corticosteroid preparations with the addition of an anticandidal agent for the flexural areas. On the scalp, sulfur and salicylic acid preparations left on overnight are usually more effective than corticosteroids. If the scale is very thick, warmed olive or paraffin oil can be used to soften it before the cream is applied. It should be emphasized that the disorder will tend to recur through infancy.

NAPKIN DERMATITIS

Napkin dermatitis encompasses various skin diseases of different etiologies. Irritant contact dermatitis is the most common due to damage to skin integrity through friction, occlusion, excessive moisture and irritants under the nappy. Secondary infection (bacterial and candidal) usually occurs. Seborrheic dermatitis and psoriasis may also affect the napkin area

The newer superabsorbent disposable napkins are often preferable to cloth napkins. A combination cream of 1% hydrocortisone and anticandidal agent is usually effective and a silicone or zinc barrier cream may be added to protect the skin against moisture. There will usually be a quick response to therapy but recurrences are to be expected.

ALLERGIC CONTACT ECZEMA

Allergic contact eczema is one of the main examples of delayed type hypersensitivity in the skin. It is much less common in children than in adults, probably due to lack of contact with sensitizing chemicals. The commonest allergen in children is nickel, which is contained in metal clips and studs (e.g. jeans studs) and in non-gold earrings. It seems likely that a number of children are sensitized following piercing of the ears and by wearing costume jewelry earrings. Other contact allergens in children include plants such as Rhus (particularly in the USA and Australia) (Fig. 30.50), chemicals used in rubber production and topical medications such as neomycin and gentamicin.

Identification of the allergen is essential, and this is carried out by patch testing the child. Interpretation requires expertise, as not all reactions are necessarily specific delayed type hypersensitivity reactions.

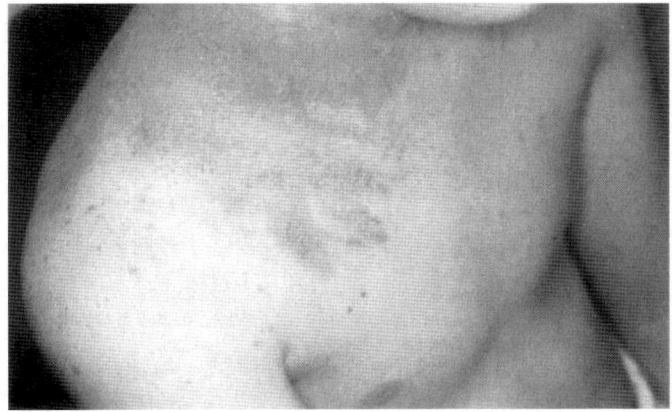

Fig. 30.50   Plant (Rhus) dermatitis.

PHYTOPHOTODERMATITIS

This is a cutaneous phototoxic inflammatory response resulting from direct contact to naturally occurring plant psoralen followed by ultraviolet (UVA) sensitization. It typically manifests in spring or summer months as painful streaky/linear erythema on exposed sites that may blister and subsequently heal with postinflammatory hyperpigmentation. The most common plants to cause this reaction are in the Umbelliferae family.

JUVENILE PLANTAR DERMATOSIS

This condition affects mainly children aged 3–14 years and is characterized by a shiny, smooth erythema affecting the plantar aspect of the weightbearing area on the foot. The forefoot and toes are typically commonly involved and the heels in about a quarter of patients. The feet are affected symmetrically and the toe webs are spared helping differentiate juvenile plantar dermatosis from tinea pedis. Pain from cracks and fissures is a major symptom. Rarely a similar pattern can be seen on the fingertips.

The exact cause is unknown but hot humid conditions caused by less porous, synthetic materials in socks and shoes are thought to contribute to the maceration process. Most cases will clear by adolescence but some are helped by changing footwear and use of emollients.

PSORIASIS

A combination of epidemiological, family and human leukocyte antigen (HLA) studies indicate that psoriasis is a genetic condition. Its mode of inheritance is probably autosomal dominant with variable penetrance. Psoriasis appears by the age of 15 years in 30% of patients. Children may present with typical adult large erythematous plaques, with a thick silvery white scale, predominantly on the knees, elbows, buttocks and scalp, but usually the plaques are smaller and with a finer scale. A common presentation is acute guttate psoriasis with the eruption of small papules in a widespread distribution, often following an intercurrent illness, particularly a streptococcal throat infection. A micropapular form of psoriasis occurs particularly in dark-skinned children with 1–2 mm papules most marked on the extensor aspects of the limbs. These lesions are usually skin colored until scratching demonstrates the white scale.

The face and intertriginous sites, such as retroauricular areas, axillae, groin, genital and perianal area, are commonly affected in children. Children presenting with vulvitis, balanitis and perianal itching may be found to have psoriasis. In these areas the typical scale is absent and the condition presents as a glazed erythema often with fissuring. Generalized pustular psoriasis is rare in children and has an explosive onset with sheets of pustules on a background of bright erythema accompanied by severe systemic toxicity. It may be the first presentation of psoriasis and settle spontaneously in a few weeks leaving

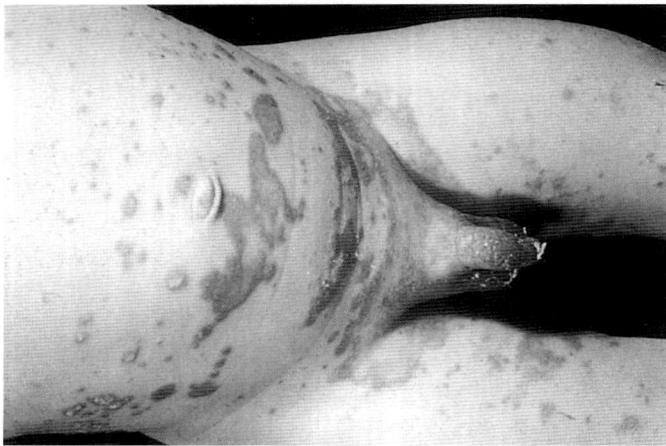

Fig. 30.51   Napkin psoriasis.

normal skin. It often recurs and usually more typical psoriasis eventually supervenes. Pustular psoriasis of the palms and soles is also very rare in children. Acropustulosis, a glazed erythema studded with pustules followed by thick scaling and fissuring, involving one or more digits, is an occasional childhood presentation. Nail involvement is usually absent or minimal with minor pitting, and psoriatic arthropathy is extremely uncommon in children.

Controversy exists over whether or not the condition called 'napkin psoriasis' or 'sebopsoriasis' (Fig. 30.51) is in fact a form of psoriasis. It occurs in the first 3 months of life with a nonspecific napkin dermatitis suddenly becoming more severe and extensive with bright, well-demarcated erythema involving most of the napkin area including the folds. Lesions resembling typical psoriasis then erupt elsewhere, usually first on face and scalp, then neck fold and axillae and finally trunk and limbs. In the scalp the lesions may appear similar to seborrhea. Evidence for this representing a form of psoriasis rather than dermatitis comes from the work of Andersen & Thomsen[61] who found a family history of psoriasis in 26% of patients compared with 4.9% of controls, and of Neville & Finn[62] who, on review of these patients at 5–13 years, found psoriasis in 17% with the expected rate being 0.4%.

In any child with a difficult napkin dermatitis responding poorly to conventional measures psoriasis should be considered, particularly if the lesions have well-defined margins and remain fairly fixed in position.

Management

Many systemic therapies (e.g. retinoids, methotrexate and ciclosporin) used in adults are inappropriate in children. As a general rule, psoriasis in children is better treated with tars than topical corticosteroids. They are often more effective, are safer for long term use, and rebound on their cessation is less of a problem. Tars may be irritant in infants, as they may be at any age when applied to the face or intertriginous areas. Useful preparations for guttate or small plaque psoriasis are coal tar and salicylic acid mixtures (equal parts 2–4%) in an aqueous cream base applied twice a day. A prospective, multicenter, double-blind study in children showed that the topical vitamin D analogue calcipotriol is effective and safe when applied to less than 30% of the body surface area.[63] Whilst oral antibiotics and tonsillectomy have been advocated for patients with recurrent guttate psoriasis following recent streptococcal infection, there are no data to show they are beneficial.[64] For large plaque psoriasis in older children the adult regimens of topical dithranol with or without ultraviolet B (UVB) (preferably narrow band) are usually tolerated.

Patients with generalized pustular psoriasis require urgent hospitalization and close monitoring of fluid and electrolyte balance and evidence of infection. Wet compresses give symptomatic relief while awaiting spontaneous recovery. Tars are contraindicated and topical steroids must be used very cautiously due to the risk of considerable absorption.

Palmoplantar pustulosis and acropustulosis usually respond slowly to tar preparations. Napkin psoriasis often clears quickly with hydrocortisone and anticandidal agents for the flexural areas and a weak corticosteroid elsewhere.

It is essential for the parents, and the child if old enough, to appreciate that psoriasis is a capricious, recurrent disease which will require varying treatments depending on the site, nature and severity of the condition at different stages. Long term follow-up, preferably with the same practitioner, is important.

CONNECTIVE TISSUE DISEASES (Ch. 29)

LUPUS ERYTHEMATOSUS (LE)

This is rare in children but neonatal lupus erythematosus is of considerable importance.

Neonatal lupus erythematosus

This occurs due to the passage of maternal antibodies through the placenta (Fig. 30.52), where the mother suffers from systemic LE, subacute cutaneous LE or the sicca syndrome. In 50% of cases the mother is asymptomatic but the vast majority have SS-A (anti-Ro) antibodies. The most important feature of neonatal LE is heart block of varying degrees. This is usually permanent, and without pacing there is a significant mortality (Ch. 21). Other features include autoimmune hemolytic anemia, thrombocytopenia, hepatitis, pneumonitis and splenomegaly.

The skin lesions resemble those of subacute cutaneous LE in the adult, occurring on the face, neck and scalp, with erythematous macules or plaques with scaling. They are often present at birth and disappear within the first year of life. There may also be photosensitivity. Treatment of the skin is with 1% hydrocortisone cream and protection from the sun.

Lupus erythematosus in the older child

This takes two main forms: systemic LE and discoid LE. It is thought that this is a spectrum of disease, as sometimes patients with discoid LE will progress to systemic LE and a proportion of those with discoid LE have circulating antinuclear antibodies, anemia, leukopenia and thrombocytopenia and other features such as Raynaud's phenomenon and arthralgia.

Discoid lupus erythematosus

This usually affects girls, who develop erythematous plaques on the face, the arms and dorsum of the hands. The most commonly affected parts of the face are the nose and the cheeks. Involvement of the scalp usually leads to scarring alopecia.

There may be mild anemia, leukopenia or thrombocytopenia and some children will have circulating antinuclear antibodies.

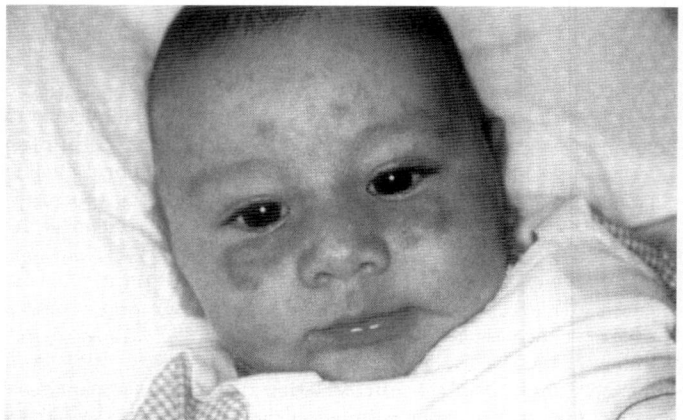

Fig. 30.52   Neonatal lupus erythematosus.

The prognosis is variable, as in some the plaques will resolve spontaneously whereas in others they tend to be persistent. Avoidance of sun exposure by the use of sunscreens and a hat is important.

Systemic lupus erythematosus

As in discoid LE, the systemic form is more common in girls. It is a multisystem connective tissue disease which often carries a poor prognosis, due to renal involvement. This is discussed fully in Chapter 29 (see p. 1427). The skin manifestations include a butterfly rash on the face, which characteristically spares the nasolabial folds, discoid plaques usually on the face, reticulate livedo most marked on the legs, panniculitis, vasculitic ulcers, cuticular hemorrhages at the fingernail folds, and alopecia. Almost half of patients will have mouth ulcers.

DERMATOMYOSITIS

This is a rare connective tissue disease affecting the skin, muscle and blood vessels. Its etiology is unknown, though in some adults there is an association with carcinomas of internal viscera and lymphomas. The histological changes in the skin may resemble those of LE, though the dermal edema is more marked. In the later stages the dermis becomes sclerotic, and the picture may be similar to the changes in scleroderma.

The clinical manifestations are extremely variable. In some children the skin signs may be very prominent with minimal myositis, whereas in others there is polymyositis with little evidence of skin involvement. Myositis is manifested by a proximal muscular weakness with difficulty in flexing the neck, climbing stairs and raising the arms above the shoulder girdle, and by a raised serum creatine phosphokinase. There may be concomitant fever and malaise.

The rash when present is very characteristic. A heliotrope (purplish-red) rash occurs on the face involving the eyelids, the forehead and upper cheeks. There may be marked edema of the hands and arms with an erythematous linear rash over the dorsum of the hands with nail fold telangiectasia. Erythema of the scalp may develop and there may be marked alopecia. Reticulate livedo is seen in some, and may lead to ulceration of the skin.

Calcification is common in children, affecting more than 50% of cases. It primarily involves the muscles, particularly around the pelvic and shoulder girdles, and may cause marked functional disability. It also occurs in the subcutaneous tissues, and there may be extrusion through the skin with ulceration.

The course of the disease is variable, but there is generally a good prognosis in children. Death may occur due to respiratory failure, difficulty in swallowing, or the side-effects of steroid therapy.

Treatment with methotrexate is now considered first line therapy in an attempt to reduce the cumulative dose of oral corticosteroids.[65] Therapy is usually necessary for months or years until the serum creatine phosphokinase returns to normal and the signs of the disease have disappeared. Physiotherapy may be useful to prevent contractures.

SCLERODERMA

In children this may take two forms: morphea (localized scleroderma), which is relatively common, and systemic sclerosis which is very rare.

Morphea

This is a localized and benign form of scleroderma, though it can cause quite marked disfigurement. On histological examination, the dermis is at first edematous with swelling and degeneration of the collagen fibrils, with later thickening of the dermis and loss of appendages. The etiology of the condition is unknown.

The areas of morphea occur usually as either plaques or linear lesions of sclerosis in the skin. These are at first purplish in color, and later become white and waxy. Hairs are lost within the area, with loss of sweating. They occur on the trunk and limbs. When they involve a limb (usually linear lesions), they may involve muscles and bone leading to shortening of the limb.

A particular disfigurement which results from morphea is the so-called 'coup de sabre', which occurs in the frontoparietal area. This starts with contraction of the skin over the affected area with development of an ivory plaque with hyperpigmentation at the edge and telangiectatic vessels coursing over it. The resulting groove may extend downwards, affecting the mouth and mandible. The tongue may be atrophic on the affected side, and there may be marked alopecia. There is marked facial asymmetry with consequent disfigurement.

A prospective, nonrandomized, open pilot study suggests that combined low dose methotrexate and high dose pulsed corticosteroids is an effective treatment (see Kreuter et al. Arch Dermatol 2005 – reference 66).[66]

Systemic sclerosis

This is very rare in children. The etiology is unknown, but as similar changes may be seen in graft versus host reactions, it may be some sort of rejection phenomenon.

In the majority of patients the condition starts with Raynaud's phenomenon which may continue for several years before other manifestations occur. These include: swelling of the hands; sclerodactyly with atrophy of the pulps of the fingers; calcinosis of the finger pulps which may be prominent; ulceration; and gangrene. In some, terminal phalangeal absorption also occurs.

Later, other features occur with beaking of the nose, radial furrowing around the mouth which becomes smaller, macroglossia, esophageal dilatation and stricture, and abnormal colonic peristalsis.

The prognosis is variable and depends on internal organ involvement, though most patients continue with the condition for many years with increasing deformity. No formal trials have evaluated the wide range of potential immunosuppressive therapies.

LICHEN SCLEROSUS

Although the precise etiology of lichen sclerosus is unknown, evidence for an autoimmune basis to the disorder is emerging. Circulating IgG autoantibodies to the glycoprotein extracellular matrix protein 1 (ECM1) have been demonstrated in the sera of about 75% of affected individuals.[67] Lichen sclerosus has a predilection for genital and perianal skin. It is more common in females and usually presents with itch although in children it may be asymptomatic. Erythema and excoriations appear in the early stages with subsequent development of well-defined pale atrophic areas. The lesions often occur in a figure of eight pattern around the vulva and anal region. Lichen sclerosus may be misdiagnosed as sexual abuse. In approximately 10% extragenital lesions are also present. In boys, the usual history is of balanitis and tightening of the foreskin which can progress to phimosis (balanitis xerotica obliterans). Potent topical steroids are the treatment of choice.[68] A Cochrane review of topical therapies is currently underway. The overall prognosis is good but for cases that persist long term follow-up is recommended because of the risk of malignant change in adults.

IDIOPATHIC PHOTOSENSITIVITY ERUPTIONS

Before considering a child to have an idiopathic photosensitivity eruption, it is important to exclude one of the hereditary diseases (q.v.), and photosensitive drug eruptions which are common and may be caused by a number of drugs (notably sulfonamides, tetracyclines and phenothiazines).

POLYMORPHIC LIGHT ERUPTION (PLE)

About 20% of patients with PLE present before the age of 10 years. A delayed reaction occurring several hours or the next day after exposure to the sun results in erythema, burning and itching, followed by papule and plaque formation. With avoidance of sun exposure this reaction will settle but will usually relapse when the child is exposed to the sun again. It usually presents during the summer, but in some children it is most marked in the spring and early summer, with remission of the symptoms in midsummer with 'hardening' of the skin. Juvenile spring eruption is probably a localized variant of PLE with papules and vesicles confined to the helices of the ears.

Most children with PLE continue into adulthood with it. Action spectrum studies are usually normal, and are therefore unhelpful. Prevention of PLE depends on adequate topical photoprotection with sunscreens. In those children with severe PLE, photochemotherapy with oral psoralen and UVA light (PUVA) may be helpful.

ACTINIC PRURIGO

This condition is clinically similar to PLE but is now recognized to be a separate entity. It is significantly associated with the haplotype HLA-DR4/DRB1*0407.[69] Actinic prurigo nearly always develops in early childhood and 80% of patients are female. There is usually progressive improvement in adolescence.

Clinically all exposed sites are affected, including face, lips, neck, ears, arms, dorsum of hands and lower legs. In the majority there is also involvement of covered skin, though to a lesser extent. It is worse during summer months but very often persists even in winter. In most cases there is a family history and there is also a strong association with atopy.

Action spectrum studies are abnormal in the majority with sensitivity to both UVA and UVB; however, in some children these studies are normal. Treatment is similar to that of PLE, but thalidomide has also been found to be particularly effective in this condition.

HYDROA VACCINIFORME

This is a very rare condition which invariably starts in childhood. On exposure to sunlight the child develops tingling and erythema followed by blistering and umbilicated papules on the face, ears, arms and dorsum of hands. These lead to crusting and varioliform scars.

Action spectrum studies are abnormal with sensitivity mainly involving UVA. Treatment is generally unsatisfactory, though broad spectrum topical sunscreens may be helpful.

DISORDERS OF HYPOPIGMENTATION

HEREDITARY DISORDERS OF HYPOPIGMENTATION

Pigmentary disorders may indicate a more serious systemic disease and the hereditary disorders of hypopigmentation are summarized in Table 30.6.

VITILIGO

This is possibly an autoimmune disease. Though specific antimelanocyte antibodies cannot be demonstrated by immunofluorescence, complement-fixing antibody to melanocytes has been shown in some patients. It is well recognized that patients with vitiligo frequently have thyroid, gastric and adrenal autoantibodies (Fig. 30.53). Vitiligo causes complete depigmentation of the skin (unlike tinea versicolor and pityriasis alba) due to absence of melanocytes and melanin in the epidermis. Vitiligo is common in adults, and is not rare in children. The depigmentation is usually symmetrical but localized, although in some patients the condition progresses to involve almost the whole body. Spontaneous repigmentation occurs more in children than in adults. In those that do not repigment topical corticosteroids can be tried although fluorinated steroids should not be used for prolonged periods. Photochemotherapy with topical or oral psoralen may be helpful in the older child although complete repigmentation rates are disappointing. The efficacy of PUVA (oral administration of psoralen and subsequent exposure to UVA) has been shown in adults to be enhanced by concurrent topical calcipotriol.[70] Several small studies and case reports have shown variable responses to topical immunomodulators (tacrolimus). Otherwise cosmetic camouflage may be applied to the depigmented skin to minimize disfiguration.

NEVUS DEPIGMENTOSUS

Usually solitary, nevoid patches of hypopigmentation are present at birth and can involve any body site. A decrease but not absence of pigment helps differentiate nevus depigmentosus (achromic nevus) from vitiligo. Furthermore, unlike vitiligo, slight darkening may be seen in the affected site following ultraviolet light exposure. The differential diagnosis also includes ash leaf macules seen in tuberous sclerosus but these are often multiple and smaller. Systemic abnormalities have only been rarely reported.[71]

HYPOMELANOSIS OF ITO

There is convincing evidence that hypomelanosis of Ito does not represent a distinct entity but is rather a symptom of many different states of mosaicism.[72] Incontinentia pigmenti type 1, which was subsequently shown to be hypomelanosis of Ito, is a sporadic condition associated with an X/autosome translocation involving Xp11.

Unilateral or bilateral macular hypopigmented whorls, streaks, and patches of hypopigmentation present at birth along the lines of Blaschko. Although some features are similar to those of classic incontinentia pigmenti the preceding inflammatory stage is absent. Abnormalities of the eyes and the musculoskeletal and central nervous systems occur in some.

DISORDERS OF HAIR LOSS

The normal transition from vellus to terminal hair in the newborn may be delayed up to 1 year giving the false impression of diffuse congenital alopecia. Genuine inability to grow normal hair can be seen in a number of genetic conditions including the ectodermal dysplasias and hair shaft abnormalities. The latter group may be detected by light microscopy of the affected hair and includes trichorrhexis nodosa which occurs as an isolated problem or in Menkes syndrome; trichothiodystrophy, characterized by sulfur-deficient, brittle hair; trichorrhexis invaginata (bamboo hair) usually associated with Netherton syndrome; monilethrix (beaded hairs due to keratin mutations); and pili torti which describes flattened and twisted hairs.

LOOSE ANAGEN SYNDROME

Diffuse or occasionally patchy hair loss is seen typically in fair-haired girls aged 2–9 years. The hair is a little unruly. Loose anagen syndrome is often familial and is diagnosed by an increased number of anagen hairs present when plucked from the scalp. The features become less prominent into adult life.

TELOGEN EFFLUVIUM

This refers to hair loss following the abrupt transformation of anagen hairs to the telogen phase during which they are shed. Normally 80–90% of hairs are in anagen but up to half may change in synchronization to telogen. This results in hair loss 3–4 months after the initiating event which may be 'stress', severe illness or certain drugs, e.g. anticoagulants, retinoids, etc.

ALOPECIA AREATA

It seems likely that at least in some patients with this condition the process is due to autoimmunity, though conclusive proof is lacking (Fig. 30.54). There is an increased incidence of autoantibodies and autoimmune diseases. There is also an increased incidence of atopy, and atopic children are more likely to develop total alopecia. A family history of alopecia areata is present in 5–25% of cases.

Most children develop discoid areas of alopecia in the scalp with peripheral exclamation hairs, and these areas regrow hair normally in due course. In some children, however, particularly those with an ophiasiform distribution of hair loss (involving the temples and occipital region), the condition is progressive to become total, and regrowth is much less likely. There are also nail changes with fine pitting and horizontal depressions known as Beau's lines. Although alopecia areata is not a life threatening condition it is obviously distressing for children and parents.

Table 30.6 Hereditary syndromes associated with hypopigmentation

	Oculocutaneous albinism (OCA types I and II)	Chediak–Higashi syndrome	Hermansky–Pudlak syndrome	Piebald trait	Waardenburg syndrome (types I–III)	Cross syndrome
Inheritance	AR	AR	AR	AD	AD	AR
Pigment loss	Type I: total, hair white. Type II: freckles in sun-exposed sites, hair yellow	Variable (patchy) oculocutaneous albinism. Silvery hair which may be sparse	Tyrosinase-positive oculocutaneous albinism	White forelock, absent pigmentation (leukoderma) ventral chest, abdomen and midportion of limbs. Pigmented macules often within affected areas	Piebaldism	Reduction in skin pigment. Variable loss of hair color
Ocular features	Nystagmus, visual loss. Type I: photophobia	Nystagmus, visual loss, photophobia pale retinae, and translucent irides	Blindness, nystagmus, strabismus, iris transillumination, foveal hypoplasia, and albinotic retinal midperiphery	Heterochromia iridis	Type I: dystopia canthorum Type II: more frequently heterochromia iridis	Nystagmus, reduced eye color
Other features		Frequent and severe pyogenic infections. Progressive neuropathy and neurodegeneration Lymphadenopathy	Bleeding tendency due to poor platelet aggregation. Cellular storage problems lead to pulmonary fibrosis, granulomatous enteropathic disease, and renal failure		Sensorineural deafness more common in type II Type III: additional severe musculoskeletal abnormalities	Mental and growth retardation, spasticity, athetoid movements
Molecular defect	Type I: tyrosinase (TYR) gene Type II: transmembrane protein (P gene)	Lysosomal trafficking regulator gene (CHS1)	Seven gene defects are associated with the four known subtypes	KIT protooncogene and occasionally zinc finger transcription factor SNA12	Types I and III: paired box homeotic gene-3 (PAX-3). Type IIA: microphthalmia-associated transcription factor gene (MITF)	Unknown
Other	Type II most common type of OCA (types I–VI) OCAIII due to TRP-1 mutations. Individuals have reddish hair and reddish-brown skin		HPS type 2 patients also have immunodeficiency	Hirschsprung disease occasionally associated	Hirschsprung disease occasionally associated	Very rare. Also referred to as oculocerebral syndrome with hypopigmentation

AR; autosomal recessive. AD; autosomal dominant.

There is no effective treatment for alopecia areata at present. Intralesional steroids may cause some local hair growth but this has no permanent effect on the course of the alopecia. In older children, short contact dithranol treatment may induce hair growth but the result is rarely cosmetically acceptable. There is no evidence as yet that topical minoxidil is helpful.

TRICHOTILLOMANIA (HAIR PULLING)

Trichotillomania is more common in girls. The alopecia is patchy with variable hair lengths in the affected region usually located on the contralateral side to the child's handedness. Hair ingestion may lead to bowel symptoms. Trichotillomania is most often an isolated symptom with a good prognosis following appropriate psychological support. However, follow-up until resolution is important to avoid missing more severe psychological disease.

THE HISTIOCYTOSES

Histiocytes include circulating monocytes and tissue macrophages as well as the dendritic cell system (antigen presenting cells). The histiocytoses

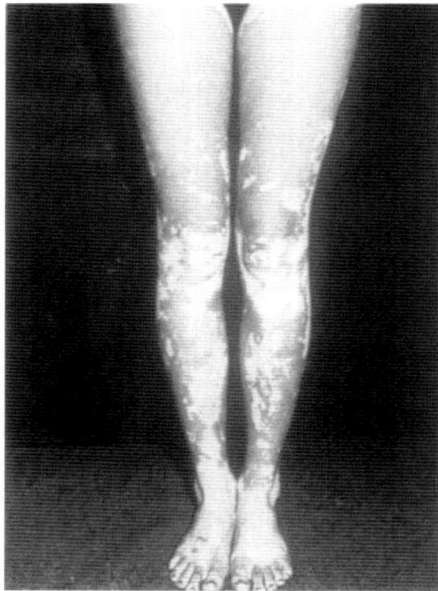

Fig. 30.53   Vitiligo.

have been classified into class I (Langerhans' cell histiocytosis), class II (proliferative histiocytoses of mononuclear phagocytes other than Langerhans' cell) and class III (malignant histiocyte disorders).[73]

CLASS I LANGERHANS' CELL HISTIOCYTOSIS (HISTIOCYTOSIS X)

This condition is rare (Ch. 24, pp. 1030) and the cells involved are Langerhans' cells which contain Birbeck granules and express the common thymocyte antigen CD1 markers. Although historically four types are recognized on the basis of clinical organ involvement, the presentations may overlap and the disease may progress from one subtype to another.[74]

Letterer–Siwe disease

This usually presents in the first year of life (Fig. 30.55). Discrete yellow–brown papules develop on the scalp, face, upper trunk and flexures, with a distribution mimicking seborrheic eczema. Purpura and crusting of the lesion may become evident. In some children mucous membranes are also involved, with gingivitis and oral and genital ulceration.

Signs of systemic involvement become manifest, with hepatosplenomegaly, lymphadenopathy and anemia. Chest X-ray shows miliary shadowing and bone scans may show osteolytic areas. Treatment with steroids and cytotoxic drugs has reduced the mortality and slowed the progression.

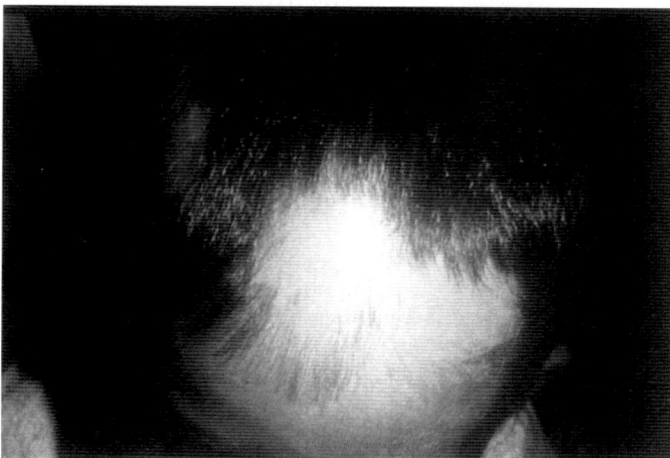

Fig. 30.54   Alopecia areata.

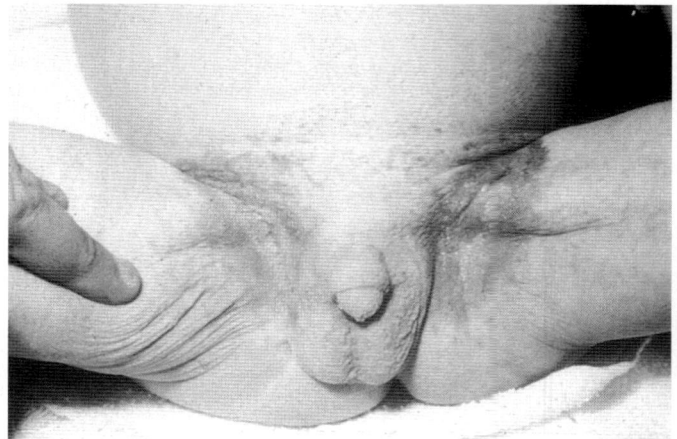

Fig. 30.55   Letterer–Siwe disease.

Hand–Schüller–Christian disease

This is a more benign form of histiocytosis X, which usually presents within the first 5 years of life and follows a chronic non-fatal course. The usual manifestations are radiological bone defects, exophthalmos and diabetes insipidus. Skin lesions similar to those in Letterer–Siwe disease are present in 30%.

Eosinophilic granuloma

This is the most benign form of histiocytosis X. It commonly presents within the first 5 years of life, and skin involvement is rare. When it does occur, yellowish or brownish papules are found on the scalp and trunk in a distribution similar to the other forms of histiocytosis X. Spontaneous resolution usually occurs.

Congenital self-healing histiocytosis

This usually affects skin only with lesions that are nodular or may mimic chickenpox. If this is the case spontaneous resolution occurs within months.

JUVENILE XANTHOGRANULOMA (JXG)

JXG is an example of a benign self-limiting non-Langerhans' cell histiocytosis (class II) (Fig. 30.56). Histologically lesions are characterized by histiocytes with foamy macrophages and multinucleated giant cells. Despite its name and appearance JXG is not associated with lipid disorders. Lesions are occasionally present at birth but typically before 1 year. They are dome-shaped nodules with a red and then orange color often located on the head and neck. Single lesions are more common but if multiple lesions are present up to 10% have ocular involvement which may lead to glaucoma.

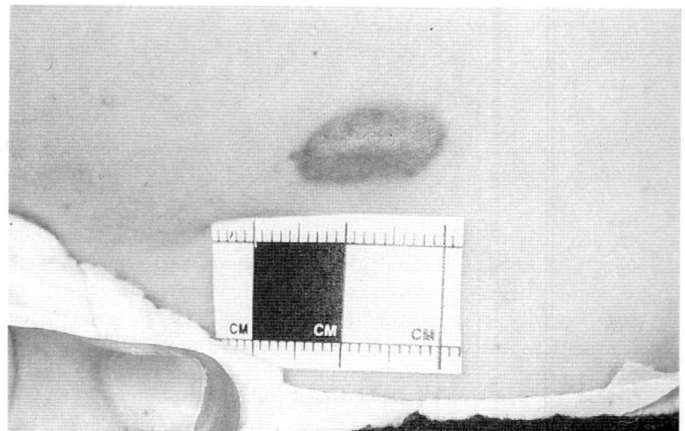

Fig. 30.56   Juvenile xanthogranuloma (XTG).

REFERENCES (* Level 1 evidence)

1. Long CC, Mills CM, Finlay AY. A practical guide to topical therapy in children. Br J Dermatol 1998; 138:293–296.

2. DeDavid M, Orlow SJ, Provost N, et al. Neurocutaneous melanosis: clinical features of large congenital melanocytic nevi in patients with manifest central nervous system melanosis. J Am Acad Dermatol 1996; 35:529–538.

3. Foster RD, Williams ML, Barkovich AJ, et al. Giant congenital melanocytic nevi: the significance of neurocutaneous melanosis in neurologically asymptomatic children. Plast Reconstr Surg 2001; 107:933–941.

4. Agero AL, Benvenuto-Andrade C, Dusza SW, et al. Asymptomatic neurocutaneous melanocytosis in patients with large congenital melanocytic nevi. A study of cases from an internet-based registry. J Am Acad Dermatol 2005; 53:959–965.

5. Bett BJ. Large or multiple congenital melanocytic nevi: Occurrence of neurocutaneous melanocytosis in 1008 persons. J Am Acad Dermatol 2006; 54: 767–777.

6. Lorentzen M, Pers M, Bretteville Jensen G. The incidence of malignant transformation in giant pigmented nevi. Scand J Plast Reconstr Surg 1977; II:163–167.

7. Illig W, Weidner F, Hundeeker M, et al. Congenital nevi < 10cms as precursors to melanoma. Arch Dermatol 1985; 121:1274–1281.

8. Rhodes AR, Sober AJ, Calvin L, et al. The malignant potential of small congenital nevocellular nevi. J Am Acad Dermatol 1982; 6:230–241.

9. Sahin S, Levin L, Kopf AW, et al. Risk of melanoma in medium-sized congenital melanocytic nevi: a follow-up study. J Am Acad Dermatol 1998; 39:428–433.

10. Goss BD, Ansell PE, Bennett V, et al. The prevalence and characteristics of congenital pigmented lesions in the newborn babies in Oxford. Paediatr Perinatal Epidemiol 1990; 4:448–457.

11. Happle R. How many epidermal nevus syndromes exist?. J Am Acad Dermatol 1991; 25:550–556.

12. Solomon LM, Esterly NM. Epidermal and other organoid nevi. Curr Probl Pediatr 1975; 6:1–56.

13. Rogers M. Epidermal nevi and the epidermal nevus syndromes: a review of 233 cases. Pediatr Dermatol 1992; 9:342–344.

14. Enjolras O, Mulliken JB. The current management of vascular birthmarks. Pediatr Dermatol 1993; 10:311–333.

15. North PE, Waner M, Mizeracki A, et al. A unique microvascular phenotype shared by juvenile hemangiomas and human placenta. Arch Dermatol 2001; 137:559–570.

*16. Bennett ML, Fleischer AB, Chamlin SL, et al. Oral corticosteroid use is effective for cutaneous hemangiomas. Arch Dermatol 2001; 137:1208–1213.

17. Dubois J, Hershon L, Carmant L, et al. Toxicity profile of interferon alfa-2b in children: a prospective evaluation. J Pediatr 1999; 135:782–785.

*18. Batta K, Goodyear HM, Moss C, et al. Randomised controlled study of early pulsed dye laser treatment of uncomplicated childhood haemangiomas: results of a 1-year analysis. Lancet 2002; 360:521–527.

19. Payarols J, Masferrer J, Gomez Bellvert C. . Treatment of life-threatening infantile hemangiomas with vincristine. N Engl J Med 1995; 333:69.

20. Krol A, MacArthur CJ. Congenital hemangiomas: rapidly involuting and noninvoluting congenital hemangiomas. Arch Facial Plast Surg 2005; 7:307–311.

21. Metry DW, Dowd CF, Barkovich AJ, et al. The many faces of PHACE syndrome. J Pediatr 2001; 139:117–123.

22. Golitz LE, Rudikoff J, O'Meara OP. Diffuse neonatal hemangiomatosis. Pediatr Dermatol 1986; 3:145–152.

23. Esterly NB, Margileth AM, Kahn G. The management of disseminated eruptive haemangiomata in infants: special symposium. Pediatr Dermatol 2001; 1:312–317.

24. Stevenson RF, Thompson HG, Marin JD. Unrecognized ocular problems associated with port wine stain of the face in children. Can Med Assoc J 1974; 11:953–955.

25. Enjolras O, Riche MC, Merland JJ. Facial port wine stains and Sturge Weber syndrome. Pediatrics 1985; 76:48–51.

26. Kelsell DP, Norgett EE, Unsworth H, et al. Mutations in ABCA12 underlie the severe congenital skin disease harlequin ichthyosis. Am J Hum Genet 2005; 76:794–803.

27. Itin PH, Fistarol SK. Ectodermal dysplasias. Am J Med Genet C Semin Med Genet 2004; 131C:45–51.

28. Cheadle JP, Reeve MP, Sampson JR, et al. Molecular genetic advances in tuberose sclerosis. Hum Genet 2000; 107:97–114.

29. Smahi A, Courtois G, Vabres P, et al. Genomic rearrangement in NEMO impairs NF-kappaB activation and is a cause of incontinentia pigmenti. The International Incontinentia Pigmenti (IP) Consortium. Nature 2000; 405:466–472.

30. Peters TJ, Sarkany R. Porphyria for the general physician. Clin Med 2005; 5:275–281.

31. Gelmetti, Schianchi R, Ermacora E. Cutis marmorata telangiectatica congenita. 4 new cases and review of the literature. Ann Dermatol Venereol 1987; 114:1517–1528.

*32. Gibbs S, Harvey I, Sterling JC, et al. Local treatments for cutaneous warts: systematic review. Br Med J 2002; 325:461–464.

33. Karabulut AA, Sahin S. Is cimetidine effective for nongenital warts: a double-blind, placebo-controlled study. Arch Dermatol 1997; 133:533–534.

34. Caputo R, Gelmetti C, Ermacora E, et al. Gianotti-Crosti syndrome: a retrospective analysis of 308 cases. J Am Acad Dermatol 1992; 26:207–210.

35. Coskey RJ, Coskey LA. Diagnosis and treatment of impetigo. J Am Acad Dermatol 1987; 17:62–63.

*36. Barton LL, Friedman AD, Portilla MG. Impetigo contagiosa: a comparison of erythromycin and dicloxacillin therapy. Pediatr Dermatol 1988; 5:88–91.

*37. McLinn S. Topical mupirocin vs. systemic erythromycin treatment for pyoderma. Pediatr Infect Dis J 1988; 7:785–790.

*38. Christensen OB, Anehus S. Hydrogen peroxide cream: an alternative to topical antibiotics in the treatment of impetigo contagiosa. Acta Derm Venereol 1994; 74:460–462.

39. Rogers M, Dorman DC, Gapes M, et al. A three year study of impetigo in Sydney. Med J Aust 1987; 147:59–62.

40. Krol AL. Perianal streptococcal dermatitis. Pediatr Dermatol 1990; 7:97–100.

41. Jones TC. Overview of the use of terbinafine (Lamisil) in children. Br J Dermatol 1995; 132:683–689.

42. Terragni L, Lasagni A, Oriani A, et al. Pityriasis versicolor in the pediatric age. Pediatr Dermatol 1991; 8:9–12.

*43. Schultz MW, Gomez M, Hansen RC, et al. Comparative study of 5% permethrin cream and 1% lindane lotion for the treatment of scabies. Arch Dermatol 1990; 126:167–170.

*44. Taplin D, Meinking TL, Chen JA, et al. Comparison on crotamiton 10% cream (Eurax) and permethrin 5% cream (Elimite) for the treatment of scabies in children. Pediatr Dermatol 1990; 7:67–73.

45. Hourihane JO, Roberts SA, Warner JO. Resolution of peanut allergy: a case control study. BMJ 1998; 316:1271–1275.

46. Sabroe RA, Greaves MW. Chronic idiopathic urticaria with functional autoantibodies: 12 years on. Br J Dermatol 2006; 154:813–819.

47. Hannaford R, Rogers M. Presentation of cutaneous mastocytosis in 173 children. Australas J Dermatol 2001; 42:15–21.

*48. Tatnall FM, Schofield JK, Leigh IM. A double-blind, placebo-controlled trial of continuous acyclovir therapy in recurrent erythema multiforme. Br J Dermatol 1995; 132:267–270.

49. Reunala T, Kosnai I, Karparti S, et al. Dermatitis herpetiformis: jejunal findings and skin response to gluten free diet. Arch Dis Child 1984; 59:517–522.

50. Barham KL, Jorizzo JL, Grattan B, et al. Vasculitis and neutrophilic vascular reactions. In: Burns DA, Breatnach S, Cox N, et al, eds. Textbook of dermatology. Oxford: Blackwell Science; 2004.49.1.

51. Brown S, Reynolds NJ. Atopic and non-atopic eczema. BMJ 2006; 332:584–588.

52. Palmer CN, Irvine AD, Terron-Kwiatkowski A, et al. Common loss-of-function variants of the epidermal barrier protein filaggrin are a major predisposing factor for atopic dermatitis. Nat Genet 2006; 38:441–446.

53. Hoare C, Li Wan Po A, Williams H. Systematic review of treatments for atopic eczema. Health Technol Assess 2000; 4:37.

54. Frequency of application of topical corticosteroids for eczema. www.nice.org.uk/TA081guidance

55. Tacrolimus and pimecrolimus for atopic eczema. www.nice.org.uk/TA082guidance

56. Zaki I, Emerson R, Allen BR. Treatment of severe atopic dermatitis in childhood with cyclosporin. Br J Dermatol 1996; 135:(suppl 48):21–24.

*57. Pei AY, Chan HH, Leung TF. Montelukast in the treatment of children with moderate-to-severe atopic dermatitis: a pilot study. Pediatr Allergy Immunol 2001; 12:154–158.

*58. Tewary M, Friedmann PS, Hotchkiss K, et al. A double blind, placebo-controlled trial of montelukast in adult atopic dermatitis. [PO02.37], EADV meeting, Rhods, October 2006.

*59. Sheehan MP, Atherton DJ. One-year follow up of children treated with Chinese medicinal herbs for atopic eczema. Br J Dermatol 1994; 130:488–493.

60. Kalliomaki M, Salminen S, Arvilommi H, et al. Probiotics in primary prevention of atopic disease: a randomised placebo-controlled trial. Lancet 2001; 357:1076–1079.

61. Andersen SL, Thomsen K. Psoriasiform napkin dermatitis. Br J Dermatol 1971; 84:316–319.

62. Neville EA, Finn OA. Psoriasiform napkin dermatitis – a follow up study. Br J Dermatol 1975; 92:279–285.

*63. Oranje AP, Marcoux D, Svensson A, et al. Topical calcipotriol in childhood psoriasis. J Am Acad Dermatol 1997; 36:203–208.

*64. Owen CM, Chalmers RJG, O'Sullivan T, et al. Antistreptococcal interventions for guttate and chronic plaque psoriasis (Cochrane review). In: The Cochrane Library. 3. Oxford: Update Software; 2001.

65. Ramanan AV, Campbell-Webster N, Ota S, et al. The effectiveness of treating juvenile dermatomyositis with methotrexate and aggressively tapered corticosteroids. Arthritis Rheum 2005; 52:3570–3578.

66. Kreuter A, Gambichler T, Breuckmann F, et al. Arch Dermatol. 2005; 141:847–852.

67. Oyama N, Chan I, Neill SM, et al. Autoantibodies to extracellular matrix protein 1 in lichen sclerosus. Lancet 2004; 362:118–123.

68. Dalziel K, Millard PR, Wojnarowska F. The treatment of vulvar lichen sclerosus with a very potent corticosteroid (clobetasol proprionate 0.05%) cream. Br J Dermatol 1991; 124:461–464.

69. Grabczynska SA, McGregor JM, Kondeatis E, et al. Actinic prurigo and polymorphic light eruption: common pathogenesis and the importance of HLA-DR4/DRB1*0407. Br J Dermatol 1999; 140:232–236.

*70. Ermis O, Alpsoy E, Cetin L, et al. Is the efficacy of psoralen plus ultraviolet A therapy for vitiligo enhanced by concurrent topical calcipotriol? A placebo-controlled double-blind study. Br J Dermatol 2001; 145:472–475.

71. Dahr S, Kanwar AJ, Kaur S. Nevus depigmentation in India: experience with 50 patients. Pediatr Dermatol 1993; 10:299–300.

72. Donnai D, Read AP, McKeown C, et al. Hypomelanosis of Ito: a manifestation of mosaicism or chimerism. J Med Genet 1988; 25:809–818.

73. Chu T, D'Angio GJ, Favara B, et al. Histiocytosis syndromes in children. Lancet 1987; i:208–209.

74. Komp DM. Concepts in staging and clinical studies for treatment of Langerhans' cell histiocytosis. Semin Oncol 1991; 18:18–23.

31

Disorders of the eye

Brian W Fleck, Alan O Mulvihill

NORMAL VISUAL DEVELOPMENT

At around 6 weeks an infant will smile in response to visual stimuli; delay of this developmental stage is significant. Visually directed reaching commences at age 2–3 months.

Preferential looking grating measurements of vision reach 6/6 level at 3 years[1] however this test is dependent on complex sensory and motor responses. Cortical VEP estimates of visual acuity give a 6/6 response by age 6–8 months.[2] Stereopsis develops between the ages of 2 and 6 months.[3]

CRITICAL PERIOD OF VISUAL DEVELOPMENT

Early visual experience is critical to the development of synaptic connections in the primary visual cortex.[4] Input from each eye 'competes' for cortical connections.[5] The visual outcome of congenital cataract surgery is poor if visual rehabilitation is delayed beyond 3 months of age. The visual outcome of surgery for uniocular cataract is less satisfactory than that for binocular cataract[6] as the normal eye dominates synaptic development.

PLASTIC PERIOD OF VISUAL DEVELOPMENT

While the critical period of visual development is at age 0–3 months, the visual system remains plastic until at least the age of 8–12 years, and probably longer.[7] Interrupted visual development below the age of about 6 years[8] may lead to permanent reduction of visual acuity even after the causative abnormality has been removed. This is termed 'amblyopia'. The younger the age at which developmental interruption happens, the greater the degree of amblyopia that may occur. Once again uniocular defects produce a greater effect than binocular defects, because of competition effects at the occipital cortex. Amblyopia may be treated during the critical and plastic period of visual development – up to approximately age 8–12 years.[7]

CLINICAL ASSESSMENT

CLINICAL HISTORY

Symptoms related to visual functions cover a wide spectrum of difficulties. Progressive bilateral visual loss in young children may go unnoticed until a relatively late stage, and may present with impairment of a wide spectrum of visually dependent behaviors. Symptoms related to consistently bumping into doorways may indicate visual field reduction on one side. Symptoms related to difficulties coming down stairs or frequent tripping may indicate inferior visual field restriction. Increased sensitivity to light (photophobia) may indicate ocular inflammation or retinal cone dysfunction. Difficulties in dim light (night blindness) may indicate poor retinal rod function. The prenatal history, birth history, developmental history, drug history, family history and educational history should always be taken.

In older children perceptual visual difficulties related to central nervous system (CNS) disease may go undetected unless a careful history is taken. Useful screening questions include:
- Does the child have difficulty identifying objects within a 'busy' or 'fast-moving' environment?
- Does the child have difficulty with coordination and movement in three-dimensional space?
- Does the child have difficulty recognizing familiar faces?
- Does the child have difficulty with orientation in familiar environments?

VISION ASSESSMENT

In infants and very young children, observed visual behavior will give useful qualitative information about visual function. A visually alert infant will fixate on and follow the movement of small objects of interest held by an examiner. Each eye is tested separately by covering one eye with a hand or eye patch. If a child will not tolerate uniocular testing then some useful information may be obtained from binocular testing. However, poor vision in one eye will not be detected by binocular testing.

QUANTITATIVE MEASUREMENTS OF VISUAL ACUITY

'Visibility' refers to the ability to identify a single object such as a sweet, thread on a carpet, or airplane in the sky. 'Resolution' refers to the ability to distinguish between two points or lines. Visual acuity tests measure resolution. Clinical tests of visibility such as Stycar balls, Catford drum, etc. may significantly overestimate results obtained with resolution tests and should be interpreted with caution.

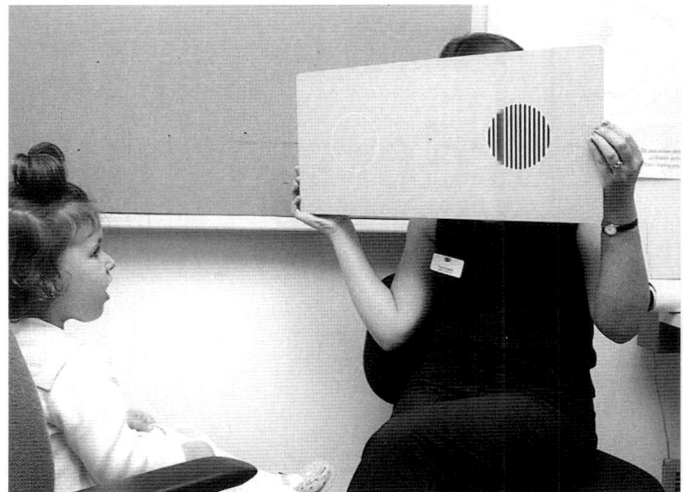

Fig. 31.1 Forced choice preferential looking test (Keeler cards). The tester looks through a hole in the card and chooses which target area the child looks at.

PREFERENTIAL LOOKING ACUITY CARDS

An infant will 'prefer' to look at an object of interest rather than at a blank background. Black and white stripes (gratings) of varying widths ('spatial frequency') are used as the stimulus (Fig. 31.1). The tester uses a series of test cards, each of which has two test areas – one blank and one a test grating. The tester observes the area the infant looks at. The test is repeated a number of times, using various stripe widths. The narrowest stripe width (lowest spatial frequency) consistently looked at by the infant is a measure of the infant's visual resolution. Preferential looking tests may be successfully used in most infants, but are of less interest to 18–24-month-old children.

Cardiff cards use black and white lines shaped into interesting pictures (Fig. 31.2). These are useful in children aged 1–3 years. The child will look at the picture if the black and white stripes are sufficiently wide to be observed (resolved).

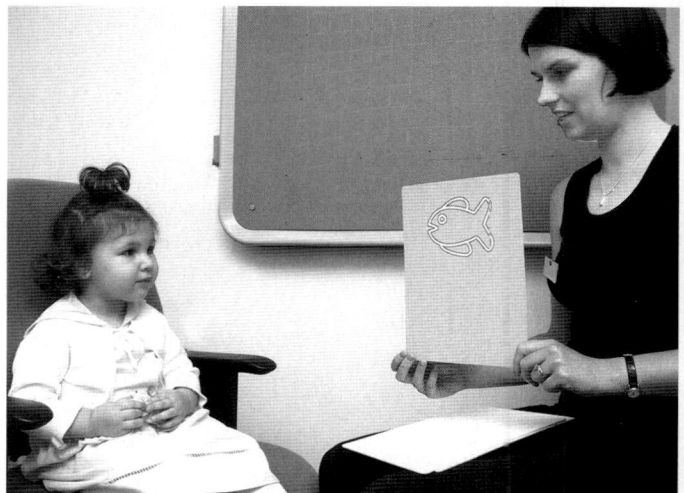

Fig. 31.2 The tester observes whether the child looks at the top or bottom half of the test card. The images are randomly distributed to the top halves and bottom halves of the test cards. The test is normally performed at 50 cm or 100 cm.

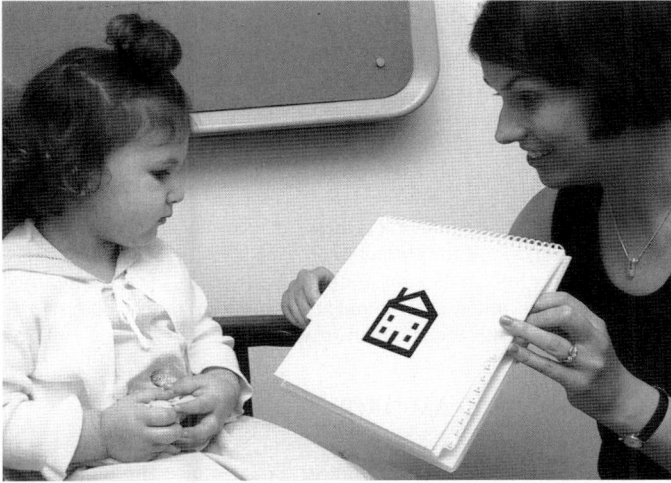

Fig. 31.3 Kay picture optotypes. The test is normally performed at 3 m or 6 m.

OPTOTYPE TESTS

From the age of 3 years upward more traditional 'optotype' visual acuity symbols may be used. Kay pictures use simple line drawings (Fig. 31.3). The Sheridan Gardiner test uses letters. A limited range of letters is used so that the child may match the shape of the letter rather than name it (Fig. 31.4). A letter placed among a line of other letters is less easily observed than a single letter. Charts that use lines of letters arranged in log unit size are preferred in children aged 4–5 years and upwards – LogMAR charts (Fig. 31.5).

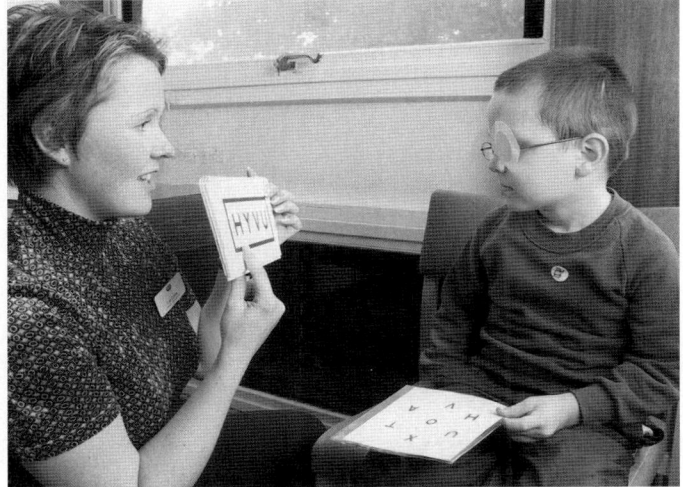

Fig. 31.4 Sheridan Gardiner optotypes. The test is usually performed at 6 m and the child matches the test letter to the key card.

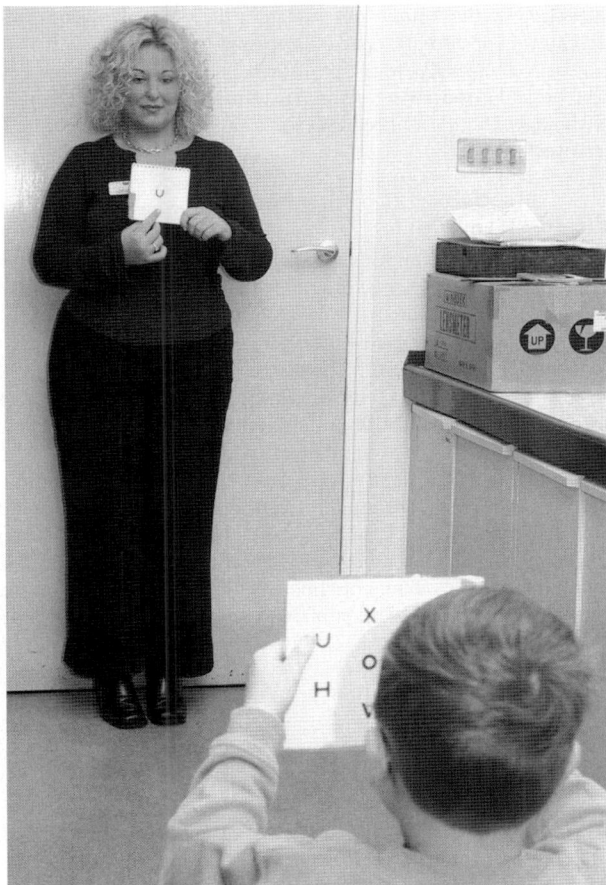

Fig. 31.5 LogMAR optotypes (Glasgow cards). The test is usually performed at 6 m and the child matches the test letter to the key card. Reduced vision due to 'crowding' is detected as the test letter is placed within a row of letters.

VISUAL FIELDS

Visual field testing may be undertaken in infants and young children by introducing an object of interest from either side and observing the response. Two observers are required (Fig. 31.6). The child sits on the lap of a carer. An observer sits approximately 1–2 m in front of the child. A second observer stands behind the parent and child. The second observer slowly brings an object of interest into the field of vision of the child. The child will turn to look at the object when it comes into the observable visual field. Binocular testing is more easily performed than uniocular testing, and will adequately detect a significant binocular visual field defect such as homonymous hemianopia or inferior visual field restriction.

In children aged 6 years upwards, Goldman visual field testing may be possible. This type of detailed visual field testing requires considerable

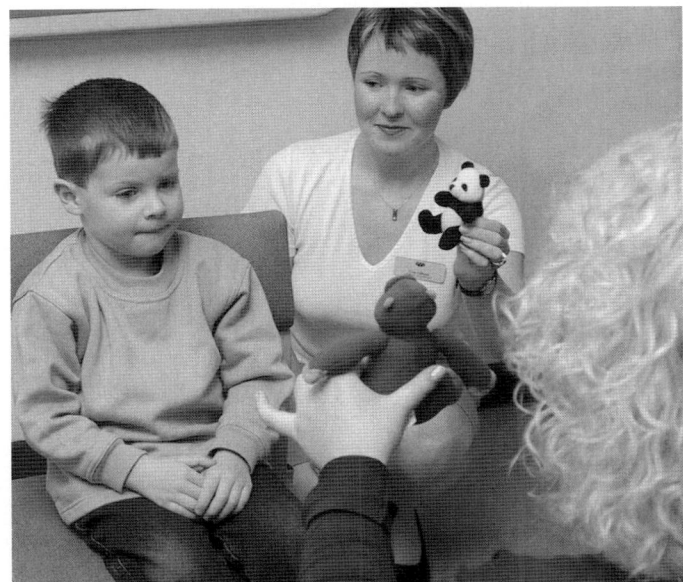

Fig. 31.6 Binocular visual field testing. Observer 1 maintains interest while observer 2 brings the test object (panda) into the child's visual field from behind. The child turns to look at the test object when it becomes visible.

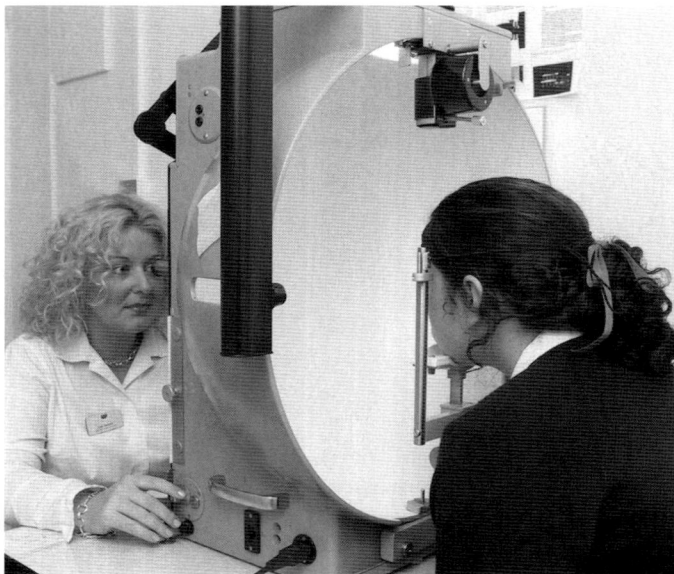

Fig. 31.7   Goldman visual field testing. The tester observes the eye fixing behavior of the child. The child fixes on the center target within the bowl and presses a buzzer when the test spot of light becomes visible in the peripheral visual field.

cooperation from the child. The child must fix on a central point in the testing bowl and a spot of light is brought in from the peripheral field of vision (Fig. 31.7). The child presses a buzzer when the spot of light comes into view. The test is very operator dependent. Testing is normally performed uniocularly, and accurate and reproducible charting of visual field defects related to optic nerve and CNS disease may be obtained.

CLINICAL EYE MOVEMENT TESTING

The cover test may be performed in order to detect a strabismus. When the straight eye is covered the strabismic eye quickly moves in order to take up fixation (Figs 31.8 and 31.9).

The range of eye movements may then be observed. The child is asked to observe an interesting target moved by the examiner. The examiner may use his or her face as the target and move from side to side and up

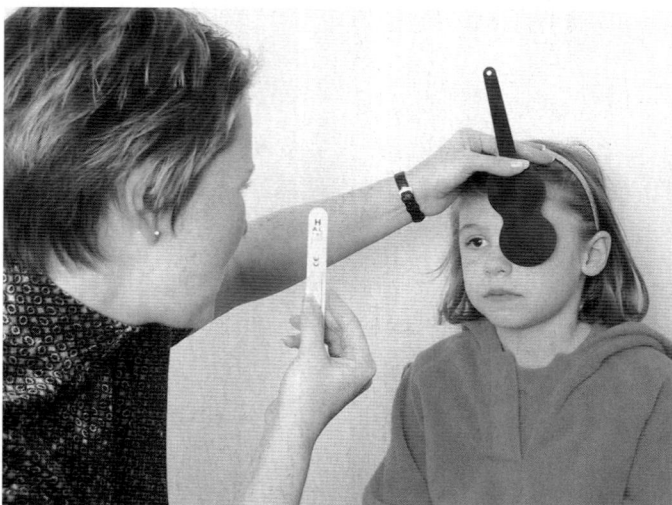

Fig. 31.8   Cover test. The child fixes on a test target at 6 m or 50 cm. The normal eye is covered. The strabismic eye then moves in order to take up fixation. Small flicks of movement may be easily detected, allowing diagnosis of small angled deviations.

and down in front of the child. Limitations of movements and changes in palpebral fissure width are observed.

Nystagmus may be described using the mnemonic 'DWARF':
Direction (horizontal or vertical)
Wave form (jerk or pendular)
Amplitude (large amplitude or small amplitude oscillations)
Rest (primary position (at rest/gaze euoked))
Frequency (rapid movements or slow movements).
The direction of nystagmus movements is recorded as the direction of the fast phase (jerk) of the oscillation.

While some information on nystagmus movements may be obtained by clinical observation, more detailed information may be obtained by analysis in an eye movement laboratory.

EXTERNAL EYE EXAMINATION

The eyelids, conjunctiva, cornea and iris may be observed using a torch. Ophthalmologists use magnification in the form of a slit lamp microscope to allow detailed examination of these structures (Fig. 31.10). Where there is a suspicion of a corneal epithelial abrasion or other corneal epithelial disease a drop of fluorescein dye may be instilled and the corneal epithelium may be observed using a blue light (Fig. 31.11). Any defects in the corneal epithelium will absorb fluorescein and these areas will fluoresce yellow.

Corneal signs such as posterior embryotoxon may be visualized with a slit lamp (Fig. 31.12).

PUPIL RED REFLEX

The transparency of the 'media' of the eye may be observed by observing the red reflex. When the media are transparent a beam of light directed from a direct ophthalmoscope will be observed to produce an orange–red reflection of the fundus, observable in the pupil area (Fig. 31.13). When cataract or vitreous opacity is present the red reflex will be dark or absent. A white reflex in the pupil area (leukocoria) is an important sign of possible underlying retinoblastoma or other significant ocular pathology. The normal red reflex is more difficult to detect in dark brown eyes.

PUPIL REACTIONS

The relative size of the pupils should be observed. Slight asymmetry of pupil size (anisocoria) may be physiological and the difference in pupil size is constant in light or dark. A torchlight may then be shone in each eye and the direct response to light observed. The light is then alternately shone in each eye, with the torch swinging backwards and forwards from eye to eye; this tests for relative afferent pupil defect. When the torch is shone in the healthy eye, the pupil constricts. However when the torch is then swung across to the eye with a sensory defect the pupil of this eye paradoxically dilates. This is because limited neural stimulation is produced by light shining in the defective eye and the dominant effect is the withdrawal of light from the healthy eye. Pupil dilatation in both eyes results and is observed in the defective eye. Motor pupil defects such as those seen following anticholinergic eye drop instillation or a III nerve palsy result in an absent pupil reaction to any stimulus.

RETINOSCOPY

The focusing of the eyes may be measured at any age using a streak retinoscope. Anticholinergic eye drops are instilled to dilate the pupil and relax the ciliary muscle so that there is no accommodation. In Caucasians cyclopentolate 1% eyedrops may be used, with measurements performed 30 min after instillation. In children with dark brown eyes it may be necessary to use atropine 1% eyedrops or ointment, instilled on two or more occasions a number of hours before the examination. A streak of light is directed into the pupil area and movement of the pupil light reflex is observed when the streak of light is moved from

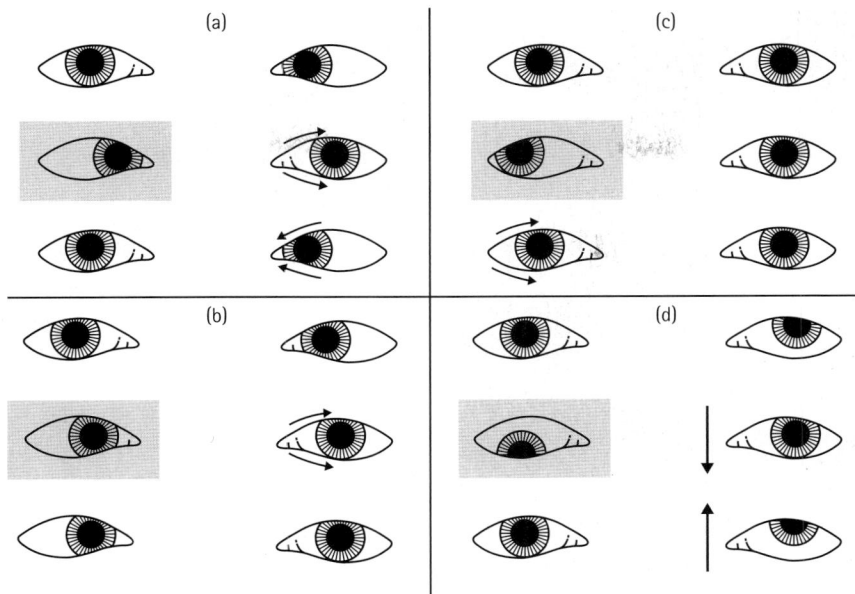

Fig. 31.9   The cover test for squint. Where there is no squint and there is normal binocular vision, both eyes maintain steady fixation on a distant object. There will be no deviation when one or other eye is covered and this is the basis of a cover test. When there is a latent or manifest squint some deviation will be observed on occluding one or other eye. (a) In manifest convergent squint the squinting eye is turned in and the nonsquinting eye maintains fixation. If the squinting eye is occluded in the cover test there will be no variation in the angle of squint, but when the nonsquinting eye ('fixing eye') is occluded it converges and the squinting eye takes up fixation. When the occluder is removed the original position of the eyes is resumed. (b) In alternating convergent squint either eye can maintain fixation while the other eye is turned in. If the squinting eye is occluded there is no alteration in the angle of deviation, but when the 'fixing eye' is occluded the opposite eye fixes the distant object and the previously straight eye converges. The former position is not resumed when the occluder is removed and the previously squinting eye maintains fixation (and the previously straight eye converges) until the occluder covers the originally squinting eye, when the originally fixing eye takes up position. (c) In latent squint both eyes will fix on a distant object but when one eye is covered it deviates. When the cover is removed the eye with the latent squint resumes fixation. The other eye does not shift or lose fixation while the opposite eye is being covered or uncovered. (d) The cover test is used to diagnose vertical squint as in horizontal squint, e.g. in left hypertropia the left eye is elevated (or the right eye depressed) and when the fixing eye is covered the opposite eye moves vertically to take up fixation.

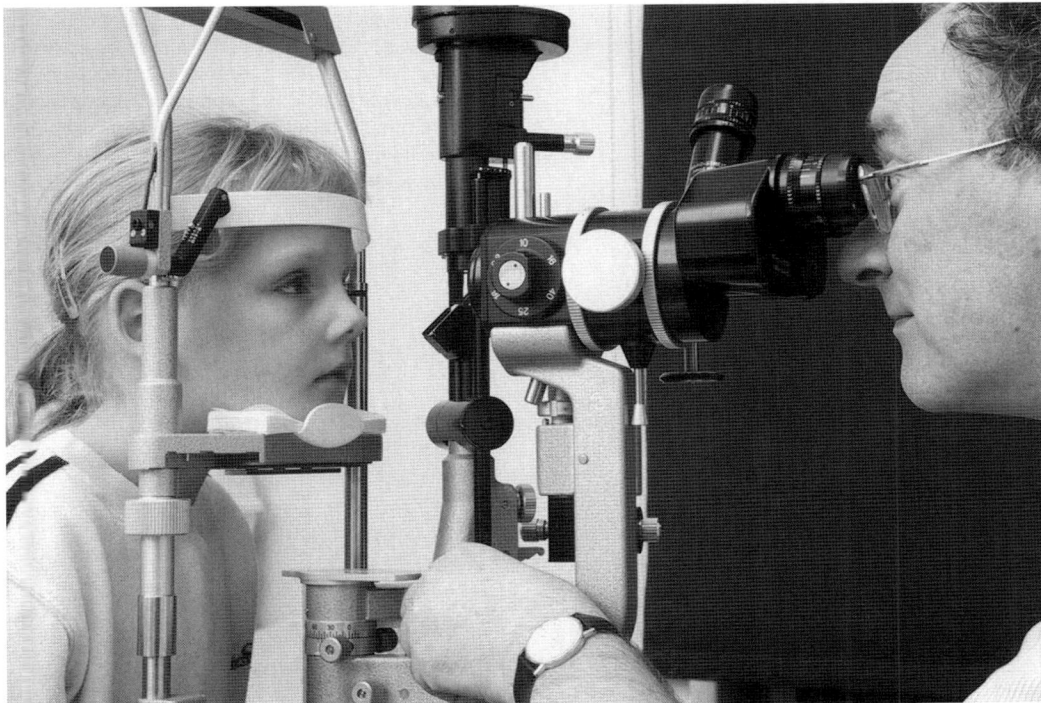

Fig. 31.10   The slit lamp is a binocular microscope with an illuminating light in the form of a slit. This enhances stereoscopic viewing of tissues.

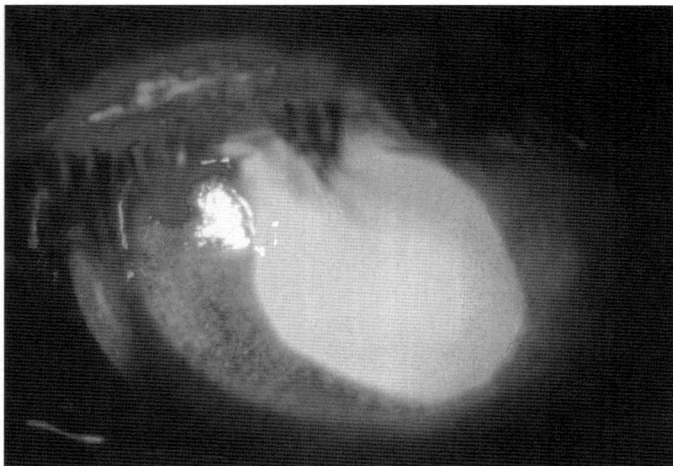

Fig. 31.11   Yellow/green fluorescein staining of an area of cornea abrasion visualized using blue light.

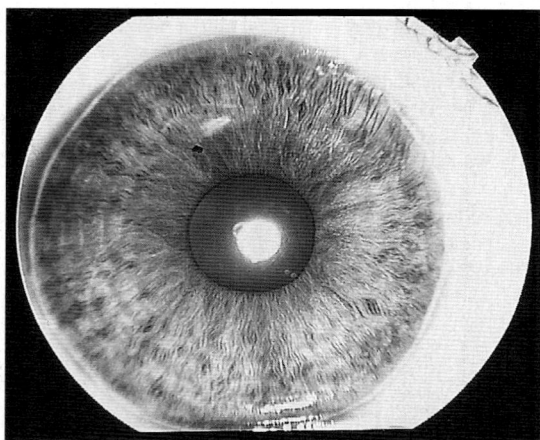

Fig. 31.12   Posterior embryotoxon. The edge of the basement membrane of the corneal endothelium is visible as a fine white line just inside the edge of the cornea. This is termed 'posterior embryotoxon'. This line is normally more peripheral, and therefore not visible.

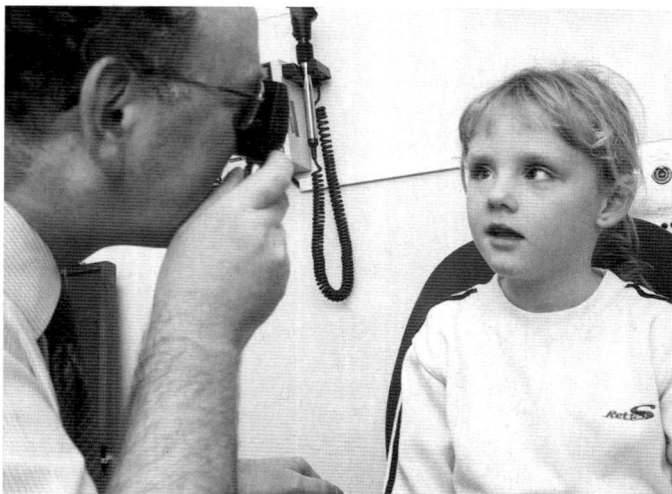

Fig. 31.13   Pupil red reflex testing using a direct ophthalmoscope. This is normally performed in a dimly lit room.

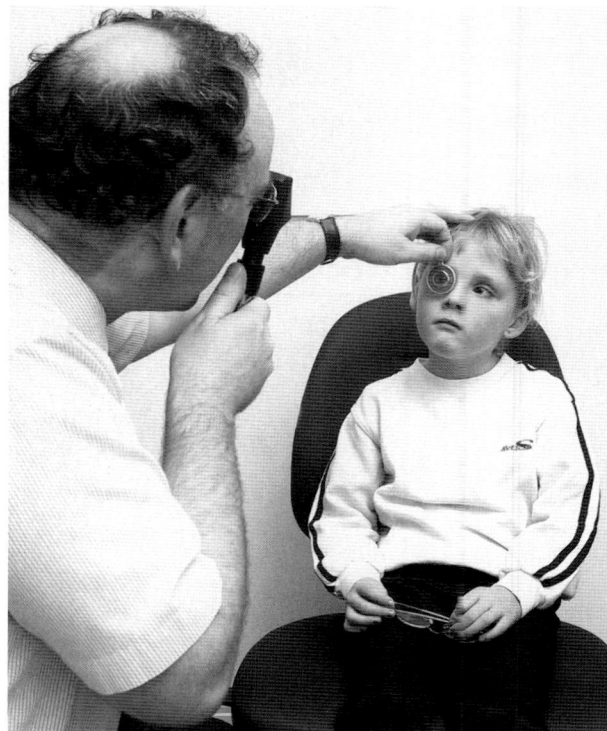

Fig. 31.14   Retinoscopy measurement of eye focusing.

side to side. A test spectacle lens is then held in front of the eye and the process is repeated (Fig. 31.14). The power of the lens that neutralizes movements of the pupil light reflex gives a measure of the focusing of the eye.

OPHTHALMOSCOPY

The fundi may be examined with the pupils dilated. Fundus examination of infants and young children is difficult with a direct ophthalmoscope. Ophthalmologists prefer to use an indirect ophthalmoscope. The light source is worn on the head and a convex lens is held in front of the eye in order to produce a focused image of the fundus (Fig. 31.15). The optic disc, macula, retinal vessels and retinal periphery may be examined. In older children, more detailed examination of the optic disc may be performed using a slit lamp microscope, in conjunction with a high powered convex lens. This allows detailed stereoscopic examination of the optic disc.

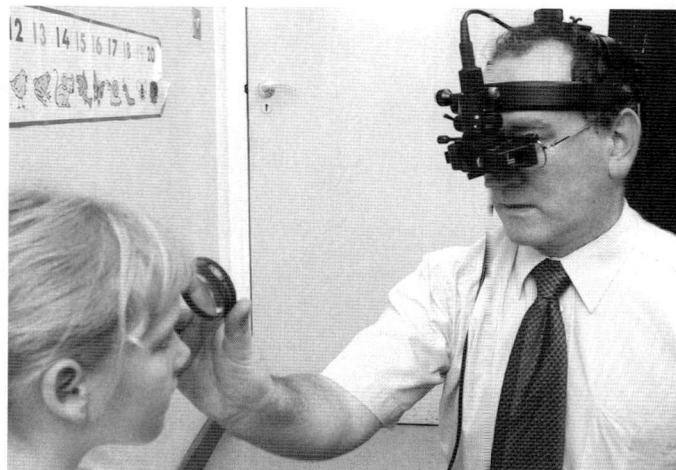

Fig. 31.15   Binocular indirect ophthalmoscope examination of the fundus.

SPECIALIZED METHODS OF EXAMINATION

ULTRASOUND

Ultrasound imaging may be used to examine the retina when the media are opaque due to cataract or other pathology (Fig. 31.16). The diameter of tumors such as retinoblastoma may be measured. High-definition ultrasound scans may be used to image the optic nerve head and optic nerve. Optic nerve head drusen may be detected. Widening of the cerebrospinal fluid (CSF) space around the optic nerve may be helpful in the diagnosis of raised intracranial pressure with papilledema.[9]

FUNDUS FLUORESCEIN ANGIOGRAPHY

Angiogram photographs of the retinal blood vessels may be obtained using i.v. or oral fluorescein dye (Fig. 31.17). This technique may be of value in assessing retinal vascular disease, retinal inflammatory disease and optic disc abnormalities. In the presence of optic disc edema, capillaries on the surface of the optic disc are dilated and leaky (Fig. 31.18). Optic nerve head drusen 'autofluoresce'–angiogram fluorescence is seen in the absence of fluorescein dye.

ELECTROPHYSIOLOGY STUDIES

Studies of the visual system using visually evoked potentials (VEPs) and of the retina using the electroretinogram may be of great diagnostic value in infants and young children with reduced vision. The stimulus for a VEP is a flash of light or a reversing pattern of black and white squares (Fig. 31.19). Pattern onset stimulation may be used as an

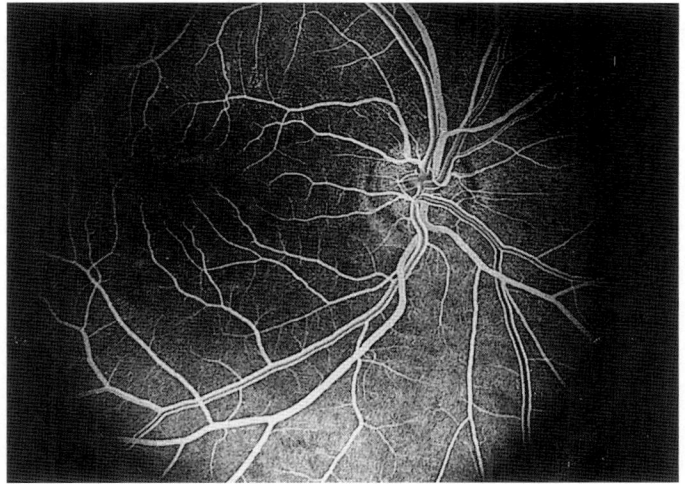

Fig. 31.18 Fluorescein dye is seen in the retinal arteries and capillaries 12 s after i.v. injection. Dye is starting to return to the veins.

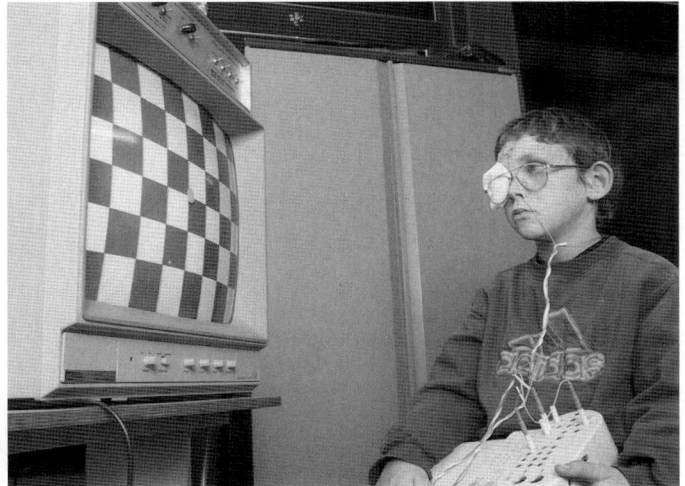

Fig. 31.19 Visually evoked potential examination using a reversing checker pattern stimulus.

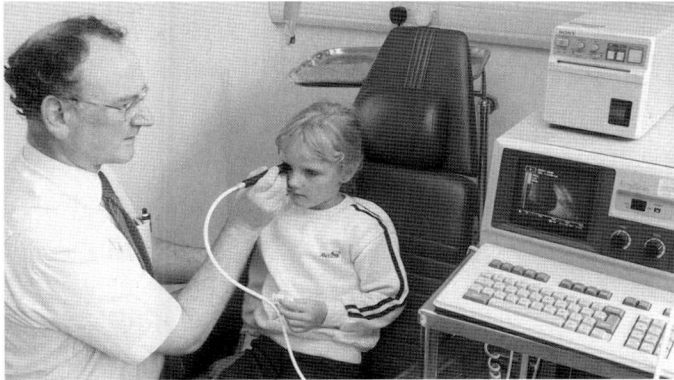

Fig. 31.16 Ocular ultrasound examination.

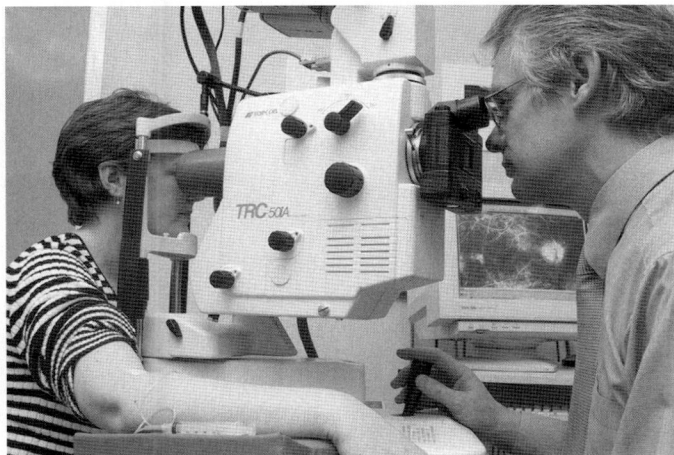

Fig. 31.17 A digital fundus camera images the retina following i.v. injection of fluorescein dye.

alternative to pattern reversal. Uniocular testing and hemifield testing may be performed. The occipital cortex response is detected using electroencephalogram (EEG) electrodes. Delayed VEP response following stimulation of one eye may indicate optic nerve demyelination on that side, while reduced amplitude may indicate reduced axonal function as in optic nerve hypoplasia (Fig. 31.20). In albinism there is increased chiasmal nerve crossing, which produces asymmetrical occipital cortex responses to uniocular stimuli.

VEPs may be used to measure visual acuity in infants. Statistical analysis of a rapid sequence ('sweep') of checker pattern sizes is used to produce an estimate of visual acuity.

The electroretinogram (ERG) gives information about retinal function. The stimulus is a flash of light. The response is detected by skin electrodes on the eyelids or by ocular contact electrodes.[10] The electrical response is generated in the retina – the 'a' wave by the photoreceptors and the 'b' wave by the inner retina. Cone function and rod function may be analyzed separately by using a range of test strategies in which the background illumination is varied and the light flash stimulation is varied. Rod responses are measured using dim flash stimuli after dark adaptation (scotopic responses). Cone responses are measured in normal lighting conditions (photopic responses) (Fig. 31.21). 30 Hz flicker stimuli are used to isolate cone responses. The individual components of

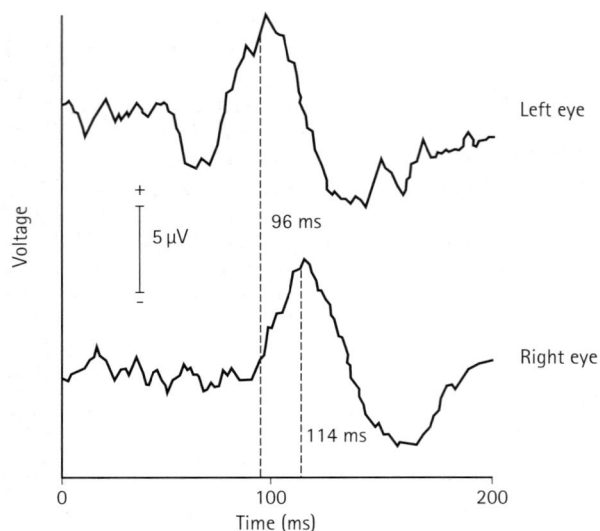

Fig. 31.20 Pattern reversal visual evoked response. The VER of two eyes where the left eye (upper trace) shows a normal pattern and there is a slight delay in the right eye (lower trace).

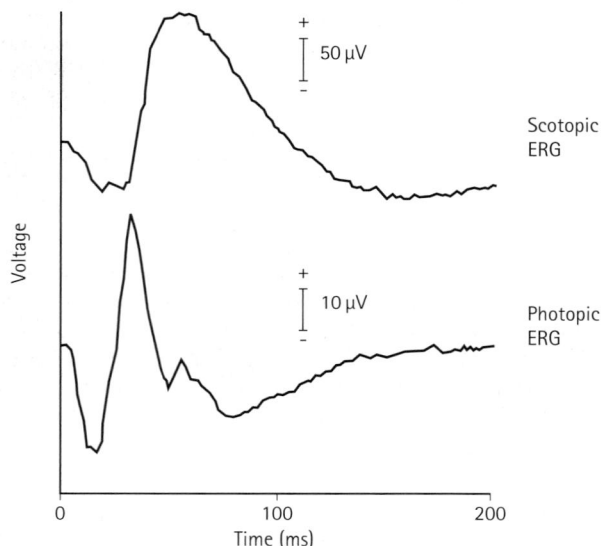

Fig. 31.21 A normal electroretinogram (ERG) showing the typical wave pattern and amplitude. The electroretinogram is taken under photopic (light adapted) conditions and scotopic (dark adapted) conditions. The wave pattern is reduced or abolished in various pathological conditions of the retina.

the ERG are best seen in the bright flash response following dark adaptation. Diseases that predominantly affect rod function produce abnormal scotopic ERG responses. Diseases that predominantly affect cone function produce abnormal photopic and 30 Hz flicker ERG responses. Diseases that predominantly affect the inner retina produce abnormal ERG b-wave responses.

REFRACTIVE ERRORS AND AMBLYOPIA

REFRACTIVE ERRORS

Refractive errors may be treated with spectacles. However the presence of a refractive error may also be of diagnostic importance. Leber's congenital amaurosis is often associated with hypermetropia,[11] and Marfan syndrome[12] with myopia.

In hypermetropia, additional accommodation is used to maintain clear focus. This may lead to excessive convergence of the eyes and is a common cause of convergent squint. In myopia, distance vision is blurred but near vision is in focus. Astigmatism causes irregular focusing due to the toric (oval) curvature of the corneal surface.

Most infants are slightly hypermetropic, which normally resolves by age 2 years – 'emmetropization'.[13] Hypermetropia present after the age of 2 years normally persists into adult life. Myopia is rare in young children. When high degrees of myopia do occur an underlying disease such as homocystinuria,[14] Marfan syndrome[12] or Stickler syndrome[15] should be considered. While refractive errors are relatively uncommon among schoolchildren in resource limited countries,[16] the incidence of myopia among schoolchildren is rapidly increasing in resource rich countries.[17,18]

AMBLYOPIA

When one eye is more hypermetropic than the other, accommodation produces a clear image in the more normal eye. However the retinal image in the more hypermetropic eye remains blurred, as accommodation amplitude is under bilateral neural drive. Untreated, occipital cortex synaptic connections related to the hypermetropic eye will remain underdeveloped.[19] This is termed 'anisometropic amblyopia'.

When a squint develops, the brain suppresses vision from the squinting eye in order to avoid diplopia. However continued suppression leads to failure of development of synaptic connections in the occipital cortex and once again the affected eye becomes amblyopic – strabismic amblyopia.[19] Anisometropic and strabismic amblyopia may coexist.[20]

The treatment of amblyopia is to first treat the underlying cause with glasses.[21] Occlusion of the normal eye is then used to drive development of synaptic connections relating to the amblyopic eye (Fig. 31.22). Atropine eyedrops may be used to blur vision in the normal eye, as an alternative to occlusion (atropine penalization).[21]

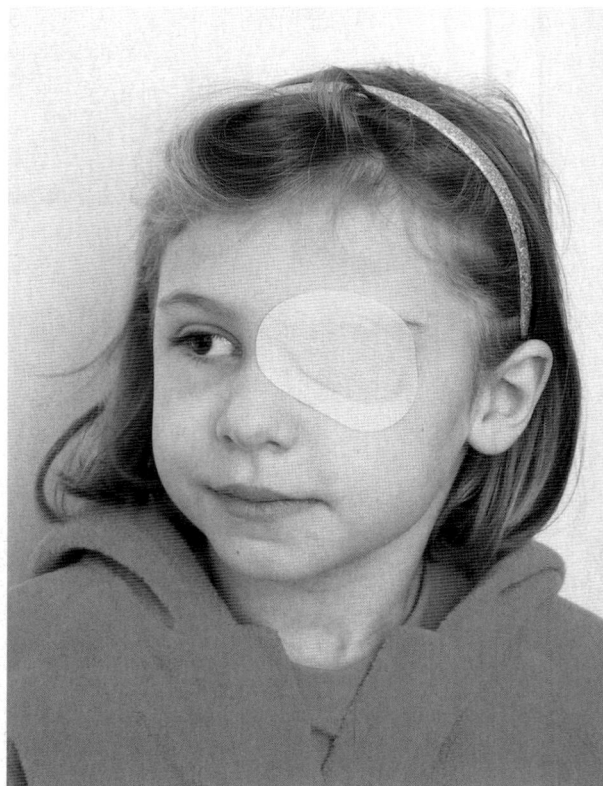

Fig. 31.22 Occlusion treatment.

Community visual screening programs are used to detect amblyopia. These are particularly necessary for the detection of anisometropic amblyopia, which is generally asymptomatic. Visual acuity measurements in each eye detect reduced vision in the amblyopic eye and lead to referral for assessment and treatment.[22] Screening may also detect small angled strabismus with amblyopia. Photographic techniques, which use pupil light reflex patterns to measure refractive errors, are an alternative approach to community screening.[23]

CEREBRAL VISUAL IMPAIRMENT

CNS disease is the most common cause of visual impairment in children.[24,25] Causes of cerebral visual impairment (CVI) in children are given in Table 31.1. A wide spectrum of severity and type of impairment may occur. Damage to the anterior visual pathways, optic radiations and occipital cortex lead to reduced visual acuity and limited visual fields. Damage to visual association areas also causes significant impairment in children, which is often under-recognized. Two key pathways associated with visual processing are the 'ventral stream' and the 'dorsal stream.'[26]

The ventral stream connects the primary visual cortex with the fusiform gyri of the inferior temporal lobes. An 'archive' of learned images is held in this area. Children with ventral stream dysfunction may have difficulty recognizing faces, shapes and objects. They may also have difficulty with orientation in familiar environments.

The dorsal stream connects the primary visual pathway with the posterior parietal lobes, and associated pathways. Dorsal stream structures subserve visual attention and visually guided motor functions. Visual attention refers to the ability to analyze complex visual scenes, concentrate on specific elements of these scenes, and suppress other elements in order to avoid distraction. Ability to suppress auditory and tactile input is an additional requirement of visual attention.

Dorsal stream structures also provide information about orientation in three-dimensional space. Connections to the motor cortex guide limb movements and connections to the frontal eye fields guide saccadic eye movements.

Timing of insult

The pattern of CVI impairment in an individual child is largely determined by the timing of the insult. Preterm infants typically sustain ischemic injury to the periventricular white matter and associated pathways (periventricular leukomalacia – PVL) following neonatal periventricular haemorrhage.[27] Symptoms emerge at about the age of 2–5 years. Reduced visual acuity, inferior visual field defects, nystagmus, and diplegia may be present. Dorsal and ventral stream impairments frequently occur. The optic discs show an enlarged physiological cup, which may be due to transsynaptic degeneration of fibers synapsing in the lateral geniculate bodies.

Damage to the visual pathways and to the dorsal and ventral streams occurs in relation to perinatal or antenatal insult in term infants. A variable combination of visual acuity, visual field and dorsal and ventral stream impairments occur. Optic atrophy may occur as a result of the primary insult or secondary to posterior visual pathway damage. Many of these infants also develop cerebral palsy.

Ischemic injury in children after infancy typically results in watershed infarcts of the cerebral cortex, especially the occipital cortex. The pupil responses are preserved. Variable degrees of optic atrophy may be present. Nystagmus is usually not present.[28] The VEP may be normal or abnormal. The visual defect may be total initially, but there is variable improvement with time, dependent on etiology and severity. Most children achieve some navigational vision. Recovery when it does occur may take from a few hours to 2 years. Full recovery has been reported after head injury and cardiac arrest, but is less likely after bacterial meningitis and does not occur in children with neurodegenerative disorders.

Ocular motor defects and CVI

Impaired eye movement control causes further visual difficulties for children with CVI. Strabismus, nystagmus, dystonic movements, impaired pursuit movements and impaired saccadic movement control may occur. In addition poor control of accommodation may lead to significant blurring of vision, especially for near tasks. Spectacles to correct hypermetropia and accommodation deficits are often helpful.[29]

Coping strategies for children with CVI

Educational approaches to help children with visual impairment are given in the section entitled 'Education of visually impaired children'. Symptoms due to inferior visual field loss may be aided by using a tilted work board so that the child may look directly at written material rather than looking down. An awareness of reduced visual field to one side will ensure that parents and teachers introduce objects of interest (including themselves) in seeing areas.

Dutton has developed behavioral strategies to reduce the impact of dorsal and ventral stream impairments, and these are given in Table 31.2.[26]

Table 31.1 Causes of cerebral visual impairment

Prenatal	Brain malformations
	Intrauterine infections
	Placental dysfunction
Preterm neonatal	Preterm neonatal periventricular haemorrhage
Perinatal	Neonatal asphyxia
	Intracerebral hemorrhage
	Meningitis
	Encephalitis
Postnatal	Trauma (accidental and non-accidental)
	Cardiac arrest
	Meningitis
	Encephalitis
	Neurodegenerative disorders

Table 31.2 Cerebral visual impairment – ventral stream and dorsal stream defects and suggested coping strategies (modified from Dutton et al.[26])

Defects	Suggested coping strategies
Ventral stream	
Impaired recognition of familiar faces	Verbal introduction; wear color/shape identifiers
Impaired orientation in familiar environment	Orientation training using cues and pathway markers
Dorsal stream	
Confused by complex ('busy') visual scenes	Store toys separately
	Store clothes separately (in transparent containers)
	Use plain carpets, bed covers and wall decoration
Difficulty identifying an individual in a group	Wave and speak
Disorientation in crowded environment	Train to use landmarks
	Visit shops when they are quiet
Reading	Mask surrounding text
Visually guide movements – upper limbs	Occupational therapy training strategies for reaching
Visually guide movements – lower limbs	Use tactile guide to height of ground – push a toy pram or bicycle, hold elbow or clothing of accompanying person
Distraction, leading to frustration at school and home	Limit visual and auditory 'clutter' in order to enhance concentration
Lose visual attention and bump or trip when talking or listening while walking	Keep quiet while walking

STRABISMUS

TERMINOLOGY

The term 'strabismus' and 'squint' are used interchangeably. 'Strabismus' is preferred. The prefix 'eso' is used for convergent deviations, and 'exo' for divergent deviations. 'Hyper' refers to upward deviation of an eye and 'hypo' to downward deviation. A 'tropia' is a manifest strabismus, which is present in binocular viewing conditions and is detected using the cover test. A 'phoria' is a latent strabismus, which is only apparent when binocular viewing is disrupted. The word 'deviation' is used to include both tropias and phorias. In 'concomitant' strabismus the deviation angle is the same in all directions of gaze. In 'incomitant' strabismus the deviation angle may be greater in one direction of gaze – for example in the direction of action of a paretic muscle. Adduction refers to medial movement of one eye, towards the nose, and abduction to lateral movement of one eye. 'Primary position' refers to the straight-ahead viewing position.

'Pseudosquint' refers to the appearance of apparent esotropia due to wide epicanthic skin folds. No true ocular deviation is present when a cover test is performed.

There are three common types of concomitant strabismus in childhood.

INFANTILE ESOTROPIA

This type of convergent strabismus becomes apparent at age 3–4 months (Fig. 31.23). Infants who have developmental neurological problems are at increased risk of developing infantile esotropia. The typical characteristics of infantile esotropia are a large angled convergent strabismus, which alternates between the eyes. There is no amblyopia as each eye is alternately used. There is no significant refractive error in most cases. Hypermetropia is present in some cases. The lateral recti may appear to be weak, as the infant habitually tends to use the right eye to look to the left side and vice versa ('cross fixation'). This may lead to the suspicion of bilateral VI cranial nerve weakness. Occlusion of one or other eye for 20–30 min will usually reveal normal abduction of the uncovered eye rather than VI palsy.

A characteristic type of nystagmus may be present, termed 'manifest latent nystagmus'. In this form of nystagmus, the nystagmus is exaggerated by covering one eye. The uncovered eye develops a jerking nystagmus with the jerk towards the side of the fixing eye.

When present, hypermetropia should be treated with spectacles.[30] Very early surgery, performed during infancy, improves binocular function outcome.[31]

ACQUIRED ESOTROPIA

Children who are hypermetropic habitually use extra accommodation in order to maintain clear focus. As accommodation and convergence reflexes are linked, this may lead to excessive convergence. Loss of control of convergence will lead to a convergent strabismus. The treatment is to promptly provide full spectacle correction.[32] This may reverse the condition. However if the strabismus does not fully reverse, occlusion treatment for amblyopia and surgical treatment may be needed. The use of preoperative prism spectacles improves the accuracy of surgical outcome.[33]

A late onset acquired esotropia may be mistakenly diagnosed as an acute VI nerve palsy. Patients with acute onset of esotropia should be assessed by an ophthalmologist as this may lead to prompt curative spectacle treatment rather than to a series of neurological investigations. Conversely concomitant convergent strabismus may be a presenting feature of VI nerve weakness due to a brainstem glioma, raised intracranial pressure or other pathology. A high index of suspicion for underlying neurological disease must therefore be maintained.

INTERMITTENT EXOTROPIA

The third common cause of strabismus in children is intermittent exotropia. In this condition binocular control is maintained at times but at other times one eye deviates laterally. The child may close the deviating eye in order to concentrate when using the straight eye. Vision is normal in each eye. Usually there is no significant refractive error and no treatment is needed unless the child is significantly symptomatic, in which case surgical correction may be undertaken.[34]

CONVERGENCE WEAKNESS

Weakness of convergence is usually an isolated abnormality, and can be treated with orthoptic convergence exercises.

STRABISMUS AS A SIGN OF UNDERLYING ORGANIC DISEASE

All cases of strabismus should be promptly assessed as both convergent and divergent strabismus may be a presenting feature of underlying neurological disease (Table 31.3). Mild VI cranial nerve weakness can cause apparently concomitant strabismus.

INCOMITANT STRABISMUS

Weak lateral rectus function is the most common cause of incomitant strabismus. VI cranial nerve weakness should be considered in all cases (Table 31.4).

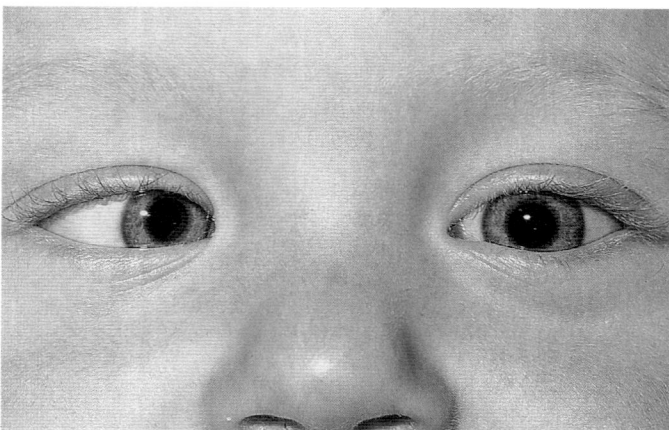

Fig. 31.23 Infantile esotropia. The right eye was converging when the photograph was taken.

Table 31.3 Conditions that may present with (apparent) concomitant strabismus

Retinoblastoma
Optic nerve hypoplasia
Optic atrophy:
Primary
Secondary to neoplasm
Unilateral cataract
Persistent fetal vasculature
VI cranial nerve weakness

Table 31.4 Causes of true or apparent VI nerve weakness in children

VI cranial nerve paresis:
Raised intracranial pressure
Brainstem glioma
Moebius syndrome
Duane's syndrome
Esotropia (abduction is usually normal)

Incomitant strabismus syndromes

Duane syndrome

In Duane syndrome VI cranial nerve innervation of the lateral rectus muscle is variably defective, and an anomalous branch of the III cranial nerve supplies the lateral rectus muscle. On attempted abduction there is variable lateral rectus weakness, which may be mistaken for VI cranial nerve palsy caused by acquired neurological disease. On attempted adduction of the eye the medial rectus and lateral rectus muscle co-contract and the eye retracts into the orbit, with narrowing of the palpebral aperture. A number of associated neurological deficits, including partial sensorineural deafness, are associated with Duane syndrome.

Surgical treatment is reserved for those children who develop a significant compensatory head turn (towards the side of the affected eye), or strabismus in primary position.[35]

Moebius syndrome

Moebius syndrome consists of congenital absence of cranial nerve nuclei, including the VI and VII nerve nuclei. Abduction is absent in each eye, and there is bilateral facial palsy.

Brown syndrome

In Brown syndrome there is a congenital anomaly of superior oblique tendon and trochlea function. When the affected eye is adducted it shoots downwards. The condition is usually treated conservatively as some spontaneous recovery may occur. In severe cases superior oblique tendon surgery may be performed.

Congenital superior oblique tendon laxity

Weakness of superior oblique function in children (and adults) is more commonly caused by congenital laxity of the superior oblique tendon than by IV cranial nerve paresis. Typically there is a compensatory head tilt to the opposite side. This may be mistaken for sternomastoid muscle induced torticollis. Eye movement examination reveals weakness of the affected superior oblique, with secondary overaction of inferior oblique function. Surgery may be performed if there is a significant compensatory head posture, or strabismus in primary position. The lax tendon may be tucked, or the overactive inferior oblique muscle may be weakened by recession surgery.

PUPIL ABNORMALITIES

Children presenting with unequal pupil size (anisocoria) tend to cause great concern to both the parents/carers and clinicians. In practice, intracranial pathology is uncommon. The most common cause is physiological anisocoria; other causes include III nerve palsy, Horner syndrome, previous blunt trauma or dilating eye drops.

The examination should be directed at determining the presence or absence of ptosis, eye movement abnormalities such as III palsy and other cranial and peripheral nerve palsies. In physiological anisocoria, the difference in pupil size is proportionately the same in bright or dim lighting.

III (OCULOMOTOR) PALSY

There is usually a marked or complete ptosis and restriction of eye movements. The eye is typically turned down and outwards. The pupil on the affected side may be enlarged. Causes include congenital (usually idiopathic), head injury, and tumors. Prompt neuroimaging is indicated in acquired cases.

HORNER SYNDROME

Horner syndrome is caused by reduced sympathetic nerve supply to the eye and comprises a partial ptosis with a small (miosed) pupil. Most cases in children are congenital. Acquired cases require prompt investigation for possible abdominal neuroblastoma. In Horner syndrome, the anisocoria is more pronounced in dim light due to failure of the affected pupil to dilate.

NYSTAGMUS

CONGENITAL IDIOPATHIC NYSTAGMUS

In congenital idiopathic nystagmus the onset of nystagmus occurs between the ages of 2 and 3 months. Some cases are familial – dominant, recessive and X-linked inheritance has been described. An underlying vision defect should be excluded. Typically the nystagmus is horizontal and the amplitude is greater on looking to one side and less on looking to the other side (null zone). Head nodding may be present. Ocular examination is otherwise normal and there are no neurological abnormalities. The ERG and VEPs are normal. On follow up, near vision develops to a relatively normal level. There is moderate reduction of distance vision and some modification of the classroom environment is often helpful. Treatment consists of spectacle correction of refractive errors. Surgical treatment may produce some benefit in selected cases,[36] and medical treatment with gabapentin is currently under investigation.[37]

SENSORY DEFECT NYSTAGMUS

Infants with congenital nystagmus may have an underlying vision defect. In most cases an ocular abnormality is present and a systematic approach to ocular and electrophysiological examination is required. A differential diagnosis is given in Table 31.5. In general, posterior visual pathway defects do not result in nystagmus.[28] Periventricular leukomalacia is an exception to this rule.[27]

ALBINISM

Albinism refers to a group of conditions that may be divided into oculocutaneous albinism (OCA) and ocular albinism (OA). The ocular abnormalities found are common to all forms of albinism. In addition to defective iris and fundus pigmentation, abnormalities include: reduced vision and photophobia; nystagmus; strabismus; delayed visual maturation; foveal hypoplasia and abnormal chiasmal crossing. More than 90% of fibers cross at the chiasm, resulting in cortical asymmetry of VEP responses. Iris translucency varies in severity and relatively minor defects of iris pigmentation may only be detected by slit lamp transillumination performed in a dark room. Most forms of OCA are autosomal recessive. Two rare forms of OCA are associated with systemic disease – increased susceptibility to infection in Chediak–Higashi disease[38] and frequent bruising due to platelet dysfunction in Hermansky–Pudlak syndrome.[39]

In ocular albinism typical ocular abnormalities are present, but skin and hair color are normal.

Refractive errors should be corrected with spectacles, and photophobia reduced with tinted spectacles and peaked hats. Mainstream education, with some attention to the classroom environment, and normal educational attainment may be anticipated in almost all cases.

ANIRIDIA

Aniridia is an autosomal dominant condition caused by mutations in the PAX 6 homeobox gene. About 30% of cases are sporadic, with deletions at 11p13. Sporadic cases have a high incidence of associated abnormalities, including Wilms tumor,[40] genitourinary abnormalities and mental retardation. Abdominal palpation and/or abdominal ultrasound examination should be performed in all new cases and as part of follow up.

Table 31.5 Causes of sensory congenital nystagmus

Albinism
Leber's amaurosis
Aniridia
Optic nerve hypoplasia
Retinal cone dystrophy

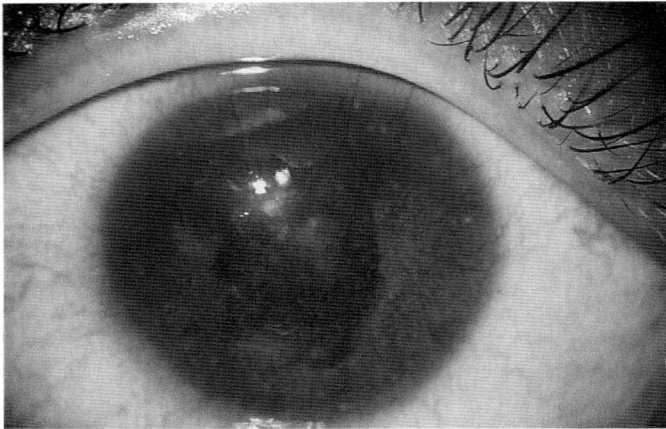

Fig. 31.24 Aniridia. No iris tissue is seen. There is fibrovascular pannus covering the peripheral cornea in this case.

Aniridia represents a defect of neural crest cell development. In addition to the striking absence of iris tissue, with only very rudimentary stubs of iris tissue present, the following ocular abnormalities are frequently seen: nystagmus, fibrovascular corneal pannus, refractive errors, glaucoma, cataract, foveal hypoplasia and optic nerve hypoplasia (Fig. 31.24). Foveal hypoplasia refers to poorly differentiated foveal structures; in extreme cases major retinal blood vessels may cross the normally avascular fovea. Corneal disease is due to defective limbal stem cell function, and responds to stem cell transplant surgery. Glaucoma surgery outcomes are limited by conjunctival scarring. Cataract surgery is also complicated, because of absent iris tissue and weak lens zonules. Progressive loss of vision over decades is usual in aniridia patients.

ACQUIRED NYSTAGMUS

Acquired nystagmus in childhood always requires prompt ophthalmic and neurological assessment. A differential diagnosis is given in Table 31.6. Vertical nystagmus may consist of downbeat nystagmus, associated with craniocervical junction abnormalities, or more rarely upbeat nystagmus, associated with brainstem and cerebellar lesions. Urgent neurological investigation, including brain imaging, is required in all cases of acquired nystagmus.

SPASMUS NUTANS

Spasmus nutans is a syndrome of infancy with nystagmus, head nodding and torticollis. Investigation to exclude an intracranial tumor is required. The syndrome resolves after 12–18 months and the diagnosis is one of exclusion, made retrospectively.

THE APPARENTLY BLIND INFANT

A carer's concern for an infant's vision is usually reliable. Infants with poor visual behavior require urgent assessment by an ophthalmologist. Treatable disease such as cataract must be dealt with promptly in order to avoid the development of irreversible amblyopia. In most cases the

Table 31.6 Causes of acquired nystagmus in children

Suprasellar tumor
Posterior fossa tumor or malformation
Neurodegenerative diseases such as:
Batten's disease
Neurolipososes
Peroxisomal disorders

Table 31.7 Ocular defects that may cause bilateral congenital blindness

Whole globe	Anophthalmos Microphthalmos
Cornea	Sclerocornea Peter's anomaly
Lens	Cataract
Retina	Retinal detachment (e.g. following retinopathy of prematurity) Retinal dysplasia (e.g. Norrie's disease) Chorioretinal coloboma Chorioretinitis scarring Cherry red spot in storage diseases (e.g. Tay–Sachs disease)

Optic atrophy	Prenatal:
	  Infection
	  Asphyxia
	  Cerebral malformations
	Perinatal:
	  Asphyxia
	Postnatal:
	Meningitis/encephalitis
	  Compression (e.g. hydrocephalus, craniopharyngioma)
	  Genetic (e.g. autosomal dominant optic atrophy)
	Secondry to retinal disease

Optic nerve hypoplasia	
Optic disc colobomas	

Table 31.8 The blind infant with apparently normal eyes

Delayed visual maturation
Cerebral visual impairment
Leber's congenital amaurosis
Retinal cone dystrophy
Optic nerve hypoplasia
Oculomotor praxia

cause is apparent following ophthalmic examination. Ocular defects that may cause bilateral congenital blindness are given in Table 31.7.

In some cases there may be no ocular abnormality evident, or only very subtle defects are found (Table 31.8). In these cases electrophysiological and neurological investigations may be required.

DELAYED VISUAL MATURATION

Delayed visual maturation (DVM) refers to visual unresponsiveness from birth that subsequently improves.[41] The diagnosis is one of exclusion and is always retrospective. The onset of visually stimulated smiling is delayed; clinical pupil responses are normal and there is no nystagmus.

LEBER'S CONGENITAL AMAUROSIS

Leber's congenital amaurosis (LCA, isolated infantile rod–cone dystrophy) is an autosomal recessive congenital retinal dystrophy.[42] Vision is absent or severely reduced from birth and the ERG is markedly reduced or absent. The pupils may show a sluggish afferent response. Refraction usually shows significant hypermetropia. The fundus appearances are normal or near normal. The term 'Leber's congenital amaurosis' should be reserved for cases of isolated infantile rod–cone dystrophy, and the diagnosis of Leber's congenital amaurosis should only be made after

Table 31.9 Syndromes associated with infantile rod–cone dystrophy

Cerebellar vermis hypoplasia, e.g. Joubert's syndrome
Deafness, e.g. Usher's syndrome type 1
Renal disease, e.g. nephronophthisis
Skeletal abnormalities
Peroxisomal disorders, e.g. Zellweger syndrome
Mitochondrial cytopathies, e.g. hydroxyacyl-CoA
   dehydrogenase deficiency
Amino acid disorders, e.g. methylmalonic aciduria

exclusion of other recognized syndromes (Table 31.9). Hearing, neurological, renal and metabolic abnormalities should be sought.

While no active treatment for LCA is possible at present, gene therapy trials are under development.[43] Genetic counseling and molecular diagnosis are therefore required.

OPTIC NERVE HYPOPLASIA

Optic nerve hypoplasia (ONH) is not inherited, and most cases are idiopathic. Insults in early embryonic development have been associated with ONH – maternal diabetes, maternal alcohol and other substance abuse. ONH may occur in isolation or in association with failure of development of the anterior midline structures of the brain (septo-optic dysplasia [SOD]), hydranencephaly, porencephaly, cerebral atrophy or leukomalacia. ONH also occurs in aniridia. A genetic basis has been identified in a small number of cases of SOD.[44] Severe bilateral cases are associated with neuroendocrine dysfunction. Hypoglycemia may occur in the neonatal period. Sudden infant death may occur as a result of an abnormal stress response to febrile illness. All cases should be referred for endocrine investigation. In addition to abnormal cortisol response, growth, thyroid and gonadotrophic hormones may be defective. Magnetic resonance imaging (MRI) is useful as a predictor of neuroendocrine dysfunction and allows assessment of optic nerve size.

There is a spectrum of severity ranging from complete blindness with very tiny optic nerve structures to virtually normal vision with very minor degrees of ONH. Cases may be unilateral, bilateral or asymmetric.

Mild cases present later in childhood. The optic disc appearances vary (Fig. 31.25) and include:

- variably small optic disc;
- peripapillary pigmented ring (double ring sign);
- slightly tortuous retinal vessels;
- associated optic atrophy;
- segmental disc hypoplasia.

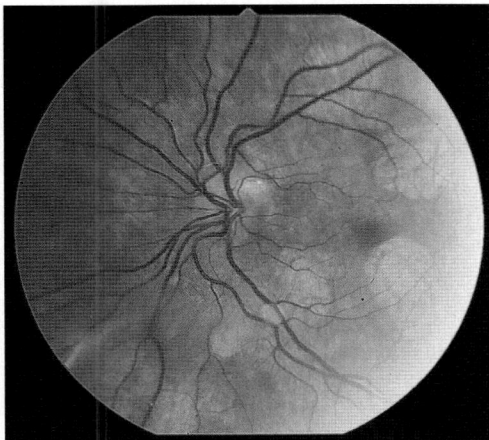

Fig. 31.25 Hypoplastic disc. Optic nerve hypoplasia. The optic disc is anatomically very small in this case, with severely reduced vision.

Mild cases present with reduced vision in one or both eyes, or with strabismus. Mild degrees of optic nerve hypoplasia may be misdiagnosed as amblyopia, and cases of amblyopia that do not respond well to occlusion treatment should always be carefully examined for the presence of subtle optic nerve hypoplasia.

OCULOMOTOR APRAXIA

Absent saccadic eye movements may be mistakenly interpreted as defective visual function. The ERG is reduced in some cases,[45] further increasing the possibility of misdiagnosing Leber's congenital amaurosis. Once the child is able to support and move their head, characteristic side-to-side head thrusting movements develop. These head movements are used as a substitute for voluntary saccadic eye movements.

ACQUIRED VISUAL LOSS IN CHILDREN

Acquired visual loss at any age requires urgent investigation. Uniocular visual loss may result in the development of strabismus. Binocular visual loss will lead to impaired visual behavior and, in older children, a complaint of reduced vision. In most cases, acquired visual loss is due to retinal, optic nerve or neurological disease (Table 31.10). When the cause is not evident on ophthalmic examination, neurological, electrophysiological, and neuro-imaging assessment will be needed.

CATARACT

Bilateral cataract developing in later childhood is rare. Metabolic disorders such as diabetes mellitus and disorders of galactose metabolism should be excluded.[46]

RETINAL DYSTROPHIES

This term refers to genetic abnormalities of the retina or retinal pigment epithelium that lead to reduced retinal function. Rod dysfunction presents with reduced vision, especially in dim lighting conditions. Cone dysfunction presents with reduced vision, photophobia, and reduced color vision. Fundus examination may show pigmentary disturbance. When the rods are predominantly affected, black spiky

Table 31.10 Causes of visual loss in children evident on ophthalmic examination.

Cataract	Metabolic disease		
Retina	Retinal dystrophies	Rod–cone dystrophies X-linked juvenile retinoschisis Stargardt's disease	
Optic atrophy	External compression	Hydrocephalus	
		Tumor	Craniopharyngioma Other suprasellar tumors
	Intrinsic tumor	Glioma	Neurofibromatosis type 1
	Retinal diseases		
	Genetic	Autosomal dominant optic atrophy	
	Demyelinating diseases		

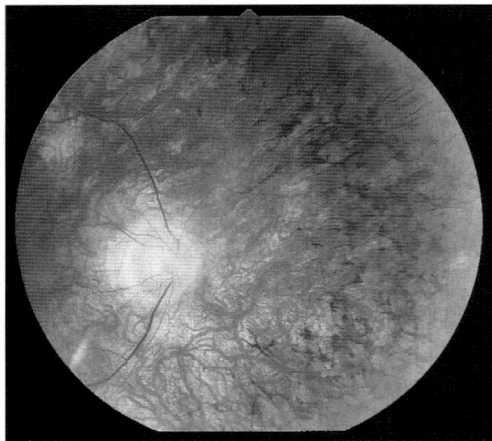

Fig. 31.26   Retinitis pigmentosa. Typical 'bone spicule' pigmentation is seen in the mid-periphery of the fundus.

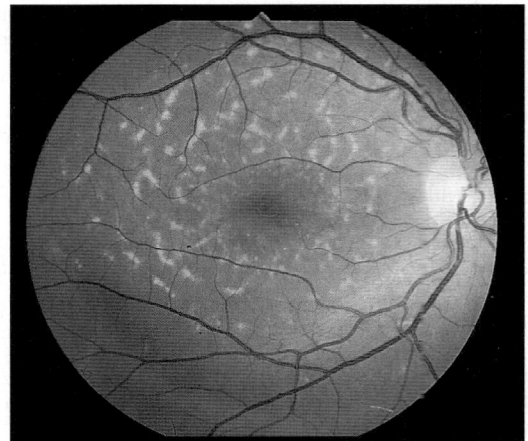

Fig. 31.28   Stargardt disease. Typical creamy fishtail-shaped flecks are seen in the fundus. There are no macular pigment changes in this case.

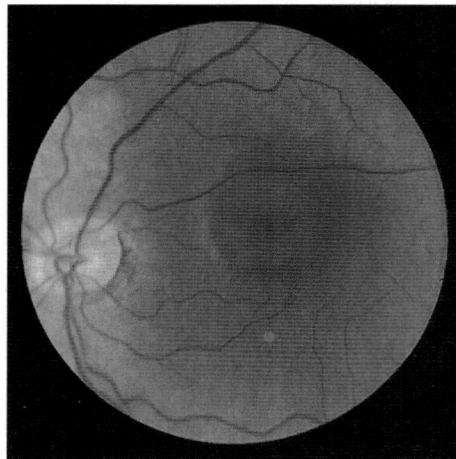

Fig. 31.27   Retinal cone dystrophy with typical 'bull's eye' pigmentation at the center of the macula.

blotches of pigment are seen in the retinal periphery (bone spicule pigmentation) (Fig. 31.26). This appearance leads to the historical term 'retinitis pigmentosa'. When the cones are affected pigmentation may be present at the macula, often in a ring shape (bull's eye) (Fig. 31.27). The diagnosis is made on clinical grounds, supported by electroretinogram abnormalities of rod and cone functions.

Most types of retinal dystrophy are currently not treatable. Two rare forms of rod-cone dystrophy of childhood are amenable to treatment. In Refsum disease serum phytanic acid levels are raised. Dietary intervention will improve the prognosis for vision and also reduce morbidity due to other systemic features of the disease. In abetalipoproteinemia, vitamin and dietary treatment improve the prognosis.

STARGARDT DISEASE

Stargardt disease is an autosomal recessive disease with onset in late childhood. Symptoms are limited to reduced visual acuity, with no symptoms of night blindness or of photophobia. Typically there are creamy fishtail-shaped flecks in the retina (fundus flavimaculatus) with additional retinal pigment epithelium atrophy at the macula (Fig. 31.28). The disease progresses until visual acuity is reduced to about 6/60.[47]

AUTOSOMAL DOMINANT OPTIC ATROPHY

The finding of reduced vision and optic atrophy should lead to prompt neurological and neuroimaging investigations. In autosomal dominant optic atrophy neurological investigations are normal. The condition is associated with defects in the OPA1 gene.[48] There is reduced visual acuity, some reduction of color vision, reduced visual field sensitivity between fixation and the blind spot ('centrocaecal scotoma'), reduced amplitude pattern VEP, and variable pallor of the temporal part of the optic disc. Visual loss is not severe, and progression is very slow.

CHILDHOOD VISUAL LOSS WITH NO ABNORMALITY ON OPHTHALMIC EXAMINATION

BATTEN DISEASE (JUVENILE NEURONAL CEROID LIPOFUSCINOSIS)

The neuronal ceroid lipofuscinoses (NCLs) are a group of autosomal recessive neurodegenerative lysosomal storage diseases. While classification by age of disease onset has been helpful in the past, more precise molecular genetic diagnosis is now possible.[49] The majority of cases of juvenile NCL have a mutation in the CLN3 gene. These cases may present with visual loss.[50] Neurological degenerative symptoms may not develop for up to 3 years later. The diagnosis must therefore be considered in any child aged 4–10 years with visual loss that cannot be explained on ophthalmic examination. The fundi may initially appear normal. The ERG is reduced, and typically shows an electronegative waveform. Later a pigmentary disturbance develops at the macula. The disease is progressive, with epileptic seizures and dementia. No treatment is currently available.

FUNCTIONAL VISUAL LOSS

A relatively common cause of apparent reduction of vision in young teenagers is 'functional' visual loss. Symptoms are precipitated by stress. Typically the child complains of blurred vision. On examination there are no objective abnormalities. The diagnosis can be made if the child is 'tricked' into giving normal visual acuity test results by using neutralizing combinations of spectacle lenses or other means. Having made the diagnosis, psychological counseling may be helpful. Underlying problems at school or in the home may be detected. The prognosis is usually good, as the underlying psychological disturbance tends to be relatively minor. When a positive diagnosis cannot be made, follow up and investigations to exclude other causes of visual loss are necessary.

DISEASES OF ORBITAL AND OCULAR TISSUES

ORBITAL DISEASE

Congenital abnormalities of skull development

A number of craniosynostoses have ocular features. Crouzon, Apert and Pfeiffer syndromes result in shallow orbits, which can lead to corneal exposure. Hydrocephalus is common in these conditions and regular optic disc examination is required. Visual loss may also occur because of amblyopia secondary to refractive errors and strabismus.[51] Complex horizontal and vertical strabismus patterns are frequently present. Strabismus surgery may be considered after corrective skull surgery has been performed.

Symptoms and signs of orbital disease

Symptoms of orbital disease include reduced vision, diplopia and altered appearance. Signs include proptosis, which may be axial (forward protrusion of the eye in the axis of the orbit) or non-axial. The pattern of non-axial proptosis gives useful clues to the site of orbital disease. For instance, if the eye is deviated laterally, it is likely that the site of orbital disease will be medial. Eye movements may be reduced. Visual acuity may be reduced and there may be sensory abnormalities of pupil reactions.

Preseptal cellulites

Preseptal cellulitis refers to eyelid cellulitis that does not extend beyond the orbital septum into the orbit. The eye appears normal and vision remains normal. While the infection may be related to local skin infection or local skin trauma, this form of cellulitis is commonly secondary to sinus infection with *Haemophilus influenzae* or *Streptococcus aureus* and is part of the spectrum of orbital cellulitis.[52] An orbital computerized tomography (CT) scan may be indicated when severe eyelid swelling prevents adequate eye examination. Treatment is with i.v. antibiotics.

Orbital cellulitis

True orbital cellulitis is much less common than preseptal cellulitis. The orbit becomes inflamed with proptosis of the eye, reduced eye movement and reduced vision. Prompt and effective treatment must be instituted as orbital cellulitis may lead to orbital or even brain abscess. Most cases are secondary to ethmoidal sinusitis. Since the advent of *H. influenzae* vaccination, streptococci sp. have become the most common organisms responsible.[53] Blood cultures should be performed and an orbital CT scan should be performed. Treatment is with broad-spectrum i.v. antibiotics covering Gram positive, Gram negative and anaerobic organisms. Visual acuity should be monitored regularly. An otolaryngologist should be involved in all cases as urgent sinus drainage may be needed in order to protect vision.[54]

Orbital tumors

Capillary hemangioma, venous-lymphatic malformations and dermoid cysts are the most common orbital masses in infants and children under the age of 2 years.

Capillary hemangiomas grow rapidly during the first 6 months of life, stabilize, and then regress at age 3–8 years. Superficial lesions are a typical 'strawberry' color (Fig. 31.29); deeper lesions have a bluish appearance. The diagnosis may be made clinically, and CT or MRI scans may be used to delineate the extent of the lesion. Visual loss is usually related to amblyopia,[55] but can be due to optic nerve compression or corneal exposure. Amblyopia may be due to occlusion of the pupil, or astigmatism in the axis of the lesion. Treatment is conservative when there is no threat of amblyopia. However lesions that occlude the pupil or cause significant astigmatism may require early intervention to prevent amblyopia. Intralesional depot steroids or even systemic steroids may be used.[55] Surgery is normally deferred until maximal spontaneous regression has occurred at about age 8 years.

Venous-lymphatic malformations present with proptosis in childhood, which may be abrupt if bleeding occurs into a cystic space. While the

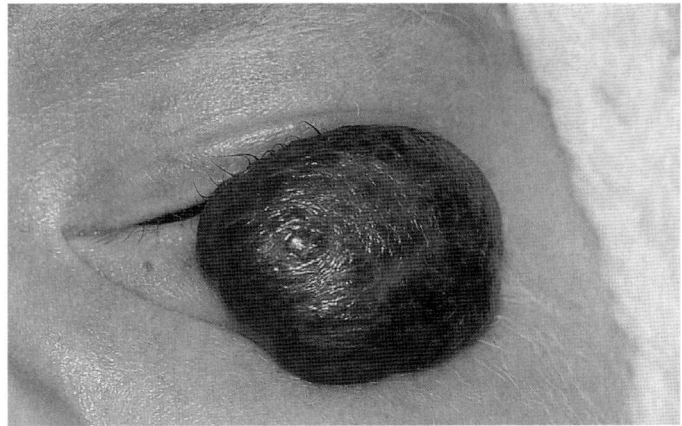

Fig. 31.29 Capillary hemangioma of the lower eyelid.

lesions consist of venous-like vascular channels they are not directly connected to the venous system.[56] They may be delineated by CT or MRI scan. Unlike capillary hemangiomas they do not regress with age. Surgical intervention is unsatisfactory and most lesions are best treated conservatively.

Dermoid cysts may be superficial or deep. Superficial lesions are most often found at the upper outer angle of the orbit. Having excluded a deeper component of the lesion by clinical examination, ultrasound examination, MRI or CT scan, excision may be performed. Deeper lesions tend to present with proptosis, at a later age. Conservative treatment is often appropriate.[57]

Rhabdomyosarcoma is the commonest malignant orbital tumor of childhood and usually develops between the ages of 4 and 12 years. The tumor enlarges rapidly with increasing proptosis, mild redness and edema of the eyelids and reduced eye movements.[58] The diagnosis is made by biopsy, and as much tissue as possible should be removed for examination. A direct approach to the lesion should be performed, as tumor seeding may occur in the biopsy track. Depending on clinical stage, chemotherapy with or without radiotherapy is the initial treatment. Orbital exenteration may be needed if primary treatment fails.

EYELID ABNORMALITIES

Epiblepharon refers to the presence of a fold of skin near the lower eyelid margin, which may cause inturning eyelashes (Fig. 31.30), most commonly affecting oriental infants. The natural history is spontaneous resolution during the first 1–2 years of life and surgery is reserved for severe cases.

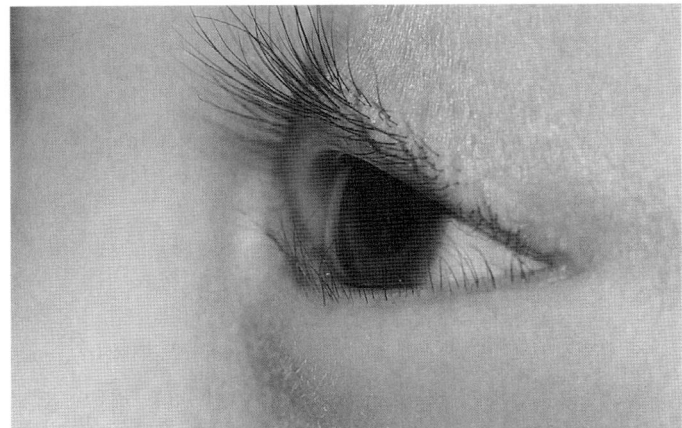

Fig. 31.30 Epiblepharon.

Blepharitis refers to inflammation of the eyelid margins. This is a relatively common condition in older children and in adults. Hot bathing and eyelid margin toilet using cotton tipped buds may be effective. When secondary staphylococcal infection is present, treatment with topical fucidic acid cream is indicated. In a small number of cases corneal inflammation with vascularization and scarring may develop, and topical steroid therapy may be needed to control this process.

A *tarsal cyst* is a retention cyst of an oil-producing meibomian gland of an eyelid. These cysts resolve spontaneously over a period of months. Surgical drainage is indicated in the minority of cases in which significant eye discomfort is present.

CONGENITAL PTOSIS

Dystrophic changes of the levator muscle of one or both upper eyelids will result in drooping of the upper eyelid, termed 'ptosis' (Fig. 31.31). Congenital III nerve palsy and Horner syndrome should be excluded. Congenital Horner syndrome is associated with neuroblastoma.[59] The jaw winking (Marcus Gunn) phenomenon should be sought – lateral movements of the jaw produce synkinetic movements of the ipsilateral upper eyelid.

If the pupil is occluded by ptosis, prompt surgery is indicated in order to prevent amblyopia. However in milder cases corrective surgery is best deferred until teenage years, when cooperation with surgery under local anesthetic may be obtained, leading to a better cosmetic result. Surgery generally involves advancement or resection of the levator aponeurosis.

LACRIMAL SYSTEM

CONGENITAL NASOLACRIMAL DUCT OBSTRUCTION

The nasolacrimal duct commonly has a persistent membranous occlusion at the distal end of the duct. This leads to watering (epiphora) of the affected eye or eyes. Epiphora is almost always first noticed during the first month of life. The fluorescein dye disappearance test is useful in diagnosis. A drop of fluorescein dye is placed in the conjunctival sac and the time taken for dye to clear is observed. Delayed drainage implies that the nasolacrimal duct is not patent. The natural history is spontaneous resolution of watering during the first 1–2 years of life. If watering persists beyond the age of 2 years, probing of the nasolacrimal duct may be undertaken.[60] While waiting for spontaneous resolution, the eyes should be bathed if they become sticky. Topical antibiotics need only be used if signs of active tissue inflammation are present.

LACRIMAL OBSTRUCTION IN OLDER CHILDREN

In some children, epiphora persists despite probing. In these cases intranasal anatomical abnormalities may be found.[61] Endoscopic exploration, with silicone intubation of the lacrimal system, is effective in 80% of cases.[62] Where severe anatomical occlusion of the nasolacrimal duct is present, dacryocystorhinostomy surgery may be required. However epiphora in older children is more often due to allergy or upper respiratory tract infection than to nasolacrimal duct occlusion.[63]

CONGENITAL ABNORMALITIES OF EYE DEVELOPMENT

The whole eye may be absent at birth (anophthalmos) (Fig. 31.32) or may be small (microphthalmos).

Orbital growth is partly stimulated by the volume effect of the eye. Orbital growth is reduced if an eye is removed during early childhood. Hydrophilic tissue expanders are therefore used to enhance orbital growth in cases of anophthalmos or severe microphthalmos.

Microphthalmos is commonly associated with coloboma due to embryonic optic fissure closure defects. Typically the inferior part of the iris is absent along with the inferior choroid and retina (Fig. 31.33). The optic disc may or may not be involved. Microphthalmos and coloboma may be isolated abnormalities, associated with chromosomal syndromes such as trisomy 13, or associated with a single gene defect such as choanal atresia with ear, eye, heart and genital defects (CHARGE) syndrome.[64]

CONJUNCTIVITIS

Neonatal conjunctivitis has been discussed in Chapter 12. Bacterial infection, viral infection, chlamydial infection and allergy may cause conjunctivitis in older infants and in children.

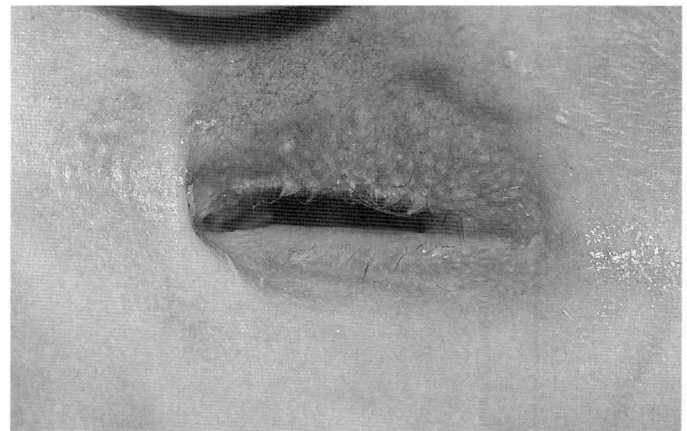

Fig. 31.32 Anophthalmos. No identifiable ocular structures are apparent.

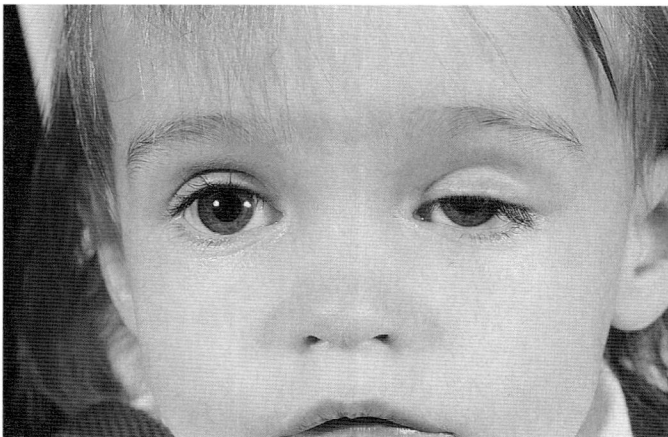

Fig. 31.31 Congenital ptosis of the left upper eyelid due to levator muscle dystrophy.

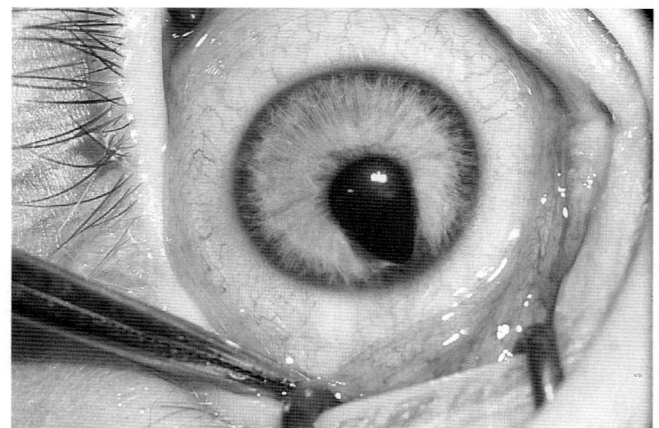

Fig. 31.33 Coloboma of the inferior iris.

Bacterial conjunctivitis produces a purulent discharge and is generally self-limiting – topical antibiotics are generally not indicated.[65] Viral conjunctivitis produces a watery discharge with a mucous component and is generally self-limiting. Chlamydial neonatal infection has been discussed in Chapter 12. In hot, dry countries with limited water supplies flies cause endemic chlamydial conjunctivitis – trachoma. Conjunctival scarring leads to dry eyes and eyelid scarring. Secondary corneal scarring follows, and remains a common avoidable cause of blindness worldwide. Prevention is by improved water supply and hygiene, and treatment of acute infection by community use of oral azithromycin.[66]

Chronic allergy in the form of vernal keratoconjunctivitis results in morbidity due to ocular discomfort and visual loss. Corneal scarring may be present along with papillary inflammation of the tarsal conjunctiva. Treatment is with mast cell stabilizers such as sodium cromoglycate, steroid eye drops, and topical cyclosporin eye drops. Topical steroid eye drops may cause glaucoma and cataract. Close supervision by an ophthalmologist is required.

Conjunctival dryness (xerosis) and corneal melting are features of vitamin A deficiency. Acute deficiency signs may be precipitated by intercurrent respiratory or gastrointestinal infection and urgent treatment with high doses of vitamin A is then needed.

CORNEAL DISEASE

Corneal scarring due to trachoma and vitamin A deficiency remains a leading cause of childhood blindness in resource poor countries.

In wealthy countries herpes simplex corneal infection is a relatively frequent cause of morbidity. Prompt treatment with topical antiviral drops or ointment (e.g. aciclovir) is usually sufficient to clear the infection, but in some cases areas of chronic inflammation and scarring of the cornea develop. Epidemics of adenovirus keratoconjunctivitis occur from time to time. While the condition is limited to viral conjunctivitis in most cases, some individuals develop inflammatory infiltrates deep to the corneal epithelium. Cautious use of topical steroids reduces symptoms, and reduces scarring.

Congenital corneal opacities due to dystrophies or as part of Peter's anomaly or sclerocornea are relatively rare. In bilateral cases corneal transplant surgery may be indicated. As with congenital cataracts, surgical treatment must be undertaken early if visual loss due to amblyopia is to be avoided. Corneal transplant surgery in infants, and the necessary intensive aftercare, are very demanding of the surgeon and the family and treatment is best undertaken in specialized referral departments.

Congenital limbal dermoids (Fig. 31.34) may occur in isolation or as part of a number of syndromes. They may be excised later in childhood. Surgery in infancy is generally not required.

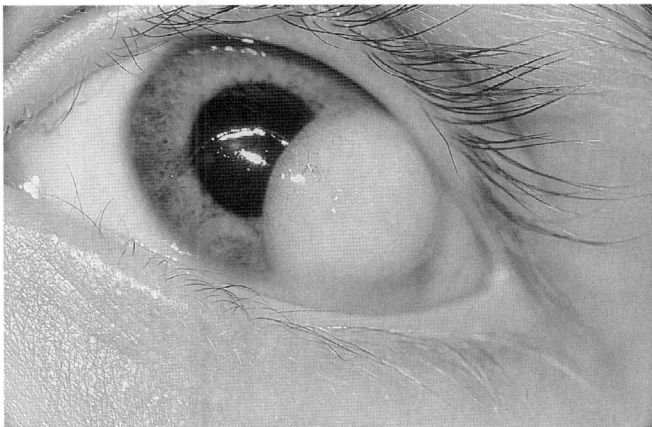

Fig. 31.34 Limbal dermoid.

UVEITIS

Uveitis screening is necessary in children with juvenile idiopathic arthritis (JIA) (Fig. 31.35). This is because the intraocular inflammation may be asymptomatic in its early stages, but untreated, may lead to glaucoma and cataract development. Slit lamp screening examination should be performed urgently when a diagnosis of JIA has been made. The groups at highest risk are those with oligoarticular disease and those who are antinuclear factor positive.[67] These children should be screened every 2–3 months initially. The children at lowest risk are children with systemic onset JIA, juvenile spondyloarthropathy and juvenile-onset rheumatoid factor positive arthritis. In these cases, screening is only required once, at disease onset. Children with other categories of JIA are at intermediate risk and should be examined every 3–4 months. Screening may generally be discontinued at age 12 years. Detailed guidelines for screening have been published by the American Academy of Pediatrics, and these are summarized in Table 31.11.[68] When iritis is detected, topical steroids and mydriatics may be used. Supervision of treatment by an ophthalmologist is needed because of the risks of glaucoma and cataract development due to steroid treatment. In more severe cases, or when there is a persisting topical steroid requirement, treatment with low-dose methotrexate, with mycophenolate or with the anti-TNF alpha agent infliximab may be required in order to reduce exposure to glucocorticoids and their side-effects.[69]

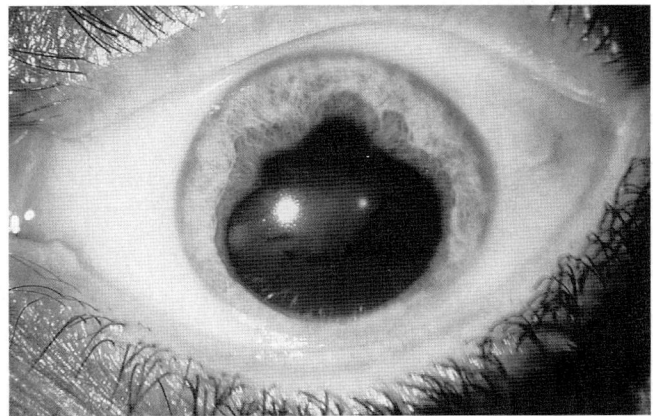

Fig. 31.35 Iritis. The pupil has been dilated and adhesions between the iris and lens (posterior synechiae) are seen.

Table 31.11 Guidelines for screening for uveitis in juvenile arthritis (taken from American Academy of Pediatrics guidelines.[68]

Juvenile arthritis subtype at onset	Age onset < 7 years	Age onset >/= 7 years
Oligoarticular, ANA positive	High	Medium
Oligoarticular, ANA negative	Medium	Medium
Polyarticular, ANA positive	High	Medium
Polyarticular, ANA negative	Medium	Medium
Systemic	Low	Low

Rules:
High risk = examinations 3–4 monthly
Medium risk = examinations 6 monthly
Low risk = examinations 12 monthly
Onset age < 7 years – risk becomes low 7 years after disease onset
Onset age >/= 7 years – risk becomes low 4 years after disease onset
All 'high risk' becomes 'Medium risk' 4 years after disease onset

CATARACT

Congenital cataract remains a major cause of childhood blindness worldwide (Fig. 31.36). In resource rich countries severe visual handicap due to congenital cataract is now rare because of improvements in surgical management.[24] The key to a satisfactory outcome is early detection and early surgery in order to avoid amblyopia.[70-72]

Two thirds of cases of congenital cataract are bilateral and one third unilateral.[73] Underlying causes or associated risk factors were present in 62% of bilateral and 8% of unilateral cases in a national UK study.[74] The causes of congenital cataract are given in Table 31.12. Every infant with congenital cataract should be examined for dysmorphic features or

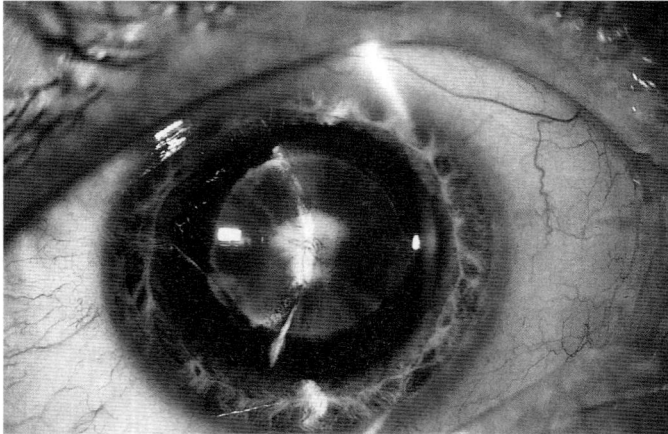

Fig. 31.36   Congenital cataract. This is a partial, lamellar cataract with relatively good vision. Surgery in infancy was not needed in this case.

Table 31.12   Causes of congenital cataracts

Idiopathic		
Isolated inherited	Dominant, recessive, X-linked	
Inherited syndrome	Chromosomal	Trisomy 21,13,18 Turner's Translocation 3;4 and 2;14 Cri du chat 5q15.2
	Mitochondrial diseases Lowe's oculocerebrorenal syndrome Ectodermal dysplasia	
Metabolic	Galactosemia Galactokinase deficiency Hypocalcemia Hypoglycemia Mannosidosis	
Prenatal infection	Rubella Toxoplasma Herpes simplex Varicella	
Trauma	Accidental Non-accidental	
Ocular associations	Microphthalmos Aniridia Persistent fetal vasculature Peter's anomaly Endophthalmitis	

evidence of metabolic disease. The parents should be examined for evidence of cataract as autosomal dominant cataracts may vary in disease expression.

Surgery should be performed within the first 6 weeks of life in order to ensure that optical rehabilitation has been completed by the age of 8–10 weeks.[73] Delayed detection and treatment will lead to irreversible visual loss due to amblyopia.[74] In bilateral cases the surgery is performed on one eye initially, with surgery to the second eye a few days later. There is uncertainty as to whether intraocular lens implants should be used at primary surgery.[76] An alternative to primary intraocular lens implantation is the use of contact lenses for primary optical correction, followed by secondary lens implantation at approximately age 2 years.

LENS SUBLUXATION

The most common cause of lens subluxation (Fig. 31.37) in children is Marfan syndrome.[75] The lenses tend to be subluxed from an early age and there is rarely any significant progression with time.[75] For this reason a single screening examination in early childhood is sufficient to detect lens subluxation and regular follow up is generally not required. The differential diagnosis includes homocystinuria [76]

When lens subluxation occurs, treatment may be either optical or surgical. Surgical treatment generally involves removing the whole lens and using contact lenses or sutured intraocular lens implants for optical correction.[78]

GLAUCOMA

PRIMARY CONGENITAL GLAUCOMA

Primary congenital glaucoma typically occurs in boys between the age of birth and 2 years. Some cases are autosomal recessive and there is a one in 20 empirical recurrence risk in siblings. The presenting signs may be present in one or both eyes. Watering, photophobia and enlargement of the corneas occur (Fig. 31.38). The diagnosis is made by performing an examination under anesthetic and measuring the intraocular pressure; i.v. or i.m. ketamine sedation is preferred for these examinations as ketamine produces a small, predictable rise in intraocular pressure. In contrast inhalational anesthetics produce a variable lowering of intraocular pressure. Treatment is surgical and demanding. Multiple operations may be required and surgical treatment is better undertaken in a pediatric glaucoma referral center.

SECONDARY GLAUCOMAS

Glaucoma may be secondary to other congenital ocular abnormalities. These include Rieger syndrome (Fig. 31.39) and aniridia. Glaucoma may develop secondary to iritis and steroid therapy in patients with JIA.

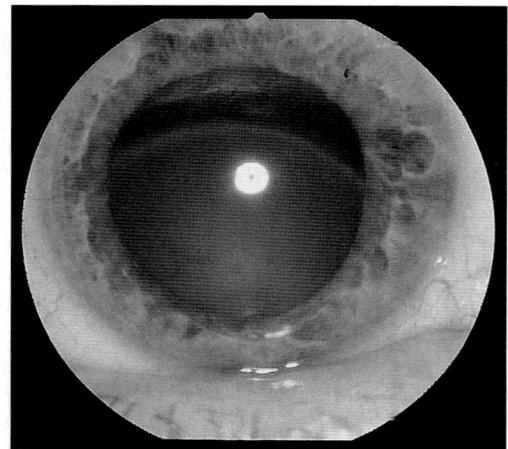

Fig. 31.37   Subluxed lens.

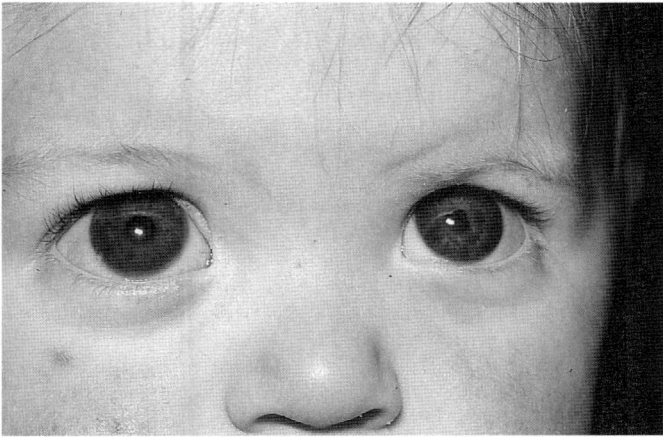

Fig. 31.38   Congenital glaucoma. Note enlarged corneas. This child had goniotomy surgery performed in infancy, which satisfactorily controlled the intraocular pressures.

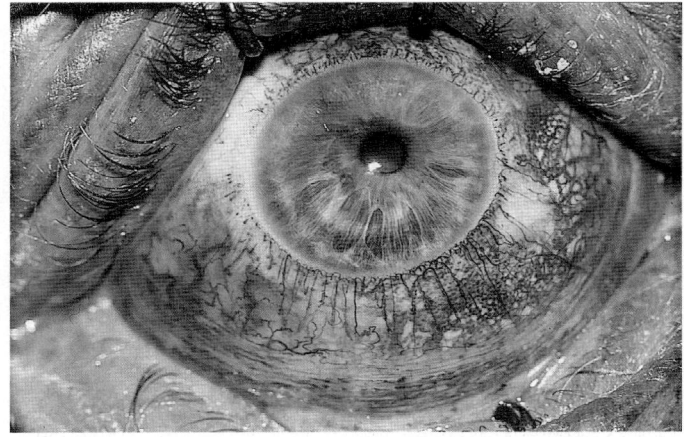

Fig. 31.39   Reiger syndrome. Note posterior embryotoxon and abnormal pupil shape and position (corectopia).

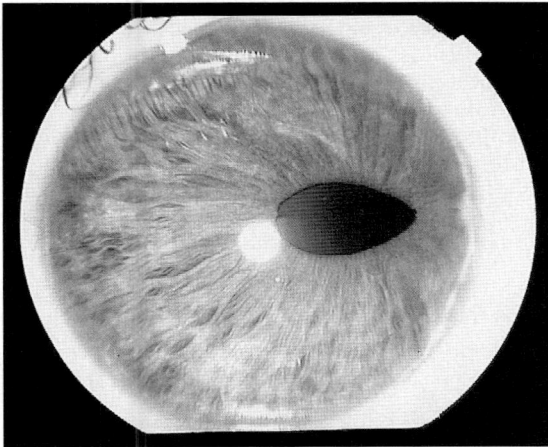

Fig. 31.40   Sturge–Weber syndrome. Note eyelid port wine stain, and abnormal scleral blood vessels.

RETINOBLASTOMA

Retinoblastoma (RB) is a malignant neuroblastic tumor of the retina, which normally develops during the first 2 years of life. Presenting signs include leukocoria (white pupil) and strabismus. Approximately 50% of cases are heritable, with a mutation of the RB1 tumor suppressor gene. In these cases, additional somatic mutations of allelic RB1 genes in retinal cells lead to loss of tumor suppressor function and neoplasia occurs. Tumors are usually multiple. Approximately 50% of heritable cases have a family history of retinoblastoma; the remainder represent new germline mutations.

In cases in which there is no germ-cell mutation, two mutations are needed to produce neoplasia in a retinal cell.[83] In these cases, the tumor is almost always solitary, with slightly later onset than heritable cases (median age 24 months compared to 12 months). However 15% of cases with solitary tumors have an underlying germ-cell mutation.

The diagnosis is made clinically. Typically the tumors have a creamy white appearance, are moderately vascular, and have areas of calcification (Fig. 31.42). The tumors tend to grow out from the retina into the vitreous ('endophytic') or grow underneath the retina ('exophytic'). Rarely the tumor diffusely infiltrates the retina. A relatively benign form of retinoblastoma – 'retinoma' – also exists. The age of onset is older, retinal pigment epithelium changes are seen surrounding the elevated gray retinal mass, and the tumor remains nonprogressive.

A particularly difficult form of childhood glaucoma is aphakic glaucoma in children who have had congenital cataract surgery.[79] Complex surgical treatment may be required.

Glaucoma may develop in Sturge–Weber syndrome, especially if the upper eyelid has a port wine stain lesion (Fig. 31.40).

RETINAL DISEASES

Retinal disorders, which cause bilateral visual loss in children, have been described earlier. Causes of unilateral retinal disease include those following.

COATS DISEASE

Coats disease is a primary retinal telangiectatic disease in which leaky vessels cause progressive accumulation of fatty deposits in the subretinal space (Fig. 31.41). Mutations in the gene for Norrie disease have been identified as the underlying cause.[81] The condition is diagnosed at a median age of 5 years, is more common in males and is almost always unilateral.[81] There are no systemic associations. Treatment with laser therapy or cryotherapy can reduce serous leakage and improve visual prognosis.[82]

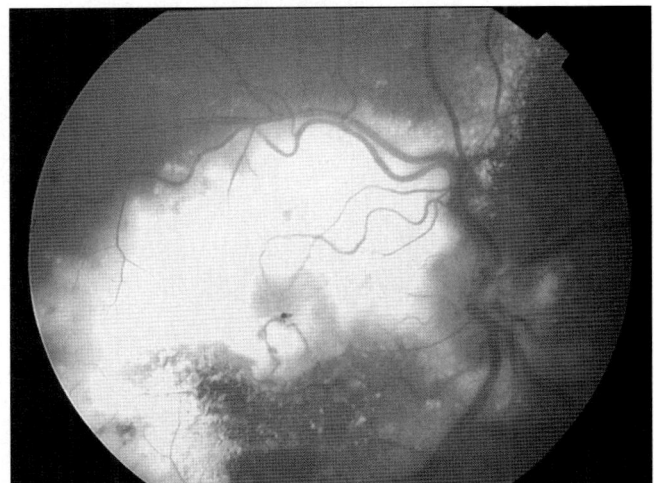

Fig. 31.41   Coats disease. Massive subretinal lipid exudation is seen at the macula, with severely reduced visual acuity.

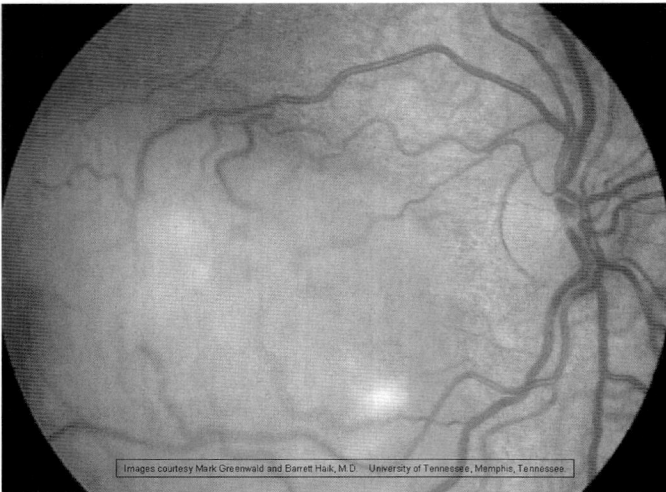

Images courtesy Mark Greenwald and Barrett Haik, M.D.   University of Tennessee, Memphis, Tennessee

Fig. 31.42   Retinoblastoma. Creamy white tumor. Image taken with 'Retcam' digital fundus camera.

The differential diagnosis includes Coats disease, tuberous sclerosis, retinal hamartomas, Norrie disease, *Toxocara* infection, and, in diffuse cases, endophthalmitis. When the optic nerve is clinically in contact with retinoblastoma tissue, assessment will include examination of the CSF and imaging of the brain and orbits. The scan will delineate the extent of the tumor, and exclude a coexisting pineal tumor ('trilateral retinoblastoma'). The most common route of spread is along the optic nerve. In advanced cases blood spread to bone marrow may occur.

An ocular oncology team in specialized referral centers should undertake management.

A range of treatment modalities may be used. Primary enucleation surgery is indicated for advanced disease (Fig. 31.43). A long length of optic nerve should be removed with the eye, and a primary orbital implant placed within the muscle cone.

Chemotherapy is now the first-line treatment for bilateral cases, though it is often necessary to enucleate one eye later. Unilateral cases that have been detected at an early stage may also be treated with chemotherapy. Six cycles of cisplatin, etoposide and vincristine are given.[84] Additional treatment modalities are required in some cases. These include retinal laser therapy, retinal cryotherapy, plaque brachytherapy and external beam radiotherapy.[85]

Frequent follow-up examinations are performed in order to detect tumor regression, and to look for new tumors, which develop in 10% of cases.[86] If there has been no evidence of local or metastatic disease for 3 years after local disease control, cure is very likely. Long-term survival is over 95%.

Heritable cases will transmit the defective RB1 gene to 50% of offspring, with 90% penetrance. The risk of disease is therefore 45%. All cases should have molecular genetic testing for an RB1 gene mutation.[88] This includes cases of solitary tumor, as 15% of these cases have an underlying germline mutation. The siblings of cases and the offspring of cases should also have molecular genetic testing.[87] If a defect is detected, or when there is uncertainty about the genetic status of an individual, regular retinal examinations must be performed. The initial examination may be performed without general anesthetic soon after birth. Examinations under anesthetic are then performed every 2–4 months until age 2 years. At each examination the peripheral retina must be fully visualized using scleral indentation. Further examinations without anesthetic are then performed 4–6 monthly until age 5 years.

All heritable cases require long-term oncology follow up. The product of the RB1 gene is the retinoblastoma protein pRB. RB1 mutations normally result in no detectable pRB production. pRB is a phosphoprotein that is involved in cell cycle control and inhibits cell proliferation. Its function is tissue specific – RB1 mutations increase the risk of retinoblastoma, pineal tumors (which presents with hydrocephalus) osteogenic sarcoma (especially in the orbit following ocular radiotherapy for retinoblastoma),[88] other sarcomas, and some carcinomas. However the RB1 gene does not predispose to other childhood neoplasias such as leukemia.

TOXOCARA INFECTION

Toxocara infection of the retina may occur in early childhood either in subclinical infection or as part of a systemic illness. The nematode dies

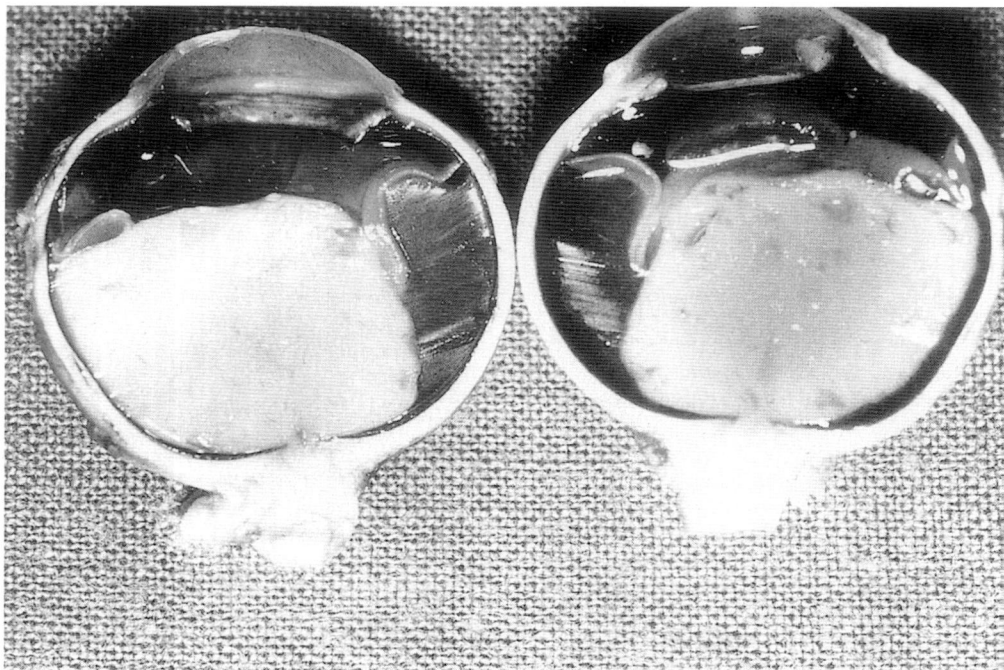

Fig. 31.43   An enucleated eye showing a large retinoblastoma causing detachment of the retina and almost filling the vitreous cavity.

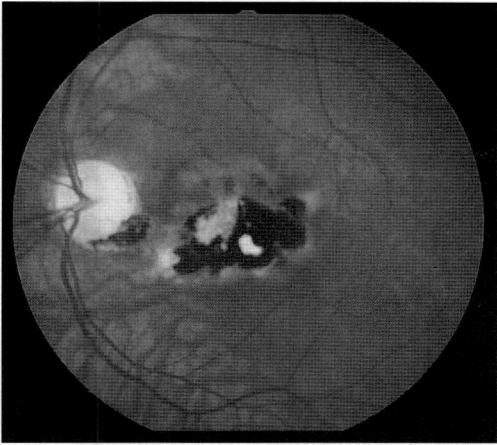

Fig. 31.44 Toxoplasmosis. Pigmented scar at macula. No active inflammation present.

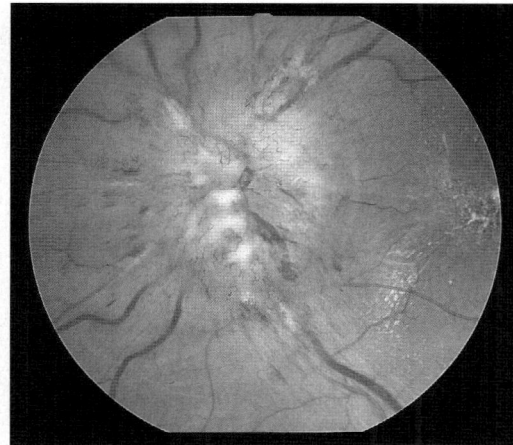

Fig. 31.45 Severe papilledema with hemorrhages and exudates.

within the eye and antigen release incites a profound inflammatory reaction. This leads to an isolated area of fibrosis with associated retinal traction. No active treatment is possible.

TOXOPLASMA INFECTION

The congenital toxoplasmosis syndrome includes chorioretinitis, intracranial calcification, seizures, hydrocephalus, microcephaly, hepatosplenomegaly, jaundice, anemia and fever.

However *Toxoplasma* infection acquired in the late prenatal period, or postnatally may remain quiescent for many years and then reactivate. The individual may have no neurological or systemic features of *Toxoplasma* infection. At the time of infection recurrence, an area of scarring of the choroid and retina is seen, with an adjacent area of retinal and vitreous inflammation (Fig. 31.44). The symptoms are reduced vision and floaters. A number of antimicrobial treatments have been used. Controlled trial evidence of efficacy is lacking.[89] Azithromycin has been used as monotherapy. Triple therapy with sulfadiazine, pyrimethamine and folinic acid has also been used. When antimicrobial therapy is given, very close follow-up is needed as death of the organisms may lead to increased inflammation due to antigen release. For this reason oral steroid treatment is often given 24–48 h after commencement of antimicrobial treatment.

DISEASES OF THE OPTIC NERVE

OPTIC ATROPHY

The causes of optic atrophy have been discussed earlier. Significant optic atrophy leads to reduced visual acuity, reduced color vision, and constricted visual fields.

OPTIC DISC EDEMA
Optic disc edema with severe visual loss

Optic disc edema due to inflammatory diseases (optic neuritis) results in profound visual loss. In children the most common pattern is bilateral optic neuritis. The discs are swollen, but hemorrhages and exudates are rare. Afferent pupil defects are present. Spontaneous, complete recovery over a period of days is usual. A neurological assessment should be carried out, including neuroimaging. There are usually no long-term neurological sequelae and the condition should be regarded as an entity separate from multiple sclerosis.

Optic disc edema without severe visual loss

The most significant cause of optic disc edema is raised intracranial pressure and the term 'papilledema' is normally used in these cases.

Papilledema may cause no visual symptoms. However in more severe cases brief periods of visual disturbance (visual obscurations) occur, and urgent investigation and control of intracranial pressure is required. Visual field examination shows enlarged blind spots in almost all cases. Paracentral scotomas may also be found. Poor intracranial pressure control leads to progressive loss of axons, with progressive constriction of the visual fields and visual impairment.

In its mildest form, papilledema causes slight blurring of the optic disc margins superiorly and inferiorly. As severity increases a larger portion of the optic disc circumference becomes blurred and the optic disc develops a pink appearance. The normal 'physiological' optic disc cup is lost, and normal venous pulsation is lost. In severe cases hemorrhages and exudates (nerve fiber layer infarcts) are seen (Fig. 31.45).

In mild cases the diagnosis may be aided by fluorescein angiography. In mild optic disc edema the capillaries on the surface of the optic disc are dilated and leak fluorescein dye (Fig. 31.46). High definition ultrasound examination of the optic disc and orbital optic nerve may allow detection of enlargement of the CSF space within the optic nerve sheath.

The differential diagnosis of papilledema includes hypermetropia and optic disc drusen. Moderately severe hypermetropia leads to small 'crowded' optic discs, which may have blurred edges and may be elevated. Optic disc drusen are deposits of amyloid tissue deep within the optic discs, leading to apparent swelling of the optic discs (Fig. 31.47). Drusen may be diagnosed using fluorescence photography or ultrasound examination.

THE EYE IN RELATION TO MEDICAL PEDIATRICS AND CLINICAL GENETICS

DIABETES MELLITUS

Diabetic retinopathy is exceptionally rare before puberty. Retinal screening examinations should be carried out annually from puberty. Cataract may develop as an acute feature of diabetes mellitus.

NEUROMETABOLIC STORAGE DISEASES – EYE SIGNS
Cherry red spot

In Tay–Sachs disease (GM2 type1) ganglioside accumulation in retinal ganglion cells leads to a 'cherry red spot' appearance (Fig. 31.48). The central fovea has no overlying ganglion cells and remains a red color due to the underlying choroidal circulation. The surrounding retina is a milky white color due to ganglioside storage in the ganglion cells. The ERG is normal, but the VEP is reduced. A cherry red spot is also seen in Niemann–Pick disease type A (sphingomyelinase deficiency) and neuraminidase deficiency (sialidosis types 1 and 2). With disease progression the cherry red spot fades as ganglion cells die and optic atrophy develops.

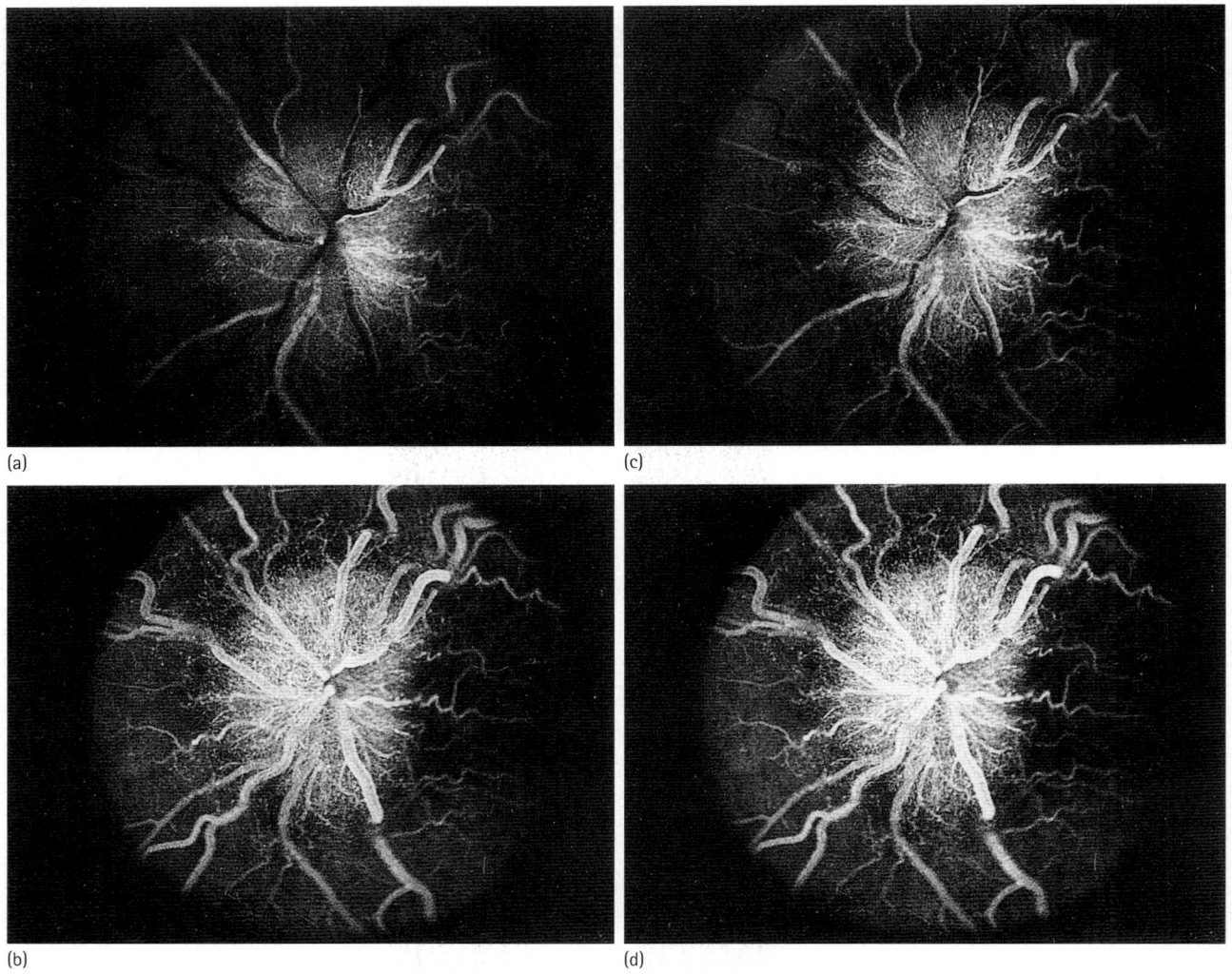

Fig. 31.46   (a–d) Fundus fluorescein angiogram showing dilated capillaries on the optic disc surface.

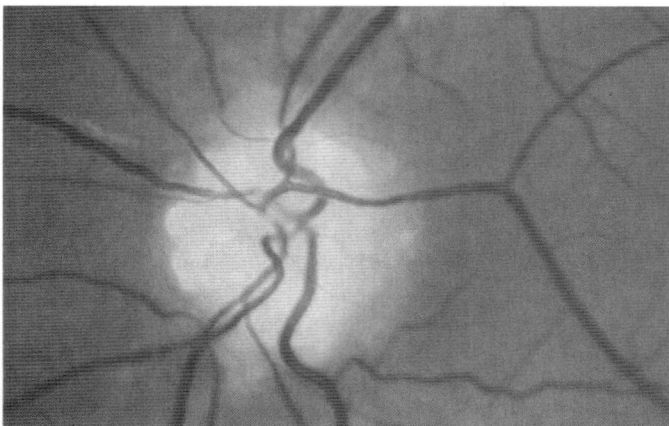

Fig. 31.47   Optic disc drusen.

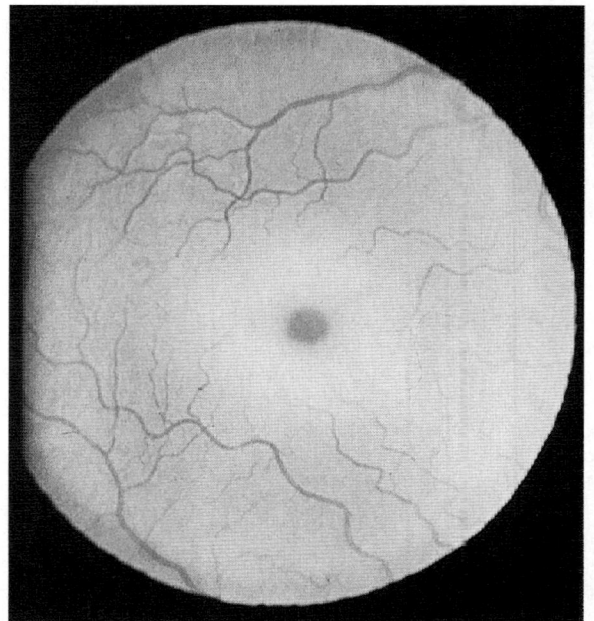

Fig. 31.48   Cherry red spot due to Tay–Sachs disease.

Corneal clouding

Corneal clouding develops in:

- mucopolysaccharidoses, all of which show corneal clouding, except MPSII and MPSIII;
- mucolipidoses;
- fucosidosis;
- mannosidosis.

WILSON DISEASE

Copper deposition in the peripheral cornea may be detected on slit lamp examination.[90]

OPHTHALMOLOGY CHANGES IN LEUKEMIA

Retinal hemorrhages may be found in severe anemia and leukemia (Fig. 31.49). The iris may act as a sanctuary site following chemotherapy for lymphoblastic leukemia. During remission periods, disease recurrence may occur in the iris, with clinical effects similar to those seen in iritis. Clinical suspicion and, if necessary, iris biopsy, will allow the correct diagnosis to be made. Treatment with further chemotherapy, and with radiotherapy to the irises, is indicated.

Opportunistic infections occur in immunosuppressed children. Infections commonly seen include herpes zoster and herpes simplex infections of the cornea or retina; and cytomegalovirus, *Toxoplasma* or *Candida* infections of the retina.

OPHTHALMOLOGY AND THE CLINICAL GENETICIST

The ophthalmologist may be asked to look for diagnostic signs in a range of inherited syndromes.

Marfan syndrome

Screening for lens subluxation may be requested. A single examination in early childhood is usually sufficient as lens subluxation develops early in life and there is rarely any significant progression with time.[78]

Neurofibromatosis

The ophthalmologist may provide diagnostic information in cases of suspected neurofibromatosis types 1 and 2 (NF1, NF2). Lisch nodules of the iris will be present in over 90% of children aged 8 years or older who have NF1 (Fig. 31.50), but are less frequent in younger children.[91] Symptomatic optic nerve gliomas are normally diagnosed by age 3 years.[91] Vision may fluctuate, deteriorate or remain stable for many years. When there is consistent deterioration of visual function, active treatment may be considered, such as chemotherapy using etoposide and cisplatin. Children with confirmed NF1 should have regular

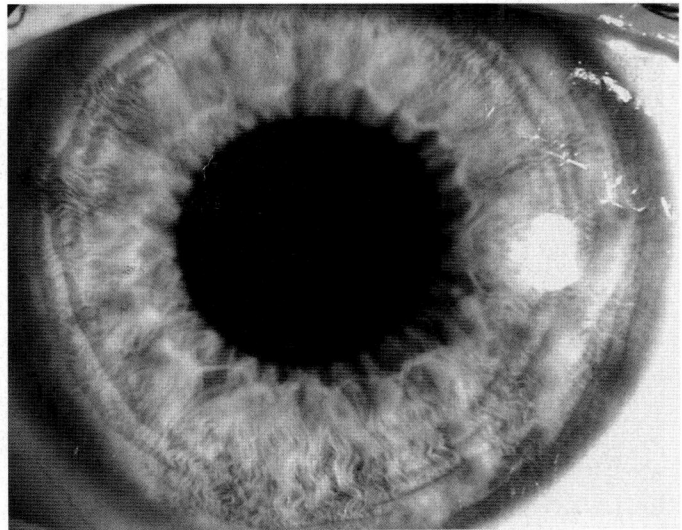

Fig. 31.50 Lisch nodules of the iris. Multiple pigmented nodules are easily visualized against the background of a lightly pigmented iris in this case.

screening examinations for anterior optic pathway gliomas. Screening examinations include measurement of visual acuity, color vision, pupil reactions, visual field measurements and optic disc examination (Fig. 31.51). Neurofibromas of the upper eyelid are associated with glaucoma in the ipsilateral eye.

In NF2, posterior subcapsular cataract is present in more than 50% of cases and is a useful diagnostic sign.[92]

Tuberous sclerosis

Fundus examination for retinal hamartomas should be performed in children with seizures and delayed cognitive development, as part of the diagnostic work-up for tuberous sclerosis. Hamartomas are found in the majority of patients with tuberous sclerosis.[93] These may appear as minimally elevated smooth translucent retinal lesions anywhere in the fundus, or as yellowish multinodular masses near the optic disc (Fig. 31.52). The lesions usually do not change significantly with time and do not cause significant visual defects, however occasional exceptions to this rule have been reported.[94]

Von Hippel–Lindau disease

Retinal angiomas are the earliest and most common clinical features of von Hippel–Lindau disease. Careful annual fundus examination is required in order to detect early lesions, which are most often found in the mid periphery.[95] The lesions tend to grow, and larger lesions leak serous fluid, which may lead to visual impairment. Early lesions should therefore be treated with laser or cryotherapy.[96]

Screening retinal examinations are needed for patients with known von Hippel–Lindau disease, and for presymptomatic family members who are known to have a mutation of the von Hippel–Lindau gene (3p25–26).

OCULAR TRAUMA

Significant ocular trauma remains a relatively common occurrence in children. Examination of an injured child requires patience, and examination under anesthetic is often preferred, especially when there is a suspicion of ocular perforation. Foreign bodies tend to lodge in the corneal epithelium, or become trapped underneath the upper eyelid. Corneal abrasions may be more easily detected by instilling a drop of fluorescein dye. A prophylactic topical broad-spectrum antibiotic should be prescribed when the corneal epithelium has been damaged. Eyelid lacerations should be carefully repaired, with particular attention to correct apposition of lacerations that involve the eyelid margins. Small ocular

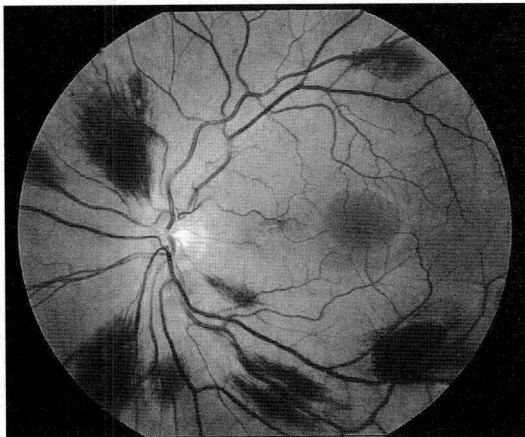

Fig. 31.49 Retinal hemorrhages related to leukemia.

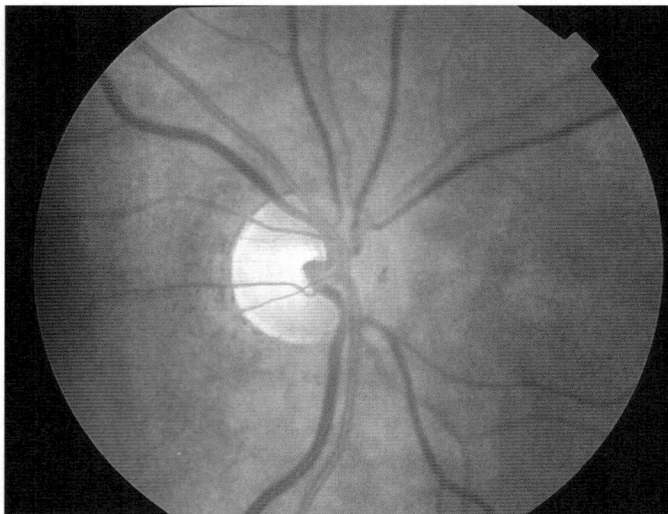
(a)

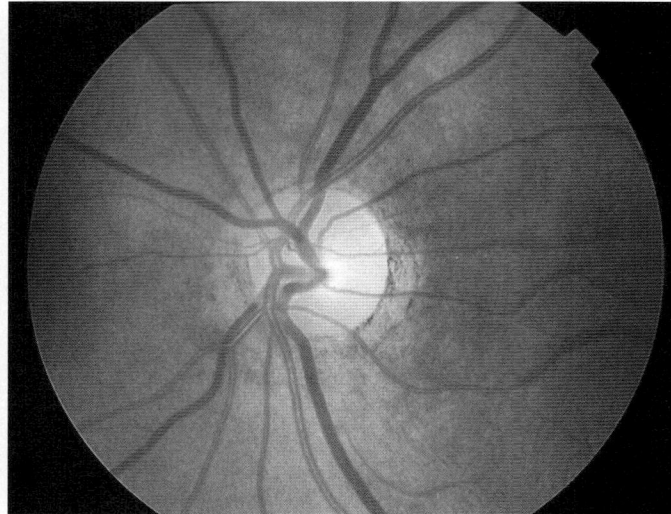
(b)

Fig. 31.51   (a) Right optic disc showing pallor on the temporal side. MRI scan showed optic nerve glioma. (b) Normal left optic disc.

lacerations may result in a distorted pupil, with prolapse of iris tissue at the perforation site.

Nonperforating blunt injuries most frequently present with hyphema – blood within the anterior chamber (Fig. 31.53). The intraocular pressure should be measured, and treated if elevated. Topical steroid and mydriatic eyedrops are given to treat associated iritis. Follow-up examinations are required in order to detect fundus abnormalities and traumatic glaucoma. Permanent visual loss is most often due to choroidal rupture (Fig. 31.54) or retinal detachment.

SHAKING INJURIES

Shaking injuries commonly produce extensive retinal hemorrhages and an ophthalmologist should be involved early in the diagnostic process.[97,98] Possible mechanisms include raised venous pressure and direct shearing forces within the retina and at the vitreoretinal interface. Typically hemorrhages are extensive, covering the whole retina from the optic disc to the ora serrata (Fig. 31.55). The hemorrhages are present deep within the retina (dot and blot hemorrhages), on the surface of the retina (flame-shaped hemorrhages within the nerve fiber layer) and on the surface of the retina (preretinal hemorrhages). Vitreous hemorrhage and traction retinal detachment may be present in more severe cases.

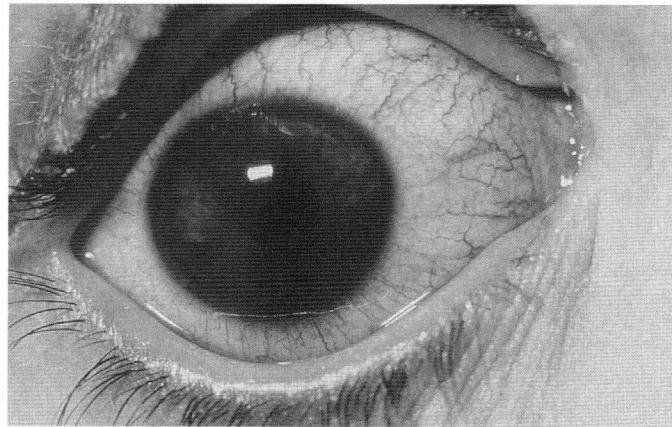
Fig. 31.53   Hyphema. Blood in the anterior chamber obscures the iris.

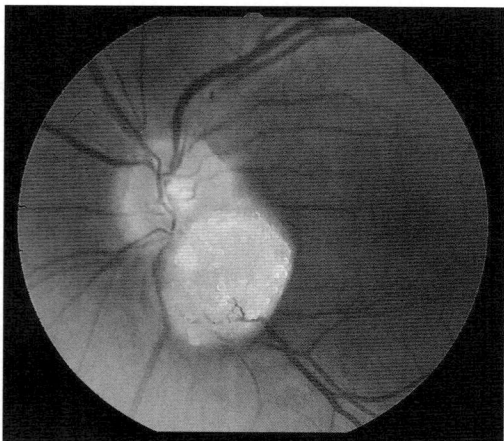
Fig. 31.52   Large multinodular retinal hamartoma adjacent to optic disc in a case of tuberous sclerosis.

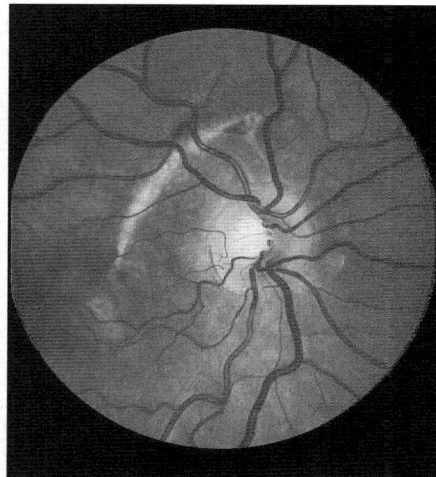
Fig. 31.54   Choroidal rupture. Blunt force has caused a curved tear in Bruch's membrane deep to the retinal pigment epithelium. There is additional pigment scarring at the macula.

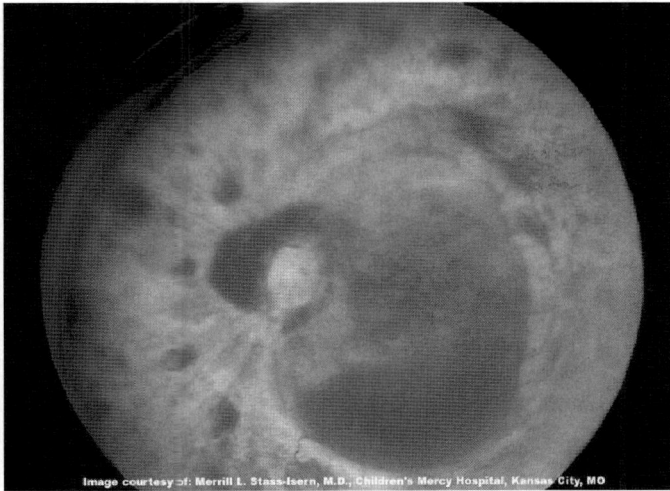

Fig. 31.55 Retinal hemorrhages following non-accidental shaking injury in an infant. Image taken with 'Retcam' digital fundus camera.

Flame-shaped surface retinal hemorrhages tend to clear within 1–2 weeks, although deep retinal hemorrhages and pre-retinal and vitreous hemorrhages may persist for a number of weeks. The differential diagnosis is given in Table 31.13 and includes birth hemorrhages and retinal hemorrhages secondary to blood clotting disorders. Retinal hemorrhages do not occur as a part of accidental head injury unless trauma is severe.[99] A few small retinal hemorrhages have been found in case series following seizures and following cardiopulmonary resuscitation.[100]

No specific treatment is indicated for retinal hemorrhages secondary to shaking injury. On follow-up, long-term visual loss is more often due to associated brain and optic nerve injury than to retinal injury.[101]

MANAGEMENT OF THE VISUALLY IMPAIRED CHILD AND THEIR FAMILY

The diagnosis of visual impairment in an infant or child may be devastating for a family. Parents are often in a state of shock when bad news is

Table 31.13 Differential diagnosis of retinal hemorrhages in an infant with suspected shaking injury (not exhaustive).

Non-accidental shaking injury
Accidental injury (severe trauma)
Leukemia
Coagulation disorders
Birth hemorrhages
Meningococcal meningitis
Glutaric aciduria type 1
Severe papilledema with raised intracranial pressure
Copper deficiency

given and an early review consultation is helpful in order to further discuss the implications of the diagnosis. Visual impairment in infants has secondary effects on general development, and appropriate use of sound and tactile stimuli by the parents will improve developmental progress. Considerable social and educational support will be needed in addition to medical interventions. Local and national parent support groups are available and should be used. Useful information may be obtained at *www.viscotland.org.uk*.

EDUCATION OF VISUALLY IMPAIRED CHILDREN

Many children with visual impairment may be satisfactorily educated in a mainstream school, provided that adequate additional teaching resources are made available. Simple measures such as satisfactory positioning of the child within the room and satisfactory lighting should be considered. Impairment due to reduced visual acuity may be helped in a wide range of ways, which include: allowing the child to observe objects of interest and text very close to their face; the use of large text (produced by photocopying with enlargement if necessary); the use of optical magnification devices and the use of computer-based technology. Braille supplemented by audiotape and speech recognition computer software enables many severely visually impaired children to progress to tertiary education. Strategies related to cerebral visual impairments are given in Table 31.2.

REFERENCES (* Level 1 evidence)

1. Teller DM. Assessment of visual acuity in infants and children: the acuity card procedure. Dev Med Child Neurol 1986; 28:770–790.
2. Norcia AM, Tyler CW. Spatial frequency sweep VEP: visual acuity during the first year of life. Vision Res 1985; 25:1399–1408.
3. Fawcett SL, Wang YZ, Birch EE. The critical period for susceptibility of human stereopsis. Invest Ophthalmol Vis Sci 2005; 46:521–525.
4. Wiesel TN, Hubel DH. Single-cell responses in striate cortex of kittens deprived of vision in one eye. J Neurophysiol 1963; 26:1003–1017.
5. Wiesel TN, Hubel DH. Comparison of the effects of unilateral and bilateral eye closure on cortical unit responses in kittens. J Neurophysiol 1965; 28:1029–1040.
6. Vaegan, Taylor D. Critical period for deprivation amblyopia in children. Trans Ophthalmol Soc UK 1979; 99:432–439.
7. Scheiman MM, Hertle RW, Beck RW, et al. Randomized trial of treatment of amblyopia in children aged 7 to 17 years. Arch Ophthalmol 2005; 123:437–447.
8. Keech RV, Kutschke PJ. Upper age limit for the development of amblyopia. J Pediatr Ophthalmol Strabismus 1995; 32:89–93.
9. Newman WD, Hollman AS, Dutton GN, et al. Measurement of optic nerve sheath diameter by

ultrasound: a means of detecting acute raised intracranial pressure in hydrocephalus. Br J Ophthalmol 2002; 86:1109–1113.
10. Kriss A. Skin ERGs: their effectiveness in paediatric visual assessment, confounding factors, and comparison with ERGs recorded using various types of corneal electrode. Int J Psychophysiol 1994; 16:137–146.
11. Dagi LR, Leys MJ, Hansen RM, et al. Hyperopia in complicated Leber's congenital amaurosis. Arch Ophthalmol 1990; 108:709–712.
12. Izquierdo NJ, Traboulsi EI, Enger C, et al. Strabismus in the Marfan syndrome. Am J Ophthalmol 1994; 117:632–635.
13. Watanabe S, Yamashita T, Ohba N. A longitudinal study of cycloplegic refraction in a cohort of 350 Japanese schoolchildren. Cycloplegic refraction. Ophthalmic Physiol Opt 1999; 19:22–29.
14. Mulvihill A, O'Keeffe M, Yap S, et al. Ocular axial length in homocystinuria patients with and without ocular changes: effects of early treatment and biochemical control. J AAPOS 2004; 8:254–258.
15. Logan NS, Gilmartin B, Marr JE, et al. Community-based study of the association of high myopia in children with ocular and systemic disease. Optom Vis Sci 2004; 81:11–13.
16. Pokharel GP, Negrel AD, Munoz SR, et al. Refractive Error Study in Children: results from Mechi Zone, Nepal. Am J Ophthalmol 2000; 129:436–444.

17. Saw SM, Shankar A, Tan SB, et al. A cohort study of incident myopia in Singaporean children. Invest Ophthalmol Vis Sci 2006; 47:1839–1844.
18. Rose K, Smith W, Morgan I, et al. The increasing prevalence of myopia: implications for Australia. Clin Experiment Ophthalmol 2001; 29:116–120.
19. Choi MY, Lee KM, Hwang JM, et al. Comparison between anisometropic and strabismic amblyopia using functional magnetic resonance imaging. Br J Ophthalmol 2001; 85:1052–1056.
20. Weakley DR Jr, Birch E, Kip K. The role of anisometropia in the development of accommodative esotropia. J AAPOS 2001; 5:153–157.
21. Holmes JM, Clarke MP. Amblyopia. Lancet 2006; 367:1343–1351.
22. Williams C, Northstone K, Harrad RA, et al. Amblyopia treatment outcomes after preschool screening v school entry screening: observational data from a prospective cohort study. Br J Ophthalmol 2003; 87:988–993.
23. Salcido AA, Bradley J, Donahue SP. Predictive value of photoscreening and traditional screening of preschool children. J AAPOS 2005; 9:114–120.
24. Fleck BW, Dangata Y. Causes of visual handicap in the Royal Blind School, Edinburgh, 1991–2. Br J Ophthalmol 1994; 78:421.
25. Bamashmus MA, Matlhaga B, Dutton GN. Causes of blindness and visual impairment in the West of Scotland. Eye 2004; 18:257–261.

26. Dutton GN, McKillop ECA, Saidkasimova S. Visual problems as a result of brain damage in children. Br J Ophthalmol 2006; 90:932–933.

27. Jacobson LK, Dutton GN. Periventricular leukomalacia: an important cause of visual and ocular motility dysfunction in children. Surv Ophthalmol 2000; 45:1–13.

28. Fielder AR, Evans NM. Is the geniculostriate system a prerequisite for nystagmus?. Eye 1988; 2:(Pt 6):628–635.

29. Ross LM, Heron G, Mackie R, et al. Reduced accommodative function in dyskinetic cerebral palsy: a novel management strategy. Dev Med Child Neurol 2000; 42:701–703.

30. Koc F, Ozal H, Firat E. Is it possible to differentiate early-onset accommodative esotropia from early-onset essential esotropia?. Eye 2003; 17:707–710.

31. Birch EE, Fawcett S, Stager DR. Why does early surgical alignment improve stereoacuity outcomes in infantile esotropia?. J AAPOS 2000; 4:10–14.

32. Mulvihill A, MacCann A, Flitcroft I, et al. Outcome in refractive accommodative esotropia. Br J Ophthalmol 2000; 84:746–749.

33. Efficacy of prism adaptation in the surgical management of acquired esotropia. Prism Adaptation Study Research Group. Arch Ophthalmol 1990; 108:1248–1256.

34. Hatt S, Gnanaraj L. Interventions for intermittent exotropia. Cochrane Database Syst Rev 2006; 3:CD003737.

35. Rosenbaum AL. Costenbader Lecture. The efficacy of rectus muscle transposition surgery in esotropic Duane syndrome and VI nerve palsy. J AAPOS 2004; 8:409–419.

36. Bagheri A, Farahi A, Yazdani S. The effect of bilateral horizontal rectus recession on visual acuity, ocular deviation or head posture in patients with nystagmus. J AAPOS 2005; 9:433–437.

37. Shery T, Proudlock FA, Sarvananthan N, et al. The effects of gabapentin and memantine in acquired and congenital nystagmus: a retrospective study. Br J Ophthalmol 2006; 90:839–843.

38. Introne W, Boissy RE, Gahl WA. Clinical, molecular, and cell biological aspects of Chediak–Higashi syndrome. Mol Genet Metab 1999; 68:283–303.

39. Wei ML. Hermansky–Pudlak syndrome: a disease of protein trafficking and organelle function. Pigment Cell Res 2006; 19:19–42.

40. Craft AW, Parker L, Stiller C, et al. Screening for Wilms' tumour in patients with aniridia, Beckwith syndrome, or hemihypertrophy. Med Pediatr Oncol 1995; 24:231–234.

41. Lambert SR, Kriss A, Taylor D. Delayed visual maturation. A longitudinal clinical and electrophysiological assessment. Ophthalmology 1989; 96:524–528.

42. Foxman SG, Heckenlively JR, Bateman JB, et al. Classification of congenital and early onset retinitis pigmentosa. Arch Ophthalmol 1985; 103:1502–1506.

43. Preising MN, Heegard S. Recent advances in early-onset severe retinal degeneration: more than just basic research. Trends Mol Med 2004; 10:51–54.

44. Rainbow LA, Rees SA, Shaikh MG, et al. Mutation analysis of POUF-1, PROP-1 and HESX-1 show low frequency of mutations in children with sporadic forms of combined pituitary hormone deficiency and septo-optic dysplasia. Clin Endocrinol (Oxf) 2005; 62:163–168.

45. Moore AT, Taylor DS. A syndrome of congenital retinal dystrophy and saccade palsy – a subset of Leber's amaurosis. Br J Ophthalmol 1984; 68:421–431.

46. Falck A, Laatikainen L. Diabetic cataract in children. Acta Ophthalmol Scand 1998; 76:238–240.

47. Kim LS, Fishman GA. Comparison of visual acuity loss in patients with different stages of Stargardt's disease. Ophthalmology 2006; 113:1748–1751

48. Wang AG, Fann MJ, Yu HY, et al. OPA1 expression in the human retina and optic nerve. Exp Eye Res 2006; 83:1171–1178

49. Ju W, Wronska A, Moroziewicz DN, et al. Genotype-phenotype analyses of classic neuronal ceroid lipofuscinosis (NCLs): genetic predictions from clinical and pathological findings. Beijing Da Xue Xue Bao 2006; 38:41–48.

50. Collins J, Holder GE, Herbert H, et al. Batten disease: features to facilitate early diagnosis. Br J Ophthalmol 2006; 90:1119–1124.

51. Newman SA. Ophthalmic features of craniosynostosis. Neurosurg Clin N Am 1991; 2:587–610.

52. Jackson K, Baker SR. Periorbital cellulitis. Head Neck Surg 1987; 9:227–234.

53. Starkey CR, Steele RW. Medical management of orbital cellulitis. Pediatr Infect Dis J 2001; 20:1002–1005.

54. Nageswaran S, Woods CR, Benjamin DK Jr, et al. Orbital cellulitis in children. Pediatr Infect Dis J 2006; 25:695–699.

55. O'Keefe M, Lanigan B, Byrne SA. Capillary haemangioma of the eyelids and orbit: a clinical review of the safety and efficacy of intralesional steroid. Acta Ophthalmol Scand 2003; 81:294–298.

56. Rootman J. Vascular malformations of the orbit: hemodynamic concepts. Orbit 2003; 22:103–120.

57. Shields JA, Shields CL. Orbital cysts of childhood – classification, clinical features, and management. Surv Ophthalmol 2004; 49:281–299.

58. Shields CL, Shields JA, Honavar SG, et al. Clinical spectrum of primary ophthalmic rhabdomyosarcoma. Ophthalmology 2001; 108:2284–2292.

59. Jeffery AR, Ellis FJ, Repka MX, et al. Pediatric Horner syndrome. J AAPOS 1998; 2:159–167.

60. Young JD, MacEwen CJ, Ogston SA. Congenital nasolacrimal duct obstruction in the second year of life: a multicentre trial of management. Eye 1996; 10(Pt 4):485–491.

61. MacEwen CJ, Young JD, Barras CW, et al. Value of nasal endoscopy and probing in the diagnosis and management of children with congenital epiphora. Br J Ophthalmol 2001; 85:314–318.

62. Lim CS, Martin F, Beckenham T, et al. Nasolacrimal duct obstruction in children: outcome of intubation. J AAPOS 2004; 8:466–472.

63. Maini R, MacEwen CJ, Young JD. The natural history of epiphora in childhood. Eye 1998; 12:(Pt 4):669–671.

64. Morrison D, FitzPatrick D, Hanson I, et al. National study of microphthalmia, anophthalmia, and coloboma (MAC) in Scotland: investigation of genetic aetiology. J Med Genet 2002; 39:16–22.

65. Everitt HA, Little PS, Smith PW. A randomised controlled trial of management strategies for acute infective conjunctivitis in general practice. BMJ 2006; 333:321.

66. Solomon AW, Mohammed Z, Massae PA, et al. Impact of mass distribution of azithromycin on the antibiotic susceptibilities of ocular Chlamydia trachomatis. Antimicrob Agents Chemother 2005; 49:4804–4806.

67. Kanski JJ. Screening for uveitis in juvenile chronic arthritis. Br J Ophthalmol 1989; 73:225–228.

68. American Academy of Pediatrics Section on Rheumatology and Section on Ophthalmology. Guidelines for ophthalmologic examinations in children with juvenile rheumatoid arthritis. Pediatrics 1993; 92:295–296.

69. Saurenmann RK, Levin AV, Rose JB, et al. Tumour necrosis factor alpha inhibitors in the treatment of childhood uveitis. Rheumatology (Oxford) 2006; 45:982–989.

70. Watts P, Abdolell M, Levin AV. Complications in infants undergoing surgery for congenital cataract in the first 12 weeks of life: is early surgery better? J AAPOS 2003; 7:81–85.

71. Lloyd IC, Goss-Sampson M, Jeffrey BG, et al. Neonatal cataract: aetiology pathogenesis and management. Eye 1992; 6:(Pt 2):184–196.

72. Rahi JS, Dezateux C. National cross sectional study of detection of congenital and infantile cataract in the United Kingdom: role of childhood screening and surveillance. The British Congenital Cataract Interest Group. BMJ 1999; 318:362–365.

73. Rahi JS, Dezateux C. Congenital and infantile cataract in the United Kingdom: underlying or associated factors. British Congenital Cataract Interest Group. Invest Ophthalmol Vis Sci 2000; 41:2108–2014.

74. Rahi JS, Dezateux C. Congenital and infantile cataract in the United Kingdom: underlying or associated factors. British Congenital Cataract Interest Group. Invest Ophthalmol Vis Sci 2000; 41: 2108–2114.

75. Lambert SR, Lynn M, Drews-Botsch C, et al. Intraocular lens implantation during infancy: perceptions of parents and the American Association for Pediatric Ophthalmology and Strabismus members. J AAPOS 2003; 7:400–405.

76. Fuchs J. Marfan syndrome and other systemic disorders with congenital ectopia lentis. A Danish national survey. Acta Paediatr 1997; 86:947–952.

77. Maumenee IH. The eye in the Marfan syndrome. Birth Defects Orig Artic Ser 1982; 18:515–524.

78. Vadala P, Capozzi P, Fortunato M, et al. Intraocular lens implantation in Marfan's syndrome. J Pediatr Ophthalmol Strabismus 2000; 37:206–208.

79. Trivedi RH, Wilson ME Jr, Golub RL. Incidence and risk factors for glaucoma after pediatric cataract surgery with and without intraocular lens implantation. J AAPOS 2006; 10:117–123.

80. Black GC, Perveen R, Bonshek R, et al. Coats' disease of the retina (unilateral retinal telangiectasis) caused by somatic mutation in the NDP gene: a role for norrin in retinal angiogenesis. Hum Mol Genet 1999; 8:2031–2035.

81. Shields JA, Shields CL, Honavar SG, et al. Clinical variations and complications of Coats' disease in 150 cases: the 2000 Sanford Gifford Memorial Lecture. Am J Ophthalmol 2001; 131:561–571.

82. Budning AS, Heon E, Gallie BL. Visual prognosis of Coats' disease. J AAPOS 1998 2:356–359.

83. Knudson AG Jr. Mutation and cancer: statistical study of retinoblastoma. Proc Natl Acad Sci USA 1971; 68:820–823.

84. Demirci H, Shields CL, Meadows AT, et al. Long-term visual outcome following chemoreduction for retinoblastoma. Arch Ophthalmol 2005; 123: 1525–1530.

85. McDaid C, Hartley S, Bagnal AM, et al. Systematic review of effectiveness of different treatments for childhood retinoblastoma. Health Technol Assess 2005; 9:145.

86. Schueler AO, Anastassiou G, Jurklies C, et al. De novo intraocular retinoblastoma development after chemotherapy in patients with hereditary retinoblastoma. Retina 2006; 26 425–431.

87. Tsai T, Fulton L, Smith BJ, et al. Rapid identification of germline mutations in retinoblastoma by protein truncation testing. Arch Ophthalmol 2004; 122:239–248.

88. Koshy M, Paulino AC, Mai WY, et al. Radiation-induced osteosarcomas in the pediatric population. Int J Radiat Oncol Biol Phys 2005; 63:1169–1174.

89. Stanford MR, See SE, Jones LV, et al. Antibiotics for toxoplasmic retinochoroiditis: an evidence-based systematic review. Ophthalmology 2003; 110:926–931.

90. Yuce A, Kocak N, Demir H, et al. Evaluation of diagnostic parameters of Wilson's disease in childhood. Indian J Gastroenterol 2003; 22:4–6.

91. DeBella K, Szudek J, Friedman JM. Use of the national institutes of health criteria for diagnosis of neurofibromatosis 1 in children. Pediatrics 2000; 105:608–614.

92. Ragge NK, Baser ME, Riccardi VM, et al. The ocular presentation of neurofibromatosis 2. Eye 1997; 11:(Pt 1):12–18.

93. Kiribuchi K, Uchida Y, Fukuyama Y, et al. High incidence of fundus hamartomas and clinical significance of a fundus score in tuberous sclerosis. Brain Dev 1986; 8:509–517.

94. Shields JA, Eagle RC Jr, Shields CL, et al. Aggressive retinal astrocytomas in four patients with tuberous sclerosis complex. Trans Am Ophthalmol Soc 2004; 102:139–147.

95. Kreusel KM, Bechrakis NE, Heinichen T, et al. Retinal angiomatosis and von Hippel–Lindau disease. Graefes Arch Clin Exp Ophthalmol 2000; 238:916–921.

96. Schmidt D, Natt E, Neumann HP. Long-term results of laser treatment for retinal angiomatosis in von Hippel–Lindau disease. Eur J Med Res 2000; 5:47–58.

97. Biron D, Shelton D. Perpetrator accounts in infant abusive head trauma brought about by a shaking event. Child Abuse Negl 2005; 29:1347–1358.

98. Adams G, Ainsworth J, Butler L, et al. Update from the ophthalmology child abuse working party: Royal College Ophthalmologists. Eye 2004; 18:795–798.

99. Pierre-Kahn V, Roche O, Dureau P, et al. Ophthalmologic findings in suspected child abuse victims with subdural hematomas. Ophthalmology 2003; 110:1718–1723.

100. Odom A, Christ E, Kerr N, et al. Prevalence of retinal hemorrhages in pediatric patients after in-hospital cardiopulmonary resuscitation: a prospective study. Pediatrics 1997; 99:E3.

101. Kivlin JD, Simons KB, Lazoritz S, et al. Shaken baby syndrome. Ophthalmology 2000; 107:1246–1254.

32

Disorders of the ear, nose and throat

Alastair IG Kerr

THE EAR

CONGENITAL ABNORMALITIES

Microtia/anotia/meatal atresia

The auricle forms from the six tubercles of His. Malformations include microtia, a misshapen auricle, or anotia, the absence of the auricle. Both may be associated with accessory auricles, which are small residual tubercles that may lie sometimes over the cheek without function. Either of these congenital abnormalities of the auricle may be associated with meatal atresia, the absence of the bony meatus. They are commonly associated together in a variety of congenital conditions and syndromes. They may present as a unilateral problem, e.g. first arch syndrome, or as a bilateral problem, e.g. craniofacial dysostosis or Treacher Collins syndrome. If the deformity is a unilateral one it is extremely important to investigate the normal ear to ensure that the hearing is normal on the unaffected side. Assuming the contralateral ear has normal hearing, then surgical or other intervention on the affected side becomes purely cosmetic. If the condition is bilateral, then the degree of conductive hearing loss should be established and, in the first instance, a bone conduction hearing aid fixed by a head band should be fitted at an early age. With the advent of osseointegrated implants, this bone conduction hearing aid should be replaced by an osseointegrated, bone-anchored hearing aid (BAHA) when the skull is thick enough to sustain this (usually ages 3–4 years). Surgical attempts to construct a patent meatus have not been successful and have been largely abandoned but reconstruction of the pinna using sculpted rib graft is becoming increasingly popular. An alternative to this is an osseointegrated prosthesis.

Meatal stenosis

Meatal stenosis may occur either as a congenital abnormality or as a result of chronic otitis externa. Down syndrome children have very narrow external auditory meati and they often have middle ear problems. This sometimes makes the fitting of grommet tubes difficult and hence careful monitoring of their hearing is important.

Ossicular abnormalities

Congenital abnormalities of the ear ossicles are rarely seen in isolation and are usually associated with some other manifest congenital abnormality. Attempts at surgical repair of ossicles in children are not normally advisable and any bilateral hearing deficit should be treated by a hearing aid.

TRAUMA AND INJURIES

Direct trauma to the auricle may produce a hematoma and is commonly seen in sporting injuries. The hematoma should be aspirated and a pressure bandage applied to avoid the cosmetic abnormality known as 'cauliflower ear'.

Perforation of tympanic membrane

This can be caused either by an object inserted into the ear or alternatively by pressure, e.g. in non-accidental injury, where a slap across the ear can cause a perforation of the drum due to the pressure of the air column in the narrow meatus. This form of injury is also seen in explosions or in diving accidents. Head injuries may be associated with perforation of the eardrum and also leakage of cerebrospinal fluid.

Treatment of perforation of the eardrum is conservative; the ear is kept dry and in the great majority of traumatic perforations the eardrum will heal spontaneously. This healing may take several months but no attempt at surgical intervention should be considered for at least 6 months.

Ninety-five percent of traumatic tympanic membrane perforations will close spontaneously and return to normal.

Foreign bodies

Aural foreign bodies are quite common and can present at any age. They usually are found in those aged 4 years or older who have the manual dexterity to put objects into their ears. They are best removed; this often requires a general anesthesia. Syringing is not recommended as this can push the object, often a bead or plastic toy, further in, potentially damaging the tympanic membrane.

Wax

It is normal for wax to be present in ears and this causes no problems unless it has been pushed into the external auditory meatus usually by the use of cotton buds. The superficial squamous epithelial cells in the external meatus have a natural flow pattern outwards, so that wax will be naturally extruded from the ear and hence, if the wax is kept soft by the use of simple olive or almond oil drops, syringing of the ears should not be required. As a general rule it is preferable not to syringe children's ears as they will find it uncomfortable and it will interfere with the natural extrusion process.

INFECTIONS OF THE EARS

Otitis externa

This condition does not occur commonly in children. The basis of treatment is aural toilet and the application of a topical antibiotic, with or without steroids, either on a small gauze dressing, which is preferable, or, alternatively, administered as eardrops. The skin of the meatus is often swollen and extremely tender and aural toilet may have to be carried out under a general anesthetic.

Furunculosis

A furuncle, or boil, in the external meatus will produce an acutely painful ear that is tender to the touch. It is often associated with a tender lymph node over the mastoid and hence the combination is often mistaken as an acute mastoiditis. The swelling in the latter is more widespread and the child is systemically unwell. Treatment of furunculosis is with oral antibiotics, usually flucloxacillin, and local dressings.

Acute otitis media

This occurs more commonly in those in the 6–36-month age range than in any other group. This is probably due to immaturity of the immune system, which can be slow in developing antibodies against bacteria with polysaccharides in their capsules, e.g. *Streptococcus pneumoniae* and *Haemophilus influenzae*. Infants also have short, wide horizontal Eustachian tubes that may allow easier passage of bacteria from the nasopharynx. Acute otitis media may occur as an accompaniment to an upper respiratory tract infection[1] but it can also occur on its own.

Clinically it will present with acute otalgia, sometimes bilateral, and the child will be fevered and may have a febrile convulsion. The eardrum, if inspected, will appear either acutely inflamed or bulging, with obvious pus behind it, the pain being due to the build-up of mucopurulent secretions in the middle ear. The first-line treatment is analgesics/antipyretics. Antibiotics provide only a small benefit for acute otitis media in children.[2] A Cochrane review[3] compared the outcome of antibiotics for 5 d with antibiotics for 8–10 d and concluded that 5 d of antibiotics (ceftriaxone or azithromycin) is effective. If the eardrum perforates, the pain will subside. In the vast majority of patients the drum will heal once the infection has settled. The treatment of infants and children with recurrent attacks of acute otitis media is either by repeated use of antibiotics or by surgical intervention. In young children, whose adenoids have not developed, the insertion of ventilation tubes (grommets) in the tympanic membranes will prevent recurrent attacks of acute otitis media. In older children who have significant adenoids, their removal may reduce further attacks of otitis media.

Acute otitis media is the commonest cause of otalgia with fever in children.

Acute mastoiditis

Acute mastoiditis still occurs but not nearly as frequently as it used to. This may be due to the use of antibiotics for acute otitis media but is more likely to be a reflection of a healthier population. Clinically, the child with acute mastoiditis will present with an acutely tender swelling in the postauricular region with the area of maximum tenderness being over the surface marking of the mastoid antrum, which is at the level of the top of the tragus. If looked at from behind, the auricle will be seen to be projecting outwards from the skull due to the loss of the postauricular sulcus and this is most commonly due to the collection of subperiosteal pus. The ear may or may not be discharging. The child will usually be in considerable pain and will be febrile. Treatment is admission, administration of i.v. antibiotics and analgesics and careful monitoring of the pulse and temperature for 24–48 h. If the postauricular swelling is increasing or if the temperature is not settling in that time, then surgical drainage of the subperiosteal pus and drilling away of the diseased cortical bone should be undertaken under general anesthesia. Acute mastoiditis rarely becomes a recurrent problem nor does it lead to chronic otitis media or cholesteatoma formation.

Postaural subperiosteal swelling with a protruding pinna is pathognomonic of acute mastoiditis.

Chronic otitis media

Chronic otitis media is associated with a permanent perforation of the tympanic membrane. There are two quite distinct groups: tubotympanic disease and attico/antral disease.

Tubotympanic disease

Usually such children have had recurrent attacks of otitis media that have either been inappropriately treated or that have resulted in a permanent residual anterior central perforation of the tympanic membrane. The clinical presentation is of intermittent, quite profuse painless mucopurulent discharge from the ear. The profuse discharge occurs in association with an upper respiratory tract infection or following the child swimming or getting the ear wet. If treated with oral antibiotics, the discharge should cease. The hearing loss will be minimal. Effective antibiotic treatment of tubotympanic disease is required and the child should keep the ear dry. Closure of the perforation by myringoplasty using a temporalis fascia graft is not advisable until the child has gone at least 6 months without any discharge from the ear and this will rarely be before the age of 8 or 9 years.

Attico/antral disease

These children have a continuous painless moderate purulent or blood-stained discharge from the ear. There may be middle ear granulations. This discharge will often be foul-smelling as the commonest organism is *Pseudomonas pyocyaneus*. This form of chronic otitis media does not usually respond to antibiotics and is more serious as it is usually associated with cholesteatoma in the mastoid antrum or mastoid air cell system, which may erode the ossicles and cause a significant hearing loss. If cholesteatoma is identified in the ear by suction clearance, under general anesthesia, then mastoid surgery is indicated as facial nerve palsy or cerebral complications can occur if the cholesteatoma is not cleared completely from the mastoid system.

REFERRED OTALGIA

Referred pain in the ear may be from the tonsils, nasopharynx or teeth, all of which must be considered in a child who has unexplained otalgia.

Otitis media with effusion

This is a very common condition in childhood that can occur at any age but is found most commonly between the ages of 4 and 6 years. It is commoner in boys. It is alternatively called 'serous otitis media', secretory otitis media, or simply 'glue ear'. Children with otitis media with effusion (OME) commonly present with a hearing loss due to the collection of fluid in their middle ears. The fluid contains polymorphonuclear leukocytes, macrophages and cell debris but no ciliated columnar cells or eosinophils. The fluid is invariably sterile and various searches for viruses have proved negative. The fluid contains glycoproteins and nucleoproteins and this gives the fluid its thick, tenacious quality.

Clinical presentation

Classically, a child with secretory OME will present with painless insidious bilateral conductive deafness that should not be greater than 40 dB. Fluid will collect without prior middle ear infections and often the child does not remark on the loss of hearing. The problem may not be identified until routine audiometric testing is done at school. The fluid collects secondary to functional blockage of the Eustachian tube. If children are left for up to 12 weeks in 30–40% of them the fluid will disappear and their hearing will return to normal. Other children present as having recurrent episodes or otalgia and hearing loss not responding completely to antibiotics or analgesics. Occasionally the ear drum may perforate. Some children can develop behavioral problems, becoming withdrawn or naughty presumably as they cannot hear properly. Others, especially toddlers, can become unsteady on their feet and start falling over, due it is thought to the vestibular system being affected by fluid in the middle ear.

Prevalence

At any one time, one child in 100 will have OME and approximately 10% of children under 10 years will have had OME.

Otitis media with effusion is the commonest cause of conductive deafness in childhood.

Diagnosis

Diagnosis is usually made by taking a careful history from the parents and/or the teachers, who are seeing the child on an everyday basis. Otoscopic examination will reveal an abnormal eardrum that may be retracted, bulging, dull, blue/yellow in color, or have an air–fluid level or bubbles visible behind it. Puretone audiometry will reveal a conductive hearing loss that is usually bilateral and worse in the lower frequencies than the higher frequencies but never greater than 40 dB. Impedance audiometry will give a flat tympanogram with a negative middle ear pressure and a greatly reduced tympanic membrane compliance.

Etiology

The underlying cause is believed to be Eustachian tube dysfunction, and certainly children with cleft palate and hence impaired Eustachian tube opening have a greatly increased risk of having OME. Children with chronic OME do have persistent negative middle ear pressure and this results in the loss of the middle fibrous layer of the tympanic membrane with atelectasis or atrophy of the membrane. Adenoids blocking the Eustachian tube orifice in the nasopharynx have long been associated with this condition and so their removal is often undertaken as a form of treatment. However, children without adenoids still get OME and therefore there must be more complex factors involved. Attempts to associate nasal allergy with OME have never been substantiated and apart from the already mentioned age and sex factors, the only other recently proven etiologic factor is passive smoking within the home environment.[4] Because the Eustachian tube is situated so centrally, it is extremely difficult to investigate its function in these children, and hence the etiology remains obscure.

Treatment

Management of OME remains controversial. The policy of 'watchful waiting' is the mainstay of treatment as over 50% of cases will spontaneously resolve in 12 weeks.[5] Medical treatment using antibiotics decongestants or nasal steroids have been shown to be ineffective.[6] Grommets offer a short-term hearing improvement only and therefore surgery is reserved for those with persisting hearing loss or those who are at increased risk of persistence at presentation.[7-9] These include those presenting in July to December and those whose hearing thresholds are worse than 30 dB in the better ear.

Surgery consists of myringotomy (drainage of the fluid) and insertion of ventilation tubes (grommets). This should be combined with adenoidectomy if a child presents with symptoms of enlarged adenoids (chronic mouth breathing, snoring, etc.) Adenoids are very small at birth but grow to a maximum size between the ages of 4 and 8 and it is in this group that adenoidectomy may be required. By ventilating the middle ear, grommet tubes reduce negative middle ear pressure and prevent the development of an effusion.

Children who have grommets can go swimming but are advised not to dive. It is sensible however to wear earplugs either customized or held in place by a headband. Grommets stay in place for 6–15 months and can cause minor scarring of the ear drums. Occasionally infections occur requiring antibiotic or removal of the grommet(s) and about 1% are associated with persisting perforations.

Surgery for otitis media with effusion should only follow 3 months of watchful waiting.

DEAFNESS

OME will produce a conductive deafness of up to 40 dB, which can affect speech and language development. If a child has a hearing loss it is important to identify whether it is conductive, sensorineural or a combination of the two. In conductive deafness the disability is not so severe and often there may be a surgical or medical method of treating it.

Sensorineural deafness in children is not uncommon. In resource rich countries, the incidence of bilateral significant sensorineural deafness is one in 1000 live births. 'Significant loss' is a loss of between 25 and 35 dB in the better ear. It is the high-frequency component of the loss that is usually important. If the loss in the better ear is at a level of 30 dB when averaged over the four frequencies 500 Hz, 1 kHz, 2 kHz and 4 kHz, then the child will require some kind of amplification to attain normal speech and language.

Significant bilateral sensorineural deafness has an incidence of one in 1000 live births.

Causes of sensorineural deafness

Only about 50% of children with significant bilateral sensorineural loss have an identifiable cause.

Hereditary prenatal causes

There are large numbers of syndromes in which deafness is a recognized factor:

Waardenburg syndrome. This autosomal dominant condition with variable expression consists of some or all of the following characteristics: unilateral or bilateral sensorineural deafness (20% of cases); hypertrichosis of the eyebrows that meet in the midline; heterochromia of the irises; or a white forelock.

Klippel–Feil syndrome. These children have short necks, which limits head movements. The hairline is low at the back, there may be paralysis of the external rectus muscle in one or both eyes and there is sensorineural hearing loss, which may be severe.

Alport syndrome. This is X-linked dominant and affects boys more severely than girls. There is severe progressive glomerulonephritis and a progressive sensorineural hearing loss, which does not show itself until the boy is about 10 years old.

Pendred syndrome. This is autosomal recessive and causes simple goiter at about the age of 4–5 years. There is an associated deafness that is often severe.

Refsum syndrome. This consists of ichthyosis, ataxia, retinitis pigmentosa, night blindness, mental retardation and sensorineural deafness.

Usher syndrome. This is autosomal recessive. There is retinitis pigmentosa with contraction of the visual fields and a severe sensorineural hearing loss that may be progressive.

Jervell and Lange–Nielsen syndrome. This is autosomal recessive with a cardiac arrhythmia secondary to a prolonged QT period, and a profound sensorineural deafness. These children may present with syncopal attacks and if untreated, these attacks can be fatal.

The inheritance of deafness is well recognized and in some children with recessive inheritance, the sensorineural hearing loss may be progressive. Nonhereditary prenatal deafness may be due to maternal illness, especially in the first trimester of pregnancy. Cytomegalovirus infections, toxoplasmosis, glandular fever and rubella are the most common, but parental syphilis and the taking of certain ototoxic drugs by the mother may also cause deafness in the baby.

Ototoxic drugs that should be specifically avoided during pregnancy are the aminoglycosides, quinine and to a lesser extent salicylates and alcohol.

Perinatal causes of deafness are usually related to prematurity or hypoxia. With the advances in neonatology, when extremely immature babies with complex neonatal problems are now surviving, the number of children with significant bilateral deafness sometimes associated with other abnormalities, and often related to hypoxia, is increasing. The cochlea is particularly sensitive to lack of oxygen. As neonatology improves further, the numbers of children with perinatal deafness will hopefully reduce.

> *Early diagnosis of sensorineural deafness is vital for acquisition of speech and language.*

Postnatal causes

Middle ear problems cause conductive deafness and the causes of these have already been discussed. Sensorineural loss may result from head injury, from the use of ototoxic drugs and as a result of specific infections. Parents whose children get repeated attacks of acute otitis media are often concerned that significant sensorineural loss may result, but this is extremely rare.

Measles and mumps. Measles and mumps remain the specific infections that can cause significant sensorineural hearing loss. Mumps, although it will sometimes cause a profound sensorineural loss, is generally only a unilateral loss. The increasing use of the measles/mumps/rubella (MMR) vaccine will reduce the incidence of deafness from these infections.

Meningitis. Meningococcal or pneumococcal meningitis may give severe bilateral sensorineural hearing loss that will be permanent and may progress in severity following recovery from the meningitis. All children who have recovered from bacterial meningitis should have their hearing tested and monitored.

Diagnosis of deafness

The first 2 years of life are vital for the acquisition of speech and language and hence the early detection of significant hearing loss in a baby is extremely important.

Neonatal hearing screening

Programs for this are now in place throughout the UK. They are based around maternity units, the aim being to test all newborns before they leave hospital. Techniques used are otoacoustic emissions then going on to automated brainstem audiometry, if necessary

> *Only 50% of children with sensorineural deafness have an identifiable cause.*

Subjective audiometry

Distraction audiometry

This is still a reliable, efficient method of testing that requires the minimum of equipment. The disadvantage is that it cannot be performed until the child is holding his head up unsupported. In the UK this is carried out by the health visitor as one of the routine screening tests at 7 or 8 months.

Conditioned audiometry

As the child gets older, he can be conditioned to perform a specific task in response to the input of sound.

Puretone audiometry

This is the main method of testing but cannot be done until the child will tolerate wearing headphones and can be relied upon to respond accurately to puretone sounds.

Objective audiometry

Brainstem evoked response audiometry

This is the most reliable form of objective audiometry and can be performed at any age. It is not, however frequency specific and young children, apart from neonates, require sedation or anesthetic.

Otoacoustic emissions

This test is based on the cochlear echo, which is an acoustic response of the cochlea when it is exposed to sound. It is easily done very quickly and gives a qualitative result as to whether the child's cochlea is working normally or not. Its disadvantage is that it does not distinguish between conductive deafness and sensorineural deafness, and any children who fail the otoacoustic emission test usually have to then progress to brainstem-evoked response audiometry.

Impedance audiometry or tympanometry

This is a simple test that measures the compliance of the eardrum and the pressure of the air in the middle ear. It is ideally suited for identifying otitis media with effusion and is useful in screening those who have failed their routine school audiometric testing.

Treatment of deafness

Treatment of conductive deafness has been discussed elsewhere in this chapter. There is no medical treatment for sensorineural deafness and management is based on prophylaxis. Genetic counseling and preventive measures such as immunization are important to avoid some causes of sensorineural hearing loss. As neonatology advances and hypoxia becomes less common, the incidence of deafness amongst ex-premature infants will be reduced. Sensorineural hearing loss is not normally progressive but in some congenital conditions it is, and so careful monitoring of the child's hearing is vital once the diagnosis has been made.

The mainstay of treatment remains amplification by some form of hearing aid. A large range of hearing aids is now available for children with sensorineural hearing loss and it is extremely important that the degree of handicap and the shape of the audiogram is known before the hearing aid is prescribed. Nowadays the hearing aid can be customized to the individual child's specific hearing loss.

The phonic ear

Teaching the deaf has been revolutionized by the advent of the phonic ear. This is a radio-aid type of hearing device where the mother or the teacher wears a microphone and a transmitter and the child wears the radio receiver. This means the child can sit anywhere in the class and be in direct radio contact with the teacher and hence the degree of amplification can be greatly enhanced. Many children with quite severe hearing handicap can therefore now be educated in their own local school rather than having to go to specific schools for the hearing impaired.

Cochlear implants

These have been used in children for nearly 20 years and are now established as the most effective way of enabling children to develop speech and language where hearing aids are not providing adequate amplification of sound. They are considered only after a thorough trial of hearing aids but experience is showing that the younger the child is implanted the better the outcome in terms of speech and language. The devices are expensive and are only available in specialized centers. Implantation is then followed by programming of the device and an intensive ongoing process of habilitation involving audiologists, teachers of the deaf, speech and language therapists, social and community workers as well as medical staff.

> *Cochlear implants are only required for a very small number of profoundly deaf children.*

THE NOSE, SINUSES AND THROAT

THE NOSE

The nose functions as an air conditioner for the lower respiratory tract. It achieves this by cleaning, warming and humidifying the inspired air. The turbinates (Fig. 32.1) project from the lateral wall, increasing the surface area and causing turbulence. This allows heat and fluid exchange and causes any particles to be deposited on the lining of the nose in the sticky mucus, which then passes posteriorly and is swallowed. The function of the paranasal sinuses is unknown.

Foreign bodies

These present as foul-smelling, sometimes bloodstained unilateral nasal discharge. They occur most often in children between the ages of 2 and 4 years, and are usually bits of foam rubber or toys that

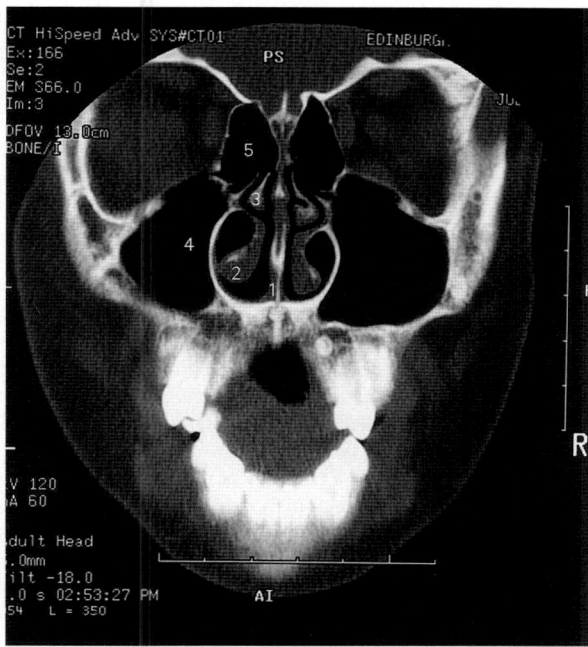

Fig. 32.1 Normal coronal CT scan of an 11-year-old boy showing: (1) nasal septum; (2) inferior turbinates; (3) middle turbinates; (4) maxillary sinuses; (5) ethmoid sinuses.

they have inserted themselves. It is rare for them to cause lower respiratory tract infections and the treatment is removal of the foreign body.

This can be done in a treatment or outpatient area sometimes by a 'parental kiss', where the parent blows into the child's mouth, the aim being to blow the foreign body out of the nose. If this is unsuccessful, and a headlight and appropriate instruments are available, and the child is cooperative, they can be removed under direct vision. Often, however, it has to be done under a general anesthetic.

Unilateral foul-smelling nasal discharge in a young child is pathognomic of a nasal foreign body.

Fracture of the nose

The nose is the commonest bone in the body to be broken. In children nasal fractures are less common than in adults as the nasal bones are smaller and the tissues more pliant.

Nasal fractures result from direct trauma. Initially, there is swelling over the bridge of the nose and around the eyes, which takes 5–7 d to subside. It is then possible to see whether the nasal bones are deviated, when manipulation under general anesthetic to straighten them is usually advised. Manipulation must be carried out within 21 d of the injury otherwise the bones become fixed.

Hematoma of the septum presents as severe blockage of the nose after an injury. This inevitably becomes infected, resulting in development of a septal abscess and destruction of cartilage and requires surgical drainage and a broad-spectrum antibiotic for 10 d.

Epistaxis

This is common after infancy. The bleeding can be spontaneous or secondary to mild trauma and usually arises from Little's area, in the anterior part of the nasal septum. Epistaxis can occur in leukemia or patients with bleeding disorders (e.g. hemophilia or thrombocytopenia) but is rarely the presenting feature of these conditions. First-aid treatment consisting of pinching the anterior cartilaginous portion of the nose with the child upright is usually successful. If there are repeated episodes, nasal cautery is indicated.

Epistaxis in a child usually comes from Little's area at the front of the nose and can be controlled by local pressure.

After identifying the source of bleeding, local anesthetic, 5% topical lidocaine (lignocaine) with 0.5% phenylephrine hydrochloride (co-phenylcaine) is applied using cotton wool or a spray. The area is then cauterized using a silver nitrate stick. In rare cases not responding to cautery, admission with nasal packing and i.v. fluid replacement may be required.

Epistaxis or oronasal hemorrhage in the first year of life is rare; coagulation disorder needs to be ruled out, and in the absence of this or obvious trauma, suffocatory child abuse should be considered.

Rhinitis

This is extremely common and is characterized by swelling and inflammation of the lining of the nose, often accompanied by clear or purulent rhinorrhea.

Viral rhinitis (the common cold or coryza)

This occurs very commonly with a pyrexial illness, runny nose, throat discomfort, sneezing and occasional earache. Treatment is symptomatic – analgesics and antipyretics as required. There is no proven place for decongestants in this condition. Viruses that have been identified as causing the common cold include rhinovirus, reovirus and adenovirus.

Viral rhinitis may be the precursor of laryngotracheobronchitis or pneumonia. A simple cold will normally last for 7–10 d and the child will not be unwell.

Bacterial rhinitis

This usually presents as purulent discharge following acute rhinitis. Antibiotics are rarely required unless the nasal blockage becomes worse or systemic symptoms such as fever and headaches occur, when adenoiditis or sinusitis should be suspected. In some children there is a constant low-grade bacterial rhinitis variable in severity, where no definitive underlying cause can be found. This can be associated with poor diet, damp housing and parental smoking. The underlying problem is thought to be lowered local nasal immunity. Antibiotics can sometimes stop persistent runny noses in children but there is no evidence of long-term benefit.[10] Most children with this condition will improve spontaneously from about the age of 8 years onwards. Immotile cilia syndrome is a rare cause and will often be associated with lower respiratory tract disease.

Allergic rhinitis

This usually occurs in children older than 5 years old. It presents as sneezing, associated with clear rhinorrhea and nasal blockage, and can be accompanied by conjunctivitis and sore throat. Seasonal rhinitis usually occurs in the summer and is caused by allergy to pollens. Perennial rhinitis can occur at any time of the year and can be associated with exposure to extrinsic allergens such as animals (e.g. cats or dogs) or housedust mite.

The diagnosis is made from the history. On examination, the nasal lining will usually be slightly pale and swollen. Confirmation of the allergic basis can be made by carrying out skin testing or serum immunoglobulin E assay.

Treatment is, if possible, by removal of the allergen but if this is not possible (e.g. seasonal rhinitis), a nonsedating antihistamine such as loratidine, supplemented by occasional use of a nasal steroid spray such as beclometasone may be helpful. Allergy to the housedust mite and housedust is increasingly recognized as a cause of rhinitis and allergic asthma. Treatment consists of cutting down the allergen in the bedroom by use of sprays or antiallergic sheeting. Nonsedating antihistamines and sometimes a short course of steroid sprays are also useful in combating this condition.

Non-allergic rhinitis (vasomotor rhinitis)

This presents as nasal blockage and catarrh and is differentiated from allergic rhinitis by negative allergy testing. Treatment is by antihistamine and decongestant combinations, and occasionally by steroid sprays for 2 months. Where there is no response to medical treatment, surgical diathermy or laser reduction of the inferior turbinate can be carried out.

NASAL SEPTAL DEVIATION

This can be traumatic but is more commonly developmental. Slight deviation is common and causes no symptoms, but more severe deviation will cause nasal obstruction, sometimes on both sides, occasionally with external nasal deformity. There may be associated allergic or vasomotor rhinitis. Surgery is only indicated for significant nasal blockage and is usually performed only in older children as surgery in young children can cause deformity, which increases with age.

DISEASES OF THE PARANASAL SINUSES

The paranasal sinuses (maxillary, ethmoid, frontal and sphenoid; Fig. 32.1) are all derived from the nasal cavity and are lined by respiratory epithelium. The maxillary sinuses are small at birth and do not attain significant size until 4 or 5 years of age. The ethmoid sinuses are well developed at birth, but the frontal sinuses do not develop until 9 or 10 years of age. The sphenoid sinuses rarely cause symptoms in childhood.

There is slight inflammation of the sinus mucosa in all forms of rhinitis and when the ostium to the sinus gets blocked, secretions are retained and purulent sinusitis develops. Treatment with antibiotics and local decongestants opens up the ostium and allows the sinuses to drain.

Maxillary sinusitis

This is rare under the age of 6 and it usually follows influenza or parainfluenza. The nose becomes very congested, there is copious purulent catarrh and there may be associated headache and fever. The commonest organisms found are *Pneumococcus* and *Haemophilus influenzae*. Diagnosis is on suspicion and the finding of purulent catarrh in the nose and throat. Treatment is by ephedrine nosedrops, combined with a broad-spectrum antibiotic such as amoxicillin or erythromycin for 1 week. X-rays are indicated only if there is no response to the appropriate antibiotics, at which time surgical drainage may occasionally be required.

Ethmoiditis

This is a potentially serious condition that occurs in children from 3 years upwards. It usually follows an upper respiratory tract infection. The symptoms are of frontal headache and pain around the eye with fever and nasal blockage. Examination shows periorbital swelling and tenderness with marked inflammation. If there is abscess formation it is usually subperiosteal and this causes lateral displacement of the globe. The clinical diagnosis is now confirmed by a computerized tomography (CT) scan. Urgent treatment with a parenteral broad-spectrum antibiotic and ephedrine nose drops is required with surgical drainage if there is abscess formation.[11] If the condition is not treated or inadequately treated, extension of the infection can result in the serious complication of cavernous sinus thrombosis or intracranial abscess.[12]

Periorbital infection often arises from infection of the ethmoid or frontal sinuses and should be treated vigorously.

Frontal sinusitis

This is less common than ethmoiditis and presents in children over 10. Like ethmoiditis, it is potentially serious with a risk of spread to involve the orbit or intracranial structures. It usually occurs after a cold or flu and causes severe frontal headache associated with inflammation and tenderness over the frontal sinus. Nasal symptoms are often minimal. Diagnosis and treatment are similar to that for ethmoiditis. Spread can occur inferiorly to involve the eye.

NASAL POLYPS

These present as unilateral or bilateral nasal blockage. Examination of the nose will show a pale, fleshy, usually mobile structure. Most common

is a unilateral antrochoanal polyp arising from the maxillary antra. These grow into the nose and down into the nasopharynx, often causing total obstruction of one side with purulent catarrh. They are benign and treatment is removal.

Ethmoidal polyps are less common and cause nasal blockage and catarrh. Ethmoidal polyps occur in children with cystic fibrosis, when the histology is different from the usual 'allergic type'. Treatment is removal under general anesthetic.

CHOANAL ATRESIA

This rare anomaly is due to failure of breakdown of the nasobuccal membrane, which normally occurs at 6 weeks' fetal development. The incidence bilaterally is one in 8000 but unilateral atresia is more common. Of these cases, 50% are associated with the choanal atresia with ear, eye, heart and genital defects (CHARGE) syndrome.

Gasping respiration in a neonate is suggestive of choanal atresia.

Bilateral choanal atresia is a neonatal emergency. The nose-breathing neonate may gasp and make significant respiratory efforts but soon becomes hypoxic and requires airway support. Some cases may mouth breathe, but then have difficulty when feeding. The diagnosis is by suspicion, by inability to pass a catheter along the nose and confirmation by endoscopic examination. The treatment consists of establishment of either an oral or orotracheal airway. A CT scan is carried out to determine the characteristics and extent of the atresia. Reviews using CT studies suggest that most atresias contain both bony and membranous components. Corrective endoscopic surgery is carried out as soon as is practicable.[13]

DISEASES OF THE NASOPHARYNX
Adenoids (nasopharyngeal tonsil)

These are part of the Waldeyer's ring of lymphoid tissue, which protects the upper airway. Adenoids are normally small at birth but enlarge from 18 months and regress normally at 8–9 years.

Adenoid hypertrophy

Since all children have adenoids, obstruction is a result of either a relatively small nasopharynx or large adenoids. Persistent enlargement causes snoring and often results in children having upper respiratory tract infections that last for 3–4 weeks instead of for 7–10 d. Such children usually mouth breathe and have hyponasal speech. There is an association between enlarged or infected adenoids and middle ear disease.

Adenoid hypertrophy is suspected with the above history and on the finding of a patent anterior nasal airway. Confirmation of adenoid size can be carried out by a lateral soft tissue X-ray of the neck (Fig. 32.2). In mild or intermittent cases, treatment is reassurance that the adenoids will go away. Surgery should be reserved for more persistent problems.

Adenoiditis

Adenoiditis occurs with viral infections and exacerbates nasal blockage. It can be quite severe in a small child with fever and purulent nasal discharge. A broad-spectrum antibiotic for 5 d is indicated in severe cases.

Adenoidectomy

Removal of the adenoids is indicated for:
1. airway obstruction in a small child (see airway obstruction, tonsillitis);
2. severe persistent nasal obstruction;
3. recurrent acute otitis media;
4. otitis media with effusion.

Primary or secondary hemorrhage occurs in about one case in 200.

Angiofibroma

This is a benign tumor of the back of the nose and nasopharynx that presents in males in their early teens. Its symptoms are of nasal blockage

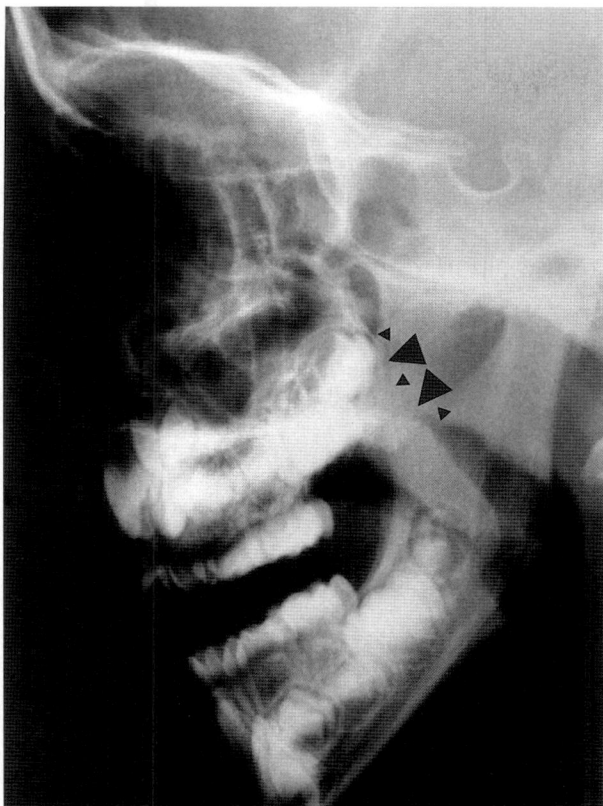

Fig. 32.2   Lateral soft tissue X-ray of a 4-year-old boy showing enlarged adenoids occluding the postnasal airway (arrowed).

with epistaxis. If expansion is rapid, cranial nerve compression can occur. The diagnosis is confirmed by endoscopy and a CT scan. Treatment is by surgery initially, radiotherapy being reserved for intracranial extension.

DISEASES OF THE PHARYNX

Pharyngitis

This is very common and usually of viral origin. It is a common presenting symptom of many upper respiratory tract infections, including the common cold, and may also precede the exanthemata of rubella or measles. There is generalized inflammation of the pharynx and often rhinitis. Treatment is supportive with antipyretics and analgesics as necessary.

Tonsils

The palatine tonsils, like the adenoids, are part of the body's defensive mechanism and serve to protect the upper airway from infection. Their removal, however causes no subsequent immunological problems, nor is it associated with any deleterious long-term effect.

Acute tonsillitis

This is commonest between the ages of 3 and 8, but can occur at any age. Of these cases, 50% are viral and 50% are bacterial, with the beta-hemolytic streptococcus being commonest, although *Staphylococcus aureus*, *Pneumococcus* and *H. influenzae* are also implicated.

The onset is abrupt, with pain in the throat, associated shivering and a pyrexia up to 39°C. The pain may be severe and radiate to the ears. Swallowing is acutely sore and solid food is refused, although fluids may be accepted. The disease progresses over 48 h, even with antibiotic therapy, and the swelling of the throat and the tonsils results in dysphagia for fluids and even for saliva that may dribble from the mouth. Speech may become thick and muffled and there is often painful enlargement of cervical glands.

On examination, the mucosa of the pillars of the fauces and soft palate are congested and as the disease progresses the tongue becomes coated and the breath become offensive. The tonsils are swollen and inflamed, with a purulent exudate. In severe cases, edema of the palate and the uvula may make the voice muffled and thick. Sometimes in streptococcal infections a scarlatiniform rash appears over the body.

Investigation

Throat cultures showing Group A beta-hemolytic *Streptococcus* may confirm the diagnosis but a negative culture does not rule it out. There is also a high asymptomatic carrier rate of this *Streptococcus*.[14] Throat swabs should not be carried out routinely in sore throats according to the Scottish Intercollegiate Guidelines Network (SIGN) guidelines.[15]

Rapid antigen testing, e.g. antistreptolysin O titer, although widely used and although showing a high specificity, shows a low sensitivity compared both with throat culture and clinical assessment.[16,17] Rapid antigen testing should therefore not be carried out routinely in the case of a sore throat.[15]

Differential diagnosis

1. *Infectious mononucleosis*. This occurs in older children and is often accompanied by marked lymphadenopathy in the neck and other areas. The child is miserable with throat discomfort due to generalized congestion of the throat and swelling of the tonsils. Serological confirmation can resolve doubt and treatment is supportive with analgesia and fluids.
2. *Viral pharyngitis*. In this condition, the child is less ill and has other symptoms, e.g. a blocked-up nose.
3. *Herpangina*. This self-limiting condition due to Coxsackie virus has papular, vesicular and ulcerative lesions on the anterior pillars of the fauces, palate and tonsils.
4. *Herpes simplex stomatitis*. This may be quite severe although it is self-limiting in the toddler, with severe pain and drooling of saliva from the pain of swallowing.
5. *Moniliasis*. White patches are present on the tongue and on the tonsils and pharynx. This is usually associated with immunodeficiency but can occur after antibiotic therapy.

Treatment

In mild tonsillitis, analgesia, usually paracetamol, and adequate fluid intake is all that is required. Antibiotics are of limited use in most people with sore throats[18] but it has been traditional in more severe cases to give penicillin V for 7–10 d. Erythromycin has been used where there is penicillin sensitivity. Amoxicillin or co-amoxiclav if given to a child with mononucleosis will result in an extensive skin rash. Parenteral penicillin may be required in persistent cases. The child should be encouraged to drink and eat a soft diet if possible. There is no clear evidence that the use of antibiotics in tonsillitis expedites symptomatic improvement, prevents rheumatic fever or glomerulonephritis or reduces the occurrence of suppurative complications, e.g. quinsy.[15]

> There is no good evidence that antibiotics for tonsillitis alter the course or severity of the acute episode.

Complications of tonsillitis

1. *Peritonsillitis*. Inflammation spreads outwith the tonsillar area and the child develops increasing pain and fever, often with significant swelling of the soft palate. Parenteral penicillin for 3–4 d can be changed to oral medication as the fever and pain subside.
2. *Peritonsillar abscess (quinsy)*. When peritonsillitis localizes, an abscess can form. Although this condition is less common in children, it still presents as a serious and potentially lethal complication. It occurs during or just after an acute attack of tonsillitis, presenting with increasing pain and swelling, usually on one side of the throat, with marked dysphagia and often otalgia. The child will have difficulty in opening his mouth. Examination can be difficult because of trismus but will show the affected tonsil to be very red, covered in pus and pushed medially. In addition,

there will be gross swelling and redness of the palate and marked cervical lymphadenopathy on the ipsilateral side. If untreated, the abscess can spread to give rise to a parapharyngeal abscess with the risk of spread to the base of the skull or even into the superior mediastinum. The treatment is drainage under general anesthetic and can be a hazardous procedure. If it is not certain that pus is present, i.v. penicillin or erythromycin is given with fluids and analgesics.

3. *Airway obstruction.* This usually occurs in children aged 2–3 as a result of chronic hypertrophy of the adenoids and tonsils. The child breathes noisily at night and often during the day. Occasionally the parents will volunteer that the child stops breathing for short periods during the night and this can cause them some understandable alarm. At other times more direct questioning is required to elicit this symptom. If untreated, this relatively common complication of tonsillitis can lead to chronic hypoxia, pulmonary hypertension and, in severe cases, cor pulmonale. Where there is any suggestion of airway obstruction, the child should undergo a sleep study with monitoring of the oxygen saturation. If there are episodes of desaturation, indicative of sleep apnea, and there is no other cause for the airway obstruction, adenotonsillectomy usually cures the condition.[19] Such children should be admitted to the high-dependency unit on the night of surgery and their breathing pattern should be monitored. In some more severe cases the respiratory drive is depressed. Oxygen may be needed until the respiratory drive returns to normal.

4. *Rheumatic fever and glomerulonephritis.* These are very rarely seen now as a complication of tonsillitis.

Indications for tonsillectomy

The following are indications for tonsillectomy (enlargement of the tonsils on their own is not an indication for their removal):

1. Airway obstruction in small children with persistent noisy breathing and suspected or proven sleep apnea. The adenoids will also be removed.
2. Suspicion of other pathology, e.g. lymphoma, is also an absolute indication. There is usually a change in the architecture of the tonsil that would suggest lymphoma.
3. Two or more attacks of peritonsillar abscess.[20]
4. Recurrent acute tonsillitis. By this is meant five or six attacks of definite tonsillitis in 1 year.[15] This number has been arrived at arbitrarily.[21] Mild symptoms do not benefit from surgery.[22]

Complications of tonsillectomy

A primary hemorrhage occurs within the first 24 h in 0.5–1.0% of children. Usually this is in the first 6 h after surgery and the child will start coughing up blood or, if unrecognized, may vomit a variable quantity of blood. After fluid replacement the child is returned to the operating room, where the bleeding vessels are identified and controlled by diathermy or ligature. A secondary hemorrhage occurs after 7–10 d. Often the child's throat will have started to become sore again and he then becomes aware of blood coming into his mouth. These children should be admitted, cross-matched and i.v. access obtained.

A broad-spectrum antibiotic such as amoxicillin is administered and local treatment consisting of hydrogen peroxide gargles and, occasionally, local adrenaline swabs can be carried out. If the bleeding persists, return to theater for ligature of the vessels or in rare cases packing of the tonsillar fossa.

DISORDERS OF PHONATION

Dysphonia

Dysphonia, or difficulty in producing sound, is usually associated with laryngeal disease (hoarseness). Some children have weakness or roughness of their voice in the course of an upper respiratory tract infection, this being a manifestation of laryngitis. Following recovery the voice usually returns to normal and no further investigation is required. Persistent hoarseness should be investigated and this can only be done by visualization of the larynx with a fiberoptic endoscope passed along the nose, into the nasopharynx. This can be done in the clinic where the child is cooperative but where this is not possible, examination under a general anesthetic is indicated to define the pathology.

The causes of hoarseness in children are as follows:

1. *Vocal nodules.* These occur at the junction between the anterior third and posterior two thirds of the vocal cords. They are usually secondary to voice abuse and in loud and noisy children are known as 'screamers' nodes. Small nodules can improve with speech therapy or if the nodules grow, surgery involving microscopic dissection is indicated. Histology shows hypertrophic squamous epithelium with underlying edema of Reinke's space.
2. *Polyps of the larynx.* These occur spontaneously or following intubation and cause variable hoarseness. They are removed under general anesthetic.
3. *Laryngeal papillomas.* These are a rare cause of hoarseness associated with maternal genital warts (papilloma virus). They present as persistent hoarseness, sometimes with aphonia and occasionally airway obstruction. Treatment is by removal and multiple operations may be required. They do not become malignant but can spread into the trachea and in rare cases, into the bronchus.
4. *Unilateral vocal cord paralysis.* This can follow surgical or nonsurgical trauma to the neck, or occur following viral infections including mononucleosis. The voice may be breathy if the cord is abducted or well maintained if the cord is medialized. The diagnosis is usually made on fiberoptic endoscopy, and treatment consists of speech therapy.

Aphonia

Complete loss of voice can occasionally occur with laryngeal pathology, e.g. papillomas, and in most cases the larynx should be visualized. Complete aphonia in an otherwise healthy child should be viewed with suspicion. Functional or 'hysterical' aphonia occurs after emotional or physical trauma, e.g. tonsillectomy. It usually affects older children and in most cases is self-correcting. Occasionally a laryngoscopy may have to be carried out to establish the diagnosis, but usually explanation of the problem together with counseling will suffice.

REFERENCES (* Level 1 evidence)

The ear

*1. Uhari M, Niemala M, Hietala J. Prediction of acute otitis media with symptoms and signs. Acta Paediatrics 1995; 84:90–92.

*2. Glasziou PP, DelMar CB, Sanders SL, et al. Antibiotics for acute otitis media in children (Cochrane Review). In: The Cochrane Library, Issue 4 Oxford: Update Software; 2002.

*3. Kozyrskyj AL, Hildes-Ripstein GE, Longstaffe SEA, et al. Short course antibiotics for otitis media (Cochrane Review). In: The Cochrane Library, 1. Oxford: Update Software; 2001.

*4. Maw AR, Parker AJ, Lance GN, et al. The effects of parental smoking on outcome after treatment for glue ear in children. Clin Otolaryngol 1992; 17:411–414.

*5. SIGN – Scottish Intercollegiate Guidelines Network. Diagnosis and management of childhood otitis media in primary care. Sign publication 66; 2003.

*6. Butler CC, van der Voort JH. Oral or topical nasal steroids for hearing loss associated with otitis media with effusion in children. In: Cochrane Library 1. Oxford; 2001.

*7. Lous J, Burton MJ, Felding JV, et al. Grommets (ventilation tubes) for hearing loss associated with otitis media with effusion in children. Cochrane Database Syst Rev. 2005. Jan 25 (1): CD001801.

*8. MRC Multicentre Otitis Media Study group. Risk factors for persistence of bilateral otitis media with effusion. Clin Otol. 2001; 26:147–156.

*9. Rovers MM, Black N, Browning GG, et al. Grommets in otitis media with effusion: an individual patient meta analysis. Arch Dis Child 2005; 90: 480–485.

The nose, sinuses and throat

*10. Morris P, Leach A. Antibiotics for persistent nasal discharge (rhonosinusitis) in children. Oxford: Cochrane Library; 2006.

*11.   Arjmand EM, Lusk RP, Muntz HR. Acute sinusitis, children and the eye. Otolaryngol Head Neck Surgery 1993; 109:886–894.

*12.   Bluestone CD, Stool SE. Paediatric otolaryngology. WB Saunders; 1982; 793–796.

*13.   Brown OE, Pownell P, Manning SC. Choanal atresia: a new anatomic classification and clinical management applications. Laryngoscope 1996; 106: 97–101.

*14.   Feery BJ, Forsell P, Guylasekharam M. Streptococcal sore throat in general practice – a controlled study. Med J Aust 1976; 1:989–991.

*15.   SIGN – Scottish Intercollegiate Guidelines Network. Management of sore throat and indications for tonsillectomy. SIGN publication 34; 1999.

*16.   Lewey S, White GB, Lieberman MM, et al. Evaluation of the throat culture as a follow up for an initially negative enzyme immunosorbent assay rapid streptococcal antigen detection test. Paediatr Infect Dis J 1988; 7:765–769.

*17.   Burke P, Bain J, Lowes A, et al. Rational decisions in managing sore throat: evaluation of a rapid test. Br Med J 1988; 296:1646–1649.

*18.   Del Mar CB, Glasziou PP, Spinks AB. Antibiotics for sore throat. Oxford: Cochrane Library; 2006.

*19.   Strading JR, Thomas G, Warley ARH, et al. Effect of adeno-tonsillectomy, on nocturnal hyponaemia, sleep disturbance and symptoms in snoring children. Lancet 1990; 335:249–253.

*20.   Wolf M, Euen-Chen I, Talmi YP, et al. Tonsillectomy following peritonsillar abscess. Int J Paediatr Otolaryngol 1995; 31:43–46.

*21.   Paradise JL, Bluestone CD, Bachman RZ, et al. Efficacy of tonsillectomy for recurrent throat infection in severely affected children. Results of parallel randomised and non-randomised clinical trials. N Engl J Med 1984; 310:674–683.

*22.   van Staaij BK, van den Akker EH, Rovers MM, et al. Effectiveness of adenotonsillectomy in children with mild symptoms of throat infections or adenotonsillar hypertrophy; open randomized trial. Br Med J 2004; 329:651–654.

33

Allergic disorders

Peter D Arkwright, Timothy J David

DEFINITIONS AND EXPLANATION OF TERMS

The widespread misuse of the word 'allergy' causes confusion. It is essential to have a definition or explanation of terms as follows.

ALLERGY

Allergy is a reproducible adverse reaction to an extrinsic substance mediated by an immunological response, irrespective of the precise mechanism. The substance provoking the reaction may have been ingested, injected, inhaled or may merely have come into contact with the skin or mucous membranes. The terms 'allergy' and 'hypersensitivity' have the same meaning and are interchangeable.

ATOPY

There is no good definition of atopy. The term was introduced to describe the 'asthma and hay fever group' of diseases. Subsequently, atopy has been redefined as a hereditary predisposition to the production of IgE antibody, an unsatisfactory oversimplification. The atopic diseases comprise atopic dermatitis, asthma, allergic rhinoconjunctivitis and some cases of urticaria. The association between food allergy and these atopic diseases is so strong that there is a case for considering food allergy as an atopic disease.[1]

ANAPHYLAXIS

The term 'anaphylaxis' is usually reserved for an allergic reaction associated with severe, life-threatening circulatory and/or respiratory compromise.

FOOD INTOLERANCE

Food intolerance is a reproducible adverse reaction to a specific food or food ingredient, and it is not psychologically based. Food intolerance occurs even when the subject cannot identify the type of food that has been given. This definition does not take into account dosage. Clearly any food in vast excess will cause a reproducible adverse reaction. Such events are not generally covered by the term 'food intolerance'.

IMMUNE MECHANISMS AND TIMING OF THE ALLERGIC RESPONSE

When the skin, airways, or conjunctivae are challenged by a single dose of allergen, an allergic reaction can be classified as immediate, delayed or dual (that is both immediate and delayed). Two main immune mechanisms determine the timing of these allergic responses (see Table 33.1). Immediate (acute) reactions usually occur within

Table 33.1   Immune mechanisms leading to allergic reactions

Mechanism	Clinical characteristics
Direct, IgE- or IgG-mediated **mast cell degranulation** with release of proinflammatory mediators (e.g. histamine, bradykinin, leukotrienes, platelet-activating factor)	Immediate/acute hypersensitivity reactions
RAST and SPT only useful if IgE mediated	Rapid onset (usually minutes)
	Urticaria/angioedema, rhinoconjunctivitis/pharyngeal edema/bronchospasm, hypotension, vomiting/diarrhea, anaphylaxis
	Mainstay of pharmacological treatment: antihistamines, adrenaline for anaphylaxis
T-lymphocyte-mediated, release of cytokines and chemokines	Delayed hypersensitivity reactions
RAST and SPT not indicated	Slower onset over hours/days
	Contact dermatitis/atopic dermatitis, chronic asthma, allergic enterocolitis
	Mainstay of pharmacological treatment: topical/local corticosteroids

minutes of contact with the allergen and are caused by mast cell degranulation usually triggered by antigen cross-linking IgE on the mast cell surface. Delayed hypersensitivity reactions may occur hours after contact with the allergen and are mediated by T-lymphocytes and the inflammatory cytokines they release. Although IgE-based allergy (skin prick tests and serum-specific IgE [RAST]) tests may be useful in the diagnostic workup of some immediate-type allergic reactions, they are not useful in delayed reactions, which are typically not IgE mediated. A summary of the types of the clinical spectrum of diseases is given in Table 33.2. The pathogenesis and mechanisms of allergic disorders are reviewed in more detail elsewhere.[2,3] It should be noted that some allergic reactions, for example reversible airway obstruction (asthma) may be mediated by both humoral and cellular immune mechanisms.

Table 33.2   Clinical spectrum of allergic disease based and immune responses aimed at allergen avoidance and removal

Body interface		
Skin	Respiratory tract	Gastrointestinal tract
A. Diseases		
Urticaria (humoral)	Rhinoconjunctivitis (humoral)	Food intolerance (humoral/cellular)
Atopic eczema (cellular)	Asthma (humoral/cellular)	
B. Protective responses against allergens		
Pruritus (rubbing/ scratching)	Copious secretions Sneezing and coughing	Vomiting and diarrhea
Hyperkeratosis (barrier)	Bronchospasm (prevent/reduce further exposure)	

HYGIENE HYPOTHESIS

The hygiene hypothesis is derived from the notion that infections and unhygienic contact might confer protection against the development of allergic illness.[4–6] The hypothesis attempts to reconcile the following facts:

- ***Increase in the prevalence of atopic diseases over the last few decades:*** The prevalence of atopic diseases (atopic dermatitis, asthma and allergic rhinitis) has doubled over the last few generations.[7] These diseases are largely a problem of developed countries such as the UK, USA, Australasia and Canada. Within these countries, the affluent within these communities (social classes I and II) are most commonly affected. Because this increase in prevalence has occurred over only a few generations, it must be due to environmental rather than genetic causes.[8]
- ***Increase in certain autoimmune conditions over the last few decades:*** What is often less appreciated is that as well as a rise in allergic diseases, there has been a parallel increase in some autoimmune conditions, such as multiple sclerosis, Crohn's disease and insulin-dependent diabetes mellitus. Other autoimmune diseases have either shown little change in prevalence (ulcerative colitis) or a reduced prevalence (rheumatoid arthritis).
- ***Reduction in exposure to certain environmental microbes, particularly those spread via the orofecal route, over the same time period:*** This evidence comes from two main sources. Firstly, a Japanese study of 867 children over the age of 12 years showed a clear negative relationship between delayed hypersensitivity responses to tuberculin and the presence of asthma.[9] Secondly, a number of studies performed in Switzerland, Austria and Germany have provided convincing evidence that growing up on a farm with regular contact with farm animals protects against allergic sensitization and the development of childhood allergic diseases.[10–12]

Based on these observations, the hygiene hypothesis proposes that certain environmental viruses and bacteria help to induce immune tolerance to normally innocuous environmental antigens (allergens) and self (autoantigens). The hypothesis is that reduced exposure to these environmental microbes, associated with modern western living has led to a lack of immune tolerance and thus an increase in immune hypersensitivity, atopy and autoimmunity.

GENETICS OF ALLERGY AND ALLERGIC DISORDERS

As well as environmental factors, there is no doubt that genetic factors are also important in the development of atopic diseases. Evidence for this comes from a number of sources:

- ***Epidemiology: family history and twin studies:*** Strong family history of atopic disease in many affected individuals, as well as twin studies point to a strong genetic influence.[13] For instance, the risk of atopic disease in the general community is approximately 10%, but this increases to 50% if one parent is affected and up to 75% if both parents are affected. Twin studies suggest that the genetic component accounts for approximately 80% of the predisposition to atopic dermatitis, asthma, allergic rhinoconjunctivitis and peanut allergy.
- ***Polygenic disease:*** In most cases, predisposition to allergic diseases is thought to be due to not one but the additive or synergistic effect of a number of genes. Rarely single gene mutations may cause allergic symptoms such as the FoxP3 gene in IPEX and the WASP gene in Wiskott–Aldrich syndrome (see Chapter 27).
- ***Specific genes largely unknown:*** The specific genes causing allergic disease in most patients are still unknown. Although numerous candidate genes have been implicated in the development of atopy, definitive evidence linking any one of these genes as a major cause of clinical atopy is lacking.[14]
- ***Candidate genes now thought to relate to molecules sensing foreign antigens and those involved in immune tolerance induction:*** Current research is focusing on genes that regulate the

innate and acquired immune responses, particularly genes that code for receptors on dendritic cells and T-lymphocytes recognizing foreign microbes (e.g. CD14, TLR 2, 4, 6, 10, TIM3).[15-17] Genetic factors that are important in regulatory immune cell function (FoxP3, TGF-β, IL-10) are also being studied.[18]

CLINICAL SPECTRUM OF DISEASE

Clinical features of allergic disease occur mainly at the three major interfaces between the body and its environment: the skin, upper and lower respiratory tract and gastrointestinal system. This subdivision, although paralleling the types of pediatric specialists to whom such patients will be referred (namely dermatologists, respiratory physicians and gastroenterologists), is artificial. Moreover in some ways it may be unhelpful to characterize allergic diseases in this way. For instance, acute allergic reactions to ingested food may manifest not only as vomiting and diarrhea, but in some cases solely as cutaneous urticaria and in others as acute pharyngeal angioedema or bronchospasm, or in yet other cases with clinical features related to all three systems. Allergic disease is primarily a systemic illness with many overlapping features.

SKIN

URTICARIA

Acute urticaria

Acute urticaria is the result of a variety of causes (often not identified) and mechanisms. The proportion of cases in which a cause is found varies; in childhood the most common is viral infection. Urticaria may develop during an illness or within 1–2 weeks after the illness, and remain a problem for a few days or weeks. Immediate allergic reactions to foods are the other major cause of acute urticaria. A parent notices, for example, that whenever a child eats fish his lips swell and he develops an urticarial rash. Fish is avoided, and the problem disappears. Occasional lapses of avoidance either demonstrate continued intolerance or, with time, loss of symptoms. Cases that come to medical attention are mostly severe (e.g. associated with pharyngeal edema), atypical, or associated with other disorders, notably atopic eczema. The common foods incriminated (cows' milk, egg, nuts, fish, tomatoes and fruit) are similar to those that cause allergic contact urticaria (see later), the difference being that children are in general more likely to touch raw foods than to eat them, and raw foods are on the whole more likely to trigger urticaria than cooked foods.

Allergic contact urticaria

This is an immediate allergic reaction, and should not be confused with contact dermatitis, which represents a delayed reaction. Although certain foods, such as cows' milk, raw eggs, raw potatoes, raw fish, apples and nuts are particularly common causes, any food containing protein could in theory cause allergic contact urticaria. The tissues and secretions of pet mammals are also common causes of allergic contact urticaria in childhood. Other causes are grass pollen, chemicals, a number of drugs applied topically, and a few vehicles contained in topical medicaments.

Irritant contact urticaria

Common causes are plants such as stinging nettles or creatures such as jellyfish, moths and caterpillars. Chemicals are a major cause of irritant contact urticaria, and the relevant chemicals are widely used in food, medicines and cosmetics.

Chronic urticaria

Chronic urticaria is defined as urticaria that has persisted for more than 6 weeks and affects the patient for several days each week. The condition can be associated with serious adverse effects on quality of life, sleep and daily activities, but is rarely associated with systemic features or life-threatening anaphylaxis.[19,20] Of these patients, 40% also have angioedema. Very few cases are caused by allergy and therefore allergy testing is rarely indicated. One half are associated with physical triggers such as cold, heat, sunlight, or stress (home or school). An autoimmune etiology should be considered, particularly in teenage girls and where there is a personal or family history of autoimmune disease, especially thyroid disease. In these cases IgG autoantibodies bind specifically to Fcε receptors on mast cells triggering degranulation. Thyroid function should be monitored in this subgroup of children, as up to one third of patients are at risk of autoimmune thyroid disease. In younger children viral or bacterial infections may also trigger the condition. Salicylates in drugs and sometimes foods can also provoke urticaria.[21] Rarely chronic urticaria may be a manifestation of cutaneous mastocytosis and therefore a careful examination of the skin is required. The natural history varies with the cause. Urticaria caused by infection or drugs is most likely to resolve, while physical and autoimmune urticaria often persists for years. Most cases respond to avoidance of obvious triggers and oral antihistamines. For refractory or more urticarial vasculitis as detailed later, immunosuppressive drugs may be required and referral to a specialist is indicated.

If urticaria persists in one location for over 48 h, or leaves residue (e.g. hyperpigmentation), or is associated with purpura or systemic manifestations (arthritis, fever, etc.) an underlying vasculitis (urticarial vasculitis) should be considered.[22,23] Skin manifestations are typically recurrent episodes of urticaria-like weals, often associated with arthralgia (50%) and angioedema (40%). In addition to the skin, the respiratory (20%), renal (5–10%) and gastrointestinal (20%) systems are most frequently involved in the disease. Urticarial vasculitis is most commonly an acquired idiopathic phenomenon but may occur in association with other disorders, most often systemic lupus erythematosus (SLE), Sjögren syndrome and serum sickness. Of these patients, 60–80% is female. Investigations should include a skin biopsy with immunofluorescent staining for immunoglobulin deposits. The most common laboratory abnormalities reported are an elevated ESR, hypocomplementemia and circulating immune complexes. Measurement of serum complement is useful prognostically, as hypocomplementemia is associated with more serious systemic involvement. There is no universally effective therapy for urticarial vasculitis but commencing treatment with antihistamines and proceeding through nonsteroidal anti-inflammatory drugs (NSAIDs), to colchicine, dapsone or hydroxychloroquine. If these medications do not achieve control, systemic steroids and azathioprine can be tried. The causes of urticaria and angioedema (see later) are listed in Table 33.3.

Table 33.3 Classification of urticaria and angioedema

Urticaria
1. Local irritants: plants, jellyfish, chemicals
2. Direct mast cell activation: opiates, antibiotics, curare, contrast media physical (cold: consider cryoglobulinemia, solar: consider SLE and porphyria, exercise, cholinergic, vibration)
3. Agents altering arachidonic acid metabolism: aspirin/NSAIDs, benzoates
4. IgE mediated: allergen mediated (pollens, dander, foods, worms, molds, *Hymenoptera* venom, drugs)
5. IgG mediated: viral infections, autoimmune (associated with other autoimmune diseases, especially thyroid disease), urticarial vasculitis
6. Idiopathic

Angioedema
1. Complement inhibitor deficiency: hereditary angioedema
2. Complement activation: vasculitis, infections, serum sickness
3. Angiotensin-converting enzyme (ACE) inhibitors

ANGIOEDEMA

Unlike urticaria, where the inflammatory edema is in the superficial dermis, in angioedema the swelling is mainly in the deeper subcutaneous and submucosal layers. Angioedema may be painful rather than pruritic, and commonly affects the face and extremities. In the upper respiratory tract it is associated with swelling of the lips, tongue, and pharyngeal tissues, which may rarely lead to life-threatening upper airway obstruction. Angioedema of the gastrointestinal tract usually manifests as abdominal pain. The major mediators of angioedema are plasma kinins (e.g. bradykinin), the activation of which is inhibited by C1 inhibitor and other protease inhibitors. Angioedema is associated with urticaria in 80% of cases; in the remaining 20% of cases angioedema occurs without any urticaria.

Hereditary angioedema

The most important differential diagnosis of allergy-induced angioedema is hereditary angioedema, because the prognosis and management of this condition is different.[24] In the past, the mortality rate for attacks involving the upper airways were around one third of patients. Subcutaneous, respiratory and gastrointestinal tract angioedema characteristic of hereditary angioedema is due to an autosomal dominantly inherited deficiency of C1 esterase inhibitor.[25] Swelling of the gastrointestinal mucosa results in nausea, vomiting, diarrhea and severe pain that can mimic a surgical emergency. The subcutaneous swellings are disfiguring but not erythematous, pruritic or painful. The angioedema is solely mediated by kinins and never associated with urticaria. That is why angioedema in combination with urticaria rules out a diagnosis of hereditary angioedema. Interestingly the pulmonary vascular tree is spared, probably because the cells lining the pulmonary vessels have surface enzymes that inactivate bradykinin and other kinins. Symptoms can last from 1–4 d. Symptom frequency may vary from very few, if any, particularly in prepubertal children, to frequent daily or weekly episodes.

The diagnosis of hereditary angioedema should be considered if: (1) angioedema occurs without urticaria; (2) there is an atypical pattern of angioedema (hands, feet, abdomen rather than face); (3) there is a family history (but 20% of cases are sporadic); (4) there are abdominal symptoms. There are two types of disease: type 1 (85% of cases) due to absent C1 inhibitor and type 2 (15% of cases) where there are normal or elevated levels of C1 inhibitor antigen, but the protein is dysfunctional.

Diagnosis in suspected cases is made by measuring C1 inhibitor levels and function as well as C4, which may be low only during acute attacks.

Unlike allergen-mediated urticaria and angioedema, antihistamines, adrenaline (epinephrine) and steroids are of little or no use in the treatment of hereditary angioedema. C1 esterase inhibitor concentrate, which should be available in all hospital emergency departments, is the treatment of choice for pharyngeal edema and severe abdominal attacks. If the concentrate is not available, fresh-frozen plasma may be used. Danazol can be used as prophylaxis in postpubertal children and non-pregnant adults. In younger children the plasmin inhibitor tranexamic acid is an alternative. Angiotensin-converting enzyme (ACE) inhibitors may precipitate attacks by blocking bradykinin degradation and should be avoided, as should estrogen-based contraceptives.

ALLERGIC ASPECTS OF ATOPIC DERMATITIS

Approximately 10% of infants attending community clinics and up to 30% of infants and young children attending specialist allergy clinics may benefit from antigen avoidance regimens.[26,27] Older children are less likely to respond to dietary manipulation, and avoidance of aeroallergens that might influence their disease is often not practical. Thus the first-line management (see also Chapter 30) is usually symptomatic treatment with emollients and topical steroids, recognition and treatment of bacterial and viral skin infection, and use of sedating H_1 antihistamines at night. The situations in which antigen avoidance should be considered are:

1. **Severe disease.** Exclusion diets are highly disruptive to family life, and are potentially nutritionally hazardous, so it makes little sense to employ a diet when the condition is mild (< 10% of the skin surface area affected) and easily controlled with simple topical therapy. Such diets are more appropriate if 25% or more of the skin surface area is affected.
2. **History.** A history of immediate urticarial or gastrointestinal reactions to foods is common. It is sensible to avoid foods for which there is a clear history of an immediate allergic reaction.
3. **Multiple atopic disorders in infancy.** The occurrence of more than one atopic disorder appears to increase the possibility of an important allergic element. This is especially true if atopic features such as eczema, asthma or rhinitis are accompanied by gastrointestinal symptoms such as persistent loose stools or vomiting.
4. **Age.** Elimination diets are simpler to administer and control in infancy and results are better at this age.
5. **Severe eczema in exclusively breast-fed infants.** In one study, in six of 37 breast-fed infants eczema improved when the mother avoided cows' milk protein and egg and relapsed when these were reintroduced.[28] It is often difficult to predict which baby would respond to maternal dietary exclusion. It is reasonable to try maternal avoidance of cows' milk and egg in an infant with eczema who is being exclusively breast-fed. Other foods can provoke eczema in this way, but their detection relies on the suspicions of a parent or doctor followed by avoidance and later challenge.

ANTIGEN AVOIDANCE IN ATOPIC DERMATITIS
Diets

The important principles underlying any elimination diet are:
1. The diet should in the first instance be tried for a defined period of time (e.g. 6 weeks in patients with eczema) and not just imposed indefinitely.
2. At the end of this period the patient should be reassessed to see if the diet has been helpful. If it has not, then the diet should be discontinued. If the diet has helped, and the parents and doctor feel that the therapeutic benefit outweighs the inconvenience of the diet, then the items omitted should be reintroduced one by one (in eczema at the rate of about one new food every 5–7 d).
3. The help of a dietitian is important to ensure that specific food items have been properly excluded from the diet, and to ensure the nutritional adequacy of the diet.

There are a variety of exclusion diets available. Infants and toddlers are far more likely to benefit than older children.

Half-hearted attempts to 'have a go'

The very small quantity of food that can provoke an adverse reaction means that the 'try cutting down his milk' type of tinkering with the diet is most unlikely to succeed. The advantage of a carefully conducted diet is that even if it fails, at least the parents will be satisfied in the knowledge that it was tried properly.

Complete avoidance of known triggers

A trial of rigorous avoidance of known or suspected triggers is a logical first step. It is common to see a child with a clear history of intolerance to a food, but where the food is being incompletely avoided. In infants with eczema, specific avoidance of cows' milk, egg and/or wheat are most often considered. These diets are unlikely to be successful in the absence of history of the eczema being made worse by these foods.

Avoidance of 10 common food triggers

The patient avoids approximately 10 common food triggers, plus foods for which there is a history of intolerance. The foods usually chosen for exclusion are cows' milk, egg, wheat, fish, legumes (pea, bean, soya, lentil), tomato, nuts, berries and currants, citrus fruit and food additives

Table 33.4 Measures that kill the house dust mite and reduce levels of mite antigen in the home

1. Reducing indoor relative humidity below 50%
   High-efficiency dehumidifiers
2. Removal of dust mites and allergens
   Washing bed linen in hot water (≥55°C)
   Adding benzyl benzoate (0.03%) to wash cycle
   Tumble drying bed linen ((≥55°C for more than 10 min)
   Dry cleaning
   Replace carpets, draperies and upholstery
   Vacuuming carpets
   Freezing toys and small items (<17°C for 24 h), then wash
   Dust with damp cloth
3. Encasements
   Mattress and pillow dust mite proof encasements

(for a discussion of these see separate section later). The chances of a useful clinical benefit are small.

The few-foods diet (so-called oligoantigenic diet)

This consists of exclusion of all foods except for five or six items. These items should not include a food for which there is a history of intolerance. Such diets comprise a meat (usually lamb or turkey), three vegetables (e.g. potato, rice, and carrot or a brassica – cauliflower, cabbage, broccoli or sprouts), a fruit (usually pear) and possibly a breakfast cereal (e.g. Rice Krispies). There are scanty data on the outcome of few-foods diets. In one study, a few-foods diet was associated with marked improvement in 50% of patients (median age 2.9 years, range 0.4–14.8) with atopic eczema, but after 12 months' follow-up, the results were the same (marked improvement) in the group that improved, the group that failed to improve, and the group that tried a diet but were unable to cope.[29] In another study, 85 children (median age 2.3 years, range 0.3–13.3 years) with atopic eczema were randomly allocated to receive a few-foods diet supplemented with either a whey hydrolysate or a casein hydrolysate formula, or to remain on their usual diet and act as controls, for a 6-week period.[30] After 6 weeks, there was a significant reduction in all three groups in the percentage of surface area involved and skin severity score. Of those who participated, 16 (73%) of the 22 controls and 15 (58%) of the 24 who received the diet showed a greater than 20% improvement in the skin severity score. This is the only controlled study of a few-foods diet, and it failed to show benefit. However, the drawback to these two studies is the relatively high median age and the wide age range, which is important because it is general experience that the best results for elimination diets are in infants. Given the tendency for most children with food hypersensitivity to grow out of the problem by the age of 3 years, the inclusion of substantial numbers of older children in these studies unintentionally biased the results against finding benefit from a diet.

Elemental diet

The application of an inpatient regimen of 4–6 weeks of a so-called elemental diet (e.g. Elemental 028, Vivonex or Tolerex) is the ultimate test of whether food intolerance is relevant or not, but until more data are available this approach must be regarded as experimental.[31] The drawbacks comprise the lack of a guarantee of success, family disruption associated with 2–3 months' hospitalization, loose stools (due to hyperosmolarity of the formula), weight loss and hypoalbuminemia.

House dust mite and pet avoidance

House dust mites and pets can trigger atopic eczema. However, the number of patients who experience benefit solely from the avoidance of pets or mites appears to be small. As with elimination diets, there is no test that predicts benefit from avoidance measures. In some children, particularly those with troublesome facial eczema and periocular irritation worse first thing in the morning, the house dust mite in pillow cases and

mattresses may be a significant factor. Even though previous trials have not shown dust-proof covers to be useful in unselected patients with eczema, they may be helpful in these selected cases. A number of additional measures are recommended to kill house dust mites and remove mite antigen from homes (Table 33.4)[32] but none of these measures have been found to significantly affect the clinical severity of eczema. Some patients with atopic eczema are worse during the pollen season or after grass has been cut, but avoidance is impossible.

RESPIRATORY TRACT

ALLERGIC ASPECTS OF ASTHMA

There is no doubt that exposure to various triggers can provoke or worsen asthma in certain patients. Observations of children with unusually severe asthma who are sent to alpine resorts, where the exposure to house dust mites and pets is greatly reduced or abolished, are that somewhere between one and two thirds become completely asymptomatic and can discontinue all therapy. Return home is followed by relapse in most patients. In the past it was believed that this improvement was due to separation from parents and 'family tension', but the current doctrine is that the benefit is due to the avoidance of inhaled allergens. A history may help identify intermittent triggers that provoke attacks (e.g. cat dander), but may not identify allergens to which the patient is regularly exposed and which are responsible for maintaining the asthmatic state (e.g. house dust mites). However, there is a lack of objective investigations to establish the qualitative importance of allergy. For example, it is impossible to state, for asthmatic children of any specific age, in what proportion exposure to an animal provokes an attack of asthma, or what proportion will benefit from removal of a household pet. Some triggers are allergens, but others are not, so it is misleading to think of asthma solely as an allergic disease. Non-allergic triggers are discussed in Chapter 20.

Trigger avoidance

It is impossible to avoid triggers such as cold weather, exercise, laughing and crying. Viral infections, pollens and fungal spores are ubiquitous, and total avoidance is impossible without unacceptable restrictions.

Avoidance of pets and pet antigens is theoretically possible but often unpopular or unacceptable to the family. Removal of the animal itself is insufficient, and if the level of pet antigen in the household is to be adequately reduced then also required are intensive carpet and furniture cleaning. Complete removal of cat antigen is especially difficult (if not impossible), and because of its adhesion to wall surfaces requires washing of the walls.

Role of antigen avoidance in management of asthma

There are no objective data upon which to base clear recommendations, with the result that there are differences of opinion about the relevance of antigen avoidance. The cornerstone of the treatment of asthma is drug therapy, supplemented where possible or relevant by the avoidance of triggers. Even with the most enthusiastic approach to the identification and avoidance of triggers, it is rare for this alone to abolish symptoms. The major triggers that are at least potentially avoidable are house dust mites and pets. Since there is no clinical or laboratory test that can accurately identify those patients who will benefit from antigen avoidance, the only logical approach is to attempt a defined trial period of avoidance, including an assessment after an agreed period of time (e.g. 3 months) as to whether there has been any benefit.

ALLERGIC RHINOCONJUCTIVITIS

Allergic rhinoconjunctivitis may be either perennial or seasonal. Important triggers of perennial disease are house dust mite and pet danders. Seasonal rhinoconjunctivitis is most frequently caused by allergy to tree (spring), grass (summer) pollens or less frequently mould spores (*Cladosporium*, *Alternaria* and *Aspergillus*). Salicylate sensitivity occurs mainly in adults and may start with symptoms of perennial rhinitis and then progress to include chronic sinusitis, nasal polyposis and asthma, which may be severe.[21]

Over 50% of patients have a combination of nasal and ocular symptoms. Nasal symptoms include sneezing, rhinorrhea and nasal blockage. Eye symptoms include itching, watering, redness, swelling and stinging. A severe seasonal form associated with cobblestoning of the conjunctiva, more common in boys is sometimes called 'vernal (spring) conjunctivitis'. During an exacerbation keratitis is common, causing photophobia and reduced visual acuity, and sometimes leading to an ulcer that may in turn cause permanent loss of vision. Asthmatic symptoms sometimes coexist with attacks of hay fever.

Avoidance of allergens is often not possible and therefore the mainstay of treatment is using medication to reduce the inflammatory effects of mast cell degranulation, particularly histamine. Nonsedating H_1 antihistamines are by far the simplest and most useful treatment for mild and moderate cases, given prophylactically during the pollen season. An advantage of H_1 antihistamines is that they help to prevent both nasal and eye symptoms.

Additional prophylactic medication for more troublesome nasal symptoms is mainly topical nasal corticosteroids. Systemic nasal decongestants are not recommended in children. Sodium cromoglycate nasal spray and oral montelukast are sometimes used, but are less effective than topical corticosteroids.

For allergic conjunctivitis, eye drops are often more effective than oral antihistamines but in more troublesome cases a combination should be used. Drops containing antihistamine, mast cell stabilizer (sodium cromoglycate), nonsteroidal anti-inflammatory agents and a combination of the above are available. Sodium cromoglycate works best if applied four times a day, which is demanding.

An exceptionally severe form of allergic conjunctivitis is known as vernal conjunctivitis, and for this steroid or cyclosporine drops may be justifiable, but these can only be prescribed under the supervision of an ophthalmologist, who can monitor for complications or adverse events side-effects such as corneal abrasions, glaucoma or cataracts.

Immunotherapy in selected children with severe allergic rhinoconjunctivitis due to grass pollen allergy can alleviate symptoms. It is worth considering where there is a poor response to oral antihistamines and topical treatments, and where the illness is having a major impact on the child's life. Referral to a specialist center for allergy testing and treatment is required.

ADVERSE REACTIONS TO FOODS AND THE GASTROINTESTINAL TRACT

All eating causes reactions, for example satiety, the urge to defecate, a feeling of warmth, and weight gain. The mechanisms for food intolerance may be immunological (food allergy), metabolic (e.g. lactase deficiency), pharmacological (e.g. vasoactive amines), toxic (e.g. lectins in red kidney beans), irritant (e.g. curry) or unknown. Individuals vary in their tolerance of events.

The prevalence of reported food intolerance in children ranges widely from 6 – 18%,[33,34] a problem with these figures being that only about one third of parental reports of food intolerance can be confirmed when tested by blind food challenge. Intolerance to most other foods can occur; these are mainly responsible for immediate allergic reactions. Where there is doubt about a specific food intolerance, the only reliable way to confirm or refute the diagnosis is to perform a food challenge. The management consists of avoidance. The prognosis for food intolerance in young children is good. A prospective study showed that the offending food or fruit was back in the diet after only 9 months in half the cases, and virtually all the offending foods were back in the diet by the third birthday.[35]

IgE-MEDIATED GASTROINTESTINAL HYPERSENSITIVITY DISORDERS

Symptoms of immediate gastrointestinal hypersensitivity are acute – usually occurring within minutes of consuming the food. Nausea and vomiting is very common in IgE-mediated food allergy and help to rid the body of the triggering allergen. Diarrhea may follow several hours after the initial symptoms. The usual offenders are milk, egg, peanut, soy, wheat and seafood. Similar to other IgE-dependent allergic disorders, allergy to milk, egg, wheat and soy general resolve, whereas allergies to peanuts, tree nuts and seafood are more likely to persist. Allergens that are enzymes, for example in some fruit and vegetables, are rapidly degrading by salivary and gastric enzymes and therefore symptoms are often localized to the lips and oral cavity (oral allergy syndrome).[36] Oral allergy syndrome may be preceded by the onset of pollen-induced allergic rhinoconjunctivitis and is sometimes secondary to cross-reactivity between allergens of similar structure (see Table 33.5). These include oral pruritus, angioedema of the lips, tongue and palate. In around 9% of cases symptoms are systemic and in 1% of cases they may be severe.

EOSINOPHILIC GASTROINTESTINAL DISORDERS

Eosinophilic gastrointestinal disorders (EGIDs) are defined as disorders that selectively effect the gut with eosinophil-rich inflammation in the absence of known causes for eosinophilia.[37,38] They need to be distinguished from drug reactions, parasitic infections (particularly strongyloides and ancylostoma), malignancies and inflammatory bowel disease. A family history of EGID was present in 10% of patients and 75% of cases are atopic. The prevalence is hard to estimate but seems to be as common as inflammatory bowel disease.

EGID is thought to have an allergic basis and the pathophysiology may involve either IgE or cell-mediated allergic responses. Clinical features and management vary depending on the segment of bowel affected (esophagus, stomach, small intestine, colon). Milk, egg, wheat, peanut and soy may trigger these disorders but in many cases multiple food allergies are involved. In 50% of cases there is a peripheral blood eosinophilia. Endoscopic appearance may be normal and the disease is often patchy. Diagnosis is dependent on the presence of an excessive eosinophilic infiltrate evaluated on multiple gut biopsies.

Eosinophilic esophagitis is associated with gastroesophageal reflux, vomiting, epigastric or chest pain, respiratory obstructive problems and dysphagia. The dysphagia, occurring in 85% of cases, may be severe enough to lead to impaction of food. Strictures and Barrett's esophagus may occur in chronic cases. Two thirds of patients are males and there is a high rate of atopic disease, particularly asthma. The condition has been thought of 'asthma of the esophagus'. Food allergens play a pathological role as dietary restriction or hydrolyzed formulae are associated with an improvement in 98% of children. Topical corticosteroids (the patient is instructed to swallow the dose from a metered-dose inhaler delivered without a spacer) provide long-term control but systemic steroids may be required for acute flares.

Eosinophilic gastritis and *gastroenteritis* are less well-defined entities and may present with vomiting, abdominal pain, anemia, failure to thrive and diarrhea, which may mimic Celiac disease. In such cases a jejunal biopsy usually shows some degree of villous atrophy. Treatment is similar to eosinophilic esophagitis with dietary restrictions and topical steroids (oral budesonide). The condition is often chronic waxing and waning.

Table 33.5   Common food allergy syndromes

Birch	Apples, cherries, peach, pear, nectarine, plum, apricot, hazelnut, walnut, almond, pecan, brazil (i.e. tree nuts), kiwi, carrot, celery, tomato, coconut, turnip, parsnip
Ragwood	Watermelon, cucumber, zucchini, banana
Mugwood	Celery, carrot, caraway, dill, parsley, fennel, green pepper
Grass	Potato, tomato, melon, peanut, orange, celery, kiwi
Latex	Banana, avocado, chestnut, kiwi

Eosinophilic colitis (including cows' milk protein intolerance) is the most common cause of bloody stools in infancy, is often due to cows' milk protein allergy and less commonly soy. Frequent loose stools occur in 25–75% of patients. In an uncommon but florid picture, infants can present with heavily bloodstained loose stools, sometimes accompanied by mucus. Acute abdominal pain (often but not always accompanied by vomiting or loose stools) can be a striking symptom. The acute presentation of blood in the stools and abdominal pain may mimic intussusception. Discomfort, crying or irritability are common and major features in infancy.

In contrast to eosinophilic esophagitis, eosinophilic colitis is a non-IgE mediated disease and thus RAST and skin prink tests are usually negative. In infants, exclusion of the offending food usually leads to resolution of the bloody diarrhea within 72 h and thus endoscopy and biopsy are reserved for refractory cases. The vast majority of infants outgrow the food intolerance by 1–3 years of age and therefore intermittent trials of reintroduction of the milk at 12 months old and then 6 monthly is advised. In older children the prognosis is similar to eosinophilic gastroenteritis with a chronic course.

Celiac disease

Celiac disease represents an immune response to a food protein (gluten in wheat, rye and barley) and therefore may be considered a food-allergic disorder.[39] Its prevalence is 1% in western populations. Symptoms include vomiting, diarrhea, anorexia and growth failure but are now recognized as often being more subtle or nonspecific. Thus the mean age of diagnosis has shifted from the first few years of life to middle adulthood. The α-gliadin peptide of gluten is presented particularly well by dendritic cells expressing HLA-DQ2 and/or DQ8 and > 95% of patients have these HLA types. α-gliadin cross-react with tissue transglutaminase 2 and stimulates the $\gamma\delta$T lymphocytic infiltrate and villous atrophy characteristic of this inflammatory enteropathy. Avoidance of dietary gluten leads to resolution of the disease, but this dietary restriction needs to be continued lifelong to prevent recurrences. Delay in removing gluten from the diet may be associated with an increased risk of other autoimmune diseases, particularly type I diabetes mellitus and autoimmune thyroid disease, as well as intestinal lymphoma. A detailed appraisal is given in Chapter 19.

BEHAVIORAL PROBLEMS

Both hospital and community-based double-blind placebo-controlled studies have repeatedly failed to confirm any validity in the idea that food or food additives cause severe behavioral problems in otherwise healthy individuals. The avoidance of food additives seems to have only a very short-lived beneficial effect on hyperkinesis and other behavior problems, and any benefit from additive avoidance diets is likely to be a placebo response. One source of confusion has been the presence of atopic disease. If a food additive makes eczema or asthma worse, then the concentration span and behavior may also be expected to suffer, but there is no evidence that this is anything other than an indirect effect.

IMPORTANT ALLERGENS IN CHILDREN

COWS' MILK PROTEIN

Cows' milk protein intolerance is a heterogeneous disorder and may present with symptoms of immediate (acute allergy, rarely even anaphylaxis) or delayed hypersensitivity reactions (EGID) (see section on the gastrointestinal tract earlier). Prevalence studies of intolerance to cows' milk protein vary from 1.9–7.5%. A most detailed study estimated a point prevalence of cows' milk protein intolerance in children with parentally perceived reactions at the age of 2.5 years at 1.1% (CI 0.8–1.6).[40]

The most common antigens in cows' milk are α-lactoglobulin, casein, α-lactalbumin, bovine serum albumin and bovine α-globulin. Digestion may result in the production of additional antigens. The marked antigenic similarity between cows' and goats' milk proteins explains why most children with cows' milk protein intolerance are intolerant to goats' milk. Intolerance to carbohydrates present in cows' milk and milk formulae is dealt with in Chapter 16.

The quantity of cows' milk required to produce an adverse reaction varies. Some patients develop anaphylaxis after ingestion of less than 1 mg of casein, α-lactoglobulin or α-lactalbumin. In contrast, Goldman et al[41] showed that 29 out of 89 children (33%) with cows' milk intolerance did not react to 100 ml of milk but only to 200 ml or more. The median reaction onset time in those who reacted to 100 ml milk challenges was 2 h, but the median reaction onset time in those who required larger amounts of milk to elicit reactions was 24 h.

Most cows' milk formula-fed infants with cows' milk protein intolerance develop symptoms in the first 3 months of life. The age of onset of the first symptoms in breast-fed babies depends on the age at which cows' milk is first introduced. A proportion of infants with cows' milk protein intolerance react adversely to traces of cows' milk protein in their mother's milk. Patients with cows' milk protein intolerance may be intolerant to other foods. In one hospital-based series of 100 children with cows' milk protein intolerance, over 50% exhibited intolerance to one or more other foods.[42] Approximately 8–14% of children with intolerance to cows' milk protein are also intolerant to soya protein.

Clues to the diagnosis of cows' milk protein intolerance in the history

1. Symptoms occur, or are made worse, soon after ingestion of cows' milk protein. Multiple affected systems (e.g. gut, chest and skin) make the diagnosis more likely; single symptoms make it most unlikely.
2. Symptoms date from the time, or soon after the time, that breast-feeding was stopped or cows' milk protein was first introduced into the diet. (NB feeding changes often coincide with the onset of atopic disease, and do not prove a cause-and-effect relationship)
3. There is a family history of cows' milk protein intolerance.
4. The presence of severe atopic disease in an infant under the age of 12 months.
5. The observation that spilling cows' milk onto non-eczematous skin causes an urticarial rash.

Making the diagnosis of cows' milk protein intolerance

Most patients whose symptoms commence within 20–30 min of cows' milk ingestion have a positive skin prick test, but most of those whose symptoms occur more slowly have negative skin prick tests. Skin prick tests and RAST tests are usually unhelpful, particularly if symptoms are delayed. A jejunal biopsy is unnecessary because it cannot replace the need for milk elimination and challenge, and the histological changes seen in the small intestine are not diagnostic for cows' milk protein intolerance.

The procedure required to diagnose cows' milk protein intolerance is:

1. a period of avoidance (2 d for those with symptoms occurring within 1 h of milk ingestion; 14–28 d for those with delayed-onset symptoms) causing loss of symptoms;
2. recurrence of symptoms on reintroduction of cows' milk protein;
3. loss of symptoms after second withdrawal of cows' milk protein;
4. Continued abatement of symptoms with continued avoidance of cows' milk protein.

This strategy must be accompanied by regular attempts to reintroduce cows' milk protein, for example yearly, to see if the patient has grown out of the intolerance.

Failure of cows' milk exclusion

The reasons why a trial period of cows' milk elimination may fail are:

1. The patient has an alternative cause for the reported symptoms.
2. The period of elimination was too short.
3. Foods containing cows' milk protein have not been fully excluded from the diet.

4. The patient is intolerant to the cows' milk substitute that has been given. This is common with goat's milk or sheep's milk. About 8–14% of patients with cows' milk protein intolerance are also intolerant to soya. An unknown proportion are intolerant to whey hydrolysate formulae (these vary in their antigenicity), and there are rare cases of intolerance to casein hydrolysate formulae (Pregestimil or Nutramigen).

5. The patient has a coexisting or intercurrent disease, e.g. gastroenteritis.

6. The patient is intolerant to other items that have not been withdrawn from the diet or the environment.

7. The patient's symptoms are trivial and have been exaggerated, or alternatively do not exist at all and have either been imagined or fabricated by the parents. Complete fabrication of symptoms by parents is rare, but the mistaken belief that a child's symptoms are attributable to food intolerance is common.

Milk challenge procedure

A challenge with cows' milk protein is carried out either to confirm the diagnosis or to see if the patient has grown out of the intolerance. If it is known that the child can tolerate small amounts of cows' milk at home then a formal challenge in hospital is not required, and the parents can continue to increase the quantity of cows' milk given at home.

It is vital to remember that during cows' milk protein challenge, symptoms may appear that had not been present previously, the most serious being anaphylactic shock. In Goldman et al's original study, three of 89 patients developed anaphylactic shock as a new symptom during milk challenge.[42] In a further five patients, anaphylaxis had been noted prior to milk challenge. Any strategy for cows' milk protein challenges has to take into account the risk of anaphylaxis.

Milk challenge procedure for patients with no history of anaphylaxis after cows' milk ingestion

The first step, prior to the oral administration of cows' milk, is the topical application of milk to the child's skin, using the back. Some cows' milk is firmly rubbed onto the patient's skin with a piece of gauze or cotton wool, and the skin observed for 15 min. A positive reaction comprises a weal, surrounded by a red flare; redness without a weal is a negative response. If there is a positive response, the challenge procedure is halted, and cows' milk protein should be avoided for a further 12 months before repeating the test.

It is acknowledged that a positive rub test may sometimes be a false positive, but the above strategy is designed to protect the child, and the need to minimize the risks of anaphylaxis. A small number of centers bypass the application of milk (or other foods) to the skin as part of the challenge procedure, and as a precaution conduct the challenge in a high dependency or intensive care facility, with an i.v. line inserted and i.v. fluids running. Reasons for the former more cautious approach are: (1) if there is a significant risk of a life-threatening adverse reaction then it is safer to avoid doing the food challenge altogether, (2) the first-line treatment of anaphylaxis is intramuscular adrenaline, and (3) i.v. fluids are not an immediate requirement.

For the first 60 min of the procedure, a nurse, doctor or parent should be present; the patient must not be left alone. The observer is looking for signs of an adverse reaction, which are:

- rash around the mouth;
- urticarial rash;
- sneezing;
- vomiting;
- irritability and pallor;
- wheezing or coughing;
- loose stools;
- **stridor;**
- **collapse**.

After the first 60 min, the patient should be checked half hourly, provided a parent is present, or quarter hourly if no parent is present. The observer needs to know that the signs above are being sought, and that it is just as important to remove the clothes and look for an urticarial rash as it is to perform the usual nursing observations of the temperature, pulse and respiration rate.

If any of the above signs appear, no further cows' milk should be given, and in the event of a rash, wheezing, stridor or collapse a doctor should be summoned.

The oral challenge procedure itself is:

1. Place one drop of ordinary cows' milk on the patient's tongue, and observe for 15 min.

2. If no reaction, give 5 ml of cows' milk and observe for 15 min.

3. If no reaction, give 10 ml of cows' milk and observe for 15 min.

4. If no reaction, give 30 ml of cows' milk and observe for 15 min.

5. If no reaction, give cows' milk freely, and give cows' milk protein-free solids as normal at meal times. Provided this does not exceed the usual intake volume, ensure the patient has taken at least 200 ml of cows' milk.

It is unclear how long observation in hospital should be continued. Rare cases are described in which severe reactions have developed late (e.g. 6 h after starting challenge) so parents must be warned that a reaction may develop later in the day, when the child is at home.

If any adverse reaction occurs, as well as stopping further cows' milk it is essential to monitor the patient very closely, as such patients are at special risk of suffering severe and possibly fatal collapse without warning. One may need to keep an infant in hospital overnight where a challenge has had to be stopped because of an adverse reaction. Such infants require close monitoring, including the use of an apnea alarm.

Procedure for patients with previous history of anaphylaxis after cows' milk ingestion

Serious consideration should be given to whether a cows' milk challenge is really necessary. If it is being carried out to confirm the diagnosis it is best omitted, because the risks of misdiagnosis are likely to be outweighed by the hazards of the challenge procedure. If the challenge is being carried out to see if the patient has grown out of cows' milk protein intolerance, then it is recommended that at least 12 months have elapse since the previous positive challenge or anaphylactic reaction. The challenge procedure is the same as detailed earlier.

Natural history of cows' milk protein intolerance

Cows' milk protein intolerance often lasts only a few months, and in many cases it has disappeared completely by the age of 12 months, hence the need for milk challenge at the age of 12 months in patients who were diagnosed in infancy. Most children become tolerant to cows' milk protein by the age of 3 years, although some degree of intolerance persists, occasionally into adult life, in a small number of patients.

Cows' milk-free diets

Cows' milk exclusion means the avoidance of all foods that contain cows' milk protein. A dietitian will be able to provide an appropriate diet sheet containing an up-to-date list of milk-free manufactured foods. Beef avoidance is unnecessary as the coexistence of intolerance to cows' milk and beef is unusual. Infants on a cows' milk-free diet require a cows' milk substitute. The choice is between formulae based on soya (bearing in mind that 8–14% of infants with cows' milk protein intolerance will also be intolerant to soya), casein hydrolysate (Pregestimil or Nutramigen) or amino acids (Neocate). The main drawback to casein hydrolysates or formulae based on amino acid is their poor palatability. The milks of other animals (goat, sheep) are inadvisable because of the high incidence of cross-sensitivity with cows' milk protein, their high solute content, and the risk of serious gastrointestinal infections due to unhygienic methods of collection and distribution. Non-infant formulae soya-based milks are unsuitable because of their low calcium, vitamin and energy content. In 2003, the UK Scientific Advisory Committee on Nutrition advised against the use of infant soya-based formulae because of their content of phytoestrogens, specifically isoflavones, which may theoretically affect reproductive health and fertility. There is currently no direct evidence from human studies to support this concern. If an infant who has not been weaned is intolerant to both soya and casein hydrolysate, the options are donated human milk, an elemental diet, or in exceptional circumstances i.v. nutrition. After weaning has commenced, if milk substitutes are unsuitable then supplementation with calcium and maybe other nutrients will be required. Even where a soya or casein hydrolysate infant milk formula is provided, the calcium intake may fall below the recommended requirements. The importance of such low intakes of calcium is unknown, but there may be special risks for patients with atopic eczema. In these children intestinal absorption may be impaired because of an associated enteropathy, the absence of lactose from the diet may impair calcium absorption, and there is a risk of vitamin D deficiency and consequently diminished gastrointestinal calcium absorption in children with atopic eczema who are kept out of sunlight.

EGG

The major allergens in egg white are ovalbumin, ovomucoid and ovotransferrin, and all three are also present in much smaller quantities in egg yolk. Cooking reduces the allergenicity of eggs by 70%. Almost all children with egg intolerance can tolerate cooked chicken. The eggs of turkeys, duck and goose contain similar allergens to hen's eggs.

Egg intolerance is very common, and one population-based study found the estimated point prevalence of intolerance to egg in children aged 2½ years was 1.6% (CI 1.3–2.0%), with an upper estimate of the cumulative incidence by this age of 2.6% (CI 1.6–3.6).[43] It is particularly common in infants with atopic dermatitis. It is most common in the first 6 months of life, and the most frequent presentation is the rapid onset of symptoms minutes after an infant is given egg for the first time. Reactions mostly occur within minutes of eating egg, and consist of an erythematous rash around the mouth, swelling and urticaria of the oral mucosa and angioedema of the face, sometimes with wheezing, stridor, conjunctivitis, rhinitis, vomiting, loose stools and in severe cases anaphylaxis. Those with immediate reactions also exhibit urticaria after skin contact with egg.

The diagnosis of egg intolerance is made from the history. Skin prick tests and RAST tests, although providing information as to whether the child is allergic to raw egg protein, may be falsely positive (e.g. in children who can tolerate cooked egg contained in cake or biscuits, and in children who have outgrown their egg allergy). When the diagnosis is in doubt it can be confirmed by challenge, which would normally comprise ingestion of increasing quantities of egg-containing biscuit, and where this is tolerated hard-boiled egg. The management is to exclude egg in a form that leads to reactions (e.g. raw egg only, partly cooked egg, or all egg) from the diet.

Egg intolerance is not a contraindication to measles or measles–mumps–rubella (MMR) vaccination because modern measles vaccines are grown on fibroblasts and do not contain detectable quantities of egg protein. The MMR vaccine can be safely given to children with egg allergy. The majority of life-threatening allergic reactions to the MMR vaccine have been reported in children who are not allergic to eggs, and these are mainly explained by IgE-mediated gelatin allergy.[44] The same may not apply to other vaccines such as the influenza vaccine, which is grown in the allantoic cavity of chick eggs and which does contain traces of egg protein.

In the majority of cases, egg intolerance has disappeared by the age of 3 years. Where the presentation is after the age of 12 months, which is unusual, the duration of intolerance may be longer, and is occasionally life-long.

SOYA

Soya protein is a permitted ingredient of flour in the UK, and this is not usually declared on manufactured food labels listing ingredients. Soya protein is widely distributed in manufactured foods including bread, pastry and sausages. Soya protein is also commonly employed as a meat extender and found in sausages, hamburgers and pie fillings.

Soya protein intolerance is less common than cows' milk protein intolerance. The clinical features and management of the two disorders are the same, but the widespread use of soya in manufactured foods means that soya protein avoidance is more difficult than cows' milk protein avoidance.

Soya and other beans can cause flatulence, abdominal pain and loose stools, which are due to the action of intestinal bacteria on poorly digestible oligosaccharides, mainly raffinose and stachyose.

FISH AND SHELLFISH

Fish allergy is common in children, whereas shellfish allergy appears to be more prevalent in adults. Fish allergens are highly cross-reactive on in vitro testing with the exception of tuna fish, in keeping with the clinical association between codfish allergy and allergy to hake, carp, pike and whiting but not tuna.

Although most reactions to fish are caused by ingestion, reactions can also occur as a result of inhalation of fish aeroallergens at fish markets or when fish is being cooked. Reactions to food aeroallergens are either respiratory (asthma) or in the skin (urticaria). The latter has been labeled as osmylogenic urticaria; 'osmyls' are minute particles given off by odoriferous substances. Aas has reported from Norway that fish antigens could be found in house dust in most homes where fish is often eaten, and he suggested that this was a possible source for sensitization to fish.[45]

Anaphylaxis caused by the unexpected presence of casein after consuming salmon has been reported. Casein has been used in the processing of salmon, posing a threat to individuals who are intolerant to cows' milk protein.

PEANUT AND TREE NUTS
What is a nut?
There is much confusion as to what does or does not constitute a nut. Whereas most nuts come from trees, peanut, the most common nut to cause allergic reactions, is in fact a legume, and the seed pod grows underground (hence an alternative name, 'groundnut'). As far as allergic reactions are concerned, the key information is not the precise botanical origin or plant family but the degree to which the nut does or does not provoke allergic reactions. Allergic reactions to peanuts, walnuts, pecans, brazil nuts, hazelnuts, cashew nuts, pistachio nuts, almonds (strictly speaking a fruit) and macadamia nuts are all well recognized. In contrast, allergic reactions to coconuts, pine nuts, oyster nuts, sweet chestnuts and horse chestnuts are only very rarely reported, and these items do not need to be avoided in children with peanut allergy.

Epidemiology and importance
Peanuts are a major cause of allergic reactions. The prevalence of peanut intolerance in western countries is approximately 0.5%. In a US survey[46] it was estimated that the prevalence of peanut and/or tree nut intolerance was 1.1% (95% CI, 1.0–1.4%). In another US survey, it was noted that peanuts and tree nuts accounted for 20 out of 32 (72%) total fatalities due to food-induced anaphylaxis.[47] Similar trends have been found in the UK.[48]

The main source of exposure to peanut and its products is consumption, but peanut oil (also known as arachis oil) has been used in some injectable, oral and topically applied pharmaceutical preparations. Because of concern that percutaneous absorption of peanut protein could cause sensitization to peanut, efforts have been made in recent years to remove arachis oil from topically applied pharmaceutical products.

The incidence of peanut intolerance is higher in siblings of affected individuals; in one study, three out of 39 siblings (7%) had peanut intolerance.[49] The concordance rate for peanut allergy in monozygotic twins is 64% compared with 7% in dizygotic twins, providing evidence for a strong genetic predisposition.[1] Nearly all patients who have had fatal or near-fatal reactions to nuts have other atopic diseases, especially asthma, but often also atopic dermatitis and allergic rhinitis. The severity of the asthma in these fatalities is variable and may be relatively mild. Asthma has in the past been thought of as a risk factor for the development of potentially severe reactions, but this is probably misleading and it is likely that asthma and peanut allergy are simply different manifestations of the same atopic disease process.

Peanut processing and its effects

The prevalence of peanut intolerance in China is low despite a high rate of peanut consumption. The method of frying or boiling peanuts, as practiced in China, reduces the allergenicity of peanuts compared with the method of dry roasting practiced widely in western countries.[50] Roasting uses higher temperatures that apparently increase the allergenic property of peanut proteins, and this may help to explain the difference in prevalence of peanut allergy observed in the two countries.

Untreated peanut oil contains peanut protein and consumption risks provoking adverse reactions in individuals with peanut intolerance. However processed and refined peanut oil, which has been subjected to degumming (separation of oil and water by centrifugation at 30–50 °C), refining with alkali and further centrifugation at 60–70 °C, bleaching with filters at 110 °C, and deodorization with steam under vacuum at 230–260 °C, does not contain peanut protein, and in one study refined peanut oil failed to provoke a reaction in any of 60 individuals with peanut intolerance.[51] However the marked variation in the degree of processing of peanut and other nut oils means that there will be marked variation in the nut protein content of various different types of refined nut oils.[52] It is worth noting that peanut oil may be used in the pharmaceutical industry, and has been used, for example, in vitamin A and D solutions.

Different cultivars of peanut are grown in many different parts of the world, but peanuts of different varieties from different parts of the world all appear to contain similar antigenic proteins.

Cross-reactivity

In a study of 122 children with allergic reactions to peanuts and tree nuts, 68 had reactions to peanuts alone, 20 to tree nuts alone, and 34 had reactions to both peanuts and at least one tree nut.[53] Of those reacting to tree nuts, 34 had reactions to one, 12 to two, and 8 to three or more different tree nuts, the most common being walnut, almond and pecan. Although there is extensive cross-reactivity between peanuts and other legumes on skin prick testing and RAST testing, clinically important cross-reactivity is uncommon. Nevertheless the risk of confusion between different nuts provides an argument for the avoidance of all nuts in a child known to be allergic to one type of nut. On the other hand, in a clear allergy to a single nut in patients known to be tolerant to others, avoidance of all nuts is not required.

Clinical features

Reactions can involve the skin (urticaria, angioedema), the respiratory tract (wheezing, throat tightness, coughing, dyspnea), and the gastrointestinal tract. Multiple organ systems may be affected. Accidental ingestion is common (30–50% over a 5-year period). In general the symptoms after accidental exposure are similar to those at an initial reaction.[54]

Modes of accidental ingestion include sharing food, hidden food ingredients,[55] cross-contamination (in kitchen utensils or in food manufacturing), and school craft projects using peanut butter.

The threshold dose required to produce a reaction varies. In one study of 14 individuals with peanut intolerance, the lowest dose of peanut to produce a convincing reaction was 2 mg, although individuals with peanut intolerance sometimes report short-lived symptoms after doses as low at 100 μg.[56] It is not uncommon for peanut-intolerant individuals to experience local urticaria after being kissed by someone who has eaten peanut. This is not specific for peanut intolerance; the same phenomenon is seen in individuals who are intolerant to other foods.

Acute allergic reactions to peanuts have been seen in neonates, and thus in some children, sensitization must occur in utero. At present there is no definitive evidence to suggest that avoidance of peanuts during pregnancy and lactation will prevent the development of peanut allergy in the child. The severity of any reaction is in part related to the quantity of nut eaten. When patients with peanut intolerance are followed-up, and experience a further reaction resulting from accidental ingestion, most follow-up reactions are less severe than the index reaction.[57]

Diagnosis

Although skin prick tests and RAST tests may provide useful supportive evidence of a peanut allergy in the absence of a clinical history, they should not be used to diagnose an allergy to peanut or any other food as false-positive reactions do occur and may inappropriately lead to children being labeled as food allergic when they are not. Furthermore, these tests cannot indicate the severity of symptoms. If the history suggests a nonlife-threatening allergy to a food but the skin prick test is negative then a food challenge should be considered as the definitive test of an allergy. If a life-threatening reaction to a food has occurred then food challenges should be avoided.

Natural history

Whilst most children fairly rapidly grow out of some food intolerances, nut allergy has always been regarded as an exception, being lifelong in most cases. Recent claims that up to 20% of patients outgrow peanut allergy have often been based on studies of patients whose original diagnosis was questionable. There probably are a few genuine cases in which nut allergy is not permanent, but they are uncommon.

Management

The management of nut allergy consists of education on avoiding the allergen, common traps being 'groundnut' (another name for peanut) and arachis oil (derived from peanuts). There are three additional treatment options – antihistamine for mild reactions, antihistamine plus inhaled adrenaline for moderate reactions, and antihistamine, adrenaline inhaler and adrenaline autoinjector for severe reactions. In the UK adrenaline inhalers (Medihaler Epi) are unavailable, and this means that adrenaline autoinjectors may need to be considered for some UK patients who have had moderately severe reactions.

Peanuts are cheap, readily available and are often used as a substitute for other nuts. For these reasons, even if there are no features of clinical cross-reactivity, patients who have peanut intolerance should in general avoid all tree nuts. Treatment of peanut allergy by immunotherapy using injections of peanut extract is not currently recommended.

FOOD-PROVOKED EXERCISE-INDUCED ANAPHYLAXIS

Exercise-induced anaphylaxis is usually associated with a combination of cholinergic urticaria (widespread tiny 1–3 mm wheals with variable erythema that last 30–60 min and occur in association with sweating) often starting in the palms and soles before spreading. Signs of autonomic dysfunction such as nausea, vomiting and diarrhea, dilated pupils and hypotension may follow. Attacks may occur spontaneously, or in association with ingestion of specific foods such as celery, shellfish, peaches or wheat.[58,59] The mechanism of this uncommon exercise-induced anaphylaxis is obscure. Management includes warm-up and moderation in exercise, avoidance of food and NSAIDs prior to exercise and making sure the patient is with someone who knows of their condition. Nonsedating antihistamines are often helpful. Hypotension should be treated by lying the patient down with their feet raised.

FOOD ADDITIVES

Food additives include coloring agents, preservatives, antioxidants, emulsifiers, stabilizers, sweeteners, other flavor modifiers and a large miscellaneous group of other agents. An obsession with food that is natural overlooks both the large number of toxic substances naturally occurring in food and the fact that most substances that provoke food intolerance are naturally occurring, such as eggs, cows' milk and nuts. There is an enormous discrepancy between the public's perception of food additive intolerance and objectively verified intolerance.[60]

Tartrazine and benzoic acid

Tartrazine is a yellow coloring agent, and one of the group of azo dyes. It is used as a coloring agent in a wide range of foods and medicines. Benzoic acid and the related benzoates retard the growth of bacteria and yeasts, and are used as food preservatives. Double-blind placebo-controlled studies have demonstrated that tartrazine can provoke urticaria, asthma or rhinitis in a small number of atopic subjects.[61] Similar studies have shown that benzoates can provoke urticaria. There is a lack of objective information about whether benzoates can provoke asthma. Tartrazine or benzoate intolerance can be identified by history (particularly unreliable in suspected food additive intolerance), elimination and challenge. It is possible that repeated administration of tartrazine or the benzoates leads to tolerance, and the severity of adverse reaction may not always be severe enough to warrant avoidance.

Sulfites

Sulfur dioxide and the sodium or potassium salts of sulfite or metabisulfite are widely used as food preservatives. Dried fruit is commonly treated with sulfur dioxide, and high levels of sulfite are sometimes found in wine, beer and salads in restaurants. Sulfites are sometimes used as preservatives in parenteral preparations of drugs, including several drugs used for the i.v. or inhalational treatment of asthma. Double-blind placebo-controlled studies have demonstrated that the oral administration of sulfite solutions can provoke bronchoconstriction in 35–70% of children with asthma.

A history of worsening of pre-existing asthma after consuming artificial drinks, eating in a restaurant or inhalation or injection of a drug containing sulfite raises the possibility of sulfite intolerance. Skin tests are unhelpful, and the diagnosis can only be confirmed by challenge, employing increasing doses of sulfite so as to establish the patient's threshold dose that can provoke asthma. Knowledge of the threshold enables the patient to avoid only those foods with a relatively high sulfite level, making a very restrictive diet unnecessary.

HOUSE DUST

House dust mites

The predominant allergens are digestive enzymes entrapped in mite fecal pellets, which are of a similar size to pollen grains. The main species of house dust mite in Europe is *Dermatophagoides pteronyssinus* and in the USA it is *Dermatophagoides farinae*. Mites feed on desquamated human skin scales, which are mainly shed in the bed and bedroom, where they can be found in mattresses, pillow cases, carpets, cuddly toys and upholstered furniture. The decisive factors that influence the number of mites are air humidity and temperature. Optimum conditions for mites are 70–80% relative humidity and an ambient temperature of 26 °C. Mites cannot reproduce when the relative humidity falls below 60%, and cannot survive for more than a few days in a relative humidity of below 40% if the temperature is above 25 °C. The relationship between the season and mite density in houses is attributable to seasonal changes in the ambient indoor humidity. In temperate areas, the number of mites is lowest in the winter, when central heating dries the indoor air. Lack of mites at higher altitudes (e.g. alpine resorts) is due to the lower relative humidity. Skin prick and RAST tests may be useful as supportive evidence where there is a history suggestive of an immediate-type hypersensitivity to house dust mite. Although it is possible to reduce levels of the house dust mite in the home (Table 33.4), these measures do not usually lead to an improvement in symptoms of eczema or asthma.

LATEX

Natural latex is produced by nearly 2000 species of plants, although only the rubber tree *Hevea brasiliensis* is commercially valuable as a source of natural rubber. Proteins or peptides, which make up 1–2% of latex are responsible for allergic reactions and different patients appear to be sensitized to different groups of latex proteins.[62] The major rubber proteins are hevamines (proteins with chitinase and lysozyme properties),

and hevein, a fungotoxic protein with considerable structural homology with wheat germ agglutinin and other plant lectins.

Latex is used in the manufacture of a number of products in general and medical use, including gloves, catheters, condoms, balloons, rubber bands, toys and tyres. About 90% of harvested rubber is processed by acid coagulation at pH 4.5–4.8 into dry sheets or crumbled particles for manufacture of extruded rubber products (rubber thread); compression, transfer, or injection molded goods (rubber seals or diaphragms); or pneumatic tyres. The remaining 10% of harvested rubber is noncoagulated and ammoniated; it is used in the manufacture of rubber gloves and other 'dipped' products, such as condoms and balloons and it is these products that are responsible for most allergic reactions to natural rubber latex (see Table 33.6).

Latex antigens can be leached from rubber gloves by normal skin moisture, with subsequent adsorption onto corn starch powder inside the gloves. Latex allergen can also be adsorbed to powder inside gloves that have not been worn. When the gloves are donned or discarded, the corn starch particles with adsorbed latex allergens become airborne and can sensitize nearby persons by inhalation or can evoke symptoms in previously sensitized persons.

Predisposing factors

Atopy is a significant risk factor in the development of latex allergy with two thirds of affected patients being atopic. Latex allergy is one disease that may affect providers of health care services more frequently than patients themselves. Other high-risk workers include housekeepers, doll manufacturers and tyre plant workers. High-risk patient groups are those requiring multiple surgical procedures, such as individuals with spina bifida, where the prevalence is reported as 18–64%.

Reasons for increased prevalence of latex allergy

Other than increased awareness, possible explanations are: (1) the increased use of gloves during medical, dental and surgical procedures, owing to the risk of hepatitis and AIDS; (2) the replacement of mineral talc powder by cornstarch powder. Mineral talc is heavy and only transiently airborne, and has a high capacity to act as an allergen eliminator by binding firmly to latex allergens.

Cross-reactions

Cross-reactions may occur between proteins in latex and various foods such as avocado, bananas, kiwi and chestnut; the so-called 'latex-fruit syndrome' (see Table 33.5).[63,64] Cross-reactions may also occur with the

Table 33.6   Relative risk of latex-containing products

High risk
Medical latex rubber gloves with powder
Latex rubber gloves for use at home
Balloons
Latex for modeling, dental impressions, etc.

Medium risk
Unpowdered gloves
Catheters
Rubber bands
Teats, dummies
Pencil erasers
Some medicines for injection in multi-dose vials

Lower risk
Tyres
Shoe soles
Hot water bottles
Squash balls, other rubber balls
Red or black rubber tubing or sheet
Condoms
Elastic threads in elasticated clothing

weeping fig *Ficus benjamani*, which is increasingly used for indoor decoration. The existence of cross-reacting allergenic structures in plant-derived products such as latex, fruit and enzymes may explain extensive allergenic reactivity.

Clinical manifestations

The most common reaction to latex products is non-immunological, *irritant contact dermatitis*, the development of dry, irritated areas on the skin caused by the effects of repeated hand washing, detergents or sanitizers, or powders added to gloves. *Allergic contact dermatitis* appears 1–2 d after contact with the offending product such as rubber gloves, shoes, sports equipment and medical devices. The dermatitis is a cell-mediated delayed-type hypersensitivity reaction to low molecular weight accelerators and antioxidants in the rubber product. Examples of rubber product components that cause contact dermatitis are thiurams, carbamates, benzothiazoles, thioureas and amine derivatives. Patients may also present with acute urticaria. Inhalation of latex allergen-coated cornstarch particles from powdered gloves can cause *rhinitis* and *asthma* in latex-allergic individuals, mainly adults who manufacture gloves and health care workers. Latex-allergic individuals can rarely experience *anaphylaxis*, occasionally fatal in a variety of medical care situations and as a result of blowing into balloons or using rubber-handled squash racquets. Finally, latex-allergic individuals can react to food that has been contaminated by latex, for example by food handlers wearing latex gloves.

Diagnosis of latex allergy

Diagnosis depends on the clinical history, coupled with examination and laboratory tests. Latex-specific IgE tests result in up to 25% false-negative and 27% false-positive results and must be interpreted with caution.

Management

The mainstay of management is avoidance, especially of powdered latex gloves, which are the major contributors of transferable allergen.[65]

STINGING INSECT VENOM

Stinging insect allergy has a prevalence of 0.3–3% within the general population. It is more common in adults than in children, and males than females. Insects of the order *Hymenoptera* (vespids [wasps] and apids [bees]) sting and these insects are most active in summer and early autumn. The venoms contain proteins such as phospholipase and hyaluronidase.

Normal local reactions consist of pain, swelling and erythema. Larger local reactions can be confused with cellulitis, which is uncommon after insect stings. These are more extensive and may peak at 48 h and last as long as 1–2 weeks. Malaise and nausea may also develop. Symptomatic treatment is with NSAIDs and antihistamines. Oral prednisolone for 2–3 d may also be helpful. People who develop large local reactions to stings typically continue to have similar reactions after subsequent stings. The risk of anaphylaxis following large local reactions is < 5% and patients do not require venom skin tests and are not candidates for immunotherapy.

The most common symptoms of acute systemic IgE-mediated reactions are dermal (urticaria and angioedema). Life-threatening symptoms include edema of the upper airway, circulatory collapse and shock, which can occur at any age.[66] There have been no deaths from insect stings in children and young adults (< 20 years old) in the UK. Deaths are most likely to occur in adults with concurrent pathology (e.g. coronary vascular disease) or those on certain drugs (ACE inhibitors; beta-blockers, tricyclic antidepressants). Just over half of deaths in the UK have been from shock, one third from upper airway obstruction, 10% from asthma.

The risk of systemic IgE-mediated reactions is highest if the second sting occurs 2–8 weeks after the first and decreases with time, being very low > 5 years after the last sting. Children who have had systemic IgE-mediated reactions (skin, respiratory or cardiovascular symptoms) should have blood taken for specific IgE to the insect and be referred to a pediatric allergist. These children should be prescribed an injectable adrenaline device and appropriate training given. They should be told that early adrenaline administration after a sting is important, as patients in established shock are unlikely to respond to this treatment. First-aid should concentrate on lying the patient down with their legs up and calling an ambulance. Venom immunotherapy typically involves a 3–5-year course of desensitizing injections and is rarely indicated in children.

DRUGS

Epidemiology

Prospective studies have estimated that the incidence of serious adverse drug reactions in hospitalized patients is 6.7% and the incidence of fatal drug reactions is 0.32%. Whereas most adverse drug reactions are non-allergic in nature, 6–10% may be attributed to an immune mechanism involving either antibodies or T cells. Drug reactions that are immunologically mediated: (1) require a period of sensitization, (2) occur in a small proportion of the population, (3) are elicited at drug doses far below the therapeutic range, and (4) in most instances subside after drug discontinuation.

The mean age of allergic drug reactions is approximately 40 years, allergic drug reactions in childhood being much less common than in adulthood. Many patients who are said to have drug allergies are not allergic to the drug. For instance, 80–90% of patients who report a penicillin allergy are not truly allergic when assessed by skin testing, and virtually all patients with a negative skin test result can take penicillin without serious sequelae.[67] In children, most of the reactions that coincide with drug administration are exanthema, which are usually due to the underlying disease.

Clinical spectrum of disease

True allergic reactions are restricted to a limited number of syndromes that are generally accepted as allergic in nature, such as anaphylaxis, Stevens–Johnson syndrome, angioedema and urticaria, contact sensitivity and various exanthema, among others. Skin reactions are the most frequent symptoms of adverse drug reactions, occurring in nearly 80% of patients and are most commonly observed with ampicillin, amoxicillin and co-trimoxazole. Beta-lactam antibiotics are the most frequent pharmacological group involved in allergic drug reactions. NSAIDs, minor analgesics and other antibiotics (e.g. co-trimoxazole) are other drugs implicated. Anesthetic agents may cause immediate-type allergic reactions: muscle relaxants are implicated in 60% of cases, suxamethonium being responsible for 39% of these.[68]

Drug antigenicity

Only a few drugs such as large peptides (e.g. insulin), papain, streptokinase and foreign antisera can directly induce an immune response. The majority of drugs are simple chemicals of low molecular weight that are not immunogenic unless combined with serum or tissue proteins to form an immunogenic complex. Thus most drugs that cause hypersensitivity reactions must first be made immunogenic by being haptenated onto proteins, a process that occurs as the drug is metabolized. The cytochrome P450-dependent oxidation pathway in the liver is an important enzyme involved in the production of these reactive drug intermediates that covalently bind to serum and membrane proteins. Penicillin is an exception, as it may haptenate proteins directly without previous metabolism. Acylation of serum proteins results from an amine bond formed from the hydrolyzed beta-lactam ring of the antibiotic.

Diagnosis and management

Diagnosis of drug allergy is largely based on history (Table 33.7) and examination. Although diagnostic testing methods exist, overall they are still of limited practical value for the clinician who is evaluating a patient with suspected drug allergy. One major problem that affects the use of diagnostic tests for drug allergies is that, except for penicillin,

Table 33.7 Important questions to ask in the history of a patient with suspected drug allergy

1. What drugs were administered, by what route and at what dose?
2. For what reason was the drug administered?
3. How long after starting the drug did the reaction commence?
4. What was the nature of the reaction?
5. What treatment if any was required for the reaction?
6. What happened when the drug was discontinued?
7. Has the patient taken the drug (or similar drugs) before and after the reaction? If so, what was the result?
8. How old was the patient at the time of the reaction?

the immunochemistry of most drugs is still not known. In most instances the definitive test for drug allergy is rechallenge; this must be approached with caution as it may precipitate anaphylactic reactions.

In children where the use of a particular drug is essential and there are no alternatives, hyposensitization can be used to induce tolerance in a highly sensitized patient.[69] The procedure is performed by the cautious administration of incremental doses of the drug to the patient over a period of hours to days. The drug can be administered either by oral or i.v. route. The starting dose for the procedure can be determined by performing intradermal skin tests with the native drug at a dose that does not cause a nonspecific reaction. Typically, doses are doubled every 15–30 min and vital signs, physical examination, and peak flow values are regularly monitored. It is critical that the individuals involved with the hyposensitization procedure understand that it can have serious consequences. While anaphylactic reactions rarely occur if conservative protocols are used, health care personnel must be prepared to treat anaphylaxis if it does happen.

Penicillin and cephalosporin allergy

Anaphylactic reactions occur in approximately 1 per 10 000 penicillin or cephalosporin courses and are mostly seen in adults between the ages of 20 and 49 years. Only 2–6% of patients with a history of acute penicillin allergy are also allergic to cephalosporins. A history of atopy does not generally place an individual at increased risk for an IgE-mediated penicillin reaction.

Degradation products of penicillin may bind with tissue or serum proteins to form an immunogenic complex that can elicit an immune response. Penicillin allergy is attributed either to the benzylpenicilloyl hapten (the so-called 'major' determinant because 95% of tissue-bound penicillin is in this form), or to a group of compounds collectively called the 'minor' determinants, which are paradoxically responsible for many of the most severe allergic reactions. Adverse reactions to penicillin can be most simply classified by the timing of their occurrence. Immediate reactions occur within 1 h of administration and are usually directed against the minor determinant antigens. Life-threatening reactions occurring beyond 1 h of penicillin administration are rare.

The clinical features include urticaria, laryngeal edema, bronchospasm and anaphylactic shock. Accelerated reactions occur 1–72 h after penicillin administration, have the same clinical features as immediate reactions, and are usually directed against the major determinant. Late reactions, the mechanisms of which are generally less well understood, occur more than 72 h after drug administration. They comprise such disorders as a maculopapular (measles-like) rash, urticaria, serum sickness, erythema multiforme, hemolytic anemia, thrombocytopenia and neutropenia. Rarely, late reactions are due to the new development of an immediate or accelerated reaction. Only 3.5% of patients with a maculopapular rash associated with penicillin administration had adverse reactions to oral challenge with penicillin.[70] Maculopapular eruptions caused by penicillin may subside spontaneously despite continuing use of the drug and may not recur on re-exposure, presumably as many of these exanthema are due to the infectious disease rather than the antibiotic.

Ampicillin can provoke the same allergic reactions as other penicillins, but in addition is associated with a particularly high incidence of a non-allergic maculopapular rash, beginning a week or more after starting therapy.

An inquiry about possible penicillin allergy is mandatory prior to an injection of penicillin. However, not all patients with penicillin allergy give a history of previous penicillin administration. In these patients either the history is incorrect and the patient has received penicillin therapy, or sensitization has occurred through inadvertent exposure to penicillin in other sources such as food, milk or even soft drinks. Almost all deaths from anaphylaxis have resulted from injection of the drug, and the oral route has only been associated with a handful of fatal cases.

The penicillin skin test has no place in the management of patients without a clinical history of an IgE-mediated penicillin allergy, and is unnecessary in the face of a bona fide history of a life-threatening acute reaction, in which case the drug should be avoided. In cases where the history is suggestive of a milder acute hypersensitivity reaction, a negative result to skin testing is associated with tolerance to penicillin in 98% of cases. In contrast, a positive skin test result should lead to avoidance of this antibiotic, or use only after hyposensitization. There are no clinically useful skin tests or IgE tests for use in patients with suspected cephalosporin allergy. On the rare occasions in childhood (e.g. endocarditis) when treatment with penicillin is essential, then it is possible to hyposensitize the patient by oral and then continuous i.v. administration, but this procedure carries a risk of fatal anaphylaxis. The protection from hyposensitization is short lived, although it is possible to maintain a state of hyposensitization by long-term administration of a low dose.

Aspirin – nonsteroidal anti-inflammatory drug intolerance

The prevalence of aspirin intolerance is around 5–6%. Up to 20% of the asthmatic population is sensitive to aspirin and other NSAIDs and present with a triad of perennial rhinitis, sinusitis and asthma when exposed to the offending drug. Chronic persistent inflammation is the hallmark of patients with aspirin-induced allergy.[21] Of the patients with aspirin-induced intolerance 50% have chronic, severe, corticosteroid-dependent asthma, 30% have moderate asthma that can be controlled with inhaled steroids, and the remaining 20% of patients have mild and intermittent asthma. Up to 25% of hospital admissions for acute asthma requiring mechanical ventilation may be due to NSAID ingestion.

Aspirin intolerance is now thought to be at least partly due to a deviation of the arachidonic acid metabolic pathway towards the production of excessive inflammatory leukotrienes (especially LTC_4 and away from the production of anti-inflammatory prostaglandins (PGE_2). Leukotriene-modifying drugs (montelukast, zileuton) have been found to attenuate but not abolish aspirin-induced bronchial reactions in aspirin-induced intolerant patients. Salmeterol, a long-acting alpha$_2$-agonist has also been found useful in the management of aspirin-induced intolerance.

Local anesthetic agents

Older amino-ester LA (e.g. cocaine) are documented to cause allergic reactions, including contact dermatitis and redness or edema of the skin or mucous membranes. These compounds are no longer used as injectable local anesthetics and modern amide anesthetics (lidocaine [Xylocaine]), mepicaine [Carbocaine], bupivacaine [Marcain], prilocaine [Citanest] and articaine [Septanest] rarely if ever cause such reactions). Symptoms suggestive of an allergic reaction may be due to vasovagal reactions, adrenaline responses, 'panic attacks' and systemic toxic reactions. These effects are compounded by the fact that patients presenting for minor surgical and dental procedures under local anesthetics are usually anxious to start with, and up to 6% of patients have a problematic fear of needles. Infrequently, reactions may be to confounding factors such as latex or the preservative in preloaded syringes. In the latter case this is due to an irritant rather than allergic reaction to benzalkonium chloride, a quaternary ammonia cationic surfactant that is also present in some skin disinfectants. If suspected, further reactions can be prevented by using preservative-free vials of the drug.

Local anesthetic agents are too small to be antigenic by themselves but are sufficiently alien to bind as haptens to tissues with antigenic properties. Large series including hundreds or thousands of patients have consistently shown that both skin prick tests and intradermal tests are negative in almost all patients referred with an adverse reaction.[71] Furthermore specific IgE in the few cases where there are reactions have been negative.

ANAPHYLAXIS

In this chapter, and in the clinical situation, the term 'anaphylaxis' or 'anaphylactic shock' is taken to mean a severe life-threatening reaction of rapid onset, with circulatory collapse or respiratory compromise. In the past the term 'anaphylaxis' was used to describe any immediate allergic reaction caused by IgE antibodies, however mild, but such usage fails to distinguish between, for example, trivial urticaria and a life-threatening event. The mechanisms are believed to be IgE mediated (e.g. penicillin or insulin allergy), the generation of immune complexes (e.g. reactions to blood products), a direct (not involving antigens or antibodies) effect on mast cells or basophils causing inflammatory mediator release (e.g. reactions to radiocontrast media) and presumed abnormalities of arachidonic acid metabolism (e.g. anaphylactoid reactions to aspirin). It is possible to theoretically differentiate between anaphylaxis (immunologically mediated reactions) and anaphylactoid (non-immunologically mediated) reactions.[72] Previous sensitization is required for the former but not the latter.

The major causes of anaphylactic shock are drugs (e.g. penicillin, muscle relaxants), heterologous antisera (used for the prophylaxis and treatment of tetanus, diphtheria, rabies, snake bites and botulism), radiographic contrast media, the administration of blood products, hyposensitization injections, venoms from stinging insects (honeybee, wasp, hornet, yellow jacket) and foods (especially nuts, cows' milk, fish, shellfish and egg).[73] Death from anaphylaxis to medicines given intravenously usually occurs within a few minutes, while in the case of stinging insect stings it is usually delayed by 15 min and with foods by 30 min, although rarely it may be delayed for up to 6 h.[73] In general, the sooner the symptoms occur the more severe is the reaction. The first symptoms are feeling unwell, feeling warm, generalized pruritus, fear, faintness and sneezing. In severe cases these early symptoms are quickly (in seconds or minutes) followed by loss of consciousness, and death from severe bronchospasm, suffocation (edema of the larynx, epiglottis and pharynx) or shock and cardiac arrhythmia.[74]

DIAGNOSIS OF ALLERGY – TAKING A HISTORY

The lack of really useful laboratory tests for allergy (see later) means that there is no substitute for a careful history.

IMPORTANT QUESTIONS WHEN TAKING A HISTORY FOR ALLERGY

The history should include questions about:
1. when symptoms occur (e.g. day or night, time of year – tree pollen allergy occurs in early spring; grass pollen allergy in summer);
2. where symptoms occur (e.g. particular place);
3. when or where the patient is free of symptoms;
4. the presence of other allergic symptoms;
5. family history of allergy or atopic disease;
6. nature and quantity of substance thought to be causing reaction;
7. timing of reaction (e.g. immediate versus delayed);
8. severity of reaction (e.g. skin, respiratory, gut, circulatory, anaphylaxis);
9. time to resolution (e.g. hours, days, weeks);
10. response to treatment (e.g. no treatment required, antihistamines, intramuscular adrenaline);
11. previous contact with trigger and reactions (e.g. has a food previously been tolerated or previously caused a similar reaction?);
12. effect of changes in environment (e.g. if it is worse in a playground this might suggest a grass pollen allergy; if it resolves on holidays this might suggest house dust mite or pet allergy).

OTHER CLUES FROM THE HISTORY

1. *The symptoms are worse at night.* Both asthma and eczema are often worse at night, but it is wrong to equate all nocturnal symptoms with house dust mite allergy, as there are other possible explanations. Circadian rhythms affecting airway caliber, bronchial reactivity[75] and cortisol secretion may account for some of the increase in symptoms at night in asthma. In eczema, heat, tiredness and low cortisol secretion may contribute to nocturnal symptoms. In theory a high concentration of house dust mite antigen found in some bedrooms could contribute to nocturnal symptoms in asthma, rhinitis or atopic eczema, but in one large study there was no association between worsening at night or on waking and the presence of house dust mite allergy.[76] Only improvement in the symptoms following the complete avoidance of house dust mites in the bedroom (very difficult to achieve – see later), and recurrence of symptoms on re-exposure, will prove the point. A study of the symptoms associated with house dust mite allergy showed that a history of symptoms being provoked during domestic activity that stirs up house dust (bed making, dusting, vacuuming, emptying a vacuum cleaner bag, sweeping, shaking out bedding) when house dust mite antigen becomes airborne, is probably the only reliable pointer to house dust mite allergy.[76]

2. *The symptoms are worse at certain times of the year.* The usual inference is that the symptoms are attributable to a seasonal allergen. Sometimes the history is convincing. For example, where sneezing and conjunctivitis occur each year in June and July on sunny days when the grass pollen count is high, it is highly probable that the symptoms are attributable to allergy to grass pollen. Often, the history is not so easy to interpret. For example, a worsening of asthma in August, September or October is often difficult to explain. Possibilities include allergy to inhaled molds, an increase in the number of house dust mites in the autumn, changes in the weather, or catching viral respiratory infections when returning to school after the summer holidays.[77,78]

3. *The symptoms are worse in certain weather conditions.* The reasons for attacks of asthma after a thunderstorm or heavy rainfall are not fully understood. Allergy to inhaled fungal spores, a fall in the barometric pressure, a sudden fall in air temperature, and release of allergenic starch granules from ruptured pollen grains are all possible explanations.

4. *The symptoms improve when the patient is away from home (e.g. on holiday).* Improvement in atopic eczema when the patient goes on holiday is frequently noted, but the reason is usually obscure. In one study[79] there was a significant correlation between improvement in eczema and a more southerly holiday location; improvement was common in holidays taken in the Mediterranean or further south (63/92 – 69%), while holidays in northern Britain were more likely to be associated with deterioration (27/100 – 27%) than improvement (13/100 – 13%). The absence of pets or house dust mites may be the explanation in some cases, although the improvement that occurs on holidays (the disease often virtually disappears) is far greater than the modest improvement that can be seen after admission to hospital in the same patients. Exposure to sea water, sunlight or lack of stress are believed by some parents to be the explanation for such improvement, but there is no evidence to support these ideas. The improvement or complete disappearance of asthma at high-altitude resorts, seen in some patients, is generally attributed to the absence of house dust mite and pet animal antigens.

5. ***The presence or absence of a family history of atopic disease.*** Patients with atopic disease often have a positive family history of atopic disease, though atopy is so common in the normal population (wheezing in 21%, eczema in 12% and hay fever in 4% of all children in the UK by the age of 5 years)[80] that a positive family history is a rather nonspecific finding. In an apparently atopic child, the absence of a positive family history is more important, and should make the physician reconsider a diagnosis of atopic disease.

6. ***Multiplicity of symptoms.*** Allergic symptoms are usually multiple. It is important to inquire if the patient has other symptoms or signs that may be allergic in origin, in addition to the presenting complaint, and these features are: wheezing, sneezing, pruritus, urticaria, perioral erythema, eczema and conjunctivitis. Several symptoms may coexist. Unilateral symptoms, whether nasal, ocular or respiratory suggest the presence of a non-allergic condition.

7. ***Symptoms occurring after exposure to pets.*** Several situations cause confusion:
   a. The patient who is noted to have an immediate allergic reaction when stroking or being licked by, for example, a dog, but who is otherwise apparently able to live in the same house as the animal without obvious immediate allergic reactions; delayed reactions or enhanced bronchial reactivity may be overlooked.
   b. The patient who apparently experiences an immediate allergic reaction to, for example, certain cats but not others; again, delayed reactions or enhanced bronchial reactivity may be overlooked.
   c. The patient whose atopic disease predates the acquisition of a pet animal; the animal could still be an important trigger continuing to provoke the disease.
   d. The patient who had a pet animal some years before the onset of symptoms; the animal could still be an important trigger.
   e. The patient's symptoms did not improve when the pet was sent to live elsewhere for a few weeks; sufficient pet antigen to provoke disease may still be present in the household.

A major source of confusion is that parents equate allergy with immediate reactions and are unaware that constant exposure to pet antigen in the home tends to cause chronic rather than acute symptoms. Many patients who are allergic to pets react to minute traces of the animal, for example a few hairs on someone's clothing, and this explains why the disease in question fails to improve after the pet is removed from the household. For therapeutic trials to be meaningful, extensive cleaning of carpets, upholstered furniture, clothing and bedding is necessary to remove the allergen.

8. ***Food intolerance.*** Food intolerance is generally associated with multiple symptoms, and it is rare for a single symptom (e.g. asthma, rhinitis, abdominal pain) to be caused by food intolerance. Parents commonly overvalue food intolerance as a cause of symptoms. In one study, double-blind food challenges provoked symptoms in only 27 of 81 (33%) of children whose parents had reported food intolerance.[81]

UNQUALIFIED REPORTS OF ALLERGY

It is unhelpful to write 'allergy' in a patient's notes without any description of the evidence for the diagnosis. Many untoward events are wrongly labeled as allergies. For example, there are several reasons why penicillin administration may be followed by an adverse event, but few justify a diagnosis of penicillin allergy. A rash during antibiotic therapy may be caused by an underlying infection, or by a coloring agent or preservative included in a liquid preparation of the antibiotic. Loose stools are likely to be due to an underlying viral infection or a disturbance of the gut flora, but it is common to find this described by parents as an allergy to the antibiotic. The incorrect and careless labeling of a child as having penicillin allergy may rob the patient of penicillin treatment for life. Common and similar examples are the patient said to be allergic to cows' milk, in whom inquiry reveals that this is based not on observation of the patient but on the fact that someone has placed the child on a cows' milk-free diet, or the patient said to be allergic to something solely on the basis of skin or blood tests.

SIMPLE CAUSE AND EFFECT

The interpretation of the observation that exposure to a single item (e.g. a cat) is followed within minutes by an obvious adverse event (e.g. sneezing and orbital edema) should be quite simple, but there are pitfalls. The history is more reliable if it is based on the parents' unprompted original observations. The parents' observations may be especially unreliable because:
1. There is a strong emotional underlay, e.g. strong attachment to a family pet, leading to underdiagnosis of allergy because the family members do not want to part with the animal.
2. In the case of food intolerance, double-blind studies have repeatedly shown parental histories to be particularly unreliable (see later).
3. In the case of behavioral symptoms, there is a widespread but mistaken belief in the importance of adverse reactions to foods or food additives.[61]
4. A parent's report of alleged allergic reactions may have been fabricated (factitious illness).

In general, the quicker the onset of the allergic reaction, the more reliable is the history. A history of the same allergic symptoms after repeated exposure to an allergen is more reliable than a report of a single episode.

DIAGNOSTIC TESTING FOR ALLERGY

There is no ideal test that will predict with certainty whether avoidance of a specific allergen will improve or abolish symptoms in an individual. Some of the problems are due to difficulties intrinsic to the test, but some are inherent in the complex nature of atopic disease. Take, for example, a child with asthma who develops sneezing, conjunctivitis and angioedema of the orbit immediately after playing with a cat, and who has a positive skin prick test and positive RAST test to cat dander. Clearly it is logical that the child should avoid cats, but there is no guarantee that cat avoidance will help the patient's asthma. The reasons for the failure of allergen avoidance are discussed later, but can be summarized as:
1. The allergen was incompletely avoided.
2. The allergen was only one of several factors provoking the patient's disease.
3. The allergen was irrelevant to the patient's symptoms.

It is unrealistic to expect any clinical or laboratory test to cope with the first two of these problems. The best that can be hoped for is that a test will help establish the potential clinical relevance of a particular allergy. Regrettably, the currently available tests, described later, all suffer from serious limitations.

SCRATCH, PRICK AND INTRADERMAL SKIN TESTS

The principle of these skin tests is that the skin wheal and flare reaction to an allergen demonstrates the presence of mast-cell-fixed antibody. This is mainly IgE antibody, although in theory it could also be IgG4 antibody. IgE is produced by plasma cells primarily in lymphoid tissue in the respiratory and gastrointestinal tract, and is distributed via the circulation to all parts of the body, so that the sensitization is generalized and therefore can be demonstrated by skin testing. Age influences the reaction, and a child under 2 years of age produces much less reaction than an older child.

Short-acting antihistamines (H_1 receptor antagonists) must be discontinued at least 5 d prior to skin testing. Because of the variability of cutaneous reactivity, it is necessary to include positive and negative controls whenever skin prick tests are performed. The negative control solution should consist of the diluent used to preserve the allergen extracts. The positive control solution usually consists of histamine, and is mainly used to detect suppression of reactivity, for example caused by H_1 antihistamine medication.

Scratch testing

A drop of allergen solution is placed on the skin, which is then scratched so as to superficially penetrate the skin. The scratch test introduces an inconstant amount of allergen through the skin and is therefore poorly standardized and produces results that are too variable for routine clinical use.[82,83]

Prick testing

A drop of allergen solution is placed on the skin, which is then pricked with a plastic lance, and the result read after 15 min. The negative control should be negative, unless the patient has dermographism. The histamine control should be positive, unless the patient has recently received H_1 antihistamines, which would invalidate negative skin test results. The flare is ignored, and the diameter of the wheal is measured. Later reactions may occur, but their significance is unclear. Prick tests can also produce variable results, but the introduction of standardized precision lances for prick testing has made the method potentially more reproducible.

The interpretation of skin prick tests is difficult. There is a lack of agreed definition about what constitutes a positive reaction.[84] Most definitions of a positive reaction are based on the absolute diameter of the wheal, with arbitrary cutoff points for positivity at 1 mm, 2 mm or 3 mm. The problems with the interpretation of prick test results in an individual patient are:

1. Skin prick test reactivity may be present in subjects with no clinical evidence of allergy.[85,86]
2. Skin prick test reactivity may persist after clinical evidence of allergy has subsided.[87]
3. Skin prick tests may be negative in some patients with allergies. For example, skin prick tests are negative in 13–17% of those with rhinitis provoked by pollen.[88]
4. False-negative results may occur in infants and toddlers. The whealing capacity of the skin is diminished in early infancy, and when wheals are produced they are smaller than in later life, so that the criteria for a positive wheal must be adjusted.[86] There are no age-related guidelines for what constitutes a positive reaction.
5. There is a poor correlation between the results of provocation tests and prick tests.
6. Skin prick tests for foods are especially unreliable.[60] A positive result using a raw food antigen does not necessarily mean that the cooked food will cause a reaction.
7. False-negative skin prick tests can occur after anaphylaxis.[89]

The results of skin tests cannot be taken alone, but need to account for the history and physical findings.[86,90] From a carefully taken history one might suspect a particular allergen, and the finding of a positive prick test would increase the likelihood that the allergen was causing symptoms. Few people, however, would be prepared to ignore a strong history of allergy in the face of a negative prick test, yet it is illogical to regard the prick test as significant when it confirms the history and to disregard it when it fails to do so. The contentious issues in clinical practice are whether a child with atopic disease will benefit from attempts to avoid household pets, house dust mites or certain foods, but skin prick tests are unreliable predictors of response to such measures.

Intradermal testing

Intradermal testing is painful, can cause fatal anaphylaxis, and is only performed for limited reasons and then only if a preliminary skin prick test is negative.[91] Intradermal tests are more sensitive than skin prick testing, and also produce more false-positive reactions. As with skin prick testing, there is a lack of agreement as to what constitutes a positive reaction. The number of false-positive reactions makes the interpretation of the results of intradermal testing even more difficult than skin prick testing.

Skin patch testing

Patch testing is used to identify causative allergens in suspected allergic contact dermatitis, and is discussed elsewhere.[92]

Measurement of circulating IgE antibody

In vitro tests for circulating allergen-specific IgE antibody (e.g. RAST tests) avoid possible confounding variables in skin testing, namely IgE affinity for mast cells, their tendency for degranulation, and skin reactivity to released mediators. Thus, in theory, the in vitro test should be more reliable than skin testing. However, the clinical interpretation of in vitro IgE antibody tests is subject to most of the same pitfalls as the interpretation of skin prick testing. Additional problems with IgE antibody tests are:

1. Cost.
2. The IgE antibody concentration in the plasma varies with allergen exposure. A few patients with allergic rhinitis are RAST negative before the pollen season, but become positive after the pollen season.
3. A very high level of total circulating IgE (e.g. in children with severe atopic eczema) may cause a false-positive result.
4. A very low level of circulating IgE may be associated with false-negative results.
5. A very high level of IgG antibody with the same allergen specificity as IgE antibody can cause a false-negative result.
6. For each allergen, the test differs in the degree to which it is influenced by elevated total serum IgE.
7. In vitro IgE assays are slightly less sensitive than skin testing.

In vitro tests for IgE antibody are only preferable to skin testing where the patient has had a very severe reaction to the allergen in question (because of the small risk of anaphylaxis with skin testing), where the patient has widespread skin disease (e.g. atopic eczema), where the skin shows dermographism, or when H_1 antihistamines cannot be discontinued.

Provocation challenge tests

With the exception of food challenges in patients with suspected food intolerance, provocation tests (bronchial, nasal, conjunctival) have little place in routine clinical practice but have been helpful in the study of the pathophysiology and pharmacology of atopic disease. The results suffer from the same major limitation as the results of skin or IgE antibody testing, which is that a positive result from an allergen challenge by no means proves that the allergen is contributing to the patient's disease.

Blinded oral food challenge

The test comprises the oral administration of a challenge substance, which is either the item under investigation or an indistinguishable inactive (placebo) substance. Neither the child, the parents nor the observers know the identity of the administered material at the time of the challenge. Food challenges are subject to a number of pitfalls:

1. There is a danger of producing anaphylactic shock, even if anaphylactic shock had not occurred on previous exposure to the food.
2. Difficulties arise if a cooked food is used for testing and the patient is only sensitive to a raw food, or vice versa. Cooking reduces the sensitizing capacity of cows' milk, and intolerance to raw but not cooked egg, potato and fish are well described.
3. It is unclear what dosage of different foods is required to exclude food intolerance. The dosage used in studies employing encapsulated foods is inevitably limited. Larger quantities of food may cause an adverse reaction when smaller quantities do not. For example, Hill et al[91] found that whereas 8–10 g of milk powder (corresponding to 60–70 ml of milk) was adequate to provoke a response in some patients with cows' milk protein intolerance, other patients (with late-onset symptoms) required up to 10 times this volume of milk daily for more than 48 h before symptoms developed.
4. Failure to randomize the order of placebo with active substance or to employ a double-blind placebo-controlled methodology are errors common to many studies, especially those of food additives in chronic urticaria.

5. A food challenge performed during a quiescent phase of the disease may fail to provoke an adverse reaction. For example, in chronic urticaria intolerance to salicylates is confined to patients with active disease.

6. The regular administration of salicylates to patients with salicylate intolerance quickly leads to a state of tolerance to salicylate. It is possible, although unproven, that a similar phenomenon occurs with certain food additives. Thus a double-blind challenge performed while a patient is regularly consuming a foodstuff may fail to provoke an adverse reaction.

7. Where food intolerance exists in children with atopic dermatitis, it is common for the patient to be intolerant to several foods. The removal of only one offending item may fail to help the patient and reintroduction may not provoke deterioration.

8. In some situations, factors other than a food are necessary for positive challenges to occur. For example, in a subgroup of patients with exercise-induced anaphylaxis, symptoms only occur if exercise follows the ingestion of a particular food.[94] Exercise or the food alone fail to provoke symptoms.

DRUG TREATMENT OF ANAPHYLAXIS AND ACUTE ALLERGIES

Anaphylaxis not associated with circulatory failure/arrest

Adrenaline 10 μg/kg (0.01 ml/kg of a 1:1000 solution), given intramuscularly is the drug and route of choice for most patients with anaphylaxis associated with life-threatening respiratory compromise (Project Team of the Resuscitation Council [UK] 1999). Subcutaneous administration results in slower rates of systemic absorption than via the intramuscular route and is therefore not recommended.

Preloaded adrenaline syringes are available for use in the community. Min-I-jet 1 ml 1:1000 epinephrine with a 6 mm needle is for s.c. injection, requires assembly before use and the dose will need to be adjusted before administration. Thus it is less suitable than the EpiPen or the Anapen, which are spring-loaded devices with a concealed needle giving a single dose of 0.3 ml of 1:1000 or 1:2000 adrenaline (0.15 or 0.30 mg) as a deep i.m. injection. The simplicity of use and concealed needle makes this the most popular option with many patients.

The junior EpiPen or Anapen (0.15 mg) are suitable for children weighing 15–30 kg; above this weight the adult EpiPen or Anapen (0.3 mg) should be used. It will rarely be appropriate to issue epinephrine for children weighing less than 15 kg.

Adrenaline has a short half-life, and if necessary the i.m. injection is repeated at 5-minute intervals. Repeated (i.e. more than one) adrenaline injections are required in approximately 10–40% of patients with anaphylaxis, and therefore it is advisable to prescribe two preloaded adrenaline syringes per patient. I.v. administration of adrenaline has been associated with acute strokes and is therefore to be avoided in most situations.

Only 20% of fatal/near-fatal anaphylactic reactions to foods occur at home. The remainder occurs at the home of friends, at school and at restaurants[95] and thus it is essential that if a pre-loaded adrenaline syringe is prescribed, it is available where the patient is and that there is someone around who is trained in its use. Thus for schoolchildren it is important that two preloaded adrenaline syringes are available at the school and that teachers have appropriate training in the recognition of anaphylaxis and the use of the adrenaline syringe.

Indications for use of preloaded adrenaline syringes

A major factor predisposing to fatalities in cases of food anaphylaxis was the delay in recognition and instigation of medical treatment. In general it is recommended that a preloaded adrenaline syringe should be given at the first signs of upper airway obstruction, wheeziness not relieved by a bronchodilator inhaler or if there is any faintness. Allergic reactions are frightening and are often associated with panic attacks, which may mimic or exacerbate the symptoms and signs of anaphylaxis. This often makes it difficult to differentiate between clinical features of allergy and acute anxiety.

Indications for preloaded adrenaline syringe prescribing

The indications for prescribing preloaded adrenaline syringes vary from center to center.[96] Some authorities recommend, for example, that all children with peanut intolerance should be issued with adrenaline syringes, however mild the previous reactions, on the basis that the next reaction could be life threatening. Others are concerned that adrenaline syringes are vastly overprescribed, and should only be used in very selected cases.[97] Unfortunately it is not possible to predict which individuals are likely to get severe reactions, except to say that those who have had previous severe reactions are those at greatest risk. The possible role of asthma as a risk factor has already been discussed earlier in relation to peanut allergy. Fatal or near-fatal anaphylactic reactions are rare (approximately 1 per million per year), often occur in places where the prescribed preloaded adrenaline syringe is not available, where there is no one trained in its use, or in some cases the reaction occurs so rapidly as to lead to circulatory arrest that is unlikely to respond to i.m. adrenaline (see section on Anaphylaxis associated with circulatory failure/arrest later).[98] Most nonvenom- and non-medication-induced allergic reactions respond to antihistamines. There is no guarantee that treatment with adrenaline will be life saving, and there are well-documented cases in which death has occurred despite the correct use of adrenaline syringes.

> **Preloaded adrenaline syringes**
> *Advantages*
> *Efficacy:* most effective acute treatment for anaphylaxis not associated with circulatory failure/arrest;
> Provides reassurance for the patient and relatives.
>
> *Disadvantages*
> *Rarity:* risk of death from anaphylaxis is approximately 1/million/y.
> *May not work:* Anaphylaxis associated with circulatory failure is not likely to respond, and some cases of anaphylaxis will prove fatal, even if adrenaline is given early.
> *Can cause anxiety:* having to carry an adrenaline syringe everywhere causes considerable anxiety to some patients, relatives, carers and teachers. Exclusion from school trips and social outings have in some cases been associated directly with prescription of a preloaded adrenaline syringe to children.
> *Lack of warning signs:* fatal reactions are sometimes not associated with warning signs.
> *Side-effects:* preloaded adrenaline syringe use for anaphylaxis has caused death from arrhythmias and strokes.
> *Availability:* preloaded adrenaline syringes are often not available at the emergency (i.e. reactions away from home, patient not carrying adrenaline).
> *Need for training:* inadequate training may prevent adequate recognition of anaphylaxis or use of preloaded adrenaline syringe.

Based on the current difficulties associated with the use of a preloaded adrenaline syringe, if it is prescribed, it is recommended that the following conditions are met:

- Appropriate training should be given to the patient, their relatives, teachers and work colleagues (see later).
- Preloaded adrenaline syringes should be available at all times, not just at home but also at school, when visiting friends and during all leisure activities.
- All trainees should undergo periodic retraining and reassessment.

Information that should be given to users of preloaded adrenaline syringes

As mentioned earlier, training of patients and their relatives in the correct use and safe handling of the preloaded adrenaline syringe as well as regular annual review of technique is essential. Table 33.8 lists the information that should be covered at training sessions.

Table 33.8 Information that should be covered at preloaded adrenaline syringe training sessions

A. Instructions should be given to the parents and if old enough the patient on the following:
   How to recognize an anaphylactic reaction
   When to use the preloaded adrenaline syringe(s)
   Where and how to inject the adrenaline
   How to dispose of the used preloaded adrenaline syringe
   What to do if the adrenaline is injected incorrectly
   When to use other medicines
   Always to seek medical help if having a reaction
   When to replace the preloaded adrenaline syringe

B. The preloaded adrenaline syringe should be checked and the parents/patient told:
   To keep the preloaded adrenaline syringe in the original pack
   Label with the patient's name
   Store safely
   Store at room temperature
   Always keep accessible for an emergency

Table 33.9 H₁ Antihistamines used in the treatment of allergic reactions

Antihistamine	Route of administration
Sedating	
Chlorpheniramine (Piriton)	Oral/parenteral
Promethazine (Phenergan)	Oral/parenteral
Trimeprazine (Vallergan)	Oral
Non-sedating	
Loratadine (Clarityn)	Oral
Desloratadine (Neoclarityn)	Oral
Fexofenadine (Telfast)	Oral
Cetirizine (Zirtek)	Oral
Mizolastine (Mistamine)	Oral
Antazoline (Otrivine-Antistin)	Eye drops
Azelastine (Optilast)	Eye drops
Levocabastine (Livostin)	Eye drops
Azelastine (Rhinolast)	Nasal spray
Levocabastine (Livostin)	Nasal spray
Antazoline (Wasp-Eze)	Topical skin ointment
Mepyramine (Anthisan)	Topical skin ointment

The date on which training was given, the people trained, the adrenaline dose and a list of the information given to the patient and the relatives should be documented in the clinical notes. Allergy clinics might use a standardized preloaded adrenaline syringe checklist form, signed and dated by the prescribing doctor, with copies added to the clinical notes, sent to the GP and given to the patient.

Nebulized adrenaline and other treatment modalities

Nebulized adrenaline is no longer recommended as treatment of anaphylaxis in the UK because the metered-dose aerosol (Medihaler-epi) has been withdrawn from the market. Bronchoconstriction is best treated with a nebulized alpha₂-agonist (e.g. salbutamol or terbutaline). I.v. fluid boluses are often required in addition to adrenaline for treatment of hypotension. A number of 20 ml/kg boluses may be required. After injection of adrenaline, an H₁ antihistamine, for example chlorphenamine should be administered, and may be continued for 48 h to prevent recurrences of the reaction. Steroids take some hours to be effective and are unhelpful in the immediate treatment of anaphylaxis, but are of possible benefit in preventing a secondary relapse. Further management consists of avoidance of the cause, and in the case of insect venom stings consideration of hyposensitization.

Anaphylaxis associated with circulatory failure/arrest

If the patient has life-threatening circulatory compromise with no palpable peripheral pulse, then i.m. adrenaline is unlikely to be effective, as it will not be adequately absorbed. In patients with circulatory failure, basic life support must be commenced, followed by the injection of i.v. adrenaline (at an initial dose of 0.1 ml/kg of a 1:10 000 solution) as per the asystole protocol for advanced pediatric life support (APLS). Great vigilance is needed to ensure that the correct strength of adrenaline is used; anaphylactic shock kits need to make a very clear distinction between the 1 in 10 000 strength normally used for i.v. use and 1 in 1000 strength used for i.m. use. I.v. administration of adrenaline for treatment of patients with anaphylaxis has been associated with death from acute strokes and ventricular fibrillation, and is therefore to be avoided in anaphylaxis not associated with circulatory failure.

Medication for nonlife-threatening allergic reactions

H₁ antihistamines are very useful in controlling symptoms of nonlife-threatening allergic reactions such as acute and chronic urticaria and allergic rhinitis and conjunctivitis. Antihistamines can be divided into two groups (Table 33.9). The older sedating antihistamines are very effective, but because they cross the blood–brain barrier they are sedative and therefore may adversely affect children's learning ability. In an effort to reduce the sedative side-effects of these drugs, a new generation of nonsedating antihistamines has been developed. Some of these nonsedating antihistamines (in particular astemizole, terfenadine) are associated with life-threatening arrhythmias (torsades de pointes) by inhibiting potassium ion channels in cardiac tissue. Astemizole and terfenadine are therefore no longer available. Mizolastine, which is still available, has been associated with an increased risk of ventricular fibrillation when given together with other drugs (analgesics, antiarrhythmics, sotalol).

Doxepin is classed as a tricyclic antidepressant, but also has anti-H₁ and H₂ antihistamine activity (75× more potent than diphenhydramine and 6× more potent than cimetidine). It may be a useful therapeutic adjunct in older children with urticaria not controlled with traditional antihistamines.

HYPOSENSITIZATION

Hyposensitization comprises the regular administration of allergen with the objective of reducing or abolishing the patient's reaction to the allergen. The basis of allergy or 'immune hypersensitivity' is increasingly recognized as an imbalance between the proinflammatory and regulatory immune responses. Although desensitization or more precisely hyposensitization, as the allergy is rarely completely abrogated, has been used for many decades, it is only now appreciated that it works by resetting the immune balance by increasing the regulatory immune response.[99] All antigens can stimulate both effector and regulatory arms of the immune system. Hyposensitization is the method of presenting the allergen in a way that the regulatory response predominates. The induction of regulatory cell memory is less robust than for proinflammatory responses and therefore regular prolonged exposure to the allergen is usually required to maintain immune tolerance. Prematurely discontinuing immunotherapy prematurely risks development of allergic reactions to the allergen, which may be severe.

Allergy immunotherapy involves exposing the patient to increasing amounts of allergen starting at a low enough dose that does not provoke a proinflammatory response (induction phase), before maintaining tolerance with continuing exposure to the allergen (maintenance phase). Allergen may be given subcutaneously (SCIT), orally, or most recently the possibility of giving it sublingually (SLIT) has been explored. There is no doubt that SCIT and oral hyposensitization can be very effective in patients where the symptoms are being provoked by specific allergens. SCIT is limited by the availability of licensed allergens, and in the UK is largely used for patients with grass and tree pollen allergen, as well as bee and wasp allergen. As SCIT requires regular injections, initially weekly and then monthly for up to 3–5 years, hyposensitization is not commonly used in children. Oral hyposensitization is almost exclusively used for drug hyposensitization.

SUBCUTANEOUS IMMUNOTHERAPY (SCIT)

Since Noon's report in 1911, controlled studies have shown that allergen immunotherapy is effective in patients with allergic rhinoconjunctivitis and allergic reactions to *Hymenoptera* venoms. Patients may be considered for immunotherapy if they have well-defined, clinically relevant allergic triggers that markedly affect their quality of life or daily function and if they do not attain adequate symptom relief with avoidance measures and pharmacotherapy. Because of the risk of death from anaphylaxis (26 deaths in the UK between 1967 and 1986), the Committee for Safety of Medicines (CSM) in the UK has concluded that SCIT should only be used for: (1) life-threatening allergy to bee or wasp venom (rare in childhood) and (2) seasonal allergic hay fever (which has not responded to anti-allergy drugs), caused by grass or tree pollen, using licensed products only. In patients with hay fever, those who also have asthma should not be treated with hyposensitizing vaccines as they are more likely to develop severe adverse reactions. Hyposensitization must only be performed in hospitals or clinics with full facilities for cardiopulmonary resuscitation, and patients need to be monitored for 30–60 min after injections. Induction of tolerance requires weekly injections of increasing doses of allergen to reach a maintenance dose of 5–20 mcg over 6 or more weeks. This is often followed by monthly injections of this maintenance dose for 3–5 years.

ORAL HYPOSENSITIZATION

Oral hyposensitization is used to induce tolerance to essential medication required and can be used for most drugs including antibiotics, anti-epilepsy medication, chemotherapeutic agents and protein, e.g. insulin. Children can be hyposensitized to most drugs using this method. This form of hyposensitization is thought to work through controlled degranulation of mast cells.[100] Clinical reactivity returns within a few days of discontinuing drug administration, implying that continuous presence of the antigen is required for continuing mast cell degranulation and thus maintaining tolerance. Oral hyposensitization has also been achieved in asthmatic patients with aspirin-exacerbated respiratory disease,[101] and in a small number of children with food intolerance, e.g. to milk, but at present must be regarded as experimental.[102,103]

The procedure is performed by the cautious administration of incremental doses of the drug to the patient over a period of hours to days. The drug can be administered either by oral or i.v. route. The starting dose for the procedure can be determined by performing intradermal skin tests with the native drug at a dose that does not cause a nonspecific reaction and may be one hundredth to one thousandth of the usual therapeutic dose. Typically, the dose is doubled every 15–30 min and vital signs, physical examination, and peak flow values are regularly monitored. It is critical that the individuals involved with the desensitization procedure understand that it can have serious consequences. While anaphylactic reactions rarely occur if conservative protocols are used, health care personnel must be prepared to treat anaphylaxis if it does occur.

SUBLINGUAL IMMUNOTHERAPY

Sublingual immunotherapy (SLIT) has been used with increasing frequency in Europe as a possible means of hyposensitization in hay fever and asthma.[104] The allergen solution or tablet is kept under the tongue for 1–2 min before either spitting it out or swallowing it. This method appears safe in that there are to date no reported severe allergic reactions, although 75% of patients may experience local symptoms in the oral cavity. At present there is no standardization of dose, timing and duration of treatment, which has varied considerably between studies.

In terms of efficacy, a 2006 Cochrane review of SLIT for hay fever concluded that in 22 double-blinded, placebo-controlled trials involving 979 patients (6 house dust mite, 5 grass pollen, 5 *Parietaria*, 2 olive, 5 other) there was a 15–69% reduction of symptoms ($P = 0.002$) and a 23–63% reduction in mediation required ($P = 0.00003$).[105] However a larger independent American review of the European studies found that in 47 randomized, controlled studies, although there was a significant improvement in symptom and medication scores in 14 (35%) of 39 studies where data was available, there was no significant improvement in either parameter in 15 (38%) trials. Of the 43 trials that provided symptom scores, 20 (46%) demonstrated no significant improvement, and a total of 20 (51%) of 39 studies that provided medication scores demonstrated no significant improvement.[82] The Cochrane review of the five studies conducted in only children found no benefit. Based on these data, routine use of SLIT cannot be recommended in children at the present time.

NOVEL TREATMENT APPROACHES

There are a number of novel approaches currently under investigation for the management of allergic diseases. These include reduction of IgE by the infusion of anti-IgE antibodies, attempts to induce tolerance by stimulating regulatory pathways with plasmid DNA, immunostimulatory sequences, cytokines and bacterial agents, as well as complementary medicines such as Chinese herbs.

ANTI-IGE THERAPY

Anti-IgE (omalizumab and TNX-901) are humanized monoclonal anti-IgE antibodies that bind to the Fc region of IgE at the same epitope that binds FcεR1. They are given subcutaneously at a dose of 0.016 mg/kg body weight 3–4 weekly. They have been well tolerated in the trials that have so far been conducted in patients over the age of 12 years and there is so far little evidence for the development of antibodies and thus resistance with repeated use. As complete neutralizing of circulating IgE is required for clinical efficacy, their use has so far been restricted to patients with total serum IgE concentrations of < 700–1000 IU/ml. Trials have shown efficacy in seasonal allergic rhinitis and moderate (but not severe) allergic asthma, significantly reducing symptoms and medication use.[83,106] In peanut-allergic patients and at a dose of 450 mg, tolerance to peanuts increases from an average of 1 peanut to 6–8 peanuts.[56] With the restrictions in use to patients with only moderately raised serum IgE levels, and an estimated average annual cost of 4–5 times that of standard asthma therapy, and the need to long-term injections, its place in the management of allergic diseases in adults and particularly children is unclear at the present time.

CHINESE HERBAL REMEDIES

Chinese herbal medicines may have a role in the treatment of allergies and atopic diseases. However the complexity of traditional Chinese herbal formulae containing many constituents makes standardization and therefore licensing of herbal products problematic. A 2005 Cochrane review of the four published randomized controlled trials of Chinese herbal remedies for eczema involving 159 participants aged 1–60 years, suggested some clinical benefit, but the conclusion was that further well-designed large-scale trials are required.[107] Attempts are ongoing to reduce the number of components within these remedies to those that are most active and least toxic but these studies are currently in the preclinical or early clinical trial stage. For example, in a murine model of peanut allergy, pretreatment of mice with a modified Chinese herbal formulae was associated with complete abrogation of clinical anaphylaxis.[108] At the present time however, patients should be warned that currently available Chinese herbal remedies are non-standardized and unlicensed and although may be efficacious have also been associated with liver and renal toxicity and therefore must be used with caution.

PREVENTION OF ATOPIC DISEASE

Since 1930, when Grulee and Sanford reported a significantly lower incidence of eczema in infants who were breast-fed babies,[109] further research has been unable to provide the definitive answer whether the development of allergic disease can be prevented by breast-feeding.[110] One explanation may be that food antigens can pass to the infant via both human milk and also via the placenta prior to birth, but breast-feeding does not necessarily lead to complete avoidance of potentially sensitizing allergens. An alternative explanation is that more children at increased risk of allergic disease may be breast-fed by their mothers.[111] Studies using hydrolyzed formulae would avoid some of these factors and may provide more conclusive data. However a Cochrane review of studies provide no support to the idea that hydrolyzed formula prevents the development of allergy any more than breast-feeding.[112]

With the recognition that early exposure to potential allergens in the gut normally induces and maintains tolerance in young children, and complete avoidance may increase the risk of allergic reactions,[113] advice on avoidance should currently be given with caution.[114] Studies looking at potential aeroallergens show that ownership of cats and dogs in early childhood may protect against rather than promote the later development of asthma. In one study of 224 28-year-olds, those who owned a cat prior to the age of 18 years had a relative risk of having asthma of 0.08 (0.01–0.46) while those who acquired a cat after the age of 18 years had a relative risk of asthma of 2.62 (0.34–19 97) compared with participants who had never owned a cat.[115,116]

The induction of oral tolerance to food allergens may be augmented by certain bacterial (e.g. environmental mycobacteria) and viral (hepatitis A virus) antigens in the gut, a concept that may help to explain the epidemiological data leading to the development of the Hygiene hypothesis.[8] There is growing interest in supplementing people's diet with normal bacterial flora, particularly *Lactobacillus* and *Bifidobacterium* strains in the form of 'probiotics' to try and prevent or treat atopic diseases. Most studies to date using probiotics have looked at their effect in children with established atopic eczema rather than the prevention[117] of the condition and therefore it is not possible to draw any firm conclusions as to the usefulness of probiotics in the prevention of atopic disease.[118] However, overall the studies detailed earlier suggest that augmentation of intestinal regulatory cell activity in early infancy might possibly help to protect against immune hypersensitivity diseases in later life.

REFERENCES (* Level 1 evidence)

*1. Sicherer SH, Furlong TJ, Maes HH, et al. Genetics of peanut allergy: a twin study. J Allergy Clin Immunol 2000; 106:53–56.

2. Church MK, Holgate ST, Lichtenstein LM. Allergy. St Louis: Elsevier Health Sciences; 2006.

3. Sampson HA, Geha RS, Leung DY. Pediatric allergy: Principles and practice. St Louis: C. V. Mosby Co.; 2003.

4. Schaub B, Lauener R, von Mutius E. The many faces of the hygiene hypothesis. J Allergy Clin Immunol 2006; 117:969–977.

5. Liu AH, Leung DYM. Renaissance of the hygiene hypothesis. J Allergy Clin Immunol 2006; 117:1063–1066.

6. Lau S, Matricardi PM. Worms, asthma, and the hygiene hypothesis. Lancet 2006; 367:1556–1558.

*7. Strachan DR. Hayfever, hygiene and household size. BMJ 1989; 299:1259–1260.

8. Arkwright PD, David TJ. Eat dirt – the hygiene hypothesis of atopic diseases. In: David TJ (ed.) Recent advances in paediatrics, vol.21. Roy Soc Med Press 2004: 197–213.

*9. Shirakawa T, Enomoto T, Shimazu S, et al. The inverse association between tuberculin responses and atopic disorder. Science 1997; 275:77–79.

*10. von Ehrenstein OS, von Mutius E, Illi SL, et al. Reduced risk of hay fever and asthma among children of farmers. Clin Exp Allergy 2000; 30:187–193.

*11. Riedler J, Braun-Fahrlander C, Eder W, et al. Exposure to farming in early life and development of asthma and allergy: a cross-sectional survey. Lancet 2001; 358:1129–1133.

*12. Braun-Fahrlander C, Riedler J, Herz U, et al. Environmental exposure to endotoxin and its relation to asthma in school-age children. N Engl J Med 2002; 347:869–877.

13. Schultz, Larsen F. Atopic dermatitis: a genetic-epidemiologic study in a population-based twin sample. J Am Acad Dermatol 1993; 28:719–723.

14. Ober C, Hoffjan S. Asthma genetics 2006: the long and winding road to gene discovery. Genes Immun 2006; 7:95–100.

*15. Arbour NC, Lorenz E, Schutte BC, et al. TLR4 mutations are associated with endotoxin hyporesponsiveness in humans. Nat Genet 2000; 25:187–191.

*16. Eder W, Klimecki W, Yu L, et al. Toll-like receptor 2 as a major gene for asthma in children of European farmers. J Allergy Clin Immunol 2004; 113:482–488.

*17. Umetsu SE, Lee WL, McIntyre JJ, et al. TIM-1 induces T cell activation and inhibits the development of peripheral tolerance. Nat Immunol 2005; 6:447–454.

18. Akbari O, Umetsu DT. Role of regulatory dendritic cells in allergy and asthma. Curr Opin Allergy Clin Immunol 2004; 4:533–538.

19. Boguniewicz M. Chronic urticaria in children. Allergy Asthma Proc 2005; 26:13–17.

20. Kaplan AP. Chronic urticaria: pathogenesis and treatment. J Allergy Clin Immunol 2004; 114:465–474.

21. Picado C. Mechanisms of aspirin sensitivity. Curr Allergy Asthma Rep 2006; 6:198–202.

22. Black AK. Urticarial vasculitis. Clinics Dermatol 1999; 17:565–569.

23. Venzor J, Lee WL, Huston DP. Urticarial vasculitis. Clin Rev Allergy Immunology 2002; 23:201–216.

24. Gompels MM, Lock RJ, Abinun M, et al. C1 inhibitor deficiency: consensus document. Clin Exp Immunol 2005; 141:189–190.

25. Davis AE. The pathophysiology of hereditary angioedema. Clin Immunol 2005; 114:3–9.

*26. Langan SM, Williams HC. What causes worsening of eczema? A systematic review. Br J Dermatol 2006; 155:504–514.

*27. Hoare C, Li Wan Po A, Williams H. Systematic review of treatments for atopic eczema. Health Technol Assess 2000; 4:1–191.

*28. Cant AJ, Bailes JA, Marsden RA, et al. Effect of maternal dietary exclusion on breast fed infants with eczema: two controlled studies. BMJ 1986; 293:231–233.

*29. Devlin J, David TJ, Stanton RHJ. Six food diet for childhood atopic dermatitis. Acta Dermatovenereologica 1991; 71:20–24.

*30. Mabin DC, Sykes AE, David TJ. Controlled trial of a few foods diet in severe atopic dermatitis. Arch Dis Child 1995; 73:202–207.

31. Devlin J, David TJ, Stanton RHJ. Elemental diet for refractory atopic eczema. Arch Dis Child 1991; 66:93–99.

32. Arlian LG, Platts-Mills TAE. The biology of dust mites and the remediation of mite allergens in allergic disease. J Allergy Clin Immunol 2001; 107:S406–S413.

33. Devereux G. Epidemiology of food intolerance and food allergy. In: Buttriss J, (ed.) Adverse reactions to food. The report of a British Nutrition Foundation task force. Oxford: Blackwell Science; 2002.57–65.

34. Venter C, Pereira B, Grundy J, et al. Incidence of parentally reported and clinically diagnosed food hypersensitivity in the first year of life. J Allergy Clin Immunol 2006; 117:1118–1124.

35. Bock SA. Prospective appraisal of complaints of adverse reactions to foods in children during the first three years of life. Pediatrics 1987; 79:683–688.

36. Mari A, Ballmer-Weber BK, Vieths S. The oral allergy syndrome: improved diagnostic and treatment methods. Curr Opin Allergy Clin Immunol 2005; 5:267–273.

37. Rothenberg ME. Eosinophilic gastrointestinal disorders (EGID). J Allergy Clin Immunol 2004; 113:11–28.

38. Liacouras CA, Spergel JM, Ruchelli E, et al. Eosinophilic esophagitis: a 10-year experience in 381 children. Clin Gastroenterol Hepatol 2005; 3:1198–1206.

39. Farrell RJ, Kelly CP. Celiac sprue. N Engl J Med 2002; 346:180–188.

40. Eggesbø M, Botten G, Halvorsen R, et al. The prevalence of CMA/CMPI in young children: the validity of parentally perceived reactions in a population-based study. Allergy 2001; 56:393–402.

41. Goldman AS, Anderson DW, Sellers WA, et al. Oral challenge with milk and isolated milk proteins in allergic children. Pediatrics 1963; 32:425–443.

42. Hill DJ, Ford RP, Shelton MJ, et al. A study of 100 infants and young children with cow's milk allergy. Clin Rev Allergy 1984; 2:125–142.

43. Eggesbø M, Botten G, Halvorsen R, et al. The prevalence of allergy to egg: a population-based study in young children. Allergy 2001; 56:403–411.

44. Khakoo GA, Lack G. Recommendations for using MMR vaccine in children allergic to eggs. BMJ 2000; 320:929–932.

45. Aas K. Fish allergy and the codfish model. In: Brostoff J, Challacombe SJ (eds). Food allergy and intolerance. London: Baillière Tindall; 1987.356–366.

46. Sicherer SH, Munoz-Furlong A, Burks AW, et al. Prevalence of peanut and tree nut allergy in the US determined by a random digit telephone survey. J Allergy Clin Immunol 1999; 103:559–562.

47. Bock SA, Munoz-Furlong A, Sampson HA. Fatalities due to anaphylactic reactions to foods. J Allergy Clin Immunol 2001; 107:191–193.

48. Pumphrey RSH, Stanworth SJ. The clinical spectrum of anaphylaxis in north-west England. Clin Exp Allergy 1996; 26:1364–1370.

49. Hourihane JOB, Dean TP, Warner JO. Peanut allergy in relation to heredity, maternal diet, and other atopic diseases: results of a questionnaire survey,

skin prick testing, and food challenges. BMJ 1996; 313:518–521.

50. Beyer K, Morrow E, Li XM, et al. Effects of cooking methods on peanut allergenicity. J Allergy Clin Immunol 2001; 107:1077–1081.

*51. Hourihane JOB, Bedwani SJ, Dean TP, et al. Randomised, double blind, crossover challenge study of allergenicity of peanut oils in subjects allergic to peanuts. BMJ 1997; 314:1084–1088.

52. Teuber SS, Brown RL, Haapanen LA. Allergenicity of gourmet nut oils processed by different methods. J Allergy Clin Immunol 1997; 99:502–506.

53. Sicherer SH, Burks AW, Sampson HA. Clinical features of acute allergic reactions to peanut and tree nuts in children. Pediatrics 1998; 102:e6.

54. Bernhisel-Broadbent J, Sampson HA. Cross-allergenicity in the legume botanical family in children with food hypersensitivity. J Allergy Clin Immunol 1989; 83:435–440.

55. Yu JW, Kagan R, Verreault N. Accidental ingestion in children with peanut allergy 2006; 118:466–472.

*56. Leung DY, Sampson HA, Yunginger JW, et al. Effect of anti-IgE therapy in patients with peanut allergy. N Engl J Med 2003; 348:986–993.

57. Ewan PW, Clark AT. Long-term prospective observational study of patients with peanut and nut allergy after participation in a management plan. Lancet 2001; 357:111–115.

58. Hosey RG, Carek PJ, Goo A. Exercise-induced anaphylaxis and urticaria. Am Fam Physician 2001; 64:1367–1372.

59. Tewari A, Du Toit G, Lack G. The difficulties of diagnosing food-dependent exercise-induced anaphylaxis in childhood – a case study and review. Pediatr Allergy Immunol 2006; 17:157–160.

60. David TJ. Food and food additive intolerance in childhood. Oxford: Blackwell Scientific; 1993.

*61. David TJ. Reactions to dietary tartrazine. Arch Dis Child 1987; 62:119–122.

62. Cullinan P, Brown R, Field A, et al. Latex allergy. A position paper of the British Society of Allergy and Clinical Immunology. Clin Exp Allergy 2003; 33:1484–1499.

63. Brehler R, Theissen U, Mohr C, et al. 'Latex-fruit syndrome'. Frequency of cross-reacting IgE antibodies. Allergy 1997; 52:404–410.

*64. Chen Z, Posch A, Cremer R, et al. Identification of hevein (Hev b 6.02) in Hevea latex as a major cross-reacting allergen with avocado fruit in patients with latex allergy. J Allergy Clin Immunol 1998; 102:476–481.

65. Heilman DK, Jones RT, Swanson MC, et al. A prospective controlled study showing that rubber gloves are the major contributor to latex aeroallergen levels in the operating room. J Allergy Clin Immunol 1996; 98:325–330.

66. Reisman RE. Stinging insect allergy. Med Clin North Am 1992; 76:883–894.

*67. Salkind AR, Cuddy PG, Foxworth JW. Is this patient allergic to penicillin? An evidence-based analysis of the likelihood of penicillin allergy. JAMA 2001; 285:2498–2505.

68. Gueant JL, Aimone-Gastin I, Namour F. Diagnosis and pathogenesis of the anaphylactic and anaphylactoid reactions to anesthetics. Clin Exp Allergy 1998; 28:(Suppl 4):65–70.

69. Gruchalla RS. Acute drug desensitization. Clin Exp Allergy 1998; 28:(Suppl 4):63–64.

70. Green GR, Rosenblum AH, Sweet LC. Evaluation of penicillin hypersensitivity: value of clinical history and skin testing with penicilloyl-polyserine and penicillin G. J Allergy Clin Immunol 1977; 60:339–345.

71. Gall H, Kaufman R, Kalveram CM. Adverse reactions to local anesthetics: analysis of 197 cases. J Allergy Clin Immunol 1996; 97:933–937.

72. Kemp SF, Lockey RF. Anaphylaxis: a review of causes and mechanisms. J Allergy Clin Immunol 2002; 110:341–381.

73. Pumphrey RS. Lessons for management of anaphylaxis from a study of fatal reactions. Clin Exp Allergy 2000; 30:1144–1150.

74. Pumphrey RS, Roberts IS. Postmortem findings after fatal anaphylactic reactions. J Clin Pathol 2000; 53:273–276.

75. Sly PD, Landau LI. Diurnal variation in bronchial responsiveness in asthmatic children. Pediatr Pulmonol 1986; 2:344–352.

76. Murray AB, Ferguson AC, Morrison BJ. Diagnosis of house dust mite allergy in asthmatic children: what constitutes a positive history?. J Allergy Clin Immunol 1983; 71:21–28.

77. Khot A, Burn R, Evans N, et al. Biometeorological triggers in childhood asthma. Clin Allergy 1988; 18:351–358.

78. Storr J, Lenney W. School holidays and admissions with asthma. Arch Dis Child 1989; 64:103–107.

79. Turner MA, Devlin J, David TJ. Holidays and atopic eczema. Arch Dis Child 1991; 66:212–215.

80. Butler NR, Golding J. A study of the health and behaviour of Britain's 5-year-olds. Oxford: Pergamon; 1986.

81. May CD, Bock SA. A modern clinical approach to food hypersensitivity. Allergy 1978; 33:166–188.

82. Lessof MH, Buisseret PD, Merrett J, et al. Assessing the value of skin tests. Clin Allergy 1980; 10:115–120.

83. Lessof MH. Skin tests. In: Lessof MH, Lee TH, Kemeny DM (eds) Allergy: An international textbook. Chichester: John Wiley; 1987:281–287.

84. Bousquet J, Michel FB. In vivo methods for study of allergy. Skin tests, techniques, and interpretation. In: Middleton E, Reed CE, Ellis EF, et al, (eds) Allergy. Principles and practice. St Louis: Mosby; 1993.573–627.

85. Ford RPK, Taylor B. Natural history of egg hypersensitivity. Arch Dis Child 1982; 57:649–652.

86. Pepys J. Skin testing. Br J Hosp Med 1975; 14:412–417.

87. Aalto-Korte K, Mökinen-Kiljunen S. False negative SPT after anaphylaxis. Allergy 2001; 56:461–462.

88. Patterson R. Allergic diseases. Diagnosis and management. 3rd edn. Philadelphia: Lippincott; 1985.

89. Bernstein IL. Proceedings of the task force guidelines for standardizing old and new techniques used for the diagnosis and treatment of allergic diseases. J Allergy Clin Immunol 1988; 82:(Suppl):487–526.985.

90. Wilkinson JD, Rycroft RJG. Contact dermatitis. In: Champion RH, Burton JL, Ebling FJG (eds) Rook/Wilkinson/Ebling textbook of dermatology. Oxford: Blackwell Scientific; 1992.611–715.

91. Hill DJ, Ball G, Hosking CS. Clinical manifestations of cows' milk allergy in childhood. I. Associations with in-vitro cellular immune responses. Clin Allergy 1988; 18:469–479.

92. Kidd JM, Cohen SH, Sosman AJ, et al. Food-dependent exercise-induced anaphylaxis. J Allergy Clin Immunol 1983; 71:407–411.

93. McLean-Tooke AP, Bethune CA, Fay AC, et al. Adrenaline in the treatment of anaphylaxis: what is the evidence?. BMJ 2003; 327:1332–1335.

94. Colver A, Hourihane J. For and against. Are the dangers of childhood food allergy exaggerated? BMJ 2006; 333:494–498.

95. Unsworth DJ. Adrenaline syringes are vastly over prescribed. Arch Dis Child 2001; 84:410–411.

96. Arkwright PD, Farragher AJ. Factors determining the ability of parents to effectively administer intramuscular adrenaline to food allergic children. Pediatr Allergy Immunol 2006; 17:227–229.

97. Jutel M, Akdis M, Blaser K, et al. Mechanisms of allergen specific immunotherapy-T-cell tolerance and more. Allergy 2006; 61:796–807.

98. Thien FC. Drug hypersensitivity. Med J Aust 2006; 185:333–338.

99. Pfaar O, Klimek L. Aspirin desensitization in aspirin intolerance: update on current standards and recent improvements. Curr Opin Allergy Clin Immunol 2006; 6:161–166.

100. Meglio P, Bartone E, Plantamura M, et al. A protocol for oral desensitization in children with IgE-mediated cow's milk allergy. Allergy 2004; 59:980–987.

101. Rolinck-Werninghaus C, Staden U, Mehl A, et al. Specific oral tolerance induction with food in children: transient or persistent effect on food allergy?. Allergy 2005; 60:1320–1322.

102. Cox LS, Linnemann DL, Nolte H, et al. Sublingual immunotherapy: a comprehensive review. J Allergy Clin Immunol 2006; 117:1021–1035.

*103. Wilson DR, Torres Lima M, et al. Sublingual immunotherapy for allergic rhinitis. Cochrane Database Systemic Rev 2006, Issue 2.

*104. Cox LS, Linnemann DL, Nolte H, et al. Sublingual immunotherapy: A comprehensive review. J Allergy Clin Immunol 2006; 117:1021–1035.

*105. Casale TB. Anti-immunoglobulin E (omalizumab) therapy in seasonal allergic rhinitis. Am J Respir Crit Care Med 2001; 164:S18–S21.

*106. Strunk RC, Bloomberg GR. Omalizumab for asthma. N Engl J Med 2006; 354:2689–2695.

*107. Zhang W, Leonard T, Bath-Hextall F, et al. Chinese herbal medicine for atopic eczema. Cochrane Database Syst Rev 2005; 2:CD002291.

108. Srivastava KD, Kattan JD, Zou ZM, et al. The Chinese herbal medicine formula FAHF-2 completely blocks anaphylactic reactions in a murine model of peanut allergy. J Allergy Clin Immunol 2005; 115:171–178.

109. Grulee CG, Sanford HN. The influence of breast and artificial feeding on infantile eczema. J Pediatr 1930; 9:223–225.

110. Chan-Yeung M, Becker A. Primary prevention of childhood asthma and allergic disorders. Curr Opin Allergy Clin Immunol 2006; 6:146–151.

111. Lowe AJ, Carlin JB, Bennett CM, et al. Atopic disease and breast-feeding – cause or consequence? J Allergy Clin Immunol 2006; 117:682–687.

*112. Osborn DA, Sinn J. Formulas containing hydrolysed protein for prevention of allergy and food intolerance in infants. Cochrane Database Syst Rev 2003; CD003664.

113. Barbi E, Gerarduzzi T, Longo G, et al. Fatal allergy as a possible consequence of long-term elimination diet. Allergy 2004; 59:668–672.

114. Strobel S, Mowat AM. Oral tolerance and allergic responses to food proteins. Curr Opin Allergy Clin Immunol 2006; 6:207–213.

*115. deMeer G, Toelle BG, Ng K, et al. Presence and timing of cat ownership by age 18 and the effect on atopy and asthma at age 28. J Allergy Clin Immunol 2004; 113:433–438.

*116. Ownby DR, Johnson CC, Peterson EL. Exposure to dogs and cats in the first year of life and risk of allergic sensitization at 6 to 7 years of age. JAMA 2002; 28:963–972.

117. Kalliomaki M, Salminen S, Poussa T, et al. Probiotics and prevenation of atopic disease: 4-year follow-up of a randomised placebo-controlled trial. Lancet 2003; 361:1869–1871.

118. Boyle RJ, Tang ML. The role of probiotics in the management of allergic disease. Clin Exp Allergy 2006; 36:568–576.

34

Psychiatric disorders in childhood

Peter Hoare

INTRODUCTION

Child psychiatry is concerned with the assessment and treatment of children's emotional and behavioral problems. These problems are common with prevalence rates of 10–20% reported in community studies. The majority of disturbed children are not seen by specialist psychiatric services, but by general practitioners, community doctors and pediatricians along with other professionals such as teachers and residential care staff. Consequently, knowledge about the range and variety of emotional and behavioral problems shown by children is important for all doctors involved in the care of children. The everyday work of the pediatrician provides clear evidence of the stressful effects of illness on the children and family's psychological well-being and adjustment.

Psychiatric disturbance in childhood is most usefully defined as an abnormality in at least one of three areas: emotions, behavior or relationships. It is *not* helpful to regard these abnormalities as strictly defined disease entities with a precise etiology, treatment and prognosis. Rather, it is preferable to regard them as deviations or departures from the norm.

which are distressing to the child or to those involved with his care (the male gender is used throughout the chapter for ease of presentation rather than from any bias or discrimination). Although child psychiatric disorders do not conform to a strict medical model of illness, it does not mean that these disorders are trivial or unimportant. Some disorders such as autism or conduct disorder have major implications for the child's development and adjustment in adult life.

In childhood, the distinction between disturbance and normality is imprecise. Isolated symptoms are common and not pathological. For example, many children will occasionally feel sad, unhappy or have temper tantrums. This does not mean that they are disturbed. Disturbance is characterized by the number, frequency, severity and duration of symptoms rather than by the type of symptomatology. In addition, disturbed children rarely present with unequivocal pathological symptoms such as hallucinations or delusions, whereas symptoms such as unhappiness and lying are common and not diagnostic. In clinical practice, it is often more important to establish why the child is the focus for concern rather than to adopt the more narrow perspective of whether the child is disturbed or not.

Another important feature of psychiatric disturbance in childhood is that several, as opposed to single, factors contribute to the development of disturbance. This makes assessment and treatment more difficult, so that an essential prerequisite for successful treatment is the correct evaluation of the relative contribution of the different etiological factors. Etiological factors are usually categorized into two groups: constitutional and environmental. The former includes heredity factors, intelligence and temperament. The three major environmental influences are the family, schooling and the community. Another factor, physical illness or disability, if present, can have a profound effect on the child's development and on his vulnerability to disturbance.

Three other considerations are of general importance in understanding children's behavior: the situation-specific nature of behavior, the impact of current stressful events, and the role of family. Children's behavior varies markedly in different situations, that is, it is situation specific. For instance, a child may be a major problem at school but not at home, or vice versa. Consequently, there may well be an apparent discrepancy between accounts of the child's behavior from the parents and from the teachers. The most likely explanation for this discrepancy is that the demands and expectations upon the child in the two situations are different. It is therefore essential to obtain several independent accounts about the child's behavior wherever possible in order to derive a more accurate and realistic assessment of the problem. This situation-specific nature of the behavior has implications for treatment, as it is important to explain to parents and to teachers the reasons for the discrepancy, thereby lessening the likelihood of misunderstanding.

Children are immature and developing individuals whose capacities and coping skills change markedly during childhood. Childhood is also a period of life characterized by change, challenge and the necessity for adaptation. Consequently it is not surprising that symptoms of disturbance may arise at times of stress when the demands on the child are excessive. Research has shown that life events are associated with an increased psychiatric morbidity among children,[1] a finding similar to that reported for adults. Some stresses such as the birth of a sibling or starting school are of course normal and inevitable, whereas others, such as marital break-up or life-threatening illness, are serious with long term implications for the child's well-being.

The child may, however, cope successfully with the stress, thereby enhancing their self-esteem and confidence. Alternatively, the child may be overwhelmed, responding with the development of symptomatic behavior. The latter may involve regressive behavior (i.e. behaving in a more immature, dependent fashion), or more specifically maladaptive (e.g. aggression, excessive anxiety or withdrawal). A crucial feature of assessment is the identification of stressful factors that may be contributing to the problem, as this will influence treatment strategies and the prognosis.

The family is the most potent force for the promotion of health as well as for the development of disturbance in the child's life. Assessment of parenting qualities, the marital relationship and the quality of family interaction are essential components of child psychiatric practice. It is a frequent observation that it is the parents who are disturbed and not the child. One consequence of this observation is that in many cases the focus of treatment is likely to be the parents, or the whole family, rather than the child. Indeed, in many instances the main emphasis of treatment is the promotion of normal healthy family interaction as much as in the amelioration of disturbed behavior.

Finally, many disturbed children do not complain about their distress nor admit to problems, but rather it is their parents or other adults involved with their care who bring the child to the attention of professionals. Disturbed children more commonly manifest their distress or unhappiness indirectly through symptoms such as abdominal pain, aggression or withdrawal. Direct questioning of the child during the initial interview is unlikely to reveal the true extent of the child's feelings or the degree of his distress. Sensitive observations during the interview and the use of indirect techniques such as play are necessary to elicit a more accurate view of the child's feelings. This is only likely to be successful once a relationship of trust has been established between the child and the clinician.

NORMAL AND ABNORMAL PSYCHOLOGICAL DEVELOPMENT

Children are developing individuals. They are not small adults. A 2-year-old is very different to a 12-year-old, whereas an adult aged 25 may not differ that much from a 35-year-old. During childhood, the child undergoes a remarkable transformation from a helpless, dependent infant to an independent self-sufficient individual with his own views and outlook, capable of embarking on a career and living separately from his family. Knowledge about the *mechanisms*, *processes* and the *sequences* underlying these events is necessary in order to understand the nature of psychological disturbance in childhood. This knowledge also helps to define more clearly what age-appropriate behavior is and to distinguish the pathological from the normal. This section has three parts: developmental theories, developmental psychopathology and personality development.

DEVELOPMENTAL THEORIES (Table 34.1)

It is useful to define some terms at the outset, as they are often used interchangeably. *Growth* refers to the incremental increase of a characteristic; *maturation* is those phases and products of development that are mainly due to innate or endogenous factors; *development* is those changes in the nature and organization of an organism's structure and behavior that are systematically related to age. Many behaviors (for example walking and talking) have a substantial maturational component, whereas others (for instance emotional and social development) are strongly influenced by environmental factors. The continuous interaction between maturational and environmental factors throughout childhood helps to mold the personality development of the child.

Developmental theories tend to focus on at least one of the following areas: cognitive, emotional or social. They differ widely in theoretical orientation, in supporting empirical evidence and in the relative importance attributed to experience in influencing development. No single theory is satisfactory, so that most clinicians utilize some parts of the various theories to explain different aspects of development. The theories are usually described as stage theories, implying that they regard development as a series of recognizable phases of increasing complexity through which the child progresses.

COGNITIVE DEVELOPMENT

In 1929, the Swiss psychologist Piaget proposed a comprehensive theory of cognitive development. Many of his conclusions were based on experiments conducted on his own children over a number of years. Piaget has had a tremendous impact on educational concepts and teaching, particularly in primary schools over the last 30 years. More recently, the

Table 34.1 Summary of cognitive, emotional and social development

	Age in years				
	0	2	6	9	12+ upwards
Cognitive (Piaget)	*Sensori-motor*	*Pre-operational*	*Concrete operational*		*Formal operational*
	Differentiates self from objects	Learns to use language and to represent objects by image and words	Thinking is more logical and less egocentric		Able to think in abstract manner about propositions and hypotheses
	Begins to act intentionally	Thinking is egocentric (unable to see other viewpoint) and animistic (everything has feelings including inanimate objects)	Achieves conservation of number (age 6), volume (age 7) mass (age 8) Able to arrange objects in rank order		
	Achieves object permanence				
Emotional (Freud)	*Oral*	*Anal*	*Phallic*	*Latency*	*Genital*
	Main concern is initially with satisfaction of basic needs such as hunger	Co-operative activity with caregiver	Learns to interact with peers, often leads to rivalry	Reduced sexual interest with main concerns about peer relationships and position within peer group	Revival of earlier conflict, especially sexual conflict
	Later on, attachment to care giver	Satisfaction with increased self-control and achievement	Aware of own sexuality causing Oedipal conflict, resolved by identification with the same sex parent Conscience begins to form		Four main tasks: separation from parents, sexual role, career choice, identity
Social & personality development	Social smiling (8 weeks) Attachment (6 months) Stranger anxiety (10 months)	Cooperative play (3 years)	Strong preference for same-sex friends with stereotyped expectations (6–7 years)	Enduring relationships (8 years onwards)	
	Erikson's stage of trust vs. mistrust	*Erikson's stage of autonomy vs. shame and doubt*	*Erikson's stage of initiative vs. guilt*	*Erikson's stage of industry vs. inferiority*	*Erikson's stage of identity vs. role diffusion*

theoretical basis and validity of Piaget's conclusions have been questioned by further empirical studies.[2] Despite these criticisms, his views remain the most useful account of cognitive development.

Piaget's theory is set within a biological framework. In order to survive, the individual must have the capacity to adapt to the demands of the environment. Cognitive development is the result of interaction between the individual and the environment. Four factors influence cognitive development: increased neurological maturation, enabling the child to appreciate new aspects of experience and to apply more complex reasoning as he gets older; the opportunity to practice newly acquired skills; the opportunity for social interaction and to benefit from schooling; and the emergence of internal psychological mechanisms or *structures* that allow the child to construct a successively more complex cognitive model based on maturation and experience.

Piaget describes two types of intellectual structure: *schemas* and *operations*. The former are present at birth, the latter arise during childhood. *Schemas* are internal representations of some specific action, for instance sucking or grasping, whereas *operations* are internal rules of a higher order that have the distinctive feature that they are *reversible*, as, for example, multiplication is reversible by division. There are two ways whereby the child adapts his cognitive structure to the demands of the environment: *assimilation* and *accommodation*. The former refers to the incorporation of new objects, thoughts and behavior into existing structures, whereas the latter describes the change of existing structures in response to novel experiences. The child attends and learns most when his environment has a degree of novelty that challenges his curiosity but is not so strange that it becomes too confusing.

Piaget describes four main phases: *sensorimotor, pre-operational, concrete operational* and *formal operational*. The age range given for each stage is the average, though this can vary considerably depending upon intelligence, cultural background and socioeconomic factors. However, the order is assumed to be the same for all children. Schemas predominate in the sensorimotor and pre-operational stages, whereas operations predominate in the concrete operational and formal operational stages.

Sensorimotor (birth–2 years). Initially, behavior is dominated by innate reflexes such as feeding, sucking and following, hence the name for this period. Gradually, the infant realizes the distinction between *self* and *non-self*, namely where his body ends and the world outside begins. The infant also realizes that his behavior can influence the environment, so that intentional and purposeful behavior begins. Finally, the infant achieves *object permanence* whereby he recognizes that an object still exists even although it is no longer visible.

Pre-operational period (2–7 years). Language development greatly facilitates cognition, so that the individual begins to represent objects by symbols and words. Thinking is, however, *egocentric* and *animistic*. The former refers to the child's tendency to regard the world solely from his own position along with an inability to see a situation from another point of view. Animistic thinking describes the child's tendency to regard everything in the world as endowed with feelings, thoughts and wishes. For instance, the moon is watching over you when you sleep, the child says 'naughty door' when he bangs into the door.

The child has problems with the principles of conservation for number, volume and mass. The essential principle underlying conservation is that the number, volume or mass of an object are not changed by any visual alteration in their display or appearance. For instance, the child readily believes that the more widely spaced of two rows of counters has more counters than a denser packed row, or that there is more water in a tall beaker when it has been poured there from a shorter, more squat beaker.

The child also believes that every event has a preceding cause, rejecting the concept of chance or coincidence. Again, the child's moral sense is rigid and inflexible, so that punishment is invariable, irrespective of the circumstances. The child's concept of illness is radically different to that of the adult, with illness seen as a consequence for misdeeds, a punishment for a misdemeanor.

Concrete operational (7–12 years). Thinking becomes more logical and less dominated by immediate perceptual experience or by changes in appearance. Conservation of number, volume and mass is successively achieved during this period. The child becomes less egocentric, capable of seeing events from another person's standpoint. The child is able to appreciate and utilize reversibility, for example if 2 and 2 equals 4, then 4 minus 2 must equal 2.

Formal operational (12 years and upwards). This stage represents the most complex mode of thinking. Its main characteristics are the ability to think in an abstract fashion, to formulate general rules and principles and to devise and test hypotheses, an approach similar to that used in mathematics or in a scientific investigation. An example of such reasoning is the following: Joan is fairer than Susan; Joan is darker than Anne. Who is the darkest? (Answer: Susan). Prior to the formal operational stage, the child would require the aid of dolls to solve this problem. It should be pointed out that not everyone achieves this stage of thinking, even as an adult! The content of thinking also alters markedly with an emphasis on the hypothetical, the future and ideological issues.

CRITICAL COMMENT ON PIAGET

Recently, the Piagetian model has been criticized extensively for the lack of evidence to support the existence of the internal structures necessary for the concrete and formal operational stages. Alternative nonPiagetian explanations for a child's inability to carry out conservation tasks successfully before a certain age have also been put forward.[3] These criticisms are substantial, but they do not detract from the major conceptual contribution that Piaget has made to knowledge about cognitive development in children.

RECENT DEVELOPMENTS IN COGNITIVE THEORY

Psychologists and psychiatrists have become increasingly interested in the development and application of cognitive theory to the understanding and treatment of psychiatric disorders.[4,5] The main principles underlying this theory are that an individual's beliefs about (1) himself, (2) the future and (3) the world influence his mood and behavior, an idea similar in some ways to the Piagetian concept of schemas. When a person is depressed, his thoughts are self-defeating and he commits certain cognitive errors. Two common types of cognitive error are *personalization* and *dichotomous thinking*. The following two statements are examples of these two errors, respectively: 'The reason my parents separated is all because of me' and 'I'm no good at tennis, so I'm bound to be useless at any other sport'.

A major extension of these ideas in childhood is the notion of the *self-concept*. By the age of 6 or 7 years, most children have very definite and clear ideas about themselves and their qualities. For example, they are able to compare themselves to other children with respect to popularity, attractiveness, scholastic ability, and so on. Self-concept is a construct similar to that of a schema in Piaget's theory. Another important facet of self-concept is the favorable or unfavorable evaluation that the child makes of himself, an aspect called *self-esteem*. Children with high self-esteem appear to do better in school, regard themselves as in control of their own destiny, have more friends and get along better with their families.[2]

EMOTIONAL AND SOCIAL DEVELOPMENT

Sigmund Freud developed the most comprehensive theory about emotional development while Erikson,[6] also a psychoanalyst, applied psychoanalytic concepts within a social and cultural framework. Freudian theory emphasizes the biological and maturational components of development with an invariable sequence to development for everyone. Like Piaget, it is a stage or phase theory with the individual progressing successively through each phase. A major criticism of Freudian theory is that its concepts do not lend themselves readily to scientific investigation, so that it is difficult to prove or disprove the validity of the theory.

Freud proposed that an individual goes through five stages prior to adulthood, namely *oral, anal, phallic, latency* and *genital*. These terms refer to the major developmental task or potential conflict that the individual has to achieve or resolve during this period. Table 34.1 describes the important features of the different stages, e.g. during the phallic stage, the Oedipal crisis arises. At this time (around 3–4 years), the child becomes aware of his own sexual feelings and also that he is attracted in a sexual manner to the parent of the opposite sex. Moreover, the child is simultaneously aware that the parent of the same sex is a rival for the attention of the other parent. The conflict arises because the child is caught between the desire for one parent and the wrath of the other. The conflict is successfully resolved by the child identifying with the parent of the same sex, thereby eliminating the rivalrous feelings.

Erikson's major contribution has been to place psychoanalytic concepts in a social and cultural dimension (see Table 34.1). For Erikson, the most important task for the individual is to achieve a coherent sense of identity, a balanced and mature appraisal of one's abilities and limitations, with recognition of the importance of previous experience and with realistic expectations for the future. Such a task occupies the individual throughout his lifetime. The individual passes through a series of developmental stages, all of which are polarized into two extremes, one successful and adaptive and the other unsuccessful and maladaptive. The two poles of the first stage are *trust* and *mistrust*. The former refers to the child's belief that the world is safe, predictable, and that he can influence events towards a favorable outcome, whereas a sense of mistrust implies a world that is cruel, erratic and unable to meet his needs. The role of the caregiver, usually the mother, is crucial to the achievement of a successful outcome. Erikson also believed that the individual carries forward the residues of earlier stages into the present, thereby giving the past an influence on contemporary behavior. Erikson's writings are a compelling and coherent account of development. A major weakness is, however, the lack of empirical evidence to support the conclusions.

Development of social relationships[2]

A characteristic of human beings is their predisposition to establish and maintain social relationships. Although Freud and Erikson refer to social relationships, it is only with the recent elaboration of *attachment theory* by Bowlby[7] and by Ainsworth[8] that a plausible theory for this phenomenon has been described. Attachment theory proposes that social relationships develop in response to the mutual biological and psychological needs of the mother and the infant. Mother–infant interaction promotes social relationships. Each member of the dyad has a repertoire of behavior that facilitates interaction: (1) the infant by crying, smiling and vocalization; (2) the mother by facial expression, vocalization and gaze. A mother can regulate the infant's state of alertness, for instance rocking or stroking to soothe the child, whilst talking or facial expressions stimulate the child.

The term *attachment* describes the infant's predisposition to seek proximity to certain people and to be more secure in their presence. Bowlby maintained that there is a biological basis for this behavior, as it has been found extensively in other primates as well as in most human societies. It has considerable survival and adaptive value for the species, as it enables the dependent infant to explore from a secure base and also to use the base as a place of safety at times of distress. From the age of 6 months onwards, infants develop selective attachment to people, usually the mother initially, but not exclusively to her. This first relationship is regarded as the prototype for subsequent relationships, so that its success or failure may have long term consequences. Clinicians distinguish between *secure attachment* and *anxious attachment*, with the former referring to healthy and the latter to potentially unsatisfactory relationships.

Bonding refers to the persistence of relationships over time, namely the child's capacity to retain the relationship despite the absence of the other individual. Much of the infant's behavior promotes the development of attachments by ensuring close proximity and interaction with the mother. These ideas have many implications for obstetric and pediatric practice, for the reduction of stress associated with hospitalization and for possibly explaining the origins of non-accidental injury to children.

Other aspects of development
Gender and sex role concepts
Gender identity is a part of self-concept, but the development of the child's understanding about 'boyness' or 'girlness', the sex role concept, is a more elaborate process. Children usually acquire *gender identity* (correctly labeling themselves and others) by about age 2 or 3 followed by *gender stability* (permanence of gender identity) by about 4. *Gender constancy* (gender identity unalterable by change in appearance) appears around 6 years, similar to other conservation-like concepts. Children show clear evidence of sex role stereotyping from an early age, with an excessively rigid concept for a brief period around 6 or 7 years. Freudian theory explains these findings on the basis of identification whereby the child imitates the same-sex parent, thus acquiring appropriate sex-typed behavior. Alternative explanations emphasize the importance of social reinforcement and of cognition whereby the child acquires a schema about the respective roles and behavior of boys and girls.

Moral development
The acquisition of moral or ethical values is an important aspect of the socialization of children. Freud and Piaget have both described how this process happens. Freudian theory maintains that the superego or conscience develops during the phallic stage around 4–5 years. At this time, the child is identifying strongly with the same-sex parent in order to resolve the Oedipal conflict and in consequence acquires parental values and prohibitions. In contrast, Piaget hypothesizes a much more gradual or stage-like sequence to the acquisition of moral values. The child around 3 years old bases his judgment on the outcome rather than the intention of an act, with an emphasis on punishment following on from a misdemeanor. Subsequently, the child adopts a more conventional morality based upon conformity with family values. Finally, the adolescent derives a personal value system that combines his own idiosyncratic values with those of his family and of society with the intention of achieving the 'greatest good for the greatest number'.

DEVELOPMENTAL PSYCHOPATHOLOGY

This long-winded phrase refers to two important dimensions necessary to evaluate children's behavior: first, whether the behavior is age appropriate (the developmental aspect); and second, whether the behavior is abnormal (the psychopathological). For example, separation anxiety is a normal phenomenon among children between 9 months and 4 years approximately, whereas it would be abnormal in a child aged 6 years.

The threefold division of disturbance into abnormalities of behavior, emotions or relationships provides a useful way to analyze disturbance. Many behavioral problems can be conceptualized in terms of deficits or excesses. For instance, children with encopresis or enuresis can be regarded as having failed to acquire the skills necessary for toileting. Similarly, the aggressive child is showing excessive belligerent or assertive behavior at an inappropriate time. This approach also has implications for treatment, as the latter is often based on behavioral techniques designed to increase certain behaviors or alternatively to eliminate others.

Anxiety is central to the understanding of emotional disturbance. It has physical manifestations such as palpitations or dry mouth as well as psychological such as fear or apprehension. Anxiety is a normal, indeed essential, part of growing up. It may occur in many situations: in response to external threat, new or strange situations, and in response to the operation of conscience. Anna Freud[9] developed the concept of *defense mechanisms* to explain how an individual dealt with excessive anxiety. This response is entirely healthy and appropriate in many situations, only becoming maladaptive when it is used exclusively or excessively, thereby preventing the individual from learning how to cope with a normal amount of anxiety. Common defense mechanisms include *denial, rationalization, regression, and displacement*. Denial is the process where the child refuses to accept the psychological implications of a particular event or situation. For instance, a child refuses to admit to stealing, even when the theft is obvious, as the resultant loss of self-esteem and the sense of guilt make this impossible. Rationalization is when the child attempts to justify or minimize the psychological consequences of an event. 'I don't really like football, so that I am not bothered about playing for the team' is an example of the way in which the child may deal with a failure to gain selection for the school team. Regression occurs when a child behaves in a more developmentally immature manner, often at times of stress, for example becoming enuretic at the start of primary school. Displacement is the transfer of hostile or aggressive feelings from their original source on to another person, for instance getting angry with a sibling rather than with an adult.

Social relationships are often impaired among disturbed children. This may be a primary failure in some instances, such as autism, or more commonly a secondary phenomenon. Children with neurotic or conduct disorders are usually isolated and unpopular with their peer group as they have either excluded themselves or have alternatively been excluded as a result of their deviant behavior. In addition, the behavior usually brings them into conflict with parents or other adults such as teachers.

PERSONALITY DEVELOPMENT

Childhood is the time during which personality is formed. Wordsworth's aphorism 'the child is father to the man' is substantially true. Personality is a broad concept referring to the enduring and uniquely individual constellation of attributes that distinguish one person from another. It comprises cognitive, emotional, motivational and temperamental attributes that determine the individual's view about himself, his world and the future. Throughout childhood, the various elements interact with each other to mold the child's personality. Moreover, this process occurs in the context of the child's life experiences, particularly within the family, and also subsequently in the world outside the family. Healthy personality formation is an important prerequisite for satisfactory adjustment during childhood and also during adult life.

Personality is influenced by two main factors – constitutional and environmental – whilst a third, illness or disability, if present, can have a profound effect on the child. Constitutional factors include intelligence and temperament. The former describes the individual's ability to think rationally about himself and his environment, while the latter refers to the individual's characteristic style or approach to new people or situations, his level of activity and prevailing mood. These temperamental traits influence the child's response to his environment and also shape the range and variety of his experiences.

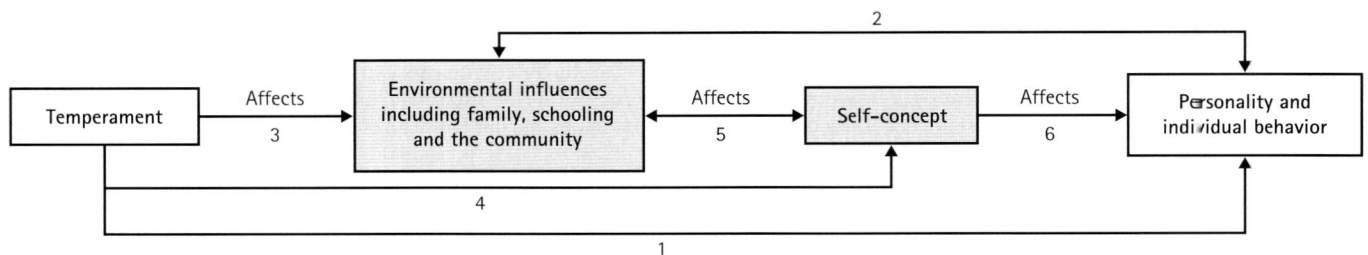

Fig. 34.1 Interactive model of personality development.

The main environmental influences are the family, schooling and the community. The family is the most powerful force for promoting healthy development as well as for causing severe disturbance in a child's life. Families fulfil many functions for children including: (1) the satisfaction of basic physical needs such as food and shelter; (2) the provision of love and security; (3) the development of social relationships with adults and peers; (4) the promotion of cognitive and language skills; (5) the experience of appropriate role models and socialization; and (6) the acquisition of ethical and moral values.

Schooling has three main roles for children: (1) the attainment of scholastic skills; (2) the promotion of peer relationships; and (3) the acceptance of adult authority outside the family. The community through the quality of housing and the availability of resources also has a considerable influence on the child's development. Finally, physical disability or illness, when present, exerts a major effect on personality development. This arises not only from the direct restrictions or limitations that they may impose on the child's abilities or activities, but more commonly and importantly, through indirect effects on the child's self-esteem, from overprotectiveness by the parents and from poor social relationships with siblings and peers.

Figure 34.1 is a diagrammatic representation of an interactive model of personality development that incorporates these ideas discussed in this section. As shown in Figure 34.1, constitutionally determined temperamental traits have a direct effect on personality and behavior, with the environment also exerting a similar impact. Environmental and temperamental factors have direct effects on the self-concept, which in turn shapes and modifies the personality as well as the environment. These interactive processes continue throughout childhood in a dynamic manner to produce a final product, an individual.

GENERAL FEATURES OF PSYCHIATRIC DISTURBANCE

DIAGNOSTIC CLASSIFICATION

A single cause is rarely responsible for the development of disturbance. The usual pattern is for several factors to be involved with a broad distinction into constitutional and environmental factors. The important constitutional factors are intelligence and temperament, whilst current life circumstances, the family, schooling and the community are the major environmental influences. One consequence of this multiple causation is that it is not possible to devise a diagnostic classification on the basis of etiology, as the relative contribution of each factor is often unclear.

Diagnostic practice is therefore descriptive or phenomenological, with three main categories of abnormality: *emotions, behavior* and *relationships*. In addition, these abnormalities should be of sufficient severity that they impair the individual in his daily activities and/or cause distress to the individual or to those responsible for his well-being. A commonly used definition of disturbance is as follows: an abnormality of emotions, behavior or relationships that is sufficiently severe and persistent to handicap the child in his social or personal functioning and/or to cause distress to the child, his parents or to people in the community.

The two commonest systems are the ICD-10[10] and DSM-IV.[11] DSM-IV is used extensively in North America, whereas ICD-10 is popular in the UK. The two systems have similar underlying principles with an emphasis on a clinical-descriptive approach to diagnosis. An important difference between ICD-10 and DSM-IV is that the latter allows for more than one diagnosis, whereas ICD-10 prefers a single diagnosis. The following list shows a convenient way to classify the important psychiatric syndromes in childhood:

1. conduct disorders;
2. emotional disorders;
3. mixed disorders of conduct and emotions;
4. hyperkinetic disorders (ICD-10) or attention deficit hyperactivity disorder (DSM-IV);
5. disorders of social functioning;
6. tic disorders;
7. pervasive developmental disorders;
8. Miscellaneous disorders – encopresis, enuresis, sleep disorders and eating disorders.

Conduct disorder is characterized by severe, persistent, socially disapproved of behavior such as aggression or stealing that often involves damage to or destruction of property and is unresponsive to normal sanctions. The main feature of emotional disorder is a subjective sense of distress, often arising in response to stress. This group is further divided into phobic, anxiety, obsessional, conversion states and severe reactions to stress. Many disturbed children show a mixture of emotional and behavioral symptoms, so that a mixed category is clinically useful. An important source of confusion between the two classification systems is the terminology relating to hyperkinetic disorders in ICD-10 and attention deficit hyperactivity disorder (ADHD) in DSM-IV. Although both systems have the same core features (overactivity, impulsivity and inattention), the different names imply the two systems regard the main abnormality differently, namely hyperactivity for ICD-10 and inattention for DSM-IV. The situation is further complicated by the popular usage of another term to describe this group of disorders: ADHD. Disorders of social functioning comprise conditions such as selective mutism and attachment disorders. Pervasive developmental disorders include autistic spectrum disorder, Rett syndrome and childhood disintegrative disorder. The miscellaneous group contains a diverse group of problems such as encopresis, enuresis and developmental disorders. Other important but uncommon conditions such as schizophrenia and mood disorders are categorized in a similar fashion to that for adults, providing that the diagnostic criteria are fulfilled.

EPIDEMIOLOGY OF DISTURBANCE

Epidemiological research has been an important research interest in the UK for the past 30 years. It has provided accurate information about the frequency and distribution of disturbance throughout childhood and adolescence,[12] the differences between urban and rural areas,[13] the effects of illness and disability on vulnerability to disturbance[14] as well as providing clues about the relative importance of various etiological factors.[13]

Most studies have shown prevalence rates of between 10% and 20% depending on the criteria for deviance. The first and most influential study was the Isle of Wight (IOW) study carried out by Rutter and colleagues.[12] Using a strict definition of disorder, they found rates of approximately 7% among 10–11-year-old children. Follow-up of these children into adolescence indicated a prevalence rate of around 7% with more than 40% of the children with conduct disorder still having major problems. Disorders arising for the first time during adolescence were more adult like in presentation, with a preponderance of females. Over 80% of the disorders were in the emotional, conduct or mixed categories. Emotional disorders were more common among girls, with anxiety the commonest type. By contrast, conduct disorders, and to an important extent mixed disorder, were more common among boys with an association with specific reading retardation. A comparative study of 10-year-olds living in London[13] showed a rate of disturbance over twice that on the IOW. This study also showed that the difference in prevalence rate was entirely accounted for by the increased frequency of predisposing factors among children and their families in London compared with those on the IOW. These factors were family discord, parental psychiatric disorder, social disadvantage and inferior quality of schooling.

The IOW study[14] also showed that children with chronic illness or disability had much higher rates of disturbance than healthy children. For instance, children with a central nervous disease such as epilepsy or cerebral palsy had a rate over five times that of the general population, while children with other illnesses such as asthma or diabetes were twice as likely to be disturbed as healthy children. A more recent epidemiological study carried out by the Department of Health in the UK[15] on 10 000 children aged 5–15 years found a very similar prevalence rate and range of disturbance as the IOW study, namely an overall prevalence rate of 10% with conduct disorder (5%), emotional disorder (4%) and attention deficit disorder (ADD) (1%) the main diagnostic categories. The survey also confirmed that adverse social circumstance, chronic illness and learning difficulties were still important risk factors for disturbance.

Studies of pre-school children, most notably by Richman et al,[16] have found that about 20% of children have significant behavior problems, with 7% classified as severe. Follow-up studies of these children indicated that about 60% persisted, most commonly among overactive boys of low ability. An important association was found between language delay and disturbed behavior. Finally, problems were more likely to persist when there was marital discord, maternal psychiatric ill health and psychosocial disadvantage such as poor housing or large family size.

ASSESSMENT PROCEDURES

Assessment is more time consuming in child psychiatry than in other branches of pediatrics. It has three components: history taking and examination, psychological assessment, and information about the child and family from other professionals.

HISTORY TAKING AND EXAMINATION

This has many similarities to traditional methods, though with important modifications. Interview skills are essential to the elucidation, understanding and treatment of emotional and behavioral problems in children. Points of general importance include: (1) clarification about the nature of the problem and the reason for referral; (2) obtaining adequate factual information; (3) observing and eliciting emotional responses and attitudes about past events and about behavior during the interview; (3) establishing trust and confidence of the child and family; and (4) providing the parents with a summary of problems and a provisional treatment plan at the end of the initial interview.

There are no absolute rules about interviewing, indeed flexibility is essential. However, the following guidelines are useful:

1. The interview room should be large enough to seat the family comfortably and also to allow the children to use the play material in a relaxed manner.
2. Avoid having a desk between the interviewer and the family, i.e. put the desk against the wall of the interview room.
3. Do not spend the interview writing down notes but rather encourage eye-to-eye contact, taking the minimal notes necessary.
4. The play material must be suitable for a wide age range and include crayons and paper, jigsaws, simple games, books (provides a rough

estimate of reading ability), doll's house, play telephones and miniature domestic and zoo animals.
5. The play material should be gradually introduced as appropriate and not left around in a haphazard manner.
6. Interview parents and young children together.
7. Older children and adolescents like to be seen separately from parents at some point during interview.
8. Older children and adolescents are able to talk about problems openly once trust in the interviewer has been established.
9. Too direct questions usually elicit denial from the child, so that open-ended questions are much more preferable.

The interview should provide information about the following (bold type indicates essential facts):

1. **Presenting problem(s). Frequency. Severity. Onset. Course. Exacerbating/ameliorating factors. Effect on family. Help given so far.**
2. Other problems or complaints:
   - general health: eating, sleeping, elimination, physical complaints, fits or faints;
   - interests, activities and hobbies;
   - **relationship with parents and siblings**;
   - relationship with other children, special friends
   - mood – happy, sad, anxious
   - level of activity, attention span, concentration
   - antisocial behavior
   - **schooling: attainments, attendance, friendships, relationship with teachers**
   - sexual knowledge, interests and behavior (when relevant).
3. **Any other problems not previously mentioned**
4. Family structure:
   a. **Parents: ages**, occupations, Current physical and psychiatric state. Previous physical and psychiatric history;
   b. siblings, ages, problems;
   c. home circumstances.
5. Family function:
   a. quality of parenting: mutual support and help, level of communication and ability to resolve problems;
   b. parent–child relationship: warmth, affection and acceptance, level of criticism, hostility and rejection;
   c. siblings' relationship;
   d. pattern of family relationships.
6. Personal history:
   a. pregnancy and delivery;
   b. early mother–child relationship, postpartum depression, early feeding patterns;
   c. temperamental characteristics: easy or difficult, irregular, restless baby and toddler;
   d. developmental milestones;
   e. **past illnesses and injuries, hospitalization;**
   f. separations greater than 1 week;
   g. Previous schooling.
7. observation of child's behavior and emotional state:
   a. appearance: nutritional state, signs of neglect or injury;
   b. activity level: involuntary movements, concentration;
   c. mood: expressions or signs of sadness, misery, anxiety;
   d. reaction to and relationship with the doctor: eye contact, spontaneous talk, inhibition and disinhibition;
   e. relationship with parents: affection/resentment, ease of separation;
   f. habits and mannerisms;
   g. presence of delusions, hallucinations, thought disorder.
8. observation of family relationships:
   a. patterns of interaction;
   b. clarity of boundaries between parents and child;
   c. communication;
   d. emotional atmosphere of family: mutual warmth/tension, criticisms.

9. physical examination:
    a. screening neurological examination:
        i.   note any facial asymmetry;
        ii. eye movements. Ask child to follow a moving finger and observe eye movement for jerkiness, uncoordination;
        iii. finger–thumb apposition. Ask child to press the tip of each finger against the thumb in rapid succession. Observe clumsiness, weakness;
        iv. copying pattern: drawing a man;
        v.   observe grip and dexterity in drawing;
        vi. observe visual competence when drawing;
        vii. jumping up and down on the spot;
        viii. hopping;
        ix. hearing. Capacity of child to repeat numbers whispered 2 m behind him.
    b. further medical examination (if relevant).

FORMULATION

At completion of the assessment, the clinician should be able to make a formulation. This is a succinct summary of the important features of the individual case. The formulation consists of the following: (1) statement of main problems; (2) diagnosis and differential diagnosis; (3) relative contribution of constitutional and environmental factors to the etiology; (4) probable short term and long term outcome; further information required (including special investigations); and (5) initial treatment plan. The formulation should be included in the case notes, thereby providing the clinician with a record of his views at referral.

PSYCHOLOGICAL ASSESSMENT

Psychological assessment carried out by a child psychologist is a valuable part of the overall assessment of a child's problems in some situations. It can provide information about three aspects of development: general intelligence, educational attainments and special skills. Assessment is usually based upon the administration of standardized assessment tests. These are either norm referenced or criterion referenced. The former compares the child's ability with other children of the same age, whereas the latter is on a pass/fail basis, for instance whether he can tie his shoelaces. Ideally, the test items should have good discriminatory value (distinguish between children of different ability), be reliable (give similar results when repeated) and valid (in agreement with other independent evidence). An important aspect of the assessment is that the tasks are carried out in a standardized fashion, thereby increasing reliability and validity.

INTELLECTUAL ABILITY

Developmental assessment in infancy and early childhood

The commonly used tests are the Bailey's Scales,[17] Griffiths Mental Development Scales[18] and the Kaufman Assessment Battery for Children (K-ABC).[19]

Assessment of general intelligence amongst school-age children

The most popular test is the Wechsler Intelligence Scale for Children – Revised Form (WISC-R).[20] This covers an age range from 6–16 years. Ten sub tests are usually used, measuring different aspects of the child's ability. Commonly, the tests are divided into 'verbal' and 'performance' categories, yielding a 'verbal IQ' and a 'performance IQ'. The 'verbal' subtests commonly used are information, comprehension, arithmetic, similarities and vocabulary, whilst the 'performance' tests are picture completion, picture arrangement, block design, object assembly and coding. Each subtest has a mean score of 10, so that combining the 10 tests gives a 'full scale' intelligence quotient (IQ) of 100 with a standard deviation of 15. The 'normal' distribution of the test scores means that it is possible to state that 66% of children will

be within the IQ range 85–115, 95% within IQ range 70–130, 99% within IQ range 55–145. Other tests used include the Stanford-Binet[21] and the British Ability Scales (BAS).[22]

EDUCATIONAL ATTAINMENT

There are two commonly used reading tests, the WORD (Wechsler Objective Reading Test)[23] and the Neale Analysis of Reading Ability.[24] The former measures basic reading, comprehension and spelling skills, whilst the latter provides information about speed, accuracy and comprehension of reading. The scores on the Neale test can be transformed into reading ages of so many years and months, for instance 6 years 11 months. The subtest scores of the WISC-R or the BAS can be used as a guide to mathematical ability.

Specific skills

Reynell development language scale,[25] Bender Motor Gestalt Test and the Vineland Social Maturity Scale are examples of tests to assess the child's acquisition of certain abilities and skills. These are often helpful with some specific problems.

Limitations of assessment

Caution should always be exercised in the interpretation of test results. It is wrong to attribute undue significance to a single result, most often done with the IQ score. Many factors influence test results including fatigue, poor testing conditions and the use of inappropriate tests. The results should be evaluated in the context of the overall assessment and the report from the child psychologist. A great deal of harm, upset and distress can arise for a child when he is incorrectly classified or labeled as too able or too dull on the basis of an unreliable psychological assessment.

Additional information

A distinctive feature of child psychiatry practice is the importance attached to obtaining independent evidence about the child's behavior. This is for two reasons: firstly, a child's behavior varies from one situation to another, so that it is helpful to have information about the child's behavior in several contexts; secondly, parental accounts of the child's behavior are likely to be distorted in many cases, as it is the parents who are disturbed rather than the child. Consequently, an important part of assessment is to obtain reports from other professionals involved with the family such as schools, health visitors or general practitioners. Another common practice is the use of questionnaires to supplement information provided by referrers and other more formal reports. Several questionnaires[16,26] have been devised to assess different age ranges and have satisfactory psychometric properties. Until recently, the most extensively used questionnaires for school-age children in the UK have been the Rutter parents' and teachers' scales, also known as Rutter A and Rutter B, respectively. These scales have established reliability and validity as well as classifying children into neurotic or emotional, conduct or antisocial and mixed categories. Over the past 5 years, the Strengths and Difficulties Questionnaire (SDQ)[27] has become more popular, as it assesses pro-social behavior as well as disturbed behavior.

DISORDERS IN PRESCHOOL CHILDREN

Except for rare but severe disorders such as childhood autism, psychiatric disorders in this age group are mostly deviations or delays from normality rather than a psychiatric illness as such. Moreover, the child's behavior and development are so influenced by the immediate surroundings that it is often the environment rather than the child that is responsible for the problems.

ETIOLOGY

Four types of factors contribute to problems in varying degrees in the individual case: temperamental factors, physical illness or handicap, family psychopathology and social disadvantage. The New York

Longitudinal Study[28] showed clearly that children with certain types of temperamental characteristics, the so-called 'difficult child' and the 'slow to warm up child' profiles, were more likely to develop problems. Again, physical illness or disability can reduce activity, directly or indirectly affect developmental progress and increase parental anxiety, all of which potentate the likelihood of behavioral disturbance. Parental psychiatric illness, marital disharmony and poor parenting skills are examples when disturbance in the parents adversely affects the child's behavior. Several authors[16,29] have shown high rates of depression among mothers with pre-school children. Social disadvantage such as poor housing or inadequate recreational facilities increases the risk of disturbance among pre-school children.[16]

FREQUENCY OF PROBLEMS

Table 34.2 shows the prevalence of common problems among 3- and 4-year-olds in the general population.[30]

Problems are mainly about eating, sleeping and elimination, with a marked decrease in wetting and soiling over the 1-year period. Affective symptoms such as unhappiness and relationship problems are much less common, but probably more significant. Community studies[16] indicate that 20% of children are regarded by their mothers as having problems, with 7% rated as severe.

COMMON PROBLEMS

This section discusses those problems that are particularly frequent among the pre-school child, whilst others such as soiling, which occur in older children as well are discussed later in the chapter.

Temper tantrums

They usually arise when the child is thwarted, angry or has hurt himself. They can occur in isolation or as part of a wider problem. They comprise a variety of behaviors, including screaming, crying, often with collapse onto the floor and banging of feet. A child can be aggressive towards other people around him, but the child rarely injures himself. Most tantrums 'burn themselves out', so that specific intervention is not necessary. If it is, then the following points are useful: if necessary, restrain from behind by folding arms around child's body; minimize any additional attention to the child; and only respond and praise when behavior is back to normal.

Feeding problems

They range in severity from a minor problem such as the finicky child to the severe disabling problem of non-organic failure to thrive. Minor problems will usually respond to patient and attentive listening to the parents' concerns, counseling and specific advice. Severe non-organic failure to thrive (prevalence 2%) is a complex problem requiring comprehensive assessment and a large amount of time and resources to remedy.[31] Several factors are responsible in most cases including a poor mother–child relationship, often in the context of more widespread emotional and social deprivation, and factors in the child, including temperamental factors and an aversion to feeding. *Pica*, the ingestion of inedible material such as dirt or rubbish, is a normal transitory phenomenon during the toddler period. Persistent ingestion is found amongst mentally retarded, psychotic or socially deprived children. Lead poisoning, though always mentioned, is a possible but uncommon danger from pica.

Sleep problems (sleep problems in older children are discussed in the miscellaneous disorders section)

These are common with up to 20% of 2-year-olds, waking at least five times per week.[16,32] The two most frequent problems are reluctance to settle at night and persistent waking up during the night. Several factors contribute to the problem including adverse temperamental characteristics in the child, perinatal problems and maternal anxiety. It is also important to distinguish between those factors responsible for the onset of the problem and those for maintaining the problem. Medication such as trimeprazine and promethazine are frequently prescribed, but side-effects often outweigh any advantages. The only real indication is to provide a brief respite for the parents as well as ensuring that the child has an uninterrupted night's sleep. The most successful management is a behavioral strategy (see Treatment section). Richman & Landsdown[30] provide a useful summary of these techniques. More recently, there have been case reports[33] suggesting the successful use of melatonin to treat sleep disorders among visually and neurologically impaired children and substantial randomized controlled trials are currently underway.

PSYCHIATRIC ASPECTS OF CHILD ABUSE[34]

Originally this was restricted to the 'battered baby syndrome', but it has now been extended to include physical abuse, sexual abuse, emotional abuse and neglect. This section will concentrate on the psychiatric aspects in childhood as other sections discuss diagnostic (see Ch. 6) and adolescent issues (see later in the chapter). It is also important to remember that the different aspects of child abuse are frequently present in the same child and family and that many comments about the detection, management and treatment apply equally to all aspects of child abuse.

PHYSICAL ABUSE

Diagnostic awareness and suspicion are the key elements in the detection and recognition of physical abuse. The following list summarizes the common characteristics of abused children and their families, although the most important factor to recognize is that child abuse can occur in any family irrespective of social class, ethnic group or religious affiliation.

Common characteristics of abused children and their families
Risk characteristics of the abused child:
1. product of unwanted pregnancy;
2. unwanted child in the family;
3. low birth weight;
4. separation from mother in neonatal period;
5. mental or physical disability;
6. habitually restless, sleeplessness or incessantly crying;
7. physically unattractive.
Risk characteristics of the parent(s):
1. single parent;
2. young;
3. abused themselves as a child;

Table 34.2 Problem behaviors in 3- and 4-year-olds[30]

Behavior	3-year-olds (%)	4-year-olds (%)
Poor appetite	19	20
Faddy eater	15	24
Difficulty settling at night	16	15
Waking at night	14	12
Overactive and restless	17	13
Poor concentration	9	6
Difficult to control	11	10
Temper	5	6
Unhappy mood	4	7
Worries	4	1
Fears	10	12
Poor relationships with siblings	10	15
Poor relationships with peers	4	6
Regular day wetting	26	8
Regular night wetting	33	19
Regular soiling	16	3

4. low self-esteem;
5. unrealistic expectations of the child and his development;
6. inconsistent or punishment-orientated discipline.

Risk characteristics of social circumstances:
1. low income or unemployment;
2. social isolation;
3. current stress such as housing crisis, domestic friction, exhaustion or ill-health;
4. large family.

Management

Most cases of child abuse do not require the involvement of a child psychiatrist, as the principal concerns are the protection of the child, practical support for the family and help with parenting skills. The child psychiatrist can make a useful contribution in two ways: firstly, to act as an outside consultant on various aspects of management and treatment to the other professionals and agencies working with the family; and secondly to provide individual and or family therapy for the child, the parents or the family depending upon the assessment.

In addition to the immediate effects, child abuse may have medium term and long term sequelae. Many abused children continue to be exposed to emotional abuse and neglect throughout their childhood, so that they often show symptoms of disturbance such as unhappiness, wariness, untrusting, low self-esteem and poor peer relationships. This childhood experience in turn predisposes abused children to become abusing parents when adults.

SEXUAL ABUSE

This has become a major public and pediatric concern over the past decade. Several factors have contributed to the increased concern: it is a common event affecting 12–17% of females and 5–8% males according to several epidemiological surveys.[35] It is traumatic for the child, giving rise to major distress at the time of its occurrence, but equally importantly acts as a predisposing factor for psychiatric disorder later on in life. Indeed, a history of sexual abuse in childhood is a very common finding among women referred to adult psychiatric services.

Complex psychological processes contribute to the development of psychopathology, as attitudes to sexuality are shaped in a dysfunctional manner by the abuse. Also, the individual has a sense of betrayal, powerlessness and stigmatization leading to shame, guilt and low self-esteem. One consequence of this process is that sexual abuse can present in a wide variety of ways from the physical, e.g. vaginal discharge to the psychological such as anxiety, aggression or encopresis. It is therefore crucial to be aware that unexplained or atypical symptoms may be the presenting complaint for a child with a current or past history of sexual abuse.

The child psychiatry team has a more clearly defined role in the management of sexual abuse, as interviewing skills, psychotherapeutic expertise and the use of specialist equipment (anatomically accurate dolls) are often necessary at the detection and also during the treatment stage of management. Detailed accounts of this work, including the use of the anatomical dolls, are well described in the several books (the Great Ormond Street child sex abuse team[36]) and the APSAC Handbook.[34]

EMOTIONAL ABUSE

This term has been introduced to describe the severe impairment of social and emotional development resulting from repeated and persistent criticism, lack of affection, rejection, verbal abuse and other similar behavior by the parent(s) to the child. Affected children display a variety of symptoms: low self-esteem; limited capacity for enjoyment; severe aggression; and impulsive behavior.

NEGLECT

This varies markedly, ranging from relative inadequacy and incompetence in providing basic shelter, love and security for the child, to a severe failure in the provision of basic essentials, often combined with emotional and social deprivation.

FACTITIOUS OR INDUCED ILLNESS[37]

This remarkable variant of physical abuse (previously called Munchausen syndrome by proxy) often occurs against the same background of parental psychopathology and social disadvantage as other forms of abuse. The role of the child psychiatrist is usually confined in most cases to offering counseling for the parents and/or family therapy when indicated.

PERVASIVE DEVELOPMENTAL DISORDERS[38,39]

Historically, these disorders were classified under childhood psychoses, as they are severe and disabling with clear-cut abnormalities. However, autistic children do not experience hallucinations or delusions, key features of a psychotic disorder, and moreover have had the abnormalities from early infancy. For these reasons, ICD-10 and DSM-IV have separated out childhood autism and related conditions from other psychotic conditions in childhood into a new diagnostic category called pervasive developmental disorders. In clinical practice, most people recognize that autistic disorders comprise a spectrum of disabilities (autistic spectrum disorders) with childhood autism at the severe end and Asperger syndrome at the mild end. Rett syndrome and disintegrative disorder are also included in the pervasive developmental disorders category.

CHILDHOOD AUTISM

Kanner's[40] original description of 11 children with 'an extreme autistic aloneness' has not been improved upon with its astute observation of 'inability to relate in an ordinary way to people and to situations' and 'an anxiously obsessive desire for the maintenance of sameness'. Subsequently, opinions have fluctuated about the diagnosis, etiology and treatment. Most authorities now agree that three features are essential to the diagnosis: general and profound failure to develop social relationships; language retardation; and ritualistic and compulsive behavior. Additionally, these abnormalities should be manifest before 30 months.

Prevalence

Previous epidemiological studies in childhood have found prevalence rates of four per 10 000 increasing to 20/10 000 when individuals with severe mental retardation and some autistic features are included. Boys are three times more affected than girls. However, a more recent study[41] reported a rate of 16 per 10 000 for autistic disorder and 64 per 10 000 for other pervasive developmental disorders. It remains to be seen whether these new findings are replicated elsewhere.

Clinical features

Impaired social relationships

Parental recollections of infancy often reveal that as an infant the child was slow to smile, unresponsive and passive with a dislike of physical contact and affection. Contemporary social deficits include the failure to use eye-to-eye gaze and facial expression for social interaction, rarely seeking others for comfort or affection, rarely initiating interaction with others, a lack of empathy (the ability to understand how others feel and think) and of cooperative play. The children are aloof and indifferent to people.

Language abnormalities

Language acquisition is delayed and deviant with many autistic children never developing language (approximately 50%). When present, language abnormalities are many and varied, including immediate and delayed echolalia (repetition of spoken word(s) or phrase(s)), poor comprehension and use of gesture, pronominal reversal (the use of the third person when 'I' is meant) and abnormalities in intonation, rhythm and pitch.

Ritualistic and compulsive behavior

Common abnormalities are rigid and restricted patterns of play, intense attachments to unusual objects such as stones, unusual preoccupations and interests (timetables, bus routes) to the exclusion of other pursuits and a marked resistance to any change in the environment or daily routine. Tantrums and explosive outbursts often occur when any change is attempted.

Other features

Autistic children often exhibit a variety of stereotypies including rocking, finger twirling, spinning and tiptoe walking. They are often overactive with a short attention span. Of autistic children 70% are in the retarded range of intelligence with only 5% having an IQ above 100. Occasionally, some have remarkable abilities in isolated areas, for instance computation, music or rote memory. About 20% will develop epilepsy during adolescence, though not usually severe.

Association with other conditions

Autistic behavior occurs in some patients with a diverse group of conditions including the fragile X syndrome, congenital rubella, phenylketonuria, tuberous sclerosis, neurolipoidoses and infantile spasms.[43] More recently, Rett syndrome, with its marked autistic features, has been described.[44]

Etiology

Most people favor an organic basis as neurological abnormalities are common, the association with epilepsy and various neurological syndromes, the increased rate of perinatal complications and a greater concordance rate among monozygotic compared with dizygotic twins.[43,45] Application of new investigative techniques such as CAT scan, MRI and positron emission tomography are beginning to reveal abnormalities in the frontal lobe region, with distinctive deficits on tests of executive function.[46] The relationship between autism and the fragile X syndrome is also unclear, as the different rates in the various studies may be a reflection of the degree of mental handicap rather than of any etiological significance. A most interesting psychological perspective on the autistic deficit is provided by the work of Baron-Cohen[47] and Hobson.[48] On the basis of sophisticated cognitive experiments with autistic children, they propose that the primary deficit in autism is a lack of empathy, namely an inability to perceive and interpret emotional cues in social situations.

Treatment

The explanation of the diagnosis is a vital first step in helping parents to accept the presence of handicap with the consequent lessening of the parental guilt about etiology. Counseling and advice are likely to be necessary throughout childhood. Lord & Rutter[43] suggested that treatment aims should have four components: (1) the promotion of normal development, (2) the reduction of rigidity and stereotypies, (3) the removal of maladaptive behavior, and (4) the alleviation of family stress. Behavioral methods, including operant conditioning and shaping (see behavioral treatment section), are the most likely ways to achieve some success with the first three aims, whilst counseling is important for the fourth. Special schooling, where the child's special social and educational needs are recognized, is very beneficial, sometimes on a residential basis. Drugs do not have an important part in management.

Outcome

Many autistic individuals are unable to live independently with only 15% looking after and supporting themselves as adults. Many were placed previously in institutions for the mentally handicapped, though government policy now favors community care. Autistic children with an IQ of at least 70, receiving proper education and coming from middle-class families do better than those in other groups. In most individuals there is some improvement in social relationships, though many are still handicapped. Parents often find it helpful to join a voluntary society such as the National Society for Autistic Children.

OTHER PERVASIVE DEVELOPMENTAL DISORDERS

Asperger syndrome/schizoid personality

This condition, originally described by Asperger,[49] shows some similarities to childhood autism in that there is an impairment of social relationships with a lack of reciprocal social interaction and a restricted repertoire of interests and activities. However, the children differ diagnostically from those with childhood autism in two important respects: there is no general intellectual retardation, and the language development is normal. Other characteristics include male preponderance and poor motor coordination with marked clumsiness. The condition is now regarded as one of the autistic spectrum disorders[39] with the impairment in social relationships persisting into adult life.

The term 'schizoid' personality of childhood was coined by Wolff & Chick[50] to describe a small number of children with unusual but distinctive personality characteristics, similar in some ways to children with Asperger syndrome. These 'schizoid' children were described as aloof, distant and lacking in empathy. Other features include: obstinate and aggressive outbursts when under pressure to conform, often at school; undue rigidity; sensitivity to criticism; and unusual interests to the exclusion of everything else. More recently, Wolff[51] has argued from follow-up studies of these children that they form a separate diagnostic category, the schizoid personality of childhood, similar to but distinct from childhood autism and Asperger syndrome. As adults, Wolff[51] found that they showed features of the schizotypal disorder.

Rett syndrome

In 1966 Rett described 22 mentally handicapped children, all girls, who had a history of regression in development and displayed strikingly repetitive movements of the hands. He thought that the children were autistic with progressive spasticity, and proposed that diffuse cerebral atrophy was the underlying cause. A more recent review[44] has indicated this syndrome is more common than previously thought with a prevalence rate of 1 per 15 000 girls.

Clinical features

The condition, which has only been described in girls, shows a characteristic clinical picture: a period of normal development up to around 18 months followed by a rapid decline in developmental progress and the rapid deterioration of higher brain functions.

Over the following 18 months, there is evidence of severe dementia, a loss of purposeful hand movements, jerky ataxia and acquired microcephaly. After this rapid decline, the condition may stabilize with no further progression for some time. Subsequently, more neurological abnormalities appear including spastic paraplegia and epilepsy.

Etiology

Rett originally believed that high levels of ammonia were responsible for the condition, though subsequent studies have not confirmed this observation. The most commonly proposed explanation is that it is due to a dominant mutation on one X chromosome, and that the condition is nonviable in the male. Genetic studies indicate that the disorder is associated with the MECP2 gene at Xq28.

Prognosis

The majority of children are left profoundly retarded with severe neurological impairments. Many succumb to intermittent infections or to the underlying neuropathological disorder.

Disintegrative disorder

Clinical features[43,52]

This term refers to a group of conditions characterized by normal development until around 4 years of age followed by profound regression and behavioral disintegration, loss of language and other skills, impairment of social relationships and the development of stereotypies. It can follow on from a minor illness or from more definite neurological disease such as measles encephalitis. The prognosis is poor due to the underlying degenerative pathology in many cases. Most individuals are left with severe learning disability.

Other related conditions

Many children with learning disabilities show some autistic features. In clinical practice, it is often difficult to know whether they fulfil the criteria for pervasive developmental disorder in addition to that for intellectual retardation. It is clear that there is a wide diversity in the severity of these 'autistic features', so that it is often arbitrary whether the label 'childhood autism' is applied to these children. Many of them also show features of hyperactivity and aggression. For these reasons, ICD-10 has made two additional categories: (1) overactive disorder associated with mental retardation and stereotyped movements and (2) pervasive developmental disorder unspecified.

EMOTIONAL DISORDERS

The primary abnormality is a subjective sense of distress due to anxiety that can be expressed overtly as in anxiety disorders or covertly as in somatization or conversion disorders. This group of disorders is similar in many respects to neurotic disorders in adults. They are further divided into the following categories: anxiety and phobic states; obsessional disorders; conversion disorders, dissociative states and somatization disorders; and reaction to severe stress and adjustment disorders. Many children often show a mixed pattern of symptoms, so that a clear-cut distinction into a single category is not possible. The DOH 2000 study[15] found a prevalence rate of 4.0% with an equal gender prevalence. Prognosis is generally favorable as many problems arise from an acute stress, so that the problems should resolve once the stressful effects lessen.

ANXIETY STATES
Clinical features

This is the commonest type of emotional disorder. Anxiety has physical and psychological components, with the former referring to palpitations and dry mouth, while the latter to the subjective sense of fear and apprehension. Somatic symptoms, particularly abdominal pain, are common. Again, many symptoms represent the persistence or exaggeration of normal developmental fears, ranging in severity from an acute panic attack to a chronic anxiety state over several months. Predisposing factors include temperamental characteristics, overinvolved and over-concerned parents and the 'special child syndrome'. The latter refers to children who are treated differently by their parents. This may arise in several circumstances, for instance the child is much wanted and previous ill health during pregnancy or infancy has resulted in an 'anxious' attachment between the child and parents. In turn, 'anxious' attachment may lead the parents to inadvertently reinforce normal fears and anxieties.

Treatment

Several approaches, including individual, behavioral and family therapy, are used, often in combination depending upon the assessment and formulation. The newer serotonin re-uptake inhibitors (SRIs) such as buspirone have been shown to be effective in clinical trials, and are preferable to benzodiazepines.

PHOBIC STATES
Clinical features

Phobias are common and normal among children. For instance, toddlers are fearful of strangers, whereas adolescents are anxious about their appearance or weight. Pathological fears often arise from ordinary fears that are exacerbated by parental and/or social reinforcement. A phobia is defined as 'a fear of specific object or situation', for instance dogs or

heights. Its characteristics are that it is out of proportion to the situation, is irrational, is beyond voluntary control and leads to avoidance of the feared situation. This avoidance behaviour is the main reason the fear is maladaptive as it leads to increasing restriction and limitation of the child's activities.

Treatment

A behavioural approach using graded exposure to the feared situation is the most commonly used treatment. The rationale for this approach is that continued exposure to the feared stimulus reduces the anxiety associated with the stimulus, thereby decreasing avoidance behaviour. The success of this method often depends on the ability of the therapist to devise a treatment program that combines gradual exposure without inducing too much anxiety. Occasionally, anxiolytic drugs are used in conjunction with this behavioral approach.

SCHOOL REFUSAL[53]

This term, also known as school phobia, refers to the child's irrational fear about school attendance. It is also known as the 'masquerade syndrome' as it can present in a variety of disguises, including abdominal pain, headaches or a viral infection. The child is reluctant to leave home in the morning to attend school, in contrast to the truant who leaves home but not arrive at school. It occurs most commonly at the commencement of schooling, change of school, or the beginning of secondary school.

Most cases can be understood in terms of the following three mechanisms, often in combination: firstly, separation anxiety, whereby the child and/or the parent are fearful of separation, of which school is an example; secondly, a specific phobia about some aspect of school such as traveling to school, mixing with other children, or some part of the school routine, for instance some subjects, gym, or assembly; and thirdly, an indication of a more general psychiatric disturbance such as depression or low self-esteem. The latter is more frequent among adolescents. Typically, most school refusers have good academic attainments and are conformist at school, but oppositional at home. School refusal can present acutely or insidiously, often becoming a chronic problem in adolescence.

Treatment

The initial essential step is to recognize the condition itself, namely to avoid unnecessary and extensive investigations for minor somatic symptoms or to advise prolonged convalescence following a minor illness. For the acute case, early return to school with firm support for the parents and liaison with the school is the most successful approach. For the more intractable cases, extensive work with the child and parents, along with a graded return to school is advisable. A specific behavioral program for the phobic aspects may be necessary as well as the use of anxiolytic drugs in some instances. The chronic problem often requires a concerted approach, sometimes involving a period of assessment and treatment at a child psychiatric day or inpatient unit. Many clinicians use family therapy to tackle the major relationship problems that exist in some cases.

Outcome

Two thirds usually return to school regularly, whilst the remainder, usually adolescents from disturbed families, only achieve erratic attendance at school at best. Follow-up studies have found that approximately one third continue with neurotic symptoms and social impairment into adult life.

OBSESSIVE–COMPULSIVE DISORDERS[54] (Fig. 34.2)
Definition

An obsession is a recurrent, intrusive thought that the individual recognizes is irrational but cannot ignore. A compulsion or ritual is the behavior(s) accompanying these ideas, the aim of which is to reduce the associated anxiety.

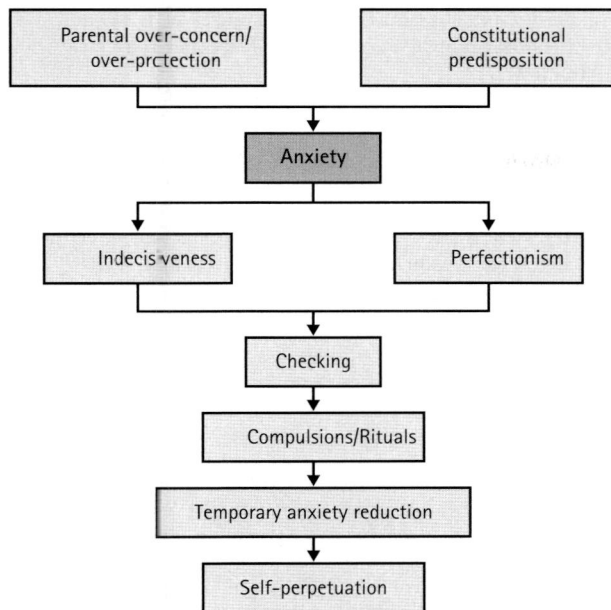

Fig. 34.2 Development of obsessional systems.

Clinical features

Most children display obsessional symptoms to a minor degree at some time, for instance avoiding cracks on paving stones or walking under ladders. They have no significance. It is when the behavior interferes with ordinary activities that it amounts to a disorder. Common obsessional rituals are hand washing and dressing. Obsessional thoughts often have a foreboding quality, for instance that 'something could happen' to a parent or sibling, that he might die, or get run over. The rituals are maintained, though maladaptive, because they produce a temporary reduction in anxiety. Commonly, the child involves other members of the family in the performance of rituals, so that the child assumes a controlling role within the family. The disorder is rare (community prevalence 0.3%) but commoner among older children and adolescents with an acute or gradual onset. In addition to anxiety symptoms, many children have depressive features.

Treatment

Behavioral methods, particularly response prevention, are successful in eliminating the obsessive–compulsive behavior. Response prevention consists of training the child to become aware of the cues that trigger the symptom and then using distraction techniques to make the performance of the ritual impossible. Recent clinical trials[54] have shown that SRIs such as paroxetine or sertraline are effective in their own right, but more importantly are very valuable as part of a combined medication – behavioral treatment package. Involvement of other members of the family, whether specifically in family therapy or to assist the child in the elimination of rituals, is necessary. Some cases require inpatient admission.

Outcome

Two thirds do well and the remainder continue to have problems, usually in a fluctuating fashion.

CONVERSION DISORDERS AND DISSOCIATIVE STATES
Clinical features

These are rare in childhood. Conversion disorder is the development of physical symptoms, usually of the special senses or limbs, without any pathological basis in the presence of identifiable stress and/or affective disturbance. The emotional conflict is said to be 'converted' into physical symptoms, which is less threatening to the individual than the under-

lying psychological conflict. A dissociative state is the restriction or narrowing of consciousness due to psychological causes, for example amnesic or fugue states. It is, however, extremely dangerous to diagnose the condition solely by the exclusion of organic disease, as follow-up studies have found that a minority subsequently develop definite organic illness. There should always be positive psychological reasons to explain the development of the symptoms. Common reasons include major life events or stresses for the child, a similar illness among other family members/peers or an underlying depressive disorder.

Minor degrees of these disorders are extremely common and frequently occur as a transitory phenomenon during the course of many illnesses. The more general term 'abnormal illness behavior', similar to the physician's phrase 'functional overlay', has been coined to describe the situation when the individual persists with or exaggerates symptoms following on from an illness.

Treatment

Successful treatment depends upon the recognition that the symptoms are 'real' for the child. Psychic pain is just as distressing as physical pain. Anger and confrontation are unhelpful. A firm sympathetic approach with little attention to the symptom per se as well as avoiding rewarding the symptom is the best strategy. Allow the child to give up the symptoms with good grace, often providing the child with some face-saving reason for improvement. Identify and treat any affective disturbance. The outcome is good for the individual episode, though other psychological problems may persist.

SOMATOFORM DISORDERS[55] (see adolescent section for chronic fatigue syndrome)
Clinical features and management

Many children complain of somatic symptoms that do not have a pathological basis. Common symptoms are abdominal pain, headaches and limb pains with community prevalence rates of approximately 10%. This condition is usually managed by general practitioners, though it sometimes results in a referral for a specialist opinion. Management involves the minimum necessary investigation to exclude any pathology, the identification of any stressful circumstances and a sensitive explanation of the basis for the symptoms. The prevention of restrictions and the active encouragement of normal activities are essential.

When the somatic symptoms are persistent, chronic and involve several systems of the body, ICD and DSM use the term *somatization disorder*. Whilst it is doubtful whether this disorder occurs in childhood, there is no doubt that persistent unexplained physical complaints are a common reason for children being taken to see the doctor. In many cases, there is clear evidence of underlying anxiety or recent stressful events.

REACTION TO SEVERE STRESS AND ADJUSTMENT DISORDERS

This group of disorders arises in response to an exceptionally stressful event or to a significantly adverse life change. The clinical features of the different syndromes vary considerably with a preponderance of affective symptoms in most cases.

Adjustment disorder
Definition

This is a maladaptive response occurring within 3 months of an identifiable psychosocial stressor. The maladaptive response must be of sufficient severity to impair daily activities such as schooling, hamper social relationships and be greater than expected given the nature of the stressor. Finally, the reaction must not last longer than 6 months.

Clinical features

By definition, the symptoms vary with ICD and DSM recognizing more than six categories. Clinical practice shows that anxiety and depressive symptoms, often combined, are the most frequent categories. Common stressors include parental divorce, unemployment, family illness or family move.

Predisposing factors

Age has different effects depending on the type of stressor. For instance, separation is more upsetting for a younger child than for an adolescent, whereas a loss of or change in a heterosexual relationship is far more important for an adolescent than for a younger child. Boys are also more vulnerable to the adverse effects of stress than girls. Temperamental characteristics such as 'difficult' or 'slow to warm up' style probably influence susceptibility as well. Again, the child's previous experience and repertoire of coping skills affect the response to the current stressor. For instance, if the child has successfully coped with adversity in the past, resilience and ability to withstand the present situation are enhanced. Finally, the family, particularly the parents, can magnify or minimize the impact of a stressor, dependent on their resourcefulness and coping style.

Outcome

By definition, the disorder can only last for 6 months, after which time the diagnostic category must change. The more important clinical consideration is not the change in diagnostic category, but the adverse effect that chronic or repeated stresses can have on the child's long term adjustment.

Post-traumatic stress disorder (PTSD)[56]

The 'epidemic' of disasters that some British children have been involved with over the past 20 years (the capsize of the Herald of Free Enterprise, the sinking of the cruise ship Jupiter, the PanAm Lockerbie air crash and the crushing disaster at the Hillsborough football stadium) have made clinicians acutely aware of this syndrome. Clinicians are now familiar with the wide symptomatology often found, and have also become involved in treatment programs to reduce the distress both in the immediate aftermath and also in the long term.

Definition

This disorder arises following exposure to a stressful event of an exceptionally threatening or catastrophic nature that would cause pervasive distress in almost anyone. The events include accidents or disasters as well as more personal traumas such as witnessing a murder, a rape or torture. In clinical practice, children who have been sexually abused commonly present with symptoms falling within the diagnostic category of PTSD.

Clinical features

These include 'flashbacks' (the repeated re-enactment of the event with intrusive memories, dreams or nightmares); a sense of detachment, 'numbness' and emotional blunting; irritability, poor concentration and memory problems. Following disasters, many survivors often experience an increased awareness of danger, a foreshortened view of the future ('only plan for today'), a feeling of 'survivor' guilt (self-reproach about own survival, whilst companions died) and acute panic reactions.

Yule[56] indicates that 30–50% of children show significant psychological morbidity following disasters with symptoms persisting for several months.

Individual vulnerability factors

Important modifying factors are probably age, previous experiences, current life situation and the availability of help. Though cognitive immaturity may protect the child from appreciating the implications of a disaster, it may also be a disadvantage, as the child may not be given the opportunity to talk about the event. The child's previous experience of stressful events and their outcome, successful or otherwise, are likely to influence the response to the disaster.

Similarly, co-existing adverse circumstances such as family disharmony or school problems reduce the child's capacity to cope with the new situation.

Management

Though most research is anecdotal rather than systematic, the available evidence[56] suggests that post-disaster 'debriefing' sessions on an individual or group basis are helpful. Specific counseling sessions to help a child deal with phobic, anxiety or depressive symptoms are frequently necessary as well. Cognitive/behavioral approaches are particularly suitable for this pattern of symptoms.

MOOD DISORDERS (See adolescent section)

CONDUCT DISORDER

Clinical features

This is usually defined as persistent antisocial or socially disapproved of behavior that often involves damage to property and is unresponsive to normal sanctions. The IOW study[14] found a prevalence rate of 4% when the mixed disorder category was included as well, with a marked male predominance (at least 3:1). There is no independent criterion for deviancy as social and cultural values determine the seriousness or otherwise attached to antisocial behavior. Consequently, most clinicians would include the criterion of impairment, namely an adverse effect on the child's daily life or development, before applying the diagnostic label of 'conduct disorder'.

Common symptoms include temper tantrums, oppositional behavior, overactivity, irritability, aggression, stealing, lying, truancy, bullying and wandering away from home/school. Delinquency (a legal term for someone committing an offence against the law) is a frequent feature among older children and adolescents. Stealing, vandalism, arson and fire setting are common forms of delinquency (male female 10:1).

Traditionally, a distinction has been made between socialized and unsocialized behavior. The former describes behavior that is in accord with peer group values, but contrary to those of society, for instance antisocial gang behavior such as stealing and vandalism. Unsocialized antisocial behavior implies more disturbed behavior as it is often done alone against a background of parental rejection or neglect and poor peer relationships. Learning difficulties, especially specific reading retardation, occur more commonly among children with conduct disorders. This is a further reason why schooling is unpopular and a source of discouragement for these children. Additionally, many children with conduct disorder have affective symptoms such as anxiety or unhappiness, as well as low self-esteem and poor peer relationships. When these symptoms are prominent, it is often appropriate to classify the disorder as mixed, implying both emotional and behavioral symptomatology.

Etiology

Four factors – the family, the peer group, the neighborhood and constitutional – make some contribution in most cases, but the family is usually the most important. Families of children with conduct disorder are characterized by having a lack of affection and rejection, marital disharmony, inconsistent and ineffective discipline, parental violence and aggression. The families are often of large size which aggravates the problems of supervision and care. Constitutional factors present in some cases include low intelligence and learning difficulties, along with adverse temperamental features such as overactivity and impulsiveness. Oppositional peer group values are an important feature in older children and adolescents. Many children with conduct disorder live in areas of urban deprivation with poor schooling. The intractable and chronic nature of these problems is a major reason for the continuation of conduct disorder into adolescence and adult life.

Treatment

Help for the family, either by counseling for the parents or by family therapy, is often used. More recently, specific intervention programs aimed at promoting positive parenting have been developed with good outcomes in the short term at least.[57] Educational support through remedial teaching or the provision of special education can be important in some cases. For many families however, the role of psychiatric services is limited, with practical support with rehousing in order to alleviate social disadvantage the most important contribution.

Prognosis

Continuity into adult life is common, with over 50% having problems as adults. Bad prognostic features are many and varied symptoms, problems at home and in the community, and anti-authority and aggressive attitudes.

HYPERACTIVITY AND ATTENTION DEFICIT SYNDROMES[39,58]

Clinical features

Considerable controversy surrounds the diagnostic terms hyperkinetic disorder (HKD), ADHD and ADD. HKD is the category used by ICD-10, which is the diagnostic system mainly used in the UK. This emphasizes the importance of pervasive overactivity (i.e. present in all situations) as a diagnostic feature. By contrast, North American psychiatrists use DSM-IV, which has the diagnostic category of ADHD. The latter stresses inattentiveness as a key symptom rather than overactivity. The different diagnostic practices probably explain the wide variation in prevalence rates (1–10%) found in epidemiological studies. Despite the difference in terminology, the two systems agree upon the same three core features: *overactivity*, *impulsivity* and *inattentiveness*.

Current UK practice has changed radically over the past 10 years, so that most UK psychiatrists use the term ADHD rather than HKD. One consequence of this change has been the dramatic increase in the prescription of methylphenidate with the annual rate in England rising from 220 000 in 1998 to 418 000 in 2004.[59]

Another controversy concerns the existence of co-morbidity among children with ADHD symptoms, which in turn is linked to the conceptual argument about whether disorders are categorical or dimensional. Traditional UK clinical practice prefers a single as opposed to several concurrent diagnoses. For instance, if a child was overactive, they would be classified as having HKD or conduct disorder, but not both. By contrast, North American practice allows, or even encourages, more than one diagnosis, namely the overactive child could have ADHD and conduct disorder. Unfortunately, current evidence is unable to provide a definite answer about the best approach. This difference in diagnostic approach is another reason for the divergent prevalence rates in epidemiological studies.

In conclusion, it is probably best to regard overactivity as a symptom rather than a diagnostic term that can occur in many clinical situations: a symptom of ADHD, HKD or ADD; a feature of many children with conduct disorder; a reflection of developmental delay on its own or in association with general intellectual retardation; one extreme of normal temperamental variation; an uncommon response to high anxiety or tension; a symptom of childhood autism; and rarely, as a reaction to some drugs, for example barbiturates or benzodiazepines.

Treatment of attention deficit hyperactivity disorder

The recent MTA Study[60] and the NICE Report[59] have provided the clearest evidence and guidance, respectively, about the most effective treatment package. Most people would advocate a multi-modal approach involving drug treatment, psycho-educational, parenting skills program and individual or group work with the child. The MTA Study showed that 80% of children improved significantly on methylphenidate with improvement persisting over the 14-month trial period. There appeared little convincing evidence that a combined approach involving drug and behavioral treatments significantly improved the outcome, but it must be remembered that the MTA study was carried out in the USA, where diagnostic practices are different.

Methylphenidate (up to 60 mg/d in divided doses) is the commonest prescribed drug in the UK, whereas dexamphetamine (up to 30 mg/d) is more popular in the USA and Australasia. Both drugs are equally effective with a similar side-effect profile, but dexamphetamine has a longer time course of effect. Stimulant drugs seem to work through an increase in dopamine levels in the frontal lobes. The common side-effects of both drugs are loss of appetite and night-time insomnia, with abdominal pain, headache, tearfulness and tics less common. It is debatable whether stimulants have any long term effect on growth or the exacerbation of tics, but careful monitoring is advisable. The last 5 years have seen important advances in the range of medications available with the licensing of extended-release preparations of methylphenidate such as Concerta XL or Equasym XL and also the availability of a once-a-day noradrenergic compound, atomoxetine. Comparative trials with these new preparations are currently underway in the UK.

Tricyclic antidepressants such as imipramine or nortriptyline are also an effective alternative treatment, and are used when the child is unresponsive to stimulants, side-effects are disabling or there is a depressive component to the child's symptoms. There are also open-label studies with clonidine, particularly for aggressive symptoms, but there have been case reports of sudden death due to cardiac arrhythmias, so that an ECG prior to commencement of treatment is essential. Pemoline, which has the considerable advantage as a once-daily dosage, has now been withdrawn in the UK on account of fears about hepatic toxicity.

Behavioral techniques, parental counseling and the alteration and manipulation of the child's environment, particularly at school, to reduce and minimize distraction are important components of most treatment programs. An alternative approach adopted by some clinicians has been the use of exclusion diets on the basis that the child is allergic to certain substances, commonly tartrazine. Evidence for the efficacy of these exclusion diets other than as a placebo response is unconvincing, though Egger et al.[61] using a sophisticated methodological design, showed that children with severe hyperactivity and mental retardation did respond. It is, however, unclear whether these results would apply to children of normal intelligence with less severe problems, who make up the majority of children with ADHD.

Outcome

Hyperactivity and attention deficits lessen considerably by adolescence, though other major problems such as learning difficulties and behavior problems persist. A substantial minority continue to have problems in adult life, mainly of an antisocial nature. There is also increasing evidence for the efficacy of methylphenidate in adults in whom the diagnosis of ADD had been missed in childhood or who have continued on treatment from childhood.[62,63]

DISORDERS OF ELIMINATION

ENURESIS

This term refers to the involuntary passage of urine in the absence of physical abnormality after the age of 5 years. It may be nocturnal and/or diurnal. Bed wetting continuously, though not usually every night, since birth is termed *primary enuresis*, whereas when there has been a 6-month period of dry beds at some stage, recurrence of bed wetting is termed *secondary* or *onset enuresis*. Diurnal enuresis is much less common than nocturnal, but more common among girls and among children who are psychiatrically disturbed. Depending upon definition, approximately 10% of 5-year-olds, 5% of 10-year-olds and 1% of 18-year-olds will have nocturnal enuresis. The majority of children with nocturnal enuresis are not psychiatrically ill, though a substantial minority, approximately 25%, have signs of psychiatric disturbance.

Etiology

A combination of individual factors such as positive family history (approximately 70%), low intelligence, psychiatric disturbance and small bladder capacity along with environmental factors such as recent stressful life events, large family size and social disadvantage are present in most cases.

Treatment

It is important to exclude any physical basis for the enuresis by history, examination and, if necessary, investigation of the renal tract. Assuming no physical pathology, the most important initial step is to minimize the handicap, namely to point out to the parents the very favorable natural outcome of the condition, and to re-label the child's enuresis as immaturity rather than laziness or wilfulness. A star chart, the accurate recording of enuresis plus positive reinforcement for dry nights, provides an accurate baseline as well as a successful treatment in its own right. An enuresis alarm is successful with older cooperative children. The success of this approach is probably because the child becomes more aware of the sensation of a full bladder along with the encouragement from parents for dry nights. The modern alarms are extremely compact and do not require a pad placed between the sheets, thereby increasing patient compliance considerably. It is useful to combine a buzzer with a star chart. Drugs such as desmopressin and imipramine are very effective at stopping enuresis, though their major limitation is that the enuresis returns when they are stopped. Most pediatricians believe it is wrong to prescribe potentially lethal drugs such as imipramine for a benign condition such as enuresis, so that desmopressin is the preferred drug treatment.

SOILING AND ENCOPRESIS

Most children are continent of feces and clean by their 4th birthday. Encopresis is usually defined as the inappropriate passage of formed feces, usually onto the underwear, in the absence of any physical pathology after 4 years of age. Soiling, the passage of semi-solid feces, is often used synonymously with encopresis. Symptoms vary widely in severity, ranging from slight staining of underwear to encopresis with the smearing of feces onto the walls. It is uncommon with a community prevalence among 8-year-olds of 1.8% for boys and of 0.7% for girls. Psychiatric disturbance is common among children with encopresis. Enuresis may also be present.

Clinical features

Figure 34.3 shows a convenient way to classify encopresis with a broad distinction between children who retain feces with eventual overflow incontinence and those who deposit feces inappropriately on a regular basis. Some children have never achieved continence, a situation called 'continuous' or 'primary encopresis', whilst others have had periods of cleanliness followed by relapse, the so-called 'discontinuous' or 'secondary encopresis'. Figure 34.3 also lists the common different patterns of interaction found among children with encopresis and their parents. For instance, children with retentive encopresis have often been subjected to coercive and obsessional toilet training practices, so that the encopresis is seen as a reaction, often of anger or aggression, towards this practice. Similarly, many children with continuous nonretentive encopresis come from disorganized, chaotic families where regular training and toileting are not the norm. Again, encopresis can arise in some children as a response to a stressful situation. Finally, encopresis can reflect poor parent–child relationship, often longstanding and usually associated with other aspects of psychiatric disturbance. The clinical picture is often, however, not as clear-cut, with the different elements each making some contribution. There may be a previous history of constipation and occasionally of anal fissure.

Treatment

A physical etiology such as Hirschsprung disease must be excluded before commencement of psychiatric treatment. The assessment must include an account of previous treatments and most importantly, the current attitude of the parents and the child to the problem. Treatment has two aims: the promotion of a normal bowel habit and the improvement of the parent–child relationship. Initially, a bowel washout and/

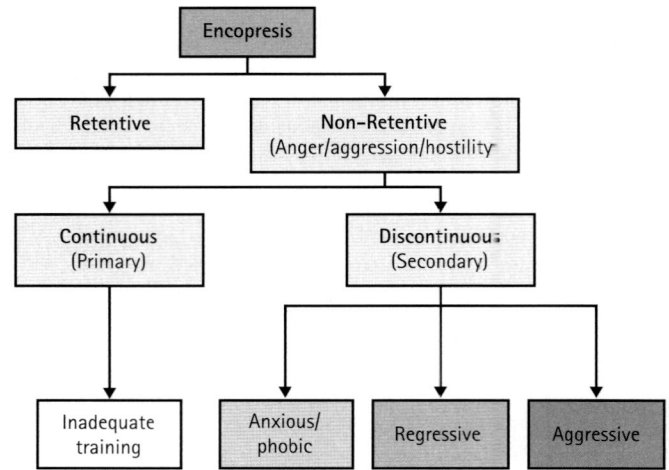

Fig. 34.3   Types of encopresis and their psychopathology. Three patterns are common in children: primary encopresis, retentive encopresis and secondary encopresis.

or microenemata may be necessary to clear out the bowel. Judicious use of bowel smooth muscle stimulants (Senokot), stool softeners (Dioctyl) and bulk agents (macrogol, lactulose) is helpful for the child with retention. Again, suppositories may be useful from time to time. This should also be combined with parent and child education about the dietary importance of fiber. The psychological component includes behavioral (star chart) and individual psychotherapy to gain the cooperation and trust of the child along with parental counseling or family therapy to modify attitudes and hostile interactions between the child and his parents.

Prognosis

It usually resolves by adolescence, though other problems may persist. Occasional case reports of persistence into adult life have been published.

MISCELLANEOUS DISORDERS

DEVELOPMENTAL DISORDERS

Language disorders (see also Ch. 23)

Children with language disorders are more vulnerable to disturbance, mainly because of the associated anxiety and embarrassment caused by the disorder. Specific language delay (5–6/1000) is twice as common in boys as in girls, with a strong association with large family size and lower social class. Richman et al[16] found that approximately 25% of 3-year-olds with specific language delay had behavioral problems.

Stuttering, an abnormality of speech rhythm consisting of hesitations and repetitions at the beginning of syllables and words is a normal, though transitory phenomenon, occurring at around 3–4 years of age. When it persists (approximately 3% of the general population), often due to inadvertent parental attention, it leads to anxiety and low self-esteem.

Selective mutism

This is not strictly a language disorder, as the main problem is the child's refusal to talk in certain situations, most commonly at school, rather than an inability to speak. Mild forms of the disorder are common but transitory, usually at the commencement of schooling, while the severe form has a prevalence rate of about 1 in 1000. Other features include a previous history of speech delay, excessively shy but stubborn temperament and parental overprotectiveness.

A combination of behavioral and family therapy techniques to promote communication and the use of speech is most commonly used, though some cases require inpatient assessment. Fluoxetine had been shown to be effective in an open trial of children with selective mutism and co-morbid anxiety disorder.[64] Prognosis is good for approximately 50%, with failure to improve by the age of 10 years a poor prognostic sign.

Reading difficulties

Though mainly of educational concern, the pediatrician or child psychiatrist may get involved because of the associated behavioral or emotional problems. The two main types are first, general reading backwardness, when the retardation is a reflection of generalized intellectual delay, and second, specific reading retardation when the attainment in reading is significantly behind the expected level after controlling for age and intelligence. The problem is 'significant' when the delay is at least 2 years. Dyslexia is a concept similar to specific reading retardation, implying a neuropsychological substrate for the specific reading difficulties. The use of this term is contentious, so that the more bland expression, 'specific reading retardation', is preferred by many clinical psychologists.

The etiology is multifactorial, involving genetic, social, perceptual and language deficits. A noteworthy feature is the strong association between specific reading retardation and conduct disorder with the behavior problem most likely arising secondary to the frustration and disillusionment associated with the reading difficulty. Treatment involves detailed psychometric assessment of the problem by a psychologist followed by an individualized remedial program carried out by a specialized teacher in collaboration with the psychologist. Help with the behavioral problem is also necessary in order to prevent more serious problems arising during adolescence.

HABIT DISORDERS

Tics and Tourette syndrome

Tics are rapid, involuntary, repetitive muscular movements, usually involving the face and neck, for instance blinks, grimaces and throat clearing. Simple tics occur as a transitory phenomenon in about 10% of the population with boys outnumbering girls three to one and with a mean age of onset around 7 years. They range in severity from simple tics involving head and neck through to complex tics extending to the limbs and trunk and finally to Tourette syndrome. The latter comprises complex tics accompanied by coprolalia (uttering obscene words and phrases) and echolalia (the repetition of sounds or words). Like stammering, tics are made worse at times of stress and may be exacerbated by undue parental concern. The differential diagnosis of tics in childhood is principally from chorea, where the movements are less coordinated and predictable, not stereotypic in form and cannot be suppressed.

Other features of tics are a positive family history and a previous history of neurodevelopmental delay. Many tics resolve spontaneously, but those that persist can be extremely disabling and difficult to treat.

Treatment

Several approaches are used singly or in combination, depending on assessment. Medication is effective, but should be reserved for severe cases. Haloperidol is the most common drug used for Tourette syndrome, but pimozide and clonidine are alternative drugs. Many children with simple tics respond to explanation and reassurance along with advice for the parents. Individual and/or family therapy may be indicated when anxiety and tension are clearly making important contributions to the problem. Behavior therapy in the form of relaxation and/or massed practice can also be helpful.

Prognosis

Simple tics have a good outcome with complete remission, whereas in Tourette syndrome the condition fluctuates in a chronic manner with 50% continuing with symptoms into adult life.

SLEEP DISORDERS (see preschool children section)

Night terrors

The usual pattern is for the child to wake up in a frightened, even terrified state, not to respond when spoken to, nor appear to see objects or people. Instead, he appears to be hallucinating, talking to and looking at people/things not actually present. The child may be difficult to comfort with the period of disturbed behavior and altered consciousness lasting up to 15 min, occasionally longer. Eventually the behavior settles, with or without comfort, and the child goes back to sleep, awakening in the morning with no recollection of the episode. The latter point is invaluable in helping to allay parental anxiety about the episodes. Night terrors arise from stage 4 or deep sleep. The peak incidence is between 4 and 7 years with a continuation of 1–3% into older children. It is also helpful to identify and ameliorate any identifiable stresses that may occasionally contribute to the problem. Lask[65] has described an apparently successful novel behavioral approach relying on waking the child 15 min prior to the expected time of the night terror. Drugs such as benzodiazepines or tricyclics have also been used successfully.

Nightmares

These are frightening or unpleasant dreams, occurring during REM (rapid eye movement) sleep. The child may or may not wake up but there will be a clear recollection of the dream if he does wake up and also in the morning. There is no period of altered consciousness or inaccessibility as in night terrors. Again, daytime anxieties and/or frightening television programs in the evening may be contributory factors.

Sleep walking (somnambulism)

The child, usually aged between 8 and 14 years, calmly arises from his bed with a blank facial expression, does not respond to attempts at communication and can only be awakened with difficulty. The child is in a state of altered consciousness at the deep level of sleep (stages 3 or 4). Any contributory anxiety should be treated as well as giving the parents some advice about the safety and protection of the child during these episodes.

PSYCHOLOGICAL EFFECTS OF ILLNESS AND DISABILITY

Approximately 15% of children have some form of chronic illness or disability. The IOW study[14] showed clearly that this group of children was much more at risk for disturbance, namely a rate of 33% for children with chronic illness affecting the central nervous system and of 12% for children with chronic illness not affecting the central nervous system compared with 7% among the general population. The IOW study also reported that children with chronic illness or handicap had the same range of disorders as other disturbed children, thereby implying that the mechanisms involved with this increased morbidity are probably indirect and nonspecific rather than direct and specific to each illness or disability. Illness or disability imposes psychological stress on the child and family not only at the time of diagnosis but also in the long term. These effects are now discussed with regard to the child himself and to other family members, though the two effects interact with each other.

Effects on the child

Three aspects are important: the acquisition of skills and outside interests, the development of self-concept, and the development of adaptive coping behavior. Many illnesses or disabilities inevitably restrict the child's ability or opportunity to acquire everyday skills and to develop interests and hobbies. For example, the child with cerebral palsy is by definition motor impaired, having the dietary restrictions of diabetes, the exercise limitations of asthma and the avoidance by children with epilepsy of some activities such as cycling or swimming. Additionally, educational problems are common among this group of children for a variety of reasons including increased absence from school, specific learning difficulties, especially among children with epilepsy, and low expectations of parents and teachers.

Illness and disability can adversely affect the child's self-concept in several ways through the effects on the child's body image and self-esteem. Many children have a distorted view of their body, believing the disability to be very prominent or disfiguring. These ideas can be reinforced by comments from parents or peers. Self-esteem can also be impaired due to a faulty cognitive appraisal of the situation and to a pessimistic attitude to the situation. This leads the child to have low self-esteem with a gloomy view about his illness and the outlook for the future. This is particularly likely and also potentially very disabling among older children and adolescents.

Successful adaptation to a disability depends on the acquisition of a range of coping behaviors and defense mechanisms to lessen anxiety to an acceptable level. Effective coping strategies include regulating the amount of stress into containable amounts, obtaining information, rehearsing the possible outcomes of treatment and assessing the situation from several viewpoints. Parents, nursing staff and pediatricians have an important role in promoting this repertoire of skills for children with a disability. Additionally, defense mechanisms such as denial, rationalization and displacement can be helpful for the child during the initial stages of adjustment to the illness or disability.

Effects on the parents

The parents can respond in various ways in the short term and also in the long term. Most parents eventually achieve some degree of adaptation, though for a minority maladaptive behavior patterns emerge and are prominent. The common reaction is overprotection whereby the parent(s) is unable to allow the child to experience the normal disappointments and upsets inevitable during childhood, so that the child leads a 'cotton wool' existence. Less frequently, the parent(s) may be rejecting and indifferent to the child because the child's disability is so damaging to the parents' self-esteem or because the disability has exacerbated an already precarious parent–child relationship. Overprotection and rejection are sometimes combined in the parental reaction.

The parents may also find it difficult to provide appropriate discipline and control, as they irrationally fear that such control may aggravate the child's illness. For example, parents of children with epilepsy may think that thwarting the child's wishes may induce an epileptic fit.

Finally, the stress of coping with the child's illness may exacerbate parental marital disharmony, though in a minority it may paradoxically unite them as they face the adversity together.

Effect on siblings

This can manifest itself in several ways: the oldest sibling may be given excessive responsibility such as looking after the disabled sibling; the siblings may lose friendships because they are reluctant to bring their friends home in case their disabled sibling is an embarrassment; and finally, the sibling's own developmental needs may be neglected with consequent resentment and frustration.

BREAKING BAD NEWS TO PARENTS

This distressing but inevitable aspect of pediatrics comes in various guises such as the birth of a child with Down syndrome or with the diagnosis of cystic fibrosis. Unfortunately, most undergraduate and postgraduate training includes very little teaching about this important subject. Though the details vary for each case, the following general principles are important:

1. Information should be given by the most senior and experienced doctor involved with the child's care.
2. Both parents must be seen together if at all possible, as this reduces misinformation and allows the parents to be mutually supportive from the outset.
3. Allow adequate time for the interview (not 10 min at the end of a ward round).

4. Privacy is essential not only as a matter of courtesy and dignity but also because it allows parents to express their emotions more freely.
5. Begin the interview by asking the parents to tell you what they know about the problems.
6. Tell parents frankly and honestly in simple and non-technical language the nature of the problem, explaining the reasons for the investigations and the basis for the diagnosis.
7. Encourage the parents to ask questions (by asking them some open-ended questions).
8. Emphasize the positive as well as the negative aspects of the diagnosis, for instance the child will be able to have physiotherapy and special equipment, will be able to go to school and to receive effective control for pain.
9. Facilitate the expression of emotions by the parents, namely respond sympathetically and sensitively to the parent(s)' distress and crying.
10. Make a definite offer of a further appointment to talk things over again.
11. Many parents find it helpful to continue the discussion with a nurse or social worker after the interview.

REACTIONS TO HOSPITALIZATION

Admission to hospital is a common experience during childhood with approximately 25% admitted by the age of 4 years. For most children, this is a short admission for a brief treatable illness whilst a minority (approximately 4%) remains in hospital for at least 1 month. While most parents and their children cope successfully with the admission, some, particularly those with repeated admissions for minor illnesses, show evidence of disturbance that may in turn have been the reason why the child was admitted in the first place.

Admission to hospital can have adverse short term and long term effects. The contributory factors can be grouped under three headings: (1) the child and family, (2) the nature of the illness, and (3) the attitudes and practices of the hospital and its staff. Important factors within the child and family include age, temperament of the child, previous experience of hospital, previous parent–child relationship and current family circumstances. Children aged between 1 and 4 years are particularly stressed by separation from familiar figures. Similarly, children with adverse temperamental characteristics, such as poor adaptability or irregularity of habits, are more vulnerable. If the child had a favorable experience when in hospital previously, this will ease the burden for any subsequent admission. If the parent–child relationship was poor prior to admission, hospitalization is likely to exacerbate this problem because of the additional stress. Adverse family circumstances, for instance financial, may also be aggravated by admission.

The nature of the illness, particularly the associated pain or the necessity for painful procedures, influences the child's response. Again, an acute admission is likely to be more stressful than an elective procedure.

The attitudes of the staff and hospital practices can minimize the distress for the child. Helpful and favorable aspects include good rooming-in facilities, adequate preparation for painful or unpleasant procedures, and nursing and medical staff trained to minimize distress and to offer comfort when required. The ward should be organized so that parents and siblings are encouraged to visit as well as ensuring the ready availability of play leaders and teachers. Medical and nursing staff should also have access to social work resources as well as to psychological and psychiatric services. Finally, joint liaison between the medical and psychiatric team and the establishment of a staff support group to enable staff to discuss their own anxieties about working in a stressful environment are likely to be beneficial.

TREATMENT METHODS

Several factors are usually responsible for the development of disturbance, so that it is unlikely that one treatment method will resolve the problem. All treatment approaches also rely upon common elements that are not only necessary but also essential for a successful outcome.

Table 34.3 Drug treatment in child psychiatry

Drug	Usage	Comment
Anxiolytics	Anxiety / phobic conditions	Short-term adjunct to behavior treatment
Neuroleptics	Phenothiazines (e.g. chlorpromazine)	Butyrophenones (e.g. haloperidol)
Newer antipsychotics	Schizophrenia/ADHD	Extrapyramidal side-effects common
(e.g. risperidone/olanzapine)	Complex tics/Tourette syndrome	Extrapyramidal side-effects common
	Schizophrenia	Fewer side-effects
Tricyclics		
Imipramine / nortriptyline	Second-line treatment for ADHD	Useful when an affective component present
clomipramine	Obsessional–compulsive disorder	Long-term usage often necessary
SRIs (fluoxetine, paroxetine, sertraline)	Probably first choice for depressive disorder	Better compliance with fewer side-effects
Stimulants		
Methylphenidate/dexamphetamine	ADHD	80% effective. Side-effects closely monitored
Hypnotics (melatonin) with ADHD	Persistent sleep disorder	Sometimes used for sleep problems associated
Lithium	Recurrent bipolar affective disorder	Close supervision of blood level and for signs of toxicity
Laxatives (e.g. bulk-forming (methylcellulose), stimulants (senna), softener (dioctyl)	Encopresis with constipation	Facilitates formation and passage of feces
Central a-agonist (e.g. clonidine)	Unresponsive Tourette syndrome	Sedation and rebound hypertension

SRIs, serotonin reuptake inhibitors.

These elements include active cooperation between the therapist and the child and family, agreement between them about the aims of treatment, and a mutual trust to enable these aims to be achieved. Again, the relative efficacy of different treatments is not clearly established, so that the choice of treatment is often a reflection of the therapist(s)' training and experience rather than an absolute indication in any particular instance. Careful analysis of the following elements is therefore necessary in order to devise an effective treatment program:

1. Individual:
   - physical illness or disability;
   - intellectual ability;
   - type of symptomatology.
2. Family
   - developmental stage (for instance a family with pre-school children or one with adolescents);
   - psychiatric health of parents;
   - marital relationship;
   - parenting qualities;
   - communication patterns within the family;
   - ability to resolve conflict;
   - support network, for instance availability of the extended family.
3. School:
   - scholastic attainments;
   - child and parents' attitude to the authority of the school;
   - peer relationships.
4. Community:
   - quality of peer relationships and of role models;
   - neighborhood and community resources.

The formulation of the problem along these four dimensions provides the basis to decide the suitable treatment program.

The three main types of treatment approach available are: (1) drug treatment, (2) the psychotherapies and (3) liaison or consultation work. The latter refers to the common practice whereby the child psychiatrist or a member of the psychiatric team does not have direct contact with the referred child, but rather helps those involved with the child to understand and modify the child's behavior. Psychotherapies are those treatments that use a variety of psychological techniques to ameliorate disturbance. They include individual therapy, behavior therapy, family therapy and group therapy as well as counseling and advice for parents.

Drug treatment[66]

This has increasing importance in child psychiatry. Table 34.3 summarizes the important indications and side-effects of various drugs used in child psychiatry.

Psychotherapies

These are a very common treatment approach in child psychiatric practice.

Individual psychotherapy[67]

Though there are several theoretical orientations, including psychoanalytic[68] and Rogerian,[69] the therapist has nevertheless the same therapeutic tasks. These are: (1) to develop a trusting, nonjudgmental relationship with the child; (2) to enable the child to express his feelings and thoughts; (3) to understand the meaning of the child's symptoms, including his behavior during the therapeutic session; and finally (4) to provide the child with some understanding and explanation for his behavior. The indications for individual psychotherapy are not clearly established, though most usually it is for children with a neurotic or reactive disorder rather than for those with a constitutionally based disorder. For younger children the medium for communication is play such as sand play or through drawing, whilst for older children verbal exchange and discussion are possible.

Behavioral psychotherapy[70]

This approach is based upon the application of the findings from experimental psychology, particularly learning theory, to a wide range of problems such as enuresis, encopresis, tantrums and aggression. Its characteristics are as follows:

1. Define problem(s) objectively with reference to the Antecedents, the Behavior itself and the Consequences (the ABC approach).
2. Place emphasis on the current behavior rather than on past events.
3. Set up hypotheses to account for the behavior.
4. Set pre-treatment baseline to determine the frequency and severity of the problem.
5. Devise behavioral program on an individual basis to test the hypothesis.
6. Evaluate outcome of treatment program.
7. Tackle one problem at a time.

As with other psychotherapies, success depends upon the establishment of a trusting relationship with the patient and the close supervision of the treatment program together with the involvement of teachers and parents in many cases.

Cognitive behavioral therapy (CBT)[71]

This is used increasingly with older children and adolescents for a variety of conditions including anxiety, depression and anorexia nervosa. The central premise is that the individual's cognitive distortions are responsible for the symptoms and the disorder, so that therapy is designed to change cognitions through a collaborative approach between the therapist and the patient. Usually the treatment lasts about 12 sessions. The early part of the treatment is devoted to teaching the patient to recognize their cognitive distortions, and then training them to devise alternative and more healthy interpretations of the situation. This is combined with 'homework tasks' between sessions in order to put into practice the new ideas or responses to situations that they find difficult.

Family therapy[72]

This is a popular treatment approach now. The rationale underlying family therapy is that the child's disturbed behavior is symptomatic of the disturbance within the family as a group. There are many different theoretical approaches and techniques,[72] but all usually involve interviewing the whole family on each occasion for about 1 h. Most family work is short term, lasting about 6 months, with approximately monthly sessions. The emphasis is on current behavior, verbal and nonverbal, observed during the session rather than on past events. The main aim is to improve communication within the family, so that dysfunctional patterns of behavior are replaced by more healthy and adaptive behavior.

Group therapy

Older children and adolescents often benefit from group therapy when the aim is to improve interpersonal relationships, particularly with the peer group, using a variety of theoretical models (for instance psychodynamic and social skills).

Supportive psychotherapy and counseling

The former is frequently used for the child with chronic illness or handicap when the focus may be the child or the parents. It is especially beneficial at the time of diagnosis and also in the long term, when the implications of the disability become more evident. Parental counseling is also used to help the parents understand their child's behavioral problems, the factors that may have led to them and that are responsible for their continuation, along with an emphasis on the parent–child relationship and the improvement of parenting skills. Counseling may therefore help the parents to devise and implement a behavioral program to modify the child's behavior as well as to promote normal development.

Liaison and consultation psychiatry[73]

This is a collaborative approach between the child psychiatry team and the professionals directly involved with the child, for instance hospital staff, teachers or residential care staff, in order to help these professionals to understand the child's disturbed behavior, their own possible contribution to the problem and to suggest ways to improve the situation. Although the child psychiatrist may see the referred child in the first instance, subsequent contact is usually with the staff rather than with the child. This approach can also include the establishment and supervision of a staff support group whose aim is to look at the attitudes and emotional responses of the staff towards the behavior shown by the children under their care.

PSYCHIATRIC DISORDERS IN ADOLESCENCE

This section has two parts: adolescent psychological development and adolescent psychiatric syndromes.

ADOLESCENT DEVELOPMENT

Adolescence is the transition between childhood and adult life. Four maturational tasks must be accomplished successfully to ensure a favorable outcome:
- attainment of independence;
- establishment of a sexual role and orientation;
- self-control of aggressive and oppositional impulses;
- achievement of self-identity.

Though these tasks are not necessarily complete nor entirely resolved by the end of adolescence, the adolescent should have made substantial progress with these tasks. Three tasks – independence, sex role and orientation, self-control of aggressive and oppositional impulses – refer to specific aspects of psychological development, whereas the fourth – self-identity – is a global term referring to that sense of uniqueness or individuality that distinguishes one person from another. Erikson[6] believed that the attainment of a stable self-identity during adolescence is the prerequisite for successful adult adjustment. Important components of self-identity for Erikson are 'sexual identity' and 'career identity'. The Eriksonian unsuccessful outcome of adolescent conflict is 'identity diffusion', with the person lacking clear goals and direction in the fulfilment of individual ambition.

Adolescent development is commonly divided into four phases:
- pre-adolescent phase (11–13 years);
- early adolescence (13–15 years);
- mid adolescence (15–17 years);
- late adolescence (18 years onwards).

The main features of the pre-adolescent phase are the onset of biological puberty and an increased interest in peer relationships and teenage pursuits. Early adolescence is characterized by the critical questioning of parental values combined with an uncritical acceptance of peer group views. The establishment of a separate sexual and social identity occurs during mid-adolescence. The individual explores and develops their own gender and sexual role. The development of social relationships outside the family enables the individual to have their own social network as well as altering the basis of their relationship with their parents. Later adolescence is focused on the career or work choice along with the expression of the sexual role through more satisfying and enduring relationships.

DETERMINANTS OF ADOLESCENT ADJUSTMENT

Though the same general factors influence development and adjustment in adolescence as in earlier periods, brief mention will be made of those that are of particular relevance.

Previous childhood experience(s)

Unsatisfactory earlier experience(s) and relationships, particularly the child–parent(s) relationship, are major factors affecting predisposition to adjustment during adolescence. The individual's capacity to withstand the inevitable stresses of adolescence and also their resilience are greatly impaired when the outcome of earlier experiences was unsatisfactory. Adverse childhood experience is an important vulnerability factor in adolescent breakdown.

Family psychopathology

Parental psychopathology such as marital disharmony or parental psychiatric illness has a powerful influence on children's behavior throughout childhood, but even more so during adolescence, when conflicts over discipline, control and autonomy are normal and unavoidable. Parental disagreements and disunity on these matters greatly exacerbate the difficulties.

Schooling

Common problems are: academic failure with scholastic subjects, poor motivation and disillusionment with schooling, conflicts over authority with teaching staff.

Peer group

Peer group values and pressure exert enormous influence on the adolescent, so that contact with and membership of a deviant peer group can lead to major problems in school, for instance truancy, or in the community, for instance delinquency or vandalism.

Chronic illness or disability

The normal adolescent drive for self-appraisal and self-identity leaves the disabled or disabled adolescent feeling isolated and different from their peers, a most distressing experience. Early childhood feelings of acceptance and tolerance by peers are replaced by those of exclusion and separateness with a reluctance or inability to gain peer group acceptance. The adolescent often deals with these feelings of anger and frustration by denial or minimalization of the seriousness of his condition. This can result in poor compliance with medication or reckless exposure to dangerous situations.

INTERVIEWING AND ASSESSMENT OF ADOLESCENTS

Though the earlier part of the chapter discussed the general principles of interviewing and assessment, it is helpful to mention some specific points relating to adolescence. Flexibility in approach is essential for successful interviewing. In general, the older the adolescent and the more serious or intimate the problem, the greater the necessity for a separate interview with the adolescent. Usually, this is combined with a family interview in order to complete the assessment.

Many adolescents are reluctant, confused or anxious attenders, so that the clinician must clarify and explain the purpose, sequence and duration of the assessment procedures at the outset. Respect for the adolescent's maturity, the right to privacy and confidentiality must be acknowledged clearly. The distinction between 'family business' and 'individual business' must be emphasized to the adolescent and to the parents. Adolescent anxieties about 'seeing the shrink' or being 'treated like a child' must be addressed and talked through. The individual interview may allow the clinician to conduct a thorough assessment of the mental state, though careful phrasing of questions about sexual or psychotic phenomena is essential in order to avoid a dismissive denial and a further increase in anxiety and confusion.

Silence and refusal to talk during the interview are common and often difficult to overcome. The clinician can use three tactics to deal with this problem: (1) it can be pointed out that the silence is just as difficult for the interviewer as it is for the adolescent; (2) there will be the opportunity and time to talk through difficult topics now or alternatively on another occasion; and finally, (3) to terminate the interview when necessary to prevent prolonged or undue tension.

Family interviews are often not only part of the assessment procedure but also of the treatment plan. Sometimes however, it is more appropriate to interview the parents and the child together rather than the whole family.

ADOLESCENT PSYCHIATRIC SYNDROMES

These are divided into three categories: those disorders persisting from earlier childhood; new disorders arising during adolescence; and those disorders with features special to adolescence. Prior to the discussion of these topics, brief comment will be made about the prevalence of psychiatric disorders in adolescence.

Prevalence

This varies widely from 10–20% depending upon the population studied, the diagnostic criteria and the age group. Most studies do however show a consistent pattern with respect to gender ratio, urban vs. rural differences and the range of clinical syndromes. In contrast to earlier childhood, when psychiatric disorder is more common among boys, the adolescent period shows a shift towards an equal gender ratio in early adolescence followed by a subsequent female preponderance in late adolescence and adult life. Prevalence rates in urban populations are at least twice that for rural populations. Schizophrenia, major affective disorder, suicide and attempted suicide, anorexia and substance abuse all begin to appear with some frequency during adolescence, whereas encopresis or enuresis decrease markedly.

PERSISTENT CHILDHOOD DISORDERS

Childhood disorders are more likely to continue into adolescence when one or more of the following are present: a major constitutional factor to the syndrome, the adverse circumstances responsible for the onset of the disorder are still present and perpetuating or maintaining factors are prominent. The follow-up study of 10-year-old children in the IOW study[13] showed that 40% of the disorders had persisted into adolescence with a strong continuity for boys with conduct disorder and associated educational problems. This section now discusses the factors responsible for the persistence of some disorders into adolescence from earlier childhood.

Conduct disorder

The oppositional and defiant character of conduct disorder means that it is very likely to be exacerbated by the rebellious and anti-authoritarian nature of ordinary adolescent behavior. Childhood predictors of persistent conduct disorder are: early onset of symptoms, extensive and varied symptomatology, and the severity of aggressive behavior. Adverse temperamental characteristics combined with continued exposure to deviant family psychopathology such as deficient and ineffective parenting, marital disharmony or parental psychiatric illness are thought to be important factors maintaining the conduct disorder. The persistence of the frequently associated learning disorders is another source of frustration and disillusionment for the adolescent, producing conflict with the teachers and reluctance to attend school.

Emotional disorders

Generally, emotional disorders have a good prognosis, often because they arise in response to some identifiable but remedial stress. Consequently, emotional disorder persisting into adolescence implies a more serious underlying cause. The school refusal syndrome is the most likely condition to show continuity from early childhood. It may reappear at the transfer from primary to secondary school, or early on during secondary schooling. Previous history of separation difficulties, for instance at the start of nursery or primary school and/or an overdependent relationship between the child and parent(s), are commonly found. The increased necessity for independence, autonomy and assertiveness at secondary school may prove too much for the vulnerable adolescent.

Childhood autism

The overt autistic-like behavior and overactivity prominent in younger children with the disorder often decrease during adolescence, but the majority are still profoundly impaired in social and communication skills with a marked apathy and lack of empathy. Educational and learning disabilities are very evident. Epilepsy also develops in about 15% of individuals with a greater risk when severe mental retardation is also present.

Attention deficit hyperactivity disorder

The overactivity usually decreases during adolescence, but persistent problems with antisocial behavior, impulsivity, recklessness, distractibility and learning disorders mean that the adolescent with ADHD is likely to remain disturbed.

NEW DISORDERS ARISING DURING ADOLESCENCE

These can be divided into two categories: those related to the stress of adolescence and major adult-like disorders arising in adolescence.

Stress-related adolescent disorders

During adolescence, the distinction between normal and abnormal behavior is often imprecise, so that it is more important to understand why the adolescent's behavior is such a cause of concern rather than whether the behavior fulfils the criteria for a disorder in a diagnostic classification system. In many cases, conflict often arises between the adolescent and the parents' overindependence and control issues. Allied with the pressure from peers, this often leads the adolescent to engage in antisocial or conduct-disordered behavior. Delinquency, vandalism and out-of-control behavior are common, sometimes mixed with a pattern of alcohol or drug abuse. Persistent antisocial disorder often culminates in criminal behavior and arrest by the police. Co-existent family problems with a limited capacity to resolve issues also contribute to the severity of the disorder. Eventually, it may be necessary for the adolescent to leave the family home and to provide him with alternative care arrangements, for instance with foster parents or community carers. Another solution sometimes adopted by the adolescent is to run away from home. Although the majority of runaways eventually return home, a minority stay away and become involved with the homeless subculture found in large cities.

The common neurotic or emotional responses to adolescent stress are affective symptoms such as irritability, liability of mood and anxiety symptoms, particularly related to social situations or mixing with peers. The latter may sometimes lead to marked social withdrawal. School refusal may sometimes present for the first time during early adolescence, when it represents a combination of adolescent stress and the revival of an earlier overdependent parent–child relationship. The increased need for independence and autonomy posed by the demands of secondary school precipitates an avoidance response to school attendance from the adolescent. The anxiety symptoms often masquerade themselves as physical complaints such as headaches or abdominal pain. The prompt exclusion of organic pathology with a minimum amount of investigation is essential in order to prevent the secondary elaboration of physical symptomatology. Delay in the recognition of the underlying psychological basis for the problem greatly exacerbates the difficulties. The prognosis is not good for a significant minority of adolescents with up to one third failing to maintain regular school attendance. Poor prognosis is usually a sign of more serious underlying family psychopathology. Follow-up studies into adult life have shown that anxiety or agoraphobic symptoms are present in about 20%.[53]

Obsessive–compulsive disorder sometimes begins during adolescence, when its occurrence can be seen as a maladaptive response to the stress of adolescence. There is often a history of earlier childhood obsessional and anxiety traits. The key element in the maintenance and exacerbation of the disorder is usually the willingness of the family to participate in the ritualistic behavior. SRIs such as sertraline and fluvoxamine have been shown to be effective in reducing OCD symptoms, but more importantly are particularly effective when combined with cognitive-behavior therapy.[74]

Major adult–like disorders arising in adolescence

Three categories of disorder – schizophrenia, mood disorders and anorexia nervosa – begin to occur with increasing frequency during adolescence.

Schizophrenia[75]

This is a rare disease during childhood. Even during adolescence, it has a frequency of less than 3 per 10 000. Symptoms are usually classified into two groups: positive and negative. Positive symptoms comprise delusions (fixed, false beliefs), hallucinations (a perceptual experience in the absence of the relevant sensory stimulus) and distortions of thinking (thought insertion and withdrawal). Negative symptoms include social withdrawal, emotional blunting, apathy, lack of motivation, poverty of speech and slowness of thought. The usual presentation is insidious rather than florid with a gradual social withdrawal and increased internal preoccupation. Dysphoric symptoms are common, so that a diagnosis of affective disorder is sometimes made. The adolescent is often able to conceal his bizarre ideas from parents and peers. However, it is the presence of increasingly unpredictable and

erratic behavior that indicates something more serious is occurring. The possibility of drug misuse is an important alternative diagnostic possibility.

Etiology

There is good evidence of a genetic component with approximately 20% of relatives having the disease.[75] The Maudsley long term follow-up study of early-onset psychosis[75] showed that one third had significant premorbid social difficulties affecting the ability to make and retain friends. There was also a downward shift in intelligence with a mean IQ of 85. The disorder tends to run a chronic course with only a minority making a full symptomatic recovery – only 12% of patients in the Maudsley study were in remission at 6 months. The best prognostic indicator was the clinical state at that time.

Treatment

It must be comprehensive including drug treatment with antipsychotics, individual and family therapy as well as help with education. Traditional antipsychotics such as chlorpromazine and haloperidol are effective, particularly for positive symptoms, but side-effects such as extrapyramidal side-effects and drowsiness adversely affect compliance. Consequently, the newer antipsychotics such as risperidone and olanzapine, with their low side-effect profile, are now the drugs of first choice. When treatment with first-line drugs is ineffective, serious consideration should be given to clozapine. This drug has been shown to be effective for treatment-resistant schizophrenia in adults, and promising case reports have been published for adolescents. There must be careful screening and monitoring for side-effects, particularly for blood dyscrasias, when clozapine is used.

Finally, bad prognostic features include poor premorbid functioning, negative symptoms and a long period of untreated illness.

MOOD DISORDERS[76,77]

This section has the following parts: depression as a symptom, depressive disorders, bipolar affective disorder, and suicide and attempted suicide.

Depression as a symptom/syndrome

Depression has been recognized as a syndrome in adults for a long time because of its characteristic constellation of symptoms, response to treatment and outcome. The depressed mood or dysphoria has qualities other than just simple sadness or unhappiness. Rather, it is the inability to derive pleasure or satisfaction from daily life (anhedonia) or to be able to respond emotionally to ordinary events. Other features of the syndrome are cognitive disturbances, behavioral changes and alterations in physiological functions. The cognitive disturbances are primarily cognitive distortions around oneself (self-blame, self-reproach, guilt and worthlessness), the world (helplessness and despair about one's life situation) and the future (hopelessness and despondency about the future). The behavioral changes range from marked agitation to withdrawal and stupor, while the physiological changes are poor appetite, weight loss and disturbed sleep pattern.

In adolescence, depression can present in the following ways: as a transient mood state; as a symptom in other psychiatric disorders, for instance anxiety states; as a symptom in physical illnesses, for instance infectious mononucleosis; and as part of a symptom complex in major depressive disorder. Epidemiological studies have shown an increasing prevalence of depressive symptomatology from childhood to adolescence. Rutter et al[78] found that many adolescents had experienced feelings of misery and depression (40%), self-deprecation (20%) and suicidal thoughts (7%) at one time or another.

Depressive disorders

Both the ICD and DSM classifications now state that depression in children and adolescents should have the same features as that in adults. They recognize the following core features: abnormal depressed mood for at least 2 weeks, marked loss of interest or pleasure in almost all activities, decreased energy or increased fatigue. Additional features include: loss of confidence and self-esteem, unreasonable feelings of guilt or self-reproach, suicidal thoughts, poor concentration and indecisiveness, psychomotor agitation or retardation, sleep disturbance, and loss of appetite.

Etiology

The etiology of child and adolescent depression is not clear but there is some support for the two main theories: genetic and environmental. Evidence for a genetic component comes from twin studies, adoption and family studies, though the size of the effect is not known. Environmental theories range from the traditional psychoanalytic perspective, to the adverse impact of life events and to the cognitive theory of Beck et al.[79] The latter regards the individual's negative view of himself, the world and the future as the cause of the depression, though clearly these cognitions could be seen as a consequence of the depressed mood rather than the cause.

Assessment

This involves detailed and sensitive interviewing of the adolescent, usually alone, as well assessment of the adolescent and the family. Family assessment is useful for two reasons: the adolescent's behavior can be seen in the context of current family functioning, and other sources of stress for the adolescent or family may be identified. Physical symptoms are frequently found among depressed adolescents, though the findings are not specific as anxious adolescents often have physical symptoms as well. The differential diagnosis must involve the distinction between normal sadness or unhappiness, other psychiatric conditions with depressive symptomatology, for instance anorexia nervosa, or physical illnesses such as infectious mononucleosis or influenza.

Treatment

A comprehensive treatment package is most likely to be most effective. Components include drug treatment, individual and family therapy and the reduction or lessening of stressful circumstances. The relative emphasis and sequence of treatments are dependent upon assessment.

Drug treatment is most likely to be effective for adolescents who are most severely affected and have a disturbance of physiological functions such as appetite, sleep or weight. Emslie et al[80] have reported the superiority of fluoxetine to placebo in a well-conducted randomized control trial. Fluoxetine is currently the only recommended SRI for the treatment of depression. This advice arose from a review of published clinical trial data of SRIs that reported that evidence of efficacy was lacking for most SRIs in this age group and they were associated with increased suicidality, namely suicidal thoughts and behavior.

The purpose of individual therapy varies widely depending on the assessment and therapeutic style of the clinician. The common aims of an individual approach are: to establish a trusting relationship with the adolescent, to enable the adolescent to feel understood and accepted, and to allow the adolescent to disclose their concerns and anxieties including suicidal thoughts. Beyond these core aims, the therapeutic approach is varied, ranging from the psychodynamically insight-orientated psychotherapy to the cognitive–behavioral.

Work with the family is often undertaken more to improve communication between members of the family rather than to specifically treat family dysfunction. Family sessions are extremely useful at the start of treatment as a way to discuss events of emotional significance that may have happened recently but have not been talked through, for instance a family illness or a bereavement. These sessions also provide the opportunity to discuss ways to reduce any overt source of stress or anxiety for the adolescent. Common sources of stress include lack of friends, bullying or teasing at school and the adolescent's sense, usually distorted, of academic failure.

Bipolar disorder or manic-depressive psychosis

ICD and DSM use similar criteria for the diagnosis of bipolar disorder whether in adolescents or adults. The following points summarize the main diagnostic criteria of ICD and DSM:

- A disorder characterized by repeated episodes (two or more) in which the subject's mood and activity are significantly disturbed. This disturbance consists on some occasions of an elevation of mood with increased energy and activity (mania or hypomania), and on others of a lowering of mood with decreased energy and activity (depression).
- Recovery is characteristically complete between episodes.
- Manic episodes usually begin abruptly, lasting from 2 weeks to 4 or 5 months, whilst depressive episodes often last longer.

Clinical features

A hypomanic or depressive episode is equally common as the first manifestation of a bipolar illness with subsequent episodes more likely to be hypomanic than depressive. A depressive episode shows similar features to other depressive illnesses except that it tends to be more severe with a pronounced disturbance in physiological functioning and frequent suicidal thoughts.

The main feature of the hypomanic episode is an elevated, expansive or irritable mood with the other aspects understandable in terms of the elevated mood. The common features are: increased physical activity or physical restlessness, increased talkativeness, difficulty in concentration and distractibility, less need for sleep, increased sexual energy, mild spending sprees or other types of reckless behavior, and increased sociability or overfamiliarity. A manic episode causes severe disruption to the individual's life. The increased talkativeness becomes a 'pressure of speech' with flight of ideas (rapid switching of ideas based on a literal rather than a logical association, for instance rhyming or punning). The social disinhibition and recklessness can have a devastating effect on the individual's life. Cases with early onset have a worse prognosis with more frequent episodes, rapid cycling and a greater risk of suicide.

Though uncommon, several organic conditions can mimic a hypomanic episode. These include infections (encephalitis), endocrine (hyperthyroidism), neurological (repeated seizures, head trauma), brain tumor (meningioma, glioma), medication (steroids) and substance misuse (alcohol and amphetamine/LSD misuse).

Management

A depressive episode should be managed in a similar manner to other depressive episodes: that is SRIs, individual and family support. ECT may need to be considered for a severely depressed and/or suicidal patient.

The hypomanic episode is often harder to manage, as it usually requires inpatient admission, measures to ensure the safety and protection of the patient and drug treatment. The most useful drug for an acute episode is haloperidol (dosage 0.05 mg/kg/d in three divided doses). It is usually necessary to supplement this medication with antiparkinsonian drugs such as benzhexol or orphenadrine. An acute dystonic reaction such as an oculogyric crisis or acute torticollis can occur when treatment is commenced. Consequently, it is essential to observe closely the initiation of the medication.

Lithium carbonate is also effective in the acute episode, though its effect has a slower onset. Lithium is more useful as a prophylactic medication for individuals who have had several episodes. Its introduction should be carefully supervised and monitored. There have however been no controlled trials of the effectiveness of lithium in the prevention of further episodes in children or adolescents. Lithium has however been shown to be less effective among individuals with a rapid cycling disorder, features common among adolescents with bipolar disorder. Other drugs such as carbamazepine and sodium valproate have been used in the treatment of previously drug-resistant manic episodes in adults, but there is insufficient evidence to evaluate their efficacy for adolescents with bipolar disorder.

Prognosis

Most individuals usually recover from an acute episode. For individuals with repeated episodes, poor prognostic features include the absence of a precipitating factor, a family history of recurrent illness and the continuation of some symptoms between acute episodes.

SUICIDE

This is extremely rare below the age of 12 years with an increase during adolescence to approximately 30 cases per million per year.[81] It is more common in males with no trend in social class. Males tend to use violent methods such as hanging or jumping from high buildings or bridges, whilst females have a preference for self-poisoning. Shaffer & Piancentini[81] identified four types of personality characteristics among adolescents who commit suicide: irritable and oversensitive to criticism; impulsive and volatile; withdrawn and uncommunicative; and perfectionist and self-critical. They also found that some evidence for an increased psychiatric disturbance in the family and that a 'disciplinary crisis' was the most common reason precipitating the suicide.

Attempted suicide

This is common with a rate of 4 per 1000 per year among 15–19-year-olds. Females are three times more likely than males to make an attempt with an excess among lower socioeconomic groups. Not surprisingly, the families show evidence of marital disharmony, maternal psychiatric ill health, particularly depression, and paternal personality disorder. About 50% of adolescents show some evidence of psychiatric disorder, usually depression. In older adolescents, there is often a history of alcohol or drug misuse and running away from home. Social isolation and poor peer relationships are also common.

The most common method is an overdose of non-opiate analgesics such as aspirin or paracetamol, probably related to their easy availability. The severity of the overdose varies markedly from a few tablets taken impulsively to swallowing the contents of a bottle of analgesics. The attempt often follows a row with a boyfriend or a serious dispute with the parents over discipline. The adolescent may have threatened to take an overdose on previous occasions, and about 50% have consulted their general practitioner in the month prior to the overdose.

A crucial part of management is the assessment of future suicide risk. This depends on three factors: the circumstances of the attempt, the patient's current mental state and their attitude to the future. Detailed questioning about events prior to the attempt are necessary as well as a 'blow-by-blow' account of the attempt. The latter includes information about the degree of planning, whether anybody else was present and any action taken after the attempt. The identification of any difficulties at home or at school is also important.

The presence of significant depressive symptoms and pessimism about the future are predictors of continued suicide risk. It is important to enquire whether the overdose has altered the adolescent's or family's attitude to their current difficulties and their resolve to improve the situation. An assessment of the coping strategies and the capacity for change within the family is important in order to make a more realistic judgment about the future. Finally, there should be some agreement about future plans and any further contact between the adolescent, the family and the relevant professional agencies.

Treatment depends on the assessment and clinical judgment. The majority of adolescents do not require specialist psychiatric follow-up, though clearly they must know how to access psychiatric services in order to arrange further help when necessary. The indications for more specialized help include: (1) the seriousness of the attempt; (2) the presence of definite depressive disorder or persistent suicidal ideas; (3) poor family circumstances and social support; and (4) the limited capacity of the family for change. A small number may require inpatient psychiatric care, particularly the older adolescent. Follow-up psychiatric contact often involves individual counseling for the adolescent as well as family sessions to improve communication and the capacity to resolve disagreements.

There have been few systematic follow-up studies, though clinical impression suggests that those with definite psychiatric disorder or adverse social or family circumstances are more likely to be 'repeaters'.

ANOREXIA NERVOSA AND RELATED DISORDERS[82]

Anorexia nervosa is a disorder of older female adolescents with a prevalence rate of 1% among 15–19-year-olds. It does however occur among prepubertal children. The core features are:

- self-induced starvation and weight loss;
- a strong desire to be thinner with a marked fear of weight gain;
- a distorted body image (for instance feeling fat when emaciated);
- a body mass index (BMI) < 17.5.

Clinical features

The presentation is varied, sometimes mimicking physical illness or the consequences of weight loss and starvation. The history is of prolonged self-imposed starvation. Dieting often begins following a chance remark about size or shape, or alternatively as a group behavior with other adolescent girls. Food portions at mealtimes are reduced, and some meals such as breakfast or lunch are skipped entirely with the total elimination of high calorific foods such as sweets, puddings or cakes. The individual derives satisfaction from the weight loss, which in turn is a further incentive for weight loss. Parents and other adults are often complimentary and pleased at this initial weight loss. More extreme and rigid dieting is then self-imposed to meet the target for further weight reduction. Appetite and hunger pains are prominent, but the prospect of further weight loss is a powerful motivator. Only when the illness is well established does the anorexia and nausea over food become apparent. Interest and participation in exercise and athletic activities often parallel the dieting in the belief that these activities will enhance weight loss. Later on, excessive laxative use begins in order to reduce weight further.

Despite an increasingly thin physique, the adolescent refuses to accept her emaciated status, still believing and perceiving herself as fat or overweight. The distorted body image is often the first indication to the parents that the adolescent has a serious illness. Increasing arguments over food and its consumption combined with an implacable refusal to eat convince the parents that urgent medical help is required. Often, the adolescent is initially referred to a pediatrician or an endocrinologist in order to exclude a physical basis to the problem rather than accepting a psychological basis for the weight loss.

Physical examination usually shows an individual who is bright and alert despite the evident emaciation. Prominent cheekbones, sunken eyes, bones protruding through the skin, dry skin and hair with blue cold hands and feet are common features. Severe emaciation is accompanied by the appearance of fine downy hair or lanugo hair on the face, limbs and trunk with a slow pulse rate, low blood pressure and hypothermia. Most biochemical investigations are normal, but low gonadotrophin levels with high growth hormone and cortisol levels are sometimes found. Although anorexia is the most likely diagnosis, other psychiatric such as depression, obsessive–compulsive disorder or schizophrenia may need to be excluded.

Etiology

Almost as many theories have been proposed as the number of people who have researched the condition with individual family or societal factors prominent in most explanations. Review of the premorbid personality characteristics of anorexics shows them to be conformist, conscientious, compliant and high achieving. Issues over autonomy and independence are core issues for anorexics with control over food intake the only available means to preserve self-identity and independence. Similar conflicts over autonomy and independence have been observed among families with an anorectic member, but whether this is cause or effect is unclear. Again, over the past 40 years, society's view about female attractiveness has veered towards the thin end of the spectrum, so that the 'pursuit of thinness' is a major issue for many women.

Management

The severity of the condition varies widely, so that treatment includes outpatient and inpatient management with an emphasis on a 'multimodal' approach. The latter implies that a variety of treatment strategies such as individual, family or cognitive therapies are used, often concurrently or sequentially, dependent on assessment. Recognition and acknowledgment of the problem are the first crucial steps in management. The nature and seriousness of the condition highlighted by the avoidance of food and the irrational ideas about eating must be explored thoroughly in order to establish a therapeutic alliance with the adolescent and the family. Only when the latter has occurred is it possible to commence a specific treatment program.

The next stage is the alteration of eating habits in order to restore weight loss and to correct nutritional deficiencies. Advice and collaboration with the dietician are important from the outset, particularly for any nutritional deficiencies. A target weight, usually around the average for the age and height, should be agreed upon along with the appropriate daily calorific intake to ensure its attainment. Only minimal concessions to food fads or preferences should be allowed with a standard protocol for regular weight checks.

If the patient is in hospital, the nursing care and support are the most important aspects of management. The nursing staff members have to win the cooperation of the adolescent for the treatment plan. They must also be vigilant about food hoarding and surreptitious vomiting. Treatment programs usually involve a graded series of privileges dependent upon satisfactory weight gain. Once the target weight is attained, the diet should be modified, so that age-appropriate weight gain continues. Inpatient programs often involve nursing staff supervising family meals at home during weekend leave.

Working with the family has two aims: to provide educational advice about the disorder and to improve communication patterns within the family. Individual and group work is also useful, but drug treatment is not indicated unless there is a specific treatable disorder such as co-morbid depression. Russell et al[83] in a randomized intervention study reported that family therapy was better than individual therapy in the prevention of relapse among anorexics under 18 years of age who had had the illness for less than 3 years. An important limitation of this study was that only 65% of the 80 patients completed the intervention program.

In many ways, the easiest part of the treatment program, particularly with inpatients, is the restoration of weight loss. A more challenging aspect is the restructuring of the adolescent's and family's attitude to food and their pattern of interaction. Regular supervision, support and contact are essential to maintain progress and keep up morale. Very often a compromise has to be made between an ideal resolution of the problem and a realistic appraisal of the adolescent's and family's capacity to change.

Outcome

Results from follow-up studies vary widely according to inclusion criteria, outcome measures and length of follow-up. Despite these problems, outcome appears to fall into three categories, one third good, one third intermediate and one third poor. There is a 10% mortality in the long term with malnutrition and suicide accounting for most deaths. Poor prognostic factors are an early age of onset, co-existent psychiatric disorder and poor family functioning.

BULIMIA NERVOSA

This has three key features: (1) recurrent binges and purges, (2) a lack of control and (3) a morbid preoccupation with weight and shape. It is rare in the prepubertal period, but becomes increasingly common in older adolescents and young adults, when it is often associated with depression. Most patients are of normal weight. The most serious medical concern is potassium depletion from frequent vomiting. The patient's lifestyle is often chaotic, so that the first aim of treatment is to establish some structure and boundaries for the patient. Dependent on assessment, a combination of individual, cognitive – behavioral and family work is appropriate in most cases.

Two new types of eating disorder have recently been described: *food avoidance emotional disorder* and *pervasive refusal syndrome*. The former is a disorder of emotions in which food avoidance is a prominent symptom along with other affective symptoms such as depression, anxiety or phobias. There is often a previous history of food fads or food restrictions, but the symptoms do not meet the criteria for anorexia nervosa. The validity and independence of this syndrome has however not yet been established.

Pervasive refusal syndrome is a severe life-threatening syndrome characterized by pervasive refusal to eat, drink, talk, walk or engage in any self-care skills. The patients are markedly underweight with an adamant refusal to eat or drink, which ultimately becomes life threatening. Although they fulfil some criteria for anorexia nervosa, the pervasiveness of the symptomatology makes this diagnosis inappropriate. They require prolonged and extensive inpatient nursing care in order to maintain vital body functions. Most patients have been girls with some suggestion that previous traumatic sexual abuse, often involving violence, may have been responsible for the precipitation of the disorder. Most make a satisfactory physical recovery, but the long term psychiatric adjustment is not yet known.

SPECIAL TOPICS

CHRONIC FATIGUE SYNDROME[84]

This has attracted widespread media coverage because of the controversy surrounding etiology and treatment. It is usually defined as a severe disabling fatigue affecting physical and mental functioning accompanied by myalgia, mood and/or sleep disturbance. Accurate prevalence figures are difficult to obtain, but are probably about 1 in 2000. Clinic samples tend to be adolescents aged between 11–15 years, with more girls and from a higher socioeconomic grouping.

Two thirds of patients have had a previous viral infection, but not usually of the Epstein–Barr type. This leads to fatigue, which results in a reduction in physical activity, leading to more fatigue on undertaking any physical activity. The situation is reinforced by parental and personal beliefs about causation, so that a state of inactivity and fatigue become established.

Management involves a thorough assessment to exclude co-morbid psychiatric disorder such as depression, but keeping investigations to an agreed minimum. The establishment of mutual trust and a collaborative approach with the adolescent and the parents are essential to a good outcome. Individual cognitive and family work combined with a structured incremental rehabilitation strategy (a graded exercise program) are the best way to make progress and limit further incapacity. A coordinated plan for school and social reintegration is also necessary.

Outcome varies depending on the initial severity, but three quarters have made a reasonable recovery after 2 years.

SUBSTANCE MISUSE

This ranges from the readily available and legal substances such as tobacco or alcohol to the more uncommon and illegal substances such as heroin or cocaine. Though the latter give rise to more public concern, there is little doubt that cigarette smoking and excessive alcohol consumption have a far more deleterious effect on the health of the population as a whole. A recent survey of over 7000 15- and 16-year-olds in the UK[85] found that almost everyone had drunk alcohol, 30% had smoked cigarettes in the previous 30 d and 43% had at some time used illicit drugs. High levels of smoking were associated with a poorer school performance, and smoking was more common among girls. Adolescents are however only rarely referred to psychiatric services because of their smoking or alcohol habits.

Solvent abuse (glue sniffing)

Ashton[86] reviewing the available literature, estimated that 5–10% of adolescents have at some time inhaled solvents, with 0.5–1% regular users. Since 1971, the death rate from solvent overdose has risen from 2 per annum to over a 100 per annum recently. Solvent abusers have the following characteristics: male gender; peak adolescent usage between 13–15 years; and more common among lower socioeconomic groupings, minority ethnic groups and disrupted families.

Inhaled substances include many everyday items such as adhesives, aerosols, dry cleaning fluids and cigarette lighter fuel. The substances are inhaled through paper bags, saturated rags or direct inhalation. It is often done as a group activity in the socioeconomically disadvantaged areas of large cities, with regular solitary sniffing a cause for more serious concern. The immediate effect is euphoria followed by confusion, perceptual distortion, hallucinations and delusions. The regular user is often able to titrate the 'sniffs', so that a pleasantly euphoric state is maintained for several hours. The characteristic appearance of red spots around the mouth is highly suggestive of solvent abuse.

Sudden death during inhalation can occur from anoxia, respiratory depression, trauma or cardiac arrhythmia. The latter accounts for over half the deaths, whilst anoxia, usually from inhalation of vomit, is responsible for over 10% of deaths. Accidents or suicide attempts during the intoxication are another cause of death, particularly with toluene adhesives. Long term effects include neurological damage (peripheral neuropathy, encephalopathy, dementia and fits) as well as renal and liver damage.

Most solvent abusers do not come into contact with psychiatric services, unless they are referred following hospital admission with acute intoxication. School-based educational program and community-resource initiatives are more likely to be beneficial in the long term. The encouragement of retailers and shop owners to enforce the restrictions on the sale of solvents is also useful. A number of solvent abusers are referred for psychiatric assessment, usually when the abuse is seen as part of more widespread individual or family psychopathology. In the long term, most adolescents do not persist with the habit, but a minority progresses onto more addictive drugs such as heroin or cocaine.

Other substances

These include 'soft' drugs such as cannabis (marijuana) or 'hard' drugs such as amphetamines, cocaine, heroin, lysergic acid diethylamide (LSD) and designer drugs such as 'Ecstasy'. The effects are euphoric and relaxing in the short term, but apathy and inertia occur with chronic use. Most individuals do not progress from cannabis to other more seriously addictive drugs, and its consumption is not indicative of underlying psychological disturbance.

Hard drug consumption is a far more serious problem with deleterious effects on physical and psychological well-being and also from the risk of physical or psychological dependence. In addition to euphoric and pleasurable effects, most of these drugs can produce acutely distressing symptoms such as panic, fright or hallucinations. This can result in suicidal behavior or an increased risk of accidents. Long term use, for example with amphetamine or cocaine, can precipitate a florid psychotic episode with hallucinations, usually visual, and paranoid delusions. Psychological withdrawal symptoms such as an unbearable craving for a 'fix' and physical withdrawal symptoms such as nausea, vomiting and diarrhea make stopping the drug extremely difficult. Physical neglect and malnutrition are also common and exacerbate the problems. The necessity for a regular supply of the drug means that the individual resorts frequently to stealing or crime to support the addiction. The practice of needle-sharing is a major health hazard with human immunodeficiency virus (HIV) infection a strong possibility. Referral of the adolescent to a specialist treatment center and support for the parents are essential to prevent the serious social and psychological problems inevitable with long term drug misuse.

SEXUAL PROBLEMS

Two topics are discussed: sexual abuse and sexual offenders in adolescence; and gender identity disorders.

Sexual abuse and sexual offenders in adolescence[34]

Sexual abuse can present in two ways, direct disclosure of abuse or indirect manifestations of abuse. The same principles of practice and management apply to adolescents as to children (see child section of the chapter), but some special features are important. Open disclosure by the adolescent is often accompanied by the plea for complete confidentiality and no further action. Clearly this guarantee cannot be given, and the adolescent must be counseled about the necessity for an open investigation and the need for a child protection conference.

Indirect manifestations of abuse are twofold, sexually related behavior and psychiatric symptomatology. Sexually related manifestations include pregnancy, venereal disease and promiscuity. The latter often arises because the adolescent relates too readily to adults in a sexual manner as a result of the earlier experience of sexual abuse by an adult. Paradoxically, the promiscuous behavior may also lead some adults to disbelieve the adolescent's claims of abuse or believe that the adolescent was responsible for the initiation of the sexual contact. Psychiatric presentations of abuse are numerous with distress a prominent feature. Common presentations include depression, deteriorating school performance or attendance, suicidal behavior and running away from home.

Help for the sexually abused adolescent has two aims: the protection of the adolescent from further abuse and the provision of therapy to lessen the psychological trauma of the abuse. The first aim is usually achieved by ensuring that the perpetrator is no longer living at home and/or does not have contact with the adolescent. A wide range of therapies is used including individual counseling and support, family therapy or group therapy. Group therapy has become extremely popular recently. This approach has several advantages: the adolescent realizes that other adolescents have had a similar experience, the adolescent has the opportunity to discuss and share their feelings with other adolescents who are in a similar predicament, and they may feel less stigmatized. The group approach is probably less successful when the predominant feeling of the adolescent is betrayal. In this instance, it is more useful to offer individual psychotherapy to enable the adolescent to establish trust with the therapist, so that disclosure and discussion can occur in a confidential setting.

A more recent development has been the provision of treatment strategies for adolescents who have committed sexual offences. The latter include exhibitionism or indecent exposure as well as sexual abuse of other, usually younger, children. The treatment program involves an assessment of the offender's sexual knowledge and attitudes as well as their social skills and relationships. Treatment programs use a variety of approaches, often in combination, including social skills training, sex education and cognitive – behavioral approaches.

GENDER IDENTITY DISORDERS[87]

Society's attitudes towards sexuality have been changing in recent years, so that a more open discussion about sexual values and behavior is possible with greater tolerance and less stigma associated with homosexuality whether in males or females. Homosexual behavior in some form or another is quite common during the pre-adolescent and adolescent years, occurring in approximately 20% of boys and 10% of girls. It appears to be a transitory pattern of behavior as adult estimates of male and female homosexuality are 3% and 1.5%, respectively. Whilst homosexuality per se is most unlikely to be a reason for psychiatric referral, occasionally anxiety and depression associated with doubts about the homosexual role are sufficiently severe to warrant referral.

Clinicians are more likely to be involved with children or adolescents who have a gender identity disorder. A core distinction is made between individuals who display anomalous gender role behavior and those with gender identity disorder. Anomalous gender role behavior is the individual's preference for interests, activities and clothes normally associated with the opposite gender. For example, effeminate boys prefer girls' style of clothing and to play with dolls, whilst 'tomboy' girls like aggressive contact games and boys' style of clothing.

By contrast, the essential feature of the gender identity disorder is the persistent wish to be of the opposite gender. This is confirmed by the frequent expression of this wish and by extensive anomalous gender role behavior including cross-dressing. During adolescence, referral is often sought for problems associated with cross-dressing, homosexual behavior and social ostracism from peers. Trans-sexualism or the wish for permanent change of gender assignment can also become an issue.

The search for etiological factors in gender identity disorder has not been fruitful with no convincing evidence for chromosomal, physiological or endocrine abnormalities. Most clinicians believe that several psychosocial factors acting in combination are responsible. The initial parental tolerance of the anomalous sexual behavior followed by subsequent acceptance and reinforcement is a common finding among referred patients together with an overdependent mother–child relationship.

Treatment strategies for gender identity disorder include individual and family therapy, parental counseling and behavior therapy. The most important aspect of treatment is to define and agree goals with the parents and the child. Clinic studies[88] indicate that the earlier treatment is commenced the better the prognosis. Behavioral programs with attainable short term goals are much more likely to be successful than more ambitious plans. Minimizing anomalous gender behavior such as cross-dressing and the promotion of gender-appropriate behavior are the basis for intervention strategies. Treatment of co-existing individual and family psychopathology is also beneficial. Finally, the long term follow-up of 66 effeminate boys[88] found that three quarters were bisexual or homosexual as adults.

PSYCHIATRIC ASPECTS OF LEARNING DISABILITY IN CHILDHOOD

INTRODUCTION

Child psychiatrists are likely to become involved with children who have learning disability in several different ways. Sometimes they are responsible for the provision of the specialist medical care for these children, but more commonly they are asked for advice from other professionals about the emotional and behavioral problems that are quite frequent in this group of children.

TERMINOLOGY

Many terms such as mental *subnormality* or/and *mental handicap* have been used in the past. ICD and DSM use IQ or mental age as the basis for classification. IQ is defined as: mental age/chronological age × 100. The mean or average IQ is therefore 100 with a standard deviation of 15. The normal or Gaussian distribution of intelligence means that approximately 2.5% of individuals are two standard deviations below the mean, corresponding to an IQ of 70. This is usually taken as the dividing point between the normal range of intelligence and learning disability/mental retardation. ICD and DSM have four categories of mental retardation: mild (IQ 50–69 approximately); moderate (IQ 35–49 approximately); severe (IQ 20–34 approximately); profound (IQ less than 20). The other important defining criterion is that there should be evidence of social impairment and limitation in the individual's daily activities and self-care skills.

PSYCHIATRIC DISORDER IN CHILDREN WITH LEARNING DISABILITY

Prevalence

The IOW study[14] found that approximately one third of children with learning disability showed signs of disturbance with the rate rising to 50% among moderate to severely learning disabled children. The children exhibited the same range of disturbance as children of normal ability but in addition three disorders were much more frequent: childhood autism, pervasive hyperkinetic disorder and severe stereotyped movement disorder. Self-injurious behavior and pica were also more frequent.

Etiology

It is important to distinguish between the factors responsible for disorders occurring in mildly learning-disabled children and those with moderate to severe learning disability. The former probably have the same risk factors as children of average ability, but to a greater extent, that is adverse temperamental characteristics, specific learning disorders and family psychopathology. The latter is particularly important, as parents of children with mild learning disability are also likely to be within the lower range of intellectual ability. Consequently, their parenting capacity may be limited with inconsistent discipline and control prominent features. In addition, this may be combined with marital disharmony

and socioeconomic disadvantage, so that the vulnerability to psychiatric disturbance is considerably increased among this group of children.

By contrast, brain damage is an important causative factor among children with severe learning disability. Several studies[12,14] have reported that half the children with moderate to severe learning disability have demonstrable brain damage. This increases the risk of psychiatric disturbance in several ways: loss of specific functions or skills; active disruption or dysfunction of normal brain activity; and the increased risk of epilepsy. These children are also more likely to have specific learning difficulties that further increase vulnerability. In addition, adverse temperamental characteristics such as impulsivity, distractibility or overactivity are more common among this group of children. The psychosocial consequences of disability for the child and the family also make a factor in some cases, though its importance is difficult to quantify.

PSYCHIATRIC SYNDROMES SPECIFICALLY ASSOCIATED WITH MODERATE TO SEVERE LEARNING DISABILITY

Childhood autism

80% of children with childhood autism have an IQ less than 70. Many clinicians distinguish between individuals who have classical childhood autism from those with severe learning disability and some autistic features. The latter include stereotypies, mannerisms and deficits in comprehension and expressive language. These symptoms, which are quite common among many retarded children, tend to occur in isolation, so that the individual does not fulfil the diagnostic criteria for childhood autism. Clinical practice and research findings do not however provide clear-cut criteria to decide the dividing line between childhood autism and severe learning disability with autistic features. Consequently, clinicians tend to have their own personal preferences in terminology and classification.

Autistic behaviors are also features of some syndromes associated with learning disability such as tuberous sclerosis, congenital rubella, fragile X syndrome and infantile spasms. In some cases, for instance congenital rubella, the autistic behavior seems to be a response to the co-existing sensory deficit rather than the separate occurrence of childhood autism. Finally, individuals with the extremely uncommon neurodegenerative diseases such as subacute sclerosing panencephalitis or with disintegrative disorder often show autistic-like stereotypic behavior.

Hyperkinetic syndrome/attention deficit hyperactivity disorder

Like autistic behavior, overactive or hyperkinetic behavior is common among children with severe learning disability. In most cases, the overactivity occurs in some situations but not others with the overactivity reflecting an immaturity in behavior and language skills. A much smaller but nevertheless significant number do show pervasive hyperactivity with other features of that syndrome including distractibility, impulsivity and aggressive behavior.

Stereotypic and self–injurious behavior

Stereotypic movements such as body rocking or hand-flapping have been reported as frequently as 40% in mild to severely learning-disabled children. Self-injurious behavior such as head banging, biting of limbs or eye gauging is much less common but more potentially harmful and also difficult to eradicate. It often arises in an individual of very limited ability whose surroundings and immediate environment provide little or minimal stimulation. The Lesch–Nyhan syndrome is particularly associated with the development of self-mutilating behavior.

Murphy[89] reviewed the treatment methods for these intractable and destructive behaviors. Protective devices such as helmets, treatment with major tranquillizers such as haloperidol and behavioral approaches have all been used with some success. A real disadvantage with drug treatment is that once started it is difficult to stop, so that the individual can remain on a drug for several years, often with an increasing dose over time. A behavioral approach is more likely to produce long-lasting benefits, but it is more time consuming to carry out and more demanding of staff cooperation.

Pica

The ingestion of inedible substances is a transitory phenomenon among normal toddlers and is even more common among children with severe learning disability. The main adverse consequence of this behavior is lead intoxication from the licking of objects. Fecal smearing and ingestion can occur among some children, particularly those with an additional sensory handicap such as blindness.

LEARNING DISABILITY SYNDROMES ASSOCIATED WITH SPECIFIC BEHAVIORAL CHARACTERISTICS

Traditionally, children with certain learning disability syndromes have been said to show a characteristic behavioral or personality profile, though contemporary opinion is more sceptical about such association.

Down syndrome

Children with this syndrome are often described as sociable, musical, contented and easy going, features they share with their siblings. Overall, these children have a slightly increased rate of disturbance with a minority showing aggressive and oppositional behavior, usually associated with Down syndrome due to a translocation trisomy.

Phenylketonuria

Untreated, these children develop severe learning disability with autistic and hyperkinetic behavior prominent. Successful dietary treatment usually results in normal growth and development, but treated children have a greater risk of psychiatric disturbance with overactivity, distractibility and restlessness common.

Lesch – Nyhan syndrome

This sex-linked disorder of purine metabolism, occurring only in boys, is associated with an extrapyramidal movement disorder including chorea and athetosis, severe mental retardation and self-injurious behavior. The latter is extremely difficult to treat and eliminate.

Prader–Willi syndrome

The main behavioral feature is the explosive outbursts associated with dietary restriction frequently imposed to control the voracious appetite and accompanying obesity.

Hydrocephalus

Children with hydrocephalus were previously described as showing the 'cocktail party' syndrome. This is characterized by a verbosity to their speech and a superficiality or shallowness to the content of their conversation. The early detection and treatment of hydrocephalus has now produced a reduction in morbidity, so that these features are less commonly seen.

Management

Many professionals including pediatricians, teachers and psychologists are likely to be involved in the provision of care for children with learning disabilities and their families. A multidisciplinary approach to assessment and treatment is vital. Different aspects of management are important at various stages during the child's life.

Breaking the news

This topic is discussed more fully in the child section of the chapter, so that only brief comments are made here. The ability to communicate bad news in a sensitive manner is a skill rarely taught to medical students or junior doctors. Many parents complain justifiably that the initial interview with the doctor was unsatisfactory and distressing. Tact, sympathy and time are essential to enable the parent(s) to begin to grasp and understand the implications of the situation. Honest discussion combined with an emphasis on the hopeful aspects are the important prerequisites for a satisfactory interview.

Promotion of normal development

Parents should be encouraged from the outset to develop the social, self-care and educational skills of their child to the maximum. A 'normalization' and 'optimalization' strategy is the basis to the approach. Specific treatment packages, for example the Portage scheme, are helpful in enabling the parents to set realistic targets for their child.

Treatment of medical and behavioral problems

Advice from neurologists, physiotherapists and occupational therapists is important in the management of the neurological deficits frequently present among this group of children. Behavioral problems are managed in a variety of ways including medication (for hyperactivity and aggressive outbursts), protective devices (for excessive head-banging) and operant or time-out procedures (for maladaptive behavior).

Educational needs

Parents need advice from an early stage about the most appropriate educational provision. A specialized pre-school nursery is vital, and should be combined with a plan for later special educational placement. Some children may benefit from attendance at schools for children with communication or autistic-like disorders.

Genetic counseling

This is clearly essential for all parents, especially when a specific syndrome is identified.

Long term casework and support

Clinical experience and practice suggest that many families find this type of help invaluable in the long term. The identification of a key professional worker who coordinates the care plan for the child is very useful. A social worker or a professional from a voluntary organization with counseling skills is often the person best placed to fulfil this role.

Outcome

Treatment programs with an emphasis on maximizing potential, minimizing adverse effects and integrating the child into the community are the best approach. Despite cognitive impairment, behavioral problems can be reduced by the treatment program, and families learn to adapt satisfactorily. The policy of the UK Government is to close institutions for individuals with learning disability and to integrate them into the community in order to promote better long term adjustment.

REFERENCES

1. Goodyer I. Life experiences. Development and childhood psychopathology. Chichester: Wiley; 1990.
2. Bee H. The developing child. 9th edn. New York: Harper; 1999.
3. Matthews S. Cognitive development. In: Bryant P, Colman A, eds. Developmental psychology. London: Longman; 1994.
4. Hawton K, Salkovskis P, Kirk J, et al. Cognitive behaviour therapy for psychiatric problems: a practical guide. 2nd edn. Oxford: Oxford University Press; 1995.

5. Johnstone E, Owens D, Lawrie S, et al. Companion to psychiatric studies. 7th edn. Edinburgh: Churchill Livingstone; 2004.
6. Erikson E. Childhood and society. London: Penguin; 1965.
7. Bowlby J. Attachment and loss, vol. 1: Attachment London: Hogarth Press; 1969.
8. Ainsworth M. Attachment: retrospect and prospect. In: Parkes CM, Stevenson-Hinde J, eds. The place of attachment in human behaviour. New York: Basic Books; 1982.
9. Freud A. The ego and the mechanisms of defence. London: Hogarth Press; 1936.

10. World Health Organization. The ICD-10 classification of mental and behaviour disorders: clinical descriptions and diagnostic guidelines. Geneva: World Health Organization; 1992.
11. American Psychiatric Association. Diagnostic and statistical manual of mental disorders. 4th edn. Washington DC: American Psychiatric Association; 1994.
12. Rutter M, Tizard J, Whitmore K. Education, health and behaviour. London: Longmans; 1970.
13. Rutter M, Yule B, Quinton D, et al. Attainment and adjustment in two geographical areas. III. Some factors accounting for area differences. Br J Psychiatry 1975; 126:520–533.

14. Rutter M, Graham P, Yule W. A neuropsychiatric study of childhood. Clinics in developmental medicine, nos. 35/36, London: SIMP/Heinemann; 1970.

15. Meltzer H, Gatward R. Mental health of children and adolescents in Great Britain. London: The Stationary Office; 2000.

16. Richman N, Stevenson J, Graham P. Pre-school to school: a behavioural study. London: Academic Press; 1982.

17. Bailey N. Bailey's Scales II. San Antonio: Psychological Corporation; 1993.

18. Huntley M. Griffiths mental development scales from birth to two years. London: Association for Research on Infant and Child Development; 1996.

19. Kaufman A, Kaufman N. Kaufman Assessment Battery for Children (K-ABC). Circle Pines: American Guidance Service; 1983.

20. Wechsler D. Manual for the Wechsler Intelligence Scale for Children – Third UK Edition (WISC-III UK). Kent: Psychological Corporation; 1992.

21. Thorndike R, Hagen E, Sattler J. Stanford Binet Intelligence Scale. 4th edn. San Antonio: Psychological Corporation; 1986.

22. Elliott C. British Ability Scales Second Edition (BASI II). Windsor: National Foundation for Educational Research/Nelson; 1996.

23. Rust J. Wechsler Individual Achievement Tests. San Antonio: Psychological Corporation; 1995.

24. Neale MD. Neale Analysis of Reading Ability Test. 2nd edn. Windsor: National Foundation for Educational Research/Nelson; 1989.

25. Reynell J. Reynell Developmental Language Scales. Windsor: Second Revision NFER; 1985.

26. Achenbach T. Integrative Guide for the 1991 CBCL/4–18, YSR and TRF Profiles. Burlington: University of Vermont; 1991.

27. Goodman R. The Strengths and Difficulties Questionnaire: a research note. J Child Psychol Psychiatry 1997; 38:581–586.

28. Thomas A, Chess S, Birch H. Temperament and behaviour disorders in childhood. New York: New York University Press; 1968.

29. Brown G, Harris T. Social origins of depression. London: Tavistock; 1978.

30. Richman N, Lansdown R. Problems of pre-school children. Chichester: Wiley; 1988.

31. Skuse D, Wolke D, Reilly S. Failure to thrive. Clinical and developmental aspects. In: Remschmidt H, Schmidt M, eds. Child and youth psychiatry, European perspectives. vol. II: Developmental psychopathology. Stuttgart: Hans Huber; 1992.

32. Morrell J. The infant sleep questionnaire: a new tool to assess infant sleep problems for clinical and research purposes. Child Psychol Psychiatry Rev 1999; 4:20–26.

33. Jan J, Espezel H, Appleton P. The treatment of sleep disorders. Develop Med Child Neurol 1994; 36:97–107.

34. Briere J, Berliner L, Buckley J, et al. The ASPAC Handbook on Child Maltreatment. Thousand Oaks: Sage Publications; 1996.

35. Stevenson J. Treatment of sequelae of child abuse. J Child Psychol Psychiatry 1999; 40:89–112.

36. Bentovim A, Elton A, Hildebrand J, et al. Sexual abuse within the family. London: Wright; 1988.

37. Eminson M, Postlethwaite R. Munchausen by proxy: a practical approach. Oxford: Butterworth-Heinemann; 1999.

38. Cohen D, Volkmar F. A handbook of autism and pervasive developmental disorders. Chichester: Wiley; 1997.

39. Gillberg C. Clinical child neuropsychiatry. Cambridge: Cambridge University Press; 1995.

40. Kanner L. Autistic disturbances of affective contact. The Nervous Child 1943; 2:217–250.

41. Chakrabarti S, Fombonne E. Pervasive developmental disorders in pre-school children. J Am Med Assoc 2001; 285:3094–3098.

42. Farrington CP, Miller E, Taylor B. MMR and autism: further evidence against a causal association. Vaccine 2001; 19:3632–3635.

43. Lord C, Rutter M. Autism and other pervasive developmental disorders. In: Rutter M, Taylor E, Hersov L, eds. Child and adolescent psychiatry: Modern approaches. 3rd edn. Oxford: Blackwell; 1994.

44. Hagberg B. Rett syndrome – clinical and biological aspects. London: MacKeith Press; 1993.

45. Rutter M, Schopler E, eds. Autism: a reappraisal of concepts and treatment. New York: Plenum Press; 1988.

46. Pennington B, Ozonoff. Executive functions and developmental psychopathology. J Child Psychol Psychiatry 1996; 37:51–88.

47. Baron-Cohen S. Mindblindness. London: MIT Press; 1995.

48. Hobson P. Autism and the development of mind. Hove: Lawrence Erlbaum Associates; 1993.

49. Asperger H. 'Die Autistischen psychopathen' im kindesalter. Archive für Psychiatrie und Nervenkrankheiten 1944; 117:76–136.

50. Wolff S, Chick J. Schizoid personality in childhood: a controlled follow-up study. Psychol Med 1980; 10:85–100.

51. Wolff S. Schizoid personality in childhood and adult life III: The childhood picture. Br J Psychiatry 1991; 159:629–635.

52. Corbett J, Harris R, Taylor E, et al. Progressive disintegrative psychosis of childhood. J Child Psychol Psychiatry 1977; 18:211–219.

53. Berg I. Absence from school and mental health. Br J Psychiatry 1992; 161:154–166.

54. Shafran R. Obsessive–compulsive disorders in children and adolescents. Child Psychology Psychiatry Rev 2001; 6:50–58.

55. Garralda E. Somatisation in children. J Child Psychol Psychiatry 1996; 37:13–33.

56. Yule W. Posttraumatic stress disorder. In: Rutter M, Taylor E, Hersov L, eds. Child and adolescent psychiatry: Modern approaches. 3rd edn. Oxford: Blackwell; 1994.

57. Webster-Stratton C, Herbert M. Troubled families – Problem children. Chichester: Wiley; 1993.

58. Taylor E, Sergeant J, Doepfner M, et al. Clinical guidelines for hyperkinetic disorder. Eur Child Adolesc Psychiatry 1998; 7:184–200.

59. NIHCE Report. Methylphenidate, atomoxetine and dexamfhetamine for attention deficit hyperactivity disorder in children and adolescents. London: NIHCE; 2006. 2006.

60. MTA Co-operative Group. Fourteen-month randomized clinical trial of treatment strategies for attention deficit hyperactivity disorder. Arch Gen Psychiatry 1999; 56:1073–1086.

61. Egger J, Stolla A, McEwan L. Controlled trial of hyposensitisation in children with food-induced hyperkinetic syndrome. Lancet 1992; 339:1150–1153.

62. Bierderman J, Faraone S, Spencer T, et al. Patterns of comorbidity, cognition, and psychosocial functioning in adults with attention deficit hyperactivity disorder. Am J Psychiatry 1993; 150:1792–1798.

63. Spencer T, Wilens T, Biederman J, et al. A double-blind crossover comparison of methylphenidate in adults with childhood-onset attention deficit hyperactivity disorder. Arch Gen Psychiatry 1995; 52:434–443.

64. Dummit E, Klein R, Tancer N, et al. Fluoxetine treatment of children with selective mutism. J Am Acad Child Adolesc Psychiatry 1996; 35:615–621.

65. Lask B. Novel and non-toxic treatment for night terrors. BMJ 1988; 297:592.

66. Kutcher S. Practical child & adolescent psychopharmacology. Cambridge: Cambridge University Press; 2002.

67. Lanyardo M, Horne A. A handbook of child and adolescent psychotherapy. London: Routledge; 1999.

68. Freud A. The psychological treatment of children. London: Imago; 1946.

69. Reisman JM. Principles of psychotherapy with children. 2nd edn. New York: Wiley; 1973.

70. Herbert M. ABC of behavioural methods. Leicester: British Psychological Society; 1996.

71. Kendall P. Child and adolescent therapy: cognitive-behavioural procedures. New York: Guilford Press; 1999.

72. Gorrell Barnes G. Family therapy. In: Rutter M, Taylor E, Hersov L, eds. Child and adolescent psychiatry: Modern approaches. 3rd edn. Oxford: Blackwell; 1994.

73. Lask B. Paediatric liaison work. In: Rutter M, Taylor E, Hersov L, eds. Child and adolescent psychiatry: Modern approaches. 3rd edn. Oxford: Blackwell; 1994.

74. King R, Leonard H, March J, et al. Practice parameters for the assessment and treatment of children and adolescents with obsessive–compulsive disorder. J Am Acad Child Adolesc Psychiatry 1998; 39 (Suppl):27S–47S.

75. Hollis C. Adolescent schizophrenia. Advances in Psychiatric Treatment 2000; 6:83–92.

76. Goodyer I. The depressed child and adolescent: developmental and clinical perspectives. Cambridge: Cambridge University Press; 1995.

77. Park R, Goodyer I. Clinical guidelines for depressive disorders in childhood and adolescence. Eur Child Adolesc Psychiatry 2000; 9:147–161.

78. Rutter M, Graham P, Chadwick O, et al. Adolescent turmoil: fact or fiction? J Child Psychol Psychiatr 1976; 17:35–56.

79. Beck A, Rush A, Shaw B, et al. Cognitive therapy of depression. New York: Wiley; 1979.

80. Emslie G, Rush J, Weinberg W, et al. A double blind, randomized, placebo-controlled trial of fluoxetine in child and adolescents with depression. Arch Gen Psychiatr 1997; 54:1031–1037.

81. Shaffer D, Piancentini J. Suicide and attempted suicide. In: Rutter M, Taylor E, Hersov L, eds. Child and adolescent psychiatry: Modern approaches. 3rd edn. Oxford: Blackwell; 1994.

82. Gowers S, Bryant-Waugh R. Management of child and adolescent eating disorders: the current evidence-base and future directions. J Child Psychol Psychiatry 2004; 45:63–83.

83. Russell G, Szmulker G, Dare C, et al. An evaluation of family therapy in anorexia nervosa and bulimia nervosa. Arch Gen Psychiatry 1987; 44: 1047–1056.

84. Gorralda E, Chalder T. Chronic fatigue in childwood. J Child Psychol Psychiatry 2005; 46:1143–1151.

85. Miller P, Platt M. Drinking, smoking and illicit drug use among 15 and 16 year olds in the United Kingdom. BMJ 1996; 313:394–397.

86. Ashton C. Solvent abuse: little progress after twenty years. BMJ 1990; 300:135–136.

87. Di Ceglie D. Gender identity disorder in young people. Advances in Psychiatric Treatment 2000; 6:458–467.

88. Zucker K, Bradley S. Gender identity disorder and psychosexual problems in children and adolescents. New York: Plenum Press; 1995.

89. Murphy G. Update–self-injuring behaviour in the mentally handicapped. Assoc Child Psychol Psychiatry Newsletter 1985; 7:2–11.

35

Adolescent medicine

Russell Viner

WHAT IS ADOLESCENCE?

Strictly speaking, adolescence is the period between childhood and adulthood. But finding a useful definition of adolescence is difficult. Biologically it is the time of sexual maturation and the completion of growth. More than mere biology, adolescence is psychosocially the period between childhood dependency and being a functionally independent autonomous adult. Theorists have viewed adolescence in different ways; Freud saw adolescence as the period of recapitulation of the childhood Oedipal complex, while Erickson claimed that the struggle between Identity and Role Confusion typified the adolescent stage of development.[1]

Chronological definitions abound and are more pragmatic for allowing us to identify who is or is not an 'adolescent'. The World Health Organization for example defines adolescence as the second decade of life, from 10 to 20 years of age, but also defines a category of 'youth' as being 10–25 years.[2] However, chronological definitions take little account of the developmental changes of adolescence and their temporal variation, failing to apply to certain cultures or to those who are early or late developers. Because of this, some have suggested that adolescence is merely a social construct, a rite of passage that is culturally and socially invented.[3] These claims ignore the biological changes of puberty and the psychological developments driven by increasing CNS maturation and myelination. The most useful definition of adolescence is that it is a period of biopsychosocial maturation between the ages of 10 and 20 years, leading to functional independence in adult life. This definition has been adopted by the Royal Medical Colleges in the UK.[4]

WHY IS A SPECIAL MEDICAL APPROACH NEEDED FOR ADOLESCENTS?

Adolescence, the period between childhood and adulthood, is increasingly recognized as a life period that poses specific challenges for treating disease and promoting health. In working with adolescents, the treatment of disease, the prevention of ill-health and the promotion of healthy behaviors are played out against a background of rapid physical, psychological and social developmental changes – changes that produce specific disease patterns, unusual symptom presentations, and above all, unique communication and management challenges. At no other time of life are the physical and the psychosocial elements of illness and behavior so inextricably intertwined as in adolescence. This can make working with adolescents difficult. However given the right skills (which can be learned!), practicing medicine with young people can be extremely rewarding and fruitful. These skills are not only for those who deal solely with young people, but are needed by all in pediatric practice. Specific skills in adolescent health are recognized as being necessary for the practice of pediatrics in the UK,[5] the USA and other countries.

The reasons for a distinct approach to medicine with adolescents are outlined below.

ADOLESCENTS ARE A LARGE CLIENT GROUP

One argument for considering adolescents differently to children is sheer numbers; young people between 10 and 20 years of age make up between 12% and 15% of the population in most resource rich countries (13% in the UK), a client group as large as children under 10 in the UK. Projections suggest that the adolescent population will grow by 8.5% between 1998 and 2011.[6] While adolescence is generally considered to be a healthy period, health resource use by young people is higher than in late childhood.[7] Most adolescents visit their general practitioner (GP) each year,[8] around 30% have a chronic condition that requires some health resource utilization,[9] mental health resource use is higher than in childhood[10] and hospital bed use is higher during adolescence than in late childhood.[11]

ADOLESCENTS HAVE A UNIQUE EPIDEMIOLOGY OF DISEASE AND HEALTH RISK

The second argument for a special approach to adolescent health is that young people have a distinct epidemiology of disease and health risk. The diseases that are unique to adolescence are small in number (Table 35.1). But both disease and health behaviors in adolescents present a unique constellation of symptoms and problems not found in children or adults. **1571**

Table 35.1   Disorders unique to adolescence or with onset predominantly in adolescence

Disorders of puberty and pubertal growth
Adolescent idiopathic scoliosis
Juvenile idiopathic arthritis – subtypes
Adolescent acne
Eating disoders (anorexia nervosa; bulimia nervosa)
Mental disorders, e.g. conduct disorder; adolescent psychosis

Those practicing with adolescents must be familiar with both persistent or late-onset 'pediatric' diseases and with early-onset 'adult' diseases. In each, ongoing adolescent development produces characteristic symptom patterns and management problems that meld the biological with the psychosocial in unique ways. For example, type 1 diabetes has its peak age of incidence around 12–14 years, and the growth hormone excess of puberty and the psychosocial challenges of chronic illness self-management produces poorer metabolic control during adolescence than at any other age.[12] Furthermore, puberty itself accelerates the progression of diabetic complications such as nephropathy.[13] Cancer during adolescence is remarkable for its threats of mortality to a personality with a newly developing sense of identity and place in the world, but also in its combination of 'late' presentations of pediatric type cancers (e.g. rhabdomyosarcoma, medulloblastoma), 'age-specific' cancers of adolescence (e.g. bone tumors) and early onset 'adult-type' carcinomas.[14]

INCREASING SURVIVAL FROM AND INCIDENCE OF CHRONIC ILLNESS IN YOUNG PEOPLE

The increase in the prevalence of chronic illness among adolescents is changing the pattern of pediatric practice, and it is likely that young people will in the future make up a larger part of the pediatric workload. This has been driven by an increasing incidence of common chronic illnesses such as asthma and diabetes, but also by increasing survival from congenital diseases previously fatal in childhood. Cohort studies in the UK report a 70% increase in the prevalence of wheezing illness at age 16 years between 1974 and 1986, with further rises apparent in the 1990s.[15] It has been reported that almost 20% of UK 12–14 year olds used asthma medications in the past 12 months.[15] Diabetes in 10–14 year olds has increased by almost 24% Europe-wide during the past 10 years,[16] and the incidence of type 2 diabetes has risen dramatically in adolescents, particularly in minority ethnic populations.[17]

Advances in the last 20 years in the treatment of metabolic conditions, cystic fibrosis and congenital heart disease has produced new cohorts of young people surviving into adolescence and early adulthood.[18–21] The prevalence of cystic fibrosis over 15 years of age in the UK more than doubled between 1977 and 1985,[21] and currently over 85% of children with chronic illness survive to adult life.[20]

HEALTH BEHAVIORS ARE LAID DOWN IN ADOLESCENCE AND CONTINUE INTO ADULT LIFE

One of the most compelling arguments for a focus on adolescent health is that adolescence is a time when new health behaviors are laid down, behaviors that track into adulthood and will influence health and morbidity life-long. Health behaviors in childhood are dominated by parental instruction and shared family values. During adolescence young people begin to explore alternative or 'adult' health behaviors, including smoking, drinking, drug use, violence and sexual intimacy. The continuities between adolescent initiation of health behaviors and adult behavior are well documented. Regular smoking rates rise from 1% at 11 years to 24% at 15 years,[22] and over 90% of adult smokers began in the teenage years.[23] Depression and its related mental health problems are rare in childhood, but rise through puberty to adult levels in late adolescence.[24]

Equally importantly, health behaviors around exercise and food are laid down in adolescence and track into adult life. Adolescent obesity

predicts adult obesity,[25] which is strongly and independently predictive of cardiovascular risk,[26,27] and cardiovascular risk in young adulthood is highly related to the degree of adiposity as early as age 13 years.[25]

ADOLESCENTS HAVE UNIQUE NEEDS IN THE MANAGEMENT OF HEALTH AND ILLNESS

Dynamic and continued development in every aspect of a young person's life during adolescence means that young people have distinct needs in the management of illness and health. In clinical interactions with younger children, management decisions are made 'adult to adult' by health professionals in consultation with parents, and day-to-day disease management is generally undertaken directly by parents. When working with adolescents, the wishes, desires, knowledge base, capabilities and rights of the young person involved must also be taken into account – as must the fact that these wishes, desires, knowledge, capabilities and rights are constantly evolving and changing! Different approaches are required to all aspects of the doctor–patient relationship. Specialized clinical communication skills are needed to take an accurate history, bearing in mind new life domains not applicable to children (sex and drugs) and adding communication and engagement of the young person to the standard pediatric communication with the family. Physical examinations of adolescents require consideration of privacy and personal integrity as well as requiring additional skills such as pubertal assessment, breast examination and possibly genital examinations. The effective treatment of illness in adolescence requires adept management of the issues regarding adherence (compliance), consent and confidentiality, and relationships between the young person and their family.

INCREASING SOCIAL MORBIDITIES AND MORTALITY LEVELS

Perhaps the most cogent argument for specific attention to adolescent health lies in the public health arena. The causes of mortality and morbidity in adolescents are distinct from both children and adults, as environmental or social causes of mortality (e.g. accidents and suicide) make up a larger proportion of total adolescent mortality than at any other age. In most public health priority areas, including cardiovascular risk (obesity, diabetes, smoking), mental health (suicide) and sexual health (teenage pregnancy and sexually transmitted diseases (STI)), the extent of problems in young people is stable or increasing rather than diminishing (Table 35.2).

Suicide rates among older male teenagers doubled over the last three decades of the 20th century and remain high.[28] Obesity has doubled among teenagers in the past 10 years, leading to the emergence of type 2 diabetes as a significant clinical and public health problem.[29,30] While smoking rates have fallen among teenage boys, rates among teenage girls have risen over the past 20 years. Earlier sexual debut and increased rates of high-risk sexual activity have lead to high rates of teenage pregnancy and STIs in countries with poor sexual and relationship education such as the UK and USA. Given explicit evidence of the continuities between adolescent and adult health risk behaviors, adolescent morbidity trends argue strongly for urgent attention to adolescent health and the development of targeted adolescent-specific interventions.

ADOLESCENT DEVELOPMENT

All clinical interactions with adolescents must be seen against the dynamic background of continued development. For example, chronic illness management issues can be quite different between a 13-year-old boy in very early puberty who has poorly developed abstract thinking and a 16-year-old girl who is sexually mature, at final height and has well-developed adult cognitive skills. The developmental tasks or events of adolescence are outlined in Table 35.3. While we group development for convenience into early, mid- and late adolescence, it

Table 35.2   Trends in indicators of adolescent health over the past two decades. (Adapted from Viner & Barker 2005[78])

Key indicator area	Outcome	Direction of change in past 30 years	Detail
Cardiovascular risk	Obesity	↑	The prevalence of adolescent obesity (defined as BMI ≥95th centile) has quadrupled in representative samples since 1970s, rising from 4–5% in 1972[72] to 8% in the mid-1990s[73] and 21–23% in 2002
	Smoking	←	There has been no significant change in prevalence of regular smoking among adolescents aged 11–15 years since 1982,[74] while smoking among adults declined significantly during the 1980s and early 1990s[75]
Sexual health	Teenage pregnancy	←	Live birth rates to women aged 15–19 years in the UK have changed little since the late 1970s, while rates have declined markedly in the same period in other European countries such as Germany and the Netherlands[76]
	STIs	↑	Rates of uncomplicated *Chlamydia* infections among 16- to 19-year-old females doubled during the 1990s in the UK (PHLS)
Mental health	Suicide	↑	In contrast to dramatic declines in suicide rates among men and women over 45 years of age between 1950 and 1998, among 15–24 year olds, suicide rates doubled in young men and remained stable in young women[28,77]

is important to remember that the timing and tempo of biological, psychological and social development each proceed independently in each individual, although each strand can influence the others. Those who are pubertally early developers may be late in developing cognitive skills or vice versa, and it is imperative to assess biological and psychosocial maturity separately. Gender issues are important here, as the timing of biological and psychosocial maturation is subtly different in boys and girls.

BIOLOGICAL CHANGES

The biological changes of adolescence are puberty, the pubertal growth spurt, and accompanying maturational changes in other organ systems. The processes and timing of puberty and pubertal assessment skills are outlined in Chapter 15. The defining event of puberty in girls is menarche. The mean age at menarche showed a dramatic decline in most resource rich countries through the first half of the 20th century, stabilizing in the 1960s at 12.8 years in the USA and 13.2 years in the

Table 35.3   Developmental tasks of adolescence

	Biological	Psychological	Social
Early adolescence	Early puberty *Girls:* Breast bud and pubic hair development (Tanner Stage II); initiation of growth spurt *Boys:* Testicular enlargement; beginning of genital growth (Stage II)	Thinking remains concrete but with development of early moral concepts Progression of sexual identity development: development of sexual orientation – possibly by experimentation Possible homosexual peer interest Reassessment and restructuring of body image in face of rapid growth	Realization of differences from parents Beginning of strong peer identification Early exploratory behaviors (smoking, violence)
Mid-adolescence	*Girls:* Mid to late puberty (Stages IV–V) and completion of growth Menarche (Stage IV event) Development of female body shape with fat deposition *Boys:* Mid-puberty (Stages III and IV) Spermarche and nocturnal emissions Voice breaking Initiation of growth spurt (Stages III–IV)	Emergence of abstract thinking although ability to imagine future applies to others rather than self (self seen as 'bullet-proof') Growing verbal abilities; adaptation to increasing educational demands Conventional morality (identification of law with morality) Development of fervently held ideology (religious/political)	Establishment of emotional separation from parents Strong peer group identification Increased health risk behaviors (smoking, alcohol, drugs, sexual exploration) Heterosexual peer interests develop Early vocational plans Development of an educational trajectory; early notions of vocational future
Late adolescence	*Boys:* Completion of pubertal development (Stage V) Continued androgenic effects on muscle bulk and body hair	Complex abstract thinking Postconventional morality (ability to recognize difference between law and morality) Increased impulse control Further completion of personal identity Further development or rejection of ideology and religion – often fervently	Further separation from parents and development of social autonomy Development of intimate relationships – initially within peer group, then separation of couples from peer group Development of vocational capability, potential or real financial independence

UK.[31] Despite recent controversy, the evidence is clear that there has been no change in the age of menarche in the USA or the UK over the past 40 years.[31]

As well as completion of linear growth and sexual maturation, other biological systems develop their final adult form during adolescence. These include maturation of enzyme systems such as cytochrome P450 systems, accretion of peak bone mass, and the development of sexually dimorphic adult patterns in blood lipids, haemoglobin and red cell indices.

PSYCHOLOGICAL DEVELOPMENT

Psychological changes in thought patterns and cognitive ability are driven by increasing maturation and myelination of the adolescent brain.[32] Between the ages of 6 and 11 years, children generally think concretely, understanding only the immediate and short-term consequence of actions or events. Ideas and concepts can only be manipulated through using concrete representations. From the age of 12 years onwards, thought patterns begin to change to formal operational or abstract thought, the ability to manipulate ideas rather than things, imagine the future, and conceive of multiple outcomes of actions. These capacities are important for the development of a settled personal and sexual identity.[33] These psychological changes, like the biological changes of puberty, are universal to all races and cultures. However, the majority of psychological and social development is culture specific, varying with social and cultural norms regarding the roles of children and adults in society.

SOCIAL DEVELOPMENT

The social changes of adolescence are outlined in Table 35.3. Biological and psychological changes occur within the context of an individual's social environment. The essential social tasks of adolescence are developing a sense of personal identity, moving from dependence to independence, and developing mature relationship with peers. These challenges exist across all cultures; however the timing of changes and the point at which successful completion is expected varies greatly between cultures.[34] In Western societies, adolescence commonly extends over many years, with its endpoints marked by relative financial independence after the completion of education. By contrast, in some societies, the social rights and responsibilities of adulthood are conferred at initiation ceremonies or rites.

IMPLICATIONS OF ADOLESCENT DEVELOPMENT FOR HEALTH

It is the reciprocal impacts of adolescent development on disease management and health-related quality of life that pose the greatest challenges of adolescent medicine. This is especially true in chronic conditions (Table 35.4). A chronic illness or disability of any type may retard normal adolescent development, producing pubertal and growth delay, delayed social independence, poor body and sexual self-image and educational and vocational failure. Doctors, including both pediatricians and adult physicians, are poor at monitoring growth and pubertal development in adolescents with chronic illness, and attention is required to growth in chronic illness well into the early twenties.[35]

Being chronically ill, having a visible disability or being required to adhere to difficult treatment regimens is difficult at all ages – but particularly so during adolescence. Alienation from the peer group and absence from school cause social isolation, failure of socialization and ultimately, educational and vocational failure. The importance of thinking proactively about helping young people with chronic illness or disability develop independent adult living and vocational skills has been shown in longitudinal follow-up studies.[36]

Conversely, adolescent development issues impact upon the management of illness and disability. Poor adherence to medical regimens and poor disease management are virtually developmentally 'appropriate' in adolescence. Immature abilities to imagine future consequences allied with a concept of themselves as 'bullet-proof' means that the prevention of long-term complications of illness is a poor motivator for compliance. Additionally, medical advice may be rejected as part of a young person's growing independence from parents, particularly in chronic pediatric illnesses where medical staff have become medical 'parents'. Adherence and disease control are also put at risk by the developmental need to explore possible modes of future behavior, no matter how dangerous (usually derogatively referred to as 'adolescent risk-taking'). Health risk behaviors such as smoking, alcohol and drug use are as common in adolescents with chronic illness or disability as in the general population.[37]

Developmental issues in adolescent medicine are becoming more important, as the burden of chronic illness in adolescence increases as larger numbers of chronically ill children survive into the second and third decades.

Table 35.4   Reciprocal effects of chronic illness or disability and adolescent development

Effects of chronic illness or disability on development	Effects of developmental issues on chronic illness or disability
Biological: Delayed puberty Short stature Reduced bone mass accretion	*Biologically:* Increased caloric requirement for growth may negatively impact on disease parameters Pubertal hormones may impact upon disease parameters (e.g. growth hormone impairs metabolic control in diabetes)
Psychological: Infantilization Adoption of sick role as personal identifier Egocentricity persists into late adolescence Impaired development of sense of sexual or attractive self	*Poor adherence and poor disease control due to:* Poorly developed abstract thinking and planning (reduced ability to plan and prepare using abstract concepts) Difficulty in imagining the future; self-concept as being 'bullet-proof' Rejection of medical professionals as part of separation from parents Exploratory (risk-taking) behaviors
Social: Reduced independence at a time when independence is normally developing Failure of peer relationships then intimate (couple) relationships Social isolation Educational failure and then vocational failure; failure of development of independent living ability	*Associated health risk behaviors:* Chaotic eating habits may result in poor nutrition Smoking, alcohol and drug use often in excess of normal population rates Sexual risk-taking, possibly in view of realization of limited life span

RESILIENCE AND RISK IN ADOLESCENT HEALTH

Morbidity in adolescence is generally understood to result from 'risk-taking', impulsivity, the rejection of parental values and the testing of boundaries. But the standard conceptions of adolescents as risk-takers with poor future thinking abilities have been shown to be largely false.[38] Most adults take as many risks and have equally poor future thinking abilities as the majority of young people. Indeed, mental health problems, drug use and sexual risk-taking is co-morbid in the same way in adults as occurs in adolescents.[39,40] That adults seem to take fewer risks is largely because they have learned to more effectively manage the consequences of their risk-taking. It is more helpful to understand so-called 'risk-taking' behaviors in young people as developmentally appropriate 'exploratory behaviors'; i.e. young people exploring the diversity of possible adult behaviors open to them – behaviors that they may or may not continue as adults.

Once these behaviors are understood to be largely developmentally motivated, it becomes unsurprising that interventions based upon education about 'risk' behaviors show very poor results.[41] Large studies of adolescent behavior and health show convincingly that health risk behaviors of all types (substance misuse, sexual risk, suicide, injuries and violence) occur together. and are strongly associated with deprivation and ethnicity.[42] Conversely, high family, community and school support ('connectedness' or 'social capital') are protective against most health risk behaviors in adolescents.[42] Identifying such 'resilience' or protective factors is now the focus of public health interventions with young people, and known protective factors for different behaviors are outlined in Table 35.5.

The search for protective factors applies equally to clinical management of acute or chronic illness in young people. In young people with poor control of a chronic illness, it is traditional to search for causes of poor control and why things go wrong. In a young person with recurrent hospital admissions with asthma, for example, causes of exacerbations may be a lack of education or lack of a crisis plan, or psychological problems including non-adherence and manipulation of the treatment regimen. In some cases, it may be more fruitful to examine 'what has helped' and what has kept the young person out of hospital between admissions. This 'solution-focused' approach, asking young people what resources they have used to stay well between exacerbations, can be very effective in treating poor chronic illness control.[42]

THE MANAGEMENT OF ILL-HEALTH IN ADOLESCENCE

Most doctors (with the notable exceptions of neonatologists and geriatricians) have adolescents in their practice. But many are not comfortable or skilled in dealing with adolescents. American studies suggest that only around a third of physicians and pediatricians actually like working with adolescents and that around another third have very little interest in adolescent care.[43]

The effective management of young people with acute or chronic illnesses requires a nonjudgemental communication style, knowledge of adolescent development and an awareness of consent and confidentiality issues, and an ethnographic approach which aims at understanding the health beliefs and contexts in which the young person manages their disease.

COMMUNICATION WITH YOUNG PEOPLE

Consultations with adolescents differ from pediatric consultations in that the young person forms a more important and more problematic third party in the decision-making process. In working with young people, we must communicate not with another adult, but with a personality undergoing rapid psychological and social changes who may or may not share an adult's understanding of society nor adult cognitive abilities to decide between treatment alternatives in the light of future risk.

Effective clinical communication is a basic health right for young people, as well as being necessary for effective disease management. Yet adolescents report that they frequently find communication with doctors unsatisfactory, with doctors often seen as remote and judgmental figures whose confidentiality cannot be trusted.[44] Communication with adolescents requires an understanding of the cognitive and social developmental level of the young person and a nonjudgmental understanding of the social contexts of that individual's health behaviors. Important elements of effective communication with young people are outlined in Table 35.6.

Table 35.5   Identified risk and protective factors for adolescent morbidities and health behaviors

Behavior	Risk factors	Protective factors
Smoking	Depression[61] Alcohol use[59] Disconnectedness from school or family[59] Difficulty talking with parents[59] Minority ethnicity[62,63] Low school achievement[42] Peer smoking and high peer popularity[64]	Family connectedness[42] Perceived healthiness[59] Higher parental expectations[42] Low school smoking prevalence[64]
Alcohol and substance use	Depression[62] Low self-esteem[42] Easy family access to alcohol[42] Ethnicity[62] Working outside school[42] Difficulty talking with parents[59] Risk factors for transition from occasional to regular use are cigarette smoking, availability, peer use and other risk behaviors[65]	Connectedness with school and family[42] Religious affiliation[42]
Teenage pregnancy	Disadvantage Urbanicity Low educational expectations[66,67] Lack of access to sexual health services[68,69] Drug and alcohol use[70]	Religious affiliation[71] Parental connectedness and expectations[42,67,68]
Sexually transmitted infections (STI)	Psychological disturbance[40] Substance use[40]	

Table 35.6   Practical points for communicating and working with adolescents

Assure confidentiality – both in the clinical interaction and in the clinical/ hospital set up
See young people by themselves as well as with their parents. The best strategy for getting the parents out of the room is warning families when you first see them that you routinely see adolescents by themselves as a way of respecting their rights as a young person
Be empathic, respectful and nonjudgemental and try to avoid taking the 'expert' position. Treat the young person as the expert in their own condition, with the doctor as the medical advisor. Find out what the young person's goals are for their treatment and health, and negotiate matching treatments to their health goals
Try to communicate and explain concepts in a developmentally appropriate fashion. This is particularly important in health promotion. For young adolescents, concentrate on concrete 'here-and-now' issues and avoid abstract discussions, particularly about possible future health risks. You may need to repeat the information in a different form as they mature cognitively
Be yourself and don't be 'cool' or use youth language. Young people don't want you as a friend, they want a knowledgeable doctor whom they can respect and trust
Provide an emotionally and physically safe environment. A gender balance among staff is important, particularly where physical examinations are undertaken
Take a full psychosocial history when seeing young people for the first time, for example using the HEADSS protocol (see Table 35.7)

Table 35.7   HEADSS psychosocial assessment interview[46]

H	Home life including relationship with parents
E	Education or employment, including achievements and financial issues
A	Activities: particularly friendships and social relationships and the existence of close friends that the young person can rely on and talk to. Also participation in sports and exercise
D	Drug use, including cigarettes and alcohol
S	Sex: information on intimate relationships and sexual risk behaviors may be important in both acute and chronic illnesses in adolescents
S	Suicide: this is short-hand for depression and other mood disturbances and self-harming behavior

The standard pediatric consultation (doctor communicates with parents) and the standard adult consultation (doctor communications solely with patient) are both inappropriate in dealing with adolescents. Best practice is to see young people both together with their parents and by themselves. While this is time consuming, it is essential for taking an accurate history, understanding the young person's motivations and goals, and for getting accurate information on health risk behaviors such as smoking, drinking, drugs and unsafe sex.[45]

Frameworks have been developed for best practice in clinical settings with young people, the most well known being the HEADSS approach which reminds clinicians to cover the important domains of Home life, Education, Activities, Drugs, Sexuality and Suicide (depression and self-harming) when interviewing any young person (Table 35.7).[46] But having a framework is not enough; the key skills required for effective communication with young people are to understand adolescent development, to be empathic, respectful and nonjudgmental, to understand the link between physical and emotional well-being, and to provide a physically and emotionally safe environment for the clinical interaction. The good news is that these skills can be learned.[47]

EXAMINING YOUNG PEOPLE

While the bulk of physical examination of adolescents is similar to that of children, new types of examinations may provide a challenge to the pediatrician, including pubertal assessments, pelvic examinations and breast and testicular examinations. Regardless of the examination, adolescents require more attention to privacy and confidentiality than children. Ensuring personal privacy is essential, and it is appropriate to ask all young people whether or not they wish their parents to be present during physical examination, especially of the genitals. Be sensitive that they may not wish their parent to be present but may have difficulty saying this in front of their parent. This can be dealt with by suggesting to the parent that the young person may now be old enough to want their privacy and then asking the young person what they wish.

The issue of the gender of the doctor and chaperones for intimate examinations is important. Many but not all adolescents prefer to be examined by a same-sex doctor, and providing a gender balance and choice of examiner is useful if this is possible. Having a chaperone for examination of adolescents of the opposite sex is obviously mandatory to protect both the patient and the doctor.

Assessment of pubertal stage is important for the management of all chronic illnesses in adolescents as well as in the assessment of endocrine disorders. These skills are easily learned, and pubertal stage should be assessed at least annually in young people with chronic illnesses during early adolescence. For those who refuse direct genital examination, pubertal self-assessment using standard Tanner photographs or drawings offers a less accurate alternative.[48] Pediatricians in most medical systems will rarely be required to undertake pelvic examinations on adolescents, although in others this is routine.

CONFIDENTIALITY AND CONSENT ISSUES

Confidentiality and consent issues are central to the management and examination of young people, who are potentially legally underage. Adolescents are very clear that the major things they want from clinicians are confidentiality, respect and clinical excellence.[49,50] Services that are not considered to be confidential are less likely to be used by young people.[51,52] Full confidentiality (including keeping confidentiality from parents) should be assured to young people unless they are found to be at risk from suicide, sexual abuse or reveal plans to harm others.[44]

In relation to issues of consent to treatment, adolescents can fall into a no-mans' land between parental rights over minors and adult rights. In most countries including the UK, adolescents are now deemed to have adult rights to consent to treatment themselves if they are legally competent, regardless of their parents' wishes. The legal criteria for competence differ between countries, but usually require the ability to give informed consent and understand the benefits and risks of treatment or nontreatment. In the UK, competence is presumed over the age of 18 years, and adolescents between 16 and 18 years can consent to treatment but cannot refuse life-saving treatment. Under 16 years of age, adolescents are legally presumed incompetent unless they show otherwise.[53] Of course, many young people under this age are competent, so in a practical sense, it is appropriate to treat adolescents from 12 to 14 years upwards as if they have full adult medical rights and responsibilities.

ADHERENCE (COMPLIANCE) AND THE CONTROL OF CHRONIC ILLNESS IN ADOLESCENCE

Adolescents are frequently poor clinic attenders and adolescence is a time of poor disease control in many chronic conditions. Because of this, adolescents are frequently labeled as 'noncompliant', [54] although there is very little evidence that young people adhere more poorly to medical regimens than adults. Many young people struggle with the organizational responsibility of managing difficult regimens; others manipulate their regimen as part of ongoing conflict with parents; but most are faithfully adherent, but adherent to a regimen of their own choosing – one that may have little relationship to that prescribed by their doctor!

Practical measures to improve adherence to medical regimens are outlined in Table 35.8. The most important aspect is to 'decriminalize' non-adherence by recognizing that some non-adherence is universal, and working with the adolescent to tailor the regimen to meet their health goals. The most effective medical regimen for adolescents is one that ensures its own success by being tailored to meet the health goals of the young person. Finding out what the young person is most worried about, what would motivate them to take their treatments, and what they would like to change about their illness, their appearance and their life, allows doctors to start a negotiation with a young person about a regimen that would maximize adherence.

When thinking about disease 'control' in adolescence, we cannot assume that control means the same thing for the young person as it does for health professionals. In diabetes for example, good medical control is defined as a low HbA1c, few hypoglycemic episodes and no admissions to hospital in diabetic ketoacidosis. But from a young person's point of view, good 'control' may mean minimizing the impact and appearance of diabetes in their lives – which may manifest as carefully running blood sugars moderately high to avoid embarrassing 'hypos' but not high enough to cause ketosis, eating a normal diet (dietary non-adherence) and doing very few blood sugar levels. Good 'control' for the young person may also include withholding insulin to control weight. This phenotype of 'careful poor control' is common in many diseases in adolescence, and is a product of young people's health goals being focused on the here-and-now and on living a normal teenage life rather than on future disease complications. The management of this form of poor control focuses on exploring the motivations and aims of the behavior, and negotiating with the young person to fulfill their aims while also producing good medical control.

Other phenotypes of poor disease control in adolescence may result from psychological problems associated with chronic illness. Perhaps more than at any other time, the developmental changes during adolescence means that the psyche and soma are inextricably interrelated. Many young people with chronic medical conditions suffer adverse psychological sequelae, particularly depression and anxiety and adjustment disorders, as well as delayed psychosocial development.[55] This can manifest as poor disease control, frequent hospital admissions and long term school absence. Assessment and management of the reciprocal psychosocial impacts of adolescence and chronic illness (Table 35.4) are a central part of medicine for adolescents. Severe or chronic illness in adolescence should be managed in the context of multidisciplinary teams that include mental health professionals, social workers, youth workers and teachers, as well as doctors and nurses. As noted above, taking a 'solution-focused' approach may help. A young person admitted for an asthma exacerbation every month has 25 days per month when their asthma is well controlled. Find out what helped them do this and identify resiliency factors that can be worked upon to help keep the young person well and their disease better controlled.

TRANSITION

The transition of adolescents with chronic illness from pediatric to adult services is now a central part of chronic illness management (Table 35.9). This transition means more than just a transfer from one clinic to another.[56] It entails a significant change from the family-centred and developmentally focused pediatric paradigm (which frequently infantilizes the adolescent) to an adult medical culture which acknowledges patient autonomy and reproduction and employment issues but neglects growth, development and family concerns. It also entails the loss of well-known and valued pediatric care-givers and the necessity of trusting new and unknown adult carers. Because this change is so significant for the young person and their family, traditional methods of transfer of care by referral letter can lead to adolescents settling poorly into the new adult service or even dropping out of medical supervision altogether for a period.[57]

This transition period is particularly dangerous in those diseases where adult services or skills are poorly developed, such as in 'pediatric' metabolic diseases or congenital heart disease. It is important for all pediatric specialist clinics to have transition guidelines and those where larger numbers of adolescents are transferring should develop an active transition program with the receiving adult service. Preparation for transition should begin in early

Table 35.8 Practical measures to improve adherence and disease control in adolescents

'Decriminalize' non-adherence. Ask: 'Most young people have trouble taking medications. How many days a week do you manage to take them all?'

Involve the adolescent as much as possible in planning the regimen, choosing the drugs (if there are alternatives), and deciding on dose timing. Young people are more likely to adhere to programs they feel responsible for

Search for motivating factors that will help the young person stick with treatment. Issues about growth, weight and appearance are often useful in chronic illness

Make a contract with the young person where each side agrees to fulfill certain conditions

Provide written instructions (in adolescent-friendly language) about the treatment regimen

Focus the regimen on the least chaotic time in the adolescent's daily life. This is usually the morning but is different for different adolescents

For complex regimens, don't assume adherence is the same for each drug. Adolescents may faithfully adhere to some and never take others because of beliefs about the drug or side-effects. Discuss compliance with each medication separately and explore beliefs and knowledge about the drug

Find ways to involve the family in ways that do not increase parent–adolescent conflict about independence; e.g. assign the parents 'checkpoints' every 2–3 days but forbid constant nagging (which usually reduces compliance!)

Don't believe that non-adherence is because of ignorance or that education will improve compliance

Take a 'solution-focused' approach. Find out when things have gone well and try to work out why. Use these

Table 35.9 Transition recommendations

Transition preparation must be seen as an essential component of high quality health care in adolescence

Every pediatric general and speciality clinic should have a specific transition policy. More formal transition programs are necessary where large numbers of young people are being transferred to adult care

Young people should not be transferred to adult services until they have the necessary skills to function in an adult service and have finished growth and puberty

An identified person within the pediatric and adult teams must be responsible for transition arrangements. The most suitable persons are nurse specialists

Management links must be developed between the two hospitals

Evaluation of transition arrangements must be undertaken

adolescence, and young people should only move to adult care when they have the necessary skill-set to survive independently in the adult service.[58]

HEALTH PROMOTION FOR YOUNG PEOPLE

The most serious health problems affecting young people are primary care issues including teenage pregnancy, drug misuse, mental health problems and violence. By 15 years of age, around 24% of adolescents in the UK are regular smokers, 38% will be regular alcohol consumers[59] and around 25% are sexually active.[60] While these problems are generally the province of general practitioners and others in primary care, all health professionals who deal with young people should possess basic health promotion skills. Over 70% of adolescents visit a doctor every year[8] and each clinical interaction with an adolescent should provide an opportunity for health promotion.

As noted above, young people with chronic illness have similar rates of risk behaviors to the general population,[37] although few pediatricians address smoking, alcohol or sex in clinical interactions with young people with chronic conditions. Health behaviors begun in adolescence continue into adult life, and health promotion during adolescence can positively influence smoking, drug use and sexual exploratory behaviors. Those looking after young people with chronic illness must begin to address smoking, alcohol and drug use and sexual health in early adolescence as this is when exploration with health behaviors begins. This is often best done by other members of the multidisciplinary team, or by the inclusion of consultation with sexual health workers, etc. as part of the multidisciplinary management of adolescents with chronic illness.

CONCLUSIONS

Adolescent health is of increasing importance in both pediatric practice and in public health. Young people require and benefit from a distinct clinical approach based upon knowledge of adolescent development in biological, psychological and social domains and the search for resiliency factors that promote health and healthy behaviors. Although chronic illness control is frequently poorer during adolescence, concepts of the 'non-adherent' or 'difficult' adolescent are based on a lack of understanding of the disparity between traditional medical goals and the health and life goals of the young person. The most effective ways to foster healthy behavior and improve disease control during adolescence are to aim for concordance between the treatment regimen and the health goals of the young person, and to focus on factors the young person finds helpful in maintaining good health/disease control.

REFERENCES

1. Cooklin A. Psychological changes of adolescence. In Brook CDG, ed. The practice of medicine in adolescence. London: Edward Arnold; 1993: 8–24.
2. World Health Organization. The health of young people. WHO: Geneva; 1993.
3. Rutter M. Changing youth in a changing society. Cambridge MA: Harvard University Press; 1980.
4. Bridging the gaps: Healthcare for adolescents. Report of the joint working party on adolescent health of the Royal medical and nursing colleges of the UK. London: Royal College of Paediatrics & Child Health; 2003.
5. Department of Health, Department for Education and Skills. National service framework for children, young people and maternity services. Gateway Ref: 3779. London: Department of Health; 2004.
6. National Statistics 2000. Social focus on young people. London: The Stationery Office; 2000.
7. MacFaul R., Werneke U. Recent trends in hospital use by children in England. Arch Dis Child 2001; 85:203–207.
8. Kari J, Donovan C, Li J, et al. Adolescents' attitudes to general practice in North London. Br J Gen Pract 1997; 47:109–110.
9. Health Survey for England: The Health of Young People '95–97. London: Stationery Office; 1998.
10. College Research Unit, Royal College of Psychiatrists. National In-patient Child and Adolescent Psychiatry Study (NICAPS). 2001.
11. Viner RM. National survey of use of hospital beds by adolescents aged 12 to 19 in the United Kingdom. BMJ 2001; 322:957–958.
12. Greene S. Diabetes in the young: Current challenges in their management. Balliere Clin Pediatr 1996; 4:563–575.
13. Lawson ML, Sochett EB, Chait PG, et al. JW, Daneman D. Effect of puberty on markers of glomerular hypertrophy and hypertension in IDDM. Diabetes 1996; 45:51–55.
14. Michelagnoli M, Viner RM. Commentary: care of the adolescent with cancer. Eur J Cancer 2001; 37:1523–1530.
15. Kaur B, Anderson HR, Austin J, et al. Prevalence of asthma symptoms, diagnosis, and treatment in 12–14 year old children across Great Britain (international study of asthma and allergies in childhood, IS AAC UK). BMJ 1998; 316:118–124.
16. Variation and trends in incidence of childhood diabetes in Europe. EURODIAB ACE Study Group. Lancet 2000; 355:873–876.
17. Fagot-Campagna A, Pettitt DJ, Engelgau MM, et al. Type 2 diabetes among North American children and adolescents: an epidemiologic review and a public health perspective. J Pediatr 2000; 136:664–672.
18. Siegel D. Adolescents and chronic illness. JAMA 1987; 257:3396–3399.
19. Newacheck P, Taylor W. Childhood chronic illness: prevalence, severity and impact. Am J Public Health 1992; 82:364–371.
20. Gortmaker S, Sappenfield W. Chronic childhood disorders: prevalence and impact. Pediatr Clin North Am 1984; 31:3–18.
21. British Paediatric Association. Working Party on Cystic Fibrosis. Report on cystic fibrosis. 1988.
22. Goddard E, Higgins V. Smoking, drinking and drug use among young teenagers in 1998. London: The Stationery Office; 1999.
23. US Department of Health and Human Services. Preventing tobacco use among young people: A report of the Surgeon General. Washington DC: US Department of Health & Human Services, Centers for Disease Control & Prevention; 1994.
24. Harrington R, Fudge H, Rutter M, et al. Adult outcomes of childhood and adolescent depression. Arch Gen Psychiatry 1990; 47:465–473.
25. Steinberger J, Moran A, Hong CP, et al. Adiposity in childhood predicts obesity and insulin resistance in young adulthood. J Pediatr 2001; 138:469–473.
26. Hubert HB, Feinleib M, McNamara PM, et al. Obesity as an independent risk factor for cardiovascular disease: a 26-year follow-up of participants in the Framingham Heart Study. Circulation 1983; 67:968–977.
27. Osmond C, Barker DJ. Fetal, infant, and childhood growth are predictors of coronary heart disease, diabetes, and hypertension in adult men and women. Environ Health Perspect 2000; 108 (suppl 3): 545–553.
28. McClure GM. Suicide in children and adolescents in England and Wales 1970–1998. Br J Psychiatry 2001; 178:469–474.
29. Reilly JJ, Dorosty AR. Epidemic of obesity in UK children. Lancet 1999; 354:1874–1875.
30. Fagot-Campagna A, Narayan KM, Imperatore G. Type 2 diabetes in children. BMJ 2001; 322:377–378.
31. Eveleth P, Tanner J. Worldwide variation in human growth. Cambridge: Cambridge University Press; 1990.
32. Paus T, Collins DL, Evans AC, et al. Maturation of white matter in the human brain: a review of magnetic resonance studies. Brain Res Bull 2001; 54:255–266.
33. Leffert N, Petersen AC. Patterns of development during adolescence. In: Rutter M, Smith DJ, eds. Psychosocial disorders in young people. London: John Wiley; 1995:67–103.
34. Muuss RE. Theories of adolescence. New York: McGraw Hill; 1996.
35. Ghosh S, Drummond H, Ferguson A. Neglect of growth and development in the clinical monitoring of children and teenagers with inflammatory bowel disease: review of case records. BMJ 1998; 317:120–121.
36. White PD. Transition to adulthood. Curr Opin Rheumatol 1999; 11:408–411.
37. Hargrave DR, McMaster C, O'Hare MM, et al. Tobacco smoke exposure in children and adolescents with diabetes mellitus. Diabet Med 1999; 16:31–34.
38. Males M. Adolescents: daughters or alien sociopaths? Lancet 1997; 349 suppl 1):I13–I16.
39. Cohen ED. An exploratory attempt to distinguish subgroups among crack-abusing African-American women. J Addict Dis 1999; 18:41–54.
40. Ramrakha S, Avshalom C, Dickson N, et al. Psychiatric disorders and risky sexual behavior in young adulthood: cross-sectional study in birth cohort. BMJ 2000; 321:66.
41. Lister-Sharp D, Chapman S, Stewart-Brown S, et al. Health promoting schools and health promotion in schools: two systematic reviews. Health Technol Assessment 2001; 3:1–6.
42. Christie D, Fredman G. Working systemically in an adolescent medical unit: collaborating with the network. Clin Psychol 2001; 3:3–11.
43. Klitsner I, Borok G, Neintstein L, et al. Adolescent health care in a large multispecialty prepaid group practice: Who provides it and how well are they doing? West J Med 1992; 156:628–632.

44. Royal College of General Practitioners and Brook. Confidentiality and young people. London: Royal College of General Practitioners; 2000.

45. MacKenzie RG. Approach to the adolescent in the clinical setting. Med Clin North Am 1990; 74:1085–1095.

46. Goldenring JM, Cohen E. Getting into adolescent heads. Contemp Pediatr 1988; July:75–90.

47. Sanci LA, Coffey CM, Veit FC, et al. Evaluation of the effectiveness of an educational intervention for general practitioners in adolescent health care: randomised controlled trial. BMJ 2000; 320:224–230.

48. Taylor SJ, Whincup PH, Hindmarsh PC, et al. Performance of a new pubertal self-assessment questionnaire: a preliminary study. Pediatr Perinat Epidemiol 2001; 15:88–94.

49. Oppong-Odiseng ACK, Heycock EG. Adolescent health services–through their eyes. Arch Dis Child 1997; 77:115–119.

50. Burack R. Young teenagers' attitudes towards general practitioners and their provision of sexual health care. Br J Gen Pract 2000; 50:550–554.

51. Ford CA, Millstein SG, Halpern-Felsher BL, et al. Influence of physician confidentiality assurances on adolescents' willingness to disclose information and seek future health care. A randomized controlled trial. JAMA 1997; 278:1029–1034.

52. Churchill R, Allen J, Denman S, et al. Do the attitudes and beliefs of young teenagers towards general practice influence actual consultation behavior? Br J Gen Pract 2000; 50:953–957.

53. British Medical Association. Consent, rights and choices in health care for children and young people. London: BMJ; 2001.

54. Kyngas HA, Kroll T, Duffy ME. Compliance in adolescents with chronic diseases: a review. J Adolesc Health 2000; 26:379–388.

55. Eiser C. Psychological effects of chronic disease. J Child Psychol Psychiatry 1990; 31:85–98.

56. Sawyer S, Blair S, Bowes G. et al. Chronic illness in adolescents: transfer or transition to adult services?. J Pediatr Child Health 1997; 33:88–90.

57. Rosen D. Between two worlds: bridging the cultures of child health and adult medicine. J Adolesc Health 1995; 17:10–16.

58. Viner RM. Transition from pediatric to adult care. Bridging the gaps or passing the buck? Arch Dis Child 1999; 81:271–275.

59. Health and health behavior among young people. Health behavior in school-aged children: A WHO cross-national study (HSBC) international report. Copenhagen: WHO; 2000.

60. Coleman J. Key data on adolescence. Brighton: Trust for the Study of Adolescence; 1999.

61. Windle M, Windle RC. Depressive symptoms and cigarette smoking among middle adolescents: prospective associations and intrapersonal and interpersonal influences. J Consult Clin Psychol 2001; 69:215–226.

62. Kelder SH, Murray NG, Orpinas P, et al. Depression and substance use in minority middle-school students. Am J Public Health 2001; 91:761–766.

63. Alexander CS, Allen P, Crawford MA, et al. Taking a first puff: cigarette smoking experiences among ethnically diverse adolescents. Ethn Health 1999; 4:245–257.

64. Alexander C, Piazza M, Mekos D, et al. Peers, schools, and adolescent cigarette smoking. J Adolesc Health 2001; 29:22–30.

65. Coffey C, Lynskey M, Wolfe R, et al. Initiation and progression of cannabis use in a population-based Australian adolescent longitudinal study. Addiction 2000; 95:1679–1690.

66. Hogan DP, Sun R, Cornwell GT. et al. Sexual and fertility behaviors of American females aged 15–19 years: 1985, 1990, and 1995. Am J Public Health 2000; 90:1421–1425.

67. Lammers C, Ireland M, Resnick M, et al. Influences on adolescents' decision to postpone onset of sexual intercourse: a survival analysis of virginity among youths aged 13 to 18 years. J Adolesc Health 2000; 26:42–48.

68. DuRant RH, Jay S, Seymore C. Contraceptive and sexual behavior of black female adolescents. A test of a social-psychological theoretical model. J Adolesc Health Care 1990; 11:326–334.

69. Porter LE, Ku L. Use of reproductive health services among young men, 1995. J Adolesc Health 2000; 27:186–194.

70. Raine TR, Jenkins R, Aarons SJ, et al. Sociodemographic correlates of virginity in seventh-grade black and Latino students. J Adolesc Health 1999; 24:304–312.

71. Coyne-Beasley T, Schoenbach VJ. The African-American church: a potential forum for adolescent comprehensive sexuality education. J Adolesc Health 2000; 26:289–294.

72. UK Data Archive. National Study of Health and Growth, Phase I: 1972–1976 (Years 1–5). Colchester: University of Essex, 2004.

73. UK Data Archive National Study of Health and Growth, Phase III : 1982–1994 (Years 11–23). Colchester: University of Essex, 1994.

74. Boreham R, Shaw A. Drug use, smoking and drinking among young people in England in 2001. London, ONS; 2002.

75. Statistics on smoking. England, 1978 onwards. Statistical Bulletin (National Statistics, UK) 2000; 17:1–36.

76. Social Exclusion Unit. Teenage pregnancy. London: Stationery Office; 1999.

77. Gunnell D, Middleton N, Whitley E, et al. Why are suicide rates rising in young men but falling in the elderly? – a time-series analysis of trends in England and Wales 1950–1998. Soc Sci Med 2003; 57:595–611.

78. Viner RM, Barker M. Young people's health: the need for action. BMJ 2005; 330 (7496):901–903.

36

Emergency care

Thomas F Beattie, Gale A Pearson

PEDIATRIC INJURY AND EMERGENCY CARE

A PEDIATRIC EMERGENCY MEDICAL SERVICE (PEMS)

Most children become critically ill or are injured in their own environment. In order to provide optimum care for these children a seamless structure of continuous care, from environment to hospital, is essential. There are few centers in the world where this seamless care exists. Where it has been achieved however, outcomes for critically ill and injured children have been positively influenced.[1,2]

The continuum of pediatric emergency care is best summarized in Figure 36.1. Within this there should be the desire to keep as many children as possible out of hospital and maintain their care within the home and community environment for as much of the time as possible.

THE HOME SETTING

For the first 5 years of life most children spend the bulk of their time within the home and local community. The majority of children coming into contact with emergency medical services do so as a result of infection or injury.

Most children will experience upper and lower respiratory tract infection with considerable frequency between the ages of 0 and 5 years. After this age it is much less frequent. Much of this illness can be treated within the home providing parents have sufficient confidence and education. Most illness in this age group will be viral and will require little more than supportive measures such as antipyretic therapy and encouraging fluid intake. However, there is an increasing demand for this type of treatment to be obtained from family doctors or emergency departments. The disintegration of the nuclear family is one factor increasing this demand on medical time, particularly in primary care. Recent evidence has indicated that attenders at emergency departments for minor illness and injury come from deprived areas of the community.[3] The reasons for this are complex but probably relate to coping mechanisms and education.

In a small number of cases bacterial infections will be present that require antibiotic therapy. In an even smaller number significant infectious disease such as meningitis, septicemia and osteomyelitis will be present. A small number of children with viral illness will get further complications such as a febrile seizure, or superimposed bacterial infection may supervene. If parents are unaware of these problems they will lose confidence in managing illness within the community.

One way to tackle such issues is to develop an educational program aimed at developing competence in minor illness and injury management. Such an education program must also alert parents to the dangers of significant illness or injury that may require further treatment with or without a stay in hospital. Within this education program it is important to differentiate the needs of the infant younger than 3 months of age from those older than 3 months of age. The response of the younger child to infection is totally different from that of older children and adults and parents should be aware of how to get advice for these children should the need arise.[4] This is a difficult task as even health professionals using clinical decision tools cannot reliably detect children with significant infection.[5-7] Similarly injury in the infant may be a harbinger of child abuse or neglect.

Despite the frequency of infections, injuries are still the leading cause of morbidity and mortality between the ages of 1 and 5 years. Most of these injuries occur within the home setting, which includes the garden and its surroundings. Burns and scalds, poisonings, falls from a height, finger tip injuries and near drowning account for the majority.

One of the means to tackle the toll wrought by injury in this age group is an integrated injury prevention program within an emergency medical system. The components of such a system include:

1. injury surveillance;
2. data analysis;
3. identification of problems;
4. development of strategies;
5. implementation of strategies;
6. injury surveillance.

In many ways this is a typical audit cycle. It relies on collaboration among emergency physicians, general practice, public health medicine, educationalists and health promotion agencies. Their respective skills should be brought together in a coordinated fashion

At present injury surveillance is patchy with much information being derived from inpatient databases. These are inaccurate and only reflect 10% of total injuries that occur.[8] Without meaningful measures of injury severity these data are at best a reflection of current medical practice. A good example of this is the documentation of poisoning. Many children who are poisoned can be safely dealt with in the home without ever coming to hospital provided adequate medical advice can be given and monitored by telephone. If this advice is not available then many children will present to hospital. They will present to the emergency room, where their treatment will depend on the experience and confidence of the staff working in that department. Junior staff, insecure or ill taught will tend to admit because they are unsure of what to do. Senior staff, experienced and confident will be able to manage many of these children on an outpatient basis. In an institution staffed in the former manner poisonings determined from inpatient stay will be at a high level whereas those in an institution managed in the latter manner will be lower. This has nothing to do with the incidence of the poisoning but all to do with medical practice. Simply by changing medical practice an apparent fall in the incidence of poisoning can be demonstrated when in fact the incidence remains high. Failure to take cognizance of these matters when developing injury surveillance will lead to inappropriate preventive measures.[9]

Effective data surveillance should start with a minimum data set. This minimum data set should aim to capture a small, important amount of information on every child who presents.[10] If too much information is to be documented staff members will tend not to collect it and parents will get irritated because they feel that their child should be treated rather than them answering questions. Typically it should include age, sex, postcode and proxies for social class and/or deprivation. Some idea as to the causation should also be included. One way of doing this is to use international classification of disease E codes;[11] this is universally accepted and is adequate for most things. This could be further

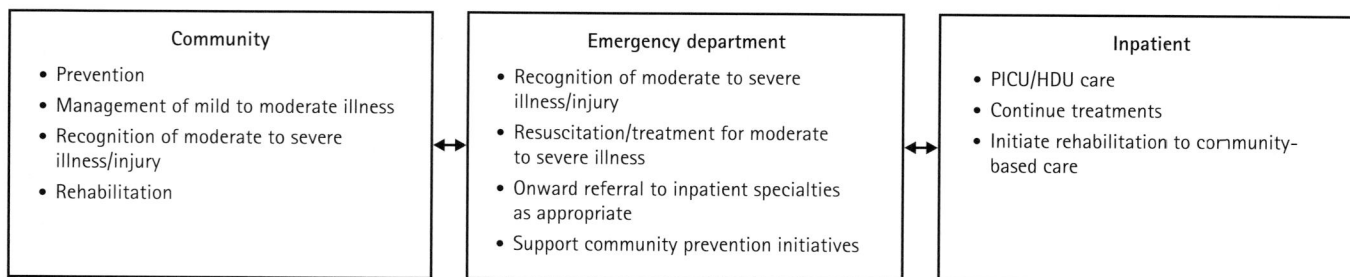

Community	Emergency department	Inpatient
• Prevention • Management of mild to moderate illness • Recognition of moderate to severe illness/injury • Rehabilitation	• Recognition of moderate to severe illness/injury • Resuscitation/treatment for moderate to severe illness • Onward referral to inpatient specialties as appropriate • Support community prevention initiatives	• PICU/HDU care • Continue treatments • Initiate rehabilitation to community-based care

Fig. 36.1   Continuum of emergency care.

refined to having the most common injuries already precoded. Similarly some ideas to the most common diagnoses using a system such as the International Classification of Disease codes (ICD) could also be included on discharge. If this information were to be collected on all children a very suitable injury surveillance system would very rapidly be developed that could be expanded as the need arose.

DATA ANALYSIS AND PROBLEM IDENTIFICATION

Once an accurate database is in place that gathers details on a substantial proportion of injury occurring within the community then problem areas can be identified. This can be on the basis of deprivation or need; clustering; type of injury, e.g. fall, poisoning; type of injury, e.g. fracture or head injury. Once analyzed this information can then be made available to the relevant health education agencies, who can then implement parts three and four of the audit cycle.

DEVISING A STRATEGY

Before any strategy can be devised to protect against childhood injury three components have to be addressed:
1. the child;
2. the family;
3. the environment.

Tackling any of these on their own will fail if it does not concomitantly address the problems inherent in the other two areas. It is well recognized that some children are more injury prone than others. Is this because the family is poor or the environment is poor? Or is it that that child is inherently more prone to injury for reasons of clumsiness, poor eyesight/coordination? Attention deficit and hyperactivity disorder is an example of a behavioral problem that might be expected to be associated with injury and this is the case.[12] To date many injury prevention programs have been simplistic with individuals working in isolation without the complete umbrella of a PEMS.

IMPLEMENTING A STRATEGY

Before a strategy can be successful the lessons from commercial advertisers have to be learned. Simply repeating the same message ad infinitum leads to message fatigue. The message must be appropriate to the target audience and must take note of all the above factors. In addition the audience must be identified and targeted effectively.

RE-AUDIT

It is important to measure any effect of the prevention campaigns against the initial database. Failure to do so may lead to inappropriate and ineffective campaigning being continued indefinitely. If there has been no diminution in the levels of injury that one has targeted then the strategies need to be re-evaluated in the light of the data analysis and message.

COMMUNITY EDUCATION

In order for the child to be cared for within the home as effectively as possible, ideally not accessing emergency medical services, a substantial amount of effort must be paid to community education. However, the target audience has not been well defined. Does the practitioner, for instance, tackle children in junior school or senior school in an effort to help future generations? Should the practitioner address the problem at antenatal classes, where there is a substantial chance of reaching an interested mother and perhaps the father? Is it appropriate to address the issue of safety in the postnatal period, when the father is almost certainly not going to be present? These issues need to be addressed as a matter of urgency if child injury prevention is to be taken forward in a meaningful manner.

COMMUNITY CARE

Within the context of a PEMS, community care should be directed at disease prevention. There will however be a significant proportion of children who have transient episodes of acute illness requiring medical intervention. Interspersed with these will be children with chronic disability who will have more sophisticated needs for emergency care than their able-bodied peers.

To work effectively there needs to be a network of experienced general practitioners and community pediatricians working alongside health visitors, district nurses, midwives and other paramedical staff. The public health system working alongside ensures good sanitation and maintenance of water supplies. Attention to housing and overcrowding is also all-important in the prevention of disease and illness. Surveillance by public health physicians and public health laboratories can identify trends in disease. Many infectious diseases, e.g. *Mycoplasma* infection, occur in a cyclical fashion over a period of years. Croup will present 2–3 times per year, one being significantly greater than the others.[13] Disease reporting can help identify when these infections are imminent and serological testing can help confirm that they have actually arrived. This will alert practitioners to the common disease that may be in the community setting at any given time and may help avoid unnecessary hospital admissions by the correct use of antibiotics.

The health professionals within the community have several roles. The first is disease prevention, primarily in terms of immunization and injury prevention. Where immunization has been effective many diseases have all but been eradicated. This is in danger of disappearing with recent changes in attitude to immunization. The recent scare regarding possible links with autism and bowel disease has led to concern about the safety of the combined measles/mumps/rubella (MMR) vaccination.[14] That this link has been convincingly disproven has not yet convinced a section of the public. This has led to a small but significant decrease in herd immunity, opening the way for a measles epidemic in particular.[15–17]

Health professionals in the community should be able to give advice to parents on disease and injury prevention. They should also be able to recognize situations where family dynamics are breaking down, making injury and child abuse more common.

Within the community one of the more vital functions is recognition of the child who has a disease process that is not suitable for treatment in the community but needs further care within a hospital setting. A good example of this is bronchiolitis. Many cases of bronchiolitis will be cared for in the community with children getting supportive care and advice. However, family practitioners should be in the position to identify the child at risk from significant airway distress, e.g. not feeding, a respiratory rate over 55 or apneic attacks.[18] In this situation the child needs to get to hospital for further treatment that may include high-dependency and/or intensive care. Equally the community services should be able to identify the child who may not be so ill but where the family circumstances mean that the child is not going to be capably looked after at home. Situations where this may occur include poverty, a mother who is not coping because of two or three other small children, and single parents or families of drug abusers. In these situations even though the child may not warrant admission for medical reasons, the social factors may indicate the child needs to be transferred for inpatient care. Community practitioners are much better placed to identify these problems than hospital-based staff.

PREHOSPITAL CARE

Prehospital care is a link between home and the community on one hand and the hospital-based services of emergency and tertiary level care on the other. The function of prehospital care is to transfer ill or injured children to places of either advanced or definitive care. Two issues predominate within the prehospital care setting:
1. access;
2. education.

To be effective prehospital care has to be easily accessed by all members of the community, e.g. in the UK dialling '999' gains access to the ambulance service. This universal national access code available to all and free of charge is probably the most effective component in the prehospital setting.

Education is also vital. The role of practitioners in prehospital care has got to be fully defined. It must be relevant to the PEMS within which the prehospital care is practiced. It will differ between urban and rural areas in terms of decisions to 'stay and play' and 'scoop and run'. It must be remembered that the absolute numbers of true pediatric emergencies (illness or trauma) is relatively rare, particularly compared to the adult population. The skills needed to carry out emergency care effectively require time to attain and practice to maintain.[19] An integrated PEMS can best evaluate the needs of its catchment area and train the prehospital care staff accordingly. Where short distances are envisaged and transfer times are rapid then training needs may be less demanding with concentration on simple airway, breathing and circulation skills. In rural areas where transport times may be prolonged advanced life support skills may be necessary.[20] Where land-based transport is adequate, training in driving skills may be required. However, should air medical transport by helicopter or fixed-wing aircraft be necessary as a routine then training in aviation medicine and the associated problems will need to be included in the training package.

There is increasing evidence that prehospital life support should include effective, simple measures. Gausche et al showed that prehospital intubation had no benefit on outcome, and worryingly might increase mortality and morbidity.[21-23] This poses a dilemma for rural practitioners in particular. Urban and semiurban situations have clear guidance that in an emergency intubation should not be attempted in the field. Rather they should concentrate on bag–valve–mask ventilation with good, simple airway-opening maneuvers and transport of the child to the nearest pediatric unit. In rural and remote areas or in situations where weather or geography make transport impossible, advanced airway care may be needed. The rarities of this, combined with the complexity of skills needed, make maintenance of skills difficult. Innovative and practical solutions have to be found, but there is no doubt that this will lead to increasing costs. Similarly the value of i.v. access has been questioned.[24] In particular the value of delaying at scene must be set against potential benefits. In this study Teach et al found no such benefit and some possible harm, either from delay at scene or inappropriate fluid administration.

Inner city areas with significant drugs problems may well have a high incidence of penetrating trauma, which will require an emphasis to be placed on treatment of such injuries within that setting.[25]

THE EMERGENCY DEPARTMENT SERVICES

Pediatric emergency departments fall into three broad categories:
1. those attached to specialist pediatric hospitals that treat only children;
2. those attached to large district or teaching hospitals that have combined pediatric and adult populations;
3. those attached to small community or cottage hospitals treating relatively small numbers of patients overall.

Within each of these three settings various problems exist.

The dedicated pediatric unit is usually situated in a large conurbation, often attached to a university or medical school. It will provide child- and family-centered care of an exceptionally high order. Major injury and illness will often be much less than that in a comparable adult population so there will have to be significant emphasis on education directed at the recognition of illness and the development of resuscitation skills to facilitate optimum care of ill and injured children. Retention of these skills is also a major issue that needs to be addressed.[26,27]

In a unit that combines pediatric and adult patients, general resuscitation skills and teamwork will be much more practiced but in contrast recognition of pediatric illness and skill in treatment may be deficient.

The ability to provide a child- and family-centered approach is often more difficult than in the purely pediatric setting.

The cottage hospital may benefit from being able to provide care closer to the patient's home but illness recognition and resuscitation skills may be poor unless teaching programs are available. This may require that staff rotate to busy units at regular intervals to update and recertify in pediatric skills.

A computer-based model of a typical region with various types of hospital postulates that all types of hospital are necessary to enable children to receive optimal care. This presupposes that skills are present and are updated regularly in each setting and that facilities for children are maintained.[28]

In all settings with the regular turnover of staff inherent with movement of junior doctors and nursing staff, regular resuscitation updates (e.g. pediatric advanced life support courses) are essential. Staffing and training in departments that have children attending should build in adequate time for training and staff development to ensure that skills are maintained at an optimum level. Within these settings certain basic concepts need to be addressed.

There should always be dedicated facilities for the reception and treatment of children, removed from the sights and sounds of the adult world. Children are often already frightened and distressed by being in hospital and every effort should be made to keep them as calm and content as possible. An attractive child-friendly environment should facilitate this. Examination rooms should have sufficient toys and pictures to enable efficient distraction therapy to be practiced. Play leaders are an invaluable resource to aid this process.

Resuscitation rooms should be fully equipped with all the various equipment that is required for pediatric resuscitation. Children change shape and size with age. A full knowledge of how this occurs and the clinical implications are important. It is almost impossible to accurately recall all the weights of children at various age groups. Drug and fluid therapy is usually done on a dose-per-weight basis. It is important to avoid calculations in 'the heat of the moment'. It is all too easy to place a decimal point in the wrong place and either over- or underdose children. For this reason charts should be available or tapes laid out on beds so that rapid determination of dosage depending on the weight/length of the child can be established. These charts will also have details of the correct size of endotracheal tube, the length to which the tube should be cut and various other parameters necessary for effective pediatric resuscitation.[29,30]

Typical equipment required in the resuscitation room is shown in Table 36.1.

The staff working within such an environment must be familiar with recognition of the sick child and similarly be comfortable with all aspects of pediatric care.

Parents often arrive at the emergency department with other siblings. The presence of play leaders will help entertain these children and enable the distressed relatives to be with the sick or injured child. Quiet rooms should be laid aside so that bereaved or distressed relatives can be alone in their time of distress though a staff member should always be available for this if required. Facilities should be available to enable nappy changing and breast-feeding to occur in private.

The function of staff in the emergency department is to receive all ill and injured children and to institute treatment in a timely and appropriate fashion depending on the urgency of the condition (triage).

The nursing staff members usually perform triage but medical staff could also perform this task. Objective triage is difficult in the pediatric population. There are few objective pediatric scales that can be related to all types of presenting problems, medical, surgical, trauma or other. Much triage therefore is subjective and will in part depend upon the volume of work. A well child presenting at a quiet time will very often get through the system more rapidly than an ill child presenting at a busy time. It is imperative that staff members working within the emergency department are able to recognize the child who has a disease process which, if left untreated, will lead to serious incapacity or death. Key recognition skills relate to respiratory and circulatory compromise.

Table 36.1   Equipment to provide emergency care for children: equipment for the resuscitation room

Airway
Guedel airways – 000→3
Endotracheal tubes – 2.5→8 uncuffed, 7→10.5 cuffed
Introducers
Laryngoscope handles
Laryngoscope blades – straight and curved
Yankauer suction catheters
Argyle suction catheters
Suction device (with backup)
Cricothyroid puncture set (this may be commercial or 'homemade')
Jet insufflation system

Breathing
Round masks
Triangular masks
Bag–valve–mask device with pressure-limiting device set at 30–40 cmH$_2$O
Reservoir bag
O$_2$ supply (with backup)
Ayres T-piece circuit (or equivalent)
Chest drains 10→32G
Drainage tubing and jars for underwater seal

Circulation
I.v. cannulae 24→14F
Central venous cannulae and Seldinger introducer wire
Intraosseous cannulae 17F
Giving sets
Blood warmer
Infusion pumps
Defibrillator with facility for synchronized DC version capable of variable energy delivery

Disability
Cervical collars
Spinal boards
Arm and leg splints

Monitoring equipment
Pulse oximeter
Cardiac monitor
Blood glucose test machines
Blood gas analyzer

Other
Tapes for i.v. lines, ETT tubes, chest drains
Syringes 1 ml, 2 ml, 5 ml, 10 ml
3-way taps
Connection tubing
Suture material

Suture packs
Chest drain packs
Urinary catheters
Nasogastric tubes
Clock
Warmth

Drugs
Epinephrine (adrenaline) – 1:10 000 and 1:1000
Atropine
Lidocaine – 1%, 2%
Sodium bicarbonate – 1.84%, 4.2%, 8.4%
Morphine
Naloxone
Glucose – 50%, 25%
Glucagon
Diazepam (as emulsion) or lorazepam
Midazolam
Phenytoin
Adenosine
Disopyramide
Beta-blocker
Thiopental
Suxamethonium
Atracurium
Mannitol – 10%, 20%
Beta 2-agonists – nebulizer solution
Ipratropium – nebulizer solution
Beta agonists – i.v. solution
Aminophylline
Hydrocortisone
Procyclidine

Fluids
Normal saline
Plasma

If neonates are expected the following equipment should also be available in addition:
Resuscitaire
Heat source
Warm towels/wraps
Umbilical catheters

In parallel, skills are needed to:
1. open and secure an airway;
2. ensure that oxygenation is maintained;
3. ensure that circulation is maintained.

The frequency with which these skills are practiced will depend on the population served and the effectiveness of the home, community and pre-hospital services. Communities that have poor home safety, poor community immunization rates and primitive public sanitation can expect to deal with large numbers of ill or injured children.

Where numbers are small maintenance of recognition skills can only be maintained by appropriate teaching programs, for example pediatric advanced life support (PALS). PALS courses were introduced into the UK in the early 1990s. Roberts et al[31] have demonstrated increased survival since these were introduced. Cause and effect have still to be reconciled.

Once a child has been received into the emergency department and the airway, breathing and circulation have been stabilized, the child needs to be transferred to a place of definitive treatment. Often this will be via an imaging facility to surgery, and from there to an intensive care setting. To complete the emergency medical system, a system of safe transfer to and from each of these areas needs to be established. Even if the emergency department is within the tertiary care center, transfer to the scanning suite or the intensive care unit can be fraught with danger if not performed expertly and efficiently. For this reason transfers should be kept to a minimum.

A transport team should be a priority development in any pediatric emergency care system so that there can be safe transfer to the tertiary care center for definitive treatment.

Both within the injury and emergency setting and the tertiary care unit rehabilitation is important. This will enable the ill or injured child to regain his place as effectively as possible within the home/community setting.

APPROACH TO THE MANAGEMENT OF THE SEVERELY ILL OR INJURED CHILD IN THE EMERGENCY DEPARTMENT

Most ill children will be brought to hospital by the prehospital services. In these situations airway care and circulatory support will have been instituted according to local training and policy guidelines. In addition there will be an element of warning so that the resuscitation team can be gathered and tasks allocated.

As it is very easy for parents or bystanders to pick up smaller children, children who are severely ill or injured will often be brought to hospital unannounced and unexpected in private transport.

Consequently the components of the resuscitation team should be established in advance. It is important that one doctor is in charge to coordinate the resuscitation and decide on the priorities for care, with other staff in complementary roles.

INITIAL ASSESSMENT

Rapid assessment of the airway, breathing and circulation is mandatory (primary survey).

AIRWAY

The airway can be described as open, maintainable or unmaintainable. An open airway is defined as one with no obstruction present. This includes the absence of secretions, stridor, gurgling or other noises. An open airway needs no further management at this stage but this should be kept under review. [32,33]

A maintainable airway is defined as one that can be kept open with simple measures such as positioning; chin lift/head tilt (or jaw-thrust only, if trauma to the cervical spine is a possibility); the use of an oropharyngeal airway or the use of gentle suction.

An unmaintainable airway is one that is still at risk despite these simple measures necessitating either intubation or the creation of a surgical airway (cricothyrotomy).

The airway should be maintained at this stage by the simplest effective measures available. Intubation must only be carried out by experienced operators who can intubate with skill in a timely fashion. Any attempt taking longer than 30 s should be abandoned and the child oxygenated with a bag–valve–mask device pending a second attempt.

All sick or injured children require high flow oxygen. This should be administered using a facemask if the airway is open and maintainable. Otherwise artificial ventilation should be established using a bag–valve–mask device (see later).

BREATHING

The efficacy of breathing can be assessed only after the airway has been opened. The rate, volume and symmetry of respiration should be assessed by observation and auscultation.

Respiratory compromise can be characterized by either an increasing or decreasing work of breathing.

Increased work of breathing
Increasing respiratory rate
Increasing heart rate
Use of accessory muscles in respiration
Flared nostrils
Intercostal/sternal recession
Grunting
Decreasing level of consciousness

Decreased work of breathing
Decreasing respiratory rate
Poor respiratory effort
Poor lung expansion

If breathing is absent or diminished, ventilation using a bag–valve–mask device should be instituted as soon as possible. Absent breath sounds and hyper-resonance to percussion on one side should lead one to consider a pneumothorax. This should be immediately drained using a needle thoracostomy. The needle should be inserted into the midclavicular line in the second intercostal space pending the insertion of a formal chest drain. Once inserted the needle should be left in place until the chest drain is working properly. If signs of respiratory compromise

are present supplemental oxygen should be administered in the highest rate available.

CIRCULATION

The adequacy of the circulation should only be assessed when Airway and Breathing are adequate. A central pulse should be palpated at this stage. The carotid pulse should be palpated lateral to the thyroid cartilage and medial to the sternocleidomastoid muscle in a child. In an infant the brachial pulse should be palpated in the upper arm.

If there is no pulse palpable (or pulse is less than 60 beats/min) cardiac massage should be started at a rate of 80–100 b.p.m. If a pulse is palpable look for other signs of circulatory embarrassment.

Physical signs of circulatory embarrassment
Rising pulse
Tachypnea
Weakening peripheral pulses
Increasing delay of capillary return (greater than 2 s)
Increasing peripheral core temperature difference
Decreased urine output
Altered level of consciousness

All children with circulatory embarrassment (and all children who are severely ill or injured) should have i.v. access established as soon as possible. Failure to establish peripheral i.v. access within a few minutes in children who are in circulatory distress should lead one to insert an intraosseous needle into the tibia or femur. If signs of circulatory embarrassment or shock are present, fluid should be administered as a 20 ml/kg bolus. Recent meta-analysis has suggested that crystalloid fluids are to be preferred. [34] Certainly UK practice has been to use colloid, e.g. plasma, but crystalloid has been widely used elsewhere. The quality of the literature makes it difficult to make a definitive decision as to best initial fluid resuscitation, but the Cochrane database review recommends avoiding albumin outwith controlled studies.

Blood pressure (BP) is an unreliable sign of circulatory compromise in children. Up to 40% of the circulating blood volume needs to be lost before the blood pressure will fall. A falling blood pressure is a late sign and indicates a failure of compensatory mechanisms to maintain perfusion to vital areas. Once BP falls, early and urgent treatment is indicated if permanent harm is to be avoided.

While the medical staff are assessing the airway, breathing and circulation, the nursing staff should help get the child undressed and should attach a cardiac monitor and a pulse oximeter.

As a result of this initial assessment, the practitioner should be dealing with one of the following:

1. a child in cardiac arrest;
2. a traumatized child who requires further trauma-orientated resuscitation; or
3. an unstable child with continuing airway, breathing or circulatory compromise associated with underlying pathology.

CARDIAC ARREST

Cardiac arrest is rare in the pediatric population. Common causes include sudden infant death syndrome, trauma, drowning and asphyxia. [35]

Cardiac arrest in children is primarily asystolic in nature. Occasionally pulseless electrical activity ([PEA] also known as electromechanical dissociation [EMD]) or ventricular fibrillation (VF) is present. [35] It is important to begin resuscitation as above but consider definitive drug and fluid therapies as indicated by the underlying rhythm.

The outcome of cardiac arrest in children is dismal, particularly when it occurs in the community. [36] Children who sustain cardiac arrest in the emergency department have a better outcome than those who arrest in the community, but worse than those who arrest in hospital. [37] Prolonged hypoxia, hypoglycemia and acidosis in addition to the underlying disease process, all contribute to cell death particularly in the myocardium and brain, making restoration of vital functions difficult. Even if cardiac function is restored the prolonged insult to the brain usually leaves the child with permanent and usually profound neurological deficit.

ASYSTOLE

Asystole is characterized by a pulseless, apneic child associated with no complexes on the cardiac monitor. It is important to confirm that this is so by going through the following procedure:

1. turning up the gain on the cardiac monitor;
2. ensuring that all the connections are made;
3. checking that the monitor is not connected to 'paddles'.

The recommended sequence for dealing with asystole is found in Figure 36.2.[38]

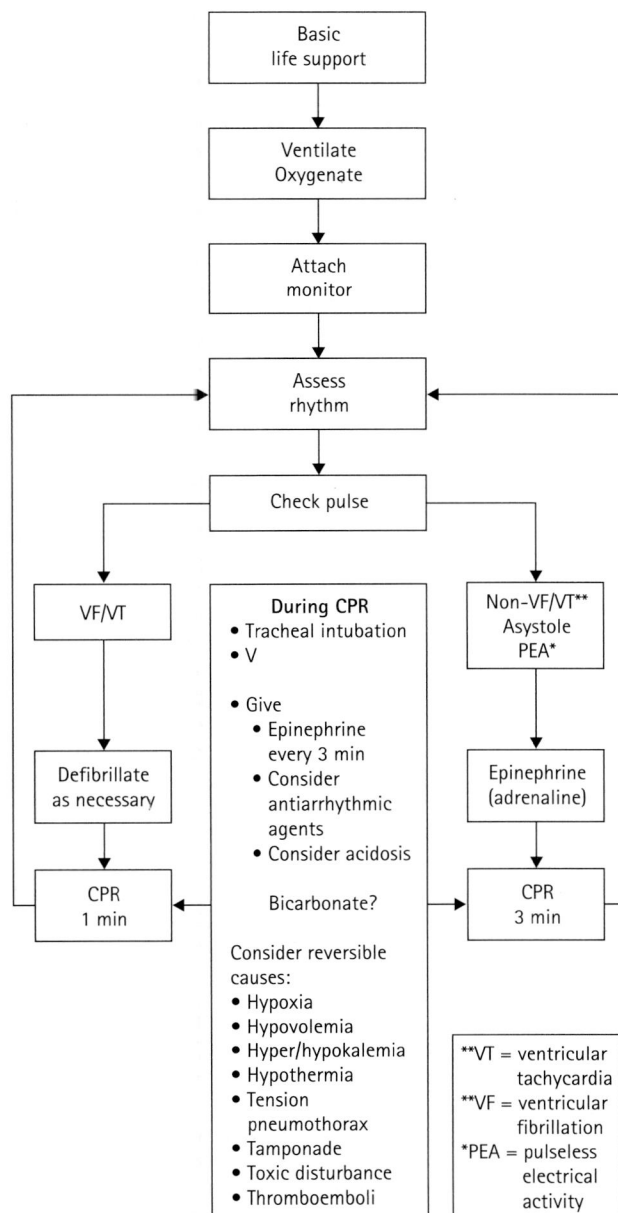

Fig. 36.2 Algorithm for management of pediatric cardiac arrest. (Adapted from Resuscitation Council (UK)[38] with permission)

PULSELESS ELECTRICAL ACTIVITY (PEA) (PREVIOUSLY KNOWN AS ELECTROMECHANICAL DISSOCIATION [EMD])

PEA is associated with a pulseless, apneic child and often bizarre complexes on a cardiac monitor. This may be associated with underlying pathology such as pneumothorax, cardiac tamponade, electrolyte imbalance, hypovolemia and hypothermia. Treatment should be aimed at correcting these underlying disorders. An algorithm for treating EMD can be seen in Figure 36.2.

VENTRICULAR FIBRILLATION

VF is much rarer in children than in adults. Recent reports have indicated that it might be more frequent than once suspected.[39,40] An algorithm for treating VF can be found in Figure 36.2.

STOPPING RESUSCITATION

The decision to terminate resuscitation can be difficult. Children who have been poisoned, drowned or who are hypothermic should have active resuscitation continued for considerable time. This will usually occur within the intensive care setting with continuing resuscitation during transit. Post-traumatic cardiac arrest has a very poor prognosis and prolonged attempts at resuscitation should be avoided. Similarly sudden infant death syndrome should not lead to unduly prolonged resuscitation attempts.

APPROACH TO THE SEVERELY INJURED CHILD

Major trauma is a relatively rare occurrence in the pediatric population compared to the adult population. Of children who die, 80% will be dead on arrival of the paramedical team at the scene, a fact which makes injury prevention all the more important. The role of paramedical intervention at the scene is crucial.

As with other forms of illness care of the airway, breathing and circulation are of paramount importance. *One of the major differences however, is that traumatized children are at risk of having damage to the spinal column, particularly the cervical spine, without radiological evidence of such injury (SCIWORA – see later).* In particular this means that one has to be able to perform airway-opening maneuvers without excessive movement being involved in the cervical spine area. Measures such as chin lift *without* head tilt are important. Oropharyngeal airways are important adjuncts to the process.

SCIWORA

SCIWORA is an acronym for *Spinal Cord Injury WithOut Radiological Abnormality*. This is a rare finding but has a potentially horrendous outcome.[41]

PATHOPHYSIOLOGY

Relative laxity of spinal ligaments associated with underdevelopment of the articular facets of the vertebrae in the spinal column allow excessive movement to take place during severe hyperflexion/extension injuries. This results in compression of the spinal cord with subsequent damage. The column will return to its normal anatomy without any evidence of fracture or subluxation being present. Normal X-rays therefore in an unconscious child should not lead one to assume that there is no possibility of spinal cord injury.

IMPLICATIONS FOR CLINICAL PRACTICE

If the child is awake and is able to move all four limbs then SCIWORA is unlikely to be present.[41] However, in those children who have an altered level of consciousness, SCIWORA must be suspected. In these children full spinal column immobilization measures must be implemented until such time as the spine can be cleared either radiologically or clinically. Simple measures to immobilize the spine will include: use of sand bags or other similar sized objects to immobilize the head, taping the head to a spinal board and immobilizing the head on the shoulders using hands and arms. The airway should be assessed and opened in the simplest way possible and this should be carried out without moving the cervical spine (see earlier).

BREATHING

Breathing abnormalities are common following trauma. Causes include pneumothorax, hemothorax, rib fractures and gastric dilatation. Children with traumatic injuries should be given supplemental oxygen and any specific underlying disease treated as appropriate. A pneumothorax should be decompressed by needle thoracostomy (above). Gastric dilatation should be decompressed by a gastric tube. If a basal skull fracture is suspected the gastric tube should be passed orally rather than nasally to avoid inadvertent placement in the brain!

CIRCULATION

Problems with circulation may be due to hypovolemia, tension pneumothorax or cardiac tamponade. Hypovolemia is the most common, particularly after intra-abdominal injuries. Small babies may become hypovolemic from an intracerebral bleed but this is unusual and other causes must be sought first. Some of the signs of hypovolemia are mimicked by trauma, in particular altered level of consciousness and poor peripheral pulses. A low blood pressure is a sign of great importance, indicating the need for urgent fluid replacement.

I.v. cannulae should be inserted into large veins, ideally avoiding fractured limbs. At the same time blood should be taken for laboratory analysis. If the child is stable and blood is not required urgently a simple 'group and save serum' is all that is required. Where the child is unstable blood will be required urgently. Ideally this blood should be fully grouped and cross-matched but occasionally O-negative blood will be needed. If sufficient blood is obtained the rest can be sent for full blood count, serum amylase and possibly urea and electrolytes. The value of each in managing the child will depend on the nature of the injury, underlying illness and local laboratory policies.

DISABILITY

Most head injuries are minor with the incidence of intracranial bleed being much less in the pediatric population than in the adult population.[42] As part of the first assessment the complete coma score, e.g. the Glasgow Coma Scale, does not need to be assessed. It is sufficient to document whether the child is *Awake*, responding to *Verbal* stimuli, responding to *Painful* stimuli or *Unresponsive* (the AVPU scale). Pupillary reflexes may be documented but at this stage they will not alter management significantly. Indeed papillary responses are often confusing. While the medical team are assessing airway, breathing, circulation and disability the nursing team should undress the child, apply a cardiac monitor and a pulse oximeter and prepare to assist with airway and i.v. access procedures. Surgical trays should be made available if required.

SECONDARY SURVEY

Once the airway, breathing and circulation have been addressed a full secondary survey of the child should be carried out. Every part of the body will be examined both visually and by palpation. Judicious use of plain X-ray, ultrasound and computed tomography (CT) will aid the diagnostic process. Minor injuries that may have been missed on the first brief survey will be detected and will lead to further treatment and investigation. Injuries that are commonly detected during the secondary survey include bleeding from the ear and nose, small pneumothoraces, gastric dilatation and minor fractures to the peripheries.

HEAD INJURY

Head injury is a significant cause of morbidity and mortality in the pediatric population.[43] The relatively large head changes the center of gravity and the head is one of the most commonly injured parts of the body in the pediatric population.

The causes of significant head injury include falls from a height, motor vehicle collisions and child abuse.

While most children who sustain significant head injury will lose consciousness it should be borne in mind that hypoxia, hypovolemia or both are significant causes of altered level of consciousness. Sharples et al[44] have shown that children transferred to a central neurosurgical unit with head injury were more likely to die as a result of associated hypoxia and/or hypovolemia due to respiratory or circulatory distress than death from the head injury. It must be questioned whether these children actually needed to be transferred at all as the head injury was often a relatively minor part of the problem. It is extremely important to exclude respiratory or circulatory problems before diagnosing intracranial problems as the cause of the altered level of consciousness.

The role of the emergency department in managing head injury is straightforward but it is important to grasp the concept of primary and secondary brain injury.

Primary brain injury occurs at the time of impact. Any damage done at this stage is usually irreversible. Secondary brain injury occurs early due to an extra insult, commonly hypoxia, hypovolemia and brain edema. Later infection, hydrocephalus and seizures may contribute substantially. The management of these later problems will fall to inpatient teams, but emergency staff members need to be aware of their role in identifying circumstances where and when they are likely to occur. There is a complex relationship between the primary injury and these other secondary factors. As a result of the initial injury there will be a degree of swelling secondary to a normal inflammatory response. Localized brain injury, which might occur if the child has been hit with a hard object such as a golf club or hammer, will result in a reasonably localized injury. Here the inflammation will be localized and will not cause generalized brain edema. At the other extreme is the small baby who is exposed to vigorous shaking (non-accidental injury). Here there will be diffuse brain injury with generalized inflammation throughout the brain. Postmortem examinations in this situation reveal multiple hemorrhages and diffuse brain edema that is often progressive and unstoppable. This malignant cerebral edema is almost impossible to treat and is usually the cause of significant morbidity and mortality associated with 'shaken baby syndrome'.[45,46] Most cases of head injury fall between these two extremes.

If the initial insult is associated with loss of consciousness then hypoxia will almost certainly follow as a result of an obstructed airway, usually from the tongue obstructing the oropharynx, or from vomitus entering the lungs. This will in turn cause cerebral anoxia with resultant cell damage and death and lead to a generalized inflammatory response with a variable degree of cerebral edema being present. The same situation will occur with other causes of hypoxia, e.g. pneumothorax, pulmonary contusion.

A decrease in perfusion pressure to the brain secondary to hemorrhage or other cause of hypovolemia will result in failure to deliver glucose and oxygen to the brain leading to an equivalent situation. Again as the inflammation increases the intracranial pressure also increases and unless there is adequate circulatory drive to perfuse the brain, a vicious circle ensues.

The primary role of the emergency department therefore is to ensure that the airway is open, that ventilation is maximized and that oxygen saturations are maintained between 95% and 100%, and to maintain circulation to enable cerebral perfusion to be normalized.

By the time the child gets to the emergency department a degree of intracranial swelling may already have taken place. In the early stages this will usually be due to an intracranial hematoma. Extradural, acute subdural or intracranial bleeds can all produce considerable pressure effects. It is important to recognize that children can sustain an extradural hematoma in the absence of fractures to the middle meningeal region, in contrast to the adult population, and normal skull X-rays therefore can be misleading.[47] The role of the emergency department is to ensure the airway, breathing and circulation are maximized and that any other life-threatening injury is identified and controlled. Only then should the child be transferred to the scanning suite, when the formal diagnosis can be made. There will often be a dilemma between surgical hemostasis (e.g. from a ruptured liver or spleen) and management of significant intracranial hematoma. It is imperative in these situations to control the circulation and to ensure brain perfusion is maximized to reduce the effect of secondary brain injury from hypoxia and/or hypovolemia. This tension is not easy to resolve and takes considerable experience and seniority to ensure the optimum sequence of events occurs.

With CT there is often evidence of raised intracranial pressure and no evidence of intracranial bleed. In this situation the practitioner is dealing with cerebral edema and several mechanisms exist to try to reduce the pressure including: hyperventilation to maintain a $PaCO_2$ of about 4 kPa, use of mannitol or furosemide (frusemide) (or other loop diuretic) and sedative techniques such as barbiturate anesthesia. It should be noted that most of these measures only work on a normal brain and are of little benefit at best. Use of these agents should be discussed with the neurosurgeon.

The emergency department is responsible for identifying basal skull fractures by clinical examination. Physical signs that indicate a basal skull fracture include 'panda eyes' (raccoon eyes), blood or cerebrospinal fluid from the nose or ears or 'Battle's sign' (bruising over the mastoid process). Basal skull fractures are open fractures and there is a high risk that infection will supervene between 12 h and 24 h, or possibly later. The use of antibiotics for the management of basal skull fractures is controversial. There is no clear evidence that antibiotics will reduce the chance of meningitis but this should be discussed with the local neurosurgical unit.[48] Many children will have seizures subsequent to the head injury. This can result in hypoxia with the inherent risks discussed earlier. After supplying oxygen and assisting ventilation the fit should be stopped using diazepam 0.2 mg/kg. Assessment of the level of consciousness is now difficult and these children should undergo CT scanning. Phenytoin 15 mg/kg may be used to reduce subsequent seizures after discussion with the neurosurgical unit.

Once a child has had a secure airway established, oxygenation is maximized and circulation and perfusion restored to normal, the child should be transferred for definitive diagnosis to the CT suite under stringent transfer conditions. Transfer from the safety of the resuscitation room should not start until full transfer protocols have been instituted. Transfer from the emergency setting to the scanning suite is just as dangerous as traveling from one center to another.

THORACOABDOMINAL INJURIES

Thoracoabdominal injury is relatively rare in the pediatric population compared with the adolescent and adult population. Most injuries are blunt although increase of firearms has meant that penetrating thoracoabdominal trauma is rising.[25] Many children with major thoracic injuries will die before reaching hospital although improvements in pre-hospital care may mean that an increasing number may survive. Injuries that fall into this category include traumatic dissection of the aorta and massive tension pneumothorax.

Traumatic dissection of the thoracic aorta is typically caused by rapid deceleration injury and most children will die in the pre-hospital phase. If they survive to reach hospital the diagnosis can be suspected by the presence of a widened mediastinum on a chest film associated with fractures of the upper ribs. It is best confirmed by either arteriography or CT. If suspected the child should be transferred to a thoracic surgical center.

Tension pneumothorax is treated by the insertion of a large-bore needle into the second intercostal space on the affected side. Signs of tension pneumothorax include signs of respiratory distress, distended neck veins and absent breath sounds on the affected side. Once the pneumothorax is drained using the needle a formal chest drain should be inserted and connected to an underwater seal as soon as possible. Drainage of a pneumothorax on one side may reveal the presence of a lesion on the other side and this should be treated appropriately.

MODERATE CHEST INJURY

The use of seat belts and seat restraints has led to an increase in chest wall bruising due to the seat belt physically restraining the child. Children who have seat belt abrasions to the chest and abdomen have been subjected to quite considerable deceleration forces. While the mostly likely thoracic injuries will be a fractured clavicle with or without a fractured sternum, it should be borne in mind that underlying myocardial contusion is possible. This is extremely difficult to detect clinically. The presence of slightly abnormal electrocardiograms (ECGs) and raised cardiac enzymes are unreliable. If there is any doubt the child should be admitted for a period of observation with continuous cardiac monitoring.

Fractured ribs are rare in the pediatric population. If seen in the infant or toddler group non-accidental injury should be suspected. Management is required for relief of pain. If there are more than three ribs fractured on one side the child should to be admitted to a high-dependency care unit for intercostal blocks to be administered. Bilateral rib fractures may lead to a flail chest but this is rare in children.

ABDOMINAL INJURY

Blunt trauma is the usual cause. Penetrating trauma increases in frequency as children get older. Blunt trauma can result in hemorrhage and loss of perfusion from rupture to solid organs such as spleen, kidney and liver; or peritonitis from injury to the bowel and pancreas. With each of these a strong index of suspicion is needed as early on the child can have minimal abdominal signs, but will subsequently develop significant problems. This is particularly so of pancreatitis and bowel perforation, where peritonitis can take between 6 h and 12 h to develop.

Intra-abdominal hemorrhage should be considered in any child who shows evidence of circulatory collapse following trauma. Clinical diagnosis is unreliable and imaging is almost certainly indicated, particularly if the child is stable. Ultrasound is a useful screening tool. In skilled hands even small amounts of free fluid can be detected. Most skilled ultrasonographers will be able to identify the site of bleeding if due to damage to solid organs, i.e. liver, spleen and kidney. If free fluid is present but no solid organ damage is identified then CT with contrast is indicated. Children who are unstable should have intra-abdominal bleeding suspected and treated according to the accompanying diagram (Fig. 36.3). Hepatic and splenic trauma will usually be treated conservatively provided the child remains stable.[49]

SEAT BELT INJURY

A seat belt ideally involves three-point fixation with a lap belt and harness. If children are restrained using a lap belt alone and are involved in a high-speed collision there is a reasonable chance they will sustain a hyperflexion injury of the torso. This will usually result in intra-abdominal injury with a significant hepatic or splenic component. This will often be associated with a degree of spinal instability with fractures occurring in the L_1, L_2 region of the lumbar spine.[50] Any child who has a significant lap belt injury to the midabdominal region should have spinal injury suspected and should have full spinal immobilization carried out until the spine has been fully cleared both radiologically and clinically (see SCIWORA as earlier).

ORTHOPEDIC INJURY

It should be stressed that orthopedic injuries are a long way down the order of treatment. Priority should be given to airway, breathing and circulation prior to doing anything with orthopedic injuries.

```
        ┌──────────────────────────┐
        │   Blunt abdominal trauma │
        └──────────────────────────┘
                     │
              ┌──────────────┐
              │    Stable    │
              └──────────────┘
              ┌──────┴────────┐
           ┌─────┐        ┌─────┐
           │ Yes │        │ No  │
           └─────┘        └─────┘
              │               │
    ┌───────────────────┐ ┌───────────────────┐
    │ Ultrasound abdomen│ │20 MLS/kg 0.9% saline│
    └───────────────────┘ └───────────────────┘
              │               │
        ┌──────────┐    ┌──────────┐
        │  Normal  │    │  Stable  │
        └──────────┘    └──────────┘
         ┌────┴────┐     ┌────┴────┐
      ┌─────┐  ┌─────┐ ┌─────┐ ┌─────┐
      │ Yes │  │ No  │ │ Yes │ │ No  │
      └─────┘  └─────┘ └─────┘ └─────┘
                 │               │
        ┌────────┴──────┐  ┌──────────┐
    ┌─────────┐ ┌─────────┐│20 MLS/kg │
    │  Solid  │ │ Hollow  ││  blood   │
    │  organ  │ │ organ   │└──────────┘
    │  injury │ │         │     │
    └─────────┘ └─────────┘ ┌──────────┐
        │           │       │  Stable  │
    ┌─────────┐ ┌─────────┐ └──────────┘
    │ Active  │ │Laparotomy│┌─────┐ ┌─────┐
    │observation││  ± CT   ││ Yes │ │Stable│
    │  ± CT   │ │         │└─────┘ └─────┘
    └─────────┘ └─────────┘         │
                              ┌─────┐
                              │ No  │
                              └─────┘
```

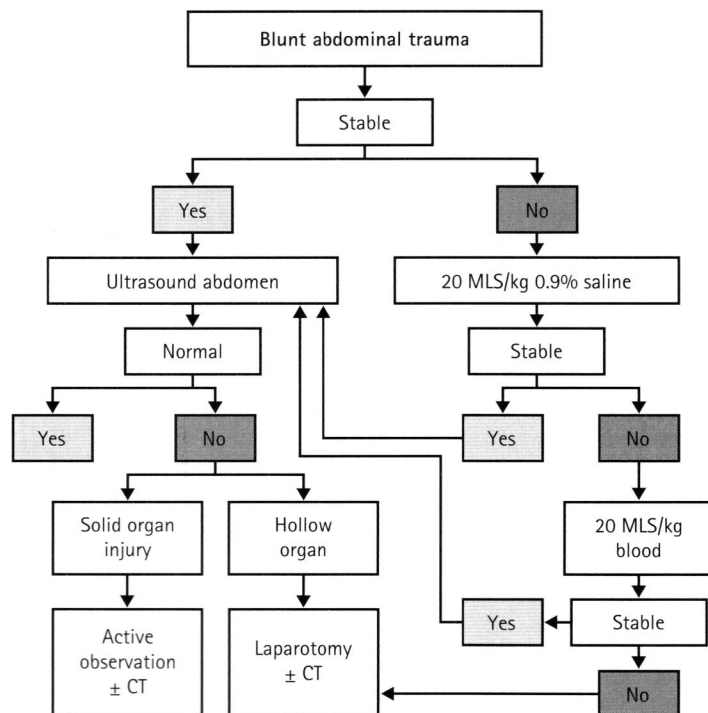

Fig. 36.3 Management of blunt abdominal trauma.

Orthopedic injury following trauma is common. Within the emergency department there are three aspects that should be considered:
1. recognition of the fracture;
2. identification of associated soft tissue injury that may cause compromise to the limb;
3. splintage and analgesia.

RECOGNITION OF THE FRACTURE

If a bone is bent, it is broken! Of more concern is the occult undisplaced fracture. Such fractures can bleed into tight fascial compartments with subsequent compartment syndrome. Vascular compromise is particularly common with fractures of the elbow, where the brachial artery may be involved, and the tibia. If there is any concern about the presence of an occult fracture the area should be X-rayed to either confirm it or rule it out.

With all fractures the distal pulses should be palpated and distal neurological function should be checked. If the perfusion is adequate distal to the fracture site then all that is needed is for the limb to be splinted until life-threatening conditions such hypoxia or hypovolemia are corrected. Nerve injuries need to be noted and examined further when the child is stable.

IDENTIFICATION OF ASSOCIATED SOFT TISSUE INJURY

Soft tissue injuries associated with fractures include:
1. tissue loss;
2. open wounds;
3. vascular damage;
4. nerve damage;
5. tendon damage.

Tissue loss and open wounds associated with fracture will lead to infection in the bone if not adequately treated and debrided. The emergency department is not the place to start this process but the wound should not be ignored. It is sufficient to assess the distal pulses and neurological function and as long as these are intact, dress the wound with a disinfectant dressing and leave further management to the orthopedic department. Broad-spectrum antibiotics effective against Gram positive, Gram negative and anaerobic organisms are important. Local policies determine which antibiotics are given. Tetanus prophylaxis is also important if the patient is not fully immunized.

ANALGESIA

Pain with a long bone fracture is severe and analgesia is greatly underused. There is often a fear of masking intra-abdominal injury or of aggravating conscious level with head injury. Both of these are inadequate reasons to withhold analgesia in a child who is in considerable pain. Two methods of analgesia exist in this situation:
1. local and peripheral nerve block;
2. i.v. opiate.

LOCAL AND PERIPHERAL NERVE BLOCK

The femur is most amenable to this management strategy. Successful block can be obtained by infiltrating a long-acting anesthetic such as levobupivacaine around the femoral nerve where it passes under the inguinal ligament lateral to the femoral artery. This will take 5–10 min to work (and can be preceded by a more fast-acting local anesthetic such as lidocaine or prilocaine). If epinephrine (adrenaline) is used great care must be taken not to inject epinephrine (adrenaline) into the femoral artery, which is adjacent to the nerve. Some authors advocate the use of sciatic nerve block for tibial fractures. To be effective however, this requires sophisticated equipment that is not always available within the emergency setting.

INTRAVENOUS OPIATE

In trauma situations opiate analgesia should always be given intravenously. Recent reports on the efficacy of intranasal diamorphine should be treated cautiously. These reports compared intranasal diamorphine against intramuscular.[51,52] There is no place for the intramuscular route as absorption is unreliable. Whether i.v. opiate will be replaced by intranasal has yet to be established.

The weight of the child should be estimated by whatever means possible and the appropriate dose of opiate obtained. This should be further diluted to 10 ml. This can then be titrated 1 ml at a time over a period of 10 min to maximal effect. As soon as the child becomes settled the administration can be stopped and a further bolus given at intervals to maintain analgesia. Usually at this stage the pain drive will be sufficient to keep the child awake and to counteract any possible diminution of level of consciousness. If there is any concern subsequently about the ability to assess either level of consciousness or the abdomen then naloxone can be used to reverse the opiate. This is rarely necessary.

Once analgesia has been administered then the fractured limb should be splinted until the child can be brought to theater by the orthopedic surgeons. Splintage is an important consideration for analgesia in injured children. One of the major challenges for pediatric emergency departments is the absence of commercially available splints suitable for all the different shapes of children. Often these have to be fashioned on an ad hoc basis from plaster of Paris or some other newer synthetic casting material.

BURN CARE

Burns are a common problem in children. Two broad issues need to be addressed:
1. the burn injury (by whatever cause);
2. complications such as smoke inhalation, hypothermia, toxic shock syndrome.

Although both issues can occur together, usually one or the other is the main problem on initial presentation to the emergency department. There are many etiologies for burn injury (Table 36.2). No matter what the cause, the approach to a burn injury is the same. The airway, breathing and circulation should be assessed and looked after as in all previous circumstances. Once these have been addressed it is important to identify the size of the burn. Management of the burn will depend on the following factors:
1. area involved;
2. depth of the burn;
3. site of the burn.

AREA OF THE BURN

Small burns, i.e. less than 5% of total body surface area (TBSA), can be managed on an outpatient basis provided that the burn is superficial, does not involve a significant area and there are no complications present.

Treatment will consist of analgesia, usually oral, and dressings according to local policy. One method of dressing the burn is to use tulle gras impregnated with mupirocin, which is an effective anti-staphylococcal agent. Once the burn is greater than 5% TBSA analgesia requirements will usually necessitate admission and an i.v. opiate will be required. Whether the wounds are dressed or left open is dependent on local practice. Once the burn is greater than 10% TBSA then the child will need i.v. rehydration according to local formulae, e.g. Parkland formula.

DEPTH OF THE BURN

Burns can be classified as superficial, partial thickness and full thickness. Superficial burns include those with erythema only or with small amounts of blistering. Partial-thickness burns are those that have a significant area of blistering, with either blisters intact or spontaneously

Table 36.2 Causes of burn injury

1. Wet heat	Scald
2. Dry heat	Flame
	Hot surface
3. Radiation	Ultraviolet (sunburn)
	Iatrogenic (as radiation treatment in oncology)
4. Chemical	Acid
	Alkali
	Corrosive
5. Electrical	

burst. Full-thickness burns present as white avascular areas that are insensitive to touch (it is unkind to touch burns in children and inspection is usually all that is required for diagnosis).

In reality a mixture of superficial, partial thickness and full thickness is usually present depending on the burning agent and the duration it has been in contact with the skin. In general all full-thickness burns should be referred to a plastic surgeon for immediate assessment and treatment. Partial-thickness burns may be suitable for outpatient care if they do not extend over a large surface area. Treatment is as discussed earlier.

SITE OF THE BURN

Burns to the face, airway, mouth, pharynx, buttock and perineum, hands and feet and any circumferential burn to either the trunk or a limb need to be treated with a great deal of caution. Burns in any of these areas need to be referred to a burns specialist for inpatient treatment. Burns to the face and airway in particular, may require admission to an intensive care unit as the risk to the airway is quite considerable.

COMPLICATIONS OF BURNS

In the emergency department it is important to identify those children with complications such as smoke inhalation, hypothermia or those with burns possibly from non-accidental injury.

SMOKE INHALATION

Smoke inhalation is a complex entity with several mechanisms:
1. inhalation of toxic fumes such as carbon monoxide and/or cyanide;
2. local action of soot and other organic particles;
3. chemical burns from acids and other compounds.

Carbon monoxide poisoning and cyanide lead to asphyxia due to red cells being unable to release oxygen. It is the leading cause of death following house fires. Children who are suspected of having carbon monoxide poisoning should be resuscitated with 100% oxygen. If cyanide poisoning is suspected then treatment with standard cyanide kits is suggested either with dicobalt edetate if the child is comatose or hydroxycobalamin if the child is comatose but still perfusing.

Bronchial lavage may be considered if particulate matter or acids are considered to be present in the airway.

The net result of the contamination is a fulminant inflammatory process leading to significant pulmonary edema. This can be of insidious onset and consequently all children who are suspected of having had smoke inhalation should be admitted for a period of observation until such time as they are proved normal.

TOXIC SHOCK

Toxic shock is a rare but significant complication of burn injury (and occasionally other minor wounds including those following minor surgery). Typically caused by staphylococcal toxins, streptococci have also been implicated. Usually the wound/burn will be colonized rather than overtly infected by the bacteria. Symptoms include fever > 38.5°C, erythematous rash, vomiting, diarrhea and malaise. If a child presents within 2–3 days of sustaining a burn/wound with any or all of these signs or symptoms toxic shock should be suspected.

Treatment consists of identifying the cause (wound swab, blood for blood culture and serology), urgent resuscitation with fluids and antibiotics (which should reflect local streptococcal and staphylococcal antibiotic sensitivities) and local wound care as appropriate. Affected children should be admitted to a critical care area for further care.

MANAGEMENT OF THE UNSTABLE CHILD WITH UNDERLYING PATHOLOGY

After securing the airway, breathing and circulation, the real challenge is to identify the actual disease process and the etiological factors that have led to the presentation so that the most appropriate therapy can be given.

The standard approach of taking a history and then doing a physical examination is often inappropriate. The history available at this stage can be scrappy and imprecise. Most information will be gained from a detailed physical examination. This is best done in a systematic fashion, excluding groups of illnesses in turn. Patterns of illness include:

1. infection and life-threatening infection;
2. seizure disorder and coma;
3. metabolic abnormalities;
4. cardiac lesions;
5. respiratory disorders;
6. surgical pathology;
7. poisoning.

INFECTION

Life-threatening infection is relatively rare in the western world where vaccination and immunization are widespread. Diseases such as diphtheria and epiglottitis have been almost eradicated with effective vaccination but in areas where vaccination is less good or has waned these diseases continue to form important causes of mortality. Meningococcemia continues to be one of the most important life-threatening infections to appear acutely to the emergency department.

When dealing with infection three broad age groups have to be considered:

1. 0–3 months;
2. 3 months–3 years;
3. 3 years and over.

Children aged 0–3 months

Neonates and young infants have many of the problems related to infection. The symptoms with which these children present are many and varied.[53,54] They include going off feeds, failure to thrive, jitteriness and irritability. While many of these children will have an infection, other causes have to be considered. These include congenital anomalies such as congenital heart disease or inborn errors of metabolism or surgical causes such as intussusception and obstructed hernia.

Physical signs such as neck stiffness and bulging fontanelles are unreliable in this age group as are blood parameters such as white cell count and preponderance of neutrophils to lymphocytes. Clinical suspicion therefore is the mainstay of diagnosis and if there is any doubt children should have blood cultures taken and antibiotic treatment started. These children are usually admitted until such time as the diagnosis is reached.

Children aged 3 months–3 years

The children at the lower end of this spectrum will still be prone to neonatal illness. Viral illness is more common than bacterial illness in this age group but underlying bacterial illness or bacteremia should still be considered. However, it is still important to recognize the child who is toxic, and who is 'not right'.[55,56] Physical signs are more precise, with these children often being pyrexial, tachycardiac and tachypneic. Signs such as neck stiffness are more reliable in the diagnosis of meningitis. Signs of chest infection, osteomyelitis and septic arthritis may be easier to detect.

Children aged 3 years and over

Significant bacterial disease is relatively rare in this age group but includes chest infection, septicemia, urinary tract infection and orthopedic infection. Meningitis and meningococcal septicemia are still relatively rare. Abdominal conditions are easier to diagnose in these children because these children are better able to communicate symptoms.

Meningococcal disease

Infection with *Neisseria meningitidis* is one of the most significant reasons for a child to be critically ill. Often starting as a vague nonspecific illness at any age this infection can kill within hours. The florid purpuric rash is often not present initially, more often developing from a subtle finding in the early stages. Limb pains are common. (In the community, treatment should consist of intramuscular benzyl penicillin and urgent transfer to hospital with supplemental oxygen by mask. In the emergency department i.v. access and fluid replacement will be added. Fluid volumes of 60 ml/kg may be needed (in 10–20 ml/kg bolus) to restore perfusion. A cephalosporin (e.g. ceftriaxone, cefuroxime or cefotaxime) will be added to penicillin to control infection. Prompt transfer to the intensive care unit should be arranged when inotropic agents may be added to the management. It is helpful to complete an assessment of the Glasgow Meningococcal Prognostic score as soon as sufficient clinical data is available.

Management of life-threatening infection

These children should be resuscitated and blood taken for full blood count, urea and electrolytes, blood glucose and culture. Capillary blood gas analysis may also help determine initial status of the child and monitor early response to resuscitation. Chest X-ray, urine culture and lumbar puncture may also be indicated. Care should be taken not to perform lumbar puncture on children who are unconscious as this may produce herniation of the brain through the tentorium with resultant brain death.

I.v. antibiotics should be administered according to local sensitivity patterns and protocols. Children should be admitted to a high dependency or intensive care unit where inotropic support may be needed.

SEIZURE DISORDER

The list of underlying pathologies for patients presenting with seizure disorders is vast. Most will either be due to idiopathic epilepsy, a febrile seizure disorder or secondary to metabolic defects such as hypoglycemia or electrolyte disorder. Trauma should also be considered. Treatment should be aimed at stopping the seizure and at the same time trying to identify underlying treatable causes such as hypoglycemia and electrolyte imbalance. If fever is present this should be reduced as rapidly as possible.

Management of seizure disorder in the emergency situation

First-line treatment is i.v. diazepam, 0.2 mg/kg to a maximum 0.6 mg/kg intravenously. Lorazepam 0.1 mg/kg is also acceptable. If i.v. access is not readily available then rectal diazepam (2.5–10 mg depending on age) or intranasal midazolam (0.2 mg/kg) are acceptable treatments. This should be followed (if the seizure is not stopped) by a slow i.v. administration of phenytoin 10–15 mg/kg under ECG control. At this stage if the child is still fitting then consideration must be given to reducing intracranial pressure, paralysis and ventilation in order to control the seizure with additional anticonvulsants. Such management will need an intensive care/high dependency unit.

Blood sugar should always be tested by strip testing. If the blood sugar is low this may reveal an underlying metabolic disorder. Further blood should be taken along with urine to help diagnose metabolic anomalies if present and the child given 10% glucose 3–5 ml/kg.

COMA

Comatose children are particularly at risk of obstructing their airway so great care must be given to maintaining this. Once the airway is secured the underlying causes such as poisoning, epilepsy, head injury or other trauma, hypoglycemia or intracranial infection should be investigated. Treatable causes should be identified and treated appropriately and the child transferred to a high-dependency area as soon as possible. This may involve transfer via CT scanning if intracranial lesion is suspected. If trauma is suspected, particularly non-accidental injury, the child should be treated as with any other trauma victim and resuscitated aggressively prior to transfer.

METABOLIC ABNORMALITIES

Diabetic abnormalities, either hypo- or hyperglycemia, are the commonest. Small babies may present critically ill as a result of an inborn error of metabolism. While these are relatively rare they should be suspected in any child who presents close to the neonatal period, particularly if there is an intercurrent infection suspected. A strong clue to this might be the presence of hypoglycemia. Diabetic emergencies should be treated as detailed under the diabetic section (Ch. 15).

CARDIAC LESIONS

Children with cardiac lesions present in one of two ways:
1. in heart failure;
2. in cardiac arrest.
Heart failure is often due to progression of cardiac abnormalities. Underlying disease processes such as renal failure with hyperkalemia may have to be considered. Previously well children may have developed myocarditis. Supraventricular tachycardia is the commonest underlying cardiac dysrhythmia to cause heart failure, particularly in the younger age groups. The treatment of heart failure should be aimed towards maximizing oxygenation and reducing the fluid load. Any underlying dysrhythmia should be treated appropriately according to local guidelines. The child should be transferred to a high dependency area as soon as possible where future treatment can be monitored and inotropic support given if necessary.

The management of cardiac arrest is described earlier (p. 1586). The underlying causes may include hypertrophic cardiomyopathy or dysrhythmia.

RESPIRATORY DISORDERS

Common respiratory disorders to present include asthma, bronchiolitis, croup and foreign body in the airway. Recognition of respiratory distress/failure has been considered earlier. All children with respiratory disease should have oxygen delivery maximized and treatment directed to the underlying cause.

If it is suspected that a foreign body is wedged in the airway, the Heimlich maneuver or chest thrust maneuver may be necessary depending on the level of consciousness of the child.

SURGICAL CAUSES

Surgical causes of collapse are often forgotten in the emergency department, particularly in those in the younger age group. Intussusception and obstructed herniae commonly cause symptoms such as vomiting. This vomiting is not typical of that of gastroenteritis; it may only consist of one or two vomits. After that the child becomes unduly collapsed. Intussusception in particular can present with a child who is deathly pale but without much else in the way of physical signs. The classic signs of redcurrant jelly stool and a palpable mass are often absent.[56]

Pyloric stenosis may present with a dehydrated alkalotic child if the vomiting has been profuse.

If a pubertal girl presents in a collapsed state, two diagnoses should be considered – drug overdose (either intentional or accidental) and ectopic pregnancy. These may be related, i.e. the pregnancy is the reason for the overdose. In both situations resuscitation is vital. Pregnancy may be the result of child sexual abuse and this should be treated, if suspected, along local guidelines.

POISONING (see Ch. 6)

Poisoning in children is commonest between the second and third year of life. Children who are poisoned usually present with minimal signs or symptoms. The role of the emergency department is to identify the child who is at risk of either airway or circulatory collapse and to deal with these problems accordingly. All doctors working in emergency departments should have a good working knowledge of pharmacology of medications that are both prescribed and bought over the counter. The knowledge of the potential side-effects will help in determining which children can be discharged and those that need to be admitted for further care.

The role of gastric decontamination in this age group is difficult. The current trend is to move away from gastric lavage, which is a particularly unpleasant process. The role of syrup of ipecacuanha has also been challenged. There is evidence to suggest that it will only be effective (if at all) if administered within 1 h of the ingestion. The current vogue is for decontamination using charcoal. Most children will actually drink charcoal despite it looking unpleasant and this probably is the method of choice for all children who actually require gastric decontamination.

Specific antidotes are available for only a few poisons. Staff working within the emergency department should be familiar with these and their usage.

CONCLUSION

The pediatric emergency medical system has many facets, all of which need to be coordinated to provide for the streamlined care of sick or injured children. The aim should be prevention if at all possible. If prevention is not possible then facilities must exist for the efficient care of all children within a seamless emergency medical structure capable of providing all aspects of emergency care and rehabilitation back to the community.

PEDIATRIC INTENSIVE CARE

INTRODUCTION

Intensive care is distinguished from high-dependency or ward care by the level of observation and the level of intervention required by the patients. Close observation is assured by:
- The numbers of staff: at least one nurse per patient and at least one doctor awake and working on the unit at all times;
- The skill level of staff: only experienced pediatric intensive care nurses are allowed to work at the bedside and the resident medical staff members have to have advanced resuscitation and airway skills. There are high levels of supervision from senior staff. Higher levels of intervention take the form of:
- Continuous physiological monitoring: this will often involve additional circulatory access such as arterial and central venous lines but may also include a variety of other techniques, for example more invasive hemodynamic monitoring, indwelling oximetric catheters, intracranial pressure monitoring;
- Intensive care dependent techniques of organ–system support: the term 'intensive care dependent' meaning that it would be inappropriate to contemplate undertaking such support for a critically ill child without the level of monitoring and supervision available on the pediatric intensive care unit. Examples include mechanical ventilation, inotropic or mechanical circulatory support and renal replacement therapies such as hemofiltration.

Pediatric intensive care units cater for critically ill children from birth to 16 years of age but the age distribution is heavily skewed towards the lower age range. The median age of admissions is frequently less than 1 year and the mean is usually around 3 years. The units are predominantly geared towards emergency admissions since typically only about 30% of admissions are booked in advance in association with elective surgery or other procedures. The case mix bears comparison with the predominant causes of death in pediatrics, which themselves change with age. Infections and congenital abnormalities along with their attendant surgery figure prominently in young patients, whereas malignancy and trauma are commoner in older patients. Of admissions, 40% occur in the context of congenital heart disease whether they are new presentations, elective admissions after surgery or emergency admissions for other causes such as respiratory infection complicating pulmonary edema. Otherwise primary respiratory problems account for about 20% of admissions with strong seasonal and geographical variations. Major trauma also displays seasonal variation (lower in winter and highest during summer holidays) but accounts for up to 15% of admissions overall. Neurological problems (other than trauma) make up less than 10%.

The contribution of other diagnostic categories is more varied, depending upon the allocation of neonatal surgical patients and other services. Survival rates amongst critically ill children are generally high (about 92% of admissions) compared to the intensive care of other age groups. The length of intensive care stay is another skewed distribution (most are of very short duration, median circa 24 h) but the mean varies from 2 to 4 d depending principally on the quality of local 'step down' (high-dependency) facilities. This average length of stay is comparatively short compared to neonatal and adult intensive care.

Many intensive care admissions are critical emergencies and decisions to admit the patient under these circumstances are not difficult or often disputed. However, the apparently abrupt decline in a patient's condition is frequently the manifest decompensation of a process or processes that have been proceeding for some time and hence could, at least in theory, have been identified in advance. The final common pathway of cellular hypoxia/ischemia and organ dysfunction that leads to death in children is initiated by circulatory or respiratory failure and ends in asystole. The potential benefits of intensive care are therefore best realized by pre-emptive intervention to avert probable further deterioration.

Hence it is important to learn to recognize the sick child. Firstly, recognize ominous diagnoses for which the likely course of the disease is known (e.g. purpura fulminans in meningococcal septicemia). Alternatively, try to realize the severity of illness from basic clinical signs. Work on a system-by-system basis taking respiration and circulation first. The two key questions are:

1. How much work is being done? Which then indicates a second question: how sustainable is this level of physiological effort? and
2. How effective is it? (since ineffective effort will need to be supplemented sooner rather than later).

For example the work of breathing can be assessed by the respiratory rate, tidal volume and the apparent ease or otherwise of chest expansion. Look for the use of accessory muscles and the strain involved. Breathing may be difficult due to poor compliance or airway obstruction (listen for inspiratory stridor or expiratory wheeze) and there may be subcostal, intercostal, costal or sternal recession, tracheal tug or head bobbing, etc. Assess the effectiveness of breathing by the adequacy of chest expansion, the amount of oxygen required to avoid desaturation, conscious level, heart rate, presence of sweating and adequacy of peripheral perfusion as well as measurements of oxygen saturation and formal blood gases. Remember that cyanosis is a preterminal sign in respiratory failure and that premature infants respond to stress (including hypoxia) with bradycardia rather than the tachycardia otherwise expected first.

Once compensatory mechanisms have been exceeded, a precipitate and rapid deterioration occurs. Hence it is also very important to use recent *trends* in physiological observations as an indication of the patient's current condition and likely progress. Early intervention is far more likely to be successful and the use of thresholds for action usually causes delay even if they are based upon age-appropriate norms and reference ranges.

In the acute presentation of critical illness, the ultimate cause (i.e. the diagnosis) may not be apparent. Hence a treatment plan may have to be devised that addresses all the possibilities until further information becomes available. The sequence of priorities is to Resuscitate, then Diagnose and Treat, i.e. *Resuscitation comes first*. If immediate resuscitation is not necessary, still concentrate on physiology/pathophysiology (in terms of work and effectiveness) to decide how and when to instigate specific organ system support and monitoring. Then proceed with investigations that may lead to more specific treatment. The ultimate diagnosis may be made over a broad timeframe and the patient may sometimes have left intensive care before the whole clinical picture is apparent.

POST-RESUSCITATION STABILIZATION AND TRANSFER

The initial resuscitation of acutely ill children is often described as being followed by a period of 'postresuscitation stabilization'. This may be prolonged and it may be found necessary to defer some aspects of

care depending upon the resuscitation priorities. For example in severe trauma the resuscitation can involve emergency surgery after which the patient is moved to the intensive care unit. At this point reassess the patient and complete a secondary survey. The resuscitation may have also created problems that need to be identified and dealt with. Studies suggest that medically significant complications due to cardiopulmonary resuscitation are rare in children (< 3%). Those complications that have been reported include retroperitoneal hemorrhage, pneumothorax, pulmonary hemorrhage, epicardial hematoma, and gastric perforation.

Once resuscitation is complete or nearing completion, prepare the patient for longer term intensive care by revision/augmentation of airway and vascular access. For example oral intubation may need changing to nasal and if necessary replace intraosseous access with a central venous line and peripheral i.v. cannulae. An arterial line may be required. Good intensive care is about doing simple things well. Hence procedures such as the style of intubation, the manner of endotracheal tube fixation and the method of securing drips should all be controlled by unit protocol unless otherwise contraindicated. For example routine, non-essential revision of the intubation is unwise if the airway was precarious initially or if intubation was difficult to achieve. But in all other circumstances, especially if the patient is to be transferred, the most stable and familiar techniques should be employed.

Oxygenation is the highest priority but adequate minute volume must be provided to clear carbon dioxide. Assess both by serial measurements of arterial blood gases. Acidosis may have metabolic consequences such as hyperkalemia (a compartment shift) or pharmacological effects such as failure to respond to catecholamines. It may aggravate symptoms of poisoning with drugs that are weak acids. Correct any respiratory acidosis by increasing minute volume particularly if the $[H^+] > 63$ nmol/L (pH < 7.2). Treat the cause of any metabolic acidosis in preference to giving bicarbonate, since without treatment of the cause the acidosis will recur. I.v. bicarbonate may be indicated to compensate for recognized bicarbonate losses (e.g. ileostomy fluid) or to recruit a pharmacodynamic response (e.g. if there is a poor response to inotrope therapy due to acidosis) but otherwise runs the risk of increasing the work of breathing (through CO_2 production) and aggravating intracellular acidosis ($CO_{2(aq)}$ and H^+ ions diffuse into cells more rapidly than bicarbonate).

A normal blood pressure is not a sufficient assessment of the cardiovascular system. Determine the adequacy of the circulation by assessing end organ (cellular) function using markers like urine output, mental state, degree of metabolic acidosis or serum lactate levels. Remember that resuscitation may have compensated for the presenting problem rather than resolved it. Furthermore a variety of other problems are common after acute resuscitation. Look for dilutional anemia, which can arise as a consequence of large intravascular volume boluses having been given during resuscitation. Give red cell transfusion priority if oxygen delivery is critical or compromised (one possible cause of metabolic acidosis). Also establish an appropriate ongoing i.v. fluid and electrolyte regime at this point that includes maintenance requirements, metered replacement of any deficit and comprehensive replacement of ongoing losses. If inotropic or chronotropic support is required then use titratable infusions of short-acting agents in preference over longer acting agents whose effects may persist when the current hemodynamic state changes. Measure the blood glucose level since hypoglycemia is common and not detectable by clinical observation in the obtunded, sedated or otherwise critically ill child. The risk of hypoglycemia is increased in smaller and younger patients as a consequence of low glycogen reserves and a high basal metabolic rate. The dose of glucose in acute hypoglycemia is 0.5 g/kg. This dose must be followed by repeated assessment of the blood glucose level to check that a therapeutic effect has been achieved and that the resulting level is maintained. The normal maintenance requirement for babies is 6 mg/kg/min.

For all but the most straightforward of resuscitation scenarios the patient then requires further management on an intensive care unit. For all but the simplest cases this should be a specialist pediatric intensive care unit particularly if it is difficult to anticipate what the length of intensive care unit stay will be or if it is likely to be more than 24 h. Transfers within hospital or between hospitals usually occur after stabilization and are conducted without undue haste by a retrieval team from the pediatric intensive care unit. The use of a skilled and trained transfer team substantially reduces critical incidents and morbidity. The need for such transfer is entirely predictable and so detailed protocols should be prepared in advance including specified indications and provision for more urgent movement. Training in intensive care transport must be practical and is best provided by supervised episodes accompanying a skilled team. Trainees must become familiar with the modes of transport used and must attain higher levels of proficiency in equipment maintenance and repair than are necessary for clinical staff within a hospital environment. This is because technical backup is not available during transfers.

RESPIRATORY SYSTEM

INDICATIONS FOR MECHANICAL VENTILATION

One of the commonest reasons for arranging intensive care admission is a decision to start mechanical ventilation. Infants and children have less respiratory reserve than adults, which leads to a relatively high incidence of respiratory failure during severe illness. Respiratory support may be indicated:

- to secure the upper airway;
- to reduce the work of spontaneous breathing;
- to supplement gas exchange in respiratory disease;
- to achieve desirable hemodynamic effects;
- as an incidental requirement during sedation or anesthesia;
- due to neurological disease with or without respiratory complications.

If the patient has adequate airway protection reflexes it may be possible to provide mechanical support with minimal sedation and without intubation.[57] Select such patients carefully on their own merits. Successful nose mask or face mask ventilation requires a degree of patient cooperation and a pressure controlled device with the capacity to deliver high flows to compensate for any leak. Negative pressure devices, whether tank or cuirass, have the disadvantage of obstructing access to the patient. So-called 'non-invasive' ventilation should only be provided in an environment where anesthetic and airway skills are readily available.

TECHNIQUE OF INTUBATION

The purpose of recognizing sick children is to enable appropriate early intervention. Hence intubation is usually performed as part of the induction of anesthesia. There are two basic approaches to the administration of an anesthetic: i.v. (usually a rapid sequence induction) and inhalation. Anesthetic skills, equipment and assistants are required for both. Rapid sequence induction is the preferred approach for most situations especially when regurgitation and aspiration of stomach contents are potential problems. It is contraindicated when the airway is compromised or when intubation may be difficult, in which case inhaled anesthetics are used.

Use a straight-bladed laryngoscope to view the larynx in infants because its position is high (at the level of the C4 vertebra) and anterior compared to the adult. The large, soft, sigma-shaped epiglottis can be kept under the blade if it obscures the laryngeal inlet. In older children, use a curved blade and lift away from you (as opposed to rotating) for a better view of the vocal cords. Once beyond puberty the larynx has assumed its adult position.

Use noncuffed tubes in prepubertal children because the larynx has a gradually tapering shape narrowest in the subglottic region (behind the cricoid cartilage). The tube should be small enough to permit a small leak of air under pressure, giving reassurance that excessive pressure is not being exerted on the subglottic tracheal mucosa where damage would otherwise lead to scarring and subsequent stenosis. After puberty the vocal cords are the narrowest part of the airway so use cuffed tubes in more mature children. The ideal position of an endotracheal tube tip is at the level of the sternoclavicular junction on the chest X-ray. In infants

the trachea bifurcates at the level of T2. The tip of the tube will move significantly when the neck is flexed (moves down) or extended (moves up).

Always attempt to preoxygenate the patient and make sure that you are proficient in airway intervention techniques because any interruption in ventilation in babies and infants very quickly leads to hypoxemia. Their high metabolic rate means faster consumption of oxygen and greater carbon dioxide production. Furthermore normal ventilator settings must include the routine use of positive end expiratory pressure because atelectasis occurs early and at a higher volume relative to the functional residual capacity of older children and adults.

CHOICE OF VENTILATOR

Ventilators differ in relation to their power source, cycling characteristics, method of generating gas flow and the provision of gas supply for spontaneous breaths. The 'cycling' label is attached to the parameter (pressure, time, volume or flow) that determines when inspiration stops and expiration starts.

The choice of cycling method will affect the behavior of the ventilator as the patient's condition changes (Table 36.3).

The method by which gas flow is generated affects the choice of 'control' mode (e.g. pressure control and volume control) and hence the pattern of pressure and flow over time during inspiration. The terms 'support' or 'assist' are applied to modes where the breath is initiated by the patient then detected and supported by the ventilator. 'Mandatory' or 'control' breaths are initiated by the ventilator and may be blended with 'support' (e.g. synchronized intermittent mandatory ventilation with pressure support).

For neonates there is a historical preference for using continuous flow, pressure-regulated, time-cycled ventilators. They are less susceptible to the fluctuations in tidal volume that are generated by the disparity between tidal volume and total gas volume in the ventilator circuit. They also do not generate large pressure fluctuations when the patient is uncoordinated with the ventilator and can function in the presence of a modest leak around the endotracheal tube. However, when compliance changes (e.g. as muscle relaxants wear off, or disease severity worsens) large changes in delivered tidal volume occur. Despite being intrinsically sensitive in the detection of circuit disruption, older models may not be capable of detecting absent tidal volume (endotracheal tube blockage). They must therefore be used in combination with an apnea monitor.

For older patients there is a historical preference for volume-controlled ventilation. Nevertheless improved technology is making it easier and sometimes more appropriate to ventilate smaller patients with such devices. However, even with newer models, when compliance changes or airway obstruction develops, airway pressure escalates and the effective tidal volume is reduced as gas is compressed in the ventilator tubing.

VENTILATOR SETTINGS

Oxygenation is critical. Since oxygen is poorly soluble in water, the important factors in oxygen uptake across the lung are:

- the amount of blood flow (e.g. the cardiac output);
- the hemoglobin concentration;

Table 36.3 Ventilator cycling

	Low compliance/high airways resistance	High compliance/low airways resistance
Volume cycled	V_T becomes a smaller % of cycled volume	i.t. becomes short
	PIP increases	PIP falls
Pressure cycled	i.t. and V_T both fall	i.t. becomes very long V_T increases
Flow cycled	i.t. and V_T both fall	i.t. and V_T both rise
Time cycled	No effect	No effect

i.t., inspiratory time; PIP, peak inspiratory pressure; V_T, tidal volume.

- the effective surface area of the lung (after the effects of shunt, deadspace and ventilation–perfusion matching);
- the diffusion gradient for oxygen.

All of the above can be manipulated independently but the ventilator is only used for the last two. To increase the diffusion gradient for oxygen, increase the inspired oxygen concentration. The effective surface area of the lung can be increased (within limits) by increases in tidal volume and mean airway pressure. Some components of shunt may be relatively fixed and not respond to changes in ventilation. It is important not to overventilate under these circumstances. Deadspace is proportionately more significant at low tidal volumes. Ventilation–perfusion matching changes with posture and positioning of the patient as well as other changes in ventilation technique.

Carbon dioxide diffuses easily across respiratory membranes and comes in and out of solution easily. Hence the rate-limiting step in removal across the lung is the speed with which equilibrated (alveolar) gas is replaced with fresh gas, i.e. the alveolar minute ventilation. Use tidal volume and respiratory rate to influence the minute volume and create responses in arterial carbon dioxide level. At low tidal volumes deadspace is more significant and reduces the effectiveness of each tidal volume in clearing carbon dioxide. There are therefore limits to how much a reduction in tidal volume can be compensated by increasing respiratory rate.

Wherever possible, choose ventilator settings that can be considered therapeutic, such as the use of higher levels of positive end expiratory pressure in pulmonary edema to reduce alveolar water content or in bronchomalacia to maintain patency of the conductance airways. Lung volume and $[H^+]$ (via carbon dioxide partial pressure; PCO_2) can also be used to manipulate pulmonary vascular resistance. The amount of work required to breathe is increased when compliance is poor or when airway resistance is high. Try to adapt ventilator settings to match the disease state and avoid complications such as gas trapping (dynamic hyperinflation), for example allow a long expiratory time if the patient has bronchospasm.

CONSEQUENCES OF VENTILATION

Endotracheal intubation and mechanical ventilation are not natural processes and are associated with hazards that can be minimized by appropriate attention to detail. Choose the correct size and length endotracheal tube. Take care to ensure that the inhaled gases are humidified to 100% relative humidity at body temperature. Avoid high pressures and tidal volumes. Any ventilator settings that induce overinflation are likely to induce or aggravate lung injury although the specific settings involved will differ between restrictive and obstructive diseases. Peak pressure is far more dangerous than end expiratory pressure and many of the problems previously associated with peak pressure are as much to do with the associated high end inflation lung volume and tidal volume as anything else. Previously injured lungs are more susceptible to ventilator-induced lung injury and if the disease is not homogenous it may be the less severely diseased segments that receive the greater insult.

NEWER VENTILATION STRATEGIES

In recent times the concept of minimizing the stress of mechanical ventilation has become pivotal in the ventilation of patients with respiratory disease. The appeal of novel approaches to ventilation is often based upon their potential (even if unproven) abilities in this respect. The simplest approaches include improved coordination between the ventilator and the patient. More complex approaches are aimed at providing increasing degrees of 'lung rest'. The conventional and best validated method of providing lung rest is extracorporeal membrane oxygenation (ECMO), which is a modified form of cardiopulmonary bypass. ECMO can be used to achieve total lung rest (gas exchange during prolonged apnea) and the circuit can be configured to provide pulmonary (venovenous cannulation) or cardiopulmonary support (venoarterial cannulation).

Examples of ventilation strategies with proposed benefits in terms of reducing ventilator-associated lung injury include:

- Permissive hypercarbia: where (pressure-limited) minute ventilation is minimized in the hope of reducing lung stress. To perform this technique, once hypoxia is overcome, allow arterial carbon dioxide levels to rise to limits dictated by the associated rise in hydrogen ion concentration (e.g. ≤ 63 nmol/L correlating with $pH \geq 7.2$). Over time, metabolic compensation allows higher and higher carbon dioxide levels to be tolerated.[57–60]
- High-frequency oscillation: these devices use the continuous distending pressure (mean airway pressure) to recruit and maintain lung volume. Gas exchange is achieved by a high-frequency vibration (6–12 Hz). Minimal tidal volumes (less than deadspace) result from the amplitude of the vibration, which itself is highly attenuated within the respiratory tract, hence minimizing shearing forces.[58] Use the amplitude (ΔP) preferentially to control the partial pressure of carbon dioxide in arterial blood ($PaCO_2$). The fall in tidal volume as frequency increases attenuates carbon dioxide removal, which is otherwise highly efficient.
- Inhaled nitric oxide[61–63]: in responsive patients, ventilation perfusion mismatch can be reduced by NO, which causes vasodilatation in ventilated areas. Some cases of pulmonary hypertension may also respond.
- Liquid ventilation (usually in the form of perfluorocarbon-assisted gas exchange)[64]: this technique involves first gradually replacing the functional residual capacity of the lung by slow instillation of perfluorocarbon during conventional ventilation. This causes bulk distention of the alveoli and considerable recruitment of lung volume. Subsequent tidal ventilation with 100% oxygen is more effective as the low surface tension at the perfluorocarbon:gas interface improves compliance.
- Intratracheal pressure release ventilation[63,65]: where expiratory flows are augmented increasing respiratory efficiency at lower tidal volumes and lower mean pressures.

WEANING VENTILATION

Improving respiratory function is reflected in the behavior of the patient and the ventilator. In the latter case the effects depend upon the mode of ventilation employed at the time. Improved compliance or airways resistance during volume-controlled ventilation causes airway pressures to fall. With pressure-controlled ventilation under the same circumstances, tidal volumes increase and the partial pressure of oxygen in arterial blood (PaO_2) may rise as the $PaCO_2$ falls. Effective tidal volume can be usefully expressed in relation to deadspace using end tidal carbon dioxide measurements. In flow-cycled ventilator modes such as pressure support, the inspiratory time decreases as compliance improves. Close observation of the patient and regular blood gas measurement allows you to respond to these changes.

Start to deliberately wean patients from mechanical ventilation when the pathology or indication for ventilation is resolving or finished. The speed of successful weaning is dictated by the adequacy of the response and the skill lies in getting the best performance out of the partially dependent patient. The patient must be able to take over ventilation without excess energy expenditure, and there must be adequate respiratory muscle strength, hemodynamic stability and a good nutritional state. Only extubate electively when the patient:

- is hemodynamically and metabolically stable;
- is making effective efforts to breathe;
- is sufficiently awake and alert;
- has protective airway reflexes.

Prior to extubation, always ensure that there is adequate provision of equipment, medication and staff to deal with complications such as laryngospasm, which might require urgent reintubation.

CARDIOVASCULAR SYSTEM

Another common reason to arrange intensive care admission is the need to perform invasive monitoring of the circulation using arterial or central venous lines. This need arises:

- as a wise precaution in case of potential instability, e.g. after major surgery or other trauma;
- in the treatment of shock such as during large volume fluid losses/replacement;
- when blood pressure is excessively high or low;
- when vasoactive drugs are being administered by infusion.

RECOGNITION OF SHOCK

Do not rely on blood pressure in the first instance or alone to assess the circulation. Shock is defined as inadequate perfusion of tissues (in particular oxygenation) and its severity is assessed in terms of end-organ function. When flow measurements are available, the global delivery of oxygen to the tissues can be calculated as the product of the oxygen content of arterial blood and the cardiac output; but not all of this oxygen is available to the tissues. Factors that influence the distribution of blood also apply and may be particularly affected by disease. The two most sensitive and clinically useful organs in the assessment of the circulation are the brain and the kidney. Altered conscious level is an important sign of shock and up to the point of acute renal failure urine output is a good marker of renal perfusion. The patient with severe cardiovascular dysfunction (shock) generally has peripheral pulses that are difficult to feel, poor capillary refill, cool extremities, decreased urine output and altered sensorium. A *low blood pressure* is a preterminal *sign* since blood pressure can be maintained by intense vasoconstriction even in the presence of a markedly reduced circulating volume. The fall in blood pressure thus represents decompensation and indicates that the patient is out of control.

It is important to monitor fluid losses and replacement accurately. In the short term this can be approximated by the fluid balance but remember to extend the comparison over days. Weigh the patient regularly and match your impressions with clinical and laboratory observations.

RECOGNITION OF HEART FAILURE

Heart failure is distinguishable from shock. It is a more chronic condition in which the heart fails to respond adequately to its preload and hence fails to obey its normal Starling relation. There may be diastolic or systolic dysfunction or both and the problem may apply to specific ventricles or regions of myocardium. Fluid retention results from 'back pressure' as well as humoral responses to a reduced cardiac output. Although true heart failure can occur in children, most patients with signs that would represent heart 'failure' in an adult are in fact displaying the manifestations of a left-to-right shunt. These patients may have positively athletic cardiac function.

RECOGNITION OF CONGENITAL HEART DISEASE

Suspect congenital heart disease especially and most importantly in neonates with shock or cyanosis but also in patients with:

- murmurs;
- pulmonary edema;
- rhythm disturbances;
- abnormally severe symptoms from respiratory disease;
- failure to thrive.

Right-to-left shunts cause cyanosis and rarely cause murmurs because they are relatively low volume shunts occurring at low pressure. Left-to-right shunts cause pulmonary and ventricular volume overload. The loudness of the murmur is to some extent inversely proportional to the size of the shunt. Sustained high pulmonary blood flow causes pulmonary hypertension. Ventricular outflow tract obstruction (pressure overload) tends to cause ventricular hypertrophy. Ventricular hypertrophy is associated with decreased ventricular compliance (diastolic dysfunction).

Congenital heart disease can produce many combinations of defects, which also evolve according to the loading forces they create.

It is essential to recognize duct-dependent lesions. These present early in the neonatal period. Duct-dependent pulmonary flow presents with cyanosis and duct-dependent systemic flow with heart failure and/or shock in the first week of life. Both require an infusion of prostaglandin (typically 20 ng/kg/min) and urgent evaluation by a pediatric cardiologist.

TREATMENT OF SHOCK

The first line in cardiovascular resuscitation and support is an intravascular volume bolus of 20 ml/kg. Such preload augmentation should increase stroke volume and therefore blood pressure even if heart failure is suspected as well as shock. The most common cause of an inadequate response to this treatment is that the magnitude of the problem has been underestimated and inadequate fluid volumes have been used, hence the protocol for repeating the boluses of i.v. fluid at least twice if there is an inadequate response. However, do not give excessive amounts of intravascular volume if heart failure is present. In rapid large volume resuscitations the central venous pressure is a useful guide to how the volume is being handled by the circulation. Palpating the liver edge can also help; hepatic engorgement suggests right ventricular volume overload.

Both myocardial contractility (and hence stroke volume) and heart rate are increased by catecholamines. The first-line inotropic support started after the second or third fluid bolus is usually adrenaline (0.05–0.5 mcg/kg/min) or dopamine (2–10 mcg/kg/min). Cardiac output can also be influenced by manipulation of afterload (end systolic ventricular wall tension) for example by agents that affect the systemic vascular resistance. The term 'systemic vascular resistance' refers to a global approximation of the resistance of the circulation to blood flow. It is calculated after measuring cardiac output by dividing the pressure drop across the circulation by the measured blood flow. Reduction of afterload may improve cardiac output in conditions where there is a left-to-right shunt. Increases in afterload (e.g. using alpha adrenergic agents) are an important component of support in shock states such as septic shock when characterized by a low systemic vascular resistance.

The intrinsic response of the cardiovascular system both to disease and resuscitation depends upon the age of the patient and the nature and stage of palliation of any congenital heart disease as well as any intercurrent disease. The fetal circulation is characterized by the fetal connections, a high pulmonary vascular resistance and a low systemic vascular resistance. The neonatal (transitional) circulation is characterized by the potential persistence of all the fetal connections other than the umbilical vessels, reactive pulmonary vasculature and limited inotropic and chronotropic reserve; that is to say reduced capacity to increase contractility in response to catecholamines and a poor return in terms of cardiac output for increases in heart rate (despite a rate-dependent cardiac output in bradycardia). The neonatal heart also displays muted (e.g. to potassium) or accentuated (e.g. to calcium) responses to various electrolytes and drugs compared to later life. In infancy and childhood the myocardium adapts progressively to its new loading conditions and develops an increased reserve to beta adrenergic stimulation.

In refractory shock, i.e. failure to respond to intravascular volume loading, it is crucially important to get accurate monitoring of the circulation. Then consider the following possible explanations:

- Overestimation of the filling pressures: both central venous and pulmonary capillary wedge pressures are heavily influenced by thoracic pressure and hence positive pressure ventilation. Use the end expiratory values in your evaluation.
- Systolic cardiac dysfunction: depression of the contractile state of the myocardium can occur with a range of common disorders, for example sepsis, acidosis, hypoglycemia, hypoxia or hypocalcemia. In addition, drugs (especially antiarrhythmics) can also decrease the contractile state. A hydrogen ion concentration greater than 63 (pH < 7.2) can decrease the effectiveness of catecholamines and may need to be corrected.

- Diastolic dysfunction: when the compliance of the myocardium is poor as can occur alongside depression of systolic function or more independently as a result of congenital heart disease, the end diastolic volume does not increase normally in response to fluid challenge, whilst the end diastolic pressure increases markedly. Poor myocardial compliance is aggravated by catecholamines.
- Extrinsic cardiac compression: tamponade can restrict atrial and therefore ventricular filling resulting in a low end diastolic volume and low cardiac output despite high measured filling pressures. Echocardiography rapidly detects pericardial fluid and in extremis, given a compatible history, a pericardial tap may be indicated as part of resuscitative efforts.

The problem may be specific to one ventricle, particularly in congenital heart disease. It is often wise to request the opinion of a pediatric cardiologist in patients with refractory shock. Left ventricular preload is commonly inferred from left atrial pressure after cardiac surgery or pulmonary capillary wedge pressure under other circumstances. Swan–Ganz catheters are available, which are small enough to use in patients as young as 18 months.

THERAPEUTIC EFFECTS OF VENTILATION IN CIRCULATORY FAILURE

Patients in significant shock should be intubated and ventilated. Since this will probably involve the induction of anesthesia, take care to pick the right moment. There is no substitute for experience in these sorts of judgments. Anesthetic agents have cardiovascular side-effects and the best approach is usually to optimize resuscitation before anesthetic induction. In contrast when patients are deteriorating rapidly and are likely to continue to do so, early ventilatory support is a priority. Patients in shock require less anesthetic to suppress the central nervous system but they take longer to respond to i.v. injections of anesthetic agents because of the reduction in effective blood flow.

Positive pressure ventilation can have a variety of hemodynamic effects, most of which are therapeutic for patients with normal anatomy but who have cardiovascular instability. The right ventricular preload is reduced by the rise in intrathoracic pressure. Left ventricular preload may be decreased as a consequence or increased as pulmonary venous blood is encouraged to leave the lung. The dominant effect can often be inferred from the systemic arterial pressure trace looking for effects reminiscent of a Valsalva maneuver or the opposite during inspiration. Left ventricular afterload is reduced by the effects of raised intrathoracic pressure on the ventricle and by encouraging diastolic arterial flow out of the thorax. The effects on right ventricular afterload depend upon the pervading pulmonary vascular resistance. Further cardiovascular benefits in terms of the treatment of shock are achieved by the decreased work of breathing and decreased oxygen consumption associated with sedation and paralysis. Reduction in alveolar water content can also improve lung compliance and oxygenation.

There are a wide variety of situations in pediatric intensive care where cardiopulmonary interactions dictate management, for example patients with high pulmonary vascular resistance and right to left ductal shunts, patients with univentricular physiology or patients with cavopulmonary connections and hence passive pulmonary blood flow as a result of cardiac surgery. Patients with low or critical pulmonary blood flow may have extraordinarily compliant lungs and experience symptomatic reductions in cardiac output during positive pressure ventilation. Patients with high pulmonary blood flow have predictably noncompliant lungs.

CENTRAL NERVOUS SYSTEM

LEVEL OF CONSCIOUSNESS

Determine the patient's level of consciousness in a reproducible fashion. Describe the stimulus required to elicit a response and then describe the organization or sophistication of that response. At lower and lower levels of consciousness, greater stimuli (voice then pain) achieve less organized reactions. The commonest nomenclature used to describe this relationship is the Glasgow coma score, which breaks the responses into three groups: 'eyes' (4-point scale), 'vocalization' (5-point scale) and 'motor' responses (6-point scale). There are a variety of adaptations for preverbal or intubated patients. The AVPU classification distinguishes patients who are Alert, respond to Voice, respond only to Pain or who are Unresponsive. Painful stimuli administered peripherally can elicit spinal reflexes and mislead the unwary as to the sophistication/localization of the response. Avoid this by causing pain in a cranial nerve distribution, e.g. by pressure under the supraorbital ridge and documenting the response particularly of any limb movement. Patients who respond only to deep pain (Glasgow coma score ≤ 8) or who are unresponsive (Glasgow coma score 3) are unlikely to have adequate airway protection reflexes and are likely to require intubation.

LEVEL OF AWARENESS

Sedation (hypnotic) agents obtund the patient, i.e. induce mental blunting often with amnesia. They are used to induce stupor so that symptoms and treatments are better tolerated. Sedation is usually provided by continuous or intermittent doses of benzodiazepines. Although these agents dull the responses they do not induce normal sleep and are not analgesics.

PAIN CONTROL

Analgesia is a high priority in intensive care and the need to provide adequate analgesia is arguably increased by the use of sedative or anesthetic agents. Conscious children naturally use distraction and play as coping mechanisms for dealing with pain and distress. They can be encouraged in their efforts by diversion therapy. Stress and anxiety amplify children's apparent distress. Anything that can minimize such stress such as the presence of a parent, a full stomach, or a degree of sedation is to be encouraged. Assessment of pain control may be difficult; first because of the patient's age and communication skills and secondly because of appropriate sedation, which impedes the response even to age-appropriate pain assessment tools. It is best to anticipate and assume that pain is present and to treat it accordingly with a morphine infusion.

TRAUMATIC BRAIN INJURY

In severe diffuse brain injury, particularly that caused by trauma, cerebral edema worsens over the first 24–48 h and is accompanied by a loss of the capacity to autoregulate cerebral blood flow. It therefore becomes highly important to keep parameters that influence cerebral blood flow as stable as possible. These include the cerebral perfusion pressure, the $PaCO_2$, the PaO_2, regional metabolic demand and autonomic activity.

'Neuroprotective' intensive care should be instigated after significant brain injury (e.g. Glasgow coma score < 12). The intention is to minimize secondary brain injury but as yet there are no therapeutic approaches outside those aimed at adequate perfusion and oxygenation of the brain. The strategy includes:

- elective sedation;
- mechanical ventilation with strict attention to adequate oxygenation and avoiding hypercarbia (keep $PaCO_2$ within the normal range);
- cranial CT scan in the early *postresuscitation* phase of management to determine the need for neurosurgery and the subsequent management of raised intracranial pressure;
- nursing with the head midline and with a 30-degree upwards head tilt and avoid stresses that increase intracranial pressure;
- circulatory support to maintain the cerebral perfusion pressure.

Maintenance of the cerebral perfusion pressure requires intracranial pressure monitoring. This enables the detection of raised intracranial pressure as well as allowing the determination of the adequacy of cerebrovascular autoregulation. Intraventricular drains are preferred for this purpose firstly because they are more reliable than the alternatives. The second advantage of an intraventricular drain is that it enables venting of cerebrospinal fluid to control recalcitrant peaks of intracranial pressure from other causes such as cerebral edema. The treatment of raised intracranial pressure depends upon the cause. Neurosurgery may be required for space-occupying lesions such as hematomata. Hydrocephalus can be treated via the intraventricular drain. However, the first-line treatments for cerebral edema are medical maneuvers designed to reduce the cerebral water content (fluid restriction or infusion of hypertonic saline or mannitol). If raised intracranial pressure is problematic or unresponsive then barbiturates (thiopental) should be used for sedation since these agents uncouple the relationship between cerebral blood flow and the metabolic consumption of oxygen. The use of barbiturates may necessitate increased use of pressors to maintain the cerebral perfusion pressure. The ultimate management for raised intracranial pressure that cannot be lowered by medical means is craniectomy (removal of bone flaps to allow cerebral expansion at lower pressure).

Anticonvulsants should be given in traumatic brain injury particularly if any component of contusion or hemorrhage is seen in the brain substance on CT scan. Breakthrough seizures may only be detected by hemodynamic or pupillary signs and should be confirmed/monitored by electroencephalogram (EEG) or alternative electrophysiological monitoring and treated aggressively. The natural tendency to become pyrexial should be countered by therapeutic cooling to normothermia in order to prevent increases in cerebral metabolic oxygen demand. The possible merits of cooling to varying degrees of hypothermia are currently under investigation.

The duration of neuroprotective intensive care is usually judged by the behavior of the intracranial pressure over time. A minimum period of 24 h after injury is wise since cerebral swelling increases over this period. Imaging techniques such as CT and magnetic resonance imaging (MRI) are insensitive when detecting raised intracranial pressure. After 10 d any opportunity to prevent secondary brain injury has probably passed and patients should be woken and weaned from support.

METABOLIC COMA

Many components of neuroprotective intensive care are routinely transferred from traumatic brain injury where their justification is far from complete, to other forms of encephalopathy where there is even less evidence of their utility. Whilst loss of cerebrovascular autoregulation may occur in both conditions, in metabolic coma the insult is cytotoxic rather than vasogenic and cerebral edema is frequently more persistent. Metabolic and infective causes of coma may also be preceded by delirium, which is not a feature of traumatic brain injury.

SEIZURES

The diagnosis of 'status epilepticus' is made on the basis of the duration of continuous or consecutive seizures (30 min or longer). The protocol for resuscitation of patients in status epilepticus culminates in barbiturate coma after a further 30 min of progressive treatment with lesser measures. This is usually achieved by i.v. induction and maintenance of anesthesia with thiopental and followed by transfer to the pediatric intensive care unit. Subsequent treatment on the intensive care unit depends upon the cause and prior duration of the seizures. Make rigorous attempts to detect potentially treatable causes such as hypoxia, fever, hypoglycemia, hypocalcemia, infection (do not perform a lumbar puncture in the acute phase after protracted seizures), poisoning, trauma, raised intracranial pressure and kernicterus.

Seizures that lasted for less than 2 h before admission are unlikely to be complicated by secondary cerebral edema and it is worth allowing sedation to wear off so that the patient can wake up and be extubated. The longer the history the greater the risk of complications such as cerebral edema, hyperthermia and rhabdomyolysis. Don't forget to perform fundoscopy to detect papilledema and to watch patients carefully for signs of hypertension or bradycardia (since the third component of Cushing's triad – hypoventilation – is masked by anesthesia and mechanical ventilation). A cranial CT may be warranted and if cerebral edema is present give mannitol and consider intracranial pressure monitoring.

Seizures that recur or persist on the intensive care unit can be highly problematic and the mortality and morbidity are appreciable. Persistent seizures imply an unresolved cause so comprehensive investigation is necessary. In recalcitrant cases it can be worthwhile monitoring the EEG during the acute phase of a new treatment to ensure that a sustained period of burst suppression has elapsed before trying to wean the dose of anticonvulsant. Trials of pyridoxine in infants with resistant seizures should also be monitored by EEG. If no diagnosis or specific treatment is forthcoming a variety of drug regimens can be tried to reach a state of seizure control without excessive obtundation. It is not appropriate to sedate patients to the point of anesthesia and nurse them on an intensive care unit when their seizures are due to an incurable or degenerative condition.

FLUIDS AND RENAL REPLACEMENT THERAPY

Fluid and electrolyte balance are covered elsewhere in the text. In general terms the tendency to fluid retention and edema in critical illness make fluid regimes on intensive care highly restrictive once intravascular volume is assured. There is also a low threshold for the use of diuretic and renal replacement therapies on the pediatric intensive care unit.

There are two approaches to conventional renal replacement therapy: peritoneal dialysis and extracorporeal circulation. In childhood the peritoneum has a greater surface area proportional to body mass, making peritoneal dialysis more effective than it would be in older patients. Short-term renal replacement therapy can also be provided by hemofiltration. The favored venovenous approach to hemofiltration minimizes the hemodynamic consequences of this approach. A variety of techniques are available. Water removal can be achieved by ultrafiltration without replacement fluid. Solute clearance is enhanced by higher ultrafiltration rates in which the solutes are removed by bulk flow. The high ultrafiltration rates are achievable when providing replacement fluid. It is this approach that is termed 'hemofiltration'. Hemodiafiltration is an attempt to increase solute removal by additional diffusion but this can be achieved with high volume hemofiltration (e.g. with prefilter administration of replacement fluid) or dialysis. The removal of larger molecules (e.g. protein bound moieties) from the circulation can be achieved by plasmafiltration.

These modalities are used in many more situations than just renal failure.[66–68] Renal replacement techniques are occasionally used electively, e.g. to allow large volume transfusions of clotting factors prior to liver transplantation in fulminant hepatic failure. They are also used therapeutically in inflammatory conditions such as the systemic inflammatory response syndrome (e.g. after cardiopulmonary bypass or in severe sepsis) and Guillain–Barré syndrome. Plasmafiltration and plasmapheresis have also been tried in a variety of 'desperate diseases' such as lupus nephritis and polymyositis, though with no evidence of benefit. The liver replacement device Molecular Adsorbents Recirculating System (MARS®) represents an alternative to plasmafiltration in the attempt to clear protein bound toxins. It uses adsorbent membranes and recycles the albumin it uses but its clearance profile has not been shown to be greater than plasmafiltration. Pediatric patients require smaller quantities of albumin replacement during plasmafiltration than adults because smaller exchange volumes are used.

HOST DEFENCE

Infections are a major cause of mortality in young children and immune-suppressed individuals such as transplant recipients and those receiving cytotoxic chemotherapy. The invasive treatments and monitoring techniques used in intensive care increase the chances of nosocomial infection as do debilitating illnesses themselves. However, liberal antibiotic policies are a major stimulus for the generation and selection of multiresistant organisms. Normal intensive care procedures do not require antibiotic prophylaxis. Reserve antibiotic treatment for patients who have had procedures that do require prophylaxis, e.g. abdominal surgery, those with proven infection or those for whom the consequences of delay in treatment pending culture results are unconscionable. Use acute phase reactants and other tests (which predict positive cultures with varying degrees of success) to aid in decisions to withhold antibiotic treatment as well as decisions to commence.

A COMBINED ORGAN SYSTEM APPROACH TO CRITICAL ILLNESS

To conclude this section there follows a logical approach, consistent with the points covered earlier, to a disease with multiple organ system problems, in this case fulminant hepatic failure.

FULMINANT HEPATIC FAILURE

The typical history of patients with fulminant hepatic failure is one of nausea and malaise, followed by jaundice and coagulopathy (unresponsive to vitamin K). The most rapidly progressive cases develop hypoglycemia, metabolic acidosis and hyperammonemia in association with coma before jaundice is detected. There is no definitive treatment available and management depends upon supportive care, with liver transplantation in selected cases. Currently most patients receive N-acetyl cysteine in the acute phase. The mortality without transplantation is 50–80% but rises to more than 90% when there is severe encephalopathy or coagulopathy. Early transfer to a specialist center with a transplant program is therefore advisable. In many patients the cause is never identified despite extensive investigation and if hepatic failure is severe enough, the diagnosis is largely academic unless it is likely to recur in a transplanted liver or contraindicate treatment by transplantation. The intensive care priorities follow the ABCD (airway, breathing, circulation, disability) approach.

Comatose patients (grade IV encephalopathy) will require intubation for airway protection and ventilation. Avoid nasotracheal intubation because of the coagulopathy. Cardiac output, blood pressure and hemoglobin concentration must all be sustained in order to preserve cerebral oxygen delivery. Ventilate with a modestly increased fractional inspired concentration of oxygen (FiO_2), even if the patient does not have pulmonary complications. Hemodynamic instability is common, often a low systemic vascular resistance and variable cardiac output. Use invasive cardiovascular monitoring (at least central venous pressure and arterial lines) and anticipate a need to use inotropic agents with alpha agonist activity (e.g. noradrenaline). Remain vigilant to detect hypovolemia due to occult/acute hemorrhage.

Identify treatable causes of coma such as hypoglycemia or subclinical status epilepticus. Hypoglycemia specifically should be anticipated, appropriately supplemented with i.v. dextrose (without compromising the fluid restriction) and closely monitored. A computed tomography (CT) scan can be useful to exclude cerebral hemorrhage as the cause of acute neurological deterioration. Cerebral edema is present in 75% of patients with grade IV encephalopathy. Assume that cerebrovascular autoregulation is impaired. It may be possible to measure intracranial pressure but intraventricular catheters and intraparenchymal

bolts both require aggressive correction of coagulopathy first and even then the risk of bleeding may not be returned to normal. Furthermore such a strategy would mask an important marker of liver function (the prothrombin time). Nevertheless ventilate to a low normal $PaCO_2$ and assume that cerebral blood flow will bear a linear relationship with cerebral perfusion pressure. Use pressor support to a level that implies that the cerebral perfusion pressure is likely to be adequate and avoid potential rises in intracranial pressure by a policy of minimal handling, nursing with head midline and a 30-degree head up position. Elective paralysis prevents coughing and straining but makes it difficult to identify status epilepticus without EEG monitoring. Minimize cerebral oxygen demand principally by recognizing and controlling seizures, and avoiding hyperthermia. Barbiturate coma may be preferred and is induced by thiopental infusion in doses sufficient to cause a burst suppression EEG.

Plasmafiltration may temporarily improve encephalopathy. Efficacy has not been proved and it has not been shown to alter outcome. In larger patients MARS will probably use less albumin but has not been formally compared to plasmafiltration. Attempts to alter gut pH and flora to reduce the number of urea splitting organisms present are also theoretically justifiable.

Impose a therapeutic fluid restriction (e.g. 50% of normal) even to the point of hypernatremia as high as 150 mmol/L. This may require the use of high concentration dextrose solutions to provide adequate carbohydrate. Mannitol is not likely to have a dramatic effect on cerebral edema since the insult is cytotoxic and therefore ongoing. Concurrent renal failure aggravates fluid overload and complicates both the management of cerebral edema and the correction of coagulopathy. Avoid mannitol if there is oliguric renal failure. Treatable causes of prerenal failure such as hypovolemia or hypotension due to hemodynamic instability should be corrected but the practitioner should have a low threshold for hemofiltration, particularly if there is a metabolic acidosis.

Since the prothrombin time is the best prognostic liver function test, only correct coagulopathy with fresh frozen plasma (± cryoprecipitate) if there is a therapeutic indication such as bleeding, the need to establish intracranial pressure monitoring or imminent surgery. Supplement the platelet count if it falls below 50 when the patient is also coagulopathic.

Treat metabolic complications as they arise. Seek the cause of metabolic acidosis rather than treating blindly with bicarbonate. Increased lactate production due to impaired oxygen delivery/extraction and impaired metabolism can impair the response to inotropes and recurs inexorably if the cause cannot be treated. Recurrent acidosis can be treated without causing hypernatremia by moderate volume hemofiltration using a bicarbonate buffered replacement fluid.

Secondary sepsis is likely as a consequence of invasive treatment, gut translocation of organisms and impaired cellular and humoral immunity. Maintain a high index of suspicion for infection if the patient's clinical condition fluctuates. This approach should be extended to starting blind therapy with broad-spectrum antimicrobial and antifungal agents when dramatic changes in clinical condition occur.

REFERENCES (* Level 1 evidence)

1. Haller JA Jr, Shorter N. Regional pediatric trauma center: does a system of management improve outcome?. Z Kinderchir 1982; 35:44–45.
2. Haller JA Jr, Shorter N, Miller D, et al. Organization and function of a regional pediatric trauma center: does a system of management improve outcome?. J Trauma 1983; 23:691–696.
3. Beattie TF, Gorman DR, Walker JJ. The association between deprivation levels, attendance rate and triage category of children attending a children's injury and emergency department. Emerg Med J 2001; 18:110–111.
4. Morley CJ, Thornton AJ, Cole TJ, et al. Baby Check: a scoring system to grade the severity of acute

systemic illness in babies under 6 months old. Arch Dis Child 1991; 66:100–105.
5. McCarthy PL, Lembo RM, Baron MA, et al. Predictive value of abnormal physical examination findings in ill-appearing and well-appearing febrile children. Pediatrics 1985; 76:167–171.
6. Baker MD, Avner JR, Bell LM. Failure of infant observation scales in detecting serious illness in febrile, 4- to 8-week-old infants. Pediatrics 1990; 85:1040–1043.
7. Wilson D. Assessing and managing the febrile child. Nurse Pract 1995; 20:59–60.68–74
8. Currie CE, Williams JM, Wright P, et al. Incidence and distribution of injury among schoolchildren aged 11–15. Inj Prev 1996; 2:21–25.
9. Beattie TF. An injury and emergency based child injury surveillance system: is it possible? J Accid Emerg Med 1996; 13:116–118.

10. Rodewald LE, Wrenn KD, Slovis CM. A method for developing and maintaining a powerful but inexpensive computer data base of clinical information about emergency department patients. Ann Emerg Med 1992; 21:41–46.
11. Ribbeck BM, Runge JW, Thomason MH, et al. Injury surveillance: a method for recording E codes for injured emergency department patients. Ann Emerg Med 1992; 21:37–40.
12. DiScala C, Lescohier I, Barthel M, et al. Injuries to children with attention deficit hyperactivity disorder. Pediatrics 1998; 102:1415–1421.
13. Segal AO, Crighton EJ, Moineddin R, et al. Croup hospitalizations in Ontario: A 14-year time-series analysis. Pediatrics 2005; 116:51–55.
14. Wakefield AJ, Murch SH, Anthony A, et al. Ileal-lymphoid-nodular hyperplasia non-specific colitis,

and pervasive developmental disorder in children. Lancet 1998; 351:637–641.

15. Anonymous. Fall in MMR vaccine coverage reported as further evidence of vaccine safety is published. Commun Dis Rep CDR Wkly 1999; 9:227.230.

16. Fombonne E, Chakrabarti S. No evidence for a new variant of measles–mumps–rubella-induced autism. Pediatrics 2001; 108:E58.

17. Anonymous CDR weekly 16 www.hpa.org.uk/cdr/archives/2006/cdr1206.pdf.

18. Isaacs D. Bronchiolitis. BMJ 1995; 310:4–5.

19. Su E, Schmidt TA, Mann NC, et al. A randomized controlled trial to assess decay in acquired knowledge among paramedics completing a pediatric resuscitation course. Acad Emerg Med 2000; 7:779–786.

20. Grossman DC, Hart LG, Rivara FP, et al. From roadside to bedside: the regionalization of trauma care in a remote rural county. J Trauma 1995; 38:14–21.

21. Gausche M, Lewis RJ, Stratton SJ, et al. Effect of out-of-hospital pediatric endotracheal intubation on survival and neurological outcome: a controlled clinical trial. JAMA 2000; 283:783–790.

22. Gausche-Hill M, Lewis RJ, Gunter CS. Design and implementation of a controlled trial of pediatric endotracheal intubation in the out-of-hospital setting. Ann Emerg Med 2000; 36:356–365.

23. Cooper A, DiScala C, Foltin G, et al. Prehospital endotracheal intubation for severe head injury in children: a reappraisal. Semin Pediatr Surg 2001; 10:3–6.

24. Teach SJ, Antosia RE, Lund DP, et al. Prehospital fluid therapy in pediatric trauma patients. Pediatr Emerg Care 1995; 11:5–8.

25. Cummings P, Grossman DC, Rivara FP, et al. State gun safe storage laws and child mortality due to firearms. JAMA 1997; 278:1084–1086.

26. Wheeler DS. Emergency medical services for children: a general pediatrician's perspective. Curr Probl Pediatr 1999; 29:221–241.

27. American Academy of Pediatrics, C o P E M, P. American College of Emergency, et al. Care of children in the emergency department: guidelines for preparedness. Pediatrics 2001; 107:777–781.

28. Sacchetti A, Brennan J, Kelly-Goodstein N, et al. Should pediatric emergency care be decentralized?: an out-of-hospital destination model for critically ill children. Acad Emerg Med 2000; 7:787–791.

29. Oakley PA. Inaccuracy and delay in decision making in paediatric resuscitation, and a proposed reference chart to reduce error. BMJ 1988; 297:817–819.

30. Luten RC, Wears RL, Broselow J, et al. Length-based endotracheal tube and emergency equipment in pediatrics. Ann Emerg Med 1992; 21:900–904.

31. Roberts I, Schierhout G, Alderson P. Absence of evidence for the effectiveness of five interventions routinely used in the intensive care management of severe head injury: a systematic review. J Neurol Neurosurg Psychiatry 1998; 65:729–733.

32. Tepas JJ 3rd, Mollitt DL, Talbert JL, et al. The pediatric trauma score as a predictor of injury severity in the injured child. J Pediatr Surg 1987; 22:14–18.

33. Tepas JJ3rd, Ramenofsky ML, Mollitt DL, et al. The Pediatric Trauma Score as a predictor of injury severity: an objective assessment. J Trauma 1988; 28:425–429.

34. Schierhout G, Roberts I. Fluid resuscitation with colloid or crystalloid solutions in critically ill patients: a systematic review of randomised trials. BMJ 1998; 316:961–964.

35. Eisenberg M, Bergner L, Hallstrom A. Epidemiology of cardiac arrest and resuscitation in children. Ann Emerg Med 1983; 12:672–674.

36. Hassan TB. Use and effect of paediatric advanced life support skills for paediatric arrest in the A&E department. J Accid Emerg Med 1997; 14:357–362.

37. Teach SJ, Moore PE, Fleisher GR. Death and resuscitation in the pediatric emergency department. Ann Emerg Med 1995; 25:799–803.

38. Resuscitation Council UK. www.resusc.org.uk.

39. Mogayzel CL, Quan L, Graves JR, et al. Out-of-hospital ventricular fibrillation in children and adolescents: causes and outcomes. Ann Emerg Med 1995; 25:484–491.

40. Quan L, Mogayzel C. Ventricular fibrillation in pediatric cardiac arrest. Ann Emerg Med 1995; 26:658–659.

41. Ferguson J, Beattie TF. Occult spinal cord injury in traumatized children. Injury 1993; 24:83–84.

42. Teasdale GM, Murray G, Anderson E, et al. Risks of acute traumatic intracranial haematoma in children and adults: implications for managing head injuries. BMJ 1990; 300:363–367.

43. Brookes M, MacMillan R, Cully S, et al. Head injuries in injury and emergency departments. How different are children from adults?. J Epidemiol Community Health 1990; 4:147–151.

44. Sharples PM, Storey A, Aynsley-Green A, et al. Avoidable factors contributing to death of children with head injury. BMJ 1990; 300:87–91.

45. Barlow KM, Milne S, Aitken K, et al. A retrospective epidemiological analysis of non-injuryal head injury in children in Scotland over a 15 year period. Scott Med J 1998; 43:112–114.

46. Barlow KM, Minns RA. The relation between intracranial pressure and outcome in non-accidentalal head injury. Dev Med Child Neurol 1999; 41:220–225.

47. Thillainayagam K, MacMillan R, Mendelow AD, et al. How accurately are fractures of the skull diagnosed in an accident and emergency department. Injury 1987; 18:319–321.

48. Villalobos T, Arango C, Kubilis P, et al. Antibiotic prophylaxis after basilar skull fractures: a meta-analysis. Clin Infect Dis 1998; 27:364–369.

49. Aseervatham R, Muller M. Blunt trauma to the spleen. Aust N Z J Surg 2000; 70:333–337.

50. Moir JS, Ashcroft GP. Lap seat-belts: still trouble after all these years. J R Coll Surg Edinb 1995; 40:139–141.

51. Wilson JA, Kendall JM, Cornelius P. Intranasal diamorphine for paediatric analgesia: assessment of safety and efficacy. J Accid Emerg Med 1997; 14:70–72.

52. Kendall JM, Reeves BC, Latter VS. Multicentre randomised controlled trial of nasal diamorphine for analgesia in children and teenagers with clinical fractures. BMJ 2001; 322:261–265.

53. Baraff LJ, Oslund SA, Schriger DL, et al. Probability of bacterial infections in febrile infants less than three months of age: a meta-analysis. Pediatr Infect Dis J 1992; 11:257–264.

54. Baraff LJ. Outpatient management of fever in selected infants. N Engl J Med 1994; 330:938–939. discussion 939–940

55. Baraff LJ, Lee SI. Fever without source: management of children 3 to 36 months of age. Pediatr Infect Dis J 1992; 11:146–151.

56. Macdonald IA, Beattie TF. Intussusception presenting to a paediatric injury and emergency department. J Accid Emerg Med 1995; 12:182–186.

57. Plant PK, Owen JL, Elliott MW. Non-invasive ventilation in acute exacerbations of chronic obstructive pulmonary disease: long term survival and predictors of in- hospital outcome. Thorax 2001; 56:708–712.

58. Bohn D. Lung salvage and protection ventilatory techniques. Pediatr Clin N Am 2001; 48:553–572.

59. Hickling KG. Low volume ventilation with permissive hypercapnia in the Adult Respiratory Distress Syndrome. Clin Intensive Care 1992; 3:67–78.

60. Laffey JG, Kavanagh BP. Carbon dioxide and the critically ill – too little of a good thing?. Lancet 1999; 354:1283–1286.

61. Finer NN, Barrington KJ. Nitric oxide for respiratory failure in infants born at or near term. Cochrane Database Syst Rev 2000; 2:CD000399.

62. Kinsella JP, Abman SH. Inhaled nitric oxide: current and future uses in neonates. Semin Perinatol 2000; 24:387–395.

63. Hirschl RB. Respiratory failure: current status of experienced therapies. Semin Pediatr Surg 1999; 8:155–170.

64. Wiedermann HP. Partial liquid ventilation for acute respiratory distress syndrome. Clin Chest Med 2000; 21:543–554.

65. Kolobow T, Giacomini M, Reali-Forster C, et al. The current status of intratracheal–pulmonary ventilation (ITPV). Int J Artif Organs 1995; 18:670–673.

66. Reeves JH, Butt WB, Sathe AS. A review of venovenous haemofiltration in seriously ill infants. J Pediatr Child Health 1994; 30:50–54.

67. Reeves JH, Butt WW, Shann F, et al. Continuous plasmafiltration in sepsis syndrome Plasmafiltration in Sepsis Study Group. Crit Care Med 1999; 27:2098–2104.

68. Schetz M. Non-renal indications for continuous renal replacement therapy. Kidney Int Suppl 1999; 72:S88–S94.

37

Surgical pediatrics

Gordon A MacKinlay

INTRODUCTION

Pediatric surgery encompasses a wider range of surgery than any other surgical specialty. It is confined to an age group rather than an organ system. In the older child, adult surgeons may deal with some commoner problems.

Congenital problems presenting in the neonatal period or later, together with other conditions peculiar to childhood, should be treated in a specialist center by trained pediatric surgeons backed by pediatric anesthetists, pediatric radiologists, pediatric pathologists and experienced nursing staff specifically trained in the care of children. In a general hospital the child should be nursed on a children's ward and if there is no pediatric surgeon, care should be provided by the surgeon who is treating the child *together* with a pediatrician.

In the case of the neonate, a particular surgical challenge is encountered not only in the requirement for a meticulous surgical technique but also in careful pre- and postoperative management. The reward is the prospect of a full three score years and ten survival compared with the commonly sought 5-year survival in many aspects of adult surgery.

The presence of an anomaly requiring surgery is often detected antenatally by ultrasound, enabling discussion with the parents, obstetrician, pediatric surgeon and neonatologist. The parents can thus be prepared and reassured, where possible, that although an abnormality has been detected it can be treated. They can visit the surgical neonatal unit, meet the staff and, where appropriate, the timing of delivery may be planned to facilitate optimal transfer of the baby to the awaiting surgical unit or direct to the operating theater. Pregnancy is a time of potential parental stress and unless great care is taken in explaining the possible consequences of an antenatally diagnosed anomaly their anxiety will be increased.

The most significant development in pediatric surgery in the last decade has been the adoption of minimally invasive surgical techniques – mainly laparoscopy and thoracoscopy. The majority of major operations in children can be accomplished through 'keyhole surgery', which results in less postoperative pain, less analgesia, less ileus, earlier postoperative feeding, fewer wound infections and reduced hospital stay.

NEONATAL SURGERY

RESPIRATORY PROBLEMS

Whilst respiratory distress in the newborn is primarily the domain of the neonatologist some causes may be surgical and early referral to a pediatric surgeon may be of lifesaving importance.

CAUSES OF RESPIRATORY DISTRESS IN THE NEWBORN

1. Upper airway:
   a. choanal atresia;
   b. nasal encephalocele;
   c. tumors of the nasopharynx;
   d. Pierre Robin syndrome;
   e. macroglossia;
   f. hemangio/lymphangiomata of oral cavity;
   g. laryngotracheoesophageal cleft;
   h. laryngeal web;
   i. laryngeal stenosis;
   j. hemangioma of larynx;
   k. laryngomalacia;

    l. tracheomalacia;
    m. tracheal stenosis;
    n. cystic hygroma;
    o. cervical teratoma;
2. Intrathoracic:
    a. congenital lobar emphysema;
    b. cystic adenomatoid lung malformation;
    c. bronchogenic and lung cysts;
    d. enterogenous cysts;
    e. pneumothorax;
    f. sequestration of lung;
    g. vascular ring;
    h. congenital heart disease;
    i. Diaphragmatic hernia;
    j. eventration of the diaphragm;
    k. esophageal atresia and tracheoesophageal fistula.

Choanal atresia is obstruction of the posterior nares by a bony or occasionally membranous septum. If bilateral it is a neonatal emergency, as babies are obligate nasal breathers. An oral airway will overcome this problem until the obstruction is relieved.

An oral airway is also of benefit in *Pierre Robin syndrome*, where there is a hypoplastic mandible and central cleft palate, the tongue falling posteriorly to occlude both the oropharynx and the nasopharynx. An airway can be maintained in position for several weeks, the baby being fed nasogastrically or via a gastrostomy. A tracheostomy may be easier to manage and is maintained until the mandible grows. It also facilitates repair of the cleft palate, which is associated in the majority of cases.

A *laryngeal web*, if complete, leads to death in utero. If partial, the symptoms may merit emergency tracheostomy. *Laryngomalacia* leads to inspiratory stridor, which usually resolves in the first 2.5 years of life. *Tracheomalacia* is commonly associated with esophageal atresia. It has been postulated that the hypertrophied upper pouch, containing swallowed liquor, compresses the developing trachea, preventing the normal growth of tracheal rings. The problem increases postoperatively, sometimes making it impossible to extubate these babies. The diagnosis may be confirmed radiologically by lateral screening of the neck, observing the anteroposterior narrowing of the trachea with inspiration. Aortopexy, suturing the aorta to the back of the sternum, thus pulling the pretracheal fascia and hence the anterior tracheal wall forward, is sometimes of benefit. Prolonged intubation may allow time for the tracheal rings to become more supportive but may itself lead to subglottic stenosis. Tracheostomy is required in some cases.

Congenital lobar emphysema leads to overexpansion of a lung lobe with compromise of ventilation. Half the cases present within days of birth, the remainder in the first few months of life. The most common cause is bronchomalacia of the associated bronchus although some cases may be caused by external compression. The baby may present with feeding difficulties due to dyspnea. The diagnosis is made radiologically and the most commonly affected lobes are the left upper lobe or the right middle lobe. Treatment is lobectomy in severe cases but in many conservative management is appropriate.

Cystic adenomatoid lung and *congenital lung cysts* can present in much the same way as lobar emphysema. Their expansion produces respiratory distress. Congenital cysts tend to be unilocular and solitary. *Cystic adenomatoid malformation* is due to excessive overgrowth of bronchioles with multiple cysts lined by cuboidal and ciliated pseudostratified columnar epithelium. The left lower lobe is commonly affected and the appearance may antenatally or even postnatally be mistaken for a diaphragmatic hernia. Treatment is resection of the affected lobe, which can now be safely performed thoracoscopically.

Pulmonary sequestration is a mass of lung tissue not communicating with the bronchial tree and which receives its blood supply from an anomalous systemic vessel. It may be within the substance of the lung (intralobar sequestration) or completely separate (extralobar). Areas of sequestration are thought to arise from an extra bronchopulmonary bud of the foregut. They most commonly occur in the left lower lobe and the blood supply comes direct from the aorta, above or below the diaphragm. The anomalous blood supply may be identified by ultrasound techniques, avoiding the need for angiography. The condition usually presents with respiratory infections, more commonly after the neonatal period. The treatment is resection.[1]

Diaphragmatic hernia

Diaphragmatic hernia may be congenital or acquired, the latter usually being traumatic in origin. Congenital diaphragmatic hernia arises due to an abnormality in the formation of the diaphragm between the fourth and tenth weeks of fetal life.

The commonest herniation is the Bochdalek type, a posterolateral defect, possibly a failure of closure of the pleuroperitoneal canal. It has been postulated that the primary anomaly is in the developing lungs that fail to induce diaphragmatic closure and this may explain hypoplasia in the contralateral lung. A hernia through the foramen of Morgagni is less common in neonates. This defect is retrosternal, to the right or left of the midline. The third site for herniation is the esophageal hiatus – the so-called hiatus hernia.

The true incidence of congenital diaphragmatic hernia is difficult to ascertain as so many die at birth; others present as live births and others after the neonatal period. This lesion represents 8% of major fatal congenital anomalies noted in a British perinatal mortality survey (present in one in 2200 of all births). In Edinburgh the incidence is one in 7000 live births, other series report 1:4000–1:10 000.

Some cases are now detected antenatally by ultrasound but the majority present with respiratory distress – cyanosis, dyspnea and tachypnea – either immediately after birth or within a few hours. Occasionally, particularly on the right side, the presentation may be later, the defect being present at birth but actual herniation of abdominal content occurring as a postnatal event. The later the onset of symptoms, the better the prognosis. Examination reveals a scaphoid abdomen, bowel sounds on auscultation of the affected side of the chest and a shift of the apex beat to the right in the case of a left-sided hernia. The right side is less common, perhaps due to plugging by the liver, but if a defect is present here it tends to be large with herniation of the liver as well as bowel.

Once air has been swallowed after birth a chest X-ray confirms the diagnosis, showing gas-filled loops of bowel on the affected side of the chest with displacement of the mediastinum to the opposite side (Fig. 37.1).

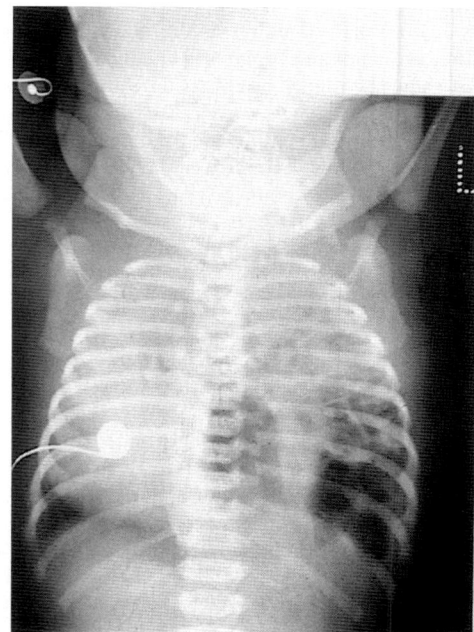

Fig. 37.1 Diaphragmatic hernia (left-sided Bochdalek defect).

Treatment

A nasogastric tube is passed to reduce the gaseous distention of the bowel with air. In the past the surgical repair of the hernia was a true emergency, it being felt that the sooner the hernia was reduced the more easily the lungs could expand. Babies were operated on virtually regardless of condition and the survival rates were poor. It has been shown that respiratory mechanics, far from improving, frequently deteriorate as a result of repair of the hernia. The role of urgent surgery has thus been re-evaluated. It has always been known that the babies with the least hypoplastic lungs fared better. These also tend to be the cases that present after hours rather than immediately at birth. Now an initial, nonsurgical approach to diaphragmatic hernia has been adopted in most centers with the aim of improving pulmonary function and reducing pulmonary vascular resistance.[2,3] After diagnosis the baby is intubated and hyperventilated to reduce the $PaCO_2$ to < 4.7 kPa (< 35 mmHg) and paralyzed. Metabolic acidosis is corrected with bicarbonate therapy. A chest X-ray is taken to verify the endotracheal tube position and exclude a pneumothorax. A preductal arterial line (radial) is sited for blood gas and pressure monitoring. The ventilatory index (mean airway pressure × respiratory rate) is calculated and this should be < 1000 with a $PaCO_2 < 5.3$ (< 40 mmHg) prior to surgery. If the index is higher, high-frequency oscillatory ventilation is instituted. Tolazoline may be administered to reduce pulmonary vascular resistance and prevent shunting through the ductus arteriosus. In some centers extracorporeal membrane oxygenation (ECMO) is used for prolonged support with variable results. Whatever the method of stabilization preoperatively, it must be carried out in a surgical unit as it is the pediatric surgeon who must be in a position to determine the timing of surgery.

Operative treatment

An abdominal approach is usually preferred with a transverse upper abdominal incision on the side of the hernia. The bowel and other organs are reduced and the defect in the diaphragm examined. If the defect is large a patch of prosthetic material may be used. Repairing a defect under tension merely reduces lung compliance. An underwater seal drain is positioned prior to completion of the repair. If the baby's condition is very stable the repair may be accomplished thoracoscopically.

Postoperatively, support is maintained until the baby can be weaned from the ventilator. A few patients who require little or no ventilatory support preoperatively may be extubated immediately. Of the remainder the mortality rate still remains around 50%, although it is hoped that the change in preoperative management will improve the outlook.

Eventration of the diaphragm

This is due to a deficiency in the muscle of the diaphragm. The thin layer becomes attenuated and bulges up into the thorax. Extensive eventrations are similar to diaphragmatic hernia presenting in the neonatal period. Smaller eventrations present later and require localized plication.

Esophageal atresia

Atresia is absence or closure of a normal body orifice or passage (Greek *a* = negative, *tresis* = hole). A fistula is an abnormal communication between two epithelial surfaces.

Esophageal atresia is a congenital defect of unknown etiology, the great majority of cases being associated with a tracheoesophageal fistula. The incidence is approximately 1 per 3000 live births. Many babies with esophageal atresia are premature and of low birth weight. The lower the birth weight, the greater the mortality. More than half the babies presenting with esophageal atresia have associated congenital abnormalities, commonly associated with vertebral, anorectal, cardiac, tracheoesophageal, renal and limb anomalies (VACTERL). This was formerly known as the VATER complex. The anatomical varieties of esophageal atresia and related disorders are illustrated in Figure 37.2.

Clinical features

Maternal hydramnios is so common that all babies born to a mother with hydramnios should have a tube passed to assess the patency of the esophagus. In cases with esophageal atresia the tube will be arrested about 10 cm from the lips. If the diagnosis is not made in this manner then the baby will be noted to froth at the mouth, choke, cough or become dyspneic and cyanosed. These symptoms will be exacerbated by attempts to feed the baby. The patency of the esophagus should then be tested by a firm tube of at least 10 or 12 FG, which should be passed orally. Acid secretions aspirated from the tube may have refluxed through the fistula so radiological confirmation of the position of the tube is necessary if suspicion is high.

A Replogle tube is a double lumen plastic catheter that can be passed via the nose into the upper esophageal pouch, enabling continuous suction to be applied without causing damage to the mucosa. Suction is applied to the end of the catheter, air passing along the finer of the two lumina as secretions are aspirated. If the latter are particularly thick, careful irrigation may be carried out via the finer lumen tube.

A plain chest X-ray with gentle pressure on the Replogle tube enables the distal extent of the pouch to be ascertained. The presence of air in the stomach and bowel confirms the presence of a distal tracheoesophageal fistula (TEF) (Fig. 37.3). In the case of atresia without a fistula there

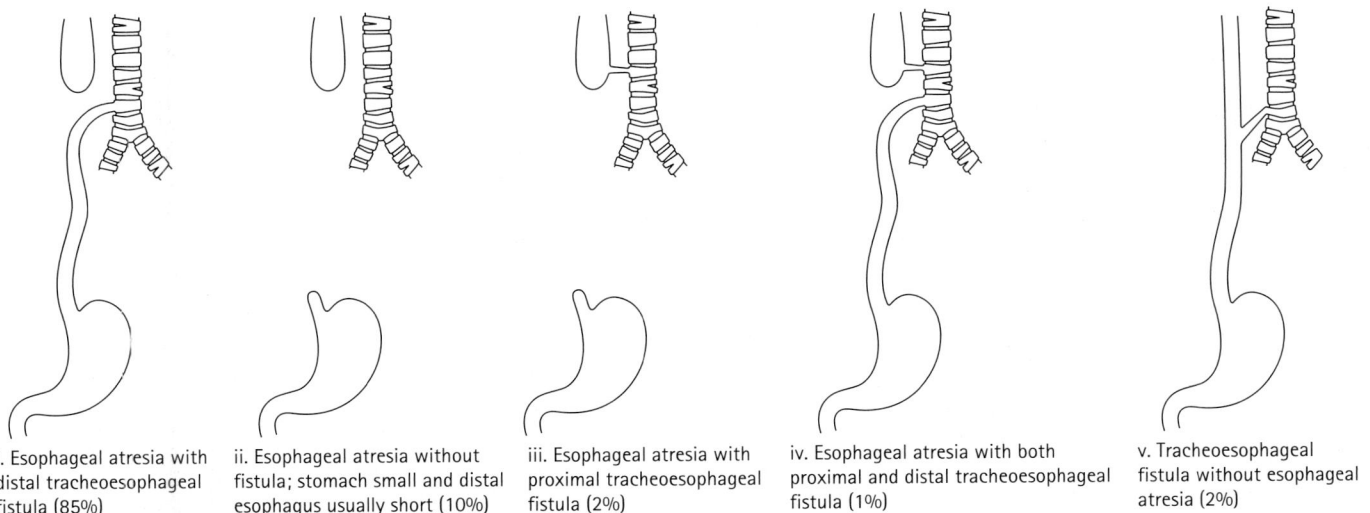

i. Esophageal atresia with distal tracheoesophageal fistula (85%)

ii. Esophageal atresia without fistula; stomach small and distal esophagus usually short (10%)

iii. Esophageal atresia with proximal tracheoesophageal fistula (2%)

iv. Esophageal atresia with both proximal and distal tracheoesophageal fistula (1%)

v. Tracheoesophageal fistula without esophageal atresia (2%)

Fig. 37.2 Esophageal atresia and tracheoesophageal fistula.

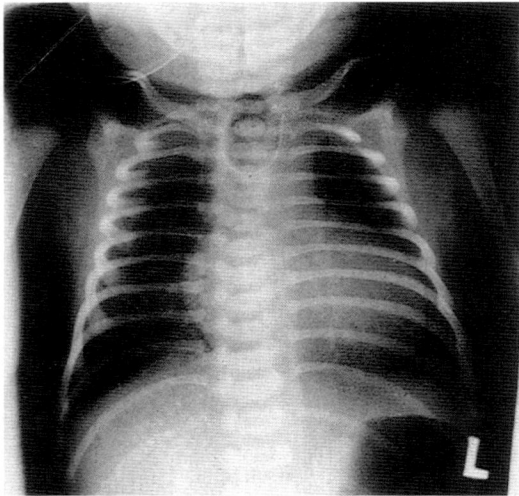

Fig. 37.3   Esophageal atresia with distal tracheoesophageal fistula.

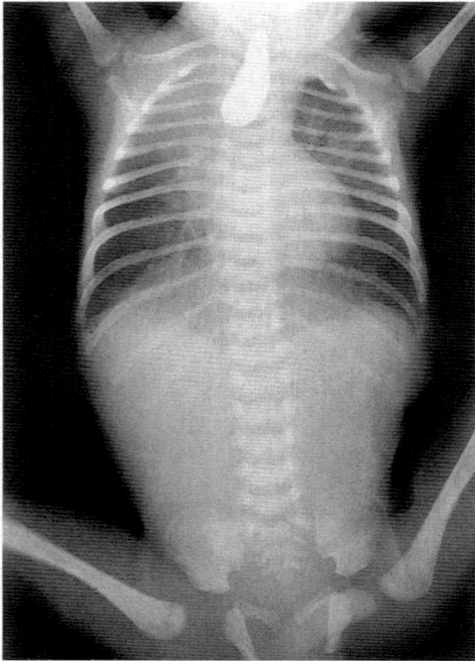

Fig. 37.4   Esophageal atresia without TEF.

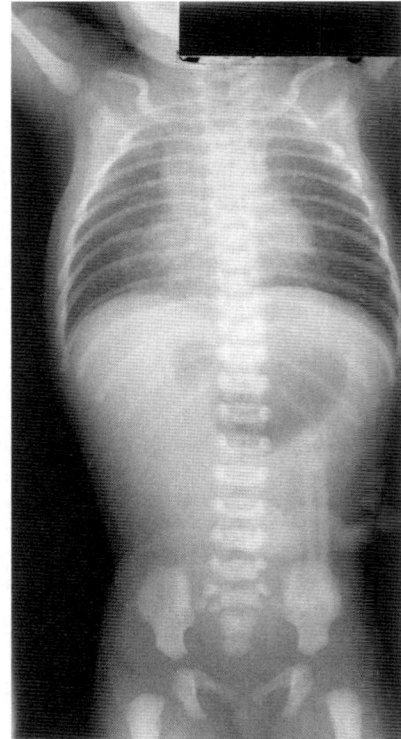

Fig. 37.5   Esophageal atresia with duodenal atresia.

is absence of air in the stomach (Fig. 37.4). Occasionally there may be associated duodenal atresia, but providing there is a TEF, then the gas pattern should clarify this (Fig. 37.5).

Some surgeons like to use 1–2 ml of contrast to define the upper pouch but there is great danger of spillage into the tracheobronchial tree and the procedure is unnecessary. Preoperatively, apart from adequate aspiration of the upper pouch, opinions differ as to the best position in which to nurse the baby. Some advocate the Trendelenburg (head down) position to prevent aspiration of secretions but this may lead to reflux of gastric content via the fistula into the lungs (especially the right upper lobe). Others, to prevent this, advise a head up position. A horizontal and semiprone position reduces the incidence of right upper lobe collapse and seems satisfactory.

Treatment

In the commonest type of anomaly (with a distal TEF), surgery does not have to be performed immediately in the middle of the night but can be safely left until the following day. If pneumonitis is present, it is justifiable to delay treatment for 24 h or more to allow chest physiotherapy and appropriate antibiotics to be administered. A right posterolateral thoracotomy is made and, via an extrapleural approach, the fistula is divided and repaired and an end-to-end anastomosis between the proximal and distal esophagus is made in a single layer. A fine transanastomotic silastic tube is passed nasogastrically prior to completion of the anastomosis so that early nasogastric feeding can be instituted. In some centers the operation can be safely performed thoracoscopically.

On the fifth postoperative day a contrast swallow is performed to confirm patency of the anastomosis and exclude leakage at this site. If leakage is present it can usually be safely managed conservatively. Anastomotic stricture, if it occurs, is treated by esophagoscopy and bougienage or balloon dilation under X-ray control. Most children, following a successful repair, have a persistent brassy cough or 'seal bark' that may last for a few years. This is probably due to a degree of tracheomalacia.

Dysphagia due to abnormal motility in the esophagus both above and below the anastomosis may be due to vagal nerve damage or, more probably, an intrinsic abnormality associated with the lesion. This, like the seal bark, usually resolves by the age of 2 years.

Cases of esophageal atresia without a fistula are best managed initially by gastrostomy and aspiration of the upper pouch via a Replogle tube. In my experience, delayed primary anastomosis can be achieved after 3 months of regular stretching of the upper pouch by the nursing staff using a Nelaton catheter at feed times. Once there is radiological evidence of a gap of less than 3 cm, as visualized with a metal bougie in the lower pouch (passed per gastrostomy) and a radiopaque tube in the upper pouch, surgery can be carried out thoracoscopically or via thoracotomy. Postoperatively, the infants are electively paralyzed and ventilated for up to 7 d to relieve the tension on the anastomosis, a technique also of value in tight anastomosis in the common type of atresia with a distal fistula.[4] Others favor construction of a cervical esophagostomy followed by gastric transposition, jejunal or colonic interposition to bridge the gap between the upper pouch and the stomach.

H-type tracheoesophageal fistula

These occasionally present in the first few weeks of life with coughing or cyanosis on feeding. More commonly they present much later with recurrent chest infections, a history of coughing on feeds, and sometimes abdominal distention. Because the fistula runs obliquely upwards from esophagus to trachea, the flow of esophageal content into the trachea is limited and intermittent. The diagnosis is made at a contrast swallow under screening. Treatment is surgical division of the fistula, usually via a cervical approach.

DUODENAL OBSTRUCTION

Duodenal obstruction may be intrinsic (atresia, membrane, stenosis or anular pancreas) or extrinsic (Ladd's bands with or without volvulus of the midgut).

Intrinsic duodenal obstruction (Fig. 37.6)

The etiology of duodenal atresias and other intrinsic duodenal obstructions differs from that of intrinsic obstructions in the remainder of the small intestine. It appears to be a failure of luminal development due to an early insult and there are often associated abnormalities. Down syndrome is present in 30% of cases. In 10% there is esophageal atresia, and a further 10% have anorectal anomalies. Cardiac and renal anomalies may also be associated. Cardiac abnormalities are particularly common in those with Down syndrome.

Atresia or stenosis usually affects the second or occasionally the third part of the duodenum.

Complete obstructions present with vomiting within 24 h after birth. The vomitus may or may not be bile stained, depending on whether the obstruction is proximal or distal to the ampulla of Vater. In those with bile-stained vomitus the meconium, if passed, may also be normally bile stained as there may be openings of the bile duct proximal and distal to the obstruction via Wirsung's and Santorini's ducts.

In maternity units where passage of a nasogastric tube is a routine soon after birth, aspiration of more than 20 ml of fluid may be indicative of a duodenal or small bowel obstruction.

Abdominal distention, if any, is confined to the upper abdomen due to obstruction of the stomach and duodenum.

The diagnosis is confirmed by a plain erect X-ray that demonstrates the characteristic 'double bubble' appearance of air–fluid levels in the stomach and duodenum (Fig. 37.7). The double bubble may also be detected antenatally, ultrasound detecting fluid distention of the stomach and duodenum.[5] An incomplete obstruction, stenosis, or membrane with a small hole in it may allow air to pass through to the rest of the bowel, thus masking the double bubble (Fig. 37.8), but a contrast study confirms the presence of obstruction (Fig. 37.9). Sometimes the diagnosis may be delayed several months or even a year or two if sufficient food can pass through.

Treatment

If there is any delay in diagnosis of a duodenal obstruction then any resulting metabolic disturbance must be corrected preoperatively. At laparotomy a duodenoduodenostomy is the procedure of choice (Fig. 37.10), or for a stenosis or membrane a duodenoplasty may be performed,

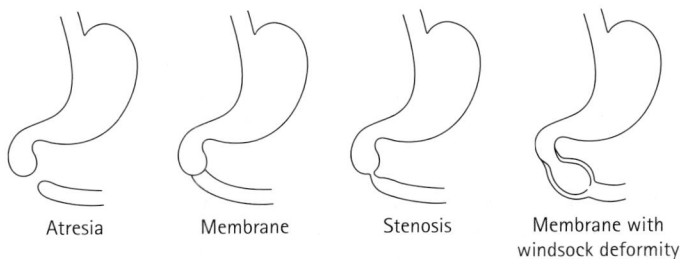

Fig. 37.7 'Double bubble' in duodenal atresia.

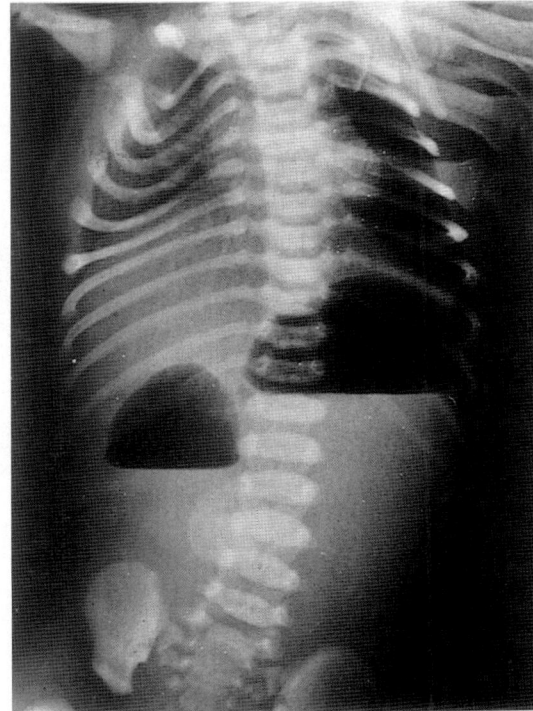

Fig. 37.8 Plain film of baby soon after birth.

opening the duodenum lengthways across the obstruction and closing it transversely. Resection of a diaphragm must be undertaken cautiously to avoid damage to the ampulla of Vater.

An anular pancreas (Fig. 37.10a) is caused by the failure of the normal migration of the ventral bud to join the dorsal one. It is rarely a true ring around the duodenum but more commonly associated with an intrinsic obstruction within the duodenum (membrane or stenosis). A duodenoduodenostomy is performed with no attempt to divide the pancreas for fear of fistula formation.

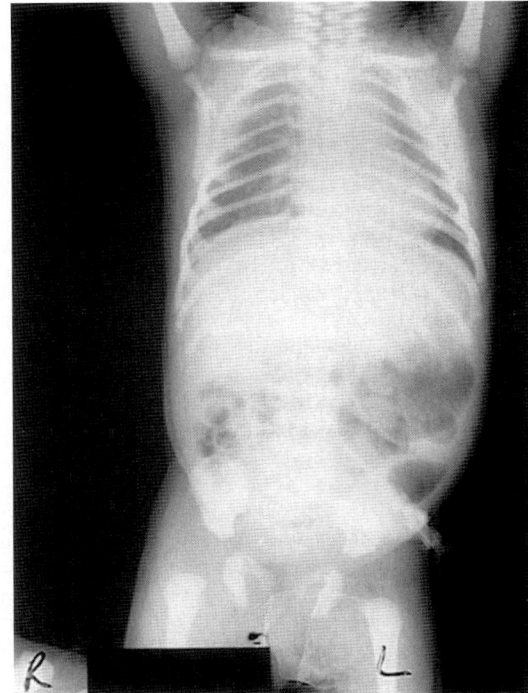

| Atresia | Membrane | Stenosis | Membrane with windsock deformity |

Fig. 37.6 Duodenal anomalies.

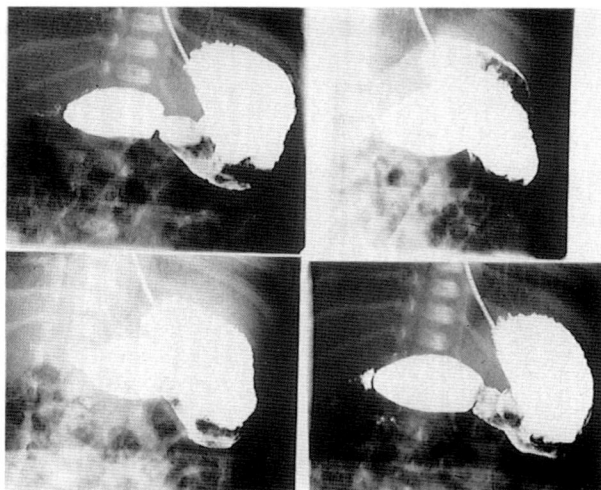

Fig. 37.9 Upper gastrointestinal contrast study on same baby as Figure 37.8.

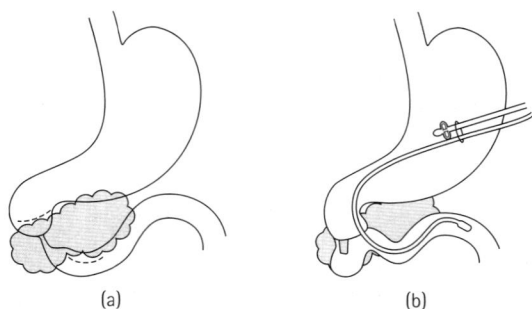

Fig. 37.10 (a) Anular pancreas with intrinsic duodenal membrane. (b) Duodenoduodenostomy with gastrostomy and transanastomotic silastic feeding tube.

Extrinsic duodenal obstruction

Ladd's bands may obstruct the duodenum, occasionally alone but more commonly in association with a midgut volvulus (volvulus neonatorum). Such a volvulus may present in the neonatal period or at any age and arises due to an incomplete, or malrotation of the bowel. By the sixth week of intrauterine life the gut tube elongates to a greater extent than can be accommodated in the developing abdominal cavity and thus herniation through the umbilical ring occurs. During the next month the bowel undergoes an anticlockwise rotation returning to the abdominal cavity by the tenth week. By the time the stomach has rotated to the left, the duodenal C-loop has formed and the small bowel, followed by the large bowel, returns to the abdomen. The cecum and ascending colon pass to the right of the abdomen, the latter becoming retroperitoneal. The small bowel mesentery is then fixed between the duodenojejunal flexure and the ileocecal region. Failure of the cecum and ascending colon to reach their normal position results in a short base to the midgut mesentery and peritoneal bands passing from the cecum (in the midline or to the left side) to the right posterior abdominal wall. These bands (Ladd's bands) obstruct the duodenum. In addition, the short base to the mesentery allows a midgut volvulus to arise, the bowel rotating in a clockwise direction, and resulting in duodenal obstruction. A plain X-ray will show a double bubble and usually a small amount of gas in the bowel more distally. Contrast studies may confirm the diagnosis. An upper gastrointestinal study may show a duodenal obstruction and a typical coiled spring sign. An enema may show an anomalous position of the cecum.

Once any electrolyte or acid–base disturbance is corrected, laparotomy must be performed without delay to avoid ischemia of the midgut.

SMALL BOWEL OBSTRUCTION

This may arise due to an abnormality directly associated with the bowel itself (intrinsic), pressure from without (extrinsic), or obstruction within the lumen (intraluminal).

Intrinsic anomalies

These are mainly atresias, membranes, stenoses and duplications of the bowel. Atresias may arise anywhere along the length of the bowel, being most common in the distal ileum and rarely seen in the colon. Their likely cause is an interruption of the mesenteric vessels in utero. These vary from membranous obstruction in continuity, those with or without an associated gap in the mesentery and multiple atresias, to the so-called apple-peel type deformity with extensive loss of mesentery and bowel, the distal small bowel receiving its blood supply from the middle colic vessels through a precarious continuity between marginal arcades (Fig. 37.11).

The bowel proximal to the obstruction is distended and hypertrophied and distally the bowel is collapsed, often with a microcolon (unused) although babies with obstructions of this kind may pass meconium of normal appearance. The latter is dependent on the timing of the vascular accident in utero.

The diagnosis is confirmed by plain X-ray, which will show a number of distended loops of small bowel with air–fluid levels in an erect view (Fig. 37.12). The level of obstruction can be estimated by the number of distended loops. There will be absence of air distal to a complete obstruction.

Contrast studies have a limited role in the diagnosis of such obstructions unless to exclude intraluminal or functional conditions.

Treatment

Preoperative treatment involves passage of a nasogastric tube and correction of electrolyte imbalance by appropriate administration of i.v. fluids. If the diagnosis is established early there is little or no requirement for i.v. resuscitation.

Operative treatment involves laparotomy, resection or tapering of grossly dilated bowel proximal to the atresia (to prevent problems of postoperative peristaltic inertia) and then anastomosis between the dilated proximal bowel and the collapsed distal bowel.

Duplications

Duplications of the alimentary tract can occur at any level from mouth to anus. A length of bowel may be duplicated, the two segments sharing a common blood supply and muscular wall yet having separate mucosal

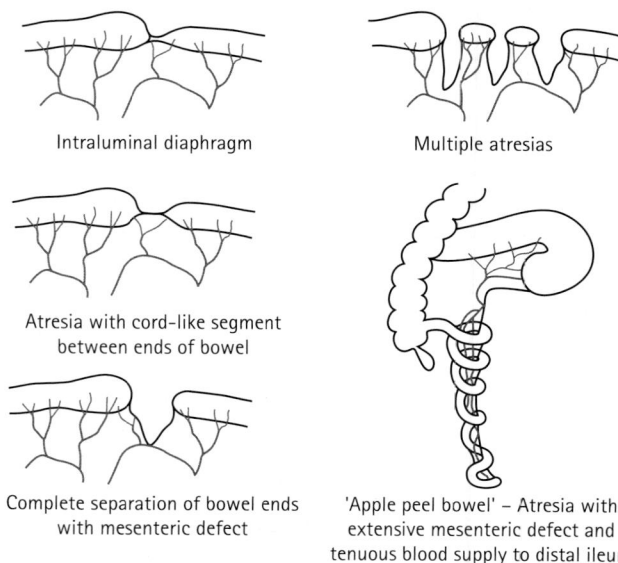

Intraluminal diaphragm

Multiple atresias

Atresia with cord-like segment between ends of bowel

Complete separation of bowel ends with mesenteric defect

'Apple peel bowel' – Atresia with extensive mesenteric defect and tenuous blood supply to distal ileum

Fig. 37.11 Small bowel atresias.

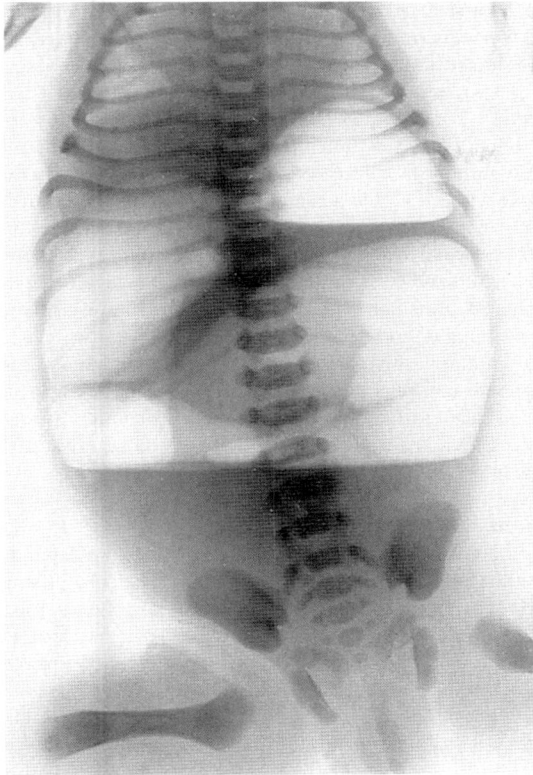

Fig. 37.12   Jejunal atresia.

linings. They may or may not communicate, and it is the noncommunicating type that tends to form a short cystic segment which, by accumulation of secretions within it, leads to intestinal obstruction. Such duplications may be palpable as a cystic intra-abdominal mass that together with the signs of intestinal obstruction lead to the diagnosis. Ultrasound and contrast studies may be of value.

Treatment. The treatment usually involves a localized bowel resection but if the duplication is extensive in length or at a site such as the ileocecal junction, the mucosa of the duplicated segment should be dissected out, thus avoiding extensive resection or loss of the ileocecal valve.

Extrinsic anomalies

Extrinsic anomalies leading to intestinal obstruction include hernias (inguinal or internal), localized volvulus, bands, vitellointestinal remnants and mesenteric cysts.

An incarcerated inguinal hernia is the commonest cause of intestinal obstruction at any age. The inguinal region must thus be carefully examined when any patient, neonate or older, presents with intestinal obstruction. Internal hernias are rare and can only be identified at laparotomy.

Localized volvulus may arise in relation to bands, duplication cysts and vitellointestinal remnants. Treatment at laparotomy varies according to the causative factor and the condition of the affected bowel. Mesenteric cysts may lead to local volvulus or may present as a palpable cystic mass. They are treated by resection.

Intraluminal anomalies

Intraluminal causes of intestinal obstruction include meconium ileus, milk curd obstruction and meconium plug syndrome.

Around 10–15% of patients with cystic fibrosis present in the neonatal period with obstruction of the distal ileum (meconium ileus). The distal few centimeters of ileum contain pale grey 'rabbit pellets' of inspissated meconium proximal to which is a segment containing hard green–black meconium and, more proximally still, distended loops containing tarry fluid meconium and air. Distal to the obstruction is a microcolon

and usually no meconium is passed, presenting signs being abdominal distention and bile-stained vomiting within a few days of birth.

Plain abdominal films show gross abdominal distention with few fluid levels and often a ground glass appearance (of air bubbles in the viscid meconium) in the right iliac fossa. Sometimes there are signs of calcification from perforation and leakage of meconium antenatally.

Volvulus of the hypertrophied distended bowel may also lead to atresia, or perforation may occur after birth.

The presence of meconium ileus has no relationship to the subsequent 'severity' of the cystic fibrosis.

Conservative management

Treatment can be either conservative or operative. Conservative management involves the administration of a Gastrografin enema under fluoroscopic control. Gastrografin with 0.1% Tween 80, a detergent, added as a wetting agent has a high osmolarity of 1900 mOsm/L and acts by drawing fluid into the bowel, thus freeing the inspissated meconium in the distal ileum. It is essential, therefore, that the baby is adequately hydrated and an i.v. infusion must be in progress. If necessary the procedure may be repeated after 24 h. If there is calcification the procedure is best avoided for fear of reperforation.

Surgical management

For cases in which there are complications such as perforation or signs of meconium peritonitis (calcification) or after failed Gastrografin enema, operative treatment is required. Laparotomy is performed via an upper transverse abdominal incision. Intestinal resection is necessary for bowel that is grossly dilated or of doubtful viability. A Bishop Koop ileostomy may be performed. This is a Roux-en-Y anastomosis between the end of the proximal limb of ileum and the side of the distal limb, bringing the end of the latter out of the abdomen as an end ileostomy in the right iliac fossa. This acts as a safety valve through which the distal ileum can be irrigated. In the case of continued obstruction the stoma will function. Once it is relieved, bowel contents pass the natural way.

Milk plug or mild curd obstruction also occurs in the distal ileum and may be due to the administration of inappropriately concentrated artificial milk feeds, or possibly a transient low bile acid excretion. The management is similar to that described earlier.

MECONIUM PLUG SYNDROME/SMALL LEFT COLON SYNDROME

Meconium plug syndrome must not be confused with meconium ileus. It is sometimes described as small left colon syndrome. The distal colon or rectum is plugged by sticky grey–white mucus distally with sticky meconium above it. The presentation is usually at about 2 d with a history of failure to pass meconium. There is evidence of low intestinal obstruction with generalized abdominal distention, frequently with a history of bile-stained vomiting and X-ray showing gaseous distention. There are multiple fluid levels present in the majority of cases.

The diagnosis is made by contrast enema. Initially barium is used to exclude Hirschsprung disease, but then changed to water-soluble contrast when the appearance of a meconium plug is seen in a narrowed left colon. The colon is usually narrow up to the splenic flexure, where it becomes dilated (Fig. 37.13). It has been postulated that there is a discrepancy in the activity of the parasympathetic supply from the vagus nerve (supplying the bowel to two thirds of the way across the transverse colon to the splenic flexure) and the sacral parasympathetics that supply the remainder. Whatever the etiology, the enema invariably proves to be therapeutic with satisfactory evacuation of meconium. The abdomen in most cases decompresses over 24 h and feeds can then be introduced. If bowel evacuation is not normal then Hirschsprung disease must be excluded.

HIRSCHSPRUNG DISEASE[6]

Hirschsprung, a Danish pediatrician, described two patients who died at 7 and 11 months from constipation associated with gross abdominal

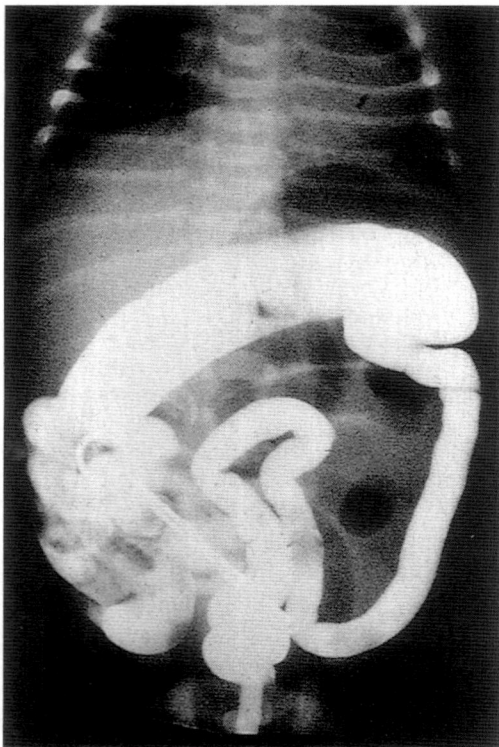

Fig. 37.13   Small left colon syndrome.

distention and a highly dilated hypertrophied colon full of feces. There is absence of ganglion cells in the myenteric plexuses (both Auerbach's and Meissner's) of the most distal bowel and extending proximally for a variable distance. Aganglionosis involving only the rectum or rectosigmoid is often termed 'short segment' Hirschsprung disease and affects males five times more commonly than females. 'Long segment' Hirschsprung disease, extending above the sigmoid, has an equal sex incidence and a greater likelihood of siblings being affected. In short segment disease there is a 1 in 20 risk that brothers will be affected and a 1 in 100 risk for sisters. In long segment disease the risk to all siblings is 1 in 10.

In a few cases there is total colonic aganglionosis with disease extending into the small bowel and in extremely rare cases involving the whole alimentary canal. At least 70% of cases are short segment, 25% long segment and about 5% total colonic.

Hirschsprung disease differs from many other alimentary tract abnormalities in that the birth weight is usually within the normal range. It is uncommon in premature and low birth weight babies. Associated congenital anomalies are uncommon apart from Down syndrome, which affects 1 in 20. The cause of the disease is unknown. It has been postulated that it is due to a failure of migration of ganglion cells from the neural crest, which normally proceeds in a craniocaudal direction having entered the upper end of the alimentary tract.[7] Differentiation of ganglion cells occurs in the wall of the gut between the seventh and eighth week of intrauterine life and proceeds in a craniocaudal direction.

Clinical features

Usually the symptoms of Hirschsprung disease are manifest within the first few days of life. This is certainly the case in all long segment or total colonic cases but some short segment cases and especially 'ultrashort' segment cases may present later, even into old age.

Failure to pass meconium within the first 24 h, abdominal distention, bile-stained vomiting and reluctance to feed are the main symptoms. Diarrhea may be the presenting feature of Hirschsprung enterocolitis, a devastating complication of the condition that has a high mortality. The etiology of Hirschsprung enterocolitis is unknown but apart from

diarrhea it is associated with gross abdominal distention and circulatory collapse. A rectal examination results in the explosive passage of flatus and loose stool, deflating the abdomen.

Diagnosis

A plain abdominal X-ray shows distended small and large bowel, sometimes with multiple fluid levels on an erect film. A barium enema is best carried out without a previous rectal examination as then the narrow aganglionic bowel with dilation proximally is demonstrated. A delayed film at 24 h, again avoiding an invasive rectal examination, shows retained barium and often a clear indication of the level of disease with a cone-shaped transition zone between normal bowel above and the narrowed aganglionic distal segment.

Definitive diagnosis is by rectal biopsy. A suction biopsy is adequate to confirm the absence of ganglion cells in the submucosal plexus, specimens being taken at 1 and 3 cm above the dentate line. Histochemical staining will demonstrate excessive acetyl cholinesterase activity in abnormal nerve trunks and absence of ganglion cells.

Treatment

Once the diagnosis is made, bowel washouts may be sufficient to maintain bowel decompression prior to a laparoscopically assisted 'pull through' procedure. Others prefer a defunctioning stoma, proximal to the diseased bowel. A definitive procedure is then carried out when the infant is 3–12 months of age, depending on the surgeon's preference. It usually consists of excision of the aganglionic bowel and a pull through procedure.

If enterocolitis supervenes (and it can even happen after a definitive procedure, especially if an aganglionic segment remains), then rapid replacement of lost fluid by a suitable electrolyte solution, often preceded by plasma, is required. This should be combined with saline bowel washouts using a two tube technique, one to run saline in, preferably above the aganglionic segment, the other at a slightly lower level to allow evacuation. Broad-spectrum antibiotics are usually administered prophylactically although infection has not been shown to be the precipitating factor. Enterocolitis is the most lethal complication of Hirschsprung disease.

UROLOGICAL PROBLEMS IN THE NEONATE

Posterior urethral valves

The commonest obstructive uropathy in male children is valvular obstruction of the posterior urethra. Occasionally the diagnosis is made on antenatal ultrasound. A large proportion of cases present in the first 2 weeks of life, the majority in the first 6 months and the remainder, whilst usually becoming apparent in the first few years, may present as late as early adult life.

The neonate may present with retention of urine or dribbling and a palpably distended bladder with or without infection or uremia. Later presentation is usually with incontinence or infection.

The valves are classically folds of mucosa attached just below the verumontanum and attempts to void lead to apposition of the valves. The obstruction leads to dilation of the posterior urethra, the bladder, the ureter and renal pelvis.

As micturition commences in the fetus in the first trimester, the back pressure on the kidneys may lead antenatally to severe damage – renal dysplasia. Occasionally the bladder hypertrophy is such that reflux no longer occurs but the ureters remain dilated and tortuous.

Diagnosis

A micturating cystourethrogram (MCU) is diagnostic in this anomaly, demonstrating the gross dilation of the posterior urethra and usually the refluxing dilated ureters and bilateral hydronephrosis.

Treatment

Disruption of the valves is required. This may be effected by pulling the inflated balloon of a Fogarty catheter across the valves or by delicately disrupting them with a Whitaker hook. A resectoscope can be used transurethrally and the valves either fulgurated or, to avoid a deep destruction of tissue, cut with a cold knife. If renal function is particularly poor, temporary drainage via bilateral cutaneous ureterostomies (preferably ring ureterostomies) may be required.

Prune belly syndrome (triad syndrome)

This consists of deficiency of the anterior abdominal wall muscles, cryptorchidism and urinary tract deformities. The abdominal muscular deficiency is mainly in the lower abdomen, the whole abdominal wall taking on the wrinkled appearance of a prune (Fig. 37.14). The ribs may be flared outwards at the lower costal margin and respiratory infections are common.

Surgery is best avoided unless there is significant renal impairment. In severe cases ring ureterostomies may be required, followed at a later date by tapering and reimplantation of the ureters, trimming of the bladder, orchidopexies and excision and repair of the lower anterior abdominal wall. Some cases have a functional urethral obstruction, which may require urethrotomy. Other cases show urethral stricture or even a diverticulum at the site of the prostatic utricle.

Urachal anomalies

The urachus in the embryo connects the bladder to the allantois. It is normally obliterated to form the median umbilical ligament. It may, however, persist as a patent urachus in the neonate, requiring repair. Occasionally the two extremities of the urachus close, leaving a cyst in the middle that becomes filled with secretions and may present as a mass or more commonly, when it becomes infected, as an abscess.

Bladder exstrophy (ectopia vesicae)

This is part of a range of lower abdominal wall defects, ranging from epispadias, through exstrophy of the bladder, to the even more catastrophic vesicointestinal fissure or cloacal exstrophy.

In bladder exstrophy there is a lower abdominal wall anomaly in which there is wide separation of the pubic bones, the bladder surface

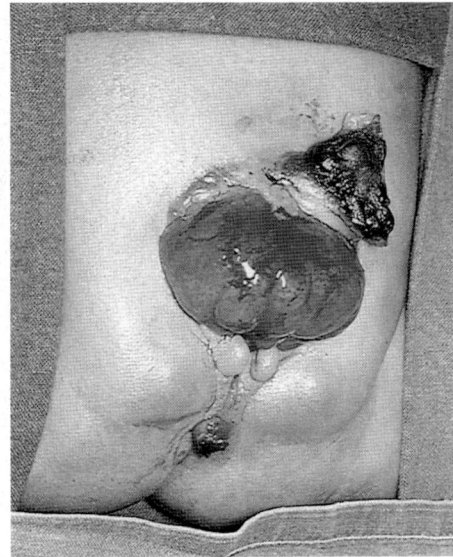

Fig. 37.15 Ectopic vesicae.

being flat and exposed with the two ureteric orifices clearly visible (Fig. 37.15). In the male there is complete epispadias with a strip of urethral mucosa on the dorsum of a short broadened, flattened penis. In the female there is also an epispadiac urethra with a bifid clitoris and separation of the labia anteriorly at the level of the vaginal orifice.

The bladder is best repaired soon after birth. If necessary, bilateral iliac osteotomies enable the pubic bones to be better approximated thus facilitating the repair. Careful construction of the bladder neck is vital to achieve subsequent continence, and in the male later repair of the severe epispadiac deformity is required. If the bladder repair is unsuccessful it may be necessary to carry out a urinary diversion procedure.

EXOMPHALOS AND GASTROSCHISIS

These are two distinct conditions of different etiology. Although formerly exomphalos was believed to be more common, gastroschisis is now seen more frequently. Antenatal diagnosis of both conditions by ultrasound examination is now almost routine. Gastroschisis also gives rise to an elevated maternal serum alpha-fetoprotein and distinction from other anomalies such as neural tube defects is by ultrasonography. Gastroschisis is not an indication for termination of pregnancy whilst exomphalos major, with its high incidence (30–40%) of associated anomalies, may be.

Exomphalos

Exomphalos (omphalocele) is a herniation of intra-abdominal contents through the umbilical ring into the umbilical cord. Defects less than 4 cm in diameter are classified as *exomphalos minor* (Fig. 37.16). There are rarely associated abnormalities in this group.

Exomphalos major (Fig. 37.17), on the other hand, commonly has coexisting abnormalities and a defect greater than 4 cm in diameter, presumably arising through failure of development of the anterior abdominal wall prior to herniation of the midgut loop. In a large defect, not only the intestines (small and large) herniate but also the liver, spleen, stomach, bladder and even ovaries and fallopian tubes in the female. Incomplete or malrotation of the bowel is common and the associated abnormalities often include cardiac defects; 20% of cases are anencephalic. In the *Beckwith–Wiedemann* syndrome there is exomphalos, macroglossia and gigantism. The baby is large for his gestational age with an exomphalos, a big tongue and large solid viscera. There is also a facial nevus flammeus in the center of the forehead and odd indentations in the ear lobe (Fig. 37.18). There may also be pancreatic hyperplasia leading to severe neonatal hypoglycemia.

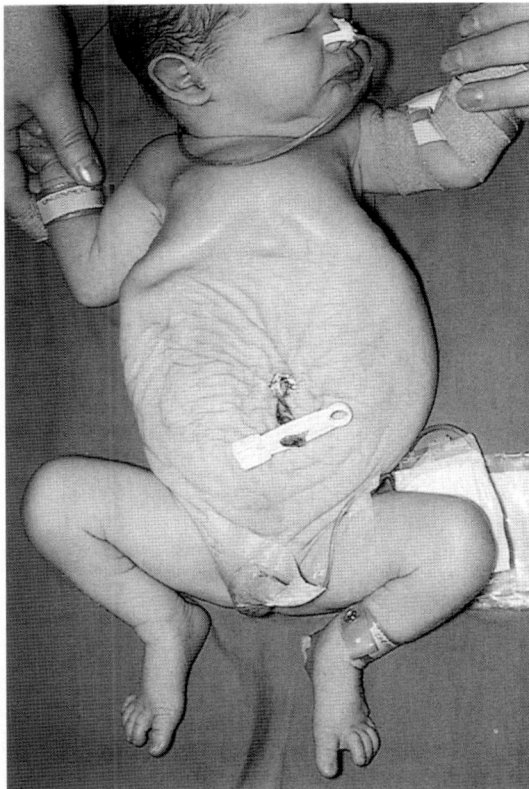

Fig. 37.14 Prune belly syndrome.

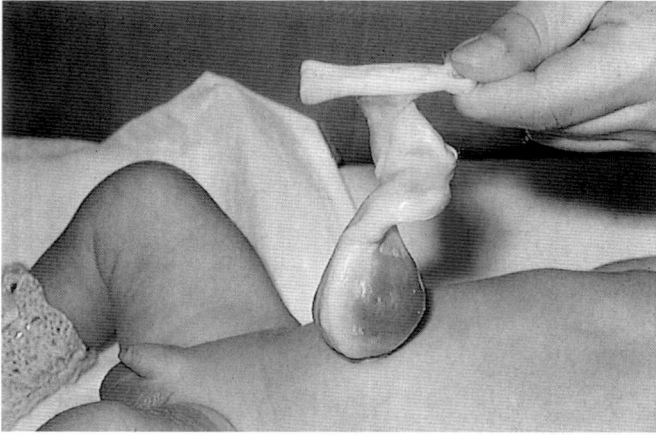

Fig. 37.16   Exomphalos minor.

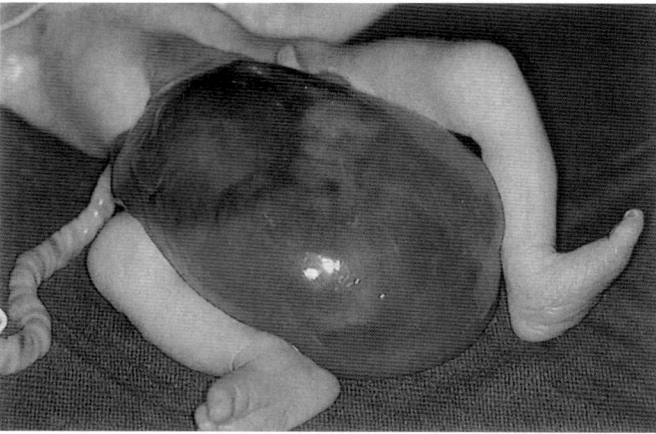

Fig. 37.17   Exomphalos major.

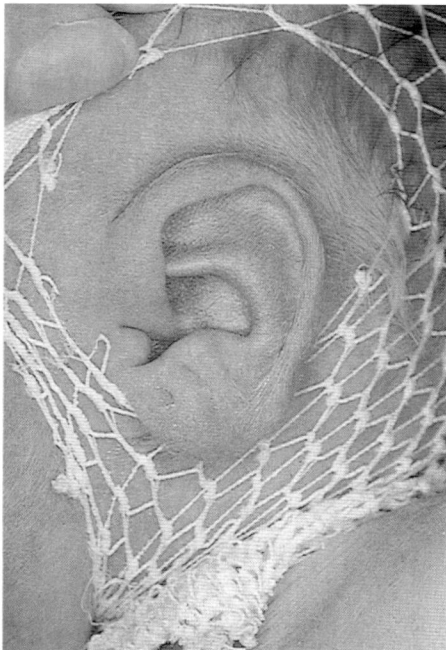

Fig. 37.18   Earlobe indentations in Beckwith–Wiedemann syndrome.

An *omphalocele* is usually covered by a sac composed of the fused layers of amniotic membrane and peritoneum. The sac may rupture ante-, intra- or postpartum.

Treatment

In a large omphalocele, conservative management may be appropriate in the neonatal period. Silver sulfadiazine dessings[8] or simple alcohol solution should be applied daily until an eschar forms. Epithelialization of the sac from the periphery results over the ensuing weeks. It may take 3–4 months before the infant can be discharged home, returning for later surgical repair of the ventral hernia. Other methods of treatment include mobilization of skin around the defect and skin coverage or coverage with prosthetic material and later repair of the ventral hernia. If the defect is small enough, with stretching of the anterior abdominal wall, primary repair may be possible as in gastroschisis (see later). In cases with an apparently simple herniation through a small defect into the umbilical cord it is tempting to twist the cord to reduce the contained bowel into the abdominal cavity, then simply ligate the cord. Such a temptation must be strongly resisted as all too frequently there is a Meckel's diverticulum or another cause of adherence of the bowel to the sac and serious damage may result. Formal surgical repair is always indicated.

Gastroschisis

Gastroschisis is a complete defect through all layers of the anterior abdominal wall extending up to about 3 cm in length and usually lying to the right of a normally attached umbilical cord (Fig. 37.19). It is almost as though a short transverse incision had been made with a scalpel antenatally. The etiology is unknown. Almost all the small and large bowel are eviscerated through the small defect – in most instances from stomach to rectum inclusive. Other organs are rarely apparent. The eviscerated bowel is markedly thickened, apparently foreshortened, matted together and often covered with a confluent gelatinous layer like 'gut in aspic'.

If possible, delivery should be in a perinatal center close to the regional pediatric surgical center. The decision whether to deliver the baby with exomphalos or gastroschisis by Cesarean section or vaginally is an obstetric one. The results of treatment of the baby are not significantly improved by cesarean delivery.

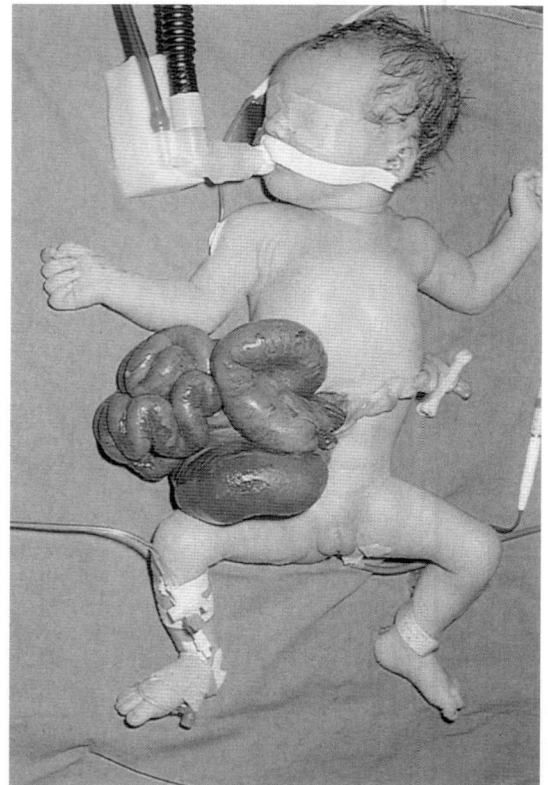

Fig. 37.19   Gastroschisis.

At delivery it is essential that the baby is placed in a plastic bag extending to above the level of the defect and leaving the head and, if necessary, the upper limbs exposed. The bowel must not be allowed to become contaminated, the baby being transferred in a transport incubator directly to the pediatric surgical operating table and the baby extracted from the bag aseptically, by the surgeon, once anesthesia is induced. The passage of a nasogastric tube prior to transfer reduces bowel distention and resulting ischemia if the anterior abdominal wall defect is very small. Transport in a polyethylene bag helps reduce hypothermia, which would otherwise result from heat loss by evaporation. These babies rapidly drop their temperature from 37°C to 35°C when exposed for even a few minutes to site an i.v. infusion. The application of warm saline soaked swabs is not a good idea as they rapidly cool, increasing the heat loss.

Treatment

Recently bedside reduction with or without a preformed silo have changed the immediate management of gastroschisis.[9,10] Providing the temperature has been adequately maintained and no significant fluid loss has occurred, direct transfer to the surgical neonatal unit and direct reduction or application of a preformed silo achieve the best results. If the bowel is particularly matted then surgical reduction in theater may be required. Leaving the cord intact and not enlarging the defect with either technique gives the best cosmetic result. The defect is usually so small that the umbilicus is not eccentric in position.

Postoperatively, no ventilatory support is required for ward reductions. A prolonged ileus however necessitates i.v. nutrition for days or in some cases even weeks. The prognosis in gastroschisis cases treated in this manner is excellent.

SACROCOCCYGEAL TERATOMA

The sacrococcygeal teratoma is the commonest teratoma presenting in the neonatal period. They tend to be large and protrude from the space between the anus and the coccyx (Fig. 37.20). The lesion is usually covered in skin but the most protuberant part may be necrotic due to vascular compromise. The tumor may also extend up into the pelvis and a large retrorectal component is palpable in all cases. In a presacral teratoma there is no protrusion behind the anus and the presentation may be later in the first year of life.

The tumor may be both solid and cystic in nature. A very large tumor may give rise to dystocia and if diagnosed antenatally is best delivered by Cesarean section.

Treatment is excision within the first few days of life. A double 'chevron' incision is made with the baby in a prone position and with careful excision and reconstruction of the pelvic floor which, despite its gross stretching, recovers normal function (Fig. 37.21). Excision of the coccyx is an essential component of the operation as failing to do so may predispose to the development of a yolk sac tumor.

There is usually an elevated alpha-fetoprotein level in the baby at birth and this should decline appropriately following excision. Even benign tumors should be followed up into adulthood as recurrence of benign or malignant elements may occur.

ANORECTAL ANOMALIES

Congenital anomalies of the anus and rectum are reported to occur in 1 in 1800 to 1 in 10 000 live births. In Edinburgh the incidence is 1 in 3100. There is a wide spectrum of anomalies and many attempts have been made to classify them. Recently a new international diagnostic classification system, operative groupings and a method of postoperative assessment of continence was developed by a large contingent of participants experienced in the management of anorectal malformations[11].

An anatomical approach simplifies matters (Table 37.1).[12] The lesions are grouped according to whether the end of the rectum is above levator ani, *high* (supralevator), or below, *low* (translevator). There is also an *intermediate*, partially translevator group. The essential component of the levator ani in these malformations is the puborectalis sling, which is the key to fecal continence.

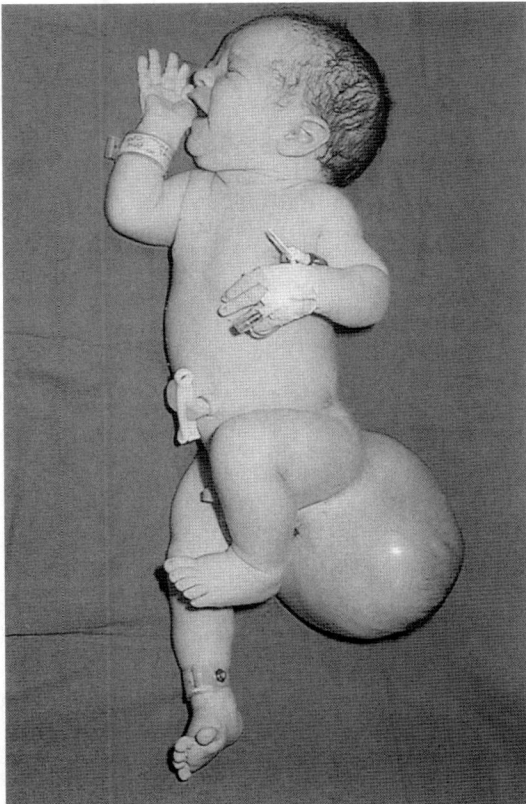

Fig. 37.20 Sacrococcygeal teratoma.

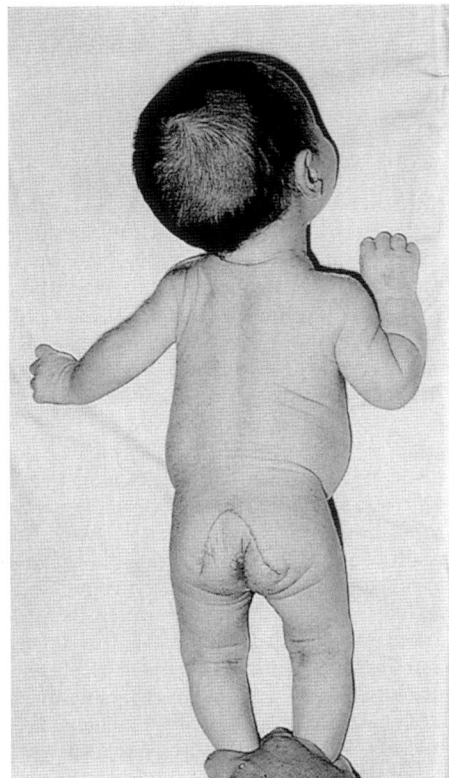

Fig. 37.21 Postoperative appearance of Figure 37.20.

Table 37.1   Classification of anorectal malformations (Stephens 1984[12])

Female	Male
High	*High*
Anorectal agenesis:	Anorectal agenesis:
With rectovaginal fistula	With recto–prostatic–urethral fistula
Without fistula	Without fistula
Intermediate	*Intermediate*
Rectovestibular fistula	Rectobulbar urethral fistula
Rectovaginal fistula	
Anal agenesis without fistula	Anal agenesis without fistula
Low	*Low*
Anovestibular fistula	
Anocutaneous fistula	Anocutaneous fistula
Anal stenosis	Anal stenosis
Cloacal malformations	
Rare malformations	Rare malformations

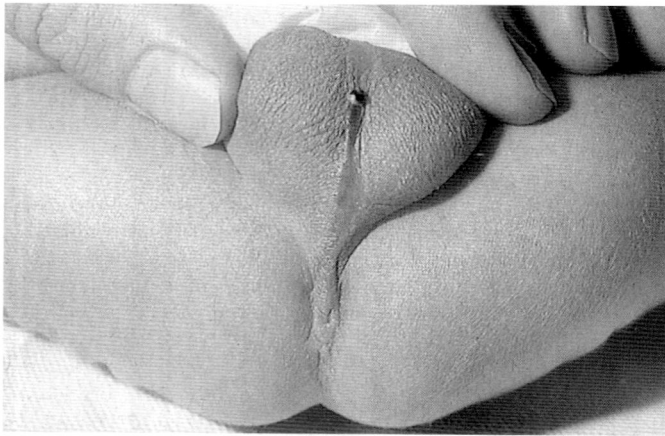

Fig. 37.22   Low anorectal anomaly.

In the male a high lesion commonly communicates with the urethra whereas in the female, with the genital tract intervening, the fistula is to the vagina. A low lesion may open onto the skin of the perineum, or in the male, track forwards along the median raphe of the scrotum (Fig. 37.22), or in the female, towards the vestibule. In addition, a severe cloacal anomaly may arise in girls with urethra, vagina and rectum opening into a common channel. Anal stenosis may arise in either sex and presents with the passage of toothpaste-like motions.

Treatment

Anal stenosis is treated by graduated anal dilation with Hegar's dilators. A low lesion with a long subcutaneous tract should have the latter opened and an anoplasty performed. An anovestibular fistula can also be managed by a cutback procedure. This may result in rather close proximity of anal and vaginal openings (shotgun perineum) but the perineum develops as the child grows, separating the orifices. To avoid this appearance some prefer to transpose the anal opening to a more normal site.

High and intermediate lesions, and low lesions where the diagnosis is not at first obvious, require a defunctioning colostomy in the neonatal period. A sigmoid colostomy will enable subsequent adequate washouts of the distal loop, a procedure that is especially important in lesions communicating with the urinary tract. Prophylactic antibiotics are also required in such cases.

Once the colostomy is established, formal contrast studies via the distal loop (distal loopogram) define the level of the lesion accurately. Definitive repair is then deferred for a few weeks or months depending on the preference of the surgeon. The procedure of choice is the posterior sagittal anorectoplasty described by de Vries and Pena,[13] requiring meticulous technique and a thorough understanding of the anatomy. Some now perform a laparoscopically assisted pull through.

NEONATAL NECROTIZING ENTEROCOLITIS (NEC)

This condition is described in detail in Chapter 12. Presenting as it does with abdominal distention and bile-stained vomiting, it is occasionally considered that the baby has intestinal obstruction but the presence of blood in the stool and pneumatosis intestinalis, often with portal venous gas, are pathognomonic of NEC. The management is conservative, wherever possible with nasogastric decompression, i.v. feeding and broad-spectrum antibiotics. The criteria for surgical management include pneumoperitoneum, persistent and increasing abdominal tenderness and continued clinical deterioration despite appropriate medical management. Operative management includes resection of necrotic bowel and stoma formation. Occasionally localized drainage under local anesthesia is of value in extremely ill babies, with appropriate intervention at a later date. Conservatively managed survivors often develop intestinal strictures requiring later resection. Asymptomatic strictures identified on contrast studies are best kept under review, reserving surgery for symptomatic cases.

BILIARY ATRESIA

Biliary atresia is a condition in which the extrahepatic bile ducts are grossly nonpatent. The condition is characterized by obstructive jaundice. There has traditionally been a division into 'correctable' biliary atresia, where only the distal ducts are occluded, and 'noncorrectable', in which the proximal ducts are occluded.

Presentation is with jaundice persisting beyond the first 2 weeks of life. Appropriate tests are carried out to exclude causes of hepatocellular disease (hepatitis A, hepatitis B, toxoplasmosis, rubella, cytomegalovirus, herpes, syphilis, listeriosis, galactosemia, fructosemia, alpha1-antitrypsin deficiency, etc.) It is vital not to waste too much time awaiting the results of all tests as delay in treatment of biliary atresia will adversely affect the progress. Suspected cases must therefore be referred early to a center capable of undertaking the necessary investigation and surgery. Ultrasound will rarely show a gallbladder and may show increased hepatic parenchymal echoes in biliary atresia. An isotope liver scan using a ^{99m}Tc iminodiacetic acid (IDA) radiopharmaceutical will demonstrate good hepatic uptake but no excretion into the bowel at 24 h. In hepatocellular jaundice there is a decrease in hepatocyte clearance.

Some surgeons prefer to do a percutaneous liver biopsy, which may be strongly indicative of biliary atresia, but others proceed directly to operative cholangiography if there is a positive IDA scan. This is carried out through a small transverse right upper abdominal incision. The gallbladder is often small and fibrotic, making a cholangiogram impossible. Occasionally patency of the cystic duct and common bile duct may be identified and, rarely, biliary hypoplasia.

Treatment

The procedure of choice for extrahepatic biliary atresia is Kasai's hepatic portoenterostomy. This was first described in Japanese in 1959 and only in 1968 in English.[14]

Kasai reports satisfactory bile drainage in 80% of cases. In other series this ranges from 35 to 75% (personal small series 75%). Many will develop portal hypertension and cholangitis (various modifications of Kasai's procedure are carried out to reduce this complication). Liver transplantation is of great value in cases that fail to achieve or maintain bile drainage following the Kasai procedure.

SURGERY OF THE INFANT AND CHILD

HEAD AND NECK, FACE AND MOUTH

Embryological abnormalities

Branchial arch–abnormalities

Sinuses, fistulae, cysts and cartilaginous elements may be apparent at birth or may be noted in infancy or later in childhood. These anomalies arise from the first and second pharyngeal arches and clefts. First cleft remnants are rare and include a tract from the external auditory canal to the upper lateral neck. They may present with recurrent abscesses in the neck, and treatment involves excision of the whole tract, usually a sinus, being blind ending at the external auditory canal. Abnormal development of the first arch results in cleft lip and palate, abnormal shape of the pinna, and deafness due to malformation of the malleus and incus.

Second branchial remnants are more common. In theory sinuses should be more common than fistulae but the reverse is true and cysts are the least common, often presenting in adult life. Fistulae have a skin opening over the anterior border of the lower third of the sternomastoid. This may be noted to discharge clear mucus. The tract passes upwards between the internal and external carotid arteries to open in the tonsillar fossa.

The length of this tract often necessitates two incisions to facilitate its removal, one being at the skin opening and the other parallel to it, at a higher level, to follow the tract through the carotid bifurcation.

Branchial cysts manifest themselves as they slowly enlarge with secretions, appearing in late childhood or young adulthood. They tend to lie deep to the anterior border of the upper third of the sternocleidomastoid muscle. They may become infected. The treatment is excision.

Cartilaginous branchial remnants may appear along the anterior border of sternocleidomastoid. They do not usually have an associated tract and are excised purely for cosmetic reasons.

Thyroglossal cysts

These are more common than branchial remnants. The thyroid develops as a diverticulum from the floor of the pharynx, leaving it attached to the foramen cecum (at the junction of the anterior two thirds, and posterior one third of the tongue) by a stalk, the thyroglossal duct, which is normally completely reabsorbed. The tract of a persistent thyroglossal duct should developmentally be ventral to the hyoid bone but differential growth results in part of the duct reaching its deep surface. A thyroglossal cyst arises typically in the midline of the neck anteriorly, or occasionally just to one or other side of the midline. By virtue of its attachment to the thyroglossal duct the cyst moves on swallowing or protrusion of the tongue (Fig. 37.23a–c). The cyst is usually at the level of or just below the hyoid bone but can be anywhere along the line of the duct. Surgery is best performed when the lesion is diagnosed, as infection may arise and lead to difficulty in complete excision. The operation involves not only removal of the cyst but the body of the hyoid and the tract must be followed up to the level of the foramen cecum. Failure to do this is likely to lead to recurrence.

Dermoid cysts

These usually occur at sites of embryological fusion. These may be in the midline. A dermoid cyst in the neck may be mistaken for a thyroglossal cyst although it will not move on swallowing or protrusion of the tongue. A common site is the external angular dermoid cyst in the eyebrow area at the outer angle of the eye. Occasionally there may be a dumbbell extension intracranially. They occur if ectodermal cells become buried beneath the skin surface during development. An inclusion dermoid cyst may similarly arise secondary to trauma.

Cystic hygroma

Commonly arising in the neck, these fluid-filled lesions of lymphatic origin may be found elsewhere, including the axilla and groin or, rarely, on the trunk. They are either present at birth, sometimes being diagnosed on antenatal ultrasonography, or may appear within the first 2 years or sometimes later. Usually arising in the posterior triangle of the neck, they may sometimes be very large indeed, extending into the floor of the mouth and tongue, where complete excision may prove difficult, leading to disfigurement and occasionally the need for a tracheostomy. Infection leads to difficulty with subsequent surgery, which is thus best performed soon after diagnosis. Aspiration of the cysts and injection of a streptococcal derivative 'OK432' (Picibanil) is a treatment that is proving to be an effective alternative to surgery.[15]

Salivary gland enlargement

This may arise secondary to a calculus in a duct (the submandibular duct in particular). Parotid duct calculi are rare but recurrent swelling of the gland may be due to sialectasis, seen on a sialogram as dilated duct radicles. The treatment is to advise the sucking of acid drop sweets to promote salivary flow and at the same time massaging the gland from back to front. If infection supervenes then antibiotics must be administered.

Ranula (Latin rana = frog)

This is a sublingual cyst that may be small or may fill the floor of the mouth. It may be related to a salivary or mucus gland. It is thin walled and contains clear viscid fluid. Care is required not to damage the submandibular duct during its excision and marsupialization is often safer.

Tongue tie

A short lingual frenum leads to maternal anxiety regarding future problems with speech. Speech therapists confirm that there will be no speech problem and others that the anterior third of the tongue will grow and a normal appearance will result. Tongue tie may lead to difficulty with breast-feeding. Division of the tongue tie in a baby prior to appearance of dentition is a simple procedure for a surgeon in the outpatient clinic. In the older child, general anesthesia is required. Tongue tie may occasionally present beyond the first 2 years and the current author personally believes in division, as all children deserve to be able to stick their tongue out – if only to lick an ice cream!

Cervical lymphadenopathy

Cervical lymph nodes are readily palpable in most children. Lymphoma is rare, but persistent painless enlargement of a cervical node is best diagnosed by excision biopsy although it is reasonable to administer an antibiotic in doubtful cases and re-examine the child in 2 weeks. Cat scratch disease, *Toxoplasma* and both tuberculosis and atypical mycobacterial infections may occur and usually affect jugulodigastric and submandibular nodes.

In mycobacterial infections, nodes may feel fixed to deeper tissues and to skin and may caseate and discharge. Sinus formation may result from abscess rupture or incomplete excision. Antituberculous chemotherapy is necessary once the diagnosis has become established.

Acute suppurative cervical lymphadenitis usually results from an upper respiratory tract infection. Early administration of antibiotics may lead to resolution without abscess formation but if an abscess does form it should be allowed to point before drainage. Kaolin poultices seem old fashioned but are still of value in this process.

Sternomastoid tumor

This is the commonest cause of torticollis in childhood (other causes include hemivertebrae, acute fasciitis, cervical adenitis and ocular muscle imbalance). The cause of this lesion is unknown. It is more common in babies born by breech presentation and was considered to be a result of trauma to the muscle during delivery. It seems likely, however, that it arises in utero, resulting in breech presentation. Within the muscle there is an area of endomysial fibrosis with atrophied muscle fibers surrounded by collagen and fibroblasts. The infant presents usually at 2–3 weeks of age with a hard swelling within the substance of sternocleidomastoid. The shortening of the muscle makes the infant look upwards and to the opposite side. It is important to commence physiotherapy as soon as the diagnosis is made. The parents are taught how to stretch the muscle by rotating the head towards the side of the tumor. These stretching exercises should be carried out twice daily and must continue

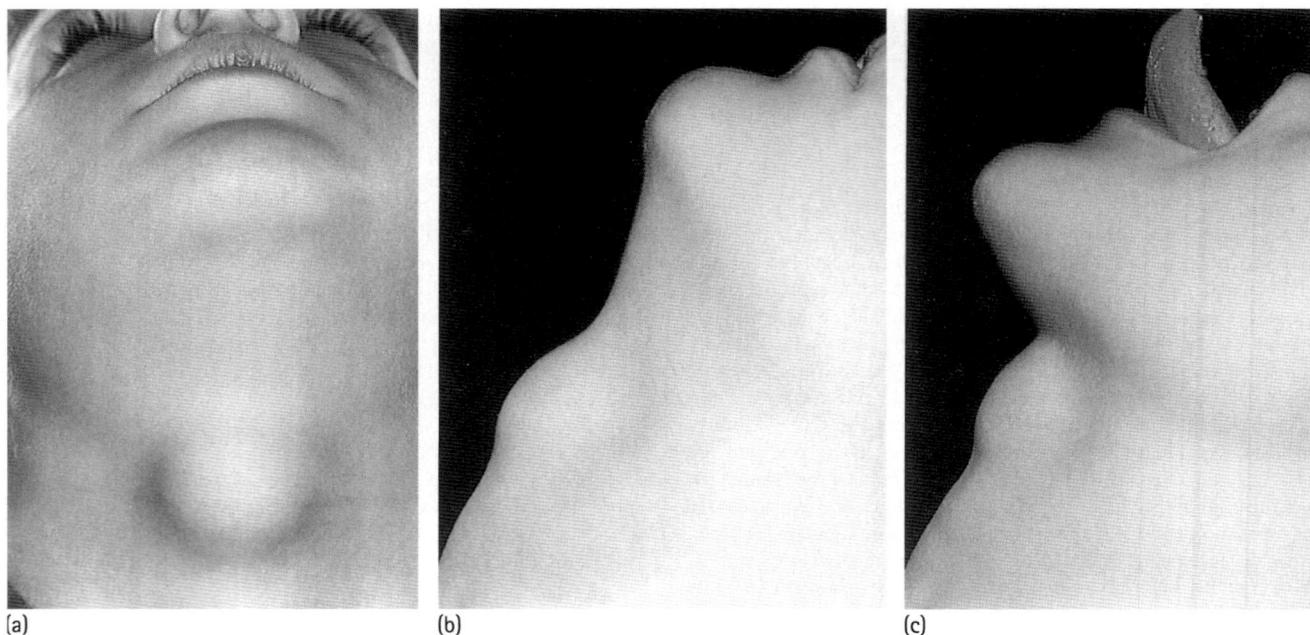

Fig. 37.23   (a) Thyroglossal cyst; (b) and (c) show elevation on tongue protrusion.

for at least the first year, diminishing in frequency thereafter. Failure to treat adequately leads to shortening of deeper cervical structures and craniofacial asymmetry. Surgical division of the muscle and deeper strictures is necessary in cases that fail to respond or are missed in the neonatal period.

Thyroid swellings
(see Chapter 15).

PYLORIC STENOSIS

Though often called congenital, hypertrophic pyloric stenosis only very rarely has its onset of symptoms at birth and has never been described in a stillbirth. Vomiting normally commences around 2–3 weeks of age, becoming more frequent and projectile. The vomitus is of gastric content (milk) and is never bile stained. It may become brownish or visibly bloodstained due either to an accompanying gastritis or to rupture of capillaries in the gastric mucosa from frequent vomiting. The baby fails to thrive, becomes constipated and dehydrated, developing a hypochloremic alkalosis from the loss of gastric acid.

Examination reveals a hungry, worried looking baby and if recently fed, visible gastric peristalsis, and a wave traveling from the left hypochondrium towards the right may be apparent (Fig. 37.24). The diagnosis is confirmed during a test feed. For this the surgeon and the nurse or mother sit facing in opposite directions, the surgeon to the left of the nurse (Fig. 37.25). The baby is fed with the bottle in the right hand or at the left breast of the nursing mother. The surgeon palpates the tumor with the left hand. It is felt as an olive-shaped mass that lies just to the right of the midline, in the right hypochondrium. Contraction of the tumor is noted with variation in palpability, thus confirming that it is not confused with a Riedel's lobe of liver, or similar anomaly. If difficulty is encountered in palpating the tumor, the passage of a nasogastric tube to wash out the stomach may facilitate the procedure (it may be that the filled gastric antrum has previously obscured the pylorus). This seemingly ritual routine not only enhances the chance of palpating the tumor but avoids the calamity of the baby vomiting over the examiner's trousers!

Most surgeons will only operate if they can palpate the tumor but if difficulty is encountered in palpation, ultrasound examination is now the diagnostic investigation of choice.

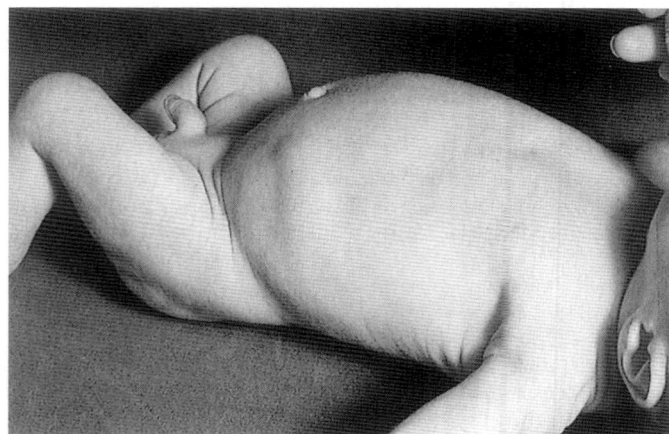

Fig. 37.24   Pyloric stenosis: visible peristalsis.

Treatment
First the hypochloremic alkalosis together with any associated hypokalemia is corrected by administering 5% dextrose in 0.45% saline with added potassium chloride if required. Although the use of 0.45% saline takes twice as long to correct the deficit as normal saline would, it is safer to administer. Preoperative gastric lavage is also performed and the nasogastric tube left in situ.

Once the electrolyte and acid–base deficit is corrected, surgery is performed under general anesthesia. The universally accepted operation of choice is the pyloromyotomy attributed to Ramstedt.[16] Actually the first recorded use of this procedure was by Sir Harold Stiles[17] in the Royal Hospital for Sick Children, Edinburgh on 3 February 1910, a year prior to Ramstedt's operation performed on 28 July 1911 and published in 1912. Unfortunately Stiles' patient died on the fourth postoperative day, either from gastroenteritis or delayed chloroform poisoning!

The pylorus can be delivered through a right transverse upper abdominal or a periumbilical incision, and an incision is made from the pyloroduodenal junction well onto the antrum of the stomach. The incision extends down into the muscle, which is then spread bluntly, all muscle fibers being ruptured, allowing the intact mucosa to bulge. The pylorus is returned to the abdomen and the wound closed.

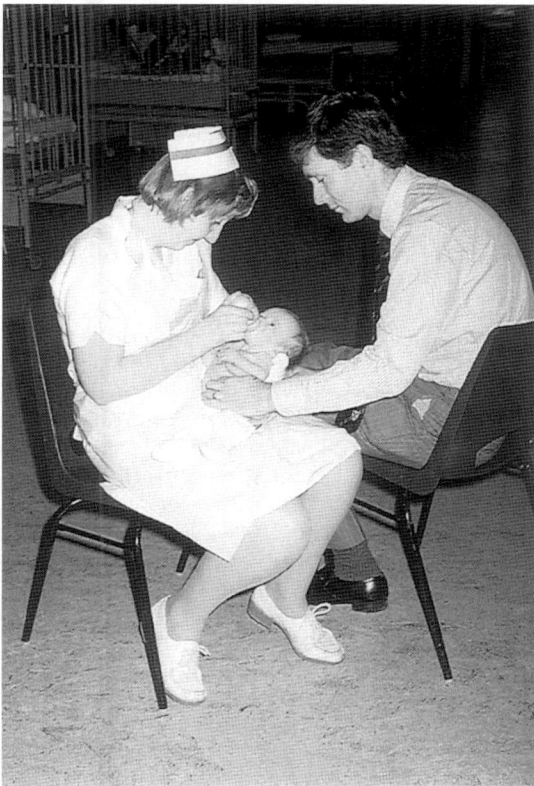

Fig. 37.25 Pyloric stenosis: test feed.

A laparoscopic approach is preferred in centers where the surgeons have the appropriate skills and is already proving to have better results with less postoperative gastric paresis.

Oral feeding can be commenced within 4 h. Some choose a graduated feeding regime of dextrose, half strength, then full strength milk introduced over 24–48 h. Others advise a more rapid return to normal feeds. Certainly breast-fed infants come to no harm from being returned to the breast initially for a short time, gradually increasing to normal feeding time.

Vomiting in the first 24 h postoperatively is not unusual and is presumably related to preoperative gastritis. If persistent it usually settles after gastric lavage. Most babies will be fit for discharge within 24–72 h after surgery.

GASTROESOPHAGEAL REFLUX

This is due to incompetence at the cardia and is another cause of vomiting that may commence as early as the neonatal period. The condition may or may not be associated with a hiatus hernia. The infant vomits effortlessly at any time, and usually appears unconcerned about the problem. The vomiting need not be related to feed times. The vomitus may be coffee ground or streaked with bright red blood if there is associated peptic esophagitis. The diagnosis is confirmed by barium studies and pH studies together with endoscopy, if indicated. Most cases respond to conservative management of thickening the feeds, sitting the baby up at all times (although there is dispute about this) and the administration of an antacid such as Gaviscon. In more severe cases an H_2 antagonist or a proton pump inhibitor is used. If, however, the infant fails to thrive, has persistent peptic esophagitis, recurrent aspiration pneumonitis or a proven large 'sliding' hiatus hernia, then a surgical antireflux procedure is required. If an esophageal stricture has already developed it will usually resolve after surgery but in some cases bougienage or balloon dilation is required. Various antireflux operations have been devised, the most popular being the Nissen fundoplication. The esophagus and the gastric fundus is mobilized, the right crus of the diaphragm tightened and wrapped around the abdominal esophagus. This operation is now best performed laparoscopically,[18] reducing postoperative discomfort and length of hospital stay.

Children with severe neurological handicap are especially prone to gastroesophageal reflux and hiatus hernia. Usually their parents or carers welcome the surgical treatment of these children, as their well-being is so obviously improved. Presumably they suffer a great deal of discomfort related to esophagitis and their frustration is increased by their inability to complain. The results of surgery in such cases is invariably rewarding.

INTUSSUSCEPTION

Intussusception is the invagination of part of the intestine into itself. An intussusception arising in the ileum may pass all the way round the large bowel to appear at the anus. The lead point is known as the *intussusceptum*, the sheath as the *intussuscipiens* and between these are the entering and returning layers of the bowel. Naturally, the mesentery with its vessels is drawn between the entering and returning layers, leading to engorgement of the vessels and diapedesis of red cells into the lumen of the bowel. Mucus is produced by the engorgement of the mucosal cells and, mixed with the red cells, creates the classic redcurrant jelly stool. Eventually a strangulating obstruction occurs and gangrene of the intussusceptum may result.

In infants the lead point is presumed to be an enlarged Peyer's patch, the lymphoid tissue presumably responding to a viral stimulant. This becomes the apex of the intussusception, which then proceeds for a variable distance into the colon. The peak incidence is in infants 3–9 months of age. The timing has been attributed to a change in the bowel flora associated with weaning. In older children the lead point may be an invaginated Meckel's diverticulum, a polyp, an enteric cyst, or hemorrhage into the bowel wall in Henoch–Schönlein purpura or leukemia. It is more common in boys than in girls, some reporting a ratio as high as 5:1, but in Edinburgh the ratio is only 1.2:1. Some report seasonal variation, possibly related to infectious agents.

The presentation is with a painful cry, drawing up the knees and going pale, presumably in relation to colic (88% in our series). The colicky pain is intermittent and occurs with increasing frequency as the condition progresses, rather like labor pains. Vomiting is a common symptom (86%) and the passage of redcurrant jelly stools is frequent (56%).

On examination, between attacks of colic, an abdominal mass is usually palpable. This is typically sausage shaped and commonly palpable in the ascending or transverse colon. A small percentage of intussusceptions present at the anus.

Investigation

Plain abdominal X-ray will often show a filling defect corresponding to the intussusception and will demonstrate any obstruction by the presence of fluid levels within the bowel. Ultrasound can identify a 'target sign' corresponding to the layers of the intussusception. Occasionally a contrast enema may be used diagnostically in frankly obstructed cases.

Treatment

First an i.v. infusion is set up. Some collapsed infants require blood or plasma for primary resuscitation, others only require isotonic fluids. A nasogastric tube may be passed, especially if vomiting has been a marked symptom at presentation. Preparation is as for a surgical reduction; the operating room is arranged in case it is required but in most cases non-operative reduction is first attempted. The only contraindications to non-operative management are a seriously ill child with a prolonged history, marked intestinal obstruction or evidence of peritonitis (rare).

Hydrostatic reduction has been intermittently popular since first advocated by Hirschsprung in 1876. A barium enema under X-ray screening is used as a therapeutic technique and is frequently successful. Recently air has been used for reduction rather than barium. (The method has for centuries found favor in China, where fire bellows have traditionally been used.) Air is an excellent contrast medium and scientific control of the pressure is by attaching the rectal Foley catheter to a sphygmomanometer, increasing the pressure to 100 mmHg if necessary. This method appears to have a greater success rate than barium and in the rare occurrence of perforation, proves safer.

Surgical reduction is required for those in whom non-operative reduction fails. The intussusception is reduced manually by stripping it back from the point the apex has reached. Pulling on the entering layer of bowel can lead to serosal splitting or rupture of the bowel. Once the intussusception is reduced appendectomy is usually performed. This may help to prevent recurrence by adherence of the cecum in the right iliac fossa. If reduction proves impossible then a limited bowel resection may be required.

Recurrence rates of 2–4% have been recorded and seem unrelated to the method of reduction.

APPENDICITIS

This is the most common condition for which emergency abdominal surgery is required in childhood. Its symptomatology and management are similar to those in adults although in the very young child there may be difficulty in making the appropriate diagnosis. Appendicitis is still a condition with significant morbidity and mortality. In a recent series, reporting on the last 5 years of the 1970s, there were four deaths related to appendicitis in children in Scotland. Delay in diagnosis can thus convert an eminently treatable condition into a lethal one.

Classically the condition presents with pain, vomiting and fever. The pain commences periumbilically, the distended appendix causing dull and poorly localized midgut pain via visceral nerve fibers to the tenth thoracic nerve root. The pathology of appendicitis is of spreading inflammation from the mucosa through the wall to the serosa. Serosal inflammation leads to peritoneal inflammation and the pain is accurately localized to the right iliac fossa – classically at McBurney's point (two thirds along a line from the umbilicus to the anterior superior iliac spine). Atypical presentation leads to difficulty in diagnosis, especially in the very young. Neonatal appendicitis is exceedingly rare and the mortality rate is high. In the preschool child the diagnosis is also difficult and a high perforation rate is encountered. The preschool child may present with anorexia, listlessness, fever, vomiting and diarrhea.

Care must be taken in the examination of the child with suspected appendicitis. The tongue may be coated and there is a classic 'fetor oris', a sweet smell on the breath perhaps partly related to ketones. The child is reluctant to climb onto the examination couch. The chest is examined to exclude a right lower lobe pneumonia, which may easily lead to a mistaken diagnosis of appendicitis. Examination of the abdomen must be very gentle, starting in the left lower quadrant and gradually working round each quadrant to finish in the right iliac fossa. Clumsy technique can lose a child's confidence and lead to voluntary guarding. Tenderness at McBurney's point remains the cardinal sign of appendicitis.

Involuntary guarding and rigidity are reliable signs of peritonism or peritonitis. There is no excuse in endeavoring to elicit rebound tenderness as, if present, the child's confidence is immediately lost, the pain being so severe, thus precluding subsequent examination. Likewise, rectal examination should be reserved for cases with negative or equivocal abdominal findings, where it may be the only means of diagnosis of a pelvic appendicitis. It may otherwise confirm a diagnosis of constipation or, in females, gynecological disease. It must be remembered that the appendix can adopt a variety of intra-abdominal positions circumferentially around the attachment to the cecum. A retrocecal appendix may have few abdominal signs initially, although psoas spasm may be apparent.

There are no investigations that can prove the presence of appendicitis. The white cell count need not be raised and an X-ray, whilst occasionally showing a fecolith, is generally unhelpful. Ultrasound is now of value in recognizing a thickened appendix with surrounding edema.

The differential diagnosis includes intestinal diseases such as gastroenteritis, Crohn disease and other causes of terminal ileitis such as *Yersinia* infection, Meckel's diverticulitis and leukemic typhlitis, mesenteric adenitis and deep iliac adenitis. In addition, gynecological problems such as salpingitis and ovarian cysts must be considered. Urinary tract infection may also be confused with appendicitis, the situation being further complicated by the possible occurrence of pyuria when an inflamed appendix is adjacent to the bladder. Finally, medical disorders such as right basal pneumonia, diabetes mellitus, Henoch–Schönlein purpura and sickle cell disease have all been misdiagnosed as appendicitis. In fact almost all causes of acute abdominal pain in childhood must be considered but appendicitis is the commonest surgical emergency.

Treatment

If necessary, preliminary resuscitation of the patient by administration of i.v. fluids should be considered. Once the patient has been adequately hydrated then appendectomy is carried out through a skin crease incision an inch or more below McBurney's point to leave a neat scar well below the 'bikini line' or preferably a laparoscopic approach is used. At induction of anesthesia a single dose of broad-spectrum antibiotics such as an aminoglycoside and metronidazole, to cover bowel flora including *Escherichia coli* and *Bacteroides fragilis*, is administered to endeavor to prevent postoperative complications such as wound infections and intra-abdominal abscesses, especially pelvic and subphrenic. If an appendix mass is palpated some prefer conservative management with bed rest, i.v. fluids and antibiotics with an interval appendectomy at 3 months. Others proceed to appendectomy appropriately covered by antibiotic therapy.

PRIMARY PERITONITIS

This has a similar presentation to appendicitis but without a history of central pain moving to the right iliac fossa. The abdominal signs are those of peritonitis especially in the lower abdomen. At operation diffuse peritonitis is found with peritoneal exudate, yet no obvious focus of infection. The commonest causative organisms are pneumococci and streptococci. The source of infection has been thought to be the genital tract, the condition being commoner in girls, but the occasional occurrence in boys leads one to suspect blood-borne spread. There may be a preceding or coexisting upper respiratory tract infection. The management is appropriate antibiotic therapy (usually penicillin).

MECKEL'S DIVERTICULUM

Meckel's diverticulum arises from the vitellointestinal duct, which leads from the primitive gut to the yolk sac. Persistence of the proximal end of the duct occurs in 2% of the population (the 2 ft from the ileocecal valve, 2 in long story is erroneous: it may be a variable length and variable distance from the ileocecal valve).

The vitellointestinal duct can lead to a number of anomalies if it persists (Fig. 37.26). The duct itself may remain patent to the umbilicus and thus present as a fistula in neonates. Partial obliteration may give rise to cyst formation or a persistent fibrous cord from the umbilicus to the ileum may act as an axis for localized volvulus or lead to bowel obstruction.

A Meckel's diverticulum may become inflamed, lead to hemorrhage or invaginate into the ileum and cause intussusception. Meckel's diverticulitis has an identical presentation to acute appendicitis and must always be considered if a normal appendix is identified at surgery.

Bleeding in relation to a Meckel's diverticulum arises because the lining often contains heterotopic gastric mucosa (35–49%). This leads to peptic ulceration of the adjacent normal ileal mucosa (Fig. 37.27). Bleeding usually occurs in preschool children, especially toddlers. It may be intermittent passage of a small amount of altered blood in the stool, although massive hemorrhage with the passage of maroon or even bright red blood is more common. After adequate resuscitation, with blood replacement, a Meckel's scan should be performed. This is a ^{99m}Tc pertechnetate isotope scan that has an affinity for parietal cells. The stomach is visualized on the scan image, together with the bladder,

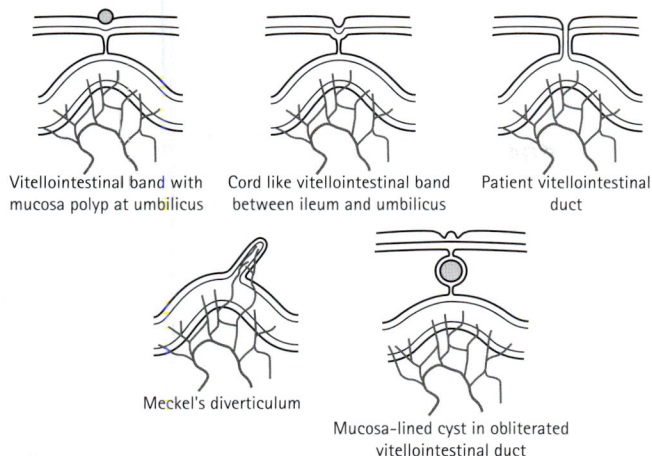

Vitellointestinal band with mucosa polyp at umbilicus

Cord like vitellointestinal band between ileum and umbilicus

Patient vitellointestinal duct

Meckel's diverticulum

Mucosa-lined cyst in obliterated vitellointestinal duct

Fig. 37.26 Vitellointestinal remnants.

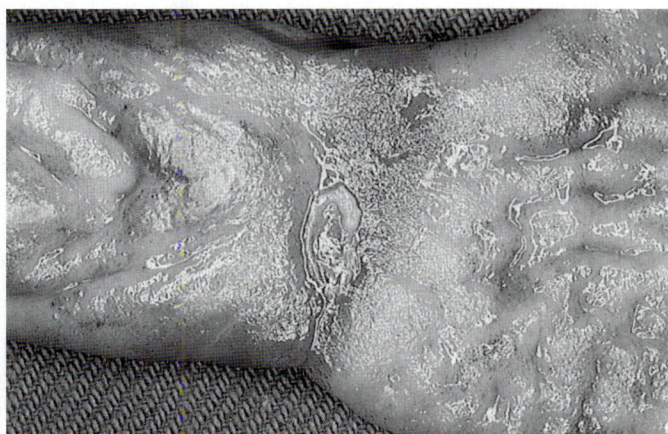

Fig. 37.27 Peptic ulcer at junction of gastric and ileal mucosa in Meckel's diverticulum.

as the isotope is excreted through the kidneys. A third 'blob' of isotope is likely to indicate ectopic gastric mucosa in a Meckel's diverticulum (or rarely in a duplicated segment of bowel). Priming the patient with cimetidine for a few days enhances the scan image. Laparoscopy can avoid the need for a scan and even in the absence of a Meckel's demonstrate the presence or absence of blood in the upper small bowel. An appropriate upper or lower gastrointestinal endoscopy can then be performed under the same anesthetic.

The treatment is in all cases Meckel's diverticulectomy, the diverticulum being found on the antimesenteric aspect of the ileum 40–100 cm proximal to the ileocecal valve.

SUPERIOR MESENTERIC ARTERY SYNDROME

This syndrome, a cause of acute and chronic abdominal pain in childhood, is due to obstruction of the third part of the duodenum by the superior mesenteric artery. It has variously been called 'Cast syndrome', 'Wilkie's syndrome', 'chronic duodenal ileus' and 'arteriomesenteric duodenal compression syndrome'. It may be congenital or acquired, the latter being due to rapid growth without associated weight gain, rapid weight loss or from hyperextension of the vertebral column in a plaster cast. The presentation may be acute or chronic with acute obstructive symptoms or intermittent abdominal pain and vomiting. Contrast studies, if performed between attacks, may show little but if performed in an acute episode will demonstrate obstruction of the third part of the duodenum. The superior mesenteric artery normally subtends an angle of 45 degrees with the aorta but under the conditions described earlier

the angle may decrease to 15 degrees, thus occluding the underlying duodenum.

Management is conservative or surgical, the former being alteration of diet, nursing prone and removing or windowing a plaster cast if present. Surgical management entails division of the ligament of Treitz and transposition of the small bowel to the right side in a position of nonrotation.[19]

CHOLEDOCHAL CYST

This is a cystic dilation of the choledochus (the common bile duct). The etiology is unknown but some believe it to be related to the reflux of pancreatic secretions into the common duct. The presentation may be in infancy with obstructive jaundice suggestive of biliary atresia, or in the older child with intermittent jaundice, abdominal pain and vomiting often associated with fever suggestive of ascending cholangitis. The diagnosis is by ultrasonography. Treatment consists of excision of the cyst and a Roux-en-Y choledochojejunostomy or hepaticojejunostomy. Failure to excise the entire cyst may result in carcinoma of the cyst wall in the long term.

CHOLELITHIASIS

Gallstones are uncommon in childhood but must be considered in children with hereditary spherocytosis. If metabolic stones develop then cholecystectomy is required, but in hemolytic disease the gallbladder is usually normal and simple cholecystotomy and removal of the stones is all that is required. This procedure should always be considered at the time of splenectomy in these children.

INGUINAL HERNIA AND HYDROCELE

These conditions have the same origin in childhood – the presence of a patent processus vaginalis. The only difference between them is the caliber of the processus (Fig. 37.28). If wide a hernia is produced, if narrow then peritoneal fluid may tract down to the tunica vaginalis. This explains the use of the term 'hydrocele' from the Greek *hydro* = water, *kele* = hernia. (A similar derivation applies to encephalocele, omphalocele, ureterocele, etc.) Frequently hydrocele is spelt, erroneously, 'coele', even in textbooks: it is not derived from coelom (Greek *koiloma* = hollow).

The processus vaginalis is an outpouching of peritoneum drawn down by the descent of the testis. The distal portion persists as the tunica

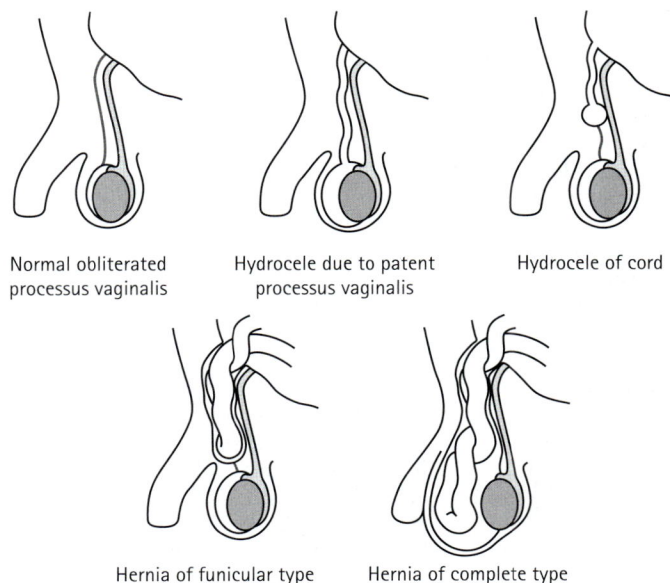

Normal obliterated processus vaginalis

Hydrocele due to patent processus vaginalis

Hydrocele of cord

Hernia of funicular type

Hernia of complete type

Fig. 37.28 Inguinal herniae and hydroceles.

vaginalis but the intervening communication with the peritoneal cavity is normally obliterated. Persistence of a widely patent processus along its whole length results in a hernia of the 'complete' type – a scrotal hernia. Obliteration of the distal portion results in a 'funicular' hernial sac. Similarly, a hydrocele of the cord can arise, the distal portion being obliterated and the proximal communication narrowed.

These conditions are more common on the right side than the left, presumably related to the later descent of the right testis. They may also arise in girls, although hernias are less common. Occasionally an ovary may prolapse into a hernia – at surgery it must be inspected to confirm that it is indeed an ovary and not a testis in testicular feminization syndrome (Fig. 37.29). Chromosomal analysis may be of value in excluding this condition in girls with bilateral hernias but the incidence is extremely low. The hydrocele equivalent in a female is a hydrocele of the canal of Nuck – a small diverticulum of peritoneum accompanying the round ligament of the uterus through the inguinal canal.

In general, hydroceles are only treated surgically if they persist beyond the age of 1 year, the majority resolving spontaneously prior to that. In toddlers there is often a history of a hydrocele increasing in size towards the end of the day – the fluid slowly returns to the peritoneum through the narrow processus when the child is recumbent at night. Surgery consists of ligation and division of the patent processus vaginalis through a small inguinal incision.

Inguinal hernias are treated with a similar operation. If the hernia is not obvious on examination, despite a typical history, tickling may increase the intra-abdominal pressure to demonstrate the hernia, but its presence can be confirmed by rolling the spermatic cord over the pubic bone with the index finger, thickening being apparent in the presence of a hernia.

If a scrotal swelling is present, a hydrocele can usually be distinguished from a hernia by the fact that the surgeon can get above it. Rarely does a hydrocele extend up into the inguinal canal. Transillumination may be misleading, as the thin bowel wall with intraluminal fluid in a young infant will also transilluminate. The surgery is a semi-urgent herniotomy. There is no requirement for herniorrhaphy (repair).

Incarceration of an inguinal hernia implies irreducibility, which will lead to strangulation of the bowel if left untreated. Gentle reduction is attempted. Force must not be applied and unless reduction is easy the child should be sedated with i.m. morphine and tipped head down; occasionally gallows traction is of benefit. If reduction is unsuccessful, immediate surgical reduction and herniotomy are necessary. If it is successfully reduced then herniotomy must be performed before the infant is discharged.

Confirmation of the previous incarceration may be made by observing an increase in testicular size on the affected side (a positive Robarts' sign). This results from venous obstruction of the pampiniform plexus, which can result in testicular infarction in cases where the hernia is not urgently reduced.

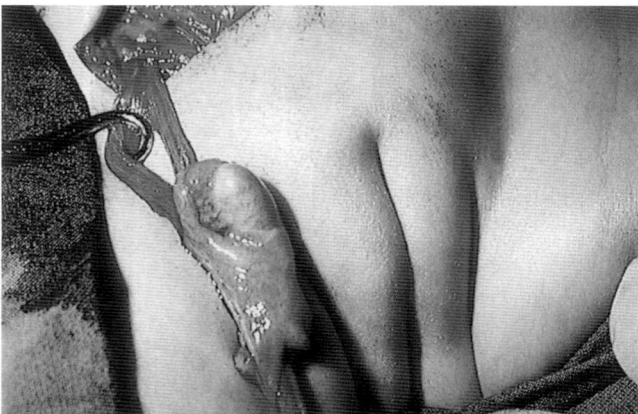

Fig. 37.29   External female genitalia and normal testis in testicular feminization syndrome.

FEMORAL HERNIA

This is uncommon in children but, as in adults, is recognized by the swelling lying below the inguinal ligament and lateral to the pubic tubercle. Femoral herniorrhaphy is required.

UMBILICAL HERNIA

By the time the umbilical cord has separated in the newborn the umbilical ring has usually closed but in a proportion of children a defect is left, resulting in an umbilical hernia. There is a higher incidence of this condition in blacks than in whites. Umbilical hernia occurs in Beckwith syndrome, Hurler syndrome, trisomy 18, and trisomy 13.

The vast majority of umbilical hernias will resolve spontaneously within the first 2 years of life. Incarceration and strangulation in umbilical hernias in childhood are so rare that they need not cause concern. Persistence of the hernia beyond the age of 2 years merits surgical repair, provided that care is taken to ensure that the incision lies within the umbilical folds.

A *paraumbilical hernia* usually lies in the linea alba immediately above the umbilical ring. This will not close spontaneously and surgical repair is required.

EPIGASTRIC HERNIA

An epigastric hernia occurs through the linea alba, usually midway between the xiphisternum and the umbilicus. It presents as a pea-sized swelling occasionally associated with pain and results from herniation of extraperitoneal fat through the defect. It is best treated surgically although it can safely be left alone.

SURGICAL ASPECTS OF THE GENITOURINARY TRACT

ANOMALIES OF TESTICULAR DESCENT

It is best to consider the following distinct entities: the testis arrested in the normal line of descent (true undescended), ectopic testes and retractile testes. In addition, testes may be atrophic or absent (anorchia).

Testes arrested along the normal line of descent

The term *cryptorchidism* (Greek *cryptos* = hidden, *orchis* = testis) should be reserved for impalpable, usually abdominal, testes. There is a higher incidence of undescended testes in premature than in full-term babies. Two thirds of undescended testes in newborn infants will descend, usually by 6 weeks in term and 3 months in preterm babies. There is an increased incidence of cryptorchidism in anencephalics and other cerebral anomalies.

Ectopic testes

These have descended as far as the external inguinal ring and then become deviated into the superficial inguinal, perineal (Fig. 37.30), suprapubic or femoral ectopic sites. The commonest by far is the superficial inguinal pouch, above and lateral to the external inguinal ring.

Retractile testes

The cremasteric reflex in young children will draw the testes into the region of the superficial inguinal pouch very readily but they can be manipulated back down to the bottom of the scrotum. The testis would normally reside in the scrotum if such a child is in a warm bath or relaxed in bed.

Anorchia

Anorchia may be on one or both sides. If on one side alone there may be ipsilateral renal agenesis. If the baby is fully masculinized but both testes are absent it must be assumed that they have atrophied subsequent to torsion or infarction during development. Absence of testicular tissue

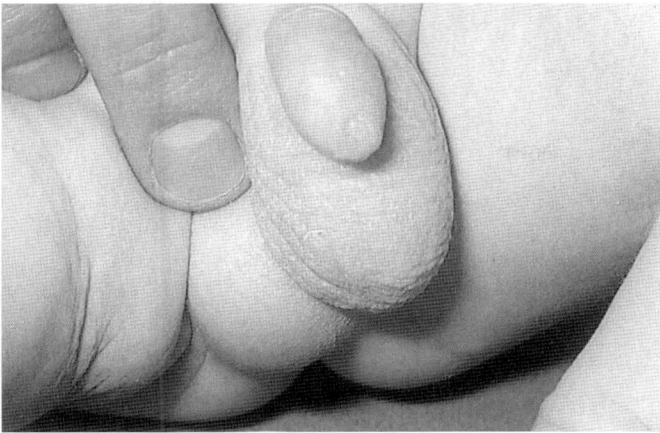

Fig. 37.30   Perineal ectopic testis.

and therefore lack of Müllerian inhibitory hormone during early gestation can lead to Müllerian development along female lines. The lack of androgenic stimulation (testosterone) from the testes leads to failure of Wolffian duct development.

'Ascending testis'

Some boys with recorded testicular descent at routine clinic checks in infancy may be found later at preschool or school medicals to have an undescended testis. This phenomenon of the 'ascending testis' was noted first by Atwell.[20] It has been suggested that this is caused by failure of elongation of the spermatic cord during differential body growth, so that the testis is drawn up by absorption of the processus vaginalis.

Treatment

It has been shown that adverse morphological changes occur in undescended testes from the second year of life onwards with a statistically significant reduction of spermatogonia and tubular growth. Most surgeons therefore choose to perform orchidopexies between 2 and 3 years of age. An associated hernia is an indication for earlier surgery. There is no place now for delaying surgery until 9 or 10 years of age. Any testis that has not descended in the first year of life will not appear later.

The treatment of the true undescended testis and the ectopic testis is orchidopexy, the testis and cord being mobilized via an inguinal approach and usually fixed in the scrotum in a subdartos pouch. Intra-abdominal testes may best be treated laparoscopically in a staged Fowler-Stephens procedure where in the first stage the testicular vessels are divided and 3–6 months later the testis may be advanced to the scrotum supplied by the artery to the vas, which has had time to hypertrophy.

Malignancy in the undescended testis

Testicular malignancy occurs in 0.0021% of adult males. Undescended testes occur in 0.28% of the population and 12% of cases of testicular malignancy are reported to occur in testes known to have been undescended. There is thus a 40 times greater incidence of malignancy in cryptorchid patients than in the general population. Orchidopexy probably does not eradicate the problem but at least the testis is placed in a position where early malignancy may be detected. In unilateral undescended testes there is also an increased risk of malignancy in the contralateral testis.

Fertility

Only one third of those following bilateral orchidopexy and two thirds of those after unilateral orchidopexy appear to have a sperm count sufficient to be potentially fertile. It is hoped, however, that these figures will be improved by the change in policy over the past few years to operate on the majority of cases in the second year of life.

THE ACUTE SCROTUM

This may result from torsion of the testis, torsion of a testicular appendage, epididymo-orchitis or idiopathic scrotal edema or, rarely, a testicular tumor.

Torsion of the testis

Torsion of the testis most commonly occurs in the neonatal period or at puberty, with a few cases presenting in the intervening years. In the neonate the torsion occurs outside the tunica vaginalis. In the neonatal period there is a plane of mobility between the tunica vaginalis and the outer layer of the scrotum. Presentation is with a reddened hemiscrotum with a hard, swollen, often indurated testis. This is not infrequently noted 24 h after birth although the torsion may have occurred at delivery. On exploration, through a groin incision, the testis is often black and infarcted but usually it is 'given the benefit of the doubt', untwisted and replaced in the scrotum, although the majority will atrophy.

After the newborn period, torsion occurs secondary to an abnormally high investment of the tunica, the testis often being described as having bell-clapper fixation. Presentation is with pain, which is usually testicular in position but theoretically, as testicular innervation is from T10, it should be felt centrally in the abdomen. Examination reveals a swollen hemiscrotum often with edema and erythema, depending on the length of history. There is exquisite tenderness on palpation. The treatment is emergency surgery as delay will affect the viability of the testis.

Preoperative isotope scanning or Doppler probing to confirm the diagnosis merely wastes time. The scrotum is explored, the testis derotated and, providing surgery is carried out within 6 h, the testis is likely to become pink under warm towels. It is then fixed in the scrotum. As the anomalous tunical attachment is likely to be bilateral, orchidopexy is also performed on the other side.

Torsion of testicular appendages

Embryological remnants are commonly attached to the testis. The hydatid of Morgagni is attached to the upper pole and is a Müllerian duct remnant. It varies in size from a pinhead to a pea or may be absent. Other remnants include the appendix epididymis (a Wolffian tubercle remnant), the paradidymis or organ of Giraldés (another mesonephric remnant) and the vas aberrans of Haller. The hydatid of Morgagni is the most common to undergo torsion, which leads to less acute pain than testicular torsion, the pain being usually at the upper pole of the testis where occasionally a bluish nodule is seen through the scrotal skin. An infarcted hydatid can give rise to considerable swelling and inflammation and doubtful cases are best explored (Fig. 37.31) to exclude testicular torsion. In any case, the necrotic hydatid is best excised as an emergency, giving instant pain relief. If treated conservatively the pain lingers on for up to 2 weeks.

Epididymo-orchitis

This is rare in children unless there is an associated renal tract anomaly. If the latter has already been established then it is safe to treat with antibiotic therapy. If, however, the clinical picture cannot be distinguished from torsion of the testis, exploration is mandatory to establish the diagnosis.

Idiopathic scrotal edema

This is a fascinating entity presenting with erythema and edema of the scrotum suggestive of a possible underlying torsion. The erythema and edema spread beyond the scrotum however into the groin and perineum (Fig. 37.32). Usually the process is confined to one side of the scrotum and the adjacent groin and perineum.

The etiology is unknown. It may be an allergic phenomenon; it is occasionally associated with an eosinophilia and may respond to antihistamine therapy. Some suggest it may be caused by an insect bite. The testis is nontender and the condition settles within a few days.

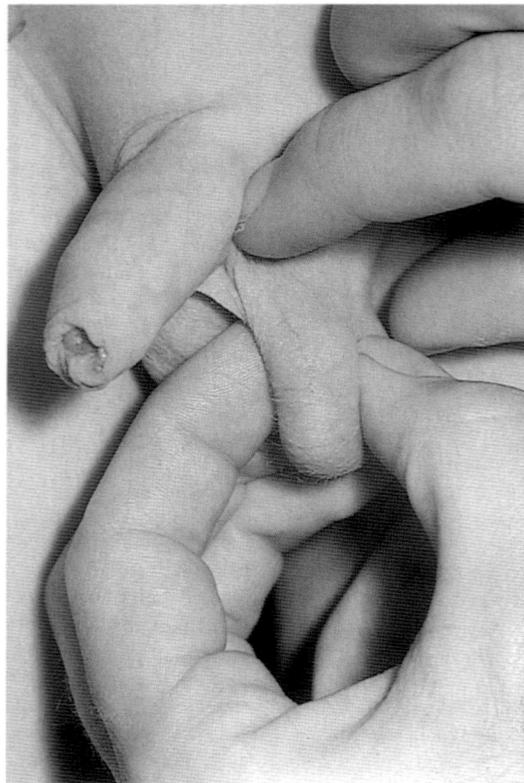

(a)

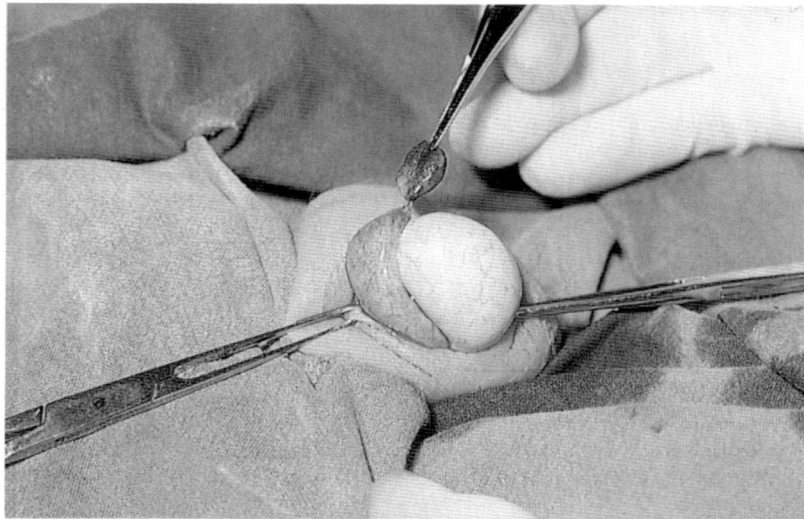

(b)

Fig. 37.31   Hydatid of Morgagni: (a) clinical appearance; (b) at operation.

CIRCUMCISION

Routine circumcision of the newborn as commonly practiced in the USA is to be condemned, the incidence of complications, including death, far outweighing the supposed advantage of avoiding such problems as carcinoma of the penis. The latter is virtually unknown in those who practice adequate hygiene. The fact that it is 'more hygienic' is often used as an excuse for circumcision but one does not chop off the ears to save washing them, or the feet because they may smell! It has been suggested that lack of carcinoma of the cervix in Jewish women is related to male circumcision but Aitken-Swan & Baird[21] showed no difference

in incidence in wives of circumcised and uncircumcised men. In 1975 a committee of the American Academy of Pediatrics stated: 'There is no absolute medical indication for the routine circumcision of the newborn. A program of good penile hygiene, simply retracting the foreskin to wash away accumulated smegma on a daily basis, would appear to offer all the advantages of circumcision without the attendant surgical risks or the increased risk of meatal stenosis'.[22]

Nonretractability of the prepuce, in childhood, should not be used as an excuse for 'lopping off an innocent and useful appendage'. Bokai[23] in 1869 was the first to draw attention to the physiological adherence

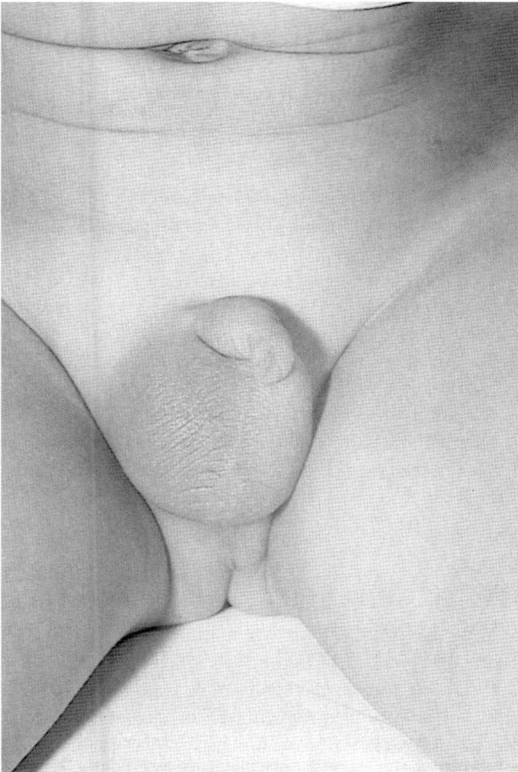

Fig. 37.32   Idiopathic scrotal edema.

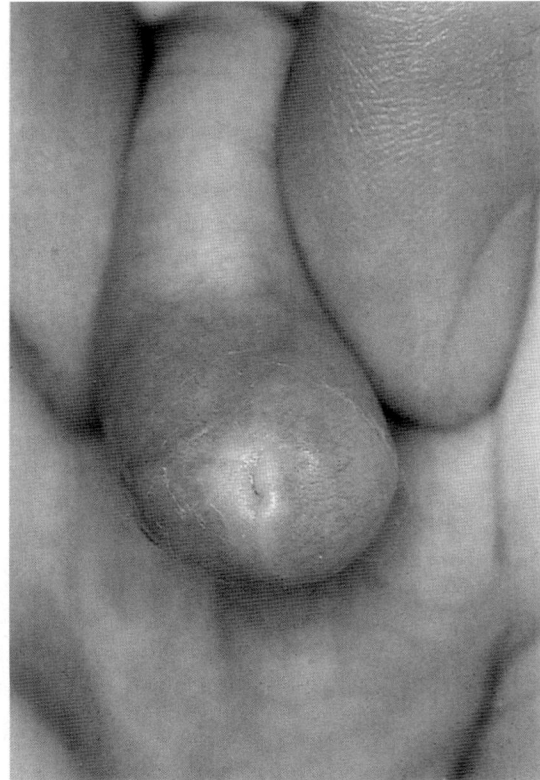

Fig. 37.33   Fibrous phimosis (balanitis xerotica obliterans).

of the foreskin, there being fusion of the glans and the prepuce developmentally. Diebert,[24] in 1933, showed that separation of the prepuce in the human penis is due to keratinization of the subpreputial epithelium, a process not complete at birth but accomplished during early childhood. Phimosis (a muzzling, from Greek *phimos* = muzzle) is thus physiological at birth.

Apart from religious or tribal reasons there are few indications for circumcision. The only valid one is a fibrous phimosis (Fig. 37.33). This may be due to inappropriate attempts at retraction at an early age, causing splitting and scarring of the preputial meatus, or perhaps is related to recurrent infections. In its most severe form it presents as balanitis xerotica obliterans with scarring of the underlying glans and urethral meatus. Meatal strictures also arise after neonatal circumcision secondary to meatitis, which arises in the absence of the protective covering of the foreskin. Ballooning of the foreskin is often seen as an indication for circumcision but it will usually resolve in time. Recurrent balanitis or balanoposthitis is possibly related to partial separation of preputial adhesion and infection of inadequately draining secretions. This can readily be resolved by separation of the adhesions. Previously this was normally carried out under general anesthesia but with the advent of EMLA cream (eutectic mixture of local anesthetics) the separation can readily be carried out painlessly and simply in the outpatient clinic or GP surgery.[25] Daily retraction with application of petroleum jelly for a few days to prevent readherence followed subsequently by normal preputial hygiene is all that is required.

In examination of the foreskin in small boys it often appears tight on attempted retraction. The simple technique advocated in 1950 by Sir James Spence[26] should be adopted: 'Retract the prepuce and you will see a pinpoint opening, but draw it forward and you will see a channel wide enough for all the purposes for which the infant needs the organ at that early age. What looks like a pinpoint opening at 7 months will become a wide channel of communication at 17 years.'

Operation

Circumcision is thus performed either for religious or tribal reasons, for fibrous phimosis or, perhaps most frequently, for remuneration! Hypospadias is a contraindication for neonatal circumcision, as is a buried penis. Neonatal circumcision is practiced, often without anesthesia using a Plastibell or a Gomco clamp. In the former, a plastic ring is placed under the foreskin and a string tied round the foreskin in a groove in the plastic device. Redundant skin together with the device separates off within a few days, leaving a very neat cosmetic result. A Gomco clamp has a similar action but rather than the string, a cutting device removes the prepuce and compresses the skin edges causing them to fuse and prevent hemorrhage. In older children a surgical cutting technique with absorbable sutures is used. In many cases of phimosis a foreskin preserving preputioplasty is sufficient.

PARAPHIMOSIS

This occurs when a narrowed foreskin is retracted behind the corona glandis penis and cannot be returned. The constriction leads to engorgement of the glans and of a cuff of foreskin distal to the tight band but behind the corona (Fig. 37.34). Firm manual compression with gauze and EMLA cream will usually reduce the edema and facilitate return of the foreskin. If this fails, injection of hyaluronidase into the swollen ring of prepuce, under general anesthesia, followed by compression, allows reduction (Fig. 37.35). Occasionally the tight constricting band needs to be incised. Circumcision is frequently advocated following paraphimosis but, surprisingly, the foreskin is usually easily retractable a fortnight after the event and recurrence is exceptional.

HYPOSPADIAS (Greek *hypo* = below, *spadon* = rent)

This is one of the commonest congenital anomalies, occurring in 1 in 400 live male births. The meatus lies in an abnormal position on the ventral aspect of the penile shaft or even scrotally or perineally. The

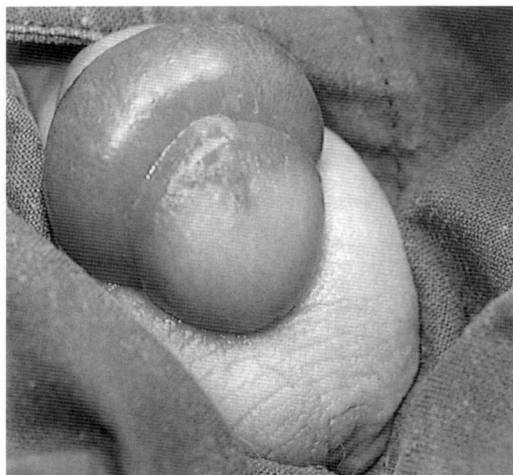

Fig. 37.34 Paraphimosis.

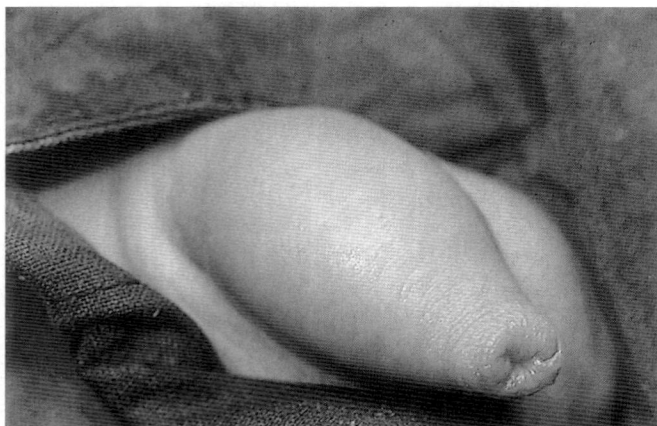

Fig. 37.35 Reduced paraphimosis.

foreskin tends to be deficient in its ventral aspect and thus is described as 'hooded'. Thirdly, there is chordee, a ventral flexion of the penis, the incidence and degree of which increases as the meatus is more proximally placed. The meatus itself may be narrowed leading to potential problems of back pressure. In the majority of cases the meatus is coronal in position; rarely it is glandular. Of the remainder, most are on the penile shaft but a few lie more proximally still in the scrotum or perineum. It is often thought that hypospadias is frequently associated with upper renal tract anomalies but in fact the incidence of these is much the same as in the general population, except perhaps in the most severe types of the deformity. In those penoscrotal and perineal types there may be associated undescended testes and the possibility of an intersex state must be investigated.

There are over 200 operations described in the literature for the correction of hypospadias. This gives some indication of the complication rate, each newly described repair aiming to be an improvement in this regard. The age for surgery is mainly the surgeon's preference. It has always been agreed that, where possible, correction should be complete by the time the boy starts school so that he may stand and pee like his peers! The more distally placed the meatus the easier it is to achieve a successful result. The essential components to the repair of the more severe varieties are release of the chordee and urethral reconstruction. The chordee is related to tight fibrous bands distal to the meatus and thought possibly to relate to atrophy of that portion of the corpus spongiosium. It is, however, possible to have chordee without hypospadias so the etiology is uncertain. Fistula formation is unfortunately common

following hypospadias repair and a few unfortunate cases require multiple interventions to achieve successful closure. The aim of all modern repairs is to create a terminal meatus on a well-formed glans and a penile shaft that is straight on erection together with a good cosmetic result (a good 'body image').

EPISPADIAS

In its most extreme form this is associated with bladder exstrophy. Otherwise it may be balanic, penile or penopubic. It may also occur in girls. In epispadias the urethra is deficient dorsally. The penis is flattened with a splayed glans and shortened, the crura being attached to often separated pubic bones. The prepuce is deficient dorsally with a ventral hood prepuce and there is dorsal chordee. Occasionally the problem is not obvious, the foreskin being complete and phimotic and the penis buried, but once the prepuce is retractable the condition is revealed. In the female the clitoris is duplicated on either side of the wide open urethra, defective dorsally (Fig. 37.36). The treatment is likewise dependent on sex and severity and the degree of continence and the success rate is variable.

URINARY TRACT INFECTION – SURGICAL ASPECTS

Medical management of urinary tract infections in neonates and in older children is discussed in Chapter 18.

The commonest cause of infection is *vesicoureteric reflux*. There remains much controversy over the role of surgery in vesicoureteric reflux.[27] Reflux in the presence of infection leads to pyelonephritis, the extension of the intrarenal reflux, if present, leading to scarring. If the child can be kept free of infection, the reflux may improve or resolve. Severe reflux should be treated surgically. This entails a transvesical operation to lengthen the submucosal tunnel of the ureter. It has a high rate of success but in a few cases leads to stenosis. More recently, a new technique involving the endoscopic injection of Teflon submucosally[28] beneath the ureteric orifice has been devised (STING – subureteric Teflon injection). This has proved very successful but long-term results have yet to be evaluated. Other substances such as Bioplastique, collagen or 'Deflux' may be used as concern has been raised that Teflon may migrate to the brain or elsewhere, although the original authors refute this concept. Deflux, a polysaccharide gel of a dextranomer and hyaluronic acid, is now the most widely used substance for this purpose.[29]

Stenosis of the lower end of the ureter requires reimplantation, the stenotic segment being excised.

Duplex ureters may be an incidental finding without causing problems in the majority of cases. If detected in investigation of a urinary tract infection, there is usually an associated anomaly. The ureter from the upper pole tends to enter the bladder at a lower level. Thus the lower pole ureter has a shorter intramural course and a tendency to reflux. The upper pole ureter has a tendency to stenosis, an association with a ureterocele and a possible tendency to open below the bladder neck, leading to incontinence. It may even open ectopically into the vagina.

If there is reflux of both ureters, reimplantation of both, in their common sheath, is usually the treatment of choice. Occasionally they join at a higher level leading to yo-yo reflux between the two and a predisposition to infection. This is treated either by heminephroureterectomy if one moiety is shown to have poor function on isotope studies, or else anastomosis at the level of the pelves may be advocated.

A *ureterocele* may arise in relation to the upper pole ureter. It represents herniation of the intramural portion of the ureter into the bladder. Its meatus may be stenosed, may open below the bladder neck or may even on occasion allow reflux. The ureterocele may obstruct the lower ureter or even lead to bladder outlet obstruction by prolapsing across the internal urethral meatus. The ureterocele may be incised endoscopically to relieve an acute problem, especially of value in the infant, or may be excised with ureteric reimplantation,

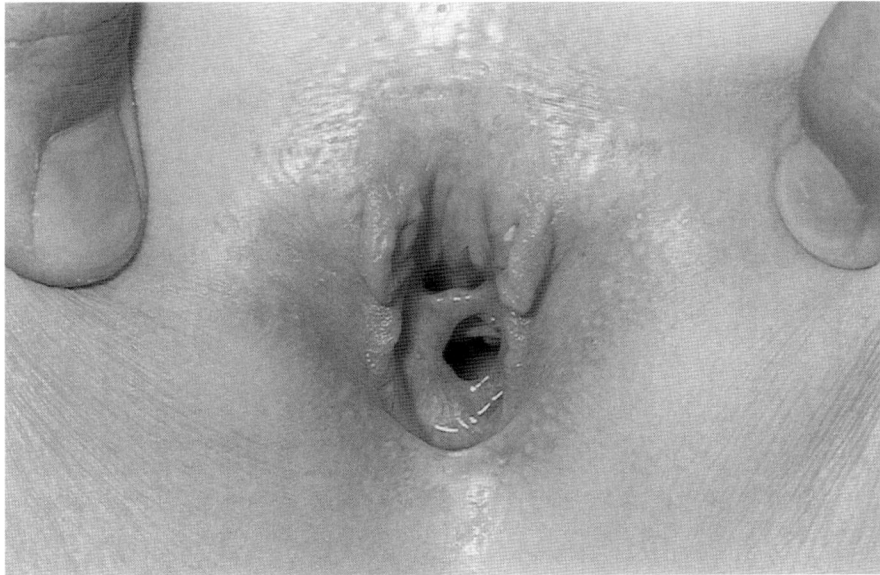

Fig. 37.36 Female epispadias.

if appropriate. If an isotope scan shows minimal function in the affected moiety then partial nephroureterectomy may be the treatment of choice.

Hydronephrosis may be due to obstruction at the pelviureteric junction (PUJ) or, if the ureter is also dilated, to vesicoureteric obstruction or vesicoureteric reflux. Obstruction at the PUJ may be due to congenital narrowing, high insertion of the ureter, or aberrant renal vessels. The presentation is usually with investigation of a urinary tract infection. It may be diagnosed antenatally or in the older child may present with a Dietl's crisis, acute obstruction at the PUJ secondary to kinking after an abnormal fluid load. This may not present until the first beer-drinking spree in a young adult! In the neonate, antenatally diagnosed hydronephrosis may be a stable condition that can be monitored with serial ultrasound examinations and isotope studies as some infants will acquire normal drainage across the PUJ as they grow. At any age an isotope study will indicate whether the kidney has already suffered major damage. If its contribution to total renal function is less than 10% then nephrectomy is the treatment of choice. If there is doubt in an acute presentation, a percutaneous nephrostomy tube may be inserted under ultrasound guidance and further isotope studies, after draining for 1–2 weeks, may show improvement. If there is reasonable function but a definite PUJ obstruction then the treatment of choice is a pyeloplasty. This involves excision of the redundant extra renal pelvis and pelviureteric junction with reanastomosis of the proximal ureter to the dependent portion of the repaired pelvis.

CONGENITAL VASCULAR MALFORMATIONS

Hemangiomas

These are malformations of developing blood vessels. They commonly appear in the skin but may develop in any organ.

Strawberry nevus

These usually appear at about a week of age and may rapidly enlarge in the first few months of life. They then stop growing and usually resolve spontaneously by intravascular thrombosis. This process is normally complete by 5–7 years of age, leaving only a minor blemish or none at all. Unless they are causing a problem such as occlusion of the eyelids, which can lead to permanent visual impairment, surgery is best avoided. The parents must be reassured that even the most unsightly

facial lesions will resolve within a year or two of the child starting school. A few involute so rapidly that they become ulcerated. This is most common in lesions subject to trauma as on the perineum or back. Scarring will result from ulceration.

Stork mark

This is a superficial capillary hemangioma that may be seen on the forehead, bridge of the nose and upper eyelids. The lesion is often v-shaped, pointing down to the nose and there is a corresponding mark on the nape of the neck. These marks presumably arise from the stork suspending the baby by the head in its beak! Again the parents can be reassured that the frontal lesion will resolve spontaneously although the nuchal one will commonly persist throughout life, usually hidden by the hair.

Port wine stain (nevus flammeus)

Unlike a strawberry nevus this is present at birth and may be very disfiguring, as it becomes darker and increasingly nodular with age. In recent years laser treatment with a pulsed tuneable dye laser has considerably improved the appearance of these lesions in childhood.[30]

Sturge–Weber syndrome is a severe form of port wine stain on the scalp and face, in the distribution of one of the branches of the trigeminal nerve, associated with an underlying vascular anomaly of the arachnoid covering the cerebral hemisphere. This leads to epilepsy, hemiplegia and mental retardation.

Cavernous hemangioma

These may occur alone or in association with a capillary lesion in the overlying skin. They increase in size after birth but usually in proportion to the growth of the infant. Most resolve spontaneously but some persist, requiring excision, if appropriate, or injection with sclerosants. Care must be taken in the latter option not to lead to ulceration of the skin. Very large lesions may lead to high output cardiac failure due to arteriovenous shunting. Embolization under radiological control may be required although some lesions regress on oral corticosteroid therapy.

Kasabach–Merritt syndrome

In the neonate, large or multiple hemangiomas are occasionally associated with a generalized bleeding disorder caused by the trapping of platelets within them, which produces a profound thrombocytopenia. A course of prednisone, 2–4 mg/kg per 24 h can effect dramatic improvement, or, if this fails, embolization of the hemangioma can be considered.

Lymphangioma

These are similar to hemangiomas but involve lymphatics. They may also occur anywhere in the body but in particular they may present as a *cystic hygroma* most commonly arising in the cervical region (see earlier under 'Head and neck').

Mixed *hamartomatous* lesions may contain hemangiomatous and lymphangiomatous elements.

CLEFT LIP AND PALATE

The main etiological factor in these anomalies is genetic. In about one third of patients there is a family history. The incidence is about 1 in 700 births. The ratio of cleft lip (with or without cleft palate) to cleft palate alone is about 2:1.

The lip, alveolus and the portion of the hard palate anterior to the incisive foramen are derived from the maxillary and medial nasal processes. These fuse by the sixth week. The remainder of the palate forms from the palatine shelves. These grow from the maxillary swellings and fuse from anterior to posterior in the ninth to twelfth weeks. At the same time the nasal septum grows down to meet the palate.

Clefts result from failure of these lines of fusion. They vary in severity from a notch in the margin of the lip to a complete cleft in the maxilla. They may be unilateral or bilateral. Figure 37.37 illustrates the major types of cleft lip and palate.

Treatment is aimed at both a good cosmetic result with normal growth as well as a functional closure to facilitate swallowing and speech. The repair of the lip and alveolus is usually performed at around 3 months of age and the palatal defect between 6 and 15 months to give the best chance of normal speech. A multidisciplinary approach is required including a plastic surgeon, orthodontist, speech therapist, ENT surgeon, audiologist, etc.

BURNS

Thermal injury is a common childhood accident in all countries. Predisposing factors include primitive, poor or overcrowded housing, families under stress, flammable clothing, ignorance and lack of insight in parents.

The toddler, exploring his world on hands and knees or with unsteady gait, is a ready victim and boys are burned more often than girls. Scalding with hot liquids is by far the commonest cause of injury in this age group. Flame burns are less common than they were, but house fires still claim victims with the added risk of smoke inhalation injury. Other causes include contact with hot objects, chemicals, friction and electric current.

Severity of injury

This depends on three main factors:

1. **Extent.** Heat damages the underlying capillaries, causing them to leak protein-rich fluid. The resulting loss from the circulation reaches a critical level when the extent of the burn exceeds about 10% of the body surface area, and the child will require i.v. resuscitation. Extent is measured by using a chart (Fig. 37.38) or by taking the area of the hand as about 1%. Erythema should be discounted when making this measurement.

2. **Depth.** Healing depends on whether epithelial elements survive in the dermis. Partial-thickness burns will heal by outgrowth of epithelial cells from hair follicles and sweat glands; they can be subdivided into superficial, which heal in less than 3 weeks and do not cause scars, and deep dermal, which take longer to heal and cause hypertrophic scars. Deep or full-thickness burns can heal only from the margins. The depth of tissue destruction is determined by the temperature of the agent, the duration of its contact, the skin thickness and the victim's age.

3. **Site.** Burns of the face and hands are particularly serious, and those of the perineum cause problems in management. While the skin is the site of injury in most instances, the epithelial linings of the respiratory and upper alimentary tracts may be damaged separately or together with a skin burn.

Pathophysiology

Local

The fluid loss from the circulation is at its maximum immediately after the burn and decreases over the following 48 h. A deep burn destroys significant numbers of red cells. The insulating and protective functions of skin are lost, and body heat, water and electrolytes pass from the body in much increased amounts. Nitrogen losses also rise.

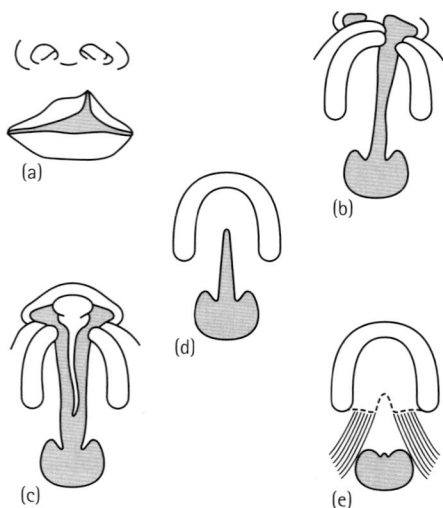

Fig. 37.37 (a) Incomplete unilateral cleft lip. (b) Complete unilateral cleft lip and palate. (c) Complete bilateral cleft lip and palate. (d) Isolated cleft of soft palate. (e) Submucous cleft palate.

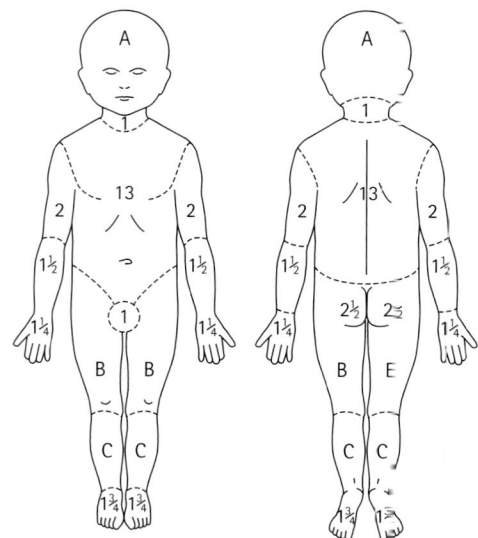

Fig. 37.38 Chart for calculating percentage area burned in childhood. A = ½ of head; B = ½ of one thigh; C = ½ of one leg. The percentages of these areas vary with age.

General

There is a massive rise in the secretion of stress hormones.[31] Urinary water and sodium excretion fall and potassium and nitrogen losses increase. The larger the burn, the more profound the reaction tends to be. The catabolic phase lasts until the burn is healed.

Treatment

First aid

After separating the child from the source of the injury, clothing should be removed and the burn cooled by immersion in lukewarm water or by use of a wet cloth (the risk of hypothermia must be remembered). The burn can then be covered with a clean cloth or clingfilm until definitive local treatment is possible.

Pain

A partial-thickness burn is very painful, while deeply burned skin is anesthetic. Potent analgesia by the i.m. or i.v. route is essential. Throughout treatment, attention must be focused on the avoidance of pain during practical procedures; analgesic or anesthetic drugs should be selected and used with precision.

Shock

Where the area burned exceeds 10% of the body surface, an i.v. infusion will be required. The restoration and maintenance of an effective circulation can be achieved with plasma, purified protein solution, dextran or balanced salt solutions. The quantities to be given vary with the weight of the child and the extent of the burn. The rate of administration is rapid initially and usually lasts for 36–48 h. Close patient observation, hourly urinary output measurement by an indwelling urethral catheter and serial hemoglobin and hematocrit estimations provide adequate control data. A central venous pressure line can be helpful in the severe case, but it has been indicted as a major source of infection if maintained for days in the burned patient.

System management

Respiratory system

Where a child has been rescued from a burning building or where clothing has burned over the face, airway problems can be anticipated. Arterial blood gases should be monitored and intubation and assisted ventilation may be necessary. Bronchopneumonia is a frequent later complication of large burns.

Central nervous system

Toddlers with even minor scalds are liable to convulse in the first 2 d with serious or even fatal outcome. The cause is thought to lie with early fluid shifts and the lag that occurs within the brain and its meninges. Papilledema is not always present. Diazepam and mannitol (1 g/kg i.v. over 20 min) gain quick control of fits and brain swelling, and phenytoin sodium and dexamethasone prolong the effect. Focal neurological deficits may occur at any time, probably as a result of septic emboli.

Urinary system

In the first 2 d after injury increased levels of antidiuretic hormone limit urinary output. Infusion should be used circumspectly and a serum sodium level of not less than 130 mmol/L should be maintained.

In deep burns, thermal damage to red blood cells causes hemoglobinuria, which may lead to tubular necrosis and renal failure. If rapid restoration of circulating fluid volume does not clear the urine, a solute diuretic such as 20% mannitol should be given without delay. A catheter may be required to monitor urine output or avoid contamination of the burn. It should be removed as soon as possible.

Cardiovascular system

Electrical current injury may cause cardiac damage and an ECG examination is advisable after such an injury. General anesthesia is best avoided until the tracing has returned to normal.

Tachycardia persists throughout recovery from a large burn and is largely a product of a high metabolic rate to offset the high evaporative heat losses. Heat regulation is disturbed and the child must be kept warm to avoid hypothermia.

Hemopoietic system

Loss of red cells, destroyed by a deep burn, must be replaced by early transfusion. Further losses take place during surgery and erythropoiesis remains depressed until a large burn has healed. The red cell mass must be maintained by transfusion if the body is to achieve quick healing.

Alimentary system

Gastric stasis is common in the early hours after a large burn but oral intake should be started as soon as possible. Ranitidine has reduced the incidence of hemorrhagic gastritis and Curling's ulcer is now rarely seen.

Accurate naked weights, obtained twice weekly from admission, guide the clinician through the early weight gain of fluid retention, diuresis, the catabolic phase, and the anabolic phase that comes more quickly and strongly in the child.

Nutrition

Daily fluid intake must take account of increased losses through the burn wound. A high calorie intake is needed to balance heat loss and minimize lean tissue breakdown. A protein intake at the upper end of the normal range is adequate. Iron and vitamins C and B complex are supplemented to combat anemia and aid wound healing. The seriously burned child cannot take food in solid form and it is kinder and more effective to give most of this as a fortified liquid feed. A fine-bore nasogastric feeding tube for this purpose should be passed in all children with burns over 15%. The planned intake should be achieved stepwise over the first 1–2 weeks. Early forcing of high food intake may predispose to a post-stress diabetes that may be resistant to insulin. Neglect of food intake will result in a profound weight loss, hypoproteinemia, and failure of the burn to heal.

Musculoskeletal system

While immobilization may be unavoidable for practical reasons, its use will increase muscle wasting and delay the recovery of an effective musculature. Regular active exercises should be performed wherever possible. Joint positioning and joint movement require constant attention if severe, and possibly permanent, joint contracture is to be avoided.

Local care

Infection is the major complication of all but the smallest burn. It can destroy surviving epithelium and penetrate a deep burn, with a risk of invasive infection. The commonest organism is *Staphylococcus aureus* but the beta-hemolytic streptococcus is feared for its destructive capabilities and *Pseudomonas aeruginosa* can be dangerous on extensive burns. Constant monitoring, scrupulous hygiene and prevention of overcrowding are essential to control infection. Large burns should be isolated. Where appropriate, early excision and grafting can lead to healing before infection can occur. Local antibacterial agents are valuable but systemic antibiotics must be used with care as they can easily lead to superinfection with resistant organisms or fungi.

A superficial burn will, if protected from infection and trauma, heal in less than 3 weeks and is usually dressed with a well-padded gauze and cotton wool dressing with a Vaseline gauze inner layer. Deeper burns need skin grafting, unless very small.

Toxic shock syndrome

This can follow even very minor burns in the child[32] and can have a mortality rate of 11%.[33] It is therefore essential to recognize and treat it on suspicion. Signs are of an unwell, irritable child, 3 d or longer after a burn, with pyrexia and three or more of the following: rash, hypotension, diarrhea or vomiting, inflamed mucous membranes, *Staphylococcus aureus* on wound swabs and occlusive dressings.

Treatment is with i.v. fluids, gammaglobulins (0.4 g/kg) or fresh blood or fresh frozen plasma (10 ml/kg over 4 h), exposure of the burn, topical antibacterial agent and i.v. antibiotics.

Scarring

A superficial burn should leave little physical trace; the healed skin will be dry and should be creamed several times a day. With deeper injuries, scarring is unavoidable. The hypertrophic scar reaction is most intense in childhood. On the face, it disfigures and distorts features. On the flexures, it limits joint movement. Unrelieved scar contracture impedes growth of that part and deforms the growing skeleton. Spontaneous resolution of the hypertrophic scar is slow, variable and incomplete. Its full development may be cut short and its regression accelerated by elastic compression, intralesional injection of steroid hormones, or application of silicone gel. Secondary surgical procedures are often required to replace the worst scars, their timing and scope being dictated by the physical, psychological and educational needs of the child.

Psychological support

A close rapport between child, nurse, parents and doctor is fundamental in such a taxing hospital stay, which can extend over months. The child deserves explanation, occupation, and freedom from recurring pain. The parents, whose guilt feelings should be appreciated, should be incorporated into the therapeutic effort. The help of an interested and experienced psychiatrist may be invaluable.

Prognosis

Intensive early therapy can resuscitate a child with the gravest of surface burns. However, long-term survival is rare where 70% or more of the skin is destroyed. A child who survives a burn with significant scarring faces the prospect of physical and psychological problems that will probably become worse during adolescence. Continued longterm support is needed for patient and family for many years.

REFERENCES (* Level 1 evidence)

1. Clements BS, Warner JO. Pulmonary sequestration and related bronchopulmonary vascular malformations: nomenclature and classification based on anatomical and embryological considerations. Thorax 1987; 42:401–408.
2. Bohn D, Tamura M, Perrin D, et al. Ventilatory predictors of pulmonary hypoplasia in congenital diaphragmatic hernia, confirmed by morphologic assessment. J Pediatr 1987; 111:423–431.
3. Sakai H, Tamura M, Hosokawa Y, et al. Effect of surgical repair on respiratory mechanics in congenital diaphragmatic hernia. J Pediatr 1987; 111:432–438.
4. MacKinlay GA, Burtles R. Oesophageal atresia: paralysis and ventilation in management of the wide gap. Pediatr Surg Int 1987; 2:10–12.
5. Hancock BJ, Wiseman NE. Congenital duodenal obstruction: the impact of an antenatal diagnosis. J Pediatr Surg 1989; 24:1027–1031.
6. Hirschsprung H. Stuhlragheit Neugeborener in Fotge von Dilation und Hypertrophie des Colons. Jahreb Kinderheilk 1887; 27:1–7.
7. Bodian M, Carter CO. A family study of Hirschsprung's disease. Ann Hum Genet 1963; 26:261–277.
8. Lee SL, Beyer TD, Kim SS, et al. Initial nonoperative management and delayed closure for treatment of giant omphaloceles. J Pediatr Surg 2006; 41:1846–1849.
9. Bianchi A, Dickson AP and Alizai NK. Elective delayed midgut reduction – No Anesthesia for Gastroschisis: Selection and Conversion criteria. J Pediatr Surg 2002; 37:1334–1336.
10. Owen A, Marven S, Jackson L, et al. Experience of bedside preformed silo staged reduction and closure for gastroschisis. J Pediatr Surg 2006; 41:1830–1835.
11. Holschneider A, Hutson J, Pena A, et al. Preliminary report on the International Conference for the Development of Standards for the Treatment of Anorectal Malformations. J Pediatr Surg 2005; 40:1521–1526.
12. Stephens FD. Wingspread Conference on Anorectal Malformations. Racine: Wisconsin; 1984.
13. de Vries PA, Pena A. Posterior sagittal anorectoplasty. J Pediatr Surg 1982; 17:638–643.
14. Kasai M, Kimura S, Asakura Y. Surgical treatment of biliary atresia. J Pediatr Surg 1968; 3:665–675.
15. Ogita S, Tsuto T, Nakamura K, et al. OK-432 therapy for lymphangioma in children: why and how does it work?. J Pediatr Surg 1996; 31:477–480.
16. Ramstedt C. Zur Operation der angeborenen Pylorusstenose. Medizinische Klinik (Berlin) 1912; 8:1702–1705.
17. Stiles HJ. (original operation note 3 February 1910 – personal possession) 1910.
18. Rothenburg SS. Experience with 220 consecutive laparoscopic Nissen fundoplications in infants and children. J Pediatr Surg 1998; 33:297–305.
19. Wilson-Storey D, MacKinlay GA. The superior mesenteric artery syndrome. J R Coll Surg Edin 1986; 31:175–178.
20. Atwell JD. Ascent of the testis: fact or fiction. Br J Urol 1985; 57:474–477.
21. Aitken-Swan J, Baird D. Circumcision and cancer of the cervix. Br J Cancer 1965; 19:217–227.
22. Report of the Ad Hoc Task Force on Circumcision. Pediatrics 1975; 56:610–611.
23. Bokai J. A fitma (preputium) sejtes adatapadasa a makkoz gyermakelnel. Orvosi Hetil 1869; 4:583–587.
24. Diebert GA. The separation of the prepuce in the human penis. Anatomical Records 1933; 54:387–393.
25. MacKinlay GA. Save the prepuce. Painless separation of preputial adhesions in the outpatient clinic. BMJ 1988; 297:590–591.
26. Spence, Sir James (1950). Spence on circumcision. Lancet 1964; ii:902.
27. White RHR, O'Donnell B. Controversies in therapeutics Management of urinary tract infection and vesico-ureteric reflux in children. 1. Operative treatment has no advantage over medical management (RHRW). 2. The case for surgery (BO'D). BMJ 1990; 300:1391–1394.
28. Puri P, Ninan GK, Sirana R. Subureteric Teflon injection (STING) Result of a European Survey. Eur Urol 1995; 27:71–73.
29. Puri P, Chertin B, Velaydham M, et al. Treatment of vesicoureteric reflux by endoscopic injection of dextranomer/hyaluronic acid copolymer: preliminary results. J Urol 2003; 170:1541–1544.
30. Tan OT, Sherwood K, Gilchrist BA. Treatment of children with port-wine stains using the flashlamp-pulsed tuneable dye laser. N Engl J Med 1989; 320:416–442.
31. Smith A, McIntosh N, Thomson M, et al. The stress effect of thermal injury on the hormones controlling fluid balance. Baillière's Clinical Paediatrics. London: Baillière; 1995.
32. Cole RP, Shakespeare PG. Toxic shock syndrome in scalded children. Burns 1990; 16:221–224.
33. de Saxe MJ, Hawtin P, Wieneke AA. Toxic shock syndrome in Britain – epidemiology and microbiology. Postgrad Med J 1985; 61:5–8.

38

Pain and palliative care

Richard F Howard, Finella Craig

INTRODUCTION

Relief from pain and suffering is a basic human right no matter what age, level of cognitive development or ability to communicate. Although children's pain is still often under-recognized around the world, in recent years there have been enormous advances in our understanding of pain in childhood.[1] Today, in the twenty-first century, it seems incredible to think that less than 20 years ago there was considerable debate about whether newborn infants were capable of feeling pain, and whether the benefits of potent analgesics outweighed their risks in young children. Since that time the study of the developmental neurobiology of pain has left little doubt that even the youngest and most premature infant is capable of pain perception, and we have learned to safely manage pain at all ages.[1,2]

Pain is a subjective experience, not necessarily proportional to any underlying physiological damage and is powerfully influenced by psychological, social and cultural factors. A common definition is that adopted by the IASP (International Association for the Study of Pain), the largest multidisciplinary international professional organization concerned with pain research and practice:

> 'Pain is an unpleasant sensory and emotional experience associated with actual or potential tissue damage, or described in terms of such damage. Note: The inability to communicate verbally does not negate the possibility that an individual is experiencing pain and is in need of appropriate pain-relieving treatment.'

Children may experience pain for many reasons, and because of its complex nature a rigid system of classification is not possible. For clinical purposes it can be helpful to consider painful experiences as acute, chronic and recurrent. Acute pain, lasting days or weeks is often clearly related to causes such as trauma or common illnesses, like accidents, ear and throat infections, appendicitis and sickle cell disease. Medical interventions are also an important cause of acute pain including immunization, diagnostic procedures and postopera-

tive pain. Chronic pain, lasting months or years may also be associated with obvious underlying disease such as chronic rheumatological disorders, orthopedic problems in cerebral palsy and progressive malignant disease. However a large group of children with chronic pain, which may be constant but is often recurrent, have much less obvious tissue damage or have pain persisting far beyond the expected normal of period recovery from injury. These pains may occur in a wide range of sites, may be associated with other diffuse symptoms including sympathetically mediated changes and are frequently associated with prominent and sometimes extreme behavioral changes.

Physiologically, pain can also be classified as either 'nociceptive' or 'neuropathic' according to the underlying neural mechanism. Nociceptive pain is that which results from a normal, intact, nervous system. It is usually self-limiting, resolving as the underlying injury resolves, and it will respond to the 'classical' analgesics such as nonsteroidal anti-inflammatory drugs (NSAIDs) and opioids. In contrast, neuropathic pain is due to damage or malfunction of the nervous system, it is particularly characterized by spontaneous pain, unpleasant abnormal painful sensations or dysesthesias and sometimes associated sensory deficits. Neuropathic pain may persist despite treatment for considerable periods, sometimes the underlying injury is not obvious, and crucially it does not respond well to classical analgesics and may require alternative treatment strategies. Both nociceptive and neuropathic pain may co-exist in the same patient, and accurate diagnosis will assist in the selection of appropriate therapy.

ASSESSMENT

A thorough assessment of pain forms the foundation for its prevention and management. There is substantial literature on pain assessment in children, and the subject has been extensively reviewed.[3–7] Children's age, developmental level and also the type of pain they are experiencing will influence the approach to assessment, and in all situations a broad picture acknowledging the complex nature of pain and the multiple factors which influence it needs to be constructed. The majority of available pain assessment tools are designed to measure pain intensity in developmentally normal individuals, mostly in acute settings. Recently tools have also been developed for use in children with severe neurological disability.[8,9] Questionnaires designed to measure functional impairment due to chronic pain are also available; see later sections of this chapter for more detail.[10,11]

SELF-ASSESSMENT

Since pain is a subjective experience the ideal or 'gold standard' approach is one of self-reporting with as much information as possible about the pain coming directly from the child. A detailed history is especially important when the pain is chronic or the cause unknown and aims to discover the sites of the pain, its nature, frequency, severity, precipitating and relieving factors and other associated symptoms. Additional wider aspects to consider include the effect of the pain on the child and family's daily life, their coping skills and the meaning of the pain for them and within their culture. A variety of formal self-report tools to measure pain intensity have now been developed and validated; the majority of these have been designed to help children quantify acute pain usually on a numerical scale, typically in the range 0–10, where 0 equals no pain and 10 the worst pain imaginable. They can also be valuable in the wider assessment of long-term pain and also to monitor the effectiveness of treatment. The type of self-report scale used will depend on age, developmental level and setting. No scale can be universally recommended and each has its advantages and limitations.[12] However there are many children in whom self-reporting cannot be used, and in whom one or more proxy measures such as behaviors or physiological parameters have to be used.

ADOLESCENTS AND SCHOOL-AGE CHILDREN

Older children are usually able to use classical visual analogue scale (VAS), and numerical rating scales (Fig. 38.1). More user-friendly scales such as those using drawings of faces depicting different degrees of

pain are suitable for this age group and can also be used for pre-school children down to the age of about 4 years.[13,14]

TODDLERS AND YOUNG CHILDREN

Toddlers and young children can provide simple information about their pain and its site but may not have the abstract concepts or verbal ability to describe its nature or intensity.[3-5] Young children tend to choose the extreme ends of the scales, and the type of face and the way it is depicted may also influence their ratings.[15,16] Another example is the poker chip tool, which uses small plastic blocks to represent 'pieces of hurt' with options of picking up between 1 and 4 to indicate pain severity.[17]

BEHAVIORAL AND MULTIDIMENSIONAL ASSESSMENT

Infants, preverbal children and children with severe developmental delay are unable to report their own pain. Assessment depends on observation of the child and knowing them well. Health care workers consistently underestimate children's pain compared with children's own self-reports and although parents' ratings are closer to the children's own they still tend to underestimate the pain.[18]

In infants indicators for pain that have been studied include facial expression, cry, motor movements and changes in behavioral state and patterns.[5] Preterm infants' responses appear to be less vigorous than those of full-term infants and their expression of pain cues are more subtle. Evaluation of pain through facial expression is best established and typical characteristics that express pain include eyes tightly closed, furrowed brows, broadened nasal root and deepened nasolabial furrow with a squared mouth and taut tongue.[19] A variety of tools to measure pain in neonates and infants are available; some 'multidimensional scales' combine behaviors and physiological parameters.[5] A number of behavioral scales have also been developed for preverbal children that may also be used in older children unable or unwilling to self-report. Two have been used extensively for postoperative pain are FLACC (Fig. 38.1), and CHEOPS, which use observation of verbal and facial

FLACC

Behavioral pain assessment

Categories	Scoring		
	0	1	2
Face	No particular expression or smile	Occasional grimace or frown, withdrawn, disinterested	Frequent to constant quivering chin, clenched jaw
Legs	Normal position or relaxed	Uneasy, restless, tense	Kicking, or legs drawn up
Activity	Lying quietly, normal position, moves easily	Squirming, shifting back and forth, tense	Arched, rigid or jerking
Cry	No cry (awake or asleep)	Moans or whimpers, occasional complaint	Crying steadily, screams or sobs, frequent complaints
Consolability	Content, relaxed	Reassured by occasional touching, hugging or being talked to, distractible	Difficult to console or comfort

Each of the five categories: (F) Face; (L) Legs; (A) Activity; (C) Cry; (C) Consolability; is scored from 0–2 which results in a total score between 0 and 10

Wong And Baker

Self-report pain assessment

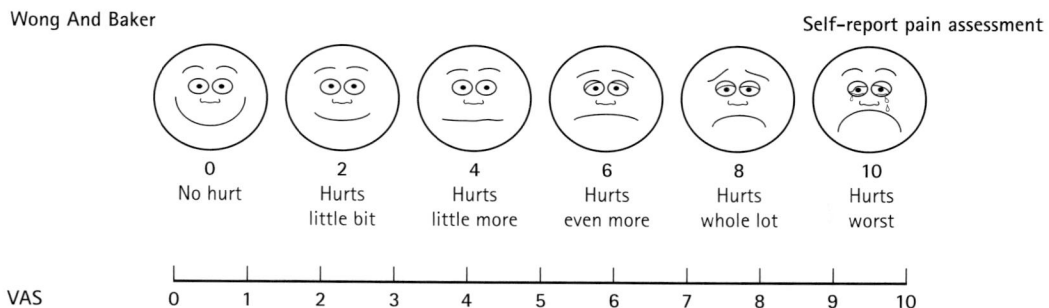

| 0 No hurt | 2 Hurts little bit | 4 Hurts little more | 6 Hurts even more | 8 Hurts whole lot | 10 Hurts worst |

VAS 0 1 2 3 4 5 6 7 8 9 10

Fig. 38.1   Behavioral and self-report pain scales (Adapted from [13,21]).

expressions of pain, behaviors, changes in muscle tone, and movement.[20,21] In intensive care settings the multi-dimensional COMFORT score has become popular.[22]

Assessment of pain in children with severe developmental delay poses a complex problem that has only recently been addressed by researchers. One approach is to document 'normal' and 'pain-related' behaviors in individual children over a period of time in order to estimate pain intensity associated with painful events such as surgery.[9]

PHYSIOLOGICAL RESPONSES

Physiological responses to pain are activated by the autonomic nervous system and include tachycardia, sweating, increasing secretion of catecholamines and adrenocorticoid hormones. These have not proved to be clinically reliable or useful as they are part of a global response to stress and not specific to pain; also, measurement of hormonal changes is invasive and slow.

CLINICAL MANAGEMENT OF PAIN

Both nonpharmacological and drug treatments of pain have a place in clinical pain management, the balance depending on the mechanism, source and circumstances of pain.

NONPHARMACOLOGICAL APPROACHES
Psychological

The unpleasant nature of pain and the many factors influencing it mean that all pain and pain management is immersed in a psychological context that needs to be taken into account.

Some approaches are very simple. Parents offer children the support children value most at times of stress, but they are still sometimes mistakenly excluded from their child's presence and care. Clinical staff need to be aware of the distress and anxiety that pain causes children, particularly in the Accident and Emergency unit, postoperatively and on the wards. Simple and honest explanations of disease processes and thorough preparation for procedures and surgery can help reassure children and families, enhance feelings of control and so reduce anxiety.[23]

A variety of more formal techniques have also been used effectively and well validated in a wide range of clinical situations, including the use of relaxation, cognitive approaches including distraction, imagery and thought blocking, and hypnosis.[24-28] Children are often very willing and co-operative subjects and enjoy the novelty of these techniques and the sense of control they engender. Such techniques are very effective for procedural pain management, and they are also used in a variety of chronic pain conditions to improve pain coping skills, with particular success in children with headache.[29]

Physiotherapy

Physiotherapy has a range of useful techniques that can contribute to pain management and are particularly important for children with chronic pain. These aim to restore optimal physical function by promoting strength and mobility, as well as to decrease pain. They include the use of active and passive exercise, often combined with goal setting and close monitoring. A number of other physical pain reduction techniques are frequently used concurrently such as desensitization of cutaneous hypersensitivity, local heat and cooling, hydrotherapy, ultrasound and TENS (transcutaneous electrical nerve stimulation).[30,31]

PHARMACOLOGICAL APPROACHES
Selection of analgesics: multi-modal analgesia

A relatively small range of analgesics is used in children. Selection of the most appropriate depends upon the cause and severity of the pain, the age and general condition of the patient, the setting and the facilities for supervision monitoring and treatment of any side-effects. The underlying neural mechanisms responsible for the clinical characteristics of both acute and chronic pain, and the influence of development on pain processing are becoming better understood. Increased pain sensitivity and tenderness (hyperalgesia and allodynia) at and near the site of injury are known to be the result of multiple changes within the CNS involving many neural and chemical mediators. The individual components of these 'pain pathways' can be targeted by combining different analgesics in order to compound their effects, thereby increasing efficacy.[32] A combination of analgesic drugs and techniques, with complimentary modes of action, maximizes the therapeutic advantage of each whilst keeping the doses and side effects to a minimum. This is the rationale underpinning the 'pain ladder' concept, in which new and more potent drugs are added as pain increases (Fig. 38.2). Whenever possible, analgesic pharmacotherapy is also combined with suitable nonpharmacological techniques in order to further reduce the pain response.

Mild analgesics
Paracetamol

Paracetamol is one of the most widely used drugs in children; it is available in oral, i.v. and rectal preparations. It is regarded as a safe and effective analgesic for mild and moderately severe pain; it can be used at all ages, including the neonate. Traditionally, paracetamol is thought to act centrally. Analgesia is attributed to inhibition of cyclo-oxygenase and thereby prostaglandin production in the CNS; other mechanisms have also been proposed including antagonism of serotonin (5HT) and possibly N-methyl D-aspartate (NMDA) receptors.[33,34]

Although several systematic reviews have demonstrated the analgesic efficacy of paracetamol for mild pain in the adult, few studies have been performed in children.[35-40] The analgesic efficacy of paracetamol is probably low; the correct dosage is important and for moderate or severe pain is probably best combined with other agents, typically opioids and nonsteroidal anti-inflammatory drugs (NSAIDs). Paracetamol does not reduce the pain response to heel lance or to circumcision in neonates although it does appear to have a small effect on late post-circumcision pain.[41,42]

Paracetamol is conjugated to glucuronide, sulphate or cysteine and excreted. In normal circumstances less than 10% is metabolized to a potentially hepatotoxic metabolite, N acetyl P amino benzoquinone imine (NAPQI). NAPQI is neutralized by combination with hepatic glutathione or with N acetyl cysteine and excreted harmlessly unless this pathway is saturated due to overdose or conjugates are in reduced supply. The p450 isoenzyme responsible for metabolism of paracetamol is developmentally regulated, with lower activity in the neonate, and this may confer some protection. However reduced clearance in neonates may lead to accumulation of the drug and its metabolites and so a reduced daily dose is usually recommended. Paracetamol hepatotoxicity is a well recognized dose-dependent complication associated with acute ingestion of more than 150 mg/kg. Long-term paracetamol treatment can also lead to toxicity at lower doses and it has been suggested that the maximum recommended dose should not be given for more than

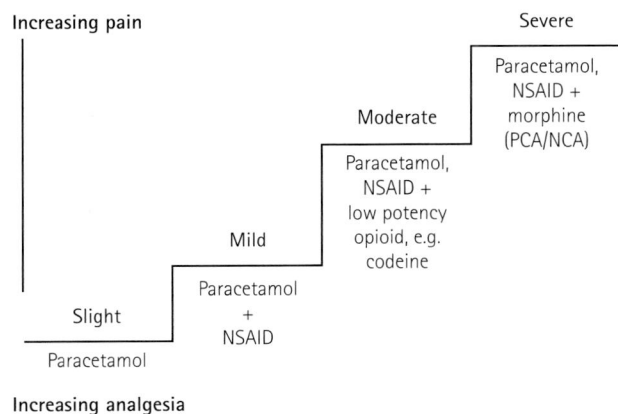

Fig. 38.2   Analgesic ladder. NCA, nurse-controlled analgesia. PCA, patient-controlled analgesia.

5 d.[43] Risk factors for toxicity include: chronic ingestion, especially in the malnourished due to reduced hepatic glutathione stores; pre-existing liver impairment (single doses are reasonably safe); hepatic enzyme induction and miscalculation or misinterpretation of commercial package labeling leading to accidental overdose.

The recommended total daily oral dose is 30 mg/kg in pre-term neonates 28–32 weeks' postmenstrual age, 60 mg/kg up to 3 months and 90 mg/kg in infants and older children.[44] This is usually given in divided doses 3 or 4 times daily. Absorption after oral paracetamol is excellent, rectal bio-availability is lower and more variable at 25–98% of the administered dose. In order to achieve therapeutic plasma levels a higher initial rectal dose is recommended (of the order of 30–40 mg/kg) followed by regular doses as above but not exceeding recommended maximum daily doses. The introduction of i.v. paracetamol has been a considerable advance, currently the recommended dose is 60 mg/kg/d for children weighing 10–50 kg and 4 g/d for those > 50 kg.[44]

Propacetamol

Propacetamol is an intravenously injectable pro-drug which is hydrolyzed to paracetamol 2:1 (1 g propacetamol yields 0.5 g paracetamol). It is useful when other preparations/routes of administration for paracetamol are not available; it is important that this preparation is not confused with i.v. paracetamol. The pharmacokinetics of propacetamol have been studied in neonates and children, and it has been used for postoperative pain.[45–47] Transient but mild platelet dysfunction after propacetamol has been described; contact dermatitis in health care workers may also occur.

Nonsteroidal anti-inflammatory drugs

This group of drugs is thought to exert their effects mainly peripherally by cyclo-oxygenase inhibition (cf paracetamol); they also inhibit the release of inflammatory mediators from neutrophils and macrophages. Cyclo-oxygenase helps to catalyze the conversion of arachidonic acid to prostaglandins, which modulate many auto-regulatory physiological processes including sensitization of normally high threshold nociceptors at sites of inflammation. The NSAIDs ibuprofen, diclofenac and ketorolac are used widely for pain due to injury, surgery and many acute and chronic disease processes. These three drugs are used interchangeably in clinical practice, but their effect and side-effect profiles may differ at an individual patient level. Table 38.1 shows doses and routes; ibuprofen is available 'over the counter' in the UK, diclofenac is presented in a convenient rectal formulation, and ketorolac is available parenterally. Piroxicam, a long-acting NSAID which can be given once daily, is useful in long-term treatment and if compliance with multiple-dosing is a problem (Table 38.1).

Side-effects and toxicity

Asthma: caution is advised in the use of NSAIDs in the presence of wheezing as they are known to be cross-reactive with aspirin-induced asthma. The risks may have been overemphasized in children and

Table 38.1 Nonsteroidal analgesics

Drug	Routes of administration	Doses	Notes
Ibuprofen (above 5 kg)	Oral	30 mg/kg/d (3–4 divided doses)	Max. 2.4 g/d
Diclofenac	Oral or rectal	3 mg/kg/d (3 divided doses)	Max.150 mg/d
Ketorolac	Oral I.v.	0.5–1 mg/kg (4 times daily) 0.5 mg/kg (4 times daily)	Dosage restrictions apply in some countries. Max. 40 mg/d
Piroxicam	Oral	0.3–0.5 mg/kg/d	Maximum dose 20 mg in children > 6 years

short-term ibuprofen treatment appears to pose very little risk.[48] Aspirin is not used in children apart from special circumstances such as Kawasaki syndrome (see Ch. 19, p. 649) because of the risk of Reye's syndrome. Aspirin-induced asthma is very rare in the young and one study in children with asthma found no deterioration in respiratory function after diclofenac administration.[49]

Renal: kidney function is regulated by prostaglandins and two mechanisms of NSAID nephrotoxicity have been described. Functional renal failure can occur in a dose-dependent fashion, disappearing on withdrawal of the drug. Pre-existing poor function and dehydration may be contributing factors. Dose-independent interstitial nephritis with or without nephritic syndrome is rare; treatment is conservative or with corticosteroids.[50,51]

Coagulopathy: Platelet function is altered by NSAIDs due to their reversible inhibition of thromboxane A2 and platelet endoperoxides. Gastrointestinal blood loss can occur particularly associated with peptic ulceration. Increased intraoperative and postoperative blood loss, which is not usually clinically significant, has also been described. Simultaneous prescription of H_2-receptor antagonists can help reduce the risk of gastrointestinal problems.[52,53]

Infants and neonates: NSAIDs are rarely given to those under the age of 3 months and are not usually used for pain indications in neonates due to fears of possible interference with cerebral blood flow autoregulation and risk to immature renal function.

Gastrointestinal: the normal protective function of the gastric mucosa is reduced by NSAIDs and this can lead to peptic ulceration. It is not usually a problem in short-term use; some newer drugs may be beneficial (see later).

NSAIDs and cyclo-oxygenase

Cyclo-oxygenase exists in two isoforms: COX-1 and COX-2. COX-1 is found in virtually all cell types; COX-2 is expressed in some organs, notably the brain and lung, but is specifically induced in inflammation in conjunction with a rapid rise in prostaglandin levels. The traditional NSAIDs are nonselective for these isoforms but individual drugs may differ slightly in their ability to depress activity. Selective COX-2 inhibitors have reputedly fewer gastrointestinal side-effects in comparison with nonselective NSAIDs and may therefore widen the indications for NSAIDs. However the exact consequences of this selectivity is not yet fully understood; for example their use in the adult has been found to be associated with increased risk of adverse cardiovascular events and the incidence of renal complications may be similar to nonselective inhibitors. The use of COX-2 selective NSAIDs has not been adequately studied in children so at present there is little evidence upon which to evaluate their use.

Opioids and related drugs

Opioids exert their effects by acting at opioid receptors primarily in the spinal cord and brain. Despite the fact that morphine is one of the oldest and most widely used analgesics, opioid pharmacology is still not fully understood and many important questions remain unanswered. Opioids are the most powerful analgesics available with high efficacy for many types of acute and chronic pain, with the notable exception of neuropathic pain. Important considerations when prescribing opioids include their unpleasant and potentially dangerous side-effects and the development of tolerance, which can be troublesome. Neonates in particular appear clinically to be more susceptible to the depressant effects of opioids; the causes of this are probably multifactorial but have not been fully explained (see later).

The doses and possible routes of administration of the commonly used opioids for children are shown in Table 38.2. Morphine has a fairly direct relationship between dose, efficacy and side effects. The same is not true for all other opioids; partial agonist drugs such as buprenorphine have a ceiling effect and others such as codeine and pethidine have unacceptable side-effect profiles at high doses, which limit their use.

Table 38.2   Opioids

Drug	Routes of administration	Doses	
Codeine	Oral	1 mg/kg (4 times daily)	
	Rectal	1–1.5 mg/kg (4 times daily)	
Oxycodone/hydrocodone	Oral	0.2 mg/kg (4 times daily)	
Morphine	Oral	0.2–0.4 mg/kg (4 times daily)	Long-acting oral preparations available
	Intravenous	0.05 mg/kg	
	Subcutaneous	0.05 mg/kg	
	Epidural	0.02–0.05 mg/kg	
Fentanyl	OTFC (oral transmucosal)	1–10 µg/kg	See relevant product
	Transdermal	1–3 µg/kg	See relevant product
	Intravenous	0.5–1.5 µg/kg/h	Loading dose (if required)
		1 µg/kg/h	Incremental dose
	Epidural		Infusion
			Infusion
Pethidine	Oral	2 mg/kg (4 times daily)	Incremental/loading dose
	Intravenous	0.5–1 mg/kg	Incremental/loading dose
	Subcutaneous	0.5–1 mg/kg	
Methadone	Oral	0.2 mg/kg (3 times daily)	Useful long acting opioid
	Intravenous	0.1–0.2 mg/kg	

Morphine

Morphine is the prototype, high potency opioid and enormous experience in its use often makes it the drug of choice for severe pain. The pharmacokinetics and clinical use of morphine in children have been studied extensively.[54,55] The pharmacokinetics and efficacy of morphine are developmentally regulated, although outside the neonatal period, which is characterized by high variability, efficacy is largely predictable and dose related.[56]

Morphine is well absorbed orally; formulations of morphine include a suspension and a slow-release compound (MST). Parenteral morphine is usually given intravenously either by intermittent dosing, continuous infusion or in a patient-controlled analgesia (PCA) or nurse-controlled analgesia (NCA) regimen see Table 38.3. Subcutaneous infusion of morphine is also used, particularly in palliative care and when i.v. access is difficult or precious. Preservative-free (as a precaution against chemical toxicity) morphine is also effective in the epidural space, usually combined with local anesthetic.

Nausea and vomiting, sedation, and respiratory depression are the most frequently seen acute adverse effects of morphine; itching also

Table 38.3   Protocols for i.v. morphine administration

1. Morphine infusion

Preparation:	Morphine sulphate 1 mg/kg in 50 ml solution	
Concentration:	20 µg/kg/ml	
Initial dose:	2.5–5.0 ml (50–100 µg/kg)	
Infusion:	0.5–1.5 ml/h (10–30 µg/kg/h)	

2. PCA

Preparation:	Morphine sulphate 1 mg/kg in 50 ml solution	
Concentration:	20 µg/kg/ml	
Initial dose:	2.5–5.0 ml (50–100µg/kg)	
Programming	Background infusion:	0–0.2 ml/h (0–4 µg/kg/h)
	PCA dose	0.5–1.0 ml (10–20 µg/kg/h)
	Lockout interval:	5 min

3. NCA

Preparation:	Morphine sulphate 1 mg/kg in 50 ml solution	
Concentration:	20 µg/kg/ml	
Initial dose:	2.5–5.0 ml (50–100 µg/kg)	
Programming	Background infusion:	0.5–1.0 ml/h (10–20 µg/kg/h)
	NCA dose	0.5–1.0 ml (10–20 µg/kg/h)
	Lockout interval:	20 min

4. Subcutaneous morphine

Preparation:	Morphine sulphate 1 mg/kg in 20 ml solution	
Concentration:	50 µg/kg/ml	
Initial dose:	Infusion:	1–2.0 ml (50–100 µg/kg)
Programming		0.2–0.4 ml/h (10–20 µg/kg/h)

Source: Pain control service, Great Ormond Street Hospital for Children.

occurs, especially after epidural morphine. Depression of gastrointestinal motility and constipation are a problem with prolonged use. In clinical practice, non-life-threatening side-effects can be treated by reducing the dosage of morphine, often in palliative care by waiting for tolerance to the side-effect to develop – drowsiness almost always wears off in a few days, or with appropriate therapy, e.g. anti-emetics, anti-pruritics and laxatives. In an emergency, adverse effects of morphine can be reversed with the opioid antagonist, naloxone 4–10 mcg/kg.

Fentanyl

Fentanyl is a synthetic, high potency (100 × morphine) lipid soluble opioid. Its main use is during general anesthesia, where its efficacy, rapid onset and short initial half-life are an advantage. Fentanyl is usually given intravenously; it is also a popular choice for ventilated neonates and infants on ICUs (see later). Postoperatively fentanyl is commonly infused into the epidural space as its high lipid solubility may limit rostral spread and reduce the incidence of some complications, notably respiratory depression, retention of urine, and itching, in comparison with morphine. Fentanyl is available as oral (transmucosal) and transdermal (fentanyl patch) preparations which can be used for procedural pain and pain in chronic conditions and palliative care.

Fentanyl is very potent with a fast onset after i.v. administration. Opioid related side-effects of sedation, respiratory depression and itching are to be expected. High doses, > 5 mcg/kg, have also been associated with chest wall rigidity and are usually only given when respiration is controlled.[57,58]

Codeine

Codeine is a low potency opioid used for mild to moderate pain including some postoperative pain and cancer pain. It is often combined with other analgesics for best effect, particularly paracetamol and NSAIDs (Fig. 38.2). Codeine is a morphine prodrug; the response to codeine is more variable than that to morphine and this may be due to genetic (and possibly developmental) differences in metabolizing capacity.[59] Of individuals from some populations, 10% or more will not benefit from codeine analgesia; despite this they may experience some adverse effects as codeine can produce these without metabolism to morphine.[60] Codeine should not be administered intravenously as it causes hypotension.

Oxycodone and hydrocodone

Oxycodone and hydrocodone are semi-synthetic opioids suitable for moderate to severe pain, especially in combination with paracetamol or NSAIDs. Oxycodone is active by oral, buccal, sublingual and i.v. routes.[61] Sustained-release formulations have also been used in children.[62]

Tramadol

Tramadol is a synthetic moderate potency analgesic which has a novel dual mode of action by a combination of inhibition of serotonin and norepinephrine reuptake and μ-opioid receptor agonism by its active metabolite o-desmethyltramadol. Metabolism of tramadol is by the same cytochrome P450 enzyme subgroup responsible for codeine metabolism, and therefore may be subject to the same drawbacks (see earlier). Tramadol has been used for early postoperative analgesia in children with good effect. It has also been used in the caudal epidural space, where it appears to have a slow onset (about 1 h) and moderate potency.

Pethidine

Pethidine is a synthetic opioid which has few advantages over morphine. Pethidine is metabolized to norpethidine, which is neurotoxic, causing tremor, twitching, agitation and even convulsions. Norpethidine is probably also the cause of abnormal neurobehavioral tests in the neonate following maternal pethidine for labor pain. High and repeated dosage and renal impairment are risk factors, but convulsions have been reported with low doses in the therapeutic range. The traditional use of pethidine in acute sickle cell pain has declined subsequent to reports of convulsions in children.

Pethidine was originally considered to induce less nausea and vomiting and to be less depressant to the respiratory center of the fetus and neonate than morphine. If it is administered in equi-analgesic dosage these differences are not apparent, although it remains popular in some centers.

Pethidine has also been recommended for use in pancreatitis as it was thought to be less likely to precipitate spasm of the sphincter of Oddi than morphine or other opioids. Evidence from adult literature does not support this hypothesis as all opioids including pethidine appear to elevate intrabiliary pressures; the question has not been examined in children.[63]

Novel systemic analgesics

Clonidine

Clonidine is an alpha-2 adrenoceptor agonist with multiple effects including analgesia, sedation, anti-hypertension, anti-sialogogue, and others. Clonidine has a direct effect on spinal pre- and postsynaptic adrenoceptors in the dorsal horn; it also has many supraspinal effects which may also contribute to analgesia. The pharmacology, use and advantages of clonidine and other alpha-2 adrenoceptor agonists appear to be particularly useful in managing postoperative pain although moderate dose-independent reductions in blood pressure have been found at doses within the therapeutic range 0.625–2.5 mg/kg. The efficacy of clonidine in the neonate is not established; severe respiratory depression after a single dose of 2 μg/kg caudal clonidine has been reported.

Ketamine

Ketamine is an antagonist at the glutamate NMDA receptor. The receptor is important in the generation of hyperalgesia and ketamine may therefore be helpful in controlling nociceptive and neuropathic pain. High doses of 1–2 mg/kg have been used for many years as a general anesthetic. At 'low dose', < 1 mg/kg, ketamine has been found to be an effective analgesic both systemically and epidurally. The use of low-dose ketamine for postoperative pain in adults is fairly commonplace, although its efficacy has not been clearly ascertained.[64] There are many reports of its use in children, including analgesia–sedation in the pediatric ICU, and for procedural pain and postoperative pain. Ketamine in high doses induces neurobehavioral and cognitive depression sometimes accompanied by psychotomimetic effects characterized by bizarre dreams or hallucinations. Ketamine has been shown to have toxic effects to the infant mouse brain, and this observation together with the potential for abuse is has lead to a reappraisal of its use in humans.[65]

Local anesthesia

Local anesthesia has a particularly important role in pediatric pain management as it is often extremely effective and avoids many of the complications of systemic analgesics.

Bupivacaine and levobupivacaine

The amide-type local anesthetic bupivacaine and its isomer levobupivacaine are popular because of their long duration of action. Bupivacaine has been used widely for most types of local anesthetic procedure in children: following trauma, wound infiltration after surgery, peripheral nerve blocks and epidural analgesia. It is almost universally the drug of choice for epidural analgesia, where it can be infused for several days for postoperative pain, and sometimes longer for other indications. The pharmacokinetics of bupivacaine and levobupivacaine in children have been studied. Neurotoxicity and cardiotoxicity have been reported, with a slightly less risk with levobupivacaine. However the incidence of these adverse events appears to be low with both drugs if dosage recommendations are not exceeded.

Local anesthetic creams and gels are widely used for procedural pain and are discussed in the relevant sections.

MANAGEMENT OF ACUTE AND POSTOPERATIVE PAIN

Pain after surgery is a largely predictable event and therefore analgesia should be planned in advance according to the expected pain and postoperative setting. Pediatric anesthetists have special training in the use of systemic analgesics and local anesthetic techniques for surgery and they should also take some responsibility for postoperative pain management. Many of the principles and techniques used for postoperative pain may also be applied to other sources of acute or acute on chronic pain. Examples are post-traumatic injury, acute sickle cell crisis, mucositis (ulceration at a mucosal surface) and many others.

ANALGESIA FOR MINOR AND AMBULATORY OR DAY-CARE SURGERY

Most routine surgery in children is relatively minor and very often undertaken on a day-case or day-stay basis. Analgesia for day surgery should be effective and not delay discharge from hospital. The objective is to maximize comfort and mobility with little sedation or other side-effects. Postoperative nausea and vomiting (PONV) is a particular problem. In practice, this means limiting or avoiding the use of sedatives and opioids whilst encouraging the use of local anesthetic techniques. Health care workers need education and training to ensure that all runs smoothly and patients are pain free at discharge. Further analgesia will usually need to be continued at home for several days managed by parents who will need information and support in order to be able to do this effectively. Postoperative pain should be mostly treatable with 'over-the-counter' analgesics, which are safe and easily obtainable by parents at home, otherwise the suitability of a procedure for day surgery must be questioned. Take home 'packs' containing analgesics and written information are often supplied to families at day-surgery centers.

Local anesthetic techniques

Infiltration of the surgical wound can be used in many situations, especially for very superficial surgery, its utility being limited mainly by the need for large volumes of local anesthetic and dosage restrictions. Infiltration is effective for a number of common pediatric procedures including herniotomy, eye surgery, dental surgery and tonsillectomy. A range of peripheral nerve blocks are frequently used. The ilioinguinal and iliohypogastric nerves, which supply the sensory innervation to the groin area, are easy to locate and block. Surgical exploration of the inguinal region includes hernia repair, ligation of patent processus vaginalis and orchidopexy. Recognized complications include quadriceps weakness due to spread of local anesthetic to the femoral nerve. The distal third of the penis is supplied by the dorsal nerves, which are easily blocked by an injection of local anesthetic at the base of the penis. Analgesia is suitable for circumcision, minor hypospadias repair and surgery on the urethral meatus. Dorsal nerve block has also been particularly advocated for neonatal circumcision, which is performed in some countries without general anesthesia.

Caudal block

There is an enormous literature extending back at least 30 years describing caudal epidural local anesthesia in children. Caudal block is effective for most operations below the level of the umbilicus; bupivacaine lasts 4–6 h by this route. Opioids, ketamine and clonidine have also been used either alone or in combination with local anesthetic, prolonging analgesia to 12 h or longer. The complications of caudal analgesia are rare but include temporary leg weakness, delayed micturition, vascular puncture, dural puncture, and inadvertent intravascular or intradural injection of local anesthetic. Epidural infection or neurological sequelae have not been reported after single caudal local anesthetic injections.

Systemic analgesia

Potent analgesia is likely to be necessary in the early postoperative period, even after minor surgery. Institution of systemic analgesia after surgery should be planned to ensure a smooth and comfortable transition from the immediate postoperative and post-anesthesia recovery phase. Drugs, timing and routes of administration selected are important. Reactive, p.r.n. or 'as required' dosing schedules are not appropriate during the period of expected postoperative pain, and if used they are likely to lead to avoidable painful intervals while drugs are taking effect.[66]

Postoperative nausea and vomiting

Nausea and vomiting is a common cause of morbidity after minor and day-care surgery; its causes are multifactorial, and it is associated with poor analgesia and not with preoperative anxiety. Risk factors for PONV include a previous history of PONV, general anesthesia, the use of opioids, early resumption of oral fluids and certain surgical procedures, notably tonsillectomy and strabismus surgery. 5HT antagonists (e.g. ondansetron) are popular for prophylaxis and first-line treatment, the synthetic corticosteroid dexamethasone, either alone or in combination has potent anti-emetic effects. Combination anti-emetic therapy is probably the most effective treatment (Table 38.4).[67]

ANALGESIA AFTER MAJOR SURGERY

As the oral route is rarely available after major surgery for at least the first postoperative day, and often much longer after gastrointestinal operations, other options must be utilized. Local anesthetic techniques, performed under general anesthesia before or after surgery can reduce analgesic requirements in the early postoperative period.[68,69] After major operations further analgesia can be accomplished by infusion of local anesthetic through a catheter located at the site of the block, e.g. continuous epidural analgesia. More commonly pain after major surgery is managed with morphine or other opioids. Paracetamol, NSAIDs, codeine and morphine are all readily available in rectal formulations, which are popular. Rectal absorption for many drugs is known to be erratic and unpredictable, and a fatality following rectal morphine in a child has been reported. Nevertheless rectal administration of less potent drugs appears to be safe and is still widespread for paracetamol and NSAIDs.

Parenteral opioid infusions

Morphine infusion has been used safely for postoperative analgesia in children for more than 20 years, the dose range in nonventilated children in general ward areas is around 10–30 mcg/kg/h. Either i.v. or s.c. routes can be used for morphine infusions, although the latter requires more concentrated solutions (Table 38.3). A wide range of morphine requirements after surgery in children has been observed and inadequate analgesia on the first postoperative day is more frequent at infusion rates < 20 mcg/kg/h.[70] Patient-controlled analgesia (PCA) is popular for children 5 years or older; there is a substantial literature describing its use and efficacy.[71–73] Nurse-controlled analgesia (NCA) is a modified continuous morphine infusion suitable for children who are unable to operate the PCA handset. Nursing staff can administer extra doses of morphine on the basis of pain assessments or before painful care or movement by operating the PCA handset. NCA increases flexibility, total morphine consumption and parent and nurse satisfaction with analgesia.[74] Protocols for morphine infusion, PCA and NCA are given in Table 38.3. Inadequate analgesia, nausea and vomiting, excessive sedation and respiratory depression can be troublesome problems in the postoperative period. Better pain assessment, appropriate dosing, multi-modal analgesia and

Table 38.4 Drug treatment of opioid side-effects

1. Respiratory depression		
Naloxone*	(Infant–12 years)	10 µg/kg i.v.
	(12–18 years)	1.5–3 µg/kg i.g.
2. Nausea and vomiting		
Cyclizine	1 mg/kg	Oral/i.v.
	3 times daily	(< 6 years max. 25 mg)
		(> 6 years max. 50 mg)
Ondansetron	0.1 mg/kg	Oral/i.v.
		(< 12 years max. 4 mg)
		(> 12 years max. 8 mg)
Dexamethasone	0.1 mg/kg	I.v.

Larger doses may be required for severe overdose. Lower doses should be used postoperatively with titration to obtain respiratory response while maintaining adequate analgesia.

clear protocols should minimize poor efficacy and side-effects. Naloxone should always be available when opioids are being infused.

MANAGEMENT OF NEONATAL PAIN

Pain in the neonatal period requires special consideration because the immaturity of many body systems has profound and often unpredictable effects on both the response to pain and analgesics. Advances in perinatal care have meant that many younger and smaller patients undergo diagnostic and therapeutic procedures and present for surgery in early life. The management of these painful situations is hindered by our inability to accurately measure pain in this group and a lack of information on the precise effects of many analgesics during early postnatal development. Research in the fields of pain assessment and the developmental neurobiology and pharmacology of pain may soon influence practice, but for the present pharmacological neonatal pain management is largely based on the empirical and judicious use of, opioids (principally codeine, morphine, and fentanyl), paracetamol, and local anesthesia.

OPIOIDS

Despite the fact that opioids are widely used in the neonatal period both for pain and sedation little is known of the thresholds for treatment or response in the term or preterm neonate.[75] The pharmacokinetics of morphine and other opioids have been investigated and clear relationships between age and volume of distribution and plasma clearance have been established.[16] Underlying medical condition is probably also important as the maturation in morphine clearance observed in infants in the first few months of life is delayed in those undergoing corrective cardiac surgery in comparison with age-matched controls after other surgical procedures.[76] The lack of sensitive pain measurement tools and failure to correlate plasma morphine levels with analgesia has led some authors to use the emergence of side-effects such as respiratory depression to quantify the response to morphine.[77] Although there is no clear dose–response relationship between plasma morphine and respiratory depression, a common threshold in neonates and infants of around 15–20 ng/ml has been suggested.[77,78] Based on this finding, the dose of morphine to reach this target level has been investigated and found to be 5–15 mcg/kg/h in the neonate, some 25–50% lower than in older children; suggested protocols are shown in Table 38.5.[54,78] Clearly, determination of the analgesic dose–response for opioids in the neonate still remains an important priority for further research.

PARACETAMOL

Paracetamol is considered to be safe and effective in the neonatal period although, as with adults and older children, the plasma level associated with analgesia is not known.

The majority of pharmacokinetic studies have assumed plasma levels associated with the antipyretic effect of paracetamol to be therapeutic, and therefore a guide to dosing schedules. The pharmacokinetics of paracetamol have been shown to be age dependent; neonates have a higher volume of distribution (174%) and lower clearance (62%) in comparison with older children.[79] Paracetamol is metabolized in the liver, where it is conjugated to glucuronide, a small amount being oxidized by cytochrome P450 to a potentially hepatotoxic product (see earlier) which is conjugated to glutathione. Both these pathways are immature in the neonate and show high variability; enhanced sulfation of paracetamol has been demonstrated, which may compensate for reduced glucuronidation.[80] The current recommended oral dose of paracetamol in the term neonate is 60 mg/kg/d with 30–45 mg/kg/d suggested for pre-term infants; there are variations between different countries regarding this. The route of administration is important as bioavailability is very variable; in term neonates 20 mg/kg rectal paracetamol 6 hourly (80 mg/kg/d) does not reliably achieve therapeutic plasma levels and an initial dose of 30 mg/kg is recommended.[81] In pre-term neonates 20 mg/kg is effective but prolonged elimination results in accumulation if the dosing interval is less than 8 h.[81] I.v. paracetamol has not yet been adequately investigated in the neonate but reports of its use are starting to appear.[82] Propacetamol, the paracetamol pro-drug has been used in the neonate; at less than 10 d old, 30 mg/kg/d of paracetamol (60 mg/kg/d of propacetamol) maintained plasma levels between 4 and 10 mg/L, whereas after 10 d double this dose was required.[45]

LOCAL ANESTHESIA IN THE NEONATE

Local anesthesia is popular in the neonate as it avoids many of the problems associated with systemic drugs. Topical local anesthesia, infiltration and nerve blocks including epidural anesthesia can be used in the newborn. Neonates may be more susceptible to toxic effects of local anesthetics so lower doses are generally recommended. Local anesthetics are extensively protein bound, the free (unbound) fraction is considered to be pharmacologically active and therefore also important for toxicity. The protein A-acid glycoprotein (AAG) and albumin are the most important plasma proteins involved and AAG levels are lower in neonates. Prilocaine is a constituent of the topical formulation eutectic mixture of local anesthetics (EMLA) and its use in the neonate has been a cause for concern. A metabolite of prilocaine, orthotoluidine is produced, which leads to the development of methemoglobin, (oxidized hemoglobin), which has a reduced oxygen carrying capacity. Methemoglobin is reduced to hemoglobin by the enzyme methemoglobin reductase, which is developmentally regulated. Neonates are also particularly susceptible because fetal hemoglobin is more easily oxidized than adult hemoglobin. Studies have shown that EMLA can be used safely in neonates provided the dose is limited proportionally.[83,84] In a systematic review of analgesia for neonatal circumcision, local anesthetic techniques were found to be the most effective and were recommended for this procedure.[85]

SUCROSE AND NONPHARMACOLOGICAL PAIN MANAGEMENT

Sweet tasting solutions such as glucose and sucrose have been found to reduce pain responses to brief procedures in the neonate.[86–88] Sucrose has become popular, and there are commercially available preparations for clinical use. The analgesic effect of sucrose is thought to be related to the release of endogenous endorphins, however administration of naloxone did not decrease the analgesic effect in one trial.[89] Non-nutritive sucking using a pacifier, breast-feeding, and tactile stimulation have all been found to reduce pain associated responses in neonates.[90–93]

MANAGEMENT OF PAIN IN THE ICU

In the intensive care unit (ICU) sources of pain include the underlying condition, the presence of endotracheal and other tubes, drains and catheters and also the many procedures which such patients frequently undergo. See section on neonatal pain for details of techniques.

Table 38.5 Suggested morphine infusion protocols in the neonate*

Neonatal morphine infusion		
Preparation:	Morphine sulphate 1.0 mg/kg in 50 ml solution	
Concentration:	20 µg/kg/ml	
Initial dose:	0.5–5.0 ml (10–100 µg/kg)	
Infusion:	0.1–0.7 ml/h (2– 14 µg/kg/h)	
Neonatal NCA		
Preparation:	Morphine sulphate	1 mg/kg in 50 ml solution.
Concentration:		20 µg/kg/ml
Initial dose:		0.5–5.0 ml (10–100 µg/kg)
Programming	Background infusion:	0.0–0.5 ml/h (0–10 µg/kg/h)
NCA dose		0.5–1.0 ml (10–20 µg/kg/h)
Lockout interval:		20 min

* With full cardiorespiratory monitoring in intensive care areas, higher doses may be appropriate when respiration is supported.

OPIOID INFUSIONS, TOLERANCE AND WITHDRAWAL

Opioid infusions provide background analgesia, sedation, improve comfort and facilitate synchronization of respiration with artificial ventilation in neonates and older children.[94,95] Morphine is the drug of choice, although fentanyl is a useful alternative, particularly if pulmonary hypertension is a concern.[96]

A characteristic feature of opioid infusions for more than a few days is progressive tolerance to both the analgesic and sedative effects and it is not uncommon for patients to receive doses far in excess of what is normally considered therapeutic. Intermittent administration is less likely to cause tolerance than continuous infusion but this can be impractical. Use of a background infusion with intermittent doses when necessary, e.g. for routine care, blood sampling, endotracheal suction and other procedures may reduce the likelihood of tolerance. This is very similar in concept to NCA (see earlier). Multi-modal analgesia may also be helpful and the use of agents such as clonidine and low-dose ketamine may reduce tolerance.

Abrupt withdrawal of opioids after 5 or more days of continuous use is very likely to result in the appearance of symptoms and signs of withdrawal. Gradual reduction of infusion rates by 10–20% per day should not delay tracheal extubation of the airway or discharge from ICU and will usually prevent unpleasant and distressing symptoms and potentially dangerous cerebral excitatory phenomena including convulsions. If necessary oral preparations can be used and weaning from high doses continued in low dependency areas, even at home. Clonidine and benzodiazepines ameliorate the withdrawal syndrome associated with opioids. High-dose infusions of benzodizepines, such as midazolam, may result in benzodizepine withdrawal, which can be avoided by substituting a long-acting benzodiazepine such as lorazepam with subsequent gradual withdrawal.

CHRONIC PAIN

There is no precise definition of when a pain becomes chronic as it is strongly influenced by patient perception. In acute pain the prevailing mood tends toward anxiety, whereas in chronic pain withdrawal from daily life and even depression can predominate. Hope remains strong in acute pain whereas despair can dominate the chronic situation. In acute pain the person is able to focus on the pain itself but with chronic pain it becomes all pervasive.[97]

Effective management depends on recognizing the need to tackle both the underlying cause for the pain and its wider manifestations. Pain may be constant, such as in progressive cancer or related to exacerbations, such as in rheumatoid and connective tissue disorders. In other disorders a combination of background chronic pain interspersed with acute episodes including from procedures such as in sickle cell disease, osteogenesis imperfecta and epidermolysis bullosa. Specific treatment aimed at reversing or relieving the underlying illness is the most effective approach accompanied by short- or long-term analgesia. Analgesics are chosen according to the severity of the pain and whether it appears to be primarily related to tissue damage to inflammatory or neuropathic elements. Psychological assessment may identify a role for cognitive and behavioral pain management skills.

SICKLE CELL DISEASE

The dual aspects of acute and chronic pain are vividly represented by sickle cell disease, where the severe pain of sickle cell crises exemplifies acute pain whereas the recurrent nature of the crises, their unpredictable nature and the lifelong and incurable nature of the disease results in aspects characteristic of chronic intractable pain.[98] Management of pain for these children and young people has a poor record, with inappropriate fears of addiction and misunderstanding of cultural aspects of the illness, resulting in analgesics being under used. Current approaches recognize the need to give patients more credence and control, by enabling a more rapid response at the start of a crisis including i.v. opioids by PCA and using nonpharmacological approaches.

CHRONIC PAIN SYNDROMES

A significant number of children present with symptoms of pain but where a physical cause is not evident, where the pain seems disproportionate to the tissue damage or where pain persists after previous damage appears to have healed.

Complex regional pain syndrome

One common picture, often occurring with limb pains is that of increasing disability and associated sympathetically mediated features such as edema, decreased temperature and pallor or cyanotic coloring of the affected part, hyper-esthesia of the skin, muscle wasting and eventually osteoporosis and atrophy. This has been called reflex sympathetic dystrophy (RSD) in the past but is now considered part of the spectrum of chronic regional pain syndrome (CRPS). Although sympathetic nervous system involvement is not invariable fatigue, widely disseminated pains and other features such as malaise, disability, school absence and family disruption are common. Significant analgesic use is usual and reported as rarely effective in relieving the pain. Sometimes these children are labeled as malingering or disbelieved, resulting in anger and frustration. CRPS is more common in girls, and in contrast to adult presentations, the lower limb is usually involved.[99] A confident diagnosis of CRPS depends on careful exclusion of an observable underlying pathology and effective intervention begins with acknowledging the reality of the pain and symptoms, of the impact on the child and family and a recognition of the complex and ill-understood nature of the problem. The causes are not clearly understood and appear to involve features of neuropathic pain, with a persistent and inappropriate upregulation of pain perception, in the wider context of a bio-behavioral response to the pain. Early diagnosis of CRPS is thought to improve prognosis, immobilization of the affected limb is strongly contraindicated and a regimen of desensitization treatment with active and passive movement should be introduced as soon as possible.[100] The most successful management is multidisciplinary.[99,100] As well as medical and nursing input it involves physiotherapy, psychological and pharmaceutical assessment followed by the development of a comprehensive treatment program, with the involvement of the child and family. Interventions should be outpatient based, but in severe situations intensive inpatient programs may be needed.[31] Care includes the gradual withdrawal of inappropriate analgesics, and cautious use of medications effective in neuropathic pain such as the sodium channel blockers gabapentin and the tricyclic antidepressants; there is little evidence to support the use of sympathetic blocks for CRPS.[99] Learning coping skills, cognitive-behavioral therapy, graded exercise, goal setting and regular support and monitoring are the mainstays of treatment. The course may be one of improvement and relapses.

PALLIATIVE CARE

Pediatric palliative care is a holistic approach to the care of children with life-limiting and life-threatening illness, where symptom management is addressed alongside the provision of practical, psychological, social and spiritual support for the whole family. It should be provided from the time of diagnosis of a life-limiting or life-threatening condition and should continue though life, death and bereavement. It is not confined to the terminal phase of an illness and can co-exist alongside life-prolonging and life-saving treatments.

WHO NEEDS PALLIATIVE CARE?

Many of the relevant illnesses are specific to children, are very rare and have a protracted course. Some are familial and may affect several children in the same family, with genetic implications for the parents and healthy siblings.

Children who may benefit from a palliative care referral can be considered in four broad groups:[101]

1. life-threatening conditions where curative treatment may be possible but may fail. Palliative care is needed in times of prognostic uncertainty or when cure becomes impossible. Cancer is an example;
2. conditions where there are long periods of intensive treatment aimed at prolonging life, but where life expectancy is significantly reduced. Cystic fibrosis and acquired immune deficiency syndrome (AIDS) fit this pattern;
3. progressive conditions where treatment is entirely palliative and may extend over many years. Neurodegenerative diseases and many inborn errors of metabolism are examples;
4. irreversible but nonprogressive conditions causing severe disability, such as severe cerebral palsy.

PROVIDING SERVICES FOR THE FAMILY

The overall needs for children and their families have been summarized in the Association for Children with life-threatening or terminal conditions and their families (ACT) Charter (Fig. 38.3).[102] These must be considered when planning and delivering palliative care services.

An increasing recognition of the need for pediatric palliative care services has resulted in an increase in the number of children's hospices and community teams and medical and nursing specialists providing these services.

- Every child shall be treated with dignity and respect and shall be afforded privacy whatever the child's physical or intellectual ability.

- Parents shall be acknowledged as the primary carers and involved as partners in all care and decisions involving their child.

- Every child shall be given the opportunity to participate in decisions affecting his or her care, according to age and understanding.

- An honest and open approach shall be the basis of all communication.

- Information shall be provided for the parent, the child, the siblings and other relatives, appropriate to age and understanding.

- The family home shall remain the center of caring whenever possible. Care away from home shall be provided in a child-centered environment by staff trained in the care of children.

- Every child shall have access to a 24-hour multidisciplinary children's palliative care team for flexible support in the home, and be in the care of a local pediatrician.

- Every child and family shall receive emotional, psychological and spiritual support to meet their needs. This shall begin at diagnosis and continue throughout the child's lifetime, death and in bereavement.

- Every family shall be entitled to a named keyworker who will enable the family to build up and maintain access to an appropriate network of support.

- Every family shall be given the opportunity of a consultation with a pediatric specialist who has particular knowledge of the child's condition.

- Every family shall have access to flexible short-term breaks (respite care) both in their own home and away from home, with appropriate children's nursing and medical support.

- Every child shall have access to education and other appropriate childhood activities.

- The needs of adolescents and young people shall be addressed and planned for well in advance.

- Every family shall have timely access to practical support, including clinical equipment, financial grants, suitable housing and domestic help.

Fig. 38.3 ACT Charter.[102]

LOCATION OF CARE

It is important that families are given choices as to where their child receives care. Many will prefer to care for their child at home,[103] whereas others will prefer hospital or hospice care. Families must be brought to a realistic expectation with regard to the needs of their child as their health deteriorates and the support that is available, particularly if they choose to be at home. They will also need access to advice and support 24 hours a day from professionals with palliative care expertise, or supported by professionals with this specialist knowledge. There should be sufficient flexibility to enable the family to move between home and/or hospice, as they choose, without care being compromised.

SYMPTOM MANAGEMENT

As parents frequently worry that their child will experience symptoms that will be difficult to control it is important to provide them with detailed and honest information about the management of their child's current and anticipated symptoms. Both they and their child need to take an active part in planning a practical and acceptable regimen of care, in order to instill a level of competence and confidence in controlling pain and discomfort and in understanding their child's management.

As death approaches parents will need and value further information, including knowledge of the possible modes of death and the physical signs that suggest death is imminent. Knowing what to expect and having a clear plan of action as the situation changes can enable families to cope better.

Almost all families can be reassured that death will be peaceful, but if there are concerns about the possibility of sudden distressing symptoms (such as convulsions, acute agitation, or bleeding) these should be discussed openly. Emergency drugs (e.g. anticonvulsants, analgesics and sedatives) should be accessible in suitable doses via appropriate routes.

PATTERN OF SYMPTOMS

Although many unpleasant and distressing symptoms are common to a number of different illnesses, their underlying cause (and therefore the approach to symptom management) may be different. For rare conditions anticipation of possible symptoms will require input from specialist pediatricians and nursing staff.

Children with malignant disease often have a relatively short final illness, lasting weeks or months, with pain from tumor progression as a predominant feature whereas in nonmalignant conditions onset may be more insidious with less prominence of pain and greater likelihood of muscle spasms, gastroesophageal reflux, seizures and respiratory distress.

ASSESSMENT OF SYMPTOMS

Thorough assessment of any symptom is essential before developing a plan of management. As much information as possible should be elicited, and this can be particularly challenging in nonverbal children and those with severe developmental impairment.[104] A range of tools are available to assess pain in children of different ages and developmental levels, but similar tools are not yet sufficiently developed to aid the assessment of other symptoms. Parents and carers should also be asked to contribute their observations to the assessment, as they will notice subtle changes that may not be apparent to health care professionals. Psychological and social factors affecting the child and family are often significant and should be considered as part of an assessment.

ROUTES OF DRUG ADMINISTRATION

The preferences of the child and family need to be taken into account. Taking a lot of medication can be difficult and complex regimens should be avoided. It is important to find the most acceptable route for the child and to be flexible to changing situations, such as a deteriorating swallow or an increasing reluctance to comply with medication regimens. Key issues in deciding routes of administration include:

- The oral route is often preferable and the child should be allowed to choose between liquids capsules and whole or crushed tablets.
- Long-acting preparations are more convenient and less intrusive.
- As the condition deteriorates the treatment plan often has to be simplified, routes of administration altered and priority given to those drugs that contribute most to the child's comfort.
- Some children prefer rectal medication to needles when the oral route is not possible and rectal preparations can also be helpful in the final hours when the child's level of consciousness has deteriorated.
- If parenteral drugs are needed they are usually given by continuous s.c. infusion, not as boluses. An i.v. line can be used if it is already in place. The transdermal route should also be considered.
- Intramuscular drugs are painful and should be avoided.

NON-DRUG MANAGEMENT

Adopting a holistic approach that addresses the psychological, social and spiritual concerns of the child and family is likely to achieve better symptom management than medication alone. Explaining the reason for the symptom agreeing a logical step-wise approach and reassuring the child and family that the situation is not going to be allowed to go 'out of control' are the foundations of successful management. Other measures that can be used alongside or in place of drug therapy include careful positioning of the child, maintaining a calm environment, distraction, imagery and relaxation techniques, play, art and music therapy.

PAIN

Pain management will include treating the underlying cause of the pain, where possible. For example, bony metastases may be treated with radiotherapy and painful muscle spasms with muscle relaxants rather than analgesics. Where treatment of the underlying cause is not possible, or does not relieve pain sufficiently, analgesics should be used alongside psychological and practical approaches. The WHO ladder of analgesia has been widely adopted, although recent evidence has shed some doubt on the routine use of codeine as up to 10% of the population may be poor metabolizers of the drug to morphine (the active metabolite). Poor efficacy is also a feature in infants because of immature enzyme systems.[105]

Opioid-sensitive pain
Strong opioids
These are used extensively in managing pain in pediatric palliative care. When prescribing strong opioids for children, the following points should be considered:
- long-acting morphine preparations are effective and convenient;
- short-acting preparations will be needed for breakthrough pain;
- where oral administration is difficult or impossible the use of transdermal patches (e.g. fentanyl) has proved invaluable;[106]
- sudden onset of severe pain may require break-through analgesia with a faster onset of action than oral morphine. Fentanyl lozenges, buccal or intranasal morphine may be appropriate in these situations.[107,108]
- studies of the pharmacokinetics of oral opioids and their metabolites suggest that in young children metabolism is more rapid than in adults and they may require relatively higher doses;
- neonates and children under 6 months old usually require a lower starting dose of opioids because of their reduced metabolism and increased sensitivity.[109]

Side-effects of opioids
Many doctors lack experience of using strong opioids in children, which can lead to unnecessary caution, underdosing and inadequate pain control. Respiratory depression with strong opioids is not usually a problem in children with severe pain and in general the side-effects from opioids tend

to be less marked than in adults. Nausea and vomiting are rare and routine anti-emetics are often not needed. Constipation is the most common side-effect of opiates and regular laxatives should always be prescribed.

Parents and children should be warned that they may become drowsy during the first few days of starting opioids but reassured that this will resolve. Itching usually responsive to antihistamines may also be a problem within the first few days. If either somnolence or pruritus remain troublesome, switching to an alternative preparation, such as fentanyl or hydromorphone is usually effective.[110]

Parental concerns about opioids
Parents may express concern that opioids will precipitate death, or worry that if they are started 'too early' they will lose efficacy as the illness and symptoms progress. Others find the transition to opioids difficult from a psychological and emotional perspective and that by agreeing to use opioids they are acknowledging that their child is going to die imminently.

Parental concerns require sensitive discussion and support. Parents must be assured that:

- their child will receive appropriate analgesia in the lowest dose needed to relieve pain;
- opioids do not precipitate death when used appropriately;
- there is no upper or ceiling dose for effective pain relief.

Musculoskeletal pain
Nonsteroidal anti-inflammatory drugs (NSAIDs) are often helpful for musculoskeletal pain, although caution is needed in the presence of bone marrow infiltration because of the increased risk of bleeding. Bisphosphonates should also be considered, particularly in children with long-term conditions associated with immobility, such as osteogenesis imperfecta.[111] Oral chemotherapy may be helpful in reducing tumor-related musculoskeletal pain.

Headaches in malignant disease
Headaches from central nervous system leukemia respond well to intrathecal methotrexate whereas those associated with raised intracranial pressure, are best managed with gradually increasing analgesics. Although steroids may seem helpful initially, the symptoms will inevitably recur as the tumor increases in size, necessitating increased doses of steroids with associated side-effects that almost always outweigh the benefits.[112]

Neuropathic pain
Neuropathic pain can often be helped by antiepileptic and antidepressant drugs. Ketamine can also be helpful, either orally or by continuous infusion.[113,114] For severe pain unresponsive to these drugs, intrathecal, epidural anesthesia and nerve blocks should be considered.

Muscle spasm and dystonia
These can be particularly problematic in children with neurological conditions and untreated can cause considerable pain and discomfort. An assessment of seating should be a priority as simple changes can have significant benefits. Muscle relaxants such as diazepam, baclofen and dantrolene may also be required.[115]

Gastro-esophageal reflux
A significant proportion of children with neurological impairment and/or disorders affecting muscle tone experience pain associated with gastro-esophageal reflux. Management should include a combination of approaches, such as attention to the feeding regimen, posture during and after feeds, as well as medical approaches including drugs to reduce acid production and to increase gastric emptying. Surgical management should also be considered for some children[116] (see Chapter 19: gastro- and hepatology chapter section GOR pp 605)

Nausea and vomiting
Nausea and vomiting can be a significant symptom in children with raised intracranial pressure and in a variety of other diseases causing metabolic disturbance or impaired gastrointestinal function. Anti-emetics

that work well in one situation (e.g. ondansetron in cancer patients undergoing chemotherapy) may be far less useful in other situations (e.g. cancer patients not having chemotherapy), so must be selected according to their site of action and the presumed cause of symptoms. This is summarized in Table 38.6.

Seizures
Children with neurodegenerative diseases often develop seizures as part of their ongoing disease with increasing problems in seizure control as the disease progresses. Other children may only develop seizures towards or during the terminal phase of their illness. Sudden acute onset of seizures can be treated with rectal diazepam or buccal midazolam.[117] Repeated severe or continuous seizures in a terminally ill child can be treated at home with a continuous subcutaneous infusion of midazolam and/or phenobarbitone.

Agitation and anxiety
Agitation and anxiety may reflect a child's need to talk about his or her fears and distress. Open communication should be encouraged throughout the child's illness, so that anxiety and fears can be addressed while the child is still able to communicate easily. If additional drugs are needed, benzodiazepines, haloperidol and levomepromazine can provide relief, especially in the final stages of life.

Respiratory symptoms
Dyspnea, cough, and excess secretions can all cause distress to children and anxiety for their parents. If the underlying cause of the symptom can be relieved, even temporarily, this may be appropriate. Palliative radiotherapy, for example, can bring good symptomatic relief to some children with primary or secondary thoracic tumors.

Breathlessness
Where treatment of the underlying cause is unlikely to be beneficial, symptom relief can be addressed by combining drugs with practical and supportive approaches. Fear is often an important element in dyspnea and reassurance and management of anxiety may help to relieve symptoms. Simple practical measures include finding the optimum body position, using a fan, and relaxation exercises. Opioids can help to relieve the sensation of breathlessness and small doses of sedatives, such as diazepam or midazolam, can relieve the associated anxiety.

Increasing hypoxemia may result in headaches, nausea, daytime drowsiness, and poor-quality sleep. Intermittent oxygen may help relieve these symptoms and can be given relatively easily at home.

Secretions
Excess secretions may occur during the terminal phase and are often a problem for children with chronic neurodegenerative diseases as they become less able to cough and swallow. Oral glycopyrronium bromide, or hyoscine hydrobromide (given transdermally or subcutaneously) can often help to reduce the secretions. For children in the terminal stage of an illness, altering the child's position to allow secretions to

Table 38.6 Medical management of nausea and vomiting

Cause of vomiting	Recommended drugs
Drug induced and metabolic	Haloperidol Levomepromazine Ondansetron
Poor gastric outflow	Metoclopramide Domperidone
Gastric outflow obstruction	Octreotide Hyoscine butylbromide
Raised intracranial pressure	Cyclizine Hyoscine Dexamethasone (in short courses of 3–5 d)

drain orally may provide temporary relief. Suction equipment may be helpful in some situations, but can stimulate increased production of secretions and also increase the burden of nursing care for the parents.

ANEMIA AND BLEEDING

The treatment of anemia by blood transfusion in the late stages of a child's life should only be used in the relief of symptoms.

Florid bleeding (e.g. severe hemoptysis or hematemesis) is extremely frightening for a child and their carers and when this occurs death is usually very rapid. If this is a serious risk both an analgesic and a sedative, such as morphine and midazolam should be readily available. In an emergency, parents can give these drugs by the buccal route and should repeat the dose every 15 min until the child is calm. Medication should be continued by continuous s.c. or i.v. infusion.

Many children with malignant diseases have widespread bone marrow infiltration and low platelets. Petechiae and minor gum bleeding are common although significant bleeding is unusual. Minor gum and nose bleeding can be managed by direct application of tranexamic acid to the bleeding point. Platelet transfusions should only be used to manage bleeding that is severe or that interferes with the child's quality of life.

IMPAIRED APPETITE AND POOR FEEDING

For many children, disease progression is associated with impaired appetite, which parents often find extremely distressing. For children, constant attempts by parents to encourage them to eat are similarly distressing.

Reasons for reduced feeding should be explored and reversible causes treated where possible. Assisted feeding, via a nasogastric tube or gastrostomy, may be necessary for children with slowly progressive disease, especially where this is associated with a declining ability to swallow but not a reduced appetite. For children with a poor appetite and rapidly progressive disease, nasogastric or gastrostomy feeding is usually inappropriate and can cause increased nausea and vomiting.

Where a child has a poor appetite or cannot tolerate amounts of food that parents consider acceptable, parents should be encouraged to relax nutritional goals and to provide only small amounts of food that the child enjoys, throughout the day. It is important to explain to parents that a reduced appetite is part of the disease progression and encouraging the child to eat more than they can manage may make them feel more unwell.

PSYCHOSOCIAL AND SPIRITUAL SUPPORT

All children and young people facing death or with a reduced life expectancy deserve help in maintaining as much normal life as possible, ensuring good access to play, education and social experiences and assistance in focusing on and achieving appropriate goals. A number of themes facing the sick child and family have been identified and these occur at diagnosis and then recur at different critical points throughout the course of the illness. Awareness and attention to these difficulties and common themes can provide valuable support for families:

- the need to be given appropriate information;
- the importance of enabling children and families to identify and express their emotions and spiritual needs;
- recognition that emotional and spiritual needs and ways of coping vary between different members of the family and at different times during the illness;
- awareness of the difficulty for families of living with uncertainty;
- acknowledging the benefits of and enabling open and honest communication both within families and between families and professionals;
- the value of empowering families and enabling them to retain choices and a sense of control.

For the parents and siblings of children with nonmalignant diseases, the prolonged time course and enormous nursing demands will increase the stress and practical difficulties. Throughout the course of a child's illness and death family members are likely to experience a huge range of feelings, such as sadness, despair, depression, hopelessness, anger, guilt, resentment of the sick child and isolation. Siblings often feel a sense of exclusion and neglect, although those who are very involved in caring for the sibling may also express positive experiences.[118,119]

Talking openly with families and with the sick child, however difficult, is usually helpful in reducing the child's level of anxiety and improving the family's later adjustment.[120] Most children are already aware, through their own interpretation of verbal and nonverbal cues, of much more about their illness and situation than most adults expect. Listening to their cues, exploring their fears and worries, responding honestly but gradually and using a range of nonverbal approaches (play, stories, art) are all skills that can help and which members of the multidisciplinary palliative care team can bring to the family and child.[121] Factors which need to be taken into account when talking with children include the child's age and developmental level, their likely understanding of their illness and of death, the child and family's past experiences and the family's normal communication pattern and culture.[122,123]

THE BEREAVED FAMILY

It is essential that the emotional support provided throughout the child's life is continued through the family's bereavement. The grief suffered after the loss of a child has been described as the most painful, enduring and difficult to survive and is associated with a high risk of pathological grief. Parents lose not only the child they have loved, but their hopes for the future and their confidence in themselves as parents. It puts an additional stress on their own relationship and alters the whole family structure. The brothers and sisters who are grieving may continue to feel isolated and neglected as their parents can spare little time or emotion for them. Ideally the professionals who know the family well and have been involved throughout the sick child's life should continue to be available through their bereavement. Grief is likely to continue over many years, and its depth and persistence is often underestimated. Parents value continuing contact with professionals who have known their child and the opportunity to talk about the child and their grief when others in the community expect them to 'have come to terms with it'.[124] This support, initially more frequent and gradually decreasing, helps facilitate the normal tasks of mourning. Most families will not need formal counseling but it is important to be able to recognize when there are signs of abnormal grief that may require referral for specialist help.

Helping to care for a child with a life-threatening illness, and for the family of such a child, is rarely easy. It presents many challenges both in terms of the professional tasks that may be required and to our own emotional resources. Though the task may seem daunting, families greatly value professionals who stay alongside them throughout their journey, providing practical help and support in an almost intolerable situation. Parents will have a lasting memory of their child's death and as professionals we have the opportunity to ensure this memory is as good as it can be.

CONCLUSION

Knowledge and skills in pain management and palliative care have been increasing in recent years. It will be essential to continue to these developments, to challenge misinformation and to work towards enhancing pain management and reducing suffering for children, throughout the world. Although little evidence-based information is available to date it is likely that employing the basic principles of pain and relief and control and good communication with children and families will ensure optimal management.

REFERENCES (* LEVEL 1 EVIDENCE)

1. Howard RF. Current status of pain management in children. JAMA 2003; 290:2464–2469.
2. Fitzgerald M. The development of nociceptive circuits. Nat Rev Neurosci 2005; 6:507–520.
3. Finley GA, McGrath PJ. Measurement of pain in infants and children. Seattle: IASP Press; 1998.
4. Clinical guidelines for the recognition and assessment of acute pain in children. London: Royal College of Nursing Institute; 1999.
5. Franck LS, Greenberg CS, Stevens B. Pain assessment in infants and children. Pediatr Clin North Am 2000; 47:487–512.
*6. Duhn LJ, Medves JM. A systematic integrative review of infant pain assessment tools. Adv Neonatal Care 2004; 4:126–140.
*7. Stinson JN, Kavanagh T, Yamada J, et al. Systematic review of the psychometric properties, interpretability and feasibility of self-report pain intensity measures for use in clinical trials in children and adolescents. Pain 2006; 125:143–157.
8. Breau LM, McGrath PJ, Camfield C, et al. Preliminary validation of an observational pain checklist for persons with cognitive impairments and inability to communicate verbally. Dev Med Child Neurol 2000; 42:609–616.
9. Hunt A, Goldman A, Seers K, et al. Clinical validation of the paediatric pain profile. Dev Med Child Neurol 2004; 46:9–18.
10. Varni JW, Thompson KL, Hanson V. The Varni/Thompson Pediatric Pain Questionnaire. I. Chronic musculoskeletal pain in juvenile rheumatoid arthritis. Pain 1987; 28:27–38.
11. Palermo TM, Witherspoon D, Valenzuela D, et al. Development and validation of the Child Activity Limitations Interview: a measure of pain-related functional impairment in school-age children and adolescents. Pain 2004; 109:461–470.
*12. von Baeyer CL, Spagrud LJ. Systematic review of observational (behavioral) measures of pain for children and adolescents aged 3 to 18 years. Pain 2007; 127:140–150.
13. Wong DL, Baker CM. Pain in children: comparison of assessment scales. Pediatr Nurs 1988; 14:9–17.
14. Hicks CL, von BCL, Spafford PA, et al. The Faces Pain Scale-Revised: toward a common metric in pediatric pain measurement. Pain 2001; 93:173–183.
15. Stanford EA, Chambers CT, Craig KD. The role of developmental factors in predicting young children's use of a self-report scale for pain. Pain 2006; 120:16–23.
16. Chambers CT, Craig KD. An intrusive impact of anchors in children's faces pain scales. Pain 1998; 78:27–37.
17. Hester NO. The preoperational child's reaction to immunizations. Nurs Res 1979; 28:250–255.
18. Chambers CT, Reid GJ, Craig KD, et al. Agreement between child and parent reports of pain. Clin J Pain 1998; 14:336–342.
19. Grunau RE, Oberlander T, Holsti L, et al. Bedside application of the Neonatal Facial Coding System in pain assessment of premature neonates. Pain 1998; 76:277–286.
20. McGrath PJ, Johnson G, Goodman JT, et al. CHEOPS: A behavioral scale for rating postoperative pain in children. Adv Pain Res Ther 1985; 9:395–402.
21. Merkel SI, Voepel-Lewis T, Shayevitz JR, et al. The FLACC: a behavioral scale for scoring postoperative pain in young children. Pediatr Nurs 1997; 23:293–227.
22. van Dijk M, Peters JW, van Deventer P, et al. The COMFORT Behavior Scale: a tool for assessing pain and sedation in infants. Am J Nurs 2005; 105:33–36.

23. Kolk AM, van Hoof R, Fiedeldij Dop MJ. Preparing children for venepuncture. The effect of an integrated intervention on distress before and during venepuncture. Child Care Health Dev 2000; 26:251–260.
24. Chen E, Joseph MH, Zeltzer L. Behavioral and cognitive interventions in the treatment of acute pain in children. Pediatr Clin North Am 2000; 47:513–525.
25. Liossi C, Hatira P. Clinical hypnosis in the alleviation of procedure-related pain in pediatric oncology patients. Int J Clin Exp Hypn 2003; 51:4–28.
26. Butler LD, Symons BK, Henderson SL, et al. Hypnosis reduces distress and duration of an invasive medical procedure for children. Pediatrics 2005; 115:e77–e85.
27. Rusy LM, Weisman SJ. Complementary therapies for acute pediatric pain management. Pediatr Clin North Am 2000; 47:589–599.
*28. Uman LS, Chambers CT, McGrath PJ, et al. Psychological interventions for needle-related procedural pain and distress in children and adolescents. Cochrane Database Syst Rev 2006; 4:CD005179.
29. Eccleston C, Yorke L, Morley S, et al. Psychological therapies for the management of chronic and recurrent pain in children and adolescents. Cochrane Database Syst Rev 2003; 1:CD003968.
30. Sherry DD, Wallace CA, Kelley C, et al. Short- and long-term outcomes of children with complex regional pain syndrome type I treated with exercise therapy. Clin J Pain 1999; 15:218–223.
31. Maillard SM, Davies K, Khubchandani R, et al. Reflex sympathetic dystrophy: a multidisciplinary approach. Arthritis Rheum 2004; 51:284–290.
32. Fitzgerald M, Howard RF. Schechter N L, Berde CB, Yaster M, eds. The neurobiologic basis of paediatric pain. In: 2nd edn. Philadelphia, PA: Lippincott Williams and Wilkins; 2003.19–42.
33. Koppert W, Wehrfritz A, Korber N, et al. The cyclooxygenase isozyme inhibitors parecoxib and paracetamol reduce central hyperalgesia in humans. Pain 2004; 108:148–153.
34. Bonnefont J, Daulhac L, Etienne M, et al. Acetaminophen recruits spinal p42/p44 MAPKs and GH/IGF-1 receptors to produce analgesia via the serotonergic system. Mol Pharmacol 2007; 71:407–415.
*35. Moore A, Collins S, Carroll D, et al. Single dose paracetamol (acetaminophen), with and without codeine, for postoperative pain. Cochrane Database Syst Rev 2000; CD001547.
36. Zhang WY, Li Wan Po A. Analgesic efficacy of paracetamol and its combination with codeine and caffeine in surgical pain – a meta-analysis. J Clin Pharm Ther 1996; 21:261–282.
37. Anderson B, Kanagasundarum S, Woollard G. Analgesic efficacy of paracetamol in children using tonsillectomy as a pain model. Anaesth Intensive Care 1996; 24:669–673.
38. Bean-Lijewski JD, Stinson JC. Acetaminophen or ketorolac for post myringotomy pain in children? A prospective, double-blinded comparison. Paediatr Anaesth 1997; 7:131–137.
*39. deCraen AJ, DiGiulio G, Lampe-Schoenmaeckers JE, et al. Analgesic efficacy and safety of paracetamol-codeine combinations versus paracetamol alone: a systematic review. BMJ 1996; 313:321–325.
40. Morton NS, O'Brien K. Analgesic efficacy of paracetamol and diclofenac in children receiving PCA morphine. Br J Anaesth 1999; 82:715–717.
41. Shah V, Taddio A, Ohlsson A. Randomised controlled trial of paracetamol for heel prick pain in neonates. Arch Dis Child Fetal Neonatal Ed 1998; 79:F209–F211.
42. Howard CR, Howard FM, Weitzman ML. Acetaminophen analgesia in neonatal circumcision: the effect on pain. Pediatrics 1994; 93:641–646.

43. Hynson JL, South M. Childhood hepatotoxicity with paracetamol doses less than 150 mg/kg per day. Med J Aust 1999; 171:497.
44. BNFC. The British National Formulary for Children. London: BMJ Publishing Group Ltd.; 2006.
45. Autret E, Dutertre JP, Breteau M, et al. Pharmacokinetics of paracetamol in the neonate and infant after administration of propacetamol chlorhydrate. Dev Pharmacol Ther 1993; 20:129–134.
46. Granry JC, Rod B, Monrigal P, et al. The analgesic efficacy of an injectable prodrug of acetaminophen in children after orthopaedic surgery. Paediatr Anaesth 1997; 7:445–449.
47. Rod B, Monrigal JP, Lepoitte vin L, et al. Treatment of postoperative pain in children in the recovery room. Use of morphine and propacetamol by the intravenous route. Cah Anesthesiol 1989; 37 525–530.
48. Lesko SM, Louik C, Vezina RM, et al. Asthma morbidity after the short-term use of ibuprofen in children. Pediatrics 2002; 109:E20.
49. Short JA, Barr CA, Palmer CD, et al. Use of diclofenac in children with asthma. Anaesthesia 2000; 55:334–337.
50. Clive DM, Stoff JS. Renal syndromes associated with nonsteroidal antiinflammatory drugs. N Engl J Med 1984; 310:563–572.
51. Robinson J, Malleson P, Lirenman D, et al. Nephrotic syndrome associated with nonsteroidal anti-inflammatory drug use in two children. Pediatrics 1990; 85:844–847.
52. Chan FK, Sung JJ. Role of acid suppressants in prophylaxis of NSAID damage. Best Pract Res Clin Gastroenterol 2001; 15:433–445.
*53. Rostom A, Wells G, Tugwell P, et al. The prevention of chronic NSAID induced upper gastrointestinal toxicity: a Cochrane collaboration metaanalysis of randomized controlled trials. J Rheumatol 2000; 27:2203–2214.
54. Kart T, Christrup LL, Rasmussen M. Recommended use of morphine in neonates, infants and children based on a literature review: Part 2 – Clinical use. Paediatr Anaesth 1997; 7:93–101.
55. Kart T, Christrup LL, Rasmussen M. Recommended use of morphine in neonates, infants and children based on a literature review: Part 1 – Pharmacokinetics. Paediatr Anaesth 1997; 7:5–11.
56. Hartley R, Levine MI. Opioid pharmacology in the newborn. In: Aynsley-Green A A, Ward Platt M P, AR L-T, eds. 3:3. London: Baillière Tindall; 1995.467–494.
57. Fahnenstich H, Steffan J, Kau N, Bartmann P. Fentanyl-induced chest wall rigidity and laryngospasm in preterm and term infants. Crit Care Med 2000; 28:836–839.
58. Streisand JB, Bailey PL, LeMaire L, et al. Fentanyl-induced rigidity and unconsciousness in human volunteers. Incidence, duration, and plasma concentrations. Anesthesiology 1993; 78:629–634.
59. William DG, Hatch DJ, Howard RF. Codeine phosphate in paediatric medicine. Br J Anaesth 2001; 86:413–421.
60. Williams DG, Patel A, Howard RF. Pharmacogenetics of codeine metabolism in an urban population of children and its implications for analgesic reliability. Br J Anaesth 2002; 89:839–845.
61. Kokki H, Rasanen I, Lasalmi M, et al. Comparison of oxycodone pharmacokinetics after buccal and sublingual administration in children. Clin Pharmacokinet 2006; 45:745–754.
62. Czarnecki ML, Jandrisevits MD, Theiler SC, et al. Controlled-release oxycodone for the management of pediatric postoperative pain. J Pain Symptom Manage 2004; 27:379–386.
63. Thompson DR. Narcotic analgesic effects on the sphincter of Oddi: a review of the data and

therapeutic implications in treating pancreatitis. Am J Gastroenterol 2001; 96:1266–1272.

64. Elia N, Tramer MR. Ketamine and postoperative pain – a quantitative systematic review of randomised trials. Pain 2005; 113:61–70.

65. Young C, Jevtovic-Todorovic V, Qin YQ, et al. Potential of ketamine and midazolam, individually or in combination, to induce apoptotic neurodegeneration in the infant mouse brain. Br J Pharmacol 2005; 146:189–197.

66. Howard RF. Planning for pain relief. In: Lindahl S G E, ed. Clinical anesthesiology: Pediatric anesthesia. London: Baillière Tindall; 1997.657–676.

67. Rose JB, Watcha MF. Postoperative nausea and vomiting in paediatric patients. Br J Anaesth 1999; 83:104–117.

68. Conroy JM, Othersen HBJ, Dorman BH, et al. A comparison of wound instillation and caudal block for analgesia following pediatric inguinal herniorrhaphy. J Pediatr Surg 1993; 28:565–567.

69. Markakis DA. Regional anesthesia in pediatrics. Anesthesiol Clin North America 2000; 18:355–381.

70. Esmail Z, Montgomery C, Courtrn C, et al. Efficacy and complications of morphine infusions in postoperative paediatric patients. Paediatr Anaesth 1999; 9:321–327.

71. Berde CB, Lehn BM, Yee JD, et al. Patient-controlled analgesia in children and adolescents: a randomized, prospective comparison with intramuscular administration of morphine for postoperative analgesia. J Pediatr 1991; 118:460–466.

72. Bray RJ, Woodhams AM, Vallis CJ, et al. Morphine consumption and respiratory depression in children receiving postoperative analgesia from continuous morphine infusion or patient controlled analgesia. Paediatr Anaesth 1996; 6:129–134.

73. Collins JJ, Geake J, Grier HE, et al. Patient-controlled analgesia for mucositis pain in children: a three-period crossover study comparing morphine and hydromorphone. J Pediatr 1996; 129:722–728.

74. Lloyd-Thomas AR, Howard RF. A pain service for children. Paediatric Anaesthesia 1994; 4:3–15.

75. Choonara I. Why do babies cry? We still know too little about what will ease babies' pain. BMJ 1999; 319:1381.

76. Lynn A, Nespeca MK, Bratton SL, et al. Clearance of morphine in postoperative infants during intravenous infusion: the influence of age and surgery. Anesth Analg 1998; 86:958–963.

77. Lynn AM, Nespeca MK, Opheim KE, et al. Respiratory effects of intravenous morphine infusions in neonates, infants, and children after cardiac surgery. Anesth Analg 1993; 77:695–701.

78. Bouwmeester NJ, van den Anker JN, Hop WC, et al. Age- and therapy-related effects on morphine requirements and plasma concentrations of morphine and its metabolites in postoperative infants. Br J Anaesth 2003; 90:642–652.

79. Anderson BJ, Woollard GA, Holford NH. A model for size and age changes in the pharmacokinetics of paracetamol in neonates, infants and children. Br J Clin Pharmacol 2000; 50:125–134.

80. Allegaert K, de Hoon J, Verbesselt R, et al. Intra- and interindividual variability of glucuronidation of paracetamol during repeated administration of propacetamol in neonates. Acta Paediatr 2005; 94:1273–1279.

81. van Lingen RA, Deinum HT, Quak CM, et al. Multiple-dose pharmacokinetics of rectally administered acetaminophen in term infants. Clin Pharmacol Ther 1999; 66:509–515.

82. Agrawal S, Fitzsimons JJ, Horn V, et al. Intravenous paracetamol for postoperative analgesia in a 4-day-old term neonate. Paediatr Anaesth 2007; 17:70–71.

83. Brisman M, Ljung BM, Otterbom I, et al. Methaemoglobin formation after the use of EMLA cream in term neonates. Acta Paediatr 1998; 87:1191–1194.

84. Taddio A, Ohlsson A, Einarson TR, et al. A systematic review of lidocaine-prilocaine cream (EMLA) in the treatment of acute pain in neonates. Pediatrics 1998; 101:E1.

85. Brady-Fryer B, Wiebe N, Lander J. Pain relief for neonatal circumcision. Cochrane Database Syst Rev 2004; 4:CD004217.

86. Stevens B, Yamada J, Ohlsson A. Sucrose for analgesia in newborn infants undergoing painful procedures. Cochrane Database Syst Rev 2004; 3:CD001069.

87. Bucher HU, Baumgartner R, Bucher N, et al. Artificial sweetener reduces nociceptive reaction in term newborn infants. Early Hum Dev 2000; 59:51–60.

88. Skogsdal Y, Eriksson M, Schollin J. Analgesia in newborns given oral glucose. Acta Paediatr 1997; 86:217–220.

89. Gradin M, Schollin J. The role of endogenous opioids in mediating pain reduction by orally administered glucose among newborns. Pediatrics 2005; 115:1004–1007.

90. Bellieni CV, Bagnoli F, Perrone S, et al. Effect of multisensory stimulation on analgesia in term neonates: a randomized controlled trial. Pediatr Res 2002; 51:460–463.

91. Shah PS, Aliwalas LI, Shah V. Breastfeeding or breast milk for procedural pain in neonates. Cochrane Database Syst Rev 2006; 3:CD004950.

92. Carbajal R, Veerapen S, Couderc S, et al. Analgesic effect of breast feeding in term neonates: randomised controlled trial. BMJ 2003; 326:313.

93. Carbajal R, Chauvet X, Couderc S, et al. Randomised trial of analgesic effects of sucrose, glucose, and pacifiers in term neonates. BMJ 1999; 319:1393–1397.

94. Tobias JD, Rasmussen GE. Pain management and sedation in the pediatric intensive care unit. Pediatr Clin North Am 1994; 41:1269–1292.

95. Dyke MP, Kohan R, Evans S. Morphine increases synchronous ventilation in preterm infants. J Paediatr Child Health 1995; 31:176–179.

96. Hickey PR, Hansen DD, Wessel DL, et al. Pulmonary and systemic hemodynamic responses to fentanyl in infants. Anesth Analg 1985; 64:483–486.

97. Palermo TM. Impact of recurrent and chronic pain on child and family daily functioning: a critical review of the literature. J Dev Behav Pediatr 2000; 21:58–69.

98. Yaster M, Kost-Byerly S, Maxwell LG. The management of pain in sickle cell disease. Pediatr Clin North Am 2000; 47:699–710.

99. Wilder RT. Management of pediatric patients with complex regional pain syndrome. Clin J Pain 2006; 22:443–448.

100. Finniss DG, Murphy PM, Brooker C, et al. Complex regional pain syndrome in children and adolescents. Eur J Pain 2006; 10:767–770.

101. Association for Children with Life-Threatening or Terminal Conditions and Their Families, and the Royal College of Paediatrics and Child Health. A guide to the development of children's palliative care services. London: RCPCH; 2003.

102. Association for Children with Life-Threatening or Terminal Conditions and their Families. ACT Charter. 1998. www.act.org.uk/dmdocuments/act_charter.pdf

103. Goldman A. Care of the dying child. Oxford: Oxford University Press; 1994.

104. Hunt A, Mastroyannopoulou K, Goldman A, et al. Not knowing – the problem of pain in children with severe neurological impairment. Int J Nurs Stud 2003; 40:171–183.

105. Williams DG, Hatch DJ, Howard RF. Codeine phosphate in paediatric medicine. Br J Anaesth 2001; 86:421–427.

106. Hunt A, Goldman A, Devine T, et al. Transdermal fentanyl for pain relief in a paediatric palliative care population. Palliat Med 2001; 15:405–412.

107. Wheeler M, Birmingham PK, Dsida RM, et al. Uptake pharmacokinetics of the Fentanyl Oralet in children scheduled for central venous access removal: implications for the timing of initiating painful procedures. Paediatr Anaesth 2002; 12:594–599.

108. Fitzgibbon D, Morgan D, Dockter D, et al. Initial pharmacokinetic, safety and efficacy evaluation of nasal morphine gluconate for breakthrough pain in cancer patients. Pain 2003; 106:309–315.

109. McGrath P, Brown S, Collins J. Paediatric palliative medicine. In: Oxford Textbook of palliative medicine, 3rd edn Oxford: Oxford University Press; 2004.775–797.

110. Goodarzi M. Comparison of epidural morphine, hydromorphone and fentanyl for postoperative pain control in children undergoing orthopaedic surgery. Paediatr Anaesth 1999; 9:419–422.

111. Devogelaer JP, Coppin C. Osteogenesis imperfecta: current treatment options and future prospects. Treat Endocrinol 2006; 5:229–242.

112. Watterson G, Goldman A, Michalski A. Corticosteroids in the palliative phase of peadiatric brain tumours. Arch Dis Child 2002; 86:A76.

113. Fitzgibbon EJ, Viola R. Parenteral ketamine as an analgesic adjuvant for severe pain: development and retrospective audit of a protocol for a palliative care unit. J Palliat Med 2005; 8:49–57.

114. Kronenberg RH. Ketamine as an analgesic: parenteral, oral, rectal, subcutaneous, transdermal and intranasal administration. J Pain Palliat Care Pharmacother 2002; 16:27–35.

115. Krach LE. Pharmacotherapy of spasticity: oral medications and intrathecal baclofen. J Child Neurol 2001; 16:31–36.

116. Hassall E. Decisions in diagnosing and managing chronic gastroesophageal reflux disease in children. J Pediatr 2005; 146:S3–S12.

117. Scott RC, Besag FM, Neville BG. Buccal midazolam and rectal diazepam for treatment of prolonged seizures in childhood and adolescence: a randomised trial. Lancet 1999; 353:623–626.

118. Foster C, Eiser C, Oades P, et al. Treatment demands and differential treatment of patients with cystic fibrosis and their siblings: patient, parent and sibling accounts. Child Care Health Dev 2001; 27:349–364.

119. Pettle Michael SA, Lansdown RG. Adjustment to the death of a sibling. Arch Dis Child 1986; 61:278–283.

120. Whittam EH. Terminal care of the dying child. Psychosocial implications of care. Cancer 1993; 71:3450–3462.

121. Wellings T. Drawings by dying and bereaved children. Paediatr Nurs 2001; 13:30–36.

122. Bluebond-Langner M. The private worlds of the dying child. Princeton: Princeton University Press; 1978.

123. Stevens M. Psychological adaptation of the dying child, 3rd edn. Oxford: Oxford University Press; 2004.775–797.

124. Laakso H, Paunonen-Ilmonen M. Mothers' experience of social support following the death of a child. J Clin Nurs 2002; 11:176–185.

Appendix

Anne Green, Rachel Webster, IA Auchterlonie, Anita MacDonald

REFERENCE RANGES FOR BIOCHEMICAL LABORATORY TESTS

INTRODUCTION

It is important to note that there are no internationally accepted world-wide reference ranges available for laboratory data. It should also be noted that it is difficult for individual laboratories to collect their own data on 'normal' subjects for ethical and logistical reasons. This problem is highlighted particularly with neonatal and pediatric reference ranges and hence many of the data available today still originate from historical studies. There are many variables which affect particular biochemical parameters and must be considered before specific data from an individual patient can be reliably used. These variables are summarized below as a prompt when considering reference data. The values detailed in this chapter are therefore a **guide only** to interpreting laboratory data for neonates, infants and children and must never be considered as absolute. They apply to the specific laboratory methods used by the individual laboratories and centers from which the assembled data has been sourced and will not necessarily apply to methods used in other laboratories.

In addition to reference ranges, many laboratories have defined 'action limits' for a number of analytes, e.g. sodium, potassium, glucose, calcium and C-reactive protein (CRP). Action limits are usually concentrations which could indicate medical emergencies and therefore need acting on promptly; values are usually agreed between laboratories and medical staff in individual units. The laboratory will usually have in place a telephoning protocol to the clinician in charge of that patient. Action limits should be differentiated from reference ranges.

Methodology

Measurement of an analyte using different technologies may significantly affect the result and hence reference ranges. This is because different methods use different characteristics of a compound to quantify the amount: this may be a chemical reaction with another molecule to produce a product which can be measured, an immunological feature or parameters based on fluorescence, light absorption or electrical activity. For example, sodium can be measured using the principle of light absorption by flame photometry or electrical activity by ion selective electrodes (ISEs). Values derived from ISEs are lower than those from flame photometry. Interference from other molecules is another factor which may be a problem for some methods used – such an example is interference by ketones in creatinine measurement. Bilirubin measurement may be interfered with by hemoglobin in some methods and therefore capillary blood samples, in which there is a greater risk of hemolysis compared to venous samples, require special attention when choosing a suitable method. Due attention must be given when a patient is referred from one hospital or clinic to another if laboratories use different analytical methods. In such circumstances apparent differences in the value of analytes may be due to the different methodologies and not to physiological changes.

Neonatal reference ranges

Providing reference range data for the neonatal period is even more difficult than for other age ranges in view of the number of physiological processes that the newborn undergoes. The birth process and subsequent rapid growth and maturation result in significant changes during the first four weeks of life for many analytes such as cortisol, TSH and thyroxine, which are all elevated immediately after birth in order to provide the newborn with the hormonal stimulation it requires to adapt to life outside the womb. Biochemical changes are also seen with different feeding regimens. Two notable examples include higher values of urea in bottle fed compared with breast fed infants, and significant differences in some amino acid levels associated with the use of formula milks.

Patient variables

Reference range data can also differ between gender, gestation, age and ethnicity. There can be marked differences in values for certain analytes, obvious examples between male and female being hormones, and differences across age range are highlighted by alkaline phosphatase. It must therefore be remembered that the cohorts of patients used to derive the reference ranges detailed in this chapter may not directly relate to the population from which the individual patient under consideration has been drawn. Where significant differences occur this has been annotated in the tables with specific text.

Specimen type

The specimen type used in the collection of the reference range data is stated in the tables where appropriate. The use of different types (plasma vs. serum) or anticoagulants (lithium heparin vs. EDTA) can greatly affect the results obtained by certain methodologies and this must be taken into account. For some analytes, such as glucose, triglycerides and amino acids, fasting is of particular importance. These features are noted in the tables where relevant.

Measurement and units

In this chapter, reference values are generally given in SI units and, where considered appropriate, a conversion factor has been given to convert from weight units. This is the number by which weight units need to be multiplied in order to convert weight units into SI (Système International d'Unités) units.

The SI unit of quantity is the mole (the molecular weight of a substance expressed in grams) and the unit of volume is the liter, therefore the SI unit used in these tables is moles/Liter or mol/L. Smaller multiples of this SI unit are generally used to convert the figure into a whole number or to reduce decimal points:

Millimole/L (mmol/L) $\times$) 10^{-3}
Micromole/L (μmol/L) $\times$) 10^{-6}
Nanomole/L (nmol/L) $\times$) 10^{-9}
Picomole/L (pmol/L) $\times$) 10^{-12}

LABORATORY REFERENCE VALUES

For enzyme measurements, where the weight and therefore molarity is often unknown, activity is measured rather than the absolute quantity of the enzyme. The International Union of Biochemistry recommended in 1964 that enzymes should be expressed in international units (IU). In this scheme 1 IU is the amount of enzyme that will catalyze the transformation of 1 micromole of substrate per minute. In addition to IU of measurement, units/liter or U/L is now in common use.

Data interpretation

The correct interpretation of laboratory results from an individual patient can only be carried out with adequate liaison with the local laboratory which should be able to provide the appropriate reference ranges taking into consideration the patient variables, methodology and sample type used.

The ranges provided in this chapter are based on literature sources, our own studies, unpublished data from specialist groups, and in some cases a combination of sources.[1-36]

Key: y = year
    m = month
    d = day

Table A.1 Blood and plasma reference ranges (common 20 analytes)

Analyte	Age	Reference range		Weight unit (where applicable)	Conversion factor	Comments
Alanine aminotransferase (ALT)	Neonate Infants Children	0–40 U/L 10–80 U/L 10–40 U/L				Gross hemolysis will cause false elevation
Alkaline phosphatase (ALP)	Preterm Neonate Infants 2–5 y 6–7 y 8–9 y	Up to 1500 U/L Up to 700 U/L 250–1000 U/L 250–850 U/L 250–1000 U/L 250–750 U/L				Alkaline phosphatase activity changes markedly through life and reference ranges are highly method dependent. These ranges should be used as a guide only and you should refer to your local laboratory for their reference ranges
		Male	*Female*			
	10–11 y 12–13 y 14–15 y 16–18 y	250–730 U/L 275–875 U/L 170–970 U/L 125–720 U/L	250–950 U/L 200–730 U/L 170–460 U/L 75–270 U/L			
Ammonia	Neonate Infants/children Preterm or sick neonate	< 100 μmol/L < 40 μmol/L < 150 μmol/L		μg/100 ml	0.54	Venous samples are preferred. Capillary concentrations are generally higher. Venous ranges are shown
Aspartate aminotransferase (AST)	Neonate Infants Children	< 120 U/L < 80 U/L 15–50 U/L				Gross hemolysis will cause false elevation
Bilirubin, total	Neonate 2–6 d Neonate 6–10 d > 1 m	Up to 217 μmol/L Up to 230 μmol/L 1.7–26 μmol/L		mg/100 ml	17.1	
Bilirubin, unconjugated	0–10 d 11d–20 y	10–180 μmol/L 3–17 μmol/L				Conjugated and unconjugated values are method dependent; older methods may measure direct and indirect bilirubin which is different

Analyte	Age	Reference range		Weight unit (where applicable)	Conversion factor	Comments
Calcium	0–5 d	1.95–2.75 mmol/L		mg/100 ml	0.25	Interpretation of calcium concentration should take into account the albumin concentration as hypoalbuminemia reduces the total calcium concentration. An equation for 'adjusted calcium', which takes into account the albumin concentration, should be available from your local hospital
	5 d – 1 y	2.15–2.75 mmol/L				
	2–5 y	2.15–2.65 mmol/L				
	>5 y	2.20–2.60 mmol/L				
Chloride		95–106 mmol/L		mEq/L	1	
Cholesterol	Birth	0.5–3.2 mmol/L		mg/100 ml	0.026	Cholesterol rises rapidly after birth and levels are higher when fed on human rather than cows' milk
	1 w	1.7–4.2 mmol/L				
	1–3 y	1.2–4.7 mmol/L				
	4–6 y	2.8–4.8 mmol/L				
	7–9 y	2.9–5.3 mmol/L				
		Male	*Female*			
	10–11 y	3.3–6.0 mmol/L	3.3–6.3 mmol/L			
	12–13 y	3.3–6.0 mmol/L	3.3–5.6 mmol/L			
	14–15 y	2.8–5.8 mmol/L	3.4–5.6 mmol/L			
Cortisol	At 9 am	180–550 nmol/L		µg/100 ml	27.6	Stress raises cortisol levels. Cortisol levels are lower in neonates but reach near adult levels by 2 m of age. Hydrocortisone and prednisolone cross react with many assays, but dexamethasone generally does not
	At midnight	<130 nmol/L				
Creatine kinase (CK)	Newborn	160–1230 U/L				Activity increases after exercise or muscle trauma
	Infant	60–305 U/L				
		Male	*Female*			
	4–6 y	75–230 U/L	75–230 U/L			
	7–9 y	60–365 U/L	60–365 U/L			
	10–11 y	55–215 U/L	80–230 U/L			
	12–13 y	60–330 U/L	50–295 U/L			
	14–15 y	60–335 U/L	50–240 U/L			
	16–19 y	55–370 U/L	45–230 U/L			
Creatinine	Neonate	20–100 µmol/L		mg/100 ml	88.4	Levels rise gradually with age, are dependent on muscle mass and are very method dependent. Values shown are based on a Jaffe method and should be used as a guide only. Contact your local laboratory for its method-related reference ranges
	>1 m and up to 2 y	20–60 µmol/L				
	Up to 5 y	20–70 µmol/L				
	5 y and over	20–80 µmol/L				
Glucose	Neonate			mg/100 ml	0.055	Symptomatic hypoglycemia is usually associated with concentrations <2.5 mmol/L. It is recommended that fasting glucose results >6.0 mmol/L should be further investigated by WHO criteria. Ranges shown are for a fasting sample
	12–24 h	2.4–5.4 mmol/L				
	25–48 h	2.9–5.2 mmol/L				
	4–7 d	3.2–5.9 mmol/L				
	Over 7 d	3.9–6.0 mmol/L				
γ-Glutamyl-transferase (γGT)	Newborns	<200 U/L				
	Infants	<120 U/L				
	Children	<35 U/L				
Magnesium	Neonate	0.48–1.05 mmol/L		mg/100 ml	0.411	
	>1 m	0.6–0.95 mmol/L				
Osmolality		275–295 mmol/kg		mosmol/kg	1	
Phosphate	Neonate	1.55–2.65 mmol/L		mg/100 ml	0.323	Hemolysis and capillary samples give elevated results
	1–3 y	1.25–2.10 mmol/L				
	4–6 y	1.3–1.75 mmol/L				
	7–11 y	1.20–1.80 mmol/L				
	12–13 y	1.05–1.75 mmol/L				
	14–15 y	0.95–1.75 mmol/L				
	16–19 y	0.90–1.50 mmol/L				

(Continued)

Table A.1 Blood and plasma reference ranges (common 20 analytes)—Cont'd

Analyte	Age	Reference range		Weight unit (where applicable)	Conversion factor	Comments
Potassium	Neonate 1 w –1 m 1–6 m 6 m – 1 y >1 y	3.2–5.5 mmol/L 3.4–6.0 mmol/L 3.5–5.6 mmol/L 3.5–5.1 mmol/L 3.3–4.6 mmol/L		mEq/L	1	Hemolysis and delayed separation can give falsely elevated results. Ranges shown are for venous samples
Total protein	Neonate 1–3 y >3 y	54–70 g/L 60–70 g/L 60–80 g/L		g/100 ml	10.0	
Triglyceride	1–3 y 4–6 y 7–9 y 10–11 y 12–13 y 14–15 y	0.33–1.48 mmol/L 0.38–1.38 mmol/L 0.34–1.53 mmol/L *Male* 0.28–1.63 mmol/L 0.28–1.72 mmol/L 0.40–1.95 mmol/L	*Female* 0.46–1.66 mmol/L 0.44–1.54 mmol/L 0.43–1.60 mmol/L	mg/100 ml	0.011	Ranges shown are for a fasting sample
Sodium	Neonate >1 m	132–145 mmol/L 135–145 mmol/L		mEq/L	1	Pseudohyponatremia can occur due to gross lipemia or hypoproteinemia when indirect ISE and flame photometry methods are used
Standard bicarbonate	Newborns >1 m	18–25 mmol/L 21–25 mmol/L		mEq/L	1	
Urea		2.5–6.6 mmol/L		mg/100 ml	0.357	Values in neonates and breast-fed infants may be lower

Table A.2 Blood and plasma reference ranges

Analyte	Age	Reference ranges		Comments
Albumin	Newborn	25–50 g/L		Albumin concentrations in the preterm infant are *normally* lower than in the term infant and are not indicative of protein deficiency
	1 y	35–50 g/L		
	4 y and older	37–50 g/L		
Adrenocorticotropic hormone (ACTH)		< 46 ng/L		There is diurnal variation with levels being higher in the morning. Samples should be taken at 10am with a serum cortisol
Aldosterone	Infants	165–2930 pmol/L		Patients should be on a normal salt diet and recumbent before blood collection
	1–4 y	70–950 pmol/L		
	5–9 y	30–620 pmol/L		
	10–15 y	70–580 pmol/L		
Amino acids		(µmol/L)		Many laboratories perform qualitative amino acid investigations looking for an abnormal pattern before undertaking quantitative investigation
Taurine		20–120		These are approximate ranges for children and are only a guide; values for the neonate and infant will differ
Aspartic acid		1.0–20		Reference values will vary with age and feeding/fasting states – consult your specialized laboratory
Threonine		40–200		
Serine		70–200		
Asparagine		15–85		
Glutamic acid		15–80		
Glutamine		330–810		
Proline		40–330		
Glycine		110–340		
Alanine		120–600		
Citrulline		10–50		
Valine		130–350		
Cystine		25–70		
Methionine		5.0–40		
Isoleucine		30–100		
Leucine		50–200		
Tyrosine		30–100		
Phenylalanine		25–100		
Ornithine		20–135		
Lysine		70–270		
Histidine		45–120		
Arginine		10–110		
Amylase	Neonates	< 50 U/L		
	> 1 m	30–100 U/L		
Androstenedione	Neonates	1.3–16.5 nmol/L		
	Prepubertal	2.0–4.2 nmol/L		
	Post puberty: male	2.8–10.5 nmol/L		
	Post puberty: female	1.7–12.9 nmol/L		
α1-antitrypsin		1.8–4.0 g/L		α1-antitrypsin is an acute phase protein
Base excess		± 2.5–2.5 mmol/L		
Bicarbonate or total CO_2	Neonates	18–23 mmol/L		
	> 1 m	20–26 mmol/L		
PCO_2		4.7–6.0 kPa		
Carboxyhemoglobin		Up to 1.5% of total Hb		
Carotenes		0.9–3.7 µmol/L		
Catecholamines (plasma)				
Noradrenaline		591–2364 pmol/L	Supine	
		1773–5320 pmol/L	Standing	
Adrenaline		< 382 pmol/L	Supine	
		< 546 pmol/L	Standing	
Dopamine		< 196 pmol/L	Supine and standing	
Ceruloplasmin	< 4 m	0.09–0.27 g/L		
	4 m – 1 y	0.14–0.41 g/L		
	1–10 y	0.24–0.47 g/L		
	10–13 y	0.18–0.27 g/L		
	> 13 y	0.24–0.71 g/L		

(Continued)

Table A.2   Blood and plasma reference ranges—Cont'd

Analyte	Age	Reference ranges		Comments
Copper	0–5 d	1.4–7.2 µmol/L		
	5 d – 6 m	4.0–11.0 µmol/L		
	>6 m	11.0–22 µmol/L		
Dehydroepiandrosterone sulfate (DHAS)		*Male*	*Female*	
	1–3 y	0.2–0.6 µmol/L	0.2–2.1 µmol/L	
	4–6 y	0.1–5.1 µmol/L	0.2–1.0 µmol/L	
	7–8 y	0.3–2.6 µmol/L	0.4–1.9 µmol/L	
	9–10 y	0.4–2.0 µmol/L	0.4–4.3 µmol/L	
	11 y	0.5–4.1 µmol/L	0.4–2.7 µmol/L	
	12 y	0.5–9.4 µmol/L	0.8–4.8 µmol/L	
	13 y	0.6–6.6 µmol/L	0.6–4.5 µmol/L	
	14 y	0.5–7.8 µmol/L	0.8–8.2 µmol/L	
	15 y	1.6–8.4 µmol/L	1.1–7.8 µmol/L	
	16 y	1.3–9.7 µmol/L	1.6–9.6 µmol/L	
Estradiol				Estradiol levels in children should only be interpreted on an individual patient basis. Reference ranges are therefore not quoted. Refer to your local laboratory for interpretation and guidance
α1-fetoprotein	>8 m	< 10 KIU/L		Falls with time and should be less than 10 KU/L by 8 m. Since a single AFP result is difficult to interpret, it is advisable to repeat the test in 2–3 weeks to look for an appropriate fall in concentration
Follicle-stimulating hormone (FSH)		*Male*	*Female*	Girls at menarche show similar typical cycle variation to adult females
	0–15 d	< 1 IU/L	0.2–3.0 IU/L	
	15 d – 6 y	0.2–3.0 IU/L	0.2–6.0 IU/L	
	7–10 y	0.2–4.0 IU/L		
	10–14 y	0.5–7.0 IU/L		
	Follicular		2–24.0 IU/L	
	Mid-cycle		0.6–11.0 IU/L	
	Luteal		0.6–9.0 IU/L	
Free fatty acids		100–300 µmol/L	If FFA > 1000 FFA:3HB < 2	Fasting sample
3-hydroxy butyrate		0–300 µmol/L		Fasting sample
Galactose-1-phosphate		Not detected in normal children		
		Treated galactosemics < 150 µmol/L		
		Untreated > 1000 µmol/L		
Growth hormone (GH)	Insulin stress test	> 17 mIU/L		Random GH is of little value. Provocative tests should be used
	GTT	< 1.0 mIU/L		
HBA1c		4.7–7.9% of total Hb		
Haptoglobins		0.3–2.0 g/L		
17 hydroxyprogesterone	Infants (unstressed)	< 13 nmol/L		There is a rapid fall from very high levels of 17-OHP (maternal source) in the first 24–48 h of life making interpretation difficult. Premature and sick infants also have 2–3 fold higher levels of 17-OHP compared with values quoted for full term well infants. Concentrations in neonates with untreated CAH are usually > 60 nmol/L
	Infants (stressed)	< 40 nmol/L		
25 OH Vitamin D		12.5–75 nmol/L		
1,25-dihydroxy vitamin D		48–120 pmol/L		

Analyte	Age	Reference ranges		Comments
Immunoglobulins				
IgG	Neonates	6.5–14.5 g/L		
	1–3 m	2.0–6.5 g/L		
	4–6 m	1.5–8.0 g/L		
	1 y	3.0–12.0 g/L		
	3 y and older	5.0–15.0 g/L		
IgA	Neonates	0–0.1 g/L		
	1–3 m	0.05–0.4 g/L		
	4–6 m	0.1–0.6 g/L		
	1 y	0.2–0.8 g/L		
	3 y and older	0.3–3.0 g/L		
IgM	Neonates	0–0.3 g/L		
	1–3 m	0.1–1.0 g/L		
	4–6 m	0.1–1.0 g/L		
	1 y	0.4–2.0 g/L		
	3 y and older	0.4–2.0 g/L		
Insulin				Insulin cannot be interpreted without a paired glucose and c-peptide result. Please refer to your local laboratory for guidance
Iron	0–4 w	10–30.0 μmol/L		The value of plasma iron is of little value in the investigation of iron deficiency as there is much within-individual variation. In addition, many conditions such as infection, trauma and chronic inflammation are associated with low plasma iron concentration but normal total body iron stores
	4 w–5 y	5–25.0 μmol/L		
	6–9 y	7–25.0 μmol/L		
		Male	*Female*	
	10–14 y	5–24.0 μmol/L	8–26.0 μmol/L	
	15–19 y	6–29.0 μmol/L	5–33.0 μmol/L	
Iron-binding capacity		*Male*	*Female*	
	1–5 y	48–79 μmol/L	48–79 μmol/L	
	6–9 y	43–91 μmol/L	43–91 μmol/L	
	10–14 y	54–91 μmol/L	57–103 μmol/L	
	14–19 y	52–102 μmol/L	52–101 μmol/L	
Lactate (plasma)	Neonates	Up to 3.0 mmol/L		Plasma lactate measurements are usually carried out as part of a timed profile and need to be interpreted with respect to glucose and other metabolites. CSF lactate: plasma lactate ratio should be calculated if a respiratory chain defect is suspected
	>1 m	1.0–1.8 mmol/L		
Lactate dehydrogenase	0–5 d	730–1650 U/L		
	1–3 y	400–720 U/L		
	4–6 y	375–700 U/L		
	7–9 y	335–590 U/L		
		Male	*Female*	
	10–11 y	345–550 U/L	305–605 U/L	
	12–13 y	375–590 U/L	305–505 U/L	
	14–15 y	290–570 U/L	315–460 U/L	
	16–19 y	275–525 U/L	275–525 U/L	
Lead		<0.5 μmol/L		
Luteinizing hormone (LH)		*Male*	*Female*	
	0–15 d	<1 I/U	<1 I/U	
	15 d–10 y	0.7–2.2 I/U	0.7–2.2 I/U	
	10–13 y	0.3–5.0 I/U		
	13–60 y	0.5–8.0 I/U		
	Follicular		1–11.0 I/U	
	Mid-cycle		15–96 I/U	
	Luteal		1–11.0 I/U	
Oxygen saturation	Umbilical artery	0.32%		
	Umbilical vein	26–73%		
	Children	86–101%		
	Newborns	30–80%		
	Older children	60–85%		

(Continued)

Table A.2 Blood and plasma reference ranges—Cont'd

Analyte	Age	Reference ranges		Comments
Parathyroid hormone (PTH)	2–15 y	13–29 ng/L		Intact PTH ranges
	> 16 y	12–65.0 ng/L		
pH		7.35–7.45		
PO₂	Neonates	9.3–13.3 kPa		
	> 1 m	11.3–14.0 kPa		
Progesterone	Male	< 2 nmol/L		
	Female	< 90 nmol/L		
Prolactin	Neonates	< 4000 mU/L		Values may rise to above the quoted ranges in response to stress
	Children	60–390 mU/L		
Renin	0–6 d	2.8–79.0 nmol/L/h		Values shown are for a recumbent patient on a normal sodium diet
	6 d – 1 y	6.4–27.2 nmol/L/h		
	2–4 y	1.5–22.6 nmol/L/h		
	5–9 y	1.8–7.2 nmol/L/h		
	10–15 y	0.7–7.8 nmol/L/h		
Testosterone	1–6 d	2.0–7.0 nmol/L	Male	
	1–9 w	< 13 nmol/L	Male	
	9–12 w	Up to 3.5 nmol/L	Male	
	12–16 w	10.0–30.0 nmol/L	Male	
	Prepubertal > 16 w	< 1 nmol/L	Male	
	Pubertal stage 2	< 8 nmol/L	Male	
	Pubertal stage 3	1.0–18 nmol/L	Male	
	Pubertal stage 4/5	4.5–25 nmol/L	Male	
	Female	< 3.5 nmol/L		
Thyroid stimulating hormone (TSH)	0–5 d	0.5–7.9 mU/L		
	5 d – 9 y	0.4–3.5 mU/L		
	10–13 y male	0.4–3.5 mU/L		
	10–13 y female	0.6–4.8 mU/L		
	14–15 y	0.4–3.5 mU/L		
	> 15 y	0.5–5.0 mU/L		
Free T4	0–5 d	21–52 pmol/L		
	5 d – 11 y	12.0–25 pmol/L		
	12–18 y	11.0–22 pmol/L		
	> 18 y	10.0–24 pmol/L		
Free T3	1–15 d	3.0–15.0 pmol/L		
	15 d – 12 y	3.6–8.5 pmol/L		
	13–19 y	3.7–7.3 pmol/L		
	> 19 y	2.7–6.5 pmol/L		
Uric acid		*Male*	*Female*	
	1–3 y	105–300 μmol/L	105–300 μmol/L	
	4–6 y	130–280 μmol/L	130–280 μmol/L	
	7–9 y	120–295 μmol/L	120–295 μmol/L	
	10–11 y	135–320 μmol/L	180–280 μmol/L	
	12–13 y	160–400 μmol/L	180–345 μmol/L	
	14–15 y	140–465 μmol/L	180–345 μmol/L	
	16–19 y	235–510 μmol/L	180–350 μmol/L	
Vitamin A	1–6 y	0.7–1.5 μmol/L		
	7–12 y	0.9–1.7 μmol/L		
	13–19 y	0.9–2.5 μmol/L		
Vitamin E	Newborn infants	5–14 μmol/L		
	2 y and older	12–28 μmol/L		
Zinc	Children	11.0–24.0 μmol/L		

Table A.3 Normal constituents of urine

Analyte	Age	Reference ranges			Comments
Amino acids					Urine amino acid concentrations vary widely with age, with high concentrations in the neonatal period and early infancy. Concentrations fall particularly over the first 6 months as the renal tubules mature
					Many laboratories perform qualitative amino acid investigations looking for an abnormal pattern before undertaking quantitative investigation
δ-aminolevulinic acid		< 5.2 µmol/mmol Creat			
Calcium	< 7 m	< 2.4 mmol/mmol Creat			These values refer to a random, spot urine taken when the overnight urine has been voided
	7–18 m	< 1.7 mmol/mmol Creat			
	19 m – 6 y	< 1.2 mmol/mmol Creat			
	> 6 y	< 0.7 mmol/mmol Creat			
Catecholamines		*Noradrenaline*	*Dopamine*	*HMMA*	These values refer to a random, spot urine
	0–6 m	0.32 mmol/mol Creat	2.2 mmol/mmol Creat	19 mmol/mmol Creat	
	6 m – 1 y	0.3 mmol/mol Creat	2 mmol/mmol Creat	16 mmol/mmol Creat	
	12–18 m	0.25 mmol/mmol Creat	1.8 mmol/mmol Creat	14 mmol/mmol Creat	
	18 m – 2 y	0.2 mmol/mmol Creat	1.6 mmol/mmol Creat	12 mmol/mmol Creat	
	2–3 y	0.17 mmol/mmol Creat	1.4 mmol/mmol Creat	11 mmol/mmol Creat	
	3–4 y	0.14 mmol/mmol Creat	1.25 mmol/mmol Creat	9 mmol/mmol Creat	
	4–5 y	0.125 mmol/mmol Creat	1.05 mmol/mmol Creat	8 mmol/mmol Creat	
	5–6 y	0.11 mmol/mmol Creat	0.9 mmol/mmol Creat	7 mmol/mmol Creat	
	6–8 y	0.09 mmol/mmol Creat	0.75 mmol/mmol Creat	6.5 mmol/mmol Creat	
	8–10 y	0.085 mmol/mmol Creat	0.65 mmol/mmol Creat	6 mmol/mmol Creat	
	10–12 y	0.08 mmol/mmol Creat	0.55 mmol/mmol Creat	5 mmol/mmol Creat	
	12–14 y	0.075 mmol/mmol Creat	0.5 mmol/mmol Creat	4.5 mmol/mmol Creat	
	14–16 y	0.07 mmol/mmol Creat	0.5 mmol/mmol Creat	4.5 mmol/mmol Creat	
	> 16 y	0.07 mmol/mmol Creat	0.5 mmol/mmol Creat	4.5 mmol/mmol Creat	
Copper		< 50 µg/24 h			Random urines are not useful as results are not interpretable in most cases
Homovanillic acid (HVA)	0–6 m	25 mmol/mol Creat			
	6 m – 1 y	25 mmol/mmol Creat			
	12–18 m	22 mmol/mmol Creat			
	18 m – 2 y	19 mmol/mmol Creat			
	2–3 y	16 mmol/mmol Creat			
	3–4 y	13 mmol/mmol Creat			
	4–5 y	12 mmol/mmol Creat			
	5–6 y	11 mmol/mmol Creat			
	6–8 y	9 mmol/mmol Creat			
	8–10 y	8 mmol/mmol Creat			
	10–12 y	7 mmol/mmol Creat			
	12–14 y	6 mmol/mmol Creat			
	14–16 y	6 mmol/mmol Creat			
	> 16 y	4.5 mmol/mmol Creat			

(Continued)

Table A.3 Normal constituents of urine—Cont'd

Analyte	Age	Reference ranges		Comments
5-hydroxyindole acetic acid (5HIAA)		<50 μmol/24 h		
Lead		<10 μg/24 h		
Magnesium	1–6 m	0.006–0.105 mmol/kg/24 h	Breast fed	
		0.006–0.132 mmol/kg/24 h	Formula fed	
	1–15 y	0.051–0.181 mmol/kg/24 h		
Magnesium/creatinine ratio	2–15 y	<1.05 mmol/mmol Creat		These values refer to a random, spot urine taken when the overnight urine has been voided
Osmolality	Newborns delivery urine	79–118 mmol/kg		
	Maximum in neonatal period	600 mmol/kg		
pH	Newborns	5.0 or higher		
	Older children	5.3–7.2		
Phosphate	% Tubular reabsorption of phosphate (TRP)	>80%		Values may be much different in the neonate
Porphobilinogen		0–10.7 μmol/L		
Potassium	Neonate	<5 mmol/kg/d		These values refer to a 24 h urine collection and are dependent on potassium intake and gestational age
	Child	25–125 mmol/24 h		
Sodium		0.08–0.16 mmol/kg/24 h		These values refer to a 24 h urine collection
Aldosterone		6–60 nmol/24 h		In children, excretion rates would increase during childhood from <1 mg/24 h in the first year
17-hydroxycorticosteroids		*Male*	*Female*	
	Adult	4.0–14 mg/24 h	2.0–12 mg/24 h	
	Children			
17-ketosteroids		*Male*	*Female*	Serum DHAS is a much better measurement
	Adult	8–20 mg/24 h	6–12 mg/24 h	
	0–1 y	0–1.0 mg/24 h	0–1.0 mg/24 h	
	1–5 y	1.0–2.0 mg/24 h	1.0–2.0 mg/24 h	
	6–10 y	1–4.4 mg/24 h	1.4–3.9 mg/24 h	
	11–12 y	1.3–8.5 mg/24 h	3.8–9.5 mg/24 h	
	13–16 y	3.4–9.8 mg/24 h	4.5–17.1 mg/24 h	
Pregnanediol			*Female*	Not a useful marker in pediatrics, measure serum progesterone
	>10 y		<50 μg/24 h	
	12 y		20–600 mg/24 h	
Pregnanetriol			*Female*	17-hydroxyprogesterone has superseded this assay
	>10 y		<50 μg/24 h	
	12 y		20–100 mg/24 h	
Vanillylmandelic acid (VMA)	0–1 y	0–18 mg/g Creat		
	2–4 y	0–11.0 mg/g Creat		
	5–9 y	0–8.3 mg/g Creat		
	10–19 y	0–8.2 mg/g Creat		
Total porphyrin		20–320 nmol/L		

Table A.4 Normal cerebrospinal fluid (CSF) values

Analyte	Age	Reference ranges	
WBC	Neonate	0–15/mm³	
	Child	0–5/mm³	
Glucose		2.5–4.5 mmol/L	
Lactate		0.8–2.4 mmol/L	CSF lactate:plasma lactate ratio should be calculated if a respiratory chain defect is suspected
Protein	0–2 m	< 1.2 g/L	
	2–4 m	< 0.6 g/L	
	5 m –10 y	< 0.25 g/L	
	10–18 y	< 0.3 g/L	

Table A.5 Normal constituents of stools

Analyte	Reference ranges
Porphyrins	0–200 nmol/g dry weight
α1-antitrypsin (AAT)	0–0.48 mg AAT/g wet weight
Elastase	
Normal exocrine function	> 200 µg/g
Mild exocrine insufficiency	100–200 µg/g
Severe exocrine deficiency	< 100 µg/g

Table A.6 Therapeutic ranges of medicines commonly used in children

Drug	Therapeutic range in blood	Comments
Caffeine	12–36.0 mg/L	1–2 h post dose
Carbamazepine	4–12.0 mg/L	Pre-dose
Digoxin	0.8–2.0 µg/L	6–24 h post dose
Ethosuximide	40–100 mg/L	Pre-dose
Gentamicin	5–10 mg/L	
Lithium	0.4–1.0 mmol/L	
Paracetamol	> 1300 µmol/L	Toxic value at 4 h
	> 650 µmol/L	Toxic value at 8 h
	> 300 µmol/L	Toxic value at 12 h
Phenobarbital	15–40 mg/L	Pre-dose
Phenytoin	10–20.0 mg/L	Pre-dose
Theophylline		
Neonates	5–10.0 mg/L	2–4 h post dose
Children	10–20.0 mg/L	
Sodium valproate	< 100 mg/L	Pre-dose
Salicylate	< 400 mg/L	Rarely causes symptoms
	> 400 mg/L	Toxic level
	> 1200 mg/L	Usually lethal

Table A.7a Normal blood count values from birth to 18 years

Age	Hb (g/dl)	RBC (×10¹²/L)	Hct	MCV (fl)	WBC (×10⁹/L)	Neutrophils (×10⁹/L)	Lympho-cytes (×10⁹/L)	Monocytes (×10⁹/L)	Eosinophils (×10⁹/L)	Basophils (×10⁹/L)	Platelets (×10⁹/L)	Reticulo-cytes (×10⁹/L)
Birth (term/ infants)	14.9–23.7	3.7–6.5	0.47–0.75	100–125	10–26	2.7–14.4	2.0–7.3	0–1.9	0–0.85	0–0.1	150–450	110–450
2 weeks	13.4–19.8	3.9–5.9	0.41–0.65	88–110	6–21	1.5–5.4	2.8–9.1	0.1–1.7	0–0.85	0–0.1	170–500	10–80
2 months	9.4–13.0	3.1–4.3	0.28–0.42	84–98	5–15	0.7–4.8	3.3–10.3	0.4–1.2	0.05–0.9	0.02–0.13	210–650	35–200
6 months	10.0–13.0	3.8–4.9	0.3–0.38	73–84	6–17	1–6	3.3–11.5	0.2–1.3	0.1–1.1	0.02–0.2	210–560	15–110
1 y	10.1–13.0	3.9–5.1	0.3–0.38	70–82	6–16	1–8	3.4–10.5	0.2–0.9	0.05–0.9	0.02–0.13	200–550	
2–6 y	11.0–13.8	3.9–5.0	0.32–0.4	72–87	6–17	1.5–8.5	1.8–8.4	0.15–1.3	0.05–1.1	0.02–0.12	210–490	
6–12 y	11.1–14.7	3.9–5.2	0.32–0.43	76–90	4.5–14.5	1.5–8.0	1.5–5.0	0.15–1.3	0.05–1.0	0.02–0.12	170–450	50–130
12–18 y												
Female	12.1–15.1	4.1–5.1	0.35–0.44	77–94	4.5–13	1.5–6	1.5–4.5	0.15–1.3	0.05–0.8	0.02–0.12	180–430	
Male	12.1–16.6	4.2–5.6	0.35–0.49	77–92								

Red cell values at birth derived from skin puncture blood; most other data from venous blood.
Adapted from Hinchliffe.[37]

Table A.7b   Reference values for coagulation tests in healthy children aged 1–16 years compared with adults

Coagulation tests	Age			
	1–5 years Mean (boundary)	6–10 years Mean (boundary)	11–16 years Mean (boundary)	Adult mean (boundary)
PT (s)	11 (10.6–11.4)	11.1 (10.1–12.1)	11.2 (10.2–12.0)	12 (11.0–14.0)
INR	1.0 (0.96–1.04)	1.01 (0.91–1.11)	1.02 (0.93–1.10)	1.10 (1.0–1.3)
APTT (s)	30 (24–36)	31 (26–36)	32 (26–37)	33 (27–40)
Fibrinogen (g/L)	2.76 (1.70–4.05)	2.79 (1.57–4.0)	3.0 (1.54–4.48)	2.78 (1.56–4.0)
Bleeding time (min)	6 (2.5–10)*	7 (2.5–13)*	5 (3–8)*	4 (1–7)
II (unit/ml)	0.94 (0.71–1.16)*	0.88 (0.67–1.07)*	0.83 (0.61–1.04)*	1.08 (0.70–1.46)
V (unit/ml)	1.03 (0.79–1.27)	0.90 (0.63–1.16)*	0.77 (0.55–0.99)*	1.06 (0.62–1.50)
VII (unit/ml)	0.82 (0.55–1.16)*	0.85 (0.52–1.20)*	0.83 (0.58–1.15)*	1.05 (0.67–1.43)
VIII (unit/ml)	0.90 (0.59–1.42)	0.95 (0.58–1.32)	0.92 (0.53–1.31)	0.99 (0.50–1.49)
vWF (unit/ml)	0.82 (0.60–1.20)	0.95 (0.44–1.44)	1.00 (0.46–1.53)	0.92 (0.50–1.58)
IX (unit/ml)	0.73 (0.47–1.04)*	0.75 (0.63–0.89)*	0.82 (0.59–1.22)*	1.09 (0.55–1.63)
X (unit/ml)	0.88 (0.58–1.16)*	0.75 (0.55–1.01)*	0.79 (0.50–1.17)*	1.06 (0.70–1.52)
XI (unit/ml)	0.97 (0.56–1.50)	0.86 (0.52–1.20)	0.74 (0.50–0.97)*	0.97 (0.67–1.27)
XII (unit/ml)	0.93 (0.64–1.29)	0.92 (0.60–1.40)	0.81 (0.34–1.37)*	1.08 (0.52–1.64)
PK (unit/ml)	0.95 (0.65–1.30)	0.99 (0.66–1.31)	0.99 (0.53–1.45)	1.12 (0.62–1.62)
HMWK (unit/ml)	0.98 (0.64–1.32)	0.93 (0.60–1.30)	0.91 (0.63–1.19)	0.92 (0.50–1.36)
XIIIa (unit/ml)	1.08 (0.72–1.43)*	1.09 (0.65–1.51)*	0.99 (0.57–1.40)	1.05 (0.55–1.55)
XIIIs (unit/ml)	1.13 (0.69–1.56)*	1.16 (0.77–1.54)*	1.02 (0.60–1.43)	0.97 (0.57–1.37)

All factors except fibrinogen are expressed as unit/ml, where pooled plasma contains 1.0 unit/ml. All data are expressed as the mean, followed by the upper and lower boundary encompassing 95% of the population. Between 20 and 50 samples were assayed for each value for each age group. Some measurements were skewed due to a disproportionate number of high values. The lower limit, which excludes the lower 2.5% of the population, is given.
APTT, activated partial thromboplastin time; HMWK, high molecular weight kininogen; INR, international normalized ratio; PK, prekallikrein; PT, prothrombin time; VIII, factor VIII procoagulant; vWF, von Willebrand factor. *Values that are significantly different from adults. From Chalmers & Gibson.[38]

NUTRIENTS AND FORMULA FEEDS

Introduction
Normal infants and children
Infant (0–12 months). Term infants with normal gastrointestinal function are fed either human breast milk or normal infant formula during the first year of life. Normal infant formula is defined as 'a food intended for nutritional use by infants in good health for the first year of life, and satisfying, by itself the nutritional requirements of such infants'. It is based on whey- or casein-dominant protein, lactose ± maltodextrin and amylose, vegetable oil and milk fat. Whey-dominant milks are the closest in composition to breast milk. Although some infant formulas contain novel nutrients such as long chain fatty acids (docosahexaenoic acid and arachidonic acid), nucleotides and prebiotics, the composition of all normal and soya infant formulas has to meet the UK's *The Infant Formula and Follow-on Formula Regulations 1995,*[39] which enact the European Community Regulations 91/321/EC.[40] The energy content by law must not be less than 60 kcal (250 kJ) and not more than 70 kcal (295 kJ) per 100 ml.

Infant (over 6 months of age). 'Follow-on formulas' are feeds designed for infants over the age of 6 months and 'constitute the principal liquid element in a progressively diversified diet'.[40] They are based on modified cows' milk. They contain less protein, calcium and phosphorus than cows' milk, but more than standard infant formula, and are fortified with other nutrients.

Children over 1 year: Growing up milk is fortified formula designed for children over 1 year. It is based on cows' milk.

Special infant formulas
It is essential that any infant or child who is intolerant of breast milk or normal infant formula, or whose condition requires nutrient specific adaptation, is prescribed a nutritional complete replacement formula in adequate volume. The composition of special infant formula has to meet the Commission Directive (1999/21/EC) on Dietary Foods for Special Medical Purposes.[41]

Soya formula. Soya infant formula is based on soya-protein isolate supplemented with L-methionine, taurine and carnitine. These formulas support normal growth, protein status and mineralization. Although they are suitable for cows' milk protein and lactose intolerance, the Committee on Toxicity of Chemicals in Food, Consumer Products and the Environment (COT) has expressed concern about the use of soya infant formula in infancy.[42] Soya infant formula contains 18–41 mg/L of phytoestrogens. This is several times higher than the quantity in human breast milk. Although the COT report concluded that there is no direct evidence that soya infant formula affects the health of infants, particularly fertility, it is believed that soya infant formula may be a potential risk to the infant. Therefore it is not recommended that soya-based infant formula is used as the first choice formula for infants with cows' milk sensitivity or lactose intolerance, but it is widely used for infants with galactosemia because of the residual lactose content of low lactose formula and protein hydrolysate formula which are both derived from cows' milk.

Protein hydrolysate formula. Based on casein, whey, meat and soya, these formulas are suitable for infants with disaccharide and/or whole protein intolerance. Protein hydrolysates are the result of heat treatment and/or enzymatic cleavage, which is used in order to produce peptides of minor antigenic activity, with a molecular weight of less than 1200 daltons. Some of the formulas contain a significant proportion of their fat source in the form of medium chain triglyceride (MCT) oil.

Low lactose formula. This type of formula is based on whole cows' milk protein. Although suitable for lactose intolerance they contain residual lactose in very small quantities. They are unsuitable for infants with cows' milk protein intolerance.

Elemental (amino acid based formula). There is only one elemental nutritionally complete formula available for infants in the UK. There is evidence to demonstrate that the feed tolerance and growth of infants taking this formula is satisfactory.

Other specialist formula. A number of specialized formulas are available for liver and renal indications. High medium chain fat based formulas for conditions such as chylothorax and long chain fatty acid disorders are available. Ketogenic, low calcium and protein free feeds are also available. These should always be used under dietetic supervision.

Complete enteral feeds

The composition of all enteral feeds has to meet the Commission Directive (1999/21/EC) on Dietary Foods for Special Medical Purposes.[41]

Infant (0–12 months). An infant with faltering growth may be given a high energy and nutrient dense feed containing between 9 and 11% energy from protein. Concentrating or supplementing normal infant formula should not be attempted without the advice of a pediatric dietitian.

Children 1–6 years (8–20 kg). A number of nutritionally complete 0.75 kcal/ml, 1.0 kcal/ml and over 1.0 kcal/ml (± fiber) ready to use feeds designed for the 1–6-year age group are available. They are all based on caseinates, maltodextrin and vegetable oils ± added medium chain tri-glyceride oil (MCT) and contain residual lactose only. These products were originally designed for 1–6-year-old (8–20 kg) children, but some products have had Advisory Committee on Borderline Substances (ACBS) extensions for children weighing up to 30 kg (approximately 10 years of age).

Children 7–12 years. Nutritionally complete 1.0 kcal/ml and 1.5 kcal/ml (± fiber) ready to use feeds designed for this age group are available. They are also based on caseinates, maltodextrin and vegetable oils and contain residual lactose only. Their formulation is in between pediatric and adult feeds.

Children 13 years and over. There are no standard enteral feeds designed for teenagers, so adult feeds are given. The intake of protein, electrolytes, vitamins and trace minerals should be carefully assessed and monitored.

Other dietary supplements

A number of dietary supplements, either based on carbohydrates, fat and/or protein, which can be used to enhance the nutrient density of the diet or nutritionally complete supplements are available. The amount and timing of supplements is important so as not to impair appetite. Ideally supplements should be administered after meals or at bedtime. Many supplements are high in sugar or maltodextrin. Care should be taken to prevent prolonged contact with teeth.

Products for phenylketonuria

There is a wide range of phenylalanine-free protein substitutes for PKU. They have a high osmolality so should be administered with extra water. Some are nutritionally incomplete and require vitamin and/or other nutrient supplementation. Protein substitutes should be taken at least 3 times daily equally distributed throughout the day.

Useful website

www.foodstandards.gov.uk/multimedia/pdfs/phtcreport0503

Notes

The Advisory Committee on Borderline Substances (ACBS) advises GPs on prescription of products that are not drugs or medical devices. The committee is an advisory nondepartmental public body (NDPB), non-statutory and UK-wide. The approved list consists of foodstuffs such as enteral feeds or foods formulated for people with medical conditions.

Table A.8a Standard infant formulas (whey dominant)

	Aptamil First	Cow and Gate First Infant Milk	Farley's First Infant Milk	Hipp Organic First Infant Milk	SMA Gold
Manufacturer	Milupa	Cow and Gate	Heinz	Hipp	SMA
kcal/100 ml	67	67*	68	68	67
kJ/100 ml	275	280	284	283	281
Protein source	Whey and skimmed milk	Whey and skimmed milk	Whey and skimmed milk	Organic whey and skimmed milk	Whey and skimmed milk
Casein: whey ratio	40:60	40:60	40:60	40:60	40:60
Protein g/100 ml	1.3	1.4	1.45	1.6	1.4
Fat source	Vegetable oils, fish oil	Vegetable oils (contains soya), fish oil	Vegetable oils, fish oil	Palm, rapeseed, sunflower oils	Vegetable fats
Fat g/100 ml	3.5	3.5	3.8	3.3	3.6
Contains LCPs	Yes	Yes	Yes	No	Yes
Carbohydrate source	Lactose	Lactose	Lactose	Lactose	Lactose
Carbohydrate g/100 ml	7.3	7.4	7.0	7.9	7.3
Fiber g/100 ml	0.8	0.8	0	0	0
Sodium mmol/100 ml	0.8	0.9	0.7	0.9	0.7
Potassium mmol/100 ml	1.6	1.6	1.5	1.7	1.7
Calcium mg/100 ml	50	50	39	65	42
Iron mg/100 ml	0.53	0.7	0.65	0.7	0.8
Nutritionally complete	Yes	Yes	Yes	Yes	Yes
% Dilution	13.7	13.9	13	13.5	12.7
Presentation	900 g powder; 200 ml carton	400 g, 900 g powder. 200 and 500 ml carton	900 g powder; 250 ml cartons	900 g powder	450 g, 900 g powder, sachets. 250 ml and 1 liter cartons
Other information	Contains prebiotics and nucleotides	Contains prebiotics and nucleotides	Contains nucleotides		Contains nucleotides, alpha-lactalbumin

*Analysis powder only.

Table A.8b   Standard infant formulas (casein dominant)

	Aptamil Extra Hungry	Cow and Gate Infant Milk for Hungrier Babies	Farley's Second Milk	SMA White
Manufacturer	Milupa	Cow and Gate	Heinz	SMA
kcal/100 ml	66*	67*	69*	67*
kJ/100 ml	275	280	289	280
Protein source	Skimmed milk	Skimmed milk	Skimmed milk	Skimmed milk
Protein g/100 ml	1.6	1.7	1.7	1.6
Casein: whey ratio	80:20	80:20	80:20	80:20
Fat source	Vegetable oils	Vegetable oils	Vegetable oils, fish oil	Vegetable oils
Fat g/100 ml	3.2	3.3	3.5	3.6
Contains LCPs	Yes	No	Yes	No
Carbohydrate source	Lactose	Lactose	Lactose	Lactose
Carbohydrate g/100 ml	7.7	7.7	7.7	7
Fiber g/100 ml	0.8	0.8	0	0
Sodium mmol/100 ml	0.9	0.9	0.8	0.90
Potassium mmol/100 ml	2.1	2.1	2.0	2.1
Calcium mg/100 ml	70	79	56	56
Iron mg/100 ml	0.53	0.68	0.73	0.8
Nutritionally complete	Yes	Yes	Yes	Yes
% Dilution	14.1	14.2	13.7	12.7
Presentation	900 g powder. 200 ml cartons	400 g, 900 g powder. 200 and 500 ml cartons	900 g; 250 ml cartons	450 g, 900 g powder. 250 ml and 500 ml cartons
Other information	Contains prebiotics and nucleotides	Contains prebiotics and nucleotides		Contains nucleotides

*Analysis powder only.

Table A.8c   Standard infant formulas (Follow-on)

	Aptamil Follow on	Cow and Gate Follow on for Hungrier Babies 6 Months	Farley's Follow on Milk	Hipp Organic Follow on Milk	SMA Progress
Manufacturer	Milupa	Cow and Gate	Heinz	Hipp	SMA
kcal/100 ml	70*	70*	68*	69	67*
kJ/100 ml	295	295	285	287	280
Protein source	Skimmed milk	Skimmed milk	Whey, skimmed milk	Organic whey and skimmed milk	Skimmed milk
Casein:whey ratio	80:20	80:20	62:38	55:45	80:20
Protein g/100 ml	1.8	1.8	1.8	2.1	1.9
Fat source	Vegetable oils	Vegetable oils (contains soya)	Vegetable oils	Palm, rapeseed, sunflower oils	Vegetable oils
Fat g/100 ml	3.4	3.4	3.4	3.5	3.3
Contains LCPs	No	No	No	No	No
Carbohydrate source	Lactose	Lactose	Lactose	Lactose	Lactose
Carbohydrate g/100 ml	8.1	8.1	7.6	7.2	7.4
Fiber g/100 ml	0.8	0.8	0	0	0
Sodium mmol/100 ml	0.9	0.95	1.3	1.6	1.3
Potassium mmol/100 ml	2.2	2.2	2.3	3.4	2.3
Calcium mg/100 ml	83	83	72	99	90
Iron mg/100 ml	1.3	1.3	1.2	1.2	1.3
Nutritionally complete	Yes	Yes	Yes	Yes	Yes
% Dilution	14.9	14.9	13.8	13.5	13.1
Presentation	900 g powder. 200 ml cartons	400 g, 900 g powder. 200 and 500 ml cartons	900 g powder; 250 ml cartons	900 g powder; 27 g sachet	450 g, 900 g powder; 250 ml, 500 ml cartons
Other information		Contains prebiotics		900 g carton	

*Analysis powder only.

Table A.8d Growing up milk

	Aptamil Growing Up Milk	Cow and Gate Growing Up Milk	Hipp Growing Up Milk
Manufacturer	Milupa	Cow and Gate	Hipp
kcal/100 ml	67	67*	79*
kJ/100 ml	280	280	330
Protein source	Skimmed milk	Skimmed milk	Organic whey and skimmed milk
Protein g/100 ml	1.9	1.9	2.5
Fat source	Canola, sunflower, and corn oil	Vegetable oils	Vegetable oil
Fat g/100 ml	3.0	3.0	3.5
Contains LCPs	No	No	No
Carbohydrate source	Lactose	Lactose	Starch, glucose, glucose syrup
Carbohydrate g/100 ml	8.1	8.1	9.2
Fiber g/100 ml	0.8	0.8	0
Sodium mmol/100 ml	1.1	1.3	1.7
Potassium mmol/100 ml	2.6	2.6	3.1
Calcium mg/100 ml	91	91	107
Iron mg/100 ml	1.2	1.2	1.0
Nutritionally complete	Yes	Yes	Yes
% Dilution	Ready made	Ready made	16.5
Presentation	200 and 500 ml bottles Contains prebiotics	200 and 500 ml bottles Contains prebiotics	600 g, 500 ml bottle 250 ml bottle

*Analysis powder only.

Table A.9a   Special infant formulas

	Pre-thickened infant formula						Infant soya formula			
	Comfort First Infant Milk from Birth	Comfort Follow-on Milk from 6 Months	Enfamil AR with Lipil	SMA Staydown	Aptamil Easy Digest	Farley's Soya Formula	InfaSoy	Isomil	Prosobee	Wysoy
Manufacturer	Cow & Gate	Cow & Gate	Mead Johnson Nutritionals	SMA	Milupa	Heinz	Cow & Gate	Abbott Laboratories	Mead Johnson Nutritionals	SMA
kcal/100 ml	70	72	68	67	70	70	66	68	68	67
kJ/100 ml	295	300	285	279	295	293	275	284	285	280
Protein source	Hydrolysed whey protein	Hydrolysed whey protein	Skimmed milk	Skimmed milk	Hydrolysed whey protein	Soya protein isolate	Soya protein isolate	Soya protein isolate	Soya protein isolate	Soya protein isolate
Protein g/100 ml	1.7	1.9	1.7	1.6	1.7	1.95	1.8	1.8	1.8	1.8
Fat source	Structured vegetable oils	Structured vegetable oils	Palm olein, coconut, soya, sunflower oil	Coconut, palm, soya, sunflower oil	Structured vegetables oils	Sunflower, palm kernel, rapeseed oil, palm olein oil	Palm, sunflower, rapeseed, coconut oil	Sunflower, coconut, soya oil	Palm olein, coconut, soya, and sunflower oil	Palm, coconut, sunflower, soya oil
Fat g/100 ml	3.3	3.3	3.5	3.6	3.3	3.8	3.6	3.7	3.7	3.6
Contains LCPs	No	No	Yes	No	No	No	No	No	No	No
Carbohydrate source	Glucose syrup, starch, lactose	Glucose syrup Starch, lactose	Glucose polymers, lactose, rice starch	Lactose, glucose syrup, corn starch	Glucose syrup, starch, lactose	Glucose syrup	Glucose syrup	Corn syrup, sucrose	Glucose syrup	Glucose syrup
Carbohydrate g/100 ml	8.4	8.7	7.6	7	8.4	7.0	6.6	6.9	6.8	6.9
Fiber g/100 ml	0.8	0.8	0	0	0.8	0	0	0	0	0
Sodium mmol/100 ml	1.0	1.6	1.0	1.0	1	1.1	0.9	1.4	1.1	0.8
Potassium mmol/100 ml	2.1	2.2	2.2	2.1	2.1	1.9	1.7	2.0	2.0	1.9
Calcium mg/100 ml	53	91	55	56	53	56	54	70	66	67
Iron mg/100 ml	0.5	1.2	0.74	0.8	0.5	0.7	0.8	1.0	1.2	0.8
Nutritionally complete	Yes	Yes	Yes	Yes	Y	Yes	Yes	Yes	Yes	Yes
Suitable for vegans	No	No	No	No	No	Yes	No	No	No	No
Lactose free	No	No	No	No	No	Yes	Yes	Yes	Yes	Yes
% Dilution	15.2	15.9	13.5		15.2	15.1	12.7	13.2	12.9	13.5
Presentation	900 g powder	900 g powder	400 g powder	900 g powder	900 g powder	450 g; 900 g powder	900 g powder	400 g powder	400 g powder	430 g, 860 g powder
ACBS listed	No	No	Yes[a]	Yes[a]	No	Yes[b]	Yes[b]	Yes[b]	Yes[b]	Yes[b]
Other information	Contains prebiotics	Contains prebiotics			Contains prebiotics					

[a] Thickened formula is ACBS listed for use in the management of significant reflux. Not for use in excess of a 6 month period. Do not use in combination with other feed thickeners or antacid products.

[b] Infant soya formula ACBS listed for proven lactose intolerance in pre-school children, galactokinase deficiency, galactosemia, and proven whole cows' milk sensitivity

Table A.9b Special infant formulas

	Infant protein hydrolysate							Infant amino acid formula	Child amino acid formula
	Nutramigen 1	Nutramigen 2	Pepti-Junior	Pepti	Pepdite	Pregestimil	Prejomin	Neocate	Neocate Advance
Manufacturer	Mead Johnson Nutritionals	Mead Johnson Nutritionals	Cow and Gate	Cow and Gate	SHS International	Mead Johnson Nutritionals	Milupa	SHS International	SHS International
kcal/100 ml	68	68	66	66	71	68	75	71	100
kJ/100 ml	280	285	275	275	297	283	315	298	420
Protein source	Enzymatically hydrolysed casein	Enzymatically hydrolysed casein	Hydrolysed whey protein	Hydrolysed whey protein	Hydrolysed pork and soya, amino acids	Enzymatically hydrolysed casein	Porcine collagen, soya hydrolysate	L-amino acids	L-amino acids
Protein g/100 ml	1.9	1.7	1.8	1.6	2.1	1.9	2.0	1.95	2.5
Fat source	Palm olein, coconut, soya, sunflower oil	Palm olein, coconut, sunflower, soya oil	MCT oil, soya, rapeseed, sunflower oil	Palm, coconut, rapeseed, sunflower oil single cell oil	Coconut, safflower, soya oil	MCT oil, corn, soya, sunflower oil	Palm, sunflower, rape seed, coconut oil	Safflower, coconut, soya oil	Safflower, coconut, canola oil
Fat g/100 ml	3.4	2.9	3.5 (50% of fat is MCT)	3.3	3.5	3.8 (55% of fat is MCT)	3.6	3.5	3.5
Contains LCPs	No	No	Yes	Yes	No	No	No	No	No
Carbohydrate source	Glucose polymer, modified corn starch	Glucose polymer, modified corn starch, fructose	Glucose syrup	Maltodextrin	Glucose syrup	Glucose polymer, dextrose, maltodextrin, modified corn starch	Maltodextrin, pre-cooked starch	Dried glucose syrup	Dried glucose syrup (glucose in flavored Neocate Advance)
Carbohydrate g/100 ml	7.5	8.6	6.8	7.1	7.8	6.9	8.6	8.1	14.6
Sodium mmol/100 ml	1.39	1.1	0.8	0.9	1.5	1.26	1.4	0.78	2.6
Potassium mmol/100 ml	2.1	2.1	1.7	1.9	1.5	1.9	2.0	1.6	3
Calcium mg/100 ml	64	94	50	47	45	78	63	49	50
Iron mg/100 ml	1.22	1.2	0.77	0.5	1	1.2	1	1.1	0.62
Nutritionally complete	Yes	Yes	Yes	Yes	Yes	Yes	Yes	Yes	Yes
Suitable for vegans	No	No	No	No	No	No	No	No, may include amino acids of animal origin. Contains fish gelatin	No, may include amino acids of animal origin. Contains fish gelatin
Lactose free	Residual lactose only	Residual lactose only	Residual lactose only	Low lactose	Yes	Residual lactose only	Yes	Yes	Yes
% Dilution	13.5	14.7	12.8	13.6	15	13.5	15	15	25
Presentation	425 g powder	425 g powder	450 g powder	900 g powder	400 g powder	450 g powder	400 g powder	400 g powder	Sachets: 100 g (unflavored); 400 g powder
ACBS listed	Yes	Yes	Yes	Yes	Yes	Yes	Yes	Yes	Yes

Nutramigen is ACBS listed for disaccharide and/or whole protein intolerance where additional medium chain triglycerides are not indicated. Nutramigen Stage 2 is ACBS listed for the same indications but for infants from 6 months onwards. Pepti-Junior and Pregestimil are ACBS listed for disaccharide and/or whole protein intolerance or where amino acids are indicated. Pepti may be prescribed for cows' milk protein intolerance with/without secondary lactose intolerance. Neocate and Neocate Advance is ACBS listed for disaccharide or dietary protein intolerance where an elemental formula is specifically indicated.

Table A.9c Special infant formulas

	Low lactose infant formula			MCT infant formula			Other special infant formula	
	Enfamil Lactofree	Galactomin 17	SMA LF	Caprilon	MCT Pepdite	Monogen	Galactomin 19	Locasol
Manufacturer	Mead Johnson Nutritionals	SNS International	SMA Nutrition	SHS International	SHS International	SHS International	SHS Inter-national	SHS International
kcal/100 ml	68	70	67	66	68	74	69	66
kJ/100 ml	280	295	281	277	286	313	288	278
Protein source	Milk protein (isolate)	Caseinate	69% whey 40% casein	Skimmed milk powder, whey	Hydrolyzed pork and soya, amino acids	Whey protein, amino acids	Caseinate, L amino acids	Demineralized whey, caseinate
Protein g/100 ml	1.4	1.7	1.5	1.5	2.0	2.0	1.9	1.9
Fat source	Palm olein, coconut, soya, sunflower oil	Palm, safflower, rapeseed, and coconut oil	Palm, coconut, soya, sunflower oil	MCT oil, soya oil	Walnut, palm kernel, coconut, maize oil	Coconut oil, walnut oil	Safflower, palm, rapeseed, coconut oil	Palm, sunflower, rapeseed, coconut oil
Fat g/100 ml	3.7	3.7	3.6	3.6 (75% MCT)	2.7 (75%) MCT	2.1 (90% MCT)	4	3.4
Contains LCPs	No	No		No	No	No	No	No
Carbohydrate source	Glucose polymers	Glucose syrup	Glucose syrup	Glucose syrup	Glucose syrup	Glucose syrup	Fructose	Lactose, dried glucose syrup
Carbohydrate g/100 ml	7.2	7.5	7.2	7	8.8	12	6.4	7
Sodium mmol/100 ml	1.35	0.9	0.7	0.88	1.5	1.5	0.9	1.2
Potassium mmol/100 ml	2.0	1.8	1.8	1.7	1.5	1.6	1.5	2
Calcium mg/100 ml	78	55	55	53	45	45	55	<7
Iron mg/100 ml	0.8	0.9	0.8	0.5	1	0.74	0.5	0.5
Nutritionally complete	Yes	Yes	Yes	Yes	Yes	Yes	Yes	Very low in calcium and vitamin D
Suitable for vegans	No	No	No	No	No	No	No	No
Lactose free	Contains residual lactose	Contains residual lactose	Contains residual lactose	No	Yes	No	Residual lactose only	No
% Dilution	12.9	13.6	13	12.7	15	17.5	12.9	13.1
Presentation	400 g powder	400 g powder	430 g powder	420 g powder	400 g powder	400 g powder	400 g powder	400 g
ACBS listed	Yes	Yes	Yes	Yes	Yes	Yes	Yes	Yes
								Prepare with distilled water as tap water may contain calcium. Monitor vitamin D levels.

Galactomin 17 is ACBS listed for proven lactose intolerance in pre-school children, galactosemia, and galactokinase deficiency. SMA LF and Enfamil Lactofree are ACBS listed for proven lactose intolerance. Caprilon and MCT Pepdite are ACBS listed for disorders in which a high intake of MCT is beneficial. Monogen ACBS listed for long chain acyl-COA dehydrogenase deficiency, carnitine palmitoyl transferase deficiency, primary and secondary lipoprotein lipase deficiency. Locasol is ACBS listed for hypercalcemia and other conditions which require extreme calcium restriction in the diet. Galactomin 19 is ACBS listed for glucose–galactose intolerance.

Table A.10a Enteral feeds for infants and children

| | Infant enteral feeds | | Post-discharge preterm formula |
	Infatrini	SMA High Energy Formula	Nutriprem 2
Manufacturer	Nutricia	SMA	Cow and Gate
kcal/100 ml	100	91	75
kJ/100 ml	420	382	315
Protein source	Skimmed milk, whey protein	60% whey, 40% casein	Whey protein, skimmed milk
Protein g/100 ml	2.6	2	2
Fat source	Vegetable oils	Coconut, palm, soya oil	Vegetable oils, egg lipid, milk fat, fish oil, sunflower oils
Fat g/100 ml	5.4	4.9	4.1
Contains LCPs	Yes	Yes	Yes
Carbohydrate source	Lactose, Maltodextrin	Lactose	Lactose, glucose syrup
Carbohydrate g/100 ml	10.3	9.8	7.4
Fiber g/100 ml	0.8 (Prebioticmix)	0	0.8 (Prebiotic mix)
Sodium mmol/100 ml	1.1	1.0	1.13
Potassium mmol/100 ml	2.4	2.3	2.0
Calcium mg/100 ml	80	57	94
Iron mg/100 ml	1.0	1.1	1.2
Nutritionally complete	Yes	Yes	Yes
Suitable for vegans	No	No	No
Lactose free	No	No	No
% Dilution	N/a	N/a	15.4
Presentation	200 ml bottle/100 ml glass bottle	200 ml carton	900 g, 200 ml carton, 100 ml glass bottle
ACBS listed	Yes	Yes	Yes
Other information			Contains prebiotics

Infant enteral feeds ACBS listed for disease-related malnutrition, malabsorption and growth failure in infancy. Both feeds are suitable for enteral and oral feeds.
Post-discharge formula ACBS listed for catch-up growth in pre-term (i.e. less than 35 weeks at birth) and small for gestational age infants, up to 6 months corrected age.

Table A10b Enteral feeds for children

	Enteral feeds: children; standard 1 kcal/ml or less					Enteral feeds: children; standard >1 kcal/ml feeds			
	Clinutren Junior	Frebini Original	Nutrini	Paediasure	Nutrini Low Energy Multi fibre	Frebini Energy	Isosource Junior	Nutrini Energy	Paediasure Plus
Manufacturer	Nestle Clinical	Fresenius Kabi	Nutricia	Abbott	Nutricia	Fresenius Kabi	Novartis	Nutricia	Abbott
kcal/100 ml	100*	100	100	101	75	150	122	150	151
kJ/100 ml	420	420	420	422	315	630	512	630	632
Protein source	Caseinate, whey	Milk proteins	Milk proteins	Milk protein	Milk proteins	Milk proteins	Milk proteins	Milk proteins	Sodium and calcium caseinates, whey protein.
Protein g/100 ml	2.97	2.5	2.8	2.8	2.1	3.75	2.7	4.1	4.2
Fat source	MCT oil, rapeseed, corn, sunflower oil	Vegetable oils (with soya oil), MCT oil, fish oil	Vegetable oils	Sunflower, soya, MCT oil	Vegetable oils	Vegetable oils (with soya oil), MCT oil, fish oil	Rapeseed, sunflower, MCT oil	Vegetable oils	Sunflower, soya, MCT oil
Fat g/100 ml	3.9	4.4	4.4	5.0	3.3	6.7	4.7	6.7	7.5
Contains LCPs	No	Yes	No	No	No	Yes	No	No	No
Carbohydrate source	Sucrose and maltodextrin (corn syrup in powder only)	Maltodextrin	Malto-dextrin	Malto-dextrin, sucrose	Malto-dextrin	Malto-dextrin	Malto-dextrin	Malto-dextrin	Malto-dextrin, sucrose
Carbohydrate g/100 ml	13.3	12.5	12.3	11.2	9.3	18.8	17	18.5	16.7
Fiber g/100 ml	0	0	0	0	0.8	0	0	0	0
Sodium mmol/100 ml	2.1	2.2	2.6	2.61	2.6	3.3	2.6	3.9	2.61
Potassium mmol/100 ml	2.8	2.6	2.8	2.8	3.4	3.8	3.0	4.2	3.5
Calcium mg/100 ml	89	60	60	56	60	90	66	90	83
Iron mg/100 ml	1	0.9	1.0	1.0	1.0	1.35	0.8	1.5	1.5
Nutritionally complete	Yes	Yes	Yes	Yes	Yes	Yes	Yes	Yes	Yes
Suitable for vegans	No	No	No	No	No	No	No	No	No
Lactose free	Residual lactose only	Residual lactose only	Residual lactose only	Residual lactose only	Residual lactose only	Residual lactose only	Residual lactose only	Residual lactose only	Residual lactose only
% Dilution	For 1 kcal per ml: 22 g powder + 85 ml water	N/a	N/a	N/a	N/a	N/a	N/a	N/a	N/a
Presentation	400 g powder	500 ml packs	200 ml bottle; 500 ml packs	250 ml cans; 500 ml packs	200 ml bottle; 500 ml packs	500 ml packs	500 ml packs	200 ml bottle; 500 ml packs	500 ml packs
ACBS listed	Yes	Yes	Yes	Yes	Yes	Yes	Yes	Yes	Yes

All children's enteral feeds are ACBS listed for the following indications: short bowel syndrome, intractable malabsorption, preoperative preparation of patients who are undernourished, dysphagia, bowel fistulas, and disease-related malnutrition and/or growth failure.
*Clinotren Junior powder can also be made up to a concentration of 1.5 kcal/ml (32 g powder; 80 ml water).

Table A.10c   Enteral feeds for children

	Enteral feeds: children; fiber enriched					Enteral feeds: children aged 7–12 years (21–45 kg)				
	Frebini Original Fibre	Frebini Energy Fibre	Nutrini Multi Fibre	Nutrini Energy Multi Fibre	Paediasure Fibre	Paediasure Plus Fibre	Tentrini	Tentrini Multi Fibre	Tentrini Energy	Tentrini Energy Multi-fibre
Manufacturer	Fresenius Kabi	Fresenius Kabi	Nutricia	Nutricia	Abbott	Abbott	Nutricia	Nutricia	Nutricia	Nutricia
kcal/100 ml	100	150	100	150	100	150	100	100	150	150
kJ/100 ml	420	630	420	630	420	629	420	420	630	630
Protein source	Milk proteins	Milk proteins	Milk proteins	Milk proteins	Milk protein	Sodium and calcium caseinate, whey protein	Milk proteins	Milk proteins	Milk proteins	Milk proteins
Protein g/100 ml	2.5	3.75	2.8	4.1	2.8	4.2	3.3	3.3	4.9	4.9
Fat source	Vegetable oils (with soya oil), MCT oil, fish oil	Vegetable oils (with soya oil), MCT oil, fish oil	Vegetable oils	Vegetable oil	Sunflower, soya, MCT oil	Sunflower, soya, MCT oil	Vegetable oils	Vegetable oils	Vegetable oils	Vegetable oils
Fat g/100 ml	4.4	6.7	4.4	6.7	5.0	7.5	4.2	4.2	6.3	6.3
Contains LCPs	Yes	Yes	No	No	No	No	No	No	No	No
Carbohydrate source	Malto-dextrin	Malto-dextrin	Malto-dextrin	Malto-dextrin	Malto-dextrin, sucrose	Malto-dextrin, sucrose	Malto-dextrin	Malto-dextrin	Malto-dextrin	Malto-dextrin
Carbohydrate g/100 ml	12.5	18.8	12.3	18.5	10.9	16.4	12.3	12.3	18.5	18.5
Fiber g/100 ml	0.75	1.13	0.8	0.8	0.73	1.1	0	1.1	0	1.1
Sodium mmol/100 ml	2.2	3.3	2.6	3.9	2.61	2.61	3.5	3.5	4.6	4.6
Potassium mmol/100 ml	2.6	3.8	2.8	4.2	2.8	3.5	3.3	3.3	4.4	4.4
Calcium mmol/100 ml	60	90	60	90	56	83	70	70	95	95
Iron mg/100 ml	0.9	1.35	1.0	1.5	1.0	1.5	1.3	1.3	2	2
Nutritionally complete	Yes	Yes	Yes	Yes	Yes	Yes	Yes	Yes	Yes	Yes
Suitable for vegans	No	No	No	No	No	No	No	No	No	No
Lactose free	Residual lactose	Residual lactose	Residual lactose	Residual lactose	Residual lactose	Residual lactose	Residual lactose	Residual lactose	Residual lactose	Residual lactose
% Dilution	N/a	N/a	N/a	N/a	N/a	N/a	N/a	N/a	N/a	N/a
Presentation	500 ml packs	500 ml packs	200 ml bottle; 500 ml packs	200 ml bottle; 500 ml packs	250 ml cans; 500 ml packs	500 ml packs	500 ml bottle; 500 ml packs	500 ml bottle; 500 ml packs	500 ml bottle; 500 ml packs	500 ml bottle; 500 ml packs
ACBS listed	Yes	Yes	Yes	Yes	Yes	Yes	Yes	Yes	Yes	Yes

All children's enteral feeds are ACBS listed for the following indications: short bowel syndrome, intractable malabsorption, preoperative preparation of patients who are undernourished, dysphagia, bowel fistulas, and disease-related malnutrition and/or growth failure.

Table A.11a   Protein substitutes for phenylketonuria (PKU)

	Infant protein substitutes for PKU				Protein substitutes for PKU				
	PKU Start	XP Analog LCP	XP Analog	Easiphen	Minaphlex	Lophlex	Lophlex LQ	Phlexy 10 Drink Mix	Phlexy 10 Bar
Analysis per 100 ml/100 g	100 ml	100 ml	100 ml	100 ml	100 g	100 g	100 ml	100 g	100 g
Manufacturer	Vitaflo International Ltd	SHS International	SHS International	SHS International	SHS International	SHS International	SHS International	SHS International	SHS International
kcal	68	72	72	65	390	326	92	343	355
kJ	282	300	300	275	1639	1384	391	1456	1496
Protein source	L-amino acids	L-amino acids	L-amino acids	L-amino acids	L-amino acids	L-amino acids	L-amino acids	L-amino acids	L-amino acids
Protein g	2.0	1.95	1.95	6.7	29	72	16	41.7	19.8
Fat source	Walnut, palm, and rapeseed oil.	Walnut, olive, coconut, tuna oil	Safflower, coconut, and soy oil	Canola, sunflower, walnut oil	Canola, safflower, coconut oil	None	None	None	Soy, palm, and peanut oil
Fat g	2.9	3.5	3.5	2	13.5	0.2	0	Nil	8.9
Contains LCPs	Yes	Yes	No	No	No	No	No	No	No
Contains essential fatty acids	Yes	Yes	Yes	Yes	Yes	No	No	No	Yes
Carbohydrate source	Maltodextrin, lactose	Glucose syrup	Glucose syrup	Glucose syrup	Glucose syrup, sugar	Glucose syrup	Maltodextrin, sugar	Glucose syrup	Glucose syrup sucrose
Carbohydrate g	8.3	8.1	8.1	5.1	38	9	7	44	48.8
Sodium mmol	1.0	0.78	0.78	4.1	30	<0.87	<5	<1	<1
Potassium mmol	1.5	1.62	1.62	3.1	25	<10	<5	<1	–
Calcium mg	60	49	49	160	945	1280	285	–	–
Iron mg	0.8	1.05	1.05	4	14	19.2	4.2	–	–

Needs vitamin and mineral supplementation	No	No	No	No	No	No	No	Yes	Yes
Suitable for vegans	No	No	No	No	No	No	No	No	No
Lactose free	No	Yes	Yes	Yes	Yes	Yes	Yes	Yes	Yes
% Dilution	N/a	15	15	N/a	N/a	N/a	N/a	N/a	N/a
Presentation	500 ml	400 g powder	400 g powder	250 ml	29 g sachet	28 g sachet	125 ml pack	20 g sachet	42 g bar
ACBS listed	Yes	Yes	Yes	Yes	Yes	Yes	Yes	Yes	Yes
Other information				Available in Forest Berries and Grapefruit flavors	Available unflavored and flavored: pineapple and vanilla flavor, chocolate, tropical twist	Available in Berry and Orange flavors	Available in Citrus, Berry and Orange flavors		Available in Citrus Burst, Apple and Blackcurrant, and tropical surprise flavors

All of these products are ACBS listed for phenylketonuria.

Table A.11b Protein substitutes

					Other protein substitutes						
Analysis per 100 ml/100 g or as specified	Phlexy 10 Capsules	Phlexy 10 Tablets	PK Aid 4	PKU 2	PKU 3	PKU Cooler 10	PKU Cooler 15	PKU Cooler 20	PKU Express	PKU Gel	XP Maxamaid
	Per 200 capsules	Per 100 capsules	Per 100 g	Per 100 g	Per 100 g	Per 100 ml	Per 100 ml	Per 100 ml	Per 100 g	Per 100 g	100 g
Manufacturer	SHS International	SHS International	SHS International	Milupa	Milupa	Vitaflo International	Vitaflo International	Vitaflo International	Vitaflo International	Vitaflo International	SHS International
kcal	333	377	334	300	288	71	71	71	302	342	309
kJ	1416	1601	1420	1275	1222	297	297	297	1260	1428	1311
Protein source	L-amino acids	L-amino acids	L-amino acids	L-amino acids	L-amino acids	L-amino acids	L-amino acids	L-amino acids	L-amino acids	L-amino acids	L-amino acids
Protein g	83.3	83.3	79	66.8	68	11.5	11.5	11.5	60	42	25
Fat source	None	Vegetable oil	0	0	0	0	0	0	0	0	0
Fat g	Nil	2	No	No	No	Trace	Trace	Trace	<0.5	<0.5	<0.5
Contains LCPs	No	No	No	No	No	No	No	No	No	No	No
Contains essential fatty acids	No	No	No	No	No	No	No	No	No	No	No
Carbohydrate source	None	Maize starch	Glucose syrup	Malto-dextrin	Malto-dextrin	Sugar, modified maize starch	Sugar, modified maize starch	Sugar, modified maize starch	Glucose syrup, maize starch	Maltodextrin, maize starch	Glucose syrup, sugar
Carbohydrate g	None	6.5	4.5	8.2	3.9	5.9	5.9	5.9	15	43	51
Sodium mmol	–	–	–	27.8	27.8	4.7	4.7	4.7	24.4	16.3	25.2
Potassium mmol	–	–	–	34.1	34.1	5.2	5.2	5.2	27.2	24.3	21.5
Calcium mg	–	–	–	1310	1310	215	215	215	1116	1085	810
Iron mg	–	–	–	15	21	4.2	4.2	4.2	21.6	10.5	12
Needs vitamin and mineral supplementation	Yes	Yes	Yes	No but does not contain selenium	No but does not contain selenium	No	No	No	No	No	No
Suitable for vegans	No	No	No	No	No	No	No	No	No	No	No
Lactose free	Yes	Yes	Yes	Yes	Yes	Yes	Yes	Yes	Yes	Yes	Yes
% Dilution	N/a	N/a	N/a	N/a	N/a	N/a	N/a	N/a	N/a	N/a	N/a
Presentation	200 capsules	75 tablets	500 g	500 g	500 g	87 ml pouch	130 ml pouch	174 ml pouch	25 g sachet	20 g sachet	500 g powder
ACBS listed	Yes	Yes	Yes	Yes	Yes	Yes	Yes	Yes	Yes	Yes	Yes
Other information						Purple and orange flavors	Purple and orange flavors	Purple and orange flavors	Orange, lemon, tropical and unflavored	Orange, raspberry, unflavored	Orange, unflavored

Table A.11c   Protein substitutes

	Other protein substitutes for PKU		Other useful special formulas			
Analysis per 100 ml/100 g	XP Maxamaid Concentrate	XP Maxamum	Kindergen	Ketocal	Heparon Junior	Energivit
	Per 100 g	Per 100 g	Per 100 ml	Per 100 ml	Per 100 ml	Per 100 ml
Manufacturer	SHS International	SHS International	SHS International	SHS International	SHS International	SHS International
kcal	239	297	101	146	86	74
kJ	1013	1260	421	602	363	309
Protein source	L-amino acids	L-amino acids	Whey protein, amino acids	Milk protein	Whey protein, skimmed milk powder	N/a
Protein g	53.5	39	1.5	3.1	2.0	0
Fat source	None	None	Safflower, coconut, soya oil.	Soya, milk fat	MCT oil, soya oil.	Safflower, coconut, and soya oil
Fat g	<0.5	<0.5	5.3	14.6	3.6	3.75
Contains LCPs	No	No	No	No	No	No
Contains essential fatty acids	No	No	Yes	Yes	Yes	Yes
Carbohydrate source	Glucose syrup, sugar	Glucose syrup, sugar	Glucose syrup	Glucose syrup, lactose	Glucose syrup	Glucose syrup
Carbohydrate g	5	34	11.8	0.6	11.6	10
Sodium mmol	54	24.3	2	4.3	0.56	0.78
Potassium mmol	46.1	17.9	0.6	4.1	1.9	1.62
Calcium mg	1733	670	22.4	86	92	48.8
Iron mg	25.7	23.5	4.8	1.5	1.3	1.05
Needs vitamin and mineral supplementation	Yes	No	Yes	Yes	Yes	Yes
Suitable for vegans	No	No	No	No	No	Yes
Lactose free	Yes	Yes	No	No	No	Yes
% Dilution	N/a	N/a	20%	20%	18%	15%
Presentation	500 g powder	500 g powder	400 g powder	300 g powder	400 g powder	400 g powder
ACBS listed	Yes	Yes	Yes	No	Yes	Yes
Other information		Available orange and unflavored	Low in calcium and phosphorus	High fat feed (73% fat calories). Can be used for classical 4:1 ketogenic diet	Nutritionally complete in recommended dilution	

Kindergen is ACBS listed for complete nutritional support or supplementary feeding for infants and children with chronic renal failure who are receiving rapid overnight peritoneal dialysis. Energivit is ACBS listed for infants with disorders of amino acid and protein metabolism on a protein-restricted diet.

Table A.12a   Milk based nutritional supplements

	Frebini Energy Drink	Frebini Energy Fibre Drink	Fortini	Fortini Multi Fibre	Paediasure Tetrapak (Children 8–30 kg)	Paediasure Fibre Tetrapak	Paediasure Plus Tetrapak	Paediasure Plus Fibre Tetrapak	Resource Junior
Manufacturer	Fresenius Kabi	Fresenius Kabi	Nutricia	Nutricia	Abbott Nutrition	Abbott Nutrition	Abbott Nutrition	Abbott Nutrition	Novartis
kcal/100 ml	150	150	150	150	101	100	151	150	150
kJ/100 ml	630	630	630	630	422	420	632	626	630
Protein source	Milk proteins	Milk proteins	Milk proteins	Milk proteins	Whey protein, calcium caseinate	Whey protein, calcium caseinate	Whey protein, calcium caseinate	Whey protein, calcium caseinate	Skimmed milk
Protein g/100 ml	3.75	3.75	3.4	3.4	2.8	2.8	4.2	4.2	3.0
Fat source	Vegetable oils (with soya oil), MCT oil, fish oil	Vegetable oils (with soya oil), MCT oil, fish oil	Veg oils	Veg oils	Sunflower oil, soya oil, MCT oil	Sunflower oil, soya oil, MCT oil	Sunflower oil, soya oil, MCT oil	Sunflower oil, soya oil, MCT oil	Cream, corn oil, rapeseed oil
Fat g/100 ml	6.7	6.7	6.8	6.8	5	5	7.5	7.5	6.2
Carbohydrate source	Maltodextrin	Maltodextrin, inulin, soya polysaccharide	Maltodextrin, sucrose	Maltodextrin, sucrose	Maltodextrin, sucrose	Maltodextrin, sucrose	Maltodextrin, sucrose	Maltodextrin, sucrose	Maltodextrin, sucrose
Carbohydrate g/100 ml	18.8	18.8	18.8	18.8	11.2	10.9	16.7	16.4	20.6
Fiber g/100 ml	0	1.1	0	1.5	0	0.73	0	1.1	–
Nutritionally complete	Yes	Yes	Yes	Yes	Yes	Yes	Yes	Yes	Yes
Presentation	Carton: 200 ml	Carton: 200 ml	Bottle 200 ml	Bottle 200 ml	Carton: 200 ml Can: 250 ml	Carton: 200 ml	Carton: 200 ml	Carton: 200 ml	Carton: 200 ml
ACBS listed	Yes	Yes	Yes	Yes	Yes	Yes	Yes	Yes	Yes
Flavors	Strawberry, banana	Chocolate	Vanilla, strawberry	Vanilla, strawberry, chocolate, banana	Carton: vanilla, strawberry, chocolate, banana Can: vanilla	Carton: vanilla, strawberry, banana	Carton: vanilla, strawberry, banana Can: vanilla	Carton: vanilla	Carton: chocolate, strawberry, vanilla

All children's nutritional supplements are ACBS listed for the following indications: short bowel syndrome, intractable malabsorption, preoperative preparation of patients who are undernourished, dysphagia, bowel fistulas, disease-related malnutrition and/or growth failure.

Table A.12b Carbohydrate based nutritional supplements

	Caloreen	Maxijul liquid	Maxijul Super Soluble	Polycal liquid	Polycal powder	Polycose powder	Vitajoule
Analysis per 100 ml/100 g	Per 100 g	Per 100 ml	Per 100 g	Per 100 ml	Per 100 g	Per 100 g	Per 100 g
Manufacturer	Nestle Clinical Nutrition	SHS International	SHS International	Nutricia	Nutricia	Abbott	Vitaflo
kcal	390	200	380	247	384	376	380
kJ	1638	850	1615	1050	1630	1598	1610
Carbohydrate source	Glucose polymer	Glucose syrup	Dried glucose syrup	Maltodextrin, glucose syrup	Maltodextrin	Glucose polymer	Glucose polymer
Carbohydrate g		50	95	61.9	96	94	96
Pack size	Can: 500 g	Carton: 200 ml	Can: 200 g Sachets: 4 × 132 g 2.5 kg tub 25 kg drum	Carton: 200 ml	Can: 400 g	Can: 350 g	Tub: 500 g 2.5 kg 25 kg
ACBS listed	Yes	Yes	Yes	Yes	Yes	Yes	Yes
Flavors	Unflavored	Orange and natural	Unflavored	Neutral, orange	Unflavored	Unflavored	Unflavored

All carbohydrate supplements are ACBS listed for disease-related malnutrition, malabsorption states, and other conditions requiring fortification with high energy or readily available carbohydrate supplements. Caution: flavored glucose polymer syrups are not suitable for use in children < 12 months of age. Liquid preparations should always be diluted at least 50% for children < 5 years of age.

Table A.12c Fat based nutritional supplements

	Calogen	Liquigen	MCT oil
Manufacturer	nutricia	SHS International	SHS International
kcal/100 ml	450	450	855
kJ/100 ml	1850	1850	3515
Fat source	Canola, sunflower	Coconut, palm kernel	Coconut oil and palm kernel oil
Fat g/100 ml	50	50 (MCT)	95 (MCT)
Pack size	Bottles: 200 ml, 500 ml ≤ C14:0; 0.01% C16; 6.3% C18: 3.4% C18:1; 59.1% C18:2; 23.7% C18:3; 4.8% > C20; 2.4%	Bottles: 250 ml C6; 0.97% C8: 80.3% C10; 14.52% C12; 0.97% C14; 0.03% C16; 1.59%	Bottle: 500 ml C6; < 2% C8; 58% C10; 38% C12; < 2% C14; < 1%
ACBS listed	Yes	Yes	Yes
Flavors	Strawberry, banana and unflavored	C18; 1.52% C20; 0.03%	

All products ACBS listed for disease-related malnutrition, malabsorption states, and other conditions requiring fortification with a high fat supplement, with or without fluid and electrolyte restrictions. MCT oil and Liquigen also ACBS listed for ketogenic diets in the management of epilepsy and type 1 hyperlipoproteinemia.

Table A.12d   Combined nutritional supplements

Analysis per 100 ml/100 g	Combined fat and carbohydrate supplements					Combined protein, fat and carbohydrate supplements		
	Duobar	Liquid Duocal	Super Soluble Duocal Powder	MCT Duocal Powder	Vitabite	Pro-cal	Quickcal	Pro-cal shot
Analysis per 100 ml/100 g	Per 100 g	Per 100 ml	Per 100 g	Per 100 g	Per 100 g	Per 100 g	Per 100 g	Per 100 ml
Manufacturer	SHS International	SHS International	SHS International	SHS International	Vitaflo International	Vitaflo International	Vitaflo International	Vitaflo International
kcal	648	166	492	497	547	667	780	334
kJ	2692	605	2061	2082	2284	2788	3260	1385
Protein source	N/a	N/a	N/a	N/a	0.12	Skimmed milk powder	N/a	Skimmed milk powder sodium carbonate
Protein g	N/a	N/a	N/a	N/a	N/a	13.5	4.6	6.7
Fat source	Palm oil, shea fat, ilipe oil	Coconut, maize, palm kernel oil	Coconut, safflower, canola oil	Coconut, walnut maize, palm kernal oil	Soya, rapeseed, and palm oil	Hydrogenated vegetable oil	Hydrogenated vegetable oil	High oleic sunflower MCT oil
Fat g	49.9	7.9	22.3	23.2 (75% MCT)	334	56	77	28.2 (17.4% MCT)
Carbohydrate source	Sucrose	Glucose syrup	Glucose syrup	Glucose syrup	Lactose, sucrose, carob flour	Lactose	Lactose	Lactose
Carbohydrate g	49.9	23.7	72.7	72	61.4	27	17	13.4
Presentation	8 × 45 g bars	Bottles: 250 ml	Can: 400 g	Can: 400 g	Bars: 7 × 25 g	25 × 15 g sachets, 200 × 15 g sachets, 510 g, 1.5 kg, 12.5 kg, 25 kg	25 × 13 g sachets	6 × 250 ml bottles
ACBS listed	Yes	Yes	Yes	Yes	Yes	Yes	Yes	Yes
Flavors	Strawberry, toffee, natural							

All combined fat and carbohydrate products ACBS listed for disease-related malnutrition, malabsorption states, and other conditions requiring fortification with fat/carbohydrate supplement.
All combined protein, fat and carbohydrate products ACBS listed for disease-related malnutrition, malabsorption states, and other conditions requiring fortification with a protein, fat and carbohydrate supplement.

Table A.12e   Protein supplements

	Casilan 90	ProMod	Protifar	Vitapro
Manufacturer	Heinz	Abbott	Nutricia	Vitaflo
kcal/100 g	370	426	373	360
kJ/100 g	1572	1798	1580	1506
Protein source	Calcium caseinate	Whey protein	Milk protein	Whey protein
Protein g/100 g	90	75.8	88.5	75
Presentation	Carton: 500 g	Can: 275 g	Can: 225 g	250 g; 2 kg
ACBS listed	Yes	Yes	Yes	Yes

All protein supplements are ACBS listed for biochemically proven hypoproteinemia.

Table A.13 Feed thickeners

Name	Instant Carobel	Nestargel	Thick and Easy	Thixo D	Vitaquick
Manufacturer	Cow and Gate	Nestle Clinical Nutrition	Fresenius Kabi	Sutherland Health	Vitaflo International
Ingredients	Carob bean gum with maltodextrin and calcium lactate	Carob seed flour and calcium lactate. It contains no metabolizable carbohydrate	Modified food starch (maize), maltodextrin	Modified waxy maize, food starch (E1442)	Modified maize starch, (E1442)
Energy kcal/100 g	251	38	373	392	380
kJ/100 g	1065	158	1567	1635	1590
CHO g/100 g	59	0	92.6	97	96
Sodium mg/100 g	8	5	175	125	<200
Potassium mg/100 g	240	350	0	10	<1.0
Calcium mg/100 g	130	640	4.5	Not declared	Not declared
Phosphorus mg/100 g	20	Not declared	24	13	20
Reconstitution	Bottle feed: add 2–3 level scoops of Carobel for every 60–90 ml (2–3 fl oz) hand-warm infant formula. Shake well and leave to thicken for 3–4 minutes. Breast feeds: add 6–7 level scoops of Carobel to 60 ml (2 fl oz) hand-warm water to form a thick gel. Feed in small quantities by spoon before and during the breast feed	Recommended concentration 0.5–1%. Bottle feed: add Nestargel in the quantity of cold water required for the feed; gently bring to the boil, stir and simmer for 1 minute; cool and add the formula powder; mix until smooth. Breast feeds: give 1 tablespoon of thickened Nestargel water (1% concentration) pre-feeds	No specific instructions given for infants. 1–3% concentration suggested.[45]		
Comments	An instant thickener 1 scoop = 0.7 g Carobel	An effective thickener; produces a smooth and stable thickened liquid. 1 scoop = 1 g Nestargel	Effective thickeners. Unsuitable for infants under 1 year, unless failing to thrive		An effective thickener. Unsuitable for infants under 1 year, unless failing to thrive. Each tub contains a 5 g scoop
Presentation	Box: 135 g	Can: 125 g	Can: 225 g, Sachets: 9 g	Tub: 375 g	Tube: 300 g, 12 kg, 6 kg
ACBS listed	Yes, for thickening feeds in the treatment of vomiting	Yes, for thickening feeds in the treatment of vomiting	Yes, for thickening of foods in the treatment of dysphagia	Yes, for thickening of foods in the treatment of dysphagia	Yes, for thickening of foods in the treatment of dysphagia
Side-effects	A minority of infants may develop loose stools. If used in galactosemia, the red cell galactose 1-phosphate should be monitored	A minority of infants may develop loose stools. If used in galactosemia, the red cell galactose 1-phosphate should be monitored	–	–	–

Table A.14 Miscellaneous

Product	Manufacturer	Description	ACBS Prescribable
Cornflour/cornstarch	Various	Maize starch BP-maize starch powder	Hypoglycemia associated with glycogen storage disease
Fructose	Various	Fructose BP Laevulose powder. 500 g	Glucose-galactose intolerance
Glucose/dextrose	Various	Glucose BP Dextrose monohydrate powder	Glycogen storage disease. Sucrose-isomaltose intolerance
SHS Module Flavour System	SHS International	Blackcurrant, orange, pineapple, tomato, *grapefruit, *cherry vanilla, *lemon and lime. Contains maltodextrin ±lactose, modified starch, sugar according to flavor. Presentation: 100 g tubs or *5 g sachets	For flavoring unflavored amino acid/peptide based products
Vitaflo Flavour Pac	Vitaflo International	Blackcurrant, lemon, orange, raspberry, tropical fruit. On a carbohydrate base containing sugar and sweeteners. Presentation 30 × 4 g sachets	For flavouring unflavoured amino acid products

Table A.15 Dietary reference values for the UK. Estimated average requirements (EARs) for energy

MJ/d (kcal/d)	Males		Females	
0–3 m	2.28	(545)	2.16	(515)
4–6 m	2.89	(690)	2.69	(645)
7–9 m	3.44	(825)	3.20	(765)
10–12 m	3.85	(920)	3.61	(865)
1–3 y	5.15	(1230)	4.86	(1165)
4–6 y	7.16	(1715)	6.46	(1545)
7–10 y	8.24	(1970)	7.28	(1740)
11–14 y	9.27	(2220)	7.72	(1845)
15–18 y	11.51	(2755)	8.83	(2110)
19–50 y	10.60	(2550)	8.10	(1940)
51–59 y	10.60	(2550)	8.00	(1900)
60–64 y	9.93	(2380)	7.99	(1900)
65–74 y	9.71	(2330)	7.96	(1900)
75+ y	8.77	(2100)	7.61	(1810)
Pregnancy			+0.80[a]	(200)
Lactation:				
1 m			+1.90	(450)
2 m			+2.20	(530)
3 m			+2.40	(570)
4–6 m (Group 1)[b]			+2.00	(480)
4–6 m (Group 2)			+2.40	(570)
>6 m (Group 1)			+1.00	(240)
>6 m (Group 2)			+2.30	(550)

Extracted from Dietary Reference Values for Food Energy and Nutrients for the United Kingdom.[46]
[a]Last trimester only.

Table A.16 Reference nutrient intakes for protein

Age	Reference nutrient intake[a] g/d
0–3 m	12.5[b]
0–4 m	12.7
7–9 m	13.7
10–12 m	14.9
1–3 y	14.5
4–6 y	19.7
7–10 y	28.3
Males	
11–14 y	42.1
15–18 y	55.2
19–50 y	55.5
51+ y	53.3
Females	
11–14 y	41.2
15–18 y	45.0
19–50 y	45.0
51+ y	46.5
Pregnancy[c]	+6
Lactation[c]	
0–4 m	+11
4+ m	+8

Extracted from Dietary Reference Values for Food Energy and Nutrients for the United Kingdom.[46]
[a]These figures, based on egg and milk protein, assume complete digestibility.
[b]No values for infants 0–3 months are given by WHO. The RNI is calculated from the recommendations of COMA.
[c]To be added to adult requirement through all stages of pregnancy and lactation.

Table A.17 Reference nutrient Intakes for vitamins

Age	Thiamin mg/d	Riboflavin mg/d	Niacin (nicotinic acid equivalent) mg/d	Vitamin B$_6$ mg/d[a]	Vitamin B$_{12}$ µg/d	Folate µg/d	Vitamin C mg/d	Vitamin A µg/d	Vitamin D µg/d
0–3 m	0.2	0.4	3	0.2	0.3	50	25	350	8.5
0–4 m	0.2	0.4	3	0.2	0.3	50	25	350	8.5
7–9 m	0.2	0.4	4	0.3	0.4	50	25	350	7
10–12 m	0.3	0.4	5	0.4	0.4	50	25	350	7
1–3 y	0.5	0.6	8	0.7	0.5	70	30	400	7
4–6 y	0.7	0.8	11	0.9	0.8	100	30	400	–
7–10 y	0.7	1.0	12	1.0	1.0	150	30	500	–
Males									
11–14 y	0.9	1.2	15	1.2	1.2	200	35	600	–
15–18 y	1.1	1.3	18	1.5	1.5	200	40	700	–
19–50 y	1.0	1.3	17	1.4	1.5	200	40	700	–
50+ y	0.9	1.3	16	1.4	1.5	200	40	700	[b]
Females									
11–14 y	0.7	1.1	12	1.0	1.2	200	35	600	–
15–18 y	0.8	1.1	14	1.2	1.5	200	40	600	–
19–50 y	0.8	1.1	13	1.2	1.5	200	40	600	–
51+ y	0.8	1.1	12	1.2	1.5	200	40	600	[b]
Pregnancy	+0.1[c]	+0.3	[d]	d	d	+100	+10[c]	+100	10
Lactation:									
0–4 m	+0.2	+0.5	+2	d	+0.5	+600	+30	+350	10
4+ m	+0.2	+0.5	+2	d	+0.5	+600	+30	+350	10

Extracted from Dietary Reference Values for Food Energy and Nutrients for the United Kingdom.[46]
[a]Based on protein providing 14.7 per cent of EAR for energy.
[b]After age 65 the RNI µg/d for men and women.
[c]For last trimester only.
[d]No increment.

Table A.18a Reference nutrient intakes for minerals (SI units)

Age	Calcium mmol/d	Phosphorus[a] mmol/d	Magnesium mmol/d	Sodium mmol/d[b]	Potassium mmol/d[c]	Chloride[d] mmol/d	Iron mmol/d	Zinc µmol/d	Copper µmol/d	Selenium µmol/d	Iodine µmol/d
0–3 m	13.1	13.1	2.2	9	20	9	30	60	5	0.1	0.4
0–4 m	13.1	13.1	2.5	12	22	12	80	60	5	0.2	0.5
7–9 m	13.1	13.1	3.2	14	18	14	140	75	5	0.1	0.5
10–12 m	13.1	13.1	3.3	15	18	15	140	75	5	0.1	0.5
1–3 y	8.8	8.8	3.5	22	20	22	120	75	6	0.2	0.6
4–6 y	11.3	11.3	4.8	30	28	30	110	100	9	0.3	0.8
7–10 y	13.8	13.8	8.0	50	50	50	160	110	11	0.4	0.9
Males											
11–14 y	25.0	25.0	11.5	70	80	70	200	140	13	0.6	1.0
15–18 y	25.0	25.0	12.3	70	90	70	200	145	16	0.9	1.0
19–50 y	17.5	17.50	12.3	70	90	70	160	145	19	0.9	1.0
50+ y	17.5	17.50	12.3	70	90	70	160	145	19	0.9	1.0
Females											
11–14 y	20.0	20.0	11.5	70	80	70	260[e]	140	13	0.6	1.0
15–18 y	20.0	20.0	12.3	70	90	70	260[e]	110	16	0.8	1.1
19–50 y	17.5	17.5	10.9	70	90	70	260[e]	110	19	0.8	1.1
51+ y	17.5	17.5	10.9	70	90	70	160	110	19	0.8	1.1
Pregnancy[f]	[g]	[g]	[g]	[g]	[g]	[g]	[g]	[g]	[g]	[g]	[g]
Lactation[f]											
0–4 m	+14.3	+14.3	+2.1	[g]	[g]	[g]	[g]	+90	+5	+0.2	[g]
4+ m	+14.3	+14.3	+2.1	[g]	[g]	[g]	[g]	+40	+5	+0.2	[g]

Extracted from Dietary Reference Values for Food Energy and Nutrients for the United Kingdom.[46]
[a]Phosphorus RNI is set equal to calcium in molar terms.
[b]1 mmol sodium = 23 mg.
[c]1 mmol potassium = 39 mg.
[d]Corresponds to sodium 1 mmol = 35.5 mg.
[e]Insufficient for women with high menstrual losses where the most practical way of meeting iron requirements is to take iron supplements.
[f]To be added to adult requirement through all stages of pregnancy and lactation.
[g]No increment.

Table A.18b Reference nutrient intakes for minerals

Age	Calcium mg/d	Phosphorus mg/d[a]	Magnesium mg/d	Sodium mg/d[b]	Potassium mg/d[c]	Chloride[d] mg/d	Iron mg/d	Zinc mg/d	Copper mg/d	Selenium µg/c	Iodine µg/d
0–3 m	525	400	55	210	800	320	1.7	4.0	0.2	10	50
0–4 m	525	400	60	280	850	400	4.3	4.0	0.3	13	60
7–9 m	525	400	75	320	700	500	7.8	5.0	0.3	10	60
10–12 m	525	400	80	350	700	500	7.8	5.0	0.3	10	60
1–3 y	350	270	85	500	800	800	6.9	5.0	0.4	15	70
4–6 y	450	350	120	700	1100	1100	6.1	6.5	0.6	20	100
7–10 y	550	450	200	1200	2000	1800	8.7	0.7	0.7	30	110
Males											
11–14 y	1000	775	280	1600	3100	2500	11.3	9.0	0.8	45	130
15–18 y	1000	775	300	1600	3500	2500	11.3	9.5	1.0	70	140
19–50 y	700	550	300	1600	3500	2500	8.7	9.5	1.2	75	140
50+ y	700	550	300	1600	3500	2500	8.7	9.5	1.2	75	140
Females											
11–14 y	800	625	280	1600	3100	2500	14.8[e]	9.0	0.8	45	130
15–18 y	800	625	300	1600	3500	2500	14.8[e]	7.0	1.0	60	140
19–50 y	700	550	270	1600	3500	2500	14.8[e]	7.0	1.2	60	140
51+ y	700	550	270	1600	3500	2500	8.7	7.0	1.2	60	140
Pregnancy[f]	g	g	g	g	g	g	g	g	g	g	g
Lactation[f]											
0–4 m	+550	+440	+50	g	g	g	g	+6.0	+0.3	+1E	g
4+ m	+550	+440	+50	g	g	g	g	+2.5	+0.3	+1E	g

Extracted from Dietary Reference Values for Food Energy and Nutrients for the United Kingdom.[46]
[a]Phosphorus RNI is set equal to calcium in molar terms.
[b]1 mmol sodium = 23 mg.
[c]1 mmol potassium = 39 mg.
[d]Corresponds to sodium 1 mmol = 35.5 mg.
[e]Insufficient for women with high menstrual losses where the most practical way of meeting iron requirements is to take iron supplements.
[f]To be added to adult requirement through all stages of pregnancy and lactation.
[g]No increment.

Table A.19 Safe intakes of vitamins and minerals

Nutrient	Safe intake
Vitamins	
Pantothenic acid	
Adults	3–7 mg/d
Infants	1.7 mg/d
Biotin	10–200 µg/d
Vitamin E	
Men	Above 4 mg/d
Women	Above 3 mg/d
Infants	0.4 mg/d polyunsaturated fatty acids
Vitamin K	
Adults	1 µg/kg/d
Infants	10 µg/d
Minerals	
Manganese	
Adults	Above 1.4 mg/dN (26 µmol/d)
Infants and children	Above 16 µg/kg/d (0.3 µmol/kg/d)
Molybdenum	
Adults	50–400 µg/d
Infants, children and adolescents	0.5–1.5 µg/kg/d
Chromium	
Adults	Above 25 µg (0.5 µmol/d)
Children and adolescents	0.1–1.0 µg (2–20 nmol/kg/d)
Fluoride	
Children over 6 years and adults	0.5 mg/kg/d (3 µmol/kg/d)
Children over 6 months	0.12 mg/kg/d (6 µmol/kg/d)
Infants under 6 months	0.22 mg/kg/d (12 µmol/kg/d)

Extracted from Dietary Reference Values for Food Energy and Nutrients for the United Kingdom.[46]

Table A.20 Multiple values proposed for adults. (Amounts per day, unless given in other items. If that for women is different from that for men, it is in parentheses)

Nutrient	Average requirement	Population reference intake	Lowest threshold intake
Protein (g)	0.6/kg body wt	0.75/kg body wt	0.45/kg body wt
Vitamin A (µg)	500 (400)	700 (600)	300 (250)
Thiamin (µg)	72/MJ	100/MJ	50/MJ
Riboflavin (mg)	1.3 (1.1)	1.6 (1.3)	0.6
Niacin (mg niacin equivalents)	1.3/MJ	1.6/MJ	1.0/MJ
Vitamin B6 (µg)	13/g protein	15/g protein	–
Folate (µg)	140	200	85
Vitamin B_{12} (µg)	1.0	1.4	0.6
Vitamin C (mg)	30	45	12
Vitamin E (mg α-tocopherol equivalents)		0.4/g PUFA	4 (3)/d regardless of PUFA intakes
n-6 PUFA (as percentage of dietary energy)	1	2	0.5
n-3 PUFA (as percentage of dietary energy)	0.2	0.5	0.1
Calcium (mg)	550	700	400
Phosphorus (mg)	400	550	300
Potassium (mg)	–	3100	1600
Iron (mg)	7 (10, 6[a])	9 (16[b], 8[a])	5 (7, 4[a])
Zinc (mg)	7.5 (5.5)	9.5 (7)	5 (4)
Copper (mg)	0.8	1.1	0.6
Selenium (µg)	40	55	20
Iodine (µg)	100	130	70
For the following, acceptable ranges of intake are given:			
Pantothenic acid (mg)	3–12		
Biotin (µg)	15–100		
Vitamin D (µg)	0–10		
Sodium (g)	0.575–3.5		
Magnesium (mg)	150–500		
Manganese (mg)	1–10		

PUFA, polyunsaturated fatty acids.
[a]Postmenopausal.
[b]PRI to cover 90% of women.
Reproduced from Nutrient and Energy Intakes for the European Community.[47]

Table A.21 EU reference intakes

Age group	Protein (g/kg body weight/d)	n-6 PUFA (% of dietary energy)	n-3 PUFA (% of dietary energy)	Vitamin A (µg/d)	Thiamin (µg/MJ)	Riboflavin (mg/d)	Niacin (mg/MJ)	Vitamin B_6 (µg/g protein)	Folate (µg/d)	Vitamin B_{12} (µg/d)	Vitamin C (mg/d)
6–11 months	1.6	4.5	0.5	350	100	0.4	1.6	15	50	0.5	20
1–3 yr	1.1	3	0.5	400	100	0.8	1.6	15	100	0.7	25
4–6 yr	1.0	2	0.5	400	100	1.0	1.6	15	130	0.9	25
7–10 yr	1.0	2	0.5	500	100	1.2	1.6	15	150	1.0	30
Males											
11–14 yr	1.0	2	0.5	600	100	1.4	1.6	15	180	1.3	35
15–17 yr	0.9	2	0.5	700	100	1.6	1.6	15	200	1.4	40
18+ yr	0.75	2	0.5	700	100	1.6	1.6	15	200	1.4	45
Females											
11–14 yr	0.95	2	0.5	600	100	1.2	1.6	15	180	1.3	35
15–17 yr	0.85	2	0.5	600	100	1.3	1.6	15	200	1.4	40
18+ yr	0.75	2	0.5	600	100	1.3	1.6	15	200[c]	1.4	45
Pregnancy	0.75 (+10 g/d)	2	0.5	700	100	1.6	1.6	15	400	1.6	55
Lactation	0.75 (+16 g/d)	2	0.5	950	100	1.7	1.6 (+2 mg/day)	15	350	1.9	70

(Continued)

Table A.21   EU reference intakes—Cont'd

Age group	Calcium (mg/d)	Phosphorus (mg/d)	Potassium (mg/d)	Iron (mg/d)	Zinc (mg/d)	Copper (mg/d)	Selenium (µg/d)	Iodine (µg/d)
6–11 months	400	300	800	6	4	0.3	8	50
1–3 yr	400	300	800	4	4	0.4	10	70
4–6 yr	450	350	1100	4	6	0.6	15	90
7–10 yr	550	450	2000	6	7	0.7	25	100
Males								
11–14 yr	1000	775	3100	100	9	0.8	35	120
15–17 yr	1000	775	3100	13	9	1.0	45	130
18+ yr	700	550	3100	9	9.5	1.1	55	130
Females								
11–14 yr	800	625	3100	22[a] 18[b]	9	0.8	35	120
15–17 yr	800	625	3100	2[a] 17[a]	7	1.0	45	130
18+ yr	700	550	3100	20[a] 16[b] 8[d]	7	1.1	55	130
Pregnancy	700	550	3100	[e]	7	1.1	55	130
Lactation	1200	950	3100	10	12	1.4	70	160

PUFA, polyunsaturated fatty acids.
[a]To cover 95% of population.
[b]To cover 90% of population.
[c]Neural tube defects have been shown to be prevented in offspring by periconceptual ingestion of 400 µg folic acid per day in the form of supplements.
[d]Postmenopausal.
[e]Supplements necessary.
Reproduced from Nutrient and Energy Intakes for the European Community.[47]

Table A.22   Daily intakes of those nutrients for which the recommendations are given in relation to body weight, energy or protein intakes[a]

Age group	Protein (g)	n-6 PUFA (g)	n-3 PUFA (g)	Thiamin (mg)	Niacin (mg)	Vitamin B_6 (mg)
6–11 months	15	4	0.5	0.3	5	0.4
1–3 yr	15	4	0.7	0.5	9	0.7
4–6 yr	20	4	1	0.7	11	0.9
7–10 yr	29	4	1	0.8	13	1.1
Males						
11–14 yr	44	5	1	1.0	15	1.3
15–17 yr	55	6	1.5	1.2	18	1.5
18+ yr (PTI)	56	6	1.5	1.1	18	1.5
(AR)	45	3	0.6	0.8	15	1.3
Females						
11–14 yr	42	4	1	0.9	14	1.1
15–17 yr	46	5	1	0.9	14	1.1
18+ yr (PRI)	47	4.5	1	0.9	14	1.1
(AR)	37	2.5	0.5	0.6	11	1.0
Pregnancy	57	5[b]	1	1.0[b]	14	1.3[c]
Lactation	63	5.5	1	1.1	16	1.4[c]

PUFA, polyunsaturated fatty acids.
[a]Population reference intakes (PRI) except where indicated as average requirements (AR) (calculated as mean group intake × PRI or AR).
[b]From 10th week of pregnancy.
[c]On protein increments in pregnancy and lactation.
Reproduced from Nutrient and Energy Intakes for the European Community.[47]

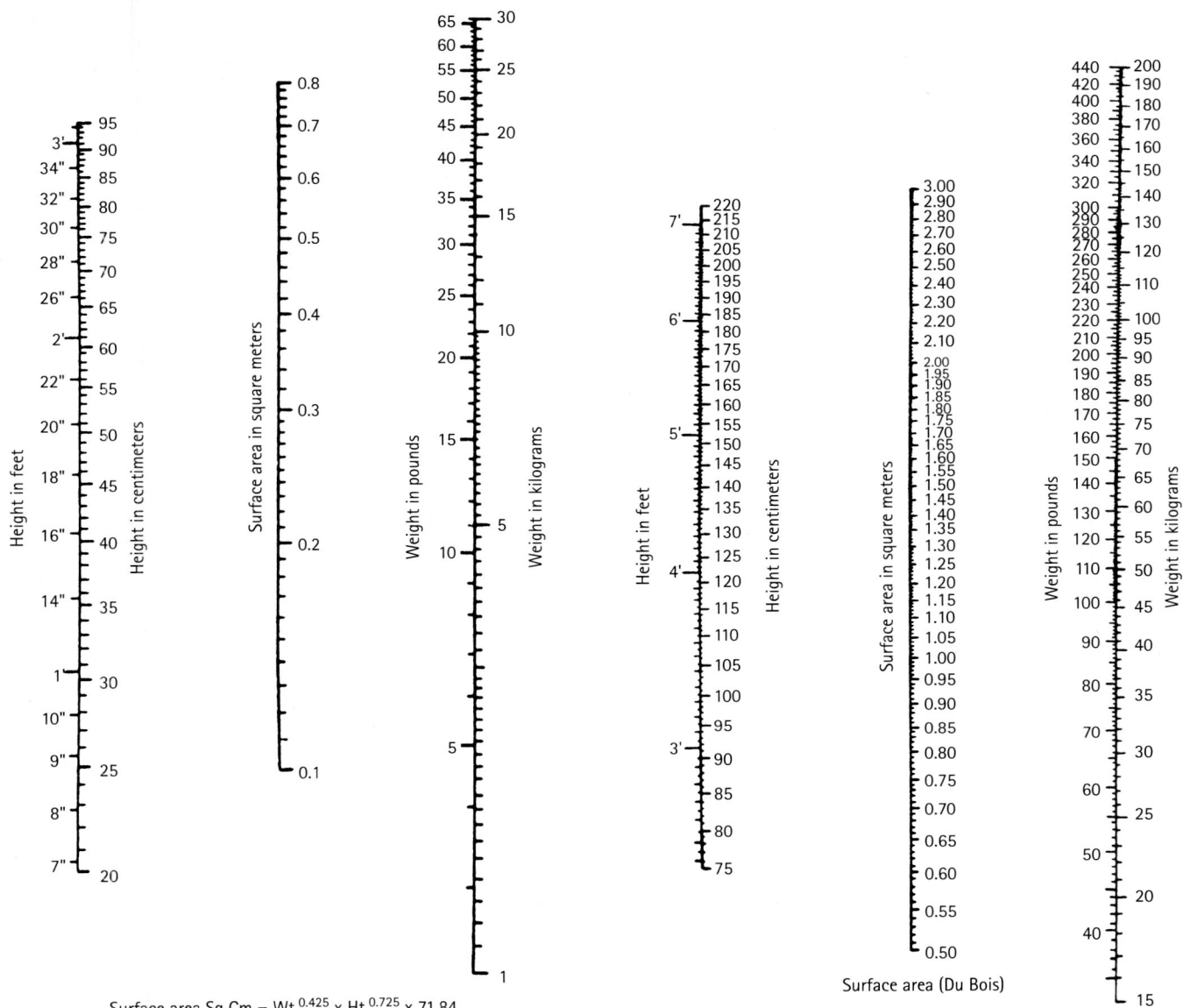

Surface area Sq Cm = Wt.$^{0.425}$ × Ht.$^{0.725}$ × 71.84

Fig. A.1 Nomograms for body surface area. After Du Bois & Du Bois 1916.[43]

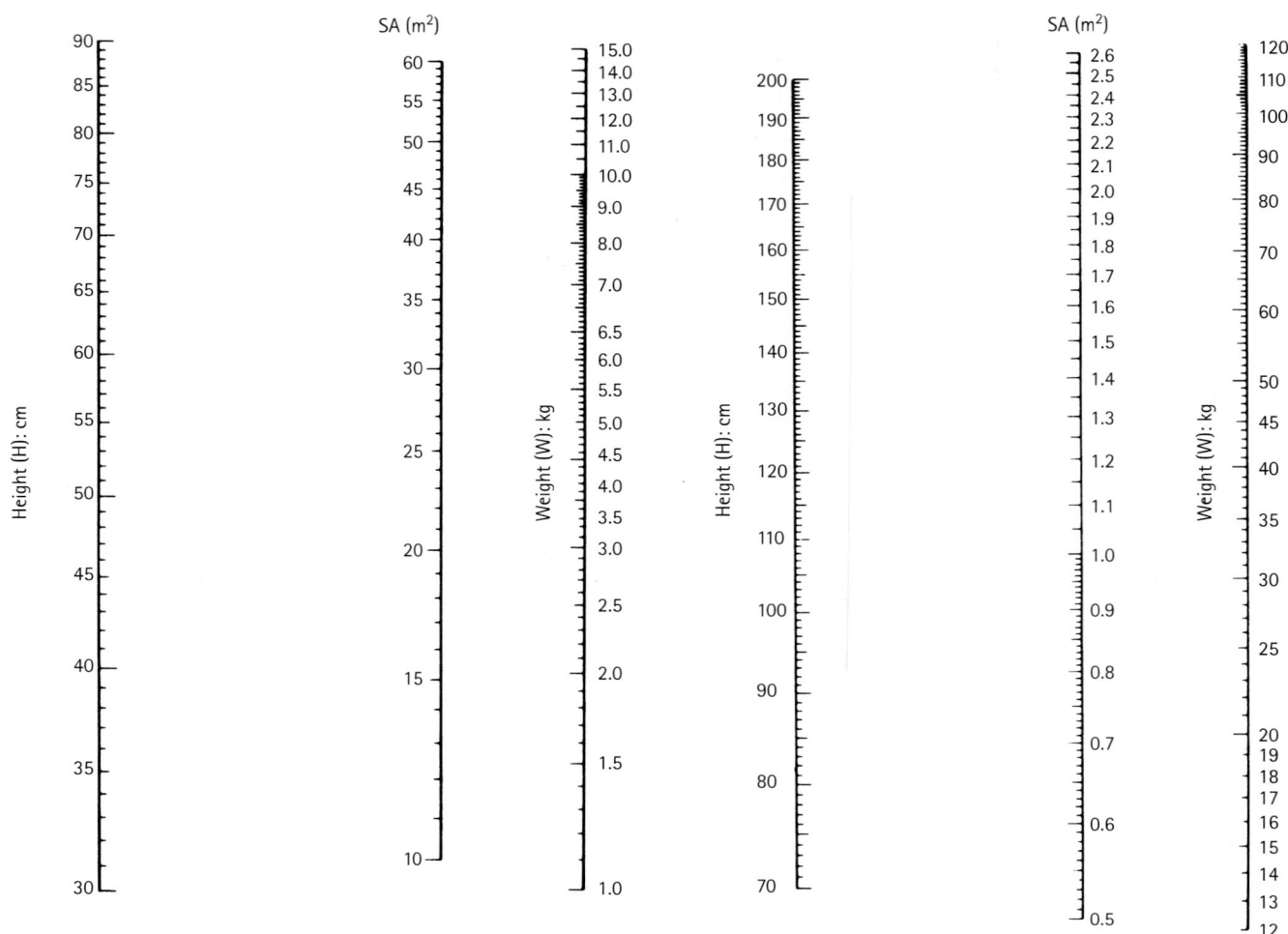

Fig. A.2   Nomograms for body surface area. After Haycock et al 1978.[44]

REFERENCES

1. Enzyme nomenclature. Report on the recommendations (1964) of the International Union of Biochemistry on Nomenclature and Classification of Enzymes. Science 1965; 150:719–721.

2. Therapeutic drug monitoring. Abbot Diagnostics Division. R 2nd edn. 2007.

3. Beddis IR, Hughes EA, Rosser E, et al. Plasma ammonia levels in newborn infants admitted to an intensive care baby unit. Arch Dis Child 1980; 55:516–520.

4. Clayton BE, Jenkins P, Round JM. Paediatric chemical pathology – clinical tests and reference ranges. Oxford: Blackwell Scientific Publications; 1980.

5. Colombo JP, Peheim E, Kretschmer R, et al. Plasma ammonia concentrations in newborns and children. Clin Chim Acta 1984; 138:283–291.

6. Deacon AC, Elder GH. Frontline tests for the investigation of suspected porphyria. J Clin Pathol 2001; 54:500–507.

7. Dillon MJ, Ryness JM. Plasma renin activity and aldosterone concentration in children. Br Med J 1975; 4:316–319.

8. Fraser C.G. Interpretation of clinical chemistry laboratory data. Oxford: Blackwell; 1986.

9. Ghazali S, Barratt TM. Urinary excretion of calcium and magnesium in children. Arch Dis Child 1974; 49:97–101.

10. Jedeikin R, Makela SK, Shennan AT, et al. Creatine kinase isoenzymes in serum from cord blood and the blood of healthy full-term infants during the first three postnatal days. Clin Chem 1982; 28:317–322.

11. Jira PE, de Jong JG, Janssen-Zijlstra FS, et al. Pitfalls in measuring plasma cholesterol in the Smith-Lemli-Opitz syndrome. Clin Chem 1997; 43:129–133.

12. Korth-Schutz S, Virdis R, Saenger P, et al. Serum androgens as a continuing index of adequacy of treatment of congenital adrenal hyperplasia. J Clin Endocrinol Metab 1978; 46:452–458.

13. Kovar I, Mayne P, Barltrop D. Plasma alkaline phosphatase activity: a screening test for rickets in preterm neonates. Lancet 1982; 1:308–310.

14. Leung AK. Carotenemia. Adv Pediatr 1987; 34:223–248.

15. Lockitch G, Halstead AC, Albersheim S, et al. Age- and sex-specific pediatric reference intervals for biochemistry analytes as measured with the Ektachem-700 analyzer. Clin Chem 1988; 34:1622–1625.

16. Lockitch G, Halstead AC, Wadsworth L, et al. Age- and sex-specific pediatric reference intervals and correlations for zinc, copper, selenium, iron, vitamins A and E, and related proteins. Clin Chem 1988; 34:1625–1628.

17. Loughrey CM, Hanna EV, McDonnell M, et al. Sodium measurement: effects of differing sampling and analytical methods. Ann Clin Biochem 2006; 43(Pt 6):488–493.

18. Mawer EB, Berry JL, Cundall JP, et al. A sensitive radioimmunoassay using a monoclonal antibody that is equipotent for ercalcitriol and calcitriol (1,25-dihydroxy vitamin D2 and D3). Clin Chim Acta 1990; 190:199–209.

19. Nelson N, Finnstrom O, Larsson L. Neonatal reference values for ionized calcium, phosphate and magnesium. Selection of reference population by optimality criteria. Scand J Clin Lab Invest 1987; 47:111–117.

20. Oberholzer VG, Schwarz KB, Smith CH, et al. Microscale modification of a cation-exchange column procedure for plasma ammonia. Clin Chem 1976; 22:1976–1981.

21. Penttila IM, Jokela HA, Viitala AJ, et al. Activities of aspartate and alanine aminotransferases and alkaline phosphatase in sera of healthy subjects. Scand J Clin Lab Invest 1975; 35:275–284.

22. Rock MJ, Mischler EH, Farrell PM, et al. Immunoreactive trypsinogen screening for cystic fibrosis: characterization of infants with a false-positive screening test. Pediatr Pulmonol 1989; 6:42–48.

23. Rock MJ, Mischler EH, Farrell PM, et al. Newborn screening for cystic fibrosis is complicated by age-related decline in immunoreactive trypsinogen levels. Pediatrics 1990; 85:1001–1007.

24. Rosler A, Belanger A, Labrie F. Mechanisms of androgen production in male pseudohermaphroditism due to 17beta-hydroxysteroid dehydrogenase deficiency. J Clin Endocrinol Metab 1992; 75:773–778.

25. Sargent JD, Stukel TA, Kresel J, et al. Normal values for random urinary calcium to creatinine ratios in infancy. J Pediatr 1993; 123:393–397.

26. Shaw NJ, Wheeldon J, Brocklebank JT. Indices of intact serum parathyroid hormone and renal excretion of calcium, phosphate, and magnesium. Arch Dis Child 1990; 65:1208–1211.

27. Shih VE. Amino acid analysis. In: Blau N, Duran M, Blaskovics M E, et al, eds. Physician's guide to the laboratory diagnosis of metabolic disease. 2007.12–14.

28. Soldin SJ, Hicks JM. Paediatric reference ranges. Washington DC: AACC Press; 1995.

29. Soldin SJ, Hill JG. Liquid-chromatographic analysis for urinary 4-hydroxy-3-methoxymandelic acid and 4-hydroxy-3-methoxyphenylacetic acid, and its use in investigation of neural crest tumors. Clin Chem 1981; 27:502–503.

30. Srinivasan G, Pildes RS, Cattamanchi G, et al. Plasma glucose values in normal neonates: a new look. J Pediatr 1986; 109:114–117.

31. Tomlinson C, Macintyre H, Dorrian CA, et al. Testosterone measurements in early infancy. Arch Dis Child Fetal Neonatal Ed 2004; 89:F558–F559.

32. Tomlinson C, Macintyre H, Dorrian CA, et al. Testosterone measurements in early infancy. Arch Dis Child Fetal Neonatal Ed 2004; 89:F558–F559.

33. Wiedemann G, Jonetz-Mentzel L, Panse R. Establishment of reference ranges for thyrotropin, triiodothyronine, thyroxine and free thyroxine in neonates, infants, children and adolescents. Eur J Clin Chem Clin Biochem 1993; 31:277–278.

34. Wilcken B, Wiley V, Sherry G, et al. Neonatal screening for cystic fibrosis: a comparison of two strategies for case detection in 1.2 million babies. J Pediatr 1995; 127:965–970.

35. Wilkins BH. Renal function in sick very low birthweight infants: 3. Sodium, potassium, and water excretion. Arch Dis Child 1992; 67(10 Spec No):1154–1161.

36. Zlotkin SH, Casselman CW. Percentile estimates of reference values for total protein and albumin in sera of premature infants (less than 37 weeks of gestation). Clin Chem 1987; 33:411–413.

37. Hinchliffe RF. Reference values. In: Lilleyman JS, Hann IM, Blanchette VS, eds. Paediatric haematology, 2nd edn. Edinburgh Churchill Livingstone; 1999:1–20.

38. Chalmers EA, Gibson BES. Acquired disorders of hemostasis during childhood. In: Lilleyman JS, Hann IM, Blanchette VS, eds. Paediatric haematology, 2nd edn. Edinburgh: Churchill Livingstone; 1999.

39. Statutory Instrument1995. The infant formula and follow-on formula regulations. 51, No 77. HMSO.

40. Commission of the European Communities Directive on infant formulae and follow-on formulae. 91/321/EEC. Off J Eur Commun 1991; L175:35–49.

41. Commission Directive 1999/21/EC. Dietary foods for special medical purposes.

42. Committee on Toxicity (COT). Phytoestrogens and health. Food Standards Agency; 2003.

43. Du Bois D, Du Bois EF. Clinical calorimetry. Tenth paper. A formula to estimate the approximate surface area if height and weight be known. Arch Intern Med 1916; 17:863.

44. Haycock GB, Schwartz GJ, Wisotsky DH. Geometric method for measuring body surface area: A height-weight formula validated in infants, children and adults. J Pediatr 1978; 93:62–66.

45. Macdonald S. The gastrointestinal tract. In: Shaw V, Lawson M, eds. Clinical paediatric dietetics, 2nd edn. Oxford: Blackwell Science; 2001.

46. Dietary reference values for food energy and nutrients for the United Kingdom. Report of the Panel on Dietary Reference Values of the Committee on Medical Aspects of Food Policy. London: HMSO; 1991. Eleventh Impression 2001.

47. Nutrient and energy intakes for the European community. Reports of the Scientific Committee for Food (thirty first series). Luxembourg: Office for Official Publications of the European Communities; 1993.

Index

Laboratory test reference ranges and nutrient and formula feeds values are in bold.